IMAGING OF THE NEWBORN, INFANT, AND YOUNG CHILD

FIFTH EDITION

IMAGING OF THE NEWBORN, INFANT, AND YOUNG CHILD

FIFTH EDITION

LEONARD E. SWISCHUK, M.D.

Professor of Radiology and Pediatrics
Director, Division of Pediatric Radiology, Children's Hospital
The University of Texas Medical Branch at Galveston
Galveston, Texas

LIPPINCOTT WILLIAMS & WILKINS
A **Wolters Kluwer** Company

Philadelphia · Baltimore · New York · London
Buenos Aires · Hong Kong · Sydney · Tokyo

Developmental Editor: Stacey L.Baze
Production Editor: Robin E. Cook
Manufacturing Manager: Benjamin Rivera
Cover Designer: Marsha Cohen
Compositor: Lippincott Williams & Wilkins Desktop Division
Printer: Maple Press

Library of Congress Cataloging-in-Publication Data

Swischuk, Leonard E., 1937-
   Imaging of the newborn infant, and young child / Leonard E. Swischuk.—5th ed.
      p. ; cm
   Includes bibliographical references and index.
   ISBN 0-7817-3458-4
      1. Infants (Newborn)—Diseases—Diagnosis. 2. Infants (Premature)—Diseases—
   Diagnosis.
   3. Pediatric radiography. 4. Pediatric diagnosic imaging. I. Title.
      [DNLM: 1. Diagnostic Imaging—Child. 2. Diagnostic Imaging—Infant.
   WN 240 S979r 2003]
   RJ255.6.R34S96 2003
   618.92′00754—dc21

                                                                    2003054514

CONTENTS

PREFACE

This is the fifth edition of this textbook. As I look back at the origins of the first edition it is difficult for me to totally comprehend the enormous changes that have occurred in imaging of children. Over the years, while the volume started as one with primary focus on the newborn infant, it slowly developed to encompass all pediatric age groups. The pressures of developing a first volume and keeping subsequent editions timely have been an enjoyable challenge for me. It is my sincere hope that I have been able to convey to the reader a balanced overall view of pediatric radiology and yet emphasize those areas which I think are of special importance. This volume is by no means meant to be totally inclusive of every entity in detail, but rather a publication which provides one with information that will get one through 80 to 90% of the day and then will provide one with enough reference information to be able to pursue further literature searches. This edition also represents considerable retooling of existing illustrations, adding new illustrations, and accomplishing significant up-to-date modifications of areas such as the acute abdomen, neurologic disease investigated with MR, childhood fractures, and an expansion of our understanding of lower respiratory tract infections.

Obviously one cannot produce a work such as this without the assistance of other individuals. First I would like to thank Mr. John Ellis, an original American of North American Indian descent—American Indiana of Tsalagiyi (Cherokee). He has helped me with the artistic side of my brain. I would also like to acknowledge and thank my former secretary Carmen Floeck who retired during the midpoint of the preparation of this manuscript. At that time my other secretary Thelma Sanchez stepped in and with great understanding and capability took over Carmen's job. She never missed a step. One cannot survive without people such as these and I am extremely indebted to them. Finally I hope that you, as a reader, will enjoy this book as much as I enjoyed preparing it. We all who enter the field of medicine have the same mission and objective.

A BUNDLE OF MOVEMENT

A bundle of movement so awkward to hold.
Crying and crying for minutes untold.
Perpetual motion, so hard to contain.
Your charisma and patience, it truly can strain.

Your very first thought may prompt a retreat.
You'll want to give up, and concede to defeat.
But before you pack up and go screaming away,
Just think for a moment, this babe needs you today.

Hold him awhile, help him adjust.
Restrain his momentum, it's almost a must.
You'll not really hurt him, if his arms you must bind.
Just stay in command, be gentle and kind.

There is nothing so fine as to take a babe home.
And nothing so hard as to leave him alone.
So help little Jack, and somebody's Jill
Their mothers and fathers sure hope that you will.

Leonard E. Swischuk, M.D.

RESPIRATORY SYSTEM

NORMAL CHEST

In most cases, complete aeration of the normal newborn infant's chest is accomplished with the first few breaths of life (1, 2). These initial respiratory efforts are rather exuberant and very adequately aerate the newborn infant's lungs. In fact, negative pressures of 20–60 cm of water are regularly generated, and tidal volumes of the first few breaths have been shown to be at least two or three times normal resting tidal volumes (1). Evidently, there is a most pronounced effort on the part of the newborn infant to accomplish initial inflation of the lungs, and while aeration still is a little uneven in that some alveoli remain unexpanded or filled with fluid (1), most of the alveolar mass is aerated. From the roentgenographic standpoint, aeration is complete (Fig. 1.1).

For the most part, the rapid sequence of neonatal lung aeration occurs in most normal infants, but in some, respiratory activity may be retarded (i.e., sedation, depressed infant, etc.), and less than complete aeration results.

With regard to the onset of respiratory activity in the newborn infant, two hypotheses generally are proposed (3).

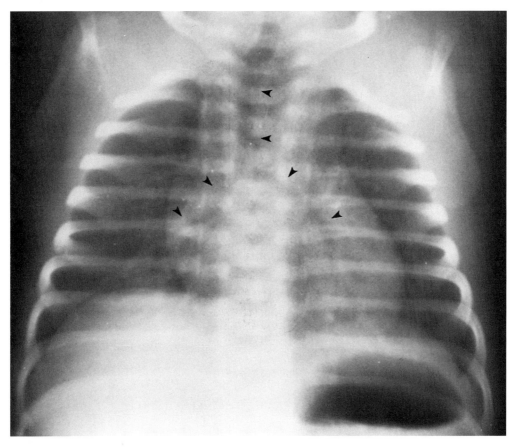

FIGURE 1.1. Normal chest. Note that the hilar and parahilar regions are less prominent than in older infants and children. A normal air bronchogram is seen in the trachea and major bronchi (arrows). Slight right-side deviation of the trachea is normal.

One suggests that the marked increase in sensory stimuli to the infant after birth results in activation of the respiratory control center, while the other suggests that respiratory activity is actively inhibited in the fetus, and at birth this inhibition is lifted and the fetus is "allowed" to breathe. However, the precise reason for this proposed inhibitory mechanism is not known, and, in truth, neither hypothesis has been totally substantiated. In terms of fetal respiratory activity, it is generally accepted that intrauterine fetal respiratory activity does occur (4–6). However, even though a variety of respiratory activity patterns have been recorded, none constitutes the equivalent of regular, deep postnatal

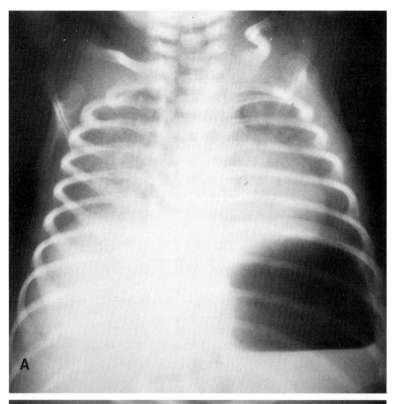

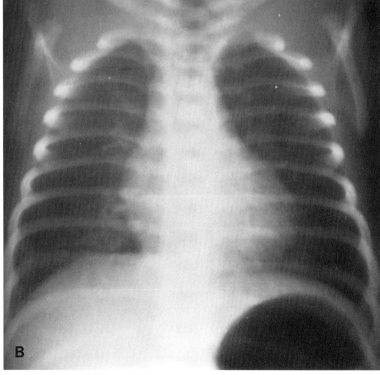

FIGURE 1.2. Normal chest: poor inspiration. A. Poor inspiration and rotation to the left produce an abnormal-appearing chest. **B.** A few minutes later, deep inspiration results in a normal chest roentgenogram.

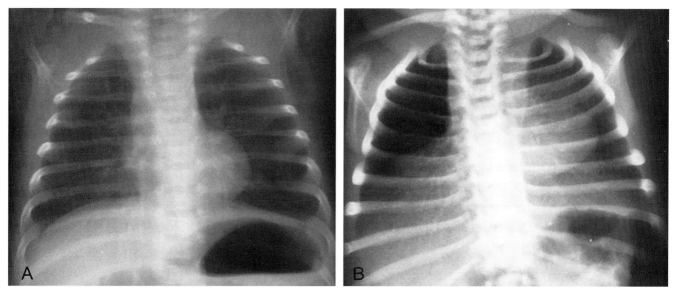

FIGURE 1.3. Normal chest. A. Lordotic position. Lordotic positioning produces a tetralogy-like configuration of the heart. Lordotic positioning is identified by the horizontal attitude of the posterior ribs. **B. Poor tube position.** When the x-ray tube is upwardly angled, gross distortion of the thorax and its contents occurs. The ribs have a bizarre fan-like configuration.

breaths. The exact significance of these fetal respiratory motions is not known, but they can be prenatally evaluated with ultrasonography, both in the normal infant and in the one subject to intrauterine distress (5, 6).

Finally, it is, of course, mandatory that chest examination be performed with adequate degrees of inspiration. An underinflated chest can suggest serious cardiac or pulmonary disease (Fig. 1.2). In addition, in young infants, the upright posteroanterior chest roentgenogram may appear as though the patient were purposely positioned for an apical lordotic view. In such cases, the cardiac apex may be thrown into such prominence that right ventricular hypertrophy,

even as in tetralogy of Fallot, is suggested (Fig. 1.3A). **With supine positioning of the patient, this does not usually occur, but at the same time with improper positioning of the x-ray tube, very peculiar and at times "grotesque" thoracic cage and mediastinal configurations result** (Fig. 1.3B).

In assessing the degree of inspiration on the chest roentgenogram, counting the number of ribs visible above the diaphragm has been frequently employed. This may be of some value in the older child and adult, but it is of no value in the infant or young child (Fig. 1.4). The reason for this is that the roentgenogram measures long volume in two dimen-

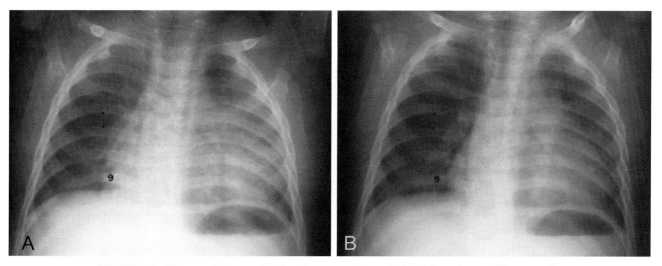

FIGURE 1.4. Rib counts in evaluating lung aeration. A. On this expiratory film, note the position of the ninth rib (black dot). **B.** With better aeration of the lungs, the lungs are blacker and the cardiomediastinal edges are sharper. Note, however, that there has been very little change in the relationship of the ninth rib (black dot) to the right diaphragmatic leaflet.

sions only, but the lungs, of course, inflate in all directions, and since in the infant, the thoracic cage is quite pliable and flexible, it expands more readily than does the thoracic cage of an older child. In addition, diaphragmatic excursion in infants is far less than in adults, and so evaluation of the degree of inspiration in infants often is more a matter of experience than science. **While many aspects of medicine are scientific, judging the degree of inspiration on a chest film is not in this category and probably never will be.**

REFERENCES

1. Fawcitt J, Lind J, Wegelius C. The first breath. Acta Paediatr Scand 1960;49(suppl 123):5–17.
2. Lind J, Tahti E, Hirvensalom M. Roentgenologic studies of the size of the lungs of the newborn baby before and after aeration. Ann Paediatr Fenn 1960;12:20.
3. Purves MJ. Onset of respiration at birth. Arch Dis Child 1974;49: 333–343.
4. Dawes GS. Revolutions and cyclical rhythms in prenatal life: fetal respiratory movements rediscovered. Pediatrics 1973;51:659–671.
5. Fox HE. Fetal breathing movements and ultrasound. Am J Dis Child 1976;130:127–129.
6. Meire HB, Fish PJ, Wheeler T. Ultrasound recording of fetal breathing. Br J Radiol 1975;48:477–480.

NORMAL VARIATIONS AND ARTIFACTS

Pleural Fissures

Visualization of the various interlobar fissures in the newborn infant is common (Fig. 1.5). This probably reflects the "wet" state of the normal neonatal lung, for fissure visualization drops rapidly after the neonatal period.

Tracheal Buckling

In the young infant, the trachea is much more flexible and mobile than in the older child. It not only shows marked changes in caliber with inspiration (dilates) and expiration (constricts), but it also is more flexible with forward or lateral movement of the neck. As a result, bizarre, but normal, tracheal configurations often are seen. Buckling, on lateral view, occurs more in the neck. On the chest film, on expiration there is normal deviation of the trachea to the right, often with an almost right angle tracheal configuration (Fig. 1.6). This is partially due to the fact that the normal left aortic arch anchors the trachea and does not allow it to deviate to the left (1). In addition, initial deviation in these cases is believed to be due to a plunger effect of the normal thymus gland being pushed upward into the cervical inlet during expiration (2).

REFERENCES

1. Chang L, Lee F, Gwinn J. Normal lateral deviation of the trachea in infants and children. AJR 1970;109:247–251.
2. Mandell GA, Bellah RD, Boulden MEC, et al. Cervical trachea: dynamics in response to herniation of the normal thymus. Radiology 1993;186:383–386.

Anterior Tracheal Indentation

Anterior indentation of the trachea, just at the level of the manubrium, generally is a normal finding and due to compression of the trachea by an anomalous innominate (Fig. 1.7), or much less commonly, left common carotid artery. **Although in a few cases, symptoms of airway obstruction can be present, in the vast majority of infants, no prob-**

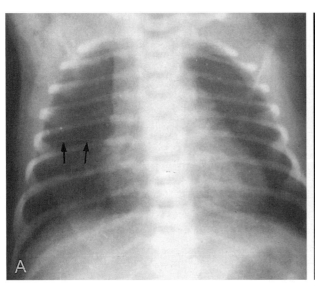
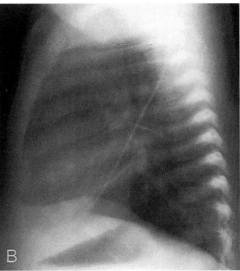

FIGURE 1.5. Normal fissures. A. Note the minor fissure (arrows) on the right. The oblique line under it is a skin fold. **B.** Lateral view in another patient demonstrates the major fissure (arrows) and numerous other fissures. The horizontal, posteriorly directed fissure is an accessory fissure.

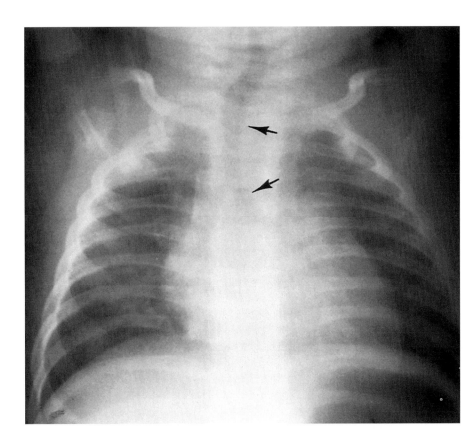

FIGURE 1.6. Normal tracheal deviation. Normal right-side deviation of the trachea (arrows), exaggerated during expiration.

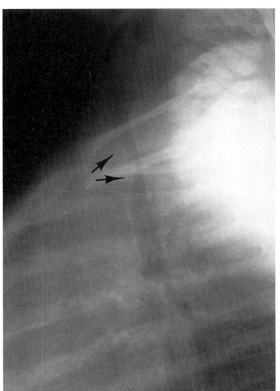

FIGURE 1.7. Anterior tracheal indentation. Note pronounced anterior tracheal indentation (arrows). This patient was symptomatic. Such indentations usually are produced by the innominate artery and can be exaggerated during expiration and flexion of the neck.

lems arise, especially when the innominate artery is the cause (1, 2). It is interesting that anterior tracheal indentation is seldom seen in the older child. In this regard, it has been suggested that because there is proportionately less space in the superior mediastinum of the young infant, there is generalized overcrowding and a greater propensity for the innominate artery to indent the trachea (1). As the infant grows older, more room develops and the indentation disappears. In addition, it may be that at the same time, the tracheal cartilages become sturdier and resist compression.

Although most infants are asymptomatic, in a few instances, airway obstruction with respiratory distress, stridor, and even apnea can result (1). In such infants, focal tracheomalacia, due to cartilage underdevelopment secondary to intrauterine tracheal compression by the anomalous artery, is present (3, 4), and actually may be the main contributing factor to the problem. Suspected tracheomalacia in these infants can be visualized with inspiratory-expiratory lateral radiographs and more vividly with dynamic computed tomography (CT) or magnetic resonance imaging (MRI) (3, 4). This small subgroup of infants is discussed in more detail in Chapter 3.

REFERENCES

1. Berdon WE, Baker DH, Bordiuk J, et al. Innominate artery compression of the trachea in infants with stridor and apnea. Method

of roentgen diagnosis and criteria for surgical treatment. Radiology 1969;92:272–278.

2. Swischuk LE. Anterior tracheal indentation in infancy and early childhood: normal or abnormal? AJR 1971;112:12–17.
3. Fletcher BD, Cohn RC. Tracheal compression and the innominate artery: MR evaluation in infants. Radiology 1989;170:103–107.
4. Vogl T, Wilimzig C, Hofmann U, et al. MRI in tracheal stenosis by innominate artery in children. Pediatr Radiol 1991;21:89–93.

Mediastinal Lines

Generally speaking, the only mediastinal line to be visualized with any regularity in the newborn and young infant is the posterior mediastinal line produced by the right pleuromediastinal reflection (1). It usually is best seen on overpenetrated chest films, and its visualization can be enhanced when the

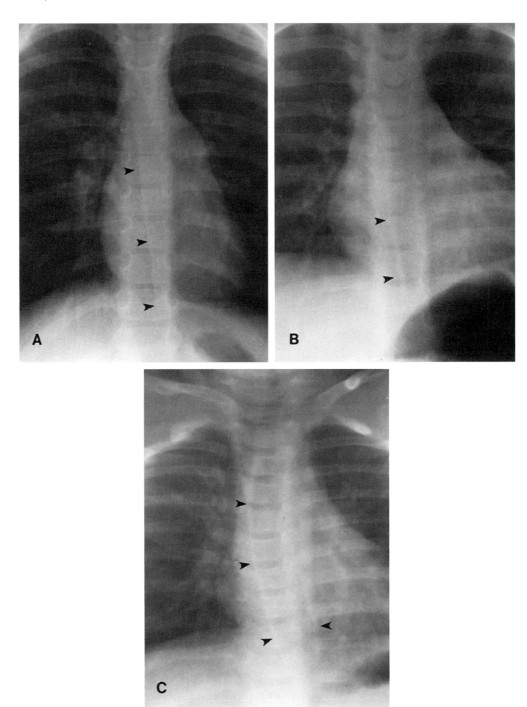

FIGURE 1.8. Posterior mediastinal line: right pleural reflection. A. Note that only the right side of the line is visualized (arrows). This is the most common configuration of this line. **B.** Both sides of the line are visualized (arrows). This probably represents the right and left pleural surfaces meeting behind the esophagus to either side of the intervening retroesophageal ligament. **C.** The esophagus is distended with swallowed air, and both walls of the esophagus are seen as individual structures (arrows).

adjacent esophagus is full of air (Fig. 1.8). Most often, only one edge of the line is visualized (Fig. 1.8A), but in some cases, both sides of the line can be visualized (Fig. 1.8B). In such cases, the findings probably represent juxtapositioning of the right and left pleural surfaces behind the esophagus (1). In older children, the posterior mediastinal line can be seen to continue upwardly as a curved line visualized through the air column of the trachea (Fig. 1.9), but this portion of the line seldom is seen in young infants. Similarly, the anterior mediastinal line (Fig. 1.9C) seldom is seen in infants.

As far as other mediastinal lines are concerned, once again, very few of these are visualized with any regularity in the neonatal and young infant, except perhaps for the left pleural reflec-

tion as it passes over the aorta. The line so produced usually is best visualized over its lower third, just adjacent to the spinal column (Fig. 1.10A). It should not be misinterpreted for a pleural effusion, but when it is markedly displaced, a paraspinal disease process or an intraabdominal tumor such as neuroblastoma or lymphoma extending into the chest should be considered. In this regard, normal width of the left paraspinal stripe has been determined to be no more than the width of the adjacent pedicle (2). Any thickening on the right should be considered abnormal and usually is due to a right descending aorta or a paraspinal tumor. In older children, the left paraspinal line may be longer and outline more of the ascending aorta (Fig. 1.10B). All of these lines also can be delineated with CT (3).

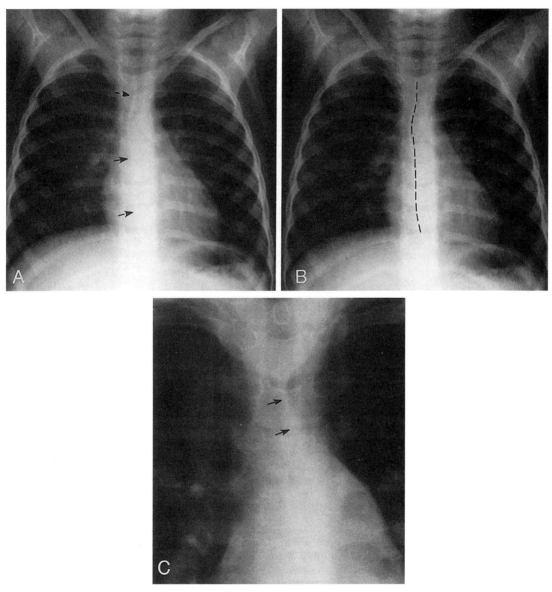

FIGURE 1.9. Posterior mediastinal line: right pleural reflection. A. Note how the posterior mediastinal line extends into the superior mediastinum (arrows). The curvature of this line, as it is projected through the tracheal air column, is typical. **B.** Dotted black line demarcates the entire extent of the line. **C. Anterior mediastinal line.** The anterior mediastinal line usually is seen in older children and is thinner (arrows) than the posterior mediastinal line. In addition, it tends to have an opposite obliquity.

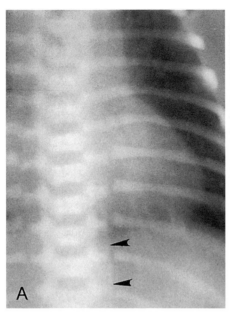
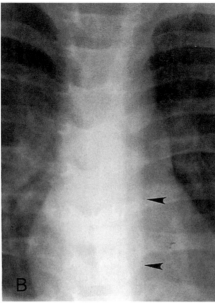

FIGURE 1.10. Left paraspinal line. A. Note the left paraspinal line (arrows), more or less paralleling the spine. In young infants, this is about as much of this line as is visible. **B.** In older children, the line, outlining the aorta, often is visible in its entirety (arrows).

REFERENCES

1. Patriquin HB, Beauregard G, Dunbar JS. The right pleuromediastinal reflection in children. J Can Assoc Radiol 1976;27: 9–15.
2. Donnelly LF, Frush DP, Zheng J-Y, et al. Differentiating normal from abnormal inferior thoracic paravertebral soft tissues on chest radiography in children. AJR 2000;175:477–483.
3. Yoon II-K, Jung KR, Han BK, et al. Mediastinal interfaces and lines in children: radiographic-CT correlation. Pediatr Radiol 2001;31:406–412.

Azygoesophageal Recess

The azygoesophageal recess in adults, when noted to be convex, is suggestive of tumor or adenopathy in the area. Normally, it is filled by the azygos vein, but as opposed to adults, it normally can appear full and convex in infants and children (1, 2). The finding is not a problem on plain films but can be a cause of erroneous diagnoses on CT scans of the chest (Fig. 1.11).

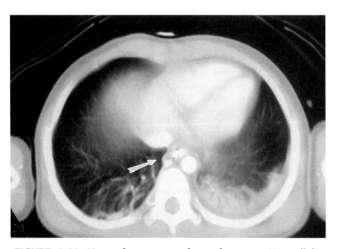

FIGURE 1.11. Normal azygoesophageal recess. Note slight convexity to the azygoesophageal recess (arrow) partially due to the azygous vein (V). Note the esophagus (E) in front of the aorta (A). This patient also has an infiltrate in the left lung posteriorly.

REFERENCES

1. Fitzgerald SW, Donaldson JS. Azygoesophageal recess: normal CT appearance in children. AJR 1992;158:1101–1104.
2. Miller FH, Fitzgerald SW, Donaldson JS. CT of the azygoesophageal recess in infants and children. Radiographics 1993;13:623–634.

Diaphragmatic Crura

Diaphragmatic crura are readily visualized in infants and children, just as they are in adults. However, it has been demonstrated that the crura are more nodular and larger relative to body size in infants and young children (1).

REFERENCE

1. Brengle M, Cohen MD, Katz B. Normal appearance and size of the diaphragmatic crura in children: CT evaluation. Pediatr Radiol 1996;26:811–814.

Normal Expiratory Tracheal Collapse

The phenomenon of tracheal collapse on expiration is normal and in some infants can be quite pronounced (Fig. 1.12). The findings in these cases should not be misinterpreted as representing those of generalized tracheomalacia. To be sure, generalized tracheomalacia is a relatively rare condition, and clinical correlation is absolutely essential in such cases. On a practical basis, this is important for the trachea also tends to narrow more than usual during expiration in patients with asthma and reactive airway disease.

Normal Tracheal and Esophageal Air

With deep inspiration, the trachea and major bronchi are clearly distended and readily identified (see Fig. 1.1). In addition, transient collections of air frequently are noted in the esophagi of newborn and young infants (Fig. 1.13).

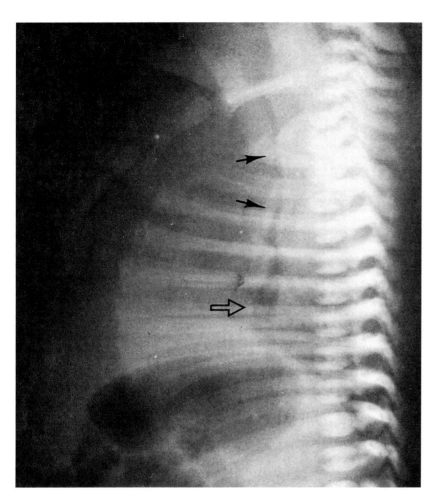

FIGURE 1.12. Normal tracheal collapse on expiration. Note extreme narrowing of the trachea during expiration (filled arrows) in this infant with no respiratory distress. Air also is present in the distal esophagus (open arrow).

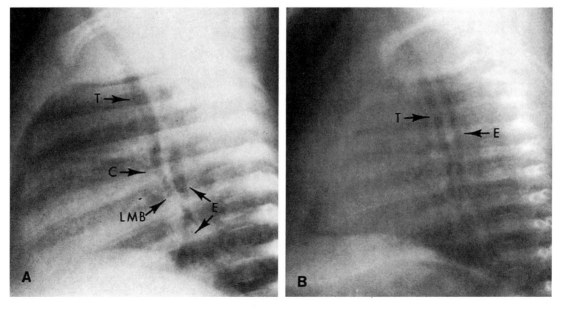

FIGURE 1.13. Normal tracheal and esophageal air. A. Note air in the trachea (T), carina (C), and left main bronchus (LMB). Also note air in the esophagus (E). **B.** Another infant demonstrating air throughout the entire trachea (T) and air in almost all of the esophagus (E).

Such collections usually are fleeting and considered normal. They result from temporary trapping of swallowed air or regurgitated air (burp). On the other hand, when esophageal air is more voluminous, and especially if it is more persistent, one must consider such problems as tracheoesophageal fistula and esophageal reflux.

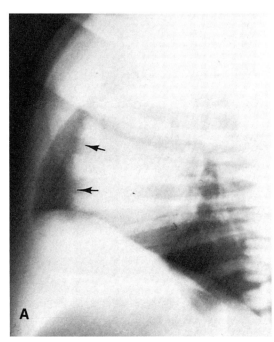

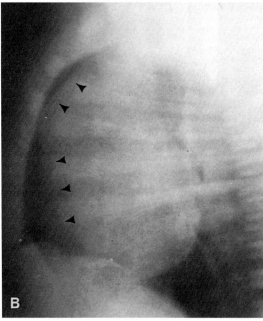

FIGURE 1.14. Pseudopneumomediastinum. A. The triangular area of hyperlucency just anterior to the heart (arrows) is normal lung. It should not be confused with pneumomediastinum, which usually collects in a more superior retrosternal location. **B.** Similar area of hyperlucency representing normal lung with extension into the upper retrosternal region (arrows).

Pseudopneumomediastinum

In some infants, on lateral projection, especially with rotation and deep inspiration, one may see a hyperlucent triangular area in the lower retrosternal space (Fig. 1.14A). Less commonly, a similar configuration is noted behind the upper sternum (Fig. 1.14B). These configurations should not be misinterpreted as representing pneumomediastinum or anterior pneumothorax, for they merely represent normally aerated lung. Generally speaking, they are not as radiolucent (black) as is true free air.

ROTATION OF THE CHEST: PSEUDOHYPERLUCENT LUNG

Rotation of the chest to one side or the other is the most common cause of apparent hyperlucency of one lung (Fig. 1.15). The hyperlucent side usually corresponds to the side of rotation, and the finding should not be misinterpreted as due to some pathologic problem. To determine whether the chest is rotated to one side or the other, it is best to check the ribs: Anteriorly the ribs will appear shorter, and posteriorly they will appear longer on the side to which the chest is rotated (Fig. 1.15).

Skin Folds

Skin folds are the most common artifact to be seen on the radiographs of newborn infants. They are especially common in premature infants and result from the folding of excessively redundant skin. It is very easy to produce folding of the skin when the infant is laid against the film cassette or radiographic table. The straight lines so produced often are misinterpreted for those of a pneumothorax, but since the obliquity of the line produced by a skin fold is opposite to that produced by the edge of the lung in pneumothorax, confusion should be fleeting (Fig. 1.16). Furthermore, the line produced by a skin fold often travels across, and outside, the chest or across the diaphragm into the abdomen. However, to establish a firm diagnosis of pneumothorax, there must be lack of visualization of vascular markings lateral to the edge of the collapsed lung, and at the same time, this space should be very black. In addition, a zone of increased density seen along the medial edge of a skin fold due to increased thickness of the skin secondary to the folding is seen. This phenomenon is not seen with pneumothorax (1). In a few cases, a skin fold may appear almost vertical, but it very rarely completely reverses its usual obliquity. Nonetheless, when it is almost vertical, it is more likely to be confused with pneumothorax (Fig. 1.17) or with the so-called "vertical fissure" (see next section and Fig. 1.18).

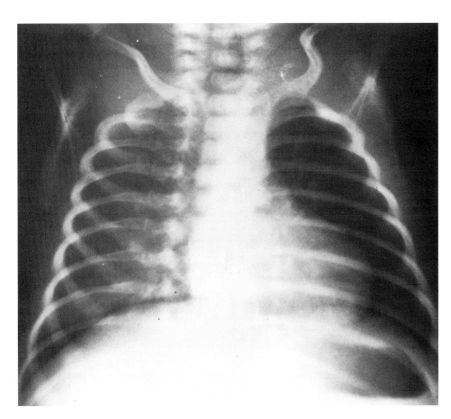

FIGURE 1.15. Hyperlucency with rotation. Rotation to the left produces asymmetry of the ribs, relative hyperlucency of the left lung, and asymmetry of the clavicles. The posterior ribs always appear longer on the side to which rotation occurs, and the anterior ribs appear longer on the opposite side.

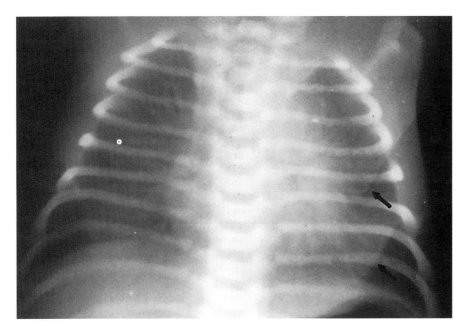

FIGURE 1.16. Skin folds. Note characteristically oblique bilateral skin folds (arrows).

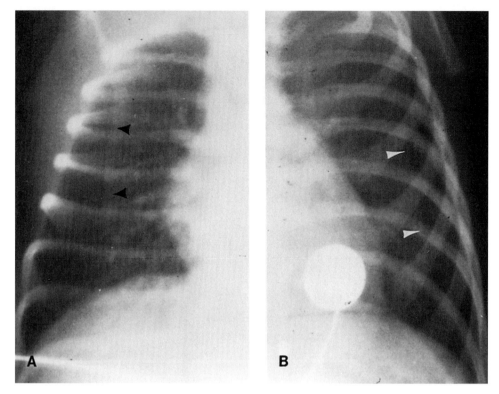

FIGURE 1.17. Vertical skin fold versus pneumothorax. A. Skin fold. Note the vertical orientation of the skin fold (arrows). In such cases, it can be confused with a pneumothorax. B. True pneumothorax. Note the near-vertical orientation of the edge of the compressed lung (arrows). No lung markings are seen lateral to the edge of the lung. In A, even though hyperlucency lateral to the skin fold is present, lung markings still are visible beyond the line of the skin fold.

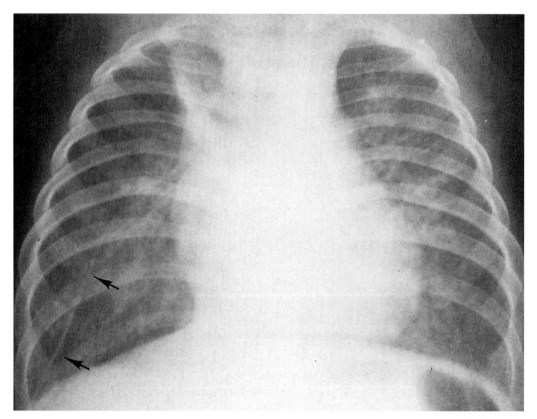

FIGURE 1.18. Vertical fissure. This fissure (arrows) can be seen on either side and is most commonly noted in patients with cardiomegaly and congestive heart failure. This infant had an ostium primum defect, congested pulmonary vascularity, and right upper lobe atelectasis. The vertical fissure represents the lower end of the major fissure.

REFERENCE

1. Fisher JK. Technical notes: skin fold vs. pneumothorax. AJR 1978; 130:791–792.

Vertical Fissure

The vertical fissure is seen as a straight line traveling vertically or obliquely from the diaphragmatic leaflet, on either side, into the corresponding lower lung field. The line is believed to represent the lower half of the major fissure (1, 2), which can be projected into this position by the presence of a partially collapsed lower lobe (3). It also is frequently seen in infants with cardiac enlargement and failure, and in such cases, fluid in the fissure enhances its visualization (Fig. 1.18). This fissure can be seen in all age groups of children.

REFERENCES

1. Davis LA. Vertical fissure line. AJR 1960;84:451–453.
2. Webber MM, O'Loughlin BJ. Variations of pleural vertical fissure line. Radiology 1964;82:461–462.
3. Friedman E. Further observations on the vertical fissure line. AJR 1966;97:171–173.

Intercostal and Apical Herniation of the Lungs

Intercostal bulging and apical herniation of the lungs can be seen in infants with diffuse air trapping (1), but it also frequently is seen as a normal variant (Fig. 1.19). In such cases, it occurs during the early expiratory phase of respiration where such expiration is accomplished against a closed glottis (e.g., crying infant). Under these circumstances, a

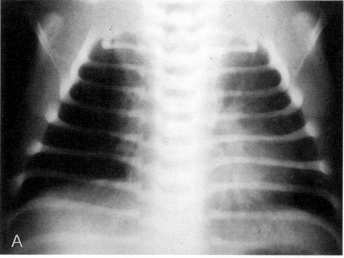

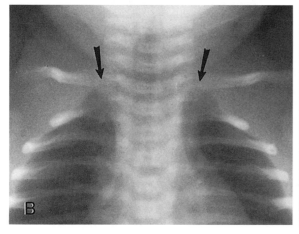
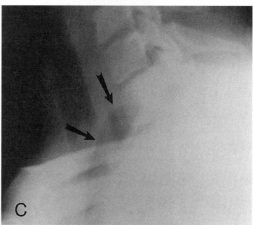

FIGURE 1.19. Intercostal bulging and apical herniation of the lungs. A. Normal intercostal bulging of the lungs in early expiration. **B. Normal expiratory apical herniation** above the first rib (arrows). **C.** Lateral view, in older child, demonstrates characteristic **normal apical herniation** of the lung (arrows).

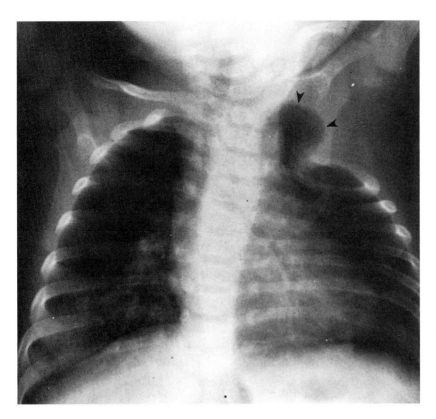

FIGURE 1.20. Apical chest wall defect and lung herniation. Note apical herniation of the left lung (arrows). Also note the spinal anomalies and absence of the first and second ribs. This patient presented with a large, but easily compressible, mass in the supraclavicular fossa. The mass became larger with crying, but the patient was otherwise asymptomatic.

momentary natural Valsalva maneuver results and leads to overdistension of the lungs.

In other cases, **herniation of the apical portion of the lung can be pathologic (2–4) and so pronounced that a mass is visible clinically.** In such cases, it is believed that herniation is due to weakness or absence of the vertebropleural (Sibson's) fascia (2). Very rarely does this condition produce any vascular or airway compression, but a case with transient venous occlusion has been reported (5). In addition, a case associated with congenital absence of the sternocleidomastoid muscle has been documented (6). Clinically, most often, the problem is that of a supraclavicular mass that tends to come and go with different phases of respiration (Fig. 1.20). Similar pathologic herniation also can be seen with extensive rib cage defects, usually congenital, but occasionally acquired.

REFERENCES

1. Schorr S, Ayalon D. Intercostal lung bulging, an early roentgen sign of emphysema in children. Radiology 1960;75:544–551.
2. Currarino G. Cervical lung protrusions in children. Pediatr Radiol 1998;28:533–538.
3. Gruenbaum M, Griscom NT. Protrusion of the lung apex through Sibson's fascia in infancy. Thorax 1978;33:290–294.
4. Thompson JS. Cervical herniation of the lung. Report of a case and review of the literature. Pediatr Radiol 1976;4:190–192.
5. Siegelman SS, Shanser JD, Attaie LA. Cervical herniation of the lung associated with transient venous occlusion. Report of a case. Dis Chest 1968;53:785–787.
6. Bayne SR, Lehman JA, Crow JP. Lung herniation into the neck associated with congenital absence of the sternocleidomastoid muscle. J Pediatr Surg 1997;32:1754–1756.

Inferior Retrosternal Density

This wedge-like lower retrosternal density (Fig. 1.21), once generally believed to represent the transverse thoracic muscle (1), probably represents the interface between the anterior aspects of the right and left lungs (2, 3). It appears that the lower left lung does not extend as far anteriorly as does the right lung (3), and because of this, the anterior edge of the aerated left lung is seen on lateral view. It forms the posterior aspect of the retrosternal density, and the density itself is believed to represent normal mediastinal soft tissues anterior to the left lung (3).

REFERENCES

1. Shopfner CE, Jansen C, O'Kell RT. Roentgen significance of the transverse thoracic muscle. AJR 1968;103:140–148.
2. Keats TE. Right parasternal stripe; a new mediastinal shadow and a contribution to the nature of the retrosternal line. AJR 1974; 120:898–900.
3. Whalen JP, Meyers MA, Oliphant M, et al. The retrosternal line: a new sign of an anterior mediastinal mass. AJR 1973;117: 861–872.

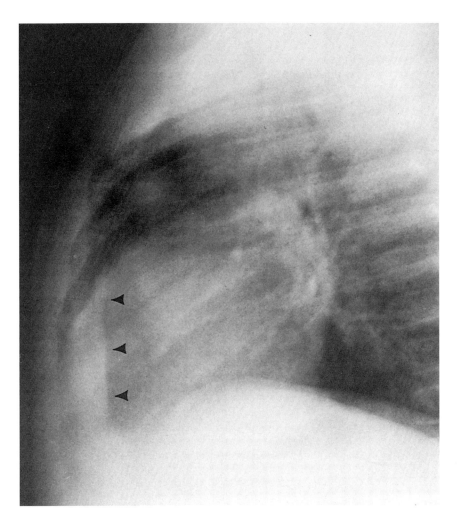

FIGURE 1.21. Inferior retrosternal density. Note the triangular-shaped inferior retrosternal density (arrows). Originally, this was thought to represent the transverse thoracic muscle, but now it generally is believed to represent the interface between the anterior aspects of the right and left lungs. It is a normal finding and should not be misinterpreted for a pleural effusion or a mass.

Scapular and Apical Pseudotumors

In some infants, on lateral views of the chest, the normal scapula, superimposed over the posterior mediastinum, produces a mass-like density (1, 2). This finding (Fig. 1.22A) should not be misinterpreted for that of a mass, and on a practical basis, it would be almost inconceivable to see a mass of such size on lateral view and not on frontal view. Another pseudotumor frequently seen on lateral chest films in young infants is that produced by the normal soft tissues projected over the apex of the thorax (Fig. 1.22B).

REFERENCES

1. Alazraki NP, Friedman PJ. Posterior mediastinal "pseudo-mass" of the newborn. AJR 1972;116:571–574.
2. Balsam D, Berdon WE, Baker DH. The scapula as a cause of a spurious posterior mediastinal mass on lateral chest films of infants. J Pediatr Surg 1974;9:501–503.

Suprasternal Fossa Artifact

In some infants, the suprasternal fossa is very deep. Most often, this occurs in infants with respiratory distress and suprasternal retractions, but it also can occur in normal infants. When the suprasternal fossa is deepened, it can present as an oval radiolucency (1), virtually indistinguishable from the dilated esophageal pouch of esophageal atresia (Fig. 1.23A). On lateral view, however, it becomes apparent that one is dealing with a deepened suprasternal fossa (Fig. 1.23B).

REFERENCE

1. Hernandez R, Kuhns LR, Holt JF. The suprasternal fossa on chest radiographs in newborns. AJR 1978;130:745–746.

Chest Magnification

Direct magnification of the chest roentgenogram has been applied in the newborn (1, 2). Some special modification,

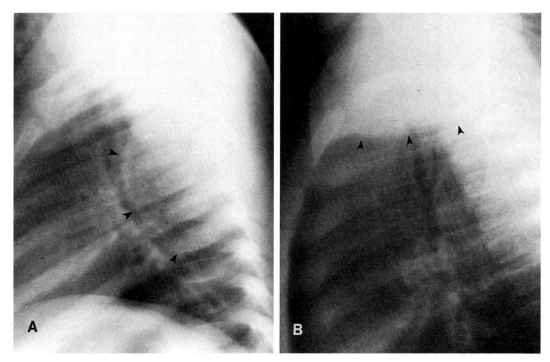

FIGURE 1.22. Scapular and apical pseudotumors. A. Note the pseudotumor (arrows) produced by the scapula and soft tissues. **B.** Another pseudotumor produced by soft tissues projected over the apex of the lungs (arrows).

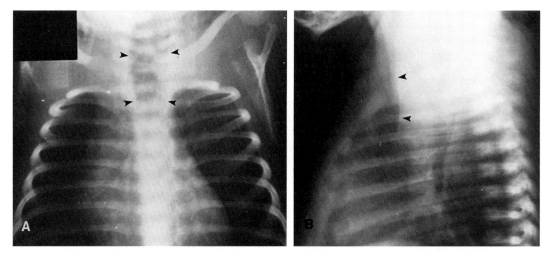

FIGURE 1.23. Suprasternal fossa. A. Note the oval radiolucency produced by the suprasternal fossa (arrows). It mimics the air-filled esophageal pouch of esophageal atresia. **B.** Lateral view demonstrating the depth of the suprasternal fossa (arrows).

notably a small focal spot, is required for this technique. The resulting roentgenogram can enhance interpretation but generally is not necessary. On the other hand, it is somewhat easier to interpret, especially for the individual not routinely engaged in the interpretation of neonatal chest roentgenograms. Currently, magnification is coming into more common use because of PACS.

REFERENCES

1. Brasch RC, Gould RG. Direct magnification radiography of the newborn infant. Radiology 1982;142:649–655.
2. Nikesch W, Kuntzier CM, Cushing FR. Neonatal magnification radiography using standard-focus x-ray tubes. AJR 1983;141: 665–669.

Chest Radiographic Technique

In a newborn infant, of course, supine chest films are obtained, and for the most part, the frontal view is the only one necessary (1). However, when frontal views are incomplete or puzzling, lateral views may be necessary (1). Oblique views are seldom obtained.

In infants beyond the neonatal period, one can obtain either supine or upright films. Supine films are favored by many (2), but there seems to be little difference in the final product. Supine films are easier to obtain in infancy, but formal, upright views are more desirable in later childhood. If upright films are obtained in infancy, some form of immobilization of the infant in the upright, sitting position is required. In our institution, we use the Pigg-o-Stat (AADCO Medical, Inc., Randolph, VT) as often as possible, and, of course, beyond the neonatal period, frontal and lateral views are standard.

Currently, standard radiographic images, more and more, are digitally acquired through PACS systems (3–5). Detail on such images is sufficiently sharp that one can accomplish accurate diagnoses. In addition, since the images can be readily manipulated to enhance viewing in many ways, they offer a great advantage to the interpreter.

Finally, a word is in order regarding dose delivered to premature infants who generally require numerous studies. It has been shown that exposure doses in these infants are well below permitted levels (6, 7). Doses are a little higher with computed radiography-acquired images (digital images) but probably still acceptable if the factors are reduced below those utilized for adult imaging. In addition, it has been determined that the numbers of studies usually obtained in pediatric intensive care units are warranted (8).

REFERENCES

1. Franken EA Jr, Yu P, Smith WL, et al. Initial chest radiography in the neonatal intensive care unit; value of the lateral view. AJR 1979;133:43–45.
2. Gyll C. Horizontal versus vertical, or lying down is better. Br J Radiol 1984;57:191–193.
3. Cohen MD, Katz BP, Kalasinski LA, et al. Digital imaging with a photostimulable phosphor in the chest of newborns. Radiology 1991;181:829–832.
4. Franken EA Jr, Smith WL, Berbaum KS, et al. Comparison of a PACS workstation with conventional film for interpretation of neonatal examinations: a paired comparison study. Pediatr Radiol 1991;21:336–340.
5. Kogutt MS, Jones JP, Perkins DD. Low-dose digital computed radiography in pediatric chest imaging. AJR 1988;151:775–779.
6. Duetting T, Foerst B, Knoch T, et al. Radiation exposure during chest x-ray examinations in a premature intensive care unit: phantom studies. Pediatr Radiol 1999;29:158–162.
7. Wilson-Costello D, Rao PS, Morrison S, et al. Radiation exposure from diagnostic radiographs in extremely low birth weight infants. Pediatrics 1996;97:369–374.
8. Valk JW, Plotz FB, Schuerman FABA, et al. The value of routine chest radiographs in a paediatric intensive care unit: a prospective study. Pediatr Radiol 2001;31:343–347.

THE THYMUS: NORMAL AND ABNORMAL

The normal thymus often plays havoc with interpretation of the young infant's chest roentgenogram, especially if one is not familiar with its varied configurations. On the other hand, once these are appreciated, the thymus is less of a problem. In this regard, the normal thymus usually is visible and identifiable at birth and, in many infants, up to the age of 2–3 years. Thereafter, while thymic tissue still is present, even into late childhood, it rapidly becomes smaller and basically invisible. However, occasionally, one may encounter an older child with normal thymic tissue visible on chest roentgenography. In such cases, the misdiagnosis of the normal thymus gland for a mediastinal tumor is more likely. In trauma cases where the film often is obtained in the supine position, a mediastinal hematoma can be erroneously suggested. In all of these cases, it should be remembered that normal thymus gland does not displace adjacent structures but merely grows in and around them.

The classic appearance of the thymus on the posteroanterior chest roentgenogram is one of bilateral, smoothly outlined superior mediastinal fullness, blending almost imperceptibly with the cardiac silhouette (Fig. 1.24). In other cases, a definite notch, unilateral or bilateral, can be seen at the junction of the inferior aspect of the normal thymus gland and cardiac silhouette (Fig. 1.25A). Another characteristic normal thymic configuration is that of the so-called "sail" sign. This configuration is most commonly seen on the right (Fig. 1.25B) but can be bilateral.

On lateral or oblique projection, the thymus fills the anterosuperior mediastinal space and often is delineated along its interior border by a distinct, relatively or slightly undulating line (Fig. 1.25C). This relatively distinct lower edge of the normal thymus is most important in differentiating it from other mediastinal masses. It is unlikely that a tumor such as a teratoma or thymoma in the same location would have such a straight inferior border. Furthermore, neoplasms tend to indent or displace the trachea and esophagus. In other instances, the thymus can extend deep into the inferior retrosternal space (1, 2). In such cases, the findings can mimic a retrosternal pleural effusion (Fig. 1.25D).

Waviness or gentle undulation of the entire lateral edge of the thymus gland also is an identifying feature of a normal gland and results from adjacent rib compression (Fig. 1.26). It is most commonly found on the left and has been termed the "wavy" thymus sign.

The normal thymus shows great variation in size and configuration with inspiration-expiration and supine or upright positioning. For example, both expiration and supine positioning tend to give the cardiothymic silhouette an extremely globular appearance (Fig. 1.27A). Indeed, it has the appearance of a large ball sitting in the center of the chest. I know of no cardiac lesion that would be likely to produce such a cardiac configuration, and it would be most unlikely that a mediastinal tumor would have such a uni-

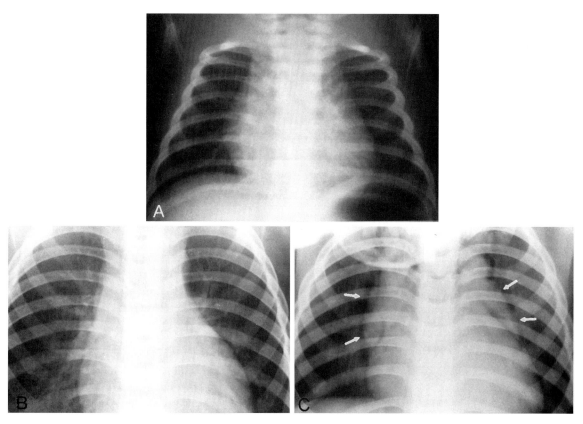

FIGURE 1.24. Normal thymus. A. Infant. Notice how the thymic silhouette blends almost imperceptibly with the cardiac silhouette (arrows). **B. Older child.** The thymus is not as evident. **C.** However, with a pneumomediastinum present, the thymic lobes (arrows) are clearly outlined.

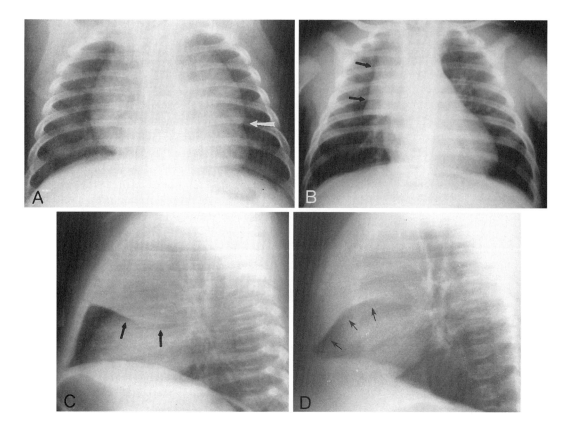

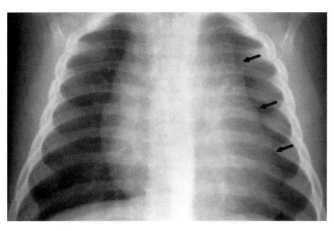

FIGURE 1.26. Wavy thymus sign. Undulation of the left lateral edge of the thymus (arrows) results from indentation by adjacent ribs.

formly spherical configuration. However, if there still is doubt, the true nature of the silhouette can easily be determined by repeating the examination in the upright position (Fig. 1.27B). Another problem resulting from positional change is the thymus mimicking upper lobe lung pathology. Usually occurring on the right, but occasionally on the left (3), rotation of the chest causes the involved lobe of the thymus gland to project into the apex of the hemithorax and mimic pneumonia or atelectasis (Fig. 1.28).

Stress atrophy of the thymus is a well-known phenomenon and usually occurs secondary to some illness or, less often, to the administration of drugs such as corticosteroids or other chemotherapeutic agents. One often can see normal thymus gland decrease in size (atrophy) with concurrent infection (i.e., pneumonia, gastroenteritis) and then return to normal size (regeneration) with clearing of the infection (Fig. 1.29). Such fluctuations in thymic size are quite common and usually closely parallel the infant's clinical course. With recovery, rebound growth can be exuberant and mass-like; contrarily, initial stress may be so pronounced that absence of the thymus erroneously is suggested. Rebound hypertrophy of the thymus also is common after cessation of chemotherapy and may be exuberant (4, 5).

In addition to the foregoing peculiarities about the thymus gland, it also is notorious for assuming bizarre configurations that, at first, might suggest a mediastinal tumor

(Fig. 1.30). In some of these cases, thymic tissue extends high into the superior mediastinum, and even into the lower neck (6). This probably represents incomplete descent of the thymus gland (Fig. 1.31), and in some cases, a lower neck mass may be present. Such a mass may be more prominent during crying, but, for the most part, even these thymus glands are not usually symptomatic. On the other hand, there have been a few reported cases of accessory or otherwise abnormally positioned thymus glands that have led to respiratory or esophageal symptoms (7). In these cases, the accessory or abnormally positioned thymus can be located almost anywhere in the neck or chest, including the posterior mediastinum (8–10).

In the latter cases, no matter which imaging modality is utilized, it is most important to appreciate that the posterior mediastinal extension of the thymus gland is contiguous with the normal portion of the gland lying in the anterior mediastinum. In many of these cases, the anterior mediastinal portion of the gland is smaller than normal, but located on the same side as the posterior mediastinal extension. Overall, MRI is probably best for identifying these eccentric glands confidently (Fig. 1.32). In addition, normal thymic tissue can extend between the brachiocephalic vein and innominate artery (11). In such cases, the finding should not be misinterpreted for a mediastinal mass, on either plain films or subsequent CT (Fig. 1.33).

In addition to the foregoing considerations, these abnormally situated thymic glands often are more prone to develop cysts or tumors, and then, of course, symptoms are more likely to arise (12). These cysts are readily demonstrable with ultrasound and may be simple fluid-filled cysts or complicated cysts with visible debris. In addition, they may be multiloculated (12) and may mimic cystic hygroma (Fig. 1.34, A–C).

Massive enlargement of the normal thymus gland, or socalled "hyperplasia of the thymus," is a benign condition that, however, can cause problems in differential diagnosis (Fig. 1.34D). Indeed, biopsy may be required for the final diagnosis (13, 14).

True tumors such as thymoma and thymolipoma (14–18) of the thymus gland are exceptionally rare in infants and young children, but it is not uncommon to encounter massive thymic enlargement secondary to infiltration by leukemia or lymphoma (19, 20). In some of these cases, the thymus gland may be enormously enlarged (Fig. 1.35) and associated with pleural effusions (20). It might

FIGURE 1.25. Normal thymus: varying configurations. A. Notch sign. Note the pronounced notch on the left (arrow). Both the right and the left thymic lobes are large but normal. The right thymic lobe blends with the heart, producing a pseudo-right atrial enlargement appearance. **B. Sail sign.** Characteristic configuration of the sail sign (arrows) of normal thymus. **C.** Lateral view, in another patient, demonstrates the slightly **undulating lower edge of the normal thymus gland** (arrow). **D.** Lateral view demonstrating **inferior retrosternal extension** (arrows) of thymus.

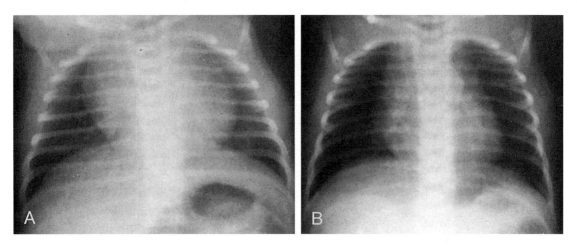

FIGURE 1.27. Normal thymus: pseudocardiomegaly. A. Supine positioning in an infant results in a round cardiothymic silhouette. Cardiomegaly or a mass might erroneously be suggested. **B.** Same patient with an upright film demonstrates a normal cardiothymic silhouette. The bulge along the upper left paraspinal region is the normal ductus bump.

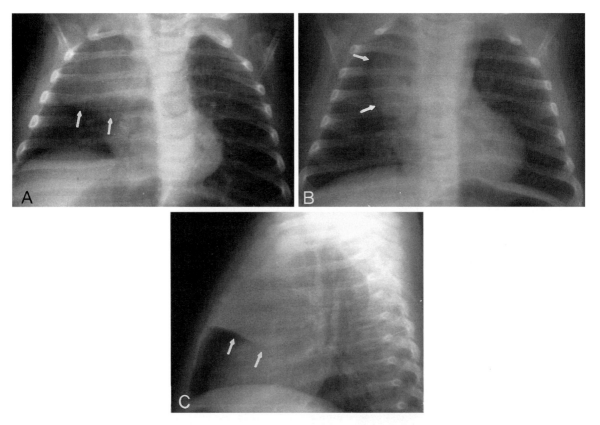

FIGURE 1.28. Normal thymus: pseudopneumonia. A. With slight rotation to the right, a prominent right thymic lobe appears as a consolidating pneumonia (arrows) of the right upper lobe. **B.** With proper positioning, the right thymic lobe (arrows) now has a more typical appearance. **C.** Lateral view demonstrates the typical undulating lower edge (arrows) of normal thymic gland.

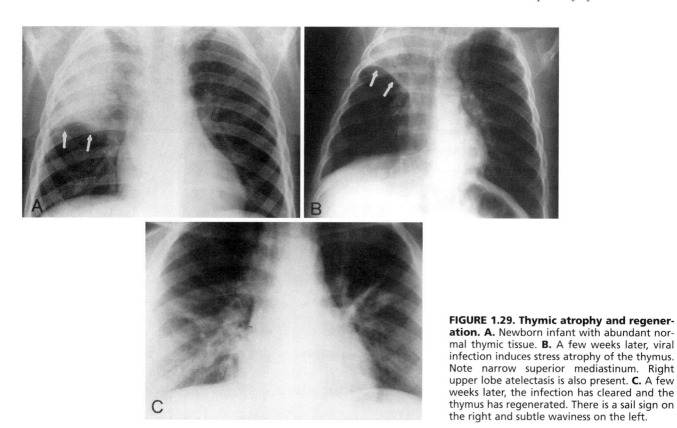

FIGURE 1.29. Thymic atrophy and regeneration. A. Newborn infant with abundant normal thymic tissue. **B.** A few weeks later, viral infection induces stress atrophy of the thymus. Note narrow superior mediastinum. Right upper lobe atelectasis is also present. **C.** A few weeks later, the infection has cleared and the thymus has regenerated. There is a sail sign on the right and subtle waviness on the left.

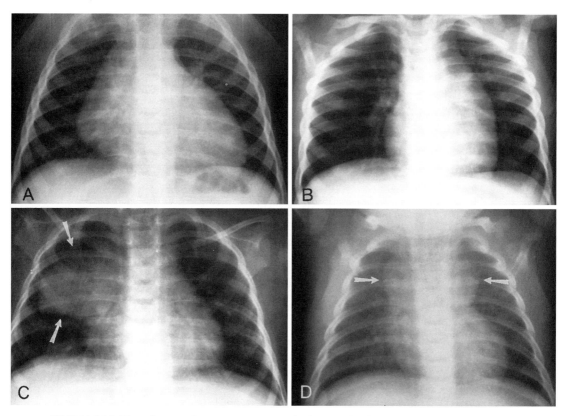

FIGURE 1.30. Thymic pseudomasses. A. Note the large right thymic lobe (arrows) producing a picture that might suggest cardiomegaly or a large mediastinal mass. **B.** Another patient with a mass-like, but normal, left thymic configuration (arrows). **C.** Eccentric thymic tissue on the right (arrows) producing a tumor-like configuration. Note that the trachea is not deviated. **D.** Bilateral prominent thymus (arrows) producing a "figure 8" heart configuration.

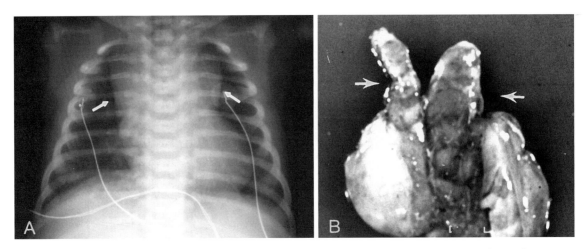

FIGURE 1.31. Incomplete descent of thymus. A. Note high position of the thymus (arrows) due to incomplete descent. This is a normal configuration but could cause one to wonder about a mass. **B.** Postmortem specimen in another patient demonstrating a thymus gland similar to that seen in **A.** Note the notches (arrows) produced by compression by the thoracic inlet.

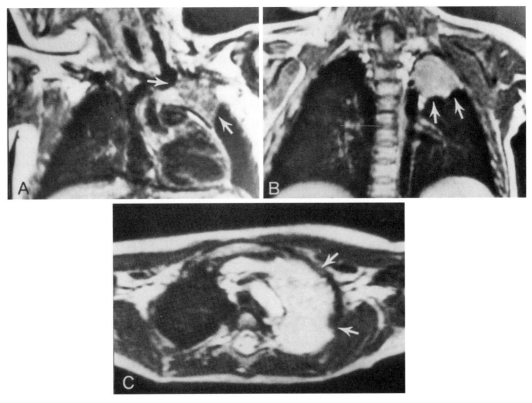

FIGURE 1.32. Normal thymus: posterior mediastinal extension. A. Anterior coronal T1-weighted image demonstrates normal thymus (arrow). **B.** More posterior coronal image demonstrates thymus (arrow) in the apex of the left hemithorax next to the spine. **C.** Coronal T1-weighted image demonstrates the thymus (arrows) to extend from its normal anterior position into the posterior paraspinal region. (Reproduced with permission from Bach AM, Hilfer CL, Holgersen LO. Left-sided posterior mediastinal thymus: MRI findings. Pediatr Radiol 1991;21:440–441).

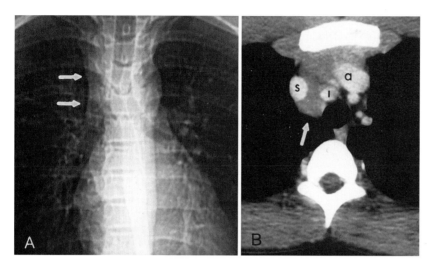

**FIGURE 1.33. Normal thymus: pseudopara-
tracheal mass. A.** Note right paratracheal
prominence in this patient whose chest x-ray
was obtained for symptoms of suspected pulmonary infection. Note that the trachea is not
indented or deviated. **B.** Computed tomography demonstrates extension of normal thymic
tissue (arrow) between the superior vena cava
(s) and innominate artery (i). a, aorta.

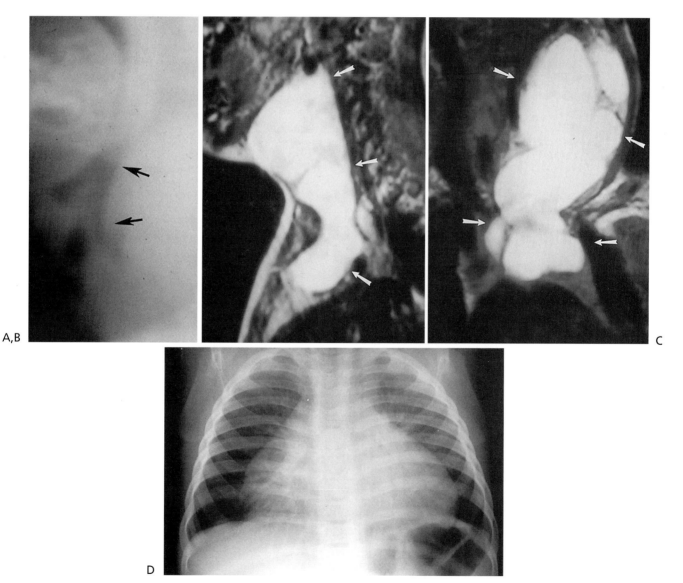

FIGURE 1.34. Thymic cyst. A. Note the mass (arrows) extending into the upper thorax. **B.** T2-
weighted magnetic resonance image demonstrates the high signal in the fluid of the cyst (arrows).
C. In another plane, the extent of the cyst is readily appreciated. **D. Thymic hyperplasia.** Note
marked bilateral enlargement of the thymus gland, resulting in what appears to be cardiomegaly.

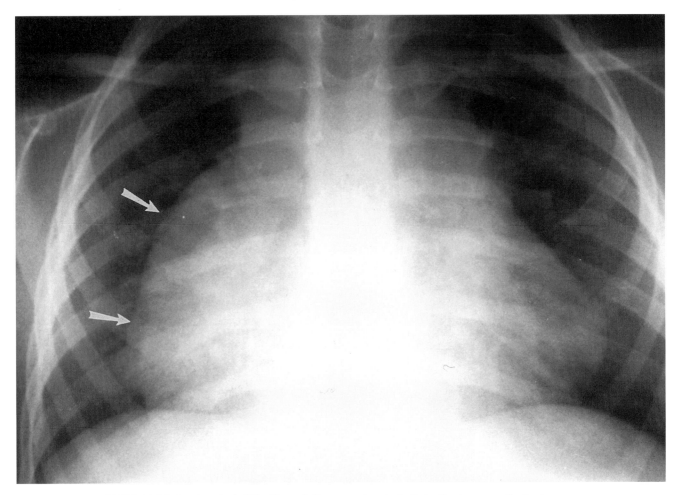

FIGURE 1.35. Leukemic infiltration of thymus gland. A. Note the large mediastinal mass (arrows), extending into the right hemithorax.

also be noted that if sonography is employed in these patients, the infiltrated gland may be so free of acoustic interfaces that a sonolucent, cystic lesion is at first suggested. This is not an uncommon phenomenon with leukemia-lymphoma in general. Other tumors generally are echogenic, and thymomas may be cystic.

Most thymomas are discovered incidentally, although a small percentage, probably less than 10%, are associated with myasthenia gravis. One might suspect the presence of a thymoma when one encounters an unusually large thymus gland in an age group where one would not expect to see such a finding. With ultrasound, CT, or MRI, if cystic structures are evident, they are relatively easily defined (Fig. 1.36), but it is not possible to determine degree of malignancy of these lesions with imaging. Thymomas may show calcification in up to 25% of cases (17, 18).

In any of these foregoing cases, and, indeed, any time one is concerned as to whether a mediastinal mass represents normal thymic tissue, a problem will exist. In this regard, since steroids induce thymic atrophy, it once was advocated that they be administered as a test, but this practice never was commonplace. Nowadays, in such cases, one's best policy probably is to perform MRI for this imaging most clearly shows the normal configuration of the thymus gland, especially on coronal views (Fig. 1.37, A and B). It is the smooth, tapering, wedge-like configuration of the thymic lobes that drape over the heart that suggests a normal gland. This finding, in addition to noting normal signal intensities, has led us to prefer MRI over CT for evaluation of the thymus. This is not to suggest that CT is not valuable, but overall we believe that one can be more confident that one is dealing with normal thymus tissue when MRI is utilized.

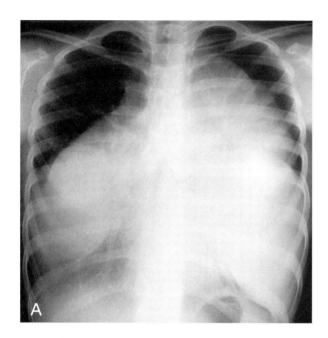

FIGURE 1.36. Thymoma. A. Plain film demonstrating large mediastinal mass. **B.** Ultrasonography shows the mass to be complex with septations, solid areas, and cystic areas. **C.** Axial computed tomography scan demonstrates the anterior position of the large mediastinal mass (arrows) and confirms its mixed cystic and solid configuration. It encircles the heart (H), and small flecks of calcium are seen on the right. (Reproduced with permission from Lam WWM, Chan FL, Lau YL, et al. Paediatric thymoma: unusual occurrence in two siblings. Pediatr Radiol 1993;23:124–126).

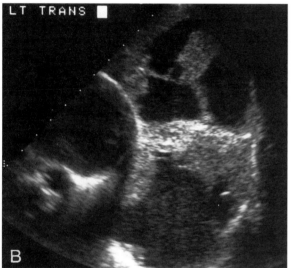

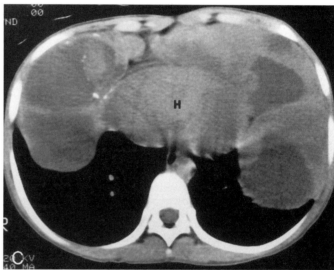

In terms of the signal characteristics of normal thymic tissue on MRI, in the infant, T1-weighted images show low signal intensity and T2-weighted images show high signal intensity. Later, as fatty replacement of the thymic tissue occurs, T1-weighted images become more signal intense. At the same time, of course, the thymic gland also becomes smaller. Ultrasonographically, the normal thymus has a uniform liver-like echotexture (21), and, once again, its location and definition of its sharp edges and pointed ends confirm its normality and presence (Fig. 1.37, C and D).

Aplasia or hypoplasia of the thymus is encountered in certain immunologic disorders, including human immunodeficiency virus (HIV) infection (22). As far as the other immunologic disorders are concerned, the most widely known association with thymic agenesis or hypoplasia occurs with the DiGeorge syndrome. These patients may demonstrate absence of the parathyroid glands and associated cardiac anomalies such as persistent truncus arteriosus and interrupted aortic arch. Absence of the parathyroid glands may lead to neonatal tetany, and

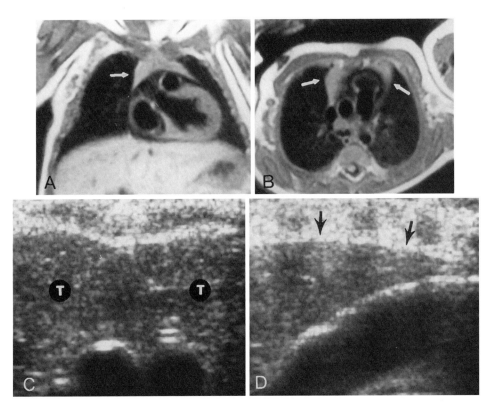

FIGURE 1.37. Normal thymus: magnetic resonance and ultrasound delineation. A. Note the normal shape and signal of the thymus (arrow) on this T2-weighted image. **B.** Axial view demonstrates the anterior position of the thymus. **C.** Ultrasonography demonstrates normal echotexture of the thymus (T) located anterior to the great vessels. **D.** Sagittal view demonstrates the typical wedge-like configuration of the thymus gland (arrows) just under the chest wall.

the entire complex results from defective development of the third and fourth pharyngeal pouches. Absence of the thymus produces a very thin superior mediastinum (Fig. 1.38, A and B), a finding, however, that can be duplicated by severe thymic atrophy (Fig. 1.38, C and D). In any of these cases, we have found that when one is searching for any residual thymic tissue, MRI is most rewarding (Fig. 1.39).

Spontaneous hemorrhage into the thymus gland causing marked mediastinal widening also can occur (23, 24). Bleeding in these cases may be the result of either vitamin K deficiency, birth trauma, or a combination of both. Bleeding also can occur into thymic cysts (23), and CT or ultrasound can delineate these suspected bleeds. Another interesting manifestation involving the thymus gland is the so-called "air cyst" of the thymus (25). Air is believed to collect under the capsule of the thymus in these infants and on roentgenographic examination is virtually indistinguishable from a loculated pneumomediastinum (Fig. 1.40). Calcification in the thymus is unusual but has been documented with histiocytosis X or Langerhans' histiocytosis (26–28).

FIGURE 1.39. Thymic agenesis and hypoplasia: magnetic resonance findings. A. Note the narrow superior mediastinum (arrows). **B.** Magnetic resonance study demonstrates no thymic tissue present in this patient with thymic agenesis. **C.** Another patient with a normal-appearing superior mediastinum. **D.** Magnetic resonance study shows a small hypoplastic thymic gland (arrow).

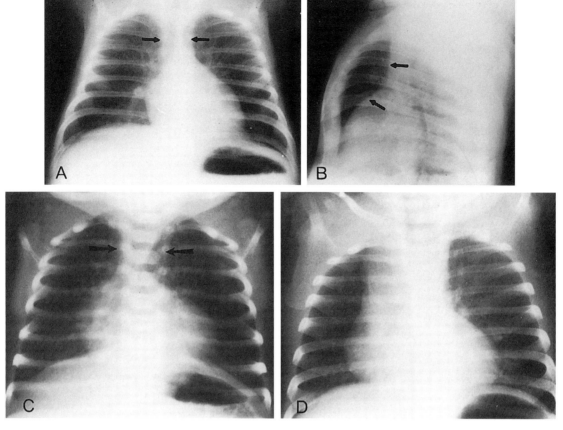

FIGURE 1.38. Thymic agenesis. A. Note the narrow superior mediastinum (arrows). B. Lateral view demonstrating an empty superior mediastinal space filled in by air-filled lung. Normally, this space should be opaque and filled by normal thymus. C. Stress atrophy. Similar findings with severe stress atrophy. The mediastinum is very narrow. D. Later, with regeneration, the mediastinum is normal.

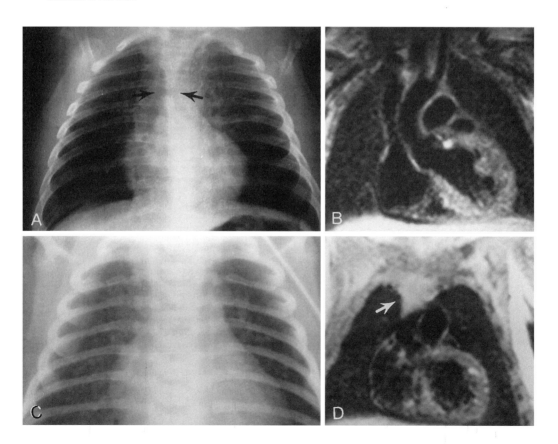

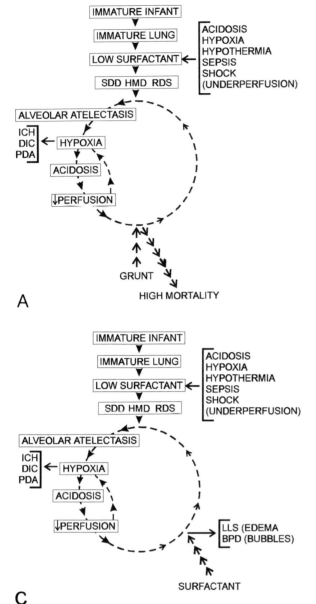

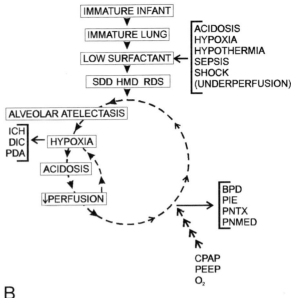

FIGURE 1.40. Surfactant deficiency disease: pathophysiologic considerations. A. Originally, in the premature infant who was inherently surfactant deficient, alveolar atelectasis leading to decreased gas exchange resulted in severe hypoxia and acidosis. Acidosis leads to decreased pulmonary perfusion, and a vicious cycle within a cycle is set in motion. Attempts to break this cycle consisted of the infant's own expiratory grunt. The result was few survivors and, of course, few pulmonary complications. **B.** With the advent of positive pressure ventilation and the delivery of high concentrations of oxygen, the number of survivors increased. However, complications also increased and took the form of pulmonary edema [leaky lung syndrome (LLS)], bronchopulmonary dysplasia (BPD), pulmonary interstitial emphysema (PIE), pneumothorax (PNTX), and pneumomediastinum (PNMED). **C.** With the advent of surfactant therapy and decreased ventilatory pressures secondary to oscillation therapy, the number of survivors again increased, and most of the previous complications decreased significantly. Current exceptions are the LSS and BPD. Complications directly related to hypoxia include shunting through a patent ductus arteriosus (PDA), disseminated intravascular coagulation (DIC), intracranial hemorrhage (ICH), and persistent fetal circulation (PFC). HMD, hyaline membrane disease; RDS, respiratory distress syndrome; CPAP, continuous positive airway pressure; PEEP, peak end-expiratory pressure.

REFERENCES

1. Fisher RM, Cremin BJ. The extent of the inferior border of the thymus: a report of two cases in infants. Br J Radiol 1975;48:814–816.
2. Mlvey RB. The thymic "wave" sign. Radiology 1963;81:834–838.
3. Lanning P, Heikkinen E. Thymus simulating left upper lobe atelectasis. Pediatr Radiol 1980;9:177–178.
4. Chertoff J, Barth RA, Dickerman JD. Rebound thymic hyperplasia five years after chemotherapy for Wilms' tumor. Pediatr Radiol 1991;21:596–597.
5. Doppman JL, Oldfield EH, Chrousos GP, et al. Rebound thymic hyperplasia after treatment of Cushing's syndrome. AJR 1986;147:1145–1147.
6. Spigland N, Bensoussan AL, Blanchard H, et al. Aberrant cervical thymus in children: three case reports and review of the literature. J Pediatr Surg 1990;25:1196–1199.
7. Shackelford GD, McAlister WH. The aberrantly positioned thymus: a cause of mediastinal or neck masses in children. AJR 1974;120:291–296.
8. Bar-Ziv J, Barki Y, Itzchak Y, et al. Posterior mediastinal accessory thymus. Pediatr Radiol 1984;14:165–167.
9. Slovis TL, Meza M, Kuhn JP. Aberrant thymus—MR assessment. Pediatr Radiol 1992;22:490–492.
10. Krysta MM, Gorecki WJ, Miezynski WH. Thymic tissue manifesting as a posterior mediastinal mass in two children. J Pediatr Surg 1998;33:632–634.
11. Swischuk LE, John SD. Case report. Normal thymus extending

between the right brachiocephalic vein and innominate artery. AJR 1996;166:1462–1464.

12. Hendrickson M, Azarow K, Ein S, et al. Congenital thymic cysts in children—mostly misdiagnosed. J Pediatr Surg 1998;33:821–825.

13. Rice HE, Flake QW, Hori T, et al. Massive thymic hyperplasia: characterization of a rare mediastinal mass. J Pediatr Surg 1994;29:1561–1564.

14. Rubb M, Keilani R, Howatson AG, et al. Benign symptomatic thymic tumors. J Pediatr Surg 2000;35:1362–1364.

15. Gregory AK, Connery CP, Resta-Flarer F, et al. A case of massive thymolipoma. J Pediatr Surg 1997;32:1780–1782.

16. Lam WWM, Chan FL, Lau YL, et al. Paediatric thymoma: unusual occurrence in two siblings. Pediatr Radiol 1993;23:124–126.

17. Kitano Y, Yokomori K, Ohkura M, et al. Giant thymolipoma in a child. J Pediatr Surg 1993;28:1622–1625.

18. Spigland N, DiLorenzo M, Youssef S, et al. Malignant thymoma in children: a 20-year review. J Pediatr Surg 1990;25:1143–1146.

19. David LA, McCreadie SR. The enlarged thymus gland in leukemia in childhood. AJR 1962;88:924.

20. Mainzer F, Taybi H. Thymic enlargement and pleural effusion; an unusual roentgenographic complex in childhood leukemia. AJR 1971;112:35–39.

21. Adam EJ, Ignotus PI. Sonography of the thymus in healthy children: frequency of visualization, size, and appearance. AJR 1993; 161:153–155.

22. Meyers A, Pep N, Cranley W, et al. Decreased thymus size on chest radiography: a sign of pediatric human immunodeficiency virus infection. Pediatrics 1992;90:99–102.

23. Urvoas E, Pariente D, Rousset A, et al. Ultrasound diagnosis of thymic hemorrhage in an infant with late-onset hemorrhagic disease. Pediatr Radiol 1994;24:96–97.

24. Walsh SV, Cooke R, Mortimer G, et al. Massive thymic hemorrhage in a neonate: an entity revisited. J Pediatr Surg 1996;31:1315–1317.

25. Raila FA, McKerchar B. Thymic cysts simulating loculated pneumomediastinum in the newborn. Br J Radiol 1977;50:286–287.

26. Junewick JJ, Fitzgerald NE. The thymus in Landerhans' cell histiocytosis. Pediatr Radiol 1999;29:904–907.

27. Heller GD, Haller JO, Berdon WE, et al. Punctate thymic calcification in infants with untreated Langerhans' cell histiocytosis: report of four new cases. Pediatr Radiol 1999;29:813–815.

28. Sumner TE, Auringer ST, Preston AA. Thymic calcifications in histiocytosis X. Pediatr Radiol 1993;23:204–205.

RESPIRATORY DISTRESS IN THE NEWBORN

Respiratory distress in the newborn infant can stem from a number of causes (Table 1.1), and yet the clinical findings may differ little from condition to condition. As a result, the chest roentgenogram still is the single most important diagnostic study that one can obtain. This is not to say that clinical data are not important, but only to emphasize the need for prompt pursuit of the radiographic examination. Most times, it is the chest radiograph that first pinpoints the correct diagnosis and, at the least, usually tells one whether pulmonary pathology is present. In this regard, **it is most unlikely that significant pulmonary disease, other than lung hypoplasia with persistent fetal circulation (PFC), is present if the chest radiograph is normal.**

TABLE 1.1. CAUSES OF NEONATAL RESPIRATORY DISTRESS

A. Surfactant Deficiency Disease
1. Hyaline membrane disease/respiratory distress syndrome
2. Retained lung fluid syndrome (transient tachypnea)
3. Meconium aspiration
4. Neonatal pneumonia
5. Leaky Lung Syndrome
6. Bronchopulmonary dysplasia, Wilson-Mikity Syndrome
7. Pulmonary hemorrhage
8. Pulmonary lymphangiectasia
9. Cystic disease of the lung (adenomatoid malformation)
10. Sequestration—bronchopulmonary foregut malformation
11. Pulmonary agenesis, hypoplasia
12. Pulmonary interstitial emphysema
13. Chronic pulmonary insufficiency of premature
14. Hyperviscosity syndrome

B. Tracheobronchial Disease
1. Tracheoesophageal fistula
2. Congenital lobar emphysema
3. Bronchobiliary fistula
4. Tracheomalacia (?)
5. Calcified tracheal cartilage (?)

C. Pleural Space Abnormalities
1. Pneumothorax, pneumomediastinum
2. Chylothorax
3. Hemothorax
4. Hydrothorax
5. Empyema

D. Tumors and Cysts
1. Neuroblastoma
2. Teratoma, thymoma
3. Various cysts
4. Cystic hygroma

E. Diaphragmatic Abnormalities
1. Diaphragmatic hernia, agenesis
2. Diaphragmatic paralysis
3. Eventration

F. Cardiac Disease
1. Various cardiac anomalies
2. Myocardial dysfunction
3. Persistent fetal circulation syndrome

G. Vascular Rings and Anomalies
1. Double aorta and other true rings
2. Anomalous innominate, left common carotid
3. Pulmonary sling

H. Chest Cage
1. Various bony dystrophies and dysplasias
2. Bony tumors
3. Myopathies

I. Gastrointestinal
1. Esophageal atresia, tracheoesophageal fistula
2. Chalasia
3. Abdominal distention
   (a) Massive pneumoperitoneum (perforation)
   (b) Ascites, chyloperitoneum, hemoperitoneum
   (c) Abdominal tumors and cysts

J. Nasopharynx, Larynx
1. Choanal atresia
2. Pharyngeal incoordination
3. Laryngomalacia
4. Laryngotracheal esophageal cleft
5. Laryngeal webs, stenosis, etc.
6. Tumors, cysts

K. Intracranial Disease
1. Intracranial hemorrhage, edema, infarction
2. Drug depression
3. Asphyxia with anoxic brain damage

L. Metabolic Disease

MEDICALLY TREATED CAUSES OF RESPIRATORY DISTRESS

Immature Lungs

Pulmonary immaturity, or "immature lung," is not truly a radiographic diagnosis, but one needs to understand the immature infant's lung before considering pulmonary conditions unique to this time of life. In terms of pulmonary immaturity, it is important to appreciate that the lung of an immature infant is both biochemically and structurally immature. In terms of biochemical immaturity, it is surfactant deficiency that is the problem, and this has led to the well-known findings of "surfactant deficiency disease" (SDD) or, in the past, "hyaline membrane disease."

The lungs of immature infants are structurally underdeveloped in terms of both number of alveoli present and integrity of the tracheobronchial tree, especially the more terminal bronchi and bronchioles. In this regard, it is generally appreciated that the number of alveoli present in immature infants is decreased (1), but it is less well appreciated that the cartilage in the peripheral bronchi and bronchioles is not as sturdy as it is in the mature infant (2). These two aspects of the immature lung are important and should be considered separately, in terms of both their embryologic development and the parts they subsequently play in the development of chronic lung disease in immature infants. All of this is discussed in later sections, but, for the time being, it is worth reiterating that they should be considered separately.

For more than two decades, attention was focused on the surfactant deficiency problem, while the structural problems associated with these lungs received less attention. However, now that intratracheal surfactant therapy so rapidly corrects the biochemical abnormality, the underlying structural immaturity problem has come into more prominence. Indeed, it is this aspect of pulmonary immaturity that most likely leads to the development of the bubbly lungs of bronchopulmonary dysplasia (BPD) (3). Once this concept is appreciated, one can understand **why some of these infants, even though showing rapid clearing of the lungs after surfactant therapy, still can go on to develop the bubbly lungs of BPD. In addition, it also can explain why some immature infants with clear lungs at birth go on to develop the same problem** (4). All of this, as previously noted, is discussed in more detail in later sections.

The lungs in immature infants, if they are not afflicted with SDD, usually appear relatively clear. They may, however, also appear slightly hazy, especially centrally, as a reflection of the abnormal ratio of solid to aerated lung parenchyma present.

REFERENCES

1. Mithal A, Emery JL. Postnatal development of alveoli in premature infants. Arch Dis Child 1961;36:449–450.
2. Burnard ED. The pulmonary syndrome of Wilson and Mikity, and respiratory function in very small premature infants. Pediatr Clin North Am 1966;13:999–1016.
3. Swischuk LE, John SD. Immature lung problems: can our nomenclature be more specific? AJR 1996;166:917–918.
4. Fitzgerald P, Donohue V, Gorman W. Bronchopulmonary dysplasia: a radiographic and clinical review of 20 patients. Br J Radiol 1990;63:444–447.

Surfactant Deficiency Disease (SDD)

SDD or, in the past, either hyaline membrane disease or idiopathic respiratory distress syndrome, still is the most common cause of respiratory distress in the immature infant. The major problem in these infants rests with biochemical (surfactant deficiency) immaturity of the lungs, but overall it should be remembered that the immaturity problem in these infants is twofold (i.e., both biochemical and structural lung immaturity). These two problems are intertwined, but it probably is best that they be considered separately (1, 2).

In terms of surfactant deficiency, the problem stems from the lack of this surface tension reducing lipoprotein in immature infants. Surfactant is believed to be produced by the alveolar cells and is essential for initial, and sustained, alveolar distention. Its absence leads to increased alveolar surface tension, decreased alveolar distensibility, and persistent collapse (atelectasis) of the alveoli. In other words, these infants cannot initially open, or thereafter normally inflate and aerate, their alveoli. As a result, gas exchange is virtually impossible. In addition, since the alveoli cannot be distended, these infants are unable to develop and maintain a significant functional residual volume. In the normal infant, after one or two breaths, a functional residual volume is established, and work for each subsequent breath is substantially decreased. In the infant with SDD, this does not occur, and it is as though the infant were taking its first, labored postnatal breath over and over again. As a result, these infants become fatigued and exhausted, and this only leads to more hypoxia, further impairment of surfactant production, and prolongation of the initial precarious condition of these infants. Postnatal surfactant therapy, now standard, has rectified this problem considerably, but in the past, it was determined that intrauterine surfactant protection could be enhanced by the presence of prenatal (maternal) stress in a variety of forms (i.e., infection, toxemia, prolonged rupture of membranes, etc.) (3, 4). Such stress is believed to result in increased steroid production by the mother and perhaps, to some extent, the fetus. As a consequence, physicians began to administer prenatal corticosteroids to mothers with suspect pregnancies. This resulted in a more favorable outcome in these patients, but this regimen of therapy is not commonly adhered to today.

The basic pathophysiology present in infants with SDD is outlined in Fig. 1.40. In this diagram, it should be noted that although the infant's lungs are immature both histologically and biochemically, it is the latter (i.e., biochemical immaturity through decreased surfactant production) that initially leads to problems. With alveolar aeration grossly impaired, increasing hypoxia and acidosis lead to spasm of the peripheral pulmonary arterioles and decreased perfusion of the lungs. This leads to further hypoxia and acidosis and the development of a vicious cycle within an already detrimental cycle of deleterious events. Unless these cycles are broken, recovery from the disease is not likely to occur, and in the more remote past hardly ever did.

In mildly afflicted infants, the cycle is slower, and the infant often survived the disease and slowly progressed to the point when normal surfactant production returned (usually by 5–7 days). In more severe cases, however, death was more or less inevitable and usually resulted from the pulmonary disease itself or from one of the complications of severe hypoxia and immaturity (i.e., intracranial hemorrhage, disseminated intravascular coagulation, pulmonary hemorrhage, and congestive heart failure from left-to-right shunting through a patent ductus arteriosus). Currently, however, intratracheal surfactant therapy has dramatically changed the entire spectrum of hyaline membrane disease or SDD (Fig. 1.40C).

In terms of coping with the problem of lack of alveolar aeration in SDD, on an innate, natural basis, such infants spontaneously develop the so-called "expiratory grunt." This grunt, tantamount to an exaggerated Valsalva maneuver, ensures that as much gas as possible is exchanged by **delivering air into the respiratory tree as deeply as possible and keeping it there for as long as possible.** Unfortunately, in more severe cases, air still reaches only the terminal bronchioles and alveolar ducts and perhaps a few alveoli. Even then, however, it still represents an improvement, for some gas exchange does occur at this level. **Artificially, the physician duplicated and exaggerated the grunt phenomenon** by the application of positive pressure assisted ventilation. Most of the severely afflicted infants required positive pressure assisted ventilation, and the advent of this form of therapy significantly improved the outcome in these infants. Unfortunately, however, it was not without problems of its own, for complications such as pneumothorax, pneumomediastinum, pulmonary interstitial emphysema (PIE), pneumoperitoneum, massive gas embolism, and BPD became commonplace (Fig. 1.40B). However, with the advent of endotracheal surfactant therapy and the general use of lower positive distending pressures or higher frequency ventilation (5–7), much of this now has been circumvented, but not completely eliminated.

Clinically, infants with SDD usually show signs of respiratory distress in the first 2 or 3 hours of life, and the very severely afflicted almost immediately after birth. **Occasionally, however, no real problem is encountered until the infant is 6–8 hours old.** These infants have "mild" hyaline membrane disease, and initially although some alveolar aeration occurs, it still is not totally normal, and unless these infants are treated, they become progressively more fatigued and hypoxic. This, of course, leads to further impairment of surfactant production and, in some cases, precipitous worsening of the infants' condition. The early radiographic changes in these infants are normal or subtly abnormal. Histologically, in SDD, the alveoli are uniformly collapsed, but the alveolar ducts and terminal bronchioles are variably distended (Fig. 1.41). These latter structures also are rimmed, on their inner aspects, by a layer of fibrin, the so-called "hyaline membrane." The membrane is believed to result from protein (serum) seepage from damaged (hypoxia) capillaries but is not specific to the disease. To be sure, hyaline membranes can be seen with other conditions such as meconium aspiration and neonatal pneumonia. Because the membranes are nonspecific, the term "hyaline membrane disease" was, in the past, replaced, with some success, by the term "respiratory distress syndrome." This term, however, is no more specific than "hyaline membrane disease" and, indeed, quite generic. To this end, it seemed appropriate to be more specific, and the name "surfactant deficiency disease" (SDD) was suggested (1).

The classic roentgenographic findings in SDD are well known and consist of pronounced pulmonary underaeration leading to small lung volumes, a finely granular (ground-glass) appearance of the pulmonary parenchyma, and peripherally extending air bronchograms (Fig. 1.42). The clarity of the air bronchogram is facilitated by air in the bronchial tree being visualized against a background of atelectatic, nonaerated alveoli. In other infants, if the roentgenogram is obtained during expiration, physiologic diminution in the caliber of the tracheobronchial tree leads to less prominent air bronchograms and more opaque, indeed even totally airless, lungs (Fig. 1.43). **This is an important physiologic point to appreciate for it will keep one from erroneously believing that the patient's condition has worsened when an expiratory film is inadvertently obtained. It is the absence of the air bronchogram in these patients that indicates that the film was obtained in total expiration.**

Granularity of the lungs in SDD results from the visualization of distended terminal bronchioles and alveolar ducts against the ever-present background of alveolar atelectasis. The variable distention of the terminal airways results in the wide spectrum of roentgenographic findings seen in these infants, and indeed, it is only when terminal bronchial and alveolar duct distention is just right that typical granularity is seen. When distention is lessened, the granularity disappears, and when distention is increased (i.e., by the infant's own grunt or assisted positive pressure ventilation), the fine granular pattern yields to a more coarse pattern and small bubble formation. These bubbles, termed type I bubbles (8), are very uniform in size, ranging from 1 to 2 mm in diameter, and often are more readily visible in the lung bases (Fig. 1.44). The bubbles result from overdistention of the terminal bronchioles and alveolar ducts (8).

The roentgenographic findings in classic hyaline membrane disease are quite characteristic, and there are few conditions that mimic them. A few congenital heart lesions man-

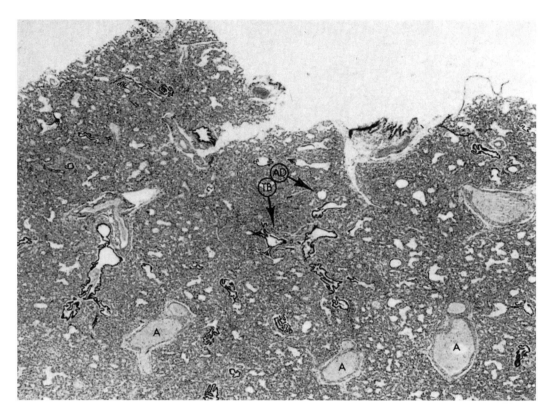

FIGURE 1.41. Surfactant deficiency disease: histologic appearance. Note that the parenchyma is underaerated and that the alveolar mass is atelectatic. Aeration occurs primarily in the terminal bronchioles (TB) and alveolar ducts (AD). The terminal bronchioles are lined by epithelium (dark border of air-filled spaces). A, arterioles.

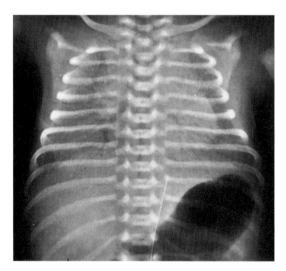

FIGURE 1.42. Surfactant deficiency disease: typical findings. Note that the lungs are underaerated and small for the overall size of the infant. In addition, note widespread peripheral air bronchograms and diffuse granularity of the lungs.

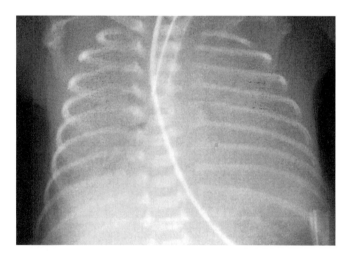

FIGURE 1.43. Surfactant deficiency disease: whiteout. On the expiratory phase, the lungs become totally opaque with little, if any, air in the tracheobronchial tree.

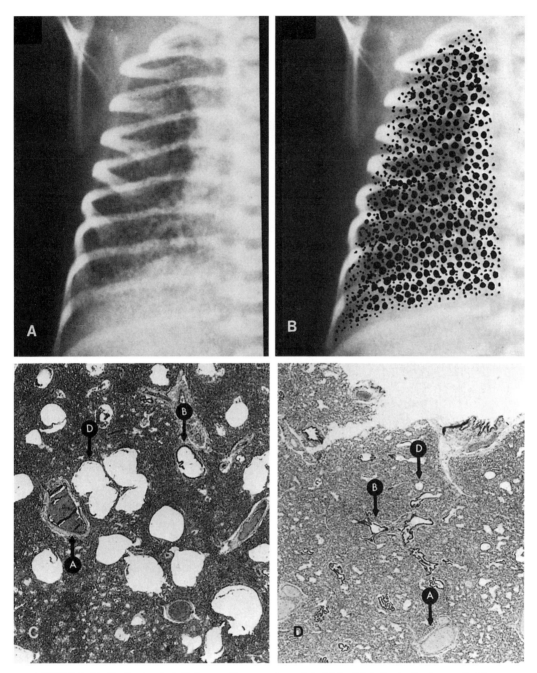

FIGURE 1.44. Surfactant deficiency disease, type I bubble: histologic features. A. Note the fine, spherical bubbles scattered throughout the right lung. **B.** Diagrammatic representation of the bubbles. **C.** Histologic appearance of overdistended terminal bronchioles (B) and alveolar ducts (D) in the same infant. A, arteriole. **D.** Another infant with more typical findings of hyaline membrane disease for comparison. Specifically compare the size of the terminal bronchioles (B) and alveolar ducts (D). The overdistended terminal airways (alveolar ducts and terminal bronchioles), as seen in **C,** are visualized as the type I bubble on the roentgenogram. (Reproduced with permission from Swischuk LE. Bubbles in hyaline membrane disease; differentiation of three types. Radiology 1977;122:417–426).

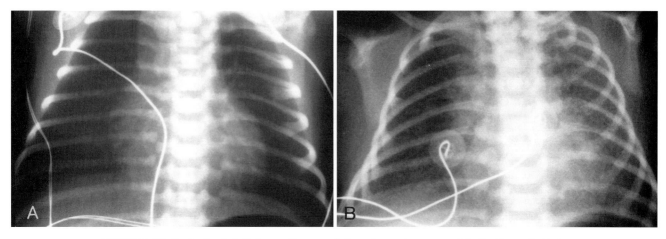

FIGURE 1.45. Surfactant deficiency disease: delayed roentgenographic findings. A. Note the completely clear lungs in this newborn infant with minimal respiratory distress. **B.** In less than 24 hours, typical granular changes of surfactant deficiency disease have developed.

ifesting in pronounced pulmonary venous obstruction (e.g., total anomalous pulmonary venous return type III, pulmonary vein atresia, and hypoplastic left heart syndrome) can produce enough interstitial pulmonary edema to mimic the granular lungs of SDD, but generally, these conditions are uncommon. In addition, some infants with pulmonary lymphangiectasia, the retained lung fluid syndrome, and neonatal pneumonia can demonstrate findings mimicking those of SDD. In these latter infants, the interstitum and/or alveoli are full of some type of fluid and thus cannot be aerated, but as opposed to infants with SDD, the lungs tend to be larger.

In the past, there have been attempts to classify severity of surfactant deficiency disease from roentgenographic findings alone, but this usually was accomplished on a gross basis only. On the other hand, those infants with the most severe disease show more profound changes and usually do so immediately after birth. The very smallest of these infants usually have a markedly reduced alveolar mass, and because of this, the lungs are very small and dense, hardly even granular. In addition, because the alveolar mass is reduced, even with surfactant therapy, clinical results are guarded. The reason for this is that there simply are not enough alveoli present, and so, surfactant or not, adequate surface area for gas exchange is not present. It is these infants that are most likely to still go on to develop complications such as pneumothorax, pneumomediastinum, PIE, and, eventually, chronic lung disease.

At the other end of the spectrum are those infants who are larger and/or have milder disease and may not meet the criteria for surfactant therapy. However, slowly but surely, they develop findings of SDD, usually over the first 6–12 hours of life. **Pathophysiologically, in these infants, surfactant is not totally absent, and considerable alveolar aeration can occur just after birth.** However, even though some alveolar aeration is present, it is not entirely normal, and hypoxia ensues. Breathing becomes more difficult, and soon fatigue sets in. As a result, ventilation becomes less efficient and increasing hypoxia takes its toll, leading to further reduction

of surfactant production and the development of typical SDD (Fig. 1.45). It is in these infants that the phenomenon (9) of more pronounced changes in the lung bases secondary to the fact that the upper lobes mature earlier is seen (Fig. 1.46).

Surfactant therapy now usually results in rapid clearing and aeration of the lungs (Fig. 1.47). However, we (2) have noted that infants most likely to be totally cured are larger, with a mean weight of 1,850 g and a mean gestational age of 32 weeks. Smaller infants are more likely to go on to develop pulmonary edema as part of the leaky lung syndrome (LLS) (Fig. 1.48), and some, the bubbly lungs of BPD.

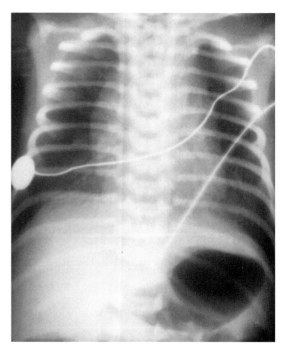

FIGURE 1.46. Surfactant deficiency disease: basal changes in larger infant. In this larger infant, note that granularity of the lungs is seen primarily in the lung bases (arrows). In addition, the lungs are nearly normal in size.

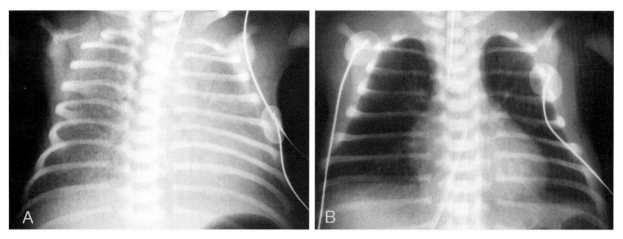

FIGURE 1.47. Surfactant deficiency disease: clearing with surfactant therapy. A. Note marked haziness/granularity of the lungs and air bronchograms consistent with surfactant deficiency disease. **B.** After surfactant therapy, the lungs are completely clear. They remained completely clear in this patient, and the patient was cured.

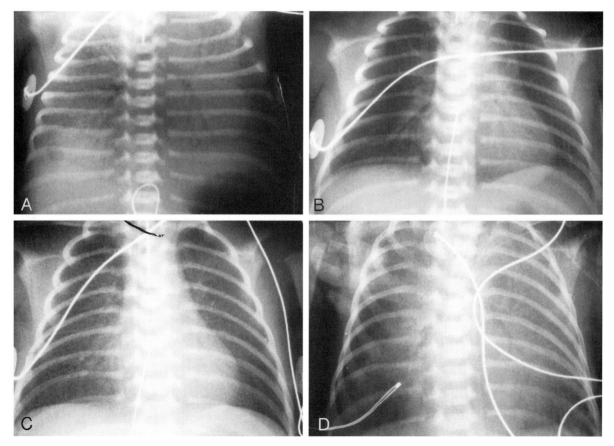

FIGURE 1.48. Leaky lung syndrome after treatment of surfactant deficiency disease. A. Note marked changes of surfactant deficiency disease with hazy to granular lungs and air bronchograms. **B.** After surfactant therapy, the lungs are completely clear. **C.** Seven to 10 days later, however, the lungs are beginning to become a little hazy, representing the development of early pulmonary edema. **D.** A few days later, extensive opacity of the lungs is seen. This is characteristic of the development of the pulmonary edema of the leaky lung syndrome.

In terms of clearing of the lungs after surfactant therapy, it has been noted that uneven aeration can occur, but it does not appear to be a clinical problem (10). Also, some infants clear their upper lobes quicker than their lung bases (11), and uneven aeration can result from uneven distribution of surfactant, predominantly having the surfactant go to one side only.

Complications of surfactant therapy are few, but some patients have been noted to develop pulmonary hemorrhage, which often is very profound (12, 13). In these patients, it is believed that the delivery of surfactant allows for hitherto-impossible free alveolar aeration, and this leads to decreased pulmonary vascular resistance, greater left-to-right shunting through the patent ductus arteriosus, and flooding of the lungs. Pulmonary hemorrhage is the consequence. When pulmonary hemorrhage develops, the roentgenographic findings consist of dense, diffuse opacification of the lungs, either nodular or very homogeneous and opaque (more often). The complication of pulmonary hemorrhage, however, is rare.

REFERENCES

1. Swischuk LE, John SD. Immature lung problems: can our nomenclature be more specific? AJR 1996;166:917–918.
2. Swischuk LE, Shetty B, John SD. The lungs in immature infants; how important is surfactant therapy in preventing chronic lung problems? Pediatr Radiol 1996;26:508–511.
3. Gould JB, Gluck L, Kulovick MV. The relationship between accelerated pulmonary maturity and accelerated neurological maturity in certain chronically stressed pregnancies. Am J Obstet Gynecol 1977;127:181–186.
4. Thibeault DW, Emmanouilides GC. Prolonged rupture of fetal membranes and decreased frequency of respiratory distress syndrome and patent ductus arteriosus in preterm infants. Am J Obstet Gynecol 1977;129:43–46.
5. Gerstmann DT, Minton SD, Stoddard RA, et al. The Provo Multicenter Early High-Frequency Oscillatory Ventilation Trial: improved pulmonary and clinical outcome in respiratory distress syndrome. Pediatrics 1996;98:1044–1057.
6. Keszler M, Modanlou HD, Brudno DS, et al. Multicenter controlled clinical trial of high-frequency jet ventilation in preterm infants with uncomplicated respiratory distress syndrome. Pediatrics 1997;100:593–599.
7. Rettwitz-Volk W, Veldman A, Roth B, et al. A prospective, randomized multicenter trial of high-frequency oscillatory ventilation compared with conventional ventilation in preterm infants with respiratory distress syndrome receiving surfactant. J Pediatr 1998;132:249–254.
8. Swischuk LE. Bubbles in hyaline membrane disease; differentiation of three types. Radiology 1977;122:417–426.
9. Ablow RC, Orzalesi MM. Localized roentgenographic pattern of hyaline membrane disease; evidence that the upper lobes of human lung mature earlier than the lower lobes. AJR 1971;112:23–27.
10. Slama M, Andre C, Huon C, et al. Radiological analysis of hyaline membrane disease after exogenous surfactant treatment. Pediatr Radiol 1999;29:56–60.
11. Edwards DK, Hilton SVW, Merrit TA, et al. Respiratory distress syndrome treated with human surfactant: radiographic findings. Radiology 1985;157:329–334.
12. Pappin A, Shenker N, Hack M, et al. Extensive intraalveolar pulmonary hemorrhage in infants dying after surfactant therapy. J Pediatr 1994;124:621–626.
13. Raju TNK, Langenberg P. Pulmonary hemorrhage and exogenous surfactant therapy: a metaanalysis. J Pediatr 1993;123:603–610.

Leaky Lung Syndrome

Infants who are severely hypoxic, and especially those who require assisted ventilator therapy with high concentrations of oxygen, sustain damage to their pulmonary capillaries in the form of "oxygen toxicity" (1, 2) and associated hypoxia. The end result is increased permeability of the capillaries, with leaking of fluid into the pulmonary interstitium. At first, this fluid is interstitial, but eventually it becomes both interstitial and intraalveolar. The resulting edema can be transient or refractory. Indeed, in many cases, it lasts for weeks.

Pulmonary edema as seen in these infants always has been considered a manifestation of BPD, but it might be better to consider the problem an entity unto itself. To this end, the term "leaky lung syndrome" (LLS) has been suggested (3, 4). This clearly separates it from the bubbly dysplastic lungs of true BPD. There is no question, of course, that pulmonary edema plays a part in the eventual development of BPD, for pulmonary edema often predisposes the infant to being placed on positive pressure ventilation for prolonged periods of time. To be sure, it is the positive pressure ventilation that eventually leads to the development of bubbly lungs, and this is discussed later in the section on BPD and the Wilson-Mikity syndrome. **The two problems, namely, LLS and BPD, although intertwined, are different, both in pathophysiology and in treatment (3, 4). Therefore, I have come to consider them different but, in some cases, inseparable.** Indeed, frequently they are seen changing from one day to another in the same patient. Overall, however, pulmonary edema is more common than the bubbles of BPD, and, indeed, pulmonary edema now is the most common abnormality seen in premature infants (5).

In regard to the development of the LLS, it should be noted that the small premature infants (under 2,500 g) developing this complication, even though demonstrating clear lungs after surfactant therapy, still have structurally immature lungs. They do not have enough alveoli, and for this reason respiratory distress continues, requiring treatment with high flows of oxygen, which, in combination with the hypoxia, lead to damage of the capillary basement membranes and leakage of fluid into the lung interstitium. This can occur in stages (Fig. 1.48) or imperceptibly pass, in very immature infants, from the findings of severe SDD to the edema of the LLS (Fig. 1.49, A and B).

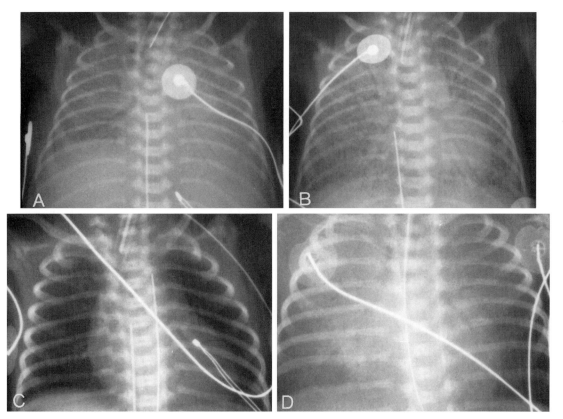

FIGURE 1.49. Leaky lung syndrome in other patients. A. Initial, severe surfactant deficiency disease. This infant had severe surfactant deficiency disease. Note that the lungs are basically opaque and that air is present only in the tracheobronchial tree. **B.** The patient was refractory to surfactant therapy and rapidly developed pulmonary edema. The lungs now are larger but still very opaque. The findings would be difficult to differentiate from pneumonia or pulmonary hemorrhage, but with clinical correlation, edema becomes the best answer. **C. Clear lungs to leaky lung syndrome.** This infant was born with clear lungs. These lungs, however, still are immature and have fewer than normal numbers.of alveoli. With persistent ventilator therapy and high concentrations of oxygen, the patient developed pulmonary edema in about 7–10 days. **D.** The lungs now are hazy but reasonably large. In all of these cases, when pulmonary edema develops, the lungs are larger in size than when surfactant deficiency disease was the problem.

The LLS also can develop in low birth weight infants who have clear lungs from the onset. They never suffer from SDD, yet these lungs are immature and similarly predispose the infant to the development of the LLS (Fig. 1.49, C and D).

Some cases of the LLS are extremely refractory to ordinary therapeutic measures. These include fluid restriction and diuretic therapy (6), but if they fail, steroids can be employed (7). Steroid therapy is aimed at curbing the inflammatory process associated with capillary wall damage. Recently, however, it has been noted that steroids may reduce gray matter brain growth (8). The pulmonary edema seen in these patients is readily visible on histologic examination (Fig. 1.50).

When one considers the pathophysiology of the LLS, it becomes apparent that it is closely related, if not the same, as that seen in the acquired respiratory distress syndrome

(ARDS). Indeed, radiographic and pathologic findings, along with complications of ventilator therapy such as interstitial emphysema, pneumothorax, and eventual development of BPD, are the same.

Finally, it should be noted that the presence of the LLS often predisposes these infants to the development of the bubbly lungs of BPD. The reason for this is that the persistent respiratory distress associated with the LLS requires longer ventilator times with higher pressures, and under such circumstances, the mechanically induced bubbles of BPD occur. This is discussed later with BPD.

Although pulmonary edema as part of the LLS is the most common cause of pulmonary edema in the immature infant, other causes of pulmonary edema also can be seen or co-exist. These include neurogenic pulmonary edema secondary to increased intracranial pressure with intracranial bleeding, left-to-right shunts through a patent ductus arte-

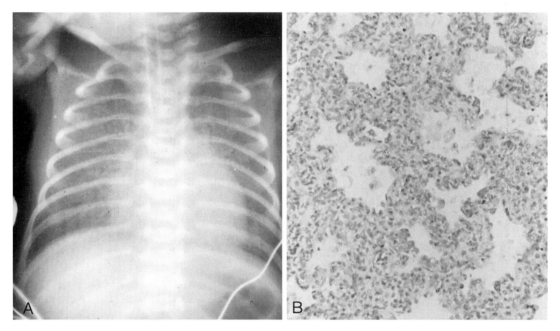

FIGURE 1.50. Leaky lung syndrome: histologic findings. A. Note diffusely hazy lungs characteristic of the leaky lung syndrome. **B.** Histologic material in this infant demonstrates the extensive edema of the pulmonary interstitium.

riosus or ventricular septal defect, renal failure, and simple fluid overload. In terms of underlying cardiac disease such as a ventricular septal defect or patent ductus arteriosus, in addition to the edema, one usually notes an increase in cardiac size.

REFERENCES

1. Brasch RC, Berthezene Y, Vexler V, et al. Pulmonary oxygen toxicity: demonstration of abnormal capillary permeability using contrast-enhanced MRI. Pediatr Radiol 1993;23:495–500.
2. Groneck P, Gotze-Speer B, Opperman M, et al. Association of pulmonary inflammation and increased microvascular permeability during the development of bronchopulmonary dysplasia: a sequential analysis of inflammatory mediators in respiratory fluids of high-risk preterm neonates. Pediatrics 1994;93:712–718.
3. Swischuk LE, John SD. Immature lung probems: can our nomenclature be more specific? AJR 1996;166:917–918.
4. Swischuk LE, Shetty B, John SD. The lungs in immature infants: how important is surfactant therapy in preventing chronic lung problems? Pediatr Radiol 1996;26:508–511.
5. Kao LC, Durand DJ, McCrea RC, et al. Randomized trial of long-term diuretic therapy for infants with oxygen-dependent bronchopulmonary dysplasia. J Pediatr 1994;124:772–781.
6. Wood BP, Davitt MA, Metlay LA. Lung disease in the very immature neonate: radiographic and microscopic correlation. Pediatr Radiol 1989;20:33–40.
7. Schrod L, Neuhaus T, Horwitz AE, et al. The effect of dexamethasone on respiratory-dependent very low birth-weight infants is best predicted by chest x-ray. Pediatr Radiol 2001;31:332–338.
8. Murphy BP, Inder TE, Huppi PS, et al. Impaired cerebral cortical gray matter growth after treatment with dexamethasone for neonatal chronic lung disease. Pediatrics 2001;107:217–221.

Retained Fluid Syndrome

Retained fluid syndrome (RFS), originally described as "transient tachypnea of the newborn" (1) and then "transient respiratory distress of the newborn" (2) or "wet lung disease" (3), simply is **a problem of retained fetal pulmonary fluid and is not a true disease.** There is an increased incidence of the condition in infants delivered by cesarean section (2, 3), and it is postulated that in these infants, absence of squeezing of the thorax (4), as experienced with delivery through the vaginal canal, leads to retention of normal fetal lung fluid. This fluid subsequently is cleared by way of the peribronchial lymphatics (5). Because of this, the lymphatics overdistend, pulmonary compliance is altered, and respiratory distress develops. However, this does not always lead to overt respiratory distress, and some infants seem to handle this fluid overload better than others. The fluid in the lungs of these infants consists primarily of fluid secreted by the fetal lung, but some amniotic fluid also is present.

In the RFS, respiratory distress usually becomes apparent by 2–4 hours of age or even earlier. Specific symptoms consist of tachypnea, nasal flaring, grunting, and retractions. Treatment is conservative and consists of supportive oxygen and maintenance of body temperature. There is no alveolar diffusion block, but rather the problem is one of a "stiff" or "splinted" lung that does not ventilate properly until the fluid is cleared. This usually occurs by 24 hours or less, although a few cases may take up to 48 hours to completely clear.

The roentgenographic findings in the RFS are rather characteristic and should lead one to suspect the diagnosis (1–3, 6). The most common and characteristic changes consist of symmetrical parahilar radiating congestion, moderate to severe overaeration of the lungs, and occasionally pleural effusions (Fig. 1.51). The parahilar radiating pattern of congestion most often is misinterpreted for vascular congestion, meconium aspiration, or neonatal pneumonia. However, as alarming as the findings can appear in some of these infants, their rapid disappearance, usually within 24–48 hours, clearly attests to the benign, transient nature of the condition. Other configurations may initially suggest cardiac failure, SDD, and, when basal, neonatal pneumonia (Fig. 1.52).

In terms of differentiating the RFS from vascular congestion secondary to heart disease, it first should be noted that **while the RFS commonly is seen in the first hours of life, congestion from cardiac disease usually is not apparent for 24 or more hours.** Cardiac problems leading to passive congestion causing problems in differentiating the findings from those of the RFS usually include total anomalous pulmonary venous return type III, the hypoplastic left heart syndrome, and pulmonary vein atresia. In total anomalous pulmonary venous return type III and pul-

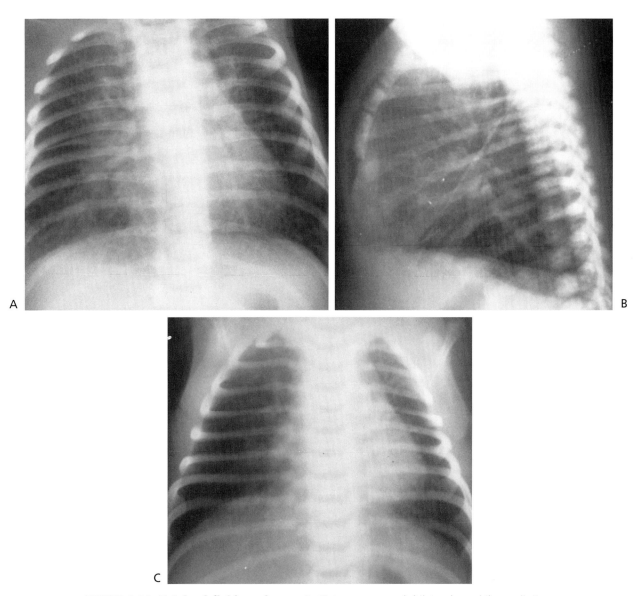

FIGURE 1.51. Retained fluid syndrome. A. Note pronounced, bilateral parahilar, radiating infiltrates and some fluid in the minor fissure. These changes often are misinterpreted for pneumonia or congestive heart failure. **B.** Lateral view demonstrates overaeration, parahilar streakiness, and fluid in the pleural fissures. **C.** Same infant 24 hours later demonstrates virtual clearing of the lungs. A little overaeration persists.

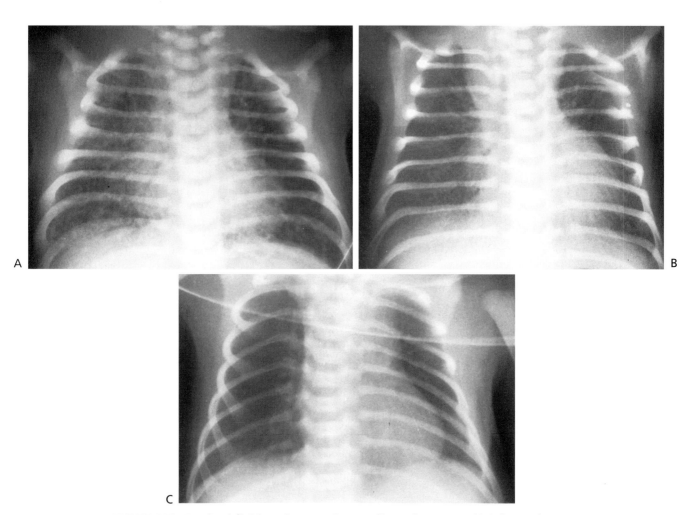

FIGURE 1.52. Retained fluid syndrome: other configurations. A. In this infant, pulmonary vascular congestion is mimicked. **B.** This patient demonstrates diffusely hazy lungs that often are misinterpreted for surfactant deficiency disease or pneumonia. **C.** In this patient, hazy to granular infiltrates are present, primarily in the lung bases. These findings also can be seen in mild cases of surfactant deficiency disease and with neonatal pneumonia.

monary vein atresia, severe cyanosis is present and there is no cardiomegaly. The presence of severe cyanosis clearly differentiates the problem from that of the RFS. In the hypoplastic left heart syndrome, cyanosis is mild or absent and the findings may be more difficult to differentiate except that pulmonary vascular congestion develops a little later and the heart becomes enlarged.

Pulmonary lymphangiectasia also can be confused with the RFS, but, once again, infants with pulmonary lymphangiectasia usually show more profound respiratory distress and cyanosis. In the end, in all cases, the benign, short, self-limiting course of the RFS serves as the final distinction from all of the more severe conditions that it can mimic.

REFERENCES

1. Avery ME, Gatewood OB, Brumley G. Transient tachypnea of the newborn; possible delayed resorption of fluid at birth. Am J Dis Child 1966;111:380–385.

2. Swischuk LE. Transient respiratory distress of the newborn—TRDN; a temporary disturbance of a normal phenomenon. AJR 1970;108:557–563.
3. Wesenberg RL, Graven SN, McCabe EB. Radiological findings in wet-lung disease. Radiology 1971;98:69–74.
4. Milner AD, Saunders RA, Hopkin IE. Effects of delivery by caesarean section on lung mechanics and lung volume in the human neonate. Arch Dis Child 1978;53:545–548.
5. Adams FH, Yanagisawa M, Kuzela D, et al. Disappearance of fetal lung fluid. J Pediatr 1971;78:837–843.
6. Kuhn JP, Fletcher BD, DeLemos RA. Roentgen findings in transient tachypnea of the newborn. Radiology 1969;92:751–757.

Opaque Right Lung Syndrome

Opaque right lung syndrome, although not common, can be problematic (1). Generally what one sees is an opaque lung, and almost invariably it is the right lung. In some cases, only a lobe of the right lung may be involved, but most often, all or most of the lung is opaque (Fig. 1.53). The findings often are misinterpreted for pneumonia,

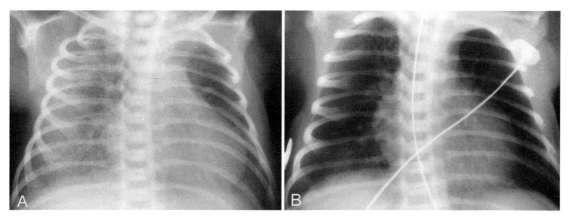

FIGURE 1.53. Opaque right lung syndrome. A. Note the opaque right lung. There is no mediastinal shift either way. **B.** One day later, both lungs are clear.

empyema, or massive atelectasis. Massive atelectasis should not be the problem as there is no volume loss with the opaque right lung syndrome. I believe the findings in the opaque right lung syndrome represent a combination of retained fetal lung fluid and an obstructed lung, probably secondary to a transient mucous plug.

Cesarean section-delivered babies are more prone to develop this condition, and impaired diaphragmatic excursion (because of the underlying liver) also could contribute to the problem (1). Whatever the cause, however, the condition is entirely benign, usually relatively asymptomatic, and clears within 24–48 hours or sooner.

REFERENCE

1. Swischuk LE, Hayden CK Jr, Richardson CJ. Neonatal opaque right lung: delayed fluid resorption. Radiology 1981;141: 671–673.

Neonatal Aspiration with and without Meconium

Although respiratory activity does occur in the fetus, it is not so exuberant that large volumes of amniotic fluid are aspirated into the lungs before birth occurs. However, when intrauterine fetal distress occurs, these normally shallow fetal respirations become deeper, and actually, fetal gasping occurs. Simultaneously, fetal distress causes the passage of meconium in utero, and thus not only is amniotic fluid aspirated, but so is meconium. The passage of meconium probably is linked to a hypoxia-induced vagal response that leads to increased gastrointestinal peristaltic activity and premature expulsion of meconium. Normally, meconium is not expelled until after birth.

Infants with meconium aspiration usually are postmature, depressed, and in severe respiratory difficulty almost immediately after birth. Tachypnea is the most prominent feature,

although retractions, grunting, and cyanosis can be seen. Widespread air trapping is the rule and results from the particles of meconium becoming lodged in the small peripheral bronchi. Complications such as pneumomediastinum and pneumothorax are common. In addition, the severe hypoxia present leads to the PFC syndrome and right-to-left shunting across the patent ductus arteriosus and/or foramen ovale (1).

Roentgenographically, the findings vary with the degree of meconium aspiration and are further influenced by the amount of amniotic fluid aspirated. In mild cases, findings may be normal, while with massive aspiration, the findings are florid. The aspirated fluid, whatever the degree of aspiration, clears quickly, but dislodging of the meconium particles takes longer, and so while the lungs may clear, respiratory distress persists. If the infant aspirates amniotic fluid primarily, the findings clear rapidly and the patient improves quickly (Fig. 1.54).

The aspirated debris can consist of squames, lanugo hair, or meconium (Fig. 1.55B). An extreme example of non-meconium debris causing serious problems is aspiration of amniotic fluid containing excessive squames from infants with congenital ichthyosis (2). In these infants, the clinical and roentgenographic features are more like those of meconium aspiration than simple amniotic fluid aspiration. A similar problem has been documented with aspiration of vernix caseosa (3).

In the classic case of meconium aspiration, findings consist of gross overaeration of the lungs and bilateral nodular infiltrates (Fig. 1.55A). The nodular infiltrates represent areas of patchy or focal alveolar atelectasis, and the overaerated spaces in between, compensatory focal alveolar overdistention. Pneumothorax and pneumomediastinum, as noted earlier, are common, and complicating chemical pneumonitis has been demonstrated to routinely occur after 48 hours or so (4). Rarely, a large piece of meconium can obstruct the bronchus and lead to obstructive emphysema or atelectasis (Fig. 1.55C).

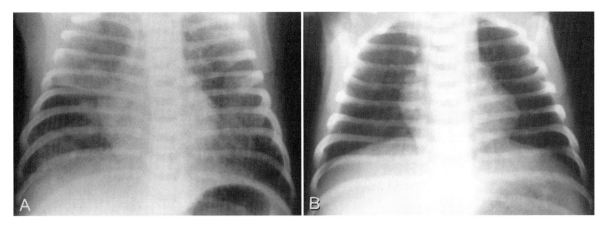

FIGURE 1.54. Amniotic fluid aspiration without significant meconium aspiration. A. Note diffuse nodular infiltrates and gross overaeration. These findings would be quite consistent with meconium aspiration. **B.** Twenty-four hours later, the lungs are completely clear. This patient could not have aspirated much in the way of meconium for the changes to have cleared so rapidly.

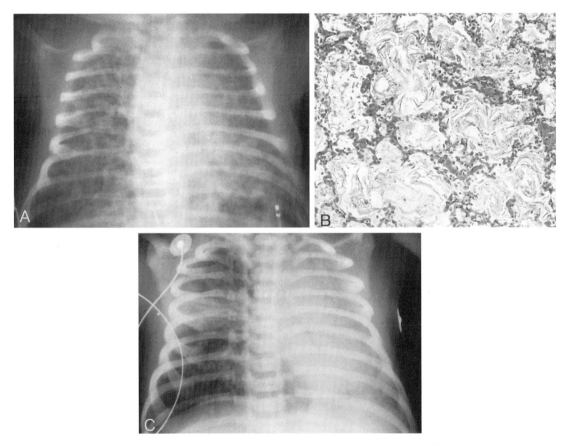

FIGURE 1.55. Meconium aspiration. A. Note typical, fluffy, nodular infiltrates scattered throughout both lungs. Overaeration is present. **B.** Histologic material from another infant demonstrates impaction of the terminal airways and alveoli with squames. **C.** In this patient with meconium aspiration, a large fragment of meconium was in the right bronchus and caused obstructive emphysema with contralateral shift of the mediastinum and compression of the left lung.

Treatment of meconium aspiration usually consists of supportive oxygen, maintenance of body temperature, humidification of the inspired air, and prophylactic antibiotics. It also is most important that suctioning of the tracheobronchial tree be performed in the delivery room as soon as fetal aspiration of meconium is suspected. This keeps the meconium from getting below the vocal cords and into the deep tracheobronchial tree where it causes symptoms. In severe cases, extracorporeal membrane oxygenation (ECMO) therapy may be required.

Routine gastric lavage also is recommended, so as to reduce the likelihood of further aspiration with vomiting, and antibiotics, as noted, are administered prophylactically. In some instances, surfactant therapy also has been employed (5, 6). In patients who recover, roentgenographic clearing is slow, often taking days. Histologic studies, in those infants who die, show particulate matter in the bronchi, cellular infiltrate, hyaline membranes, and areas of focal atelectasis interspersed with areas of alveolar overdistention. Long-term sequelae of meconium aspiration primarily are those of bronchospasm or reactive airway disease (7, 8).

REFERENCES

1. Fox WF, Gewitz MH, Dinwiddie R, et al. Pulmonary hypertension in the perinatal aspiration syndromes. Pediatrics 1977;59: 205–211.
2. Perlman M, Bar-Ziv J. Congenital ichthyosis and neonatal pulmonary disease. Pediatrics 1974;53:573–575.
3. Ohlsson A, Cumming WA, Najiar H. Neonatal aspiration syndrome due to vernix caseosa. Pediatr Radiol 1985;15:193–195.
4. Tyler DC, Murphy J, Cheney FW. Mechanical and chemical damage to lung tissue caused by meconium aspiration. Pediatrics 1978; 62:454–459.
5. Dargaville PA, South M, McDougall PN. Surfactant and surfactant inhibitors in meconium aspiration syndrome. J Pediatr 2001; 138:113–115.
6. Findlay RD, Taeusch HW, Walther FJ. Surfactant replacement therapy for meconium aspiration syndrome. Pediatrics 1996;97: 48–52.
7. Macfarlane PI, Heaf DP. Pulmonary function in children after neonatal meconium aspiration syndrome. Arch Dis Child 1988; 63:368–372.
8. Swaminathan S, Quinn J, Stabile MW, et al. Long-term pulmonary sequelae of meconium aspiration syndrome. J Pediatr 1989;114:356–361.

Neonatal Pneumonia

Although a number of pulmonary infections can develop in the first 4 weeks of life, this section deals with those pneumonias developing at, or soon after, birth. Most of these are of bacterial origin, and the common organisms include nonhemolytic *Streptococcus, Staphylococcus aureus,* and *Escherichia coli.* Other gram-negative and -positive organisms also are encountered, and even *Candida albicans* has been documented to result in widespread fulminant neonatal pneumonia (1). In addition, viral infections can occur, and causative agents include adenovirus (2, 3), herpes simplex (4, 5), influenza, and parainfluenza (6). In addition, even pertussis (7) and syphilis (8) as causes have been documented. In syphilis, the disease process is interstitial, as it is with pertussis, and for the most part, diffusely hazy lungs are seen. The lungs in infants with syphilis infection are pale pink to white, and hence the term "pneumonia alba" has been applied.

It is more difficult to distinguish between the patterns of bacterial and viral infections in neonates than in older infants and children, but bacterial infections still tend to be more alveolar and viral infections more interstitial (Figs 1.56 and 1.57). For this reason, radiating parahilar streakiness and diffuse, hazy, or reticulonodular lungs favor viral disease. Contrarily, coarse, patchy parenchymal infiltrates and consolidations (rare in neonates) favor bacterial disease. In addition, pleural effusions are relatively common with bacterial infections but quite rare with viral infections. Rarely, viral infections can produce pulmonary calcifications later in life (9).

In any neonatal pulmonary infection, the infant can become infected in utero, during passage through the birth canal, or just after birth. The first two modes, however, are most common, and predisposing factors include prolonged, premature rupture of the membranes, ascending infection from the vagina, placental infection, and contamination of the infant with maternal fecal material or bacteria from a poorly prepared perineum. Septicemia is a commonly associated feature, and, actually, most of these infants are frankly septic.

If the infection is derived in utero, the infant is often stillborn or premature. On the other hand, if the infant is born alive, marked respiratory distress with tachypnea, retractions, and cyanosis usually is apparent shortly after birth. In spite of this, it is interesting that these infants often are afebrile or even hypothermic. Consequently, diagnosis depends upon a high index of suspicion and the roentgenographic demonstration of pulmonary infiltrates.

The roentgenographic findings in neonatal pneumonia are quite varied, but overall solitary lobar consolidations are uncommon. With group B *Streptococcus,* there is a propensity for the roentgenographic findings to mimic the granularity of the lungs seen in SDD (Fig. 1.58). In some cases, these changes are more pronounced in the lung bases. Although group B streptococcal infections account for most of the cases demonstrating this roentgenographic pattern, other bacterial infections and even *Listeria* pneumonia can also be the cause. In these cases, the alveoli, as opposed to the collapsed alveoli in SDD, are distended and filled with purulent exudate. This results in an increase in lung volume, and so the lungs are granular, but large. This is very different from the lungs of SDD, where they are granular, but small.

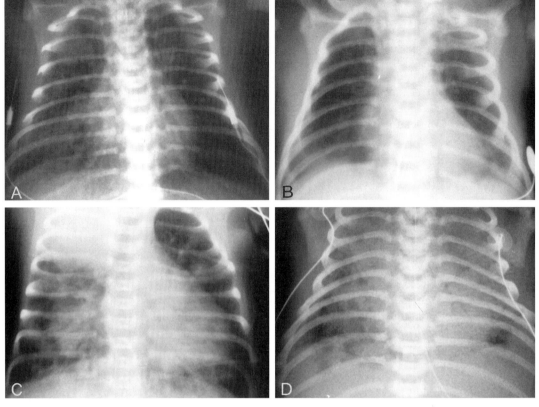

FIGURE 1.56. Neonatal pneumonia: alveolar patterns. A. Note coarse nodularity throughout both lungs, but more pronounced on the right. The upper lobe is beginning to consolidate, and there is a little fluid in the costophrenic angle. **B.** This patient demonstrates early bilateral, hazy basal consolidations. **C.** In this patient, there is a well-developed consolidation in the right upper lobe and another one developing in the right lower lobe. Similar early changes are present in the left lower lobe behind the heart. **D.** Opaque, totally opacified lungs in severe streptococcal pneumonia.

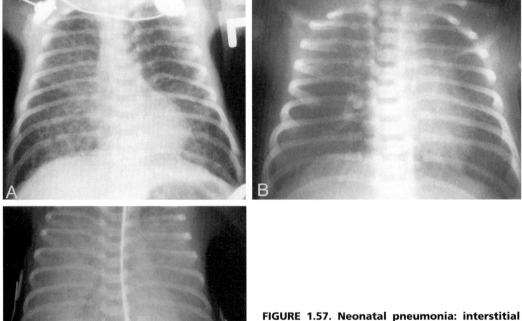

FIGURE 1.57. Neonatal pneumonia: interstitial patterns. A and B. Diffuse reticulonodularity is present throughout both lungs, but there also is a diffuse underlying haziness. Both patterns are characteristic of interstitial pneumonitis. **C.** Another patient with herpes demonstrating totally consolidated (pseudoconsolidation) lungs.

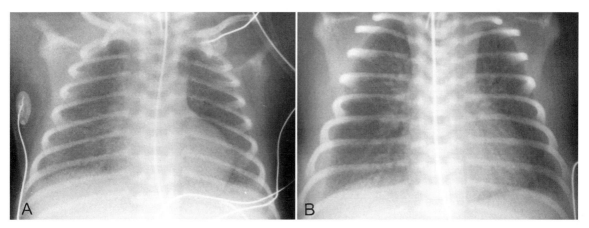

FIGURE 1.58. Group B streptococcal pneumonia mimicking hyaline membrane disease. **A.** Note diffuse granularity throughout both lung fields virtually indistinguishable from that seen with hyaline membrane disease. **B.** Another patient with hazy to granular lungs with some parahilar streakiness. Also note pleural fluid bilaterally but much more pronounced on the right.

An interesting feature of neonatal pneumonia, almost always group B streptococcal in origin, is the delayed onset of right diaphragmatic hernia (10–12). Just why these infants are prone to this complication is not known, but it has been postulated that the presence of pneumonia reduces pulmonary compliance and thus inspiratory intrathoracic pressures. This being the case, herniation of an otherwise stable hernia might occur.

Complications in neonatal pneumonia are not particularly common and for the most part occur with bacterial infections. They include empyema (Fig. 1.59), abscesses (13), and pneumatoceles (Fig. 1.60). These pneumatoceles have been documented with *E. coli* pneumonias (14) but

can occur with any infection. Pleural effusions, as mentioned earlier, are relatively common with bacterial infections but rare with viral infections.

Listeria infection of the newborn, as has been noted earlier, can produce granular-appearing lungs, but overall the infection is more common in Europe. Clinically, in *Listeria* infection, the presenting problems frequently are septicemia and meningitis. Roentgenographically, the findings in the lungs can vary from bilateral miliary pulmonary infiltrates (granulomas), through patchy parenchymal infiltrates, to streaky or hazy interstitial fibrosis.

Tuberculosis and fungal infections, acquired on a congenital basis, are rather rare. Furthermore, while the patient

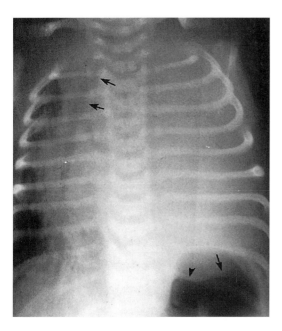

FIGURE 1.59. Empyema. Large left streptococcal empyema producing pronounced contralateral shift of the mediastinum and trachea (upper arrows) and downward displacement of the diaphragm (lower arrows). There is complete opacification of the left hemithorax.

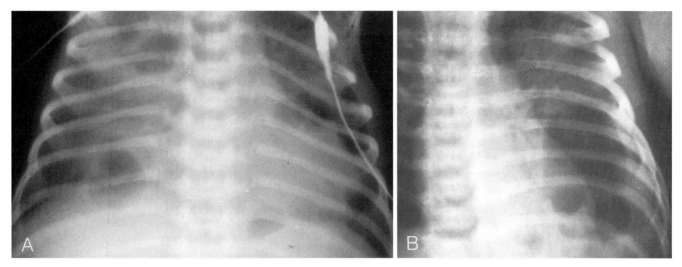

FIGURE 1.60. Neonatal pneumonia with pneumatoceles. A. Note numerous small air-filled cystic structures (pneumatoceles) in this patient with widespread pneumonia. **B.** Infant with *Escherichia coli* pneumonia and a large pneumatocele in the left lower lung.

may be infected in the perinatal period, infiltrates may not develop until later. Tubercular and fungal infections after the neonatal period are discussed later.

REFERENCES

1. Dixon BL, Houston CS. Radiographic exhibit; fatal neonatal pulmonary candidiasis. Radiology 1978;129:132.
2. Abzug MJ, Levin MJ. Neonatal adenovirus infection: four patients and review of the literature. Pediatrics 1991;87:890–896.
3. Pinto A, Beck R, Jadavji T. Fatal neonatal pneumonia caused by adenovirus type 35: report of one case and review of the literature. Arch Pathol Lab Med 1992;116:95–99.
4. Anderson RD. Herpes simplex virus infection of the neonatal respiratory tract. Am J Dis Child 1987;141:274–276.
5. Dominguez R, Rivero H, Gaisie G, et al. Neonatal herpes simplex pneumonia: radiographic findings. Radiology 1984;153:395–399.
6. Joshi VV, Escobar MR, Stewart L, et al. Fatal influenza A2 viral pneumonia in a newborn infant. Am J Dis Child 1973;126:839–840.
7. Christie CDC, Baltimore RS. Pertussis in neonates. Am J Dis Child 1989;143:1199–1202.
8. Austin R, Melhem RE. Pulmonary changes in congenital syphilis. Pediatr Radiol 1991;21:404–405.
9. Mannhardt W, Schumacher R. Progressive calcifications of lung and liver in neonatal herpes simplex virus infection. Pediatr Radiol 1991;21:236–237.
10. Giacoia GP, Jegathesen S. "Acquired" congenital diaphragmatic hernia following early onset group B streptococcal pneumonia. Clin Pediatr 1981;19:662–664.
11. Handa N, Suite S, Shono T, et al. Right-sided diaphragmatic hernia following group B streptococcal pneumonia and sepsis. J Pediatr Surg 1992;27:764–766.
12. Harris MC, Moskowitz WB, Engle WD, et al. Group B streptococcal septicemia and delayed-onset diaphragmatic hernia. Am J Dis Child 1981;135:723–725.
13. Siegel JD, McCracken GH Jr. Neonatal lung abscess. Am J Dis Child 1979;133:947–949.
14. Kuhn JP, Lee SB. Pneumatoceles associated with *Escherichia coli* pneumonias in the newborn. Pediatrics 1973;51:1008–1011.

Neonatal Atelectasis

Stillborn infants show total atelectasis of the lungs. The term "anectasis" might more properly be used, but nonetheless the lungs are small in volume and totally airless. Segmental, lobar, or even total atelectasis of a lung is a different problem and not at all uncommon in the newborn infant. In these cases, there is usually mechanical obstruction of a bronchus, either extrinsic (mass or vessel) or intrinsic (mucous or meconium plug). Because collapse is usually unilateral, the mediastinal structures often shift to the affected side, the shift being proportional to the degree of atelectasis (Fig. 1.61). Right upper lobe atelectasis has been noted to occur after extubation of infants on assisted respiratory therapy (1). Right upper lobe atelectasis also can be atypical in its configuration and, as such, mimic a pleural effusion (2). This phenomenon is not unique to the neonate and can occur with right upper lobe atelectasis in any age group. When total atelectasis of one lung occurs, there may be some difficulty in differentiating the findings from those of unilateral pulmonary agenesis. Another common cause of atelectasis in the neonate is obstruction of a bronchus by the tip of the endotracheal tube entering the contralateral bronchus (Fig. 1.62).

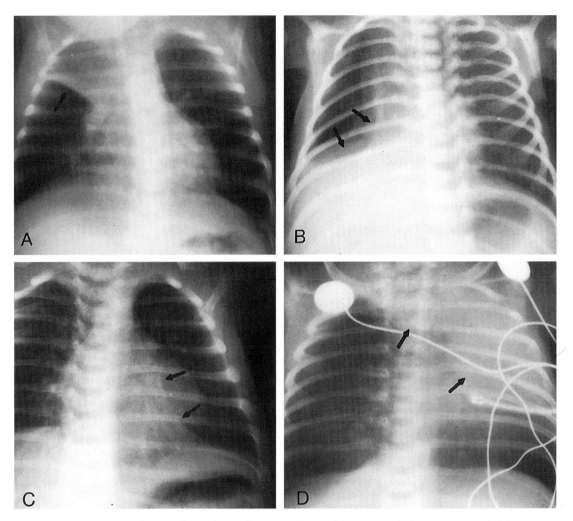

FIGURE 1.61. Lobar atelectasis: various configurations. A. Typical appearance of right upper lobe atelectasis (arrow). **B.** Peculiar but characteristic configuration of right middle and lower lobe atelectasis (arrows). Note that the diaphragmatic leaflet on the right is elevated. **C.** Typical left lower lobe atelectasis (arrows). **D.** Typical appearance of left upper lobe and lingular atelectasis (arrows). Note how this produces opacity of the left hemithorax and virtual disappearance of the left side of the cardiac silhouette. This is associated with leftward and upward displacement of the mediastinum. Also note compensatory overaeration of the right lung.

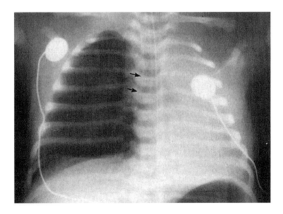

FIGURE 1.62. Atelectasis due to improper endotracheal tube positioning. Note complete atelectasis of the left lung. The endotracheal tube (arrows) is in the right bronchus.

REFERENCES

1. Odita JC, Kayyali M, Ammari A. Post-extubation atelectasis in ventilated newborn infants. Pediatr Radiol 1993;23:183–185.
2. Tamaki Y, Pandit R, Godding CA. Neonatal atypical peripheral atelectasis. Pediatr Radiol 1994;24:589–591.

Bronchopulmonary Dysplasia and the Wilson-Mikity Syndrome: The Focal Hyperaeration Syndromes

There always has been a problem in separating the Wilson-Mikity from the BPD syndrome, primarily because both occur in premature infants and both end up with bubbly lungs. To this end, I have always considered them more similar than different (1), for, indeed, they both result in focal hyperaeration of some alveolar groups interspersed with atelectasis of others. Initially, this leads to a reticular appearance of the lungs and then to frankly bubbly lungs.

The Wilson-Mikity syndrome (2) was described before BPD was recognized, but shortly thereafter BPD became much more common and virtually became synonymous with SDD. Prior to ventilator therapy, infants developing the Wilson-Mikity syndrome did so on their own. After the arrival of ventilator therapy, however, these infants quickly and routinely were placed on such therapy and thus did not develop the pattern of bubbly lungs on their own. Rather, they did so while on the ventilator and, this being the case, were clumped under the umbrella of the newly described syndrome of BPD.

In the classic Wilson-Mikity syndrome, the lungs usually were normally aerated for the first few days of life, but with subsequent respiratory distress, a coarse, nodular appearance resulted (Fig. 1.63). These changes probably were due to early uneven aeration of alveolar groups. This was the so-called "stage I" abnormality, and then, as the uneven aeration of the alveolar groups became more pronounced, especially in the lung bases, large cystic areas developed, and the bubbly lungs of stage II of the disease were seen. The findings at this stage of the disease are exactly the same as the ones seen in stages III and IV of the BPD syndrome. Currently, the Wilson-Mikity syndrome, as a pure entity, is uncommonly seen, but the phenomenon of bubbly lungs developing in infants with initially clear lungs still occurs. Indeed, in some of these patients, either spontaneously or as the result of ventilator therapy, bubbly changes can develop very rapidly, even within days (Fig. 1.64) (3, 4).

In contradistinction to infants with the Wilson-Mikity syndrome, infants with BPD classically first suffered from

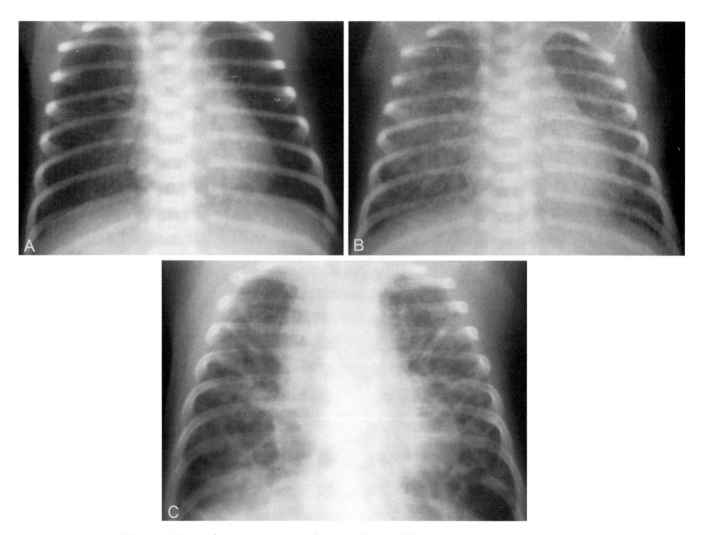

FIGURE 1.63. Focal overaeration syndrome: Wilson-Mikity type. A. Chest roentgenogram obtained at 1 day of age. The lungs basically are clear. **B.** A few days later, note widespread coarse nodularity with early cyst formation. **C.** Two months later, classic findings consisting of numerous emphysematous blebs, most pronounced in the lung bases, are present.

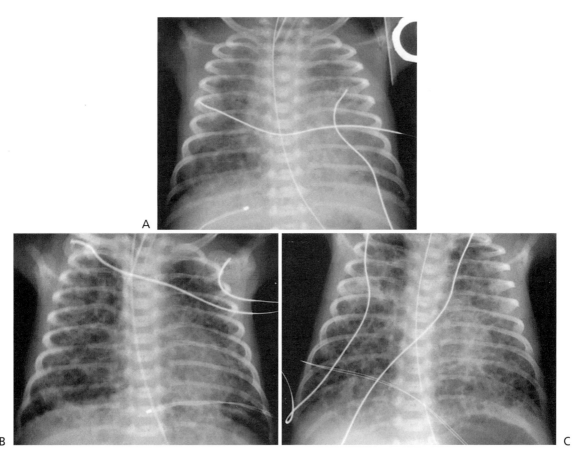

FIGURE 1.64. Focal hyperaeration syndrome: rapid onset. A. On day 1, the changes of SDD are present. **B.** One day later, early bubbly changes of focal hyperaeration, bronchopulmonary dysplasia, develop. **C.** Two days later, profound cystic changes consistent with advanced bronchopulmonary dysplasia are seen.

SDD and thus were placed on oxygen and ventilator therapy (5). It is now accepted that SDD need not always be the primary precipitator of the need for ventilator-assisted therapy. Nonetheless, it still is the most common condition leading to placement of infants on positive pressure ventilation and hence the subsequent development of the bubbly lungs of BPD. Furthermore, with the delivery of excessive concentrations of oxygen, oxygen toxicity also became an important factor (6) and at first was difficult to separate from the mechanical injury (barotrauma) of positive pressure ventilators. However, the former leads to damage of the basement membrane of the pulmonary arterioles, resulting in the leakage of fluid into the pulmonary interstitium. This results in edema and the so-called "leaky lung syndrome" (LLS) (1), and the presence of the edema almost always preordains these infants to prolonged ventilator-assisted therapy and its resultant barotrauma. The end result is the superimposed development of the bubbly lungs of BPD.

Once all the foregoing is realized, it also should be noted that not all these infants go on to develop the bubbly lungs of BPD. Indeed, some retain pulmonary edema for prolonged periods of time and never go on to develop bubbly lung changes. This probably has to do with the currently accepted regimens of less positive pressure applied to the airway and high-frequency, low-amplitude ventilator assistance.

In terms of the development of the bubbly lungs of BPD, it was demonstrated long ago that if distending pressures could be lessened, there was far less chance of the bubbly pattern appearing. This was attempted with negative pressure ventilation, but this form of therapy was controversial and never very successful. In addition, while, early on, the bubbles were believed to result from expiratory obstruction of small bronchioles, it subsequently was demonstrated that the bubbles actually collapsed and emptied on expiration (7). This was most important for it demonstrated that the lung, albeit still abnormal, could be inflated and deflated (Fig. 1.65). Because of this, even though less than normal, gas exchange still could be accomplished. All of this pointed to the fact that the most important factor in the development of these bubbles was positive pressure ventilation and overdistention of alveolar groups, that is, barotrauma and not pulmonary edema. Longstanding BPD is characterized by submucosal bronchial fibrosis,

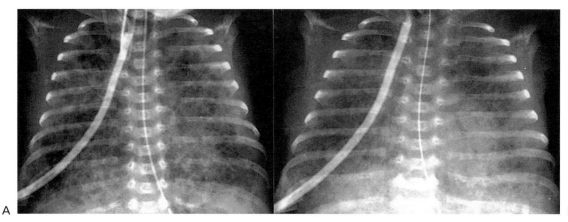

FIGURE 1.65. Focal hyperaeration syndrome, bronchopulmonary dysplasia type: inspiratory-expiratory sequence. A. Note extensive bubbly changes in this patient with bronchopulmonary dysplasia. **B.** With expiration, almost all of the bubbles collapse and empty. A baseline of pulmonary edema remains (i.e., leaky lung syndrome).

septal fibrosis, chronic inflammation, and squamous metaplasia (8). In addition, arteriolar changes reflecting the presence of pulmonary hypertension also can be seen.

It is not known just why uneven alveolar aeration occurs in these patients and those with the Wilson-Mikity syndrome. However, it might be that because the terminal bronchioles are immature, they lack normal structural mural support and thus could collapse on expiration and cause air trapping. On the other hand, because of Bernoulli's principle, as high-velocity air is forced through

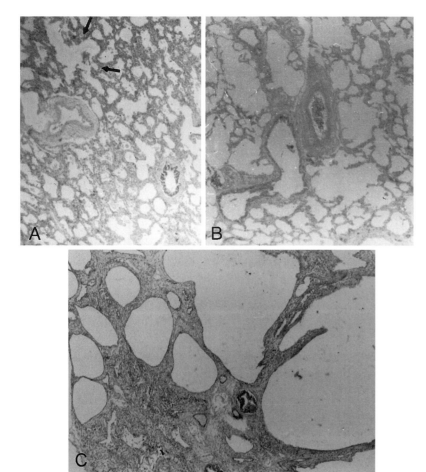

FIGURE 1.66. Focal hyperaeration syndrome, bronchopulmonary dysplasia type: development of bubbles. A. Histologic material in the early stages shows the development of the uneven aeration pattern with some alveolar clusters coalescing and becoming overaerated cystic structures (arrows). **B.** More advanced stage demonstrates large bubbles. **C.** Extreme late stage shows large well-defined bubbles.

them during inspiration, intraluminal pressures become negative, and this could lead to collapse of some of the softer bronchial walls. This being the case, air would be diverted from the collapsed bronchioles to bronchioles that did not collapse. The end result would be uneven aeration of alveolar groups, and as these alveolar groups receiving more air would dilate, expand, and conglomerate, bubbles would develop. In addition, it has been suggested that with septal fibrosis of the alveoli, those alveoli injured to a greater degree lose their distensibility and thus remain underaerated, while the others overdistend and form bubbles (9). In the end, however, no definite cause for the bubble formation (Fig. 1.66) has been determined.

The roentgenographic appearance of the bubbly lungs of BPD is quite variable. The findings depend on the size of the bubbles and the degree of associated interstitial inflammatory change and fibrosis. As a consequence, some patients may show large bubbles (Fig. 1.67C), especially in the lung bases, while others may show more interstitial scarring, fibrosis, and segmental atelectasis (Fig. 1.67A). Still others will show overlap of the findings of BPD and the LLS (Fig. 1.67B), and some infants may even develop pneumatoceles (Fig. 1.67C). Actually, overlap of the LLS with BPD is very common and can change from day to day, depending on the overall fluid load and the degree of positive pressure respiratory tract distention. Finally, even though BPD can develop in immature infants who do not suffer from SDD, most often the scenario is as follows: SDD, surfactant therapy, the development of the LLS, and then the development of BPD (Fig. 1.68).

In well-established BPD, the lungs are significantly injured (8), and healing takes up to 2 years (10, 11). Dur-

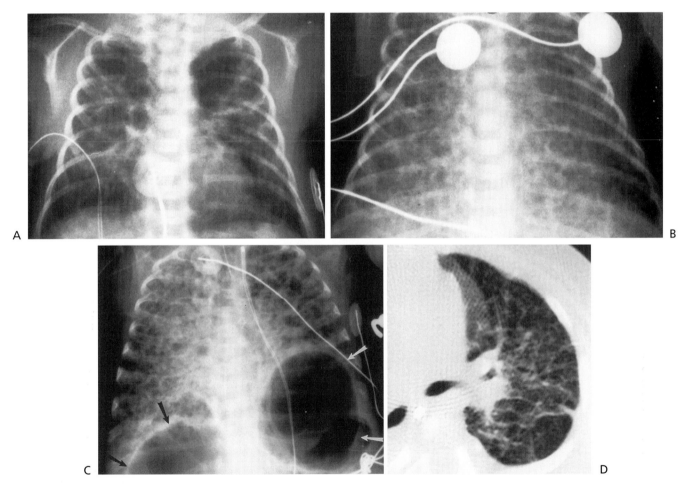

FIGURE 1.67. Focal hyperaeration syndrome, bronchopulmonary dysplasia type: variability of radiographic findings. A. In this patient, little in the way of bubble formation is seen, but rather one sees widespread, central, streaky, and wedge-like segmental atelectasis and fibrosis. **B.** In this patient, there is overlap of changes of bronchopulmonary dysplasia and the leaky lung syndrome. The bubbles in this patient are not as distinct as in other cases of bronchopulmonary dysplasia because of overlapping pulmonary edema from the leaky lung syndrome. **C.** In this patient, bubble formation predominates, but there also are two large pneumatoceles (arrows) present. **D.** CT study demonstrates the same findings.

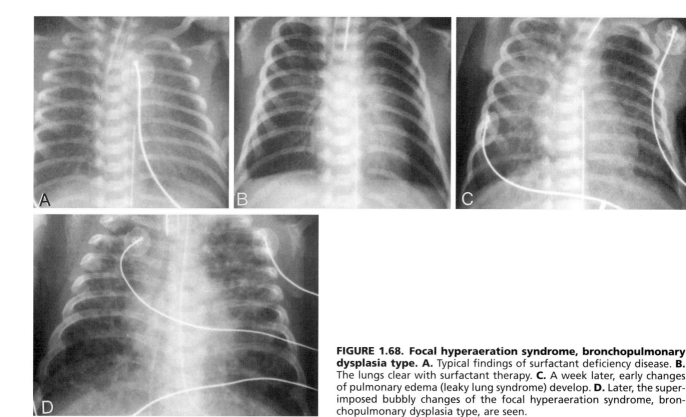

FIGURE 1.68. Focal hyperaeration syndrome, bronchopulmonary dysplasia type. A. Typical findings of surfactant deficiency disease. **B.** The lungs clear with surfactant therapy. **C.** A week later, early changes of pulmonary edema (leaky lung syndrome) develop. **D.** Later, the superimposed bubbly changes of the focal hyperaeration syndrome, bronchopulmonary dysplasia type, are seen.

ing the interval, these infants suffer from hyperactive airways and are very susceptible to viral infections, especially respiratory syncytial virus (12). After the 2 years, pulmonary function is mildly affected, but no serious sequelae

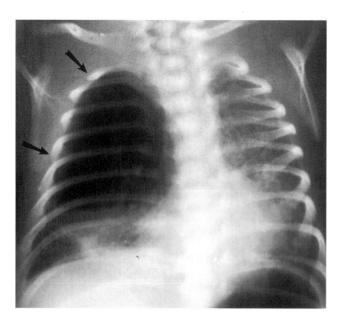

FIGURE 1.69. Obstructive emphysema in bronchopulmonary dysplasia. Note emphysema of the right upper lobe (arrows).

have been documented (13–15). Other complicating problems encountered in BPD are focal areas of tracheomalacia (10, 12), tracheal stenosis, and acquired lobar emphysema (16, 17) (Fig. 1.69). The latter usually is treated conservatively.

Chronic imaging changes in BPD are readily demonstrable with CT and consist of the same changes seen on plain films. There are alternating areas of alveolar group overdistention and atelectasis, bronchial wall thickening, air trapping, and areas of decreased perfusion (18–20).

Generally, however, CT evaluation of the lungs is not required in these infants and does not add a great deal to their clinical care or eventual outcome. Nuclear scintigraphy (21) also has been utilized for evaluation of BPD but has a very limited practical role.

REFERENCES

1. Swischuk LE, John SD. Immature lung problems: can our nomenclature be more specific? AJR 1996;166:917–918.
2. Wilson MG, Mikity VG. A new form of respiratory disease in premature infants. Am J Dis Child 1960;99:489–499.
3. Fitzgerald P, Donohue V, Gorman W. Bronchopulmonary dysplasia: a radiographic and clinical review of 20 patients. Br J Radiol 1990;63:444–447.
4. Swischuk LE, Shetty BP, John SD. The lungs in immature infants: how important is surfactant therapy in preventing chronic lung problems? Pediatr Radiol 1996;26:508–511.

5. Northway WH Jr, Rosan RC, Porter DY. Pulmonary disease following respiratory therapy of hyaline membrane disease; bronchopulmonary dysplasia. N Engl J Med 1967;276:358–368.

6. Northway WH Jr, Rosan RC. The radiographic features of pulmonary oxygen toxicity in the newborn; bronchopulmonary dysplasia. Radiology 1968;91:49–58.

7. Swischuk LE. Bubbles in hyaline membrane disease, differentiation of three types. Radiology 1977;122:417—426.

8. Stocker JT. The pathology of longstanding "healed" bronchopulmonary dysplasia. Hum Pathol 1986;17:959.

9. Cilley RE, Wang JY, Coran AG. Lung injury produced by moderate lung over-inflation in rats. J Pediatr Surg 1993;28: 488–495.

10. Northway WH Jr, Moss RB, Carlisle KB, et al. Late pulmonary sequelae of bronchopulmonary dysplasia. N Engl J Med 1990; 323:1793–1799.

11. Smyth JA, Tabachnik E, Duncan WJ, et al. Pulmonary function and bronchial hyperactivity in long-term survivors of bronchopulmonary dysplasia. Pediatrics 1981;68:336–340.

12. Groothuis JR, Gutierrez KM, Lauer BA. Respiratory syncytial virus infection in children with bronchopulmonary dysplasia. Pediatrics 1988;82:199–203.

13. Griscom NT, Wheeler WB, Sweezey NB, et al. Bronchopulmonary dysplasia: radiographic appearance in middle childhood. Radiology 1989;171:811–814.

14. Giacoia GP, Venkataraman PS, West-Wilson KI, et al. Follow-up of school age children with bronchopulmonary dysplasia. J Pediatr 1997;130:400–408.

15. Jacob SV, Coates AL, Lands L, et al. Long-term pulmonary sequelae of severe bronchopulmonary dysplasia. J Pediatr 1998; 133:193–200.

16. Miller RW, Woo P, Kellman RK, et al. Tracheobronchial abnormalities in infants with bronchopulmonary dysplasia. J Pediatr 1987;111:779–782.

17. Miller KE, Edwards DK, Hilton S, et al. Acquired lobar emphysema in premature infants with bronchopulmonary dysplasia: an iatrogenic disease? Radiology 1981;138:589–592.

18. Aquino SL, Schechter MS, Chiles C, et al. High-resolution inspiratory and expiratory CT in older children and adults with bronchopulmonary dysplasia. AJR 1999;173:963–967.

19. Oppenheim C, Mamou-Mani T, Sayegh N, et al. Bronchopulmonary dysplasia: value of CT in identifying pulmonary sequelae. AJR 1994;163:169–172.

20. Howling SJ, Northway WH Jr, Hansell DM, et al. Pulmonary sequelae of bronchopulmonary dysplasia survivors: high-resolution CT findings. AJR 2000;174:1323–1326.

21. Soler C, Figueras J, Roca I, et al. Pulmonary perfusion scintigraphy in the evaluation of the severity of bronchopulmonary dysplasia. Pediatr Radiol 1997;27:32–35.

Pulmonary Hemorrhage

Microscopic hemorrhage into the lungs, into either the interstitium or the alveoli, is not an uncommon finding at necropsy, but the premortem identification of such hemorrhage is uncommon. It results from hypoxia and subsequent capillary damage as seen with conditions such as SDD, meconium aspiration, neonatal pneumonia, BPD, and congenital heart disease. Massive pulmonary hemorrhage (1, 2), on the other hand, is more readily identified, both clinically and roentgenographically. In terms of the latter, the lungs appear somewhat homogeneously opaque and airless (Fig. 1.70), and clinically, respiratory distress develops suddenly. In addition, blood may be seen to ooze from the nose, mouth, or endotracheal tube, and so the roentgenographic findings are hardly ever a surprise to the clinician. The etiology of such hemorrhage is related to prematurity and severe hypoxia, and the outcome usually is fatal. Shunting through a patent ductus arteriosus with resultant high flow through the pulmonary circulation also is believed to contribute to pulmonary hemorrhage in some cases (3).

REFERENCES

1. Esterly JR, Oppenheimer EH. Massive pulmonary hemorrhage in the newborn. I. Pathologic considerations. J Pediatr 1966;69: 3–11.

2. Trompeter R, Yu VYH, Aynsley-Green A, et al. Massive pulmonary haemorrhage in the newborn infant. Arch Dis Child 1975;50:123–127.

3. Kluckow M, Evans N. Ductal shunting, high pulmonary blood flow, and pulmonary hemorrhage. J Pediatr 2000;137:68–72.

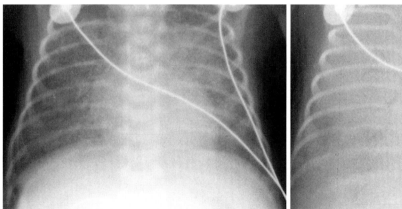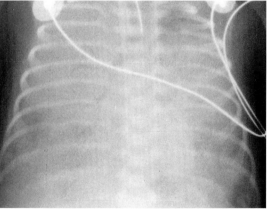

FIGURE 1.70. Pulmonary hemorrhage. A. This infant shows mild pulmonary edema as part of the leaky lung syndrome. **B.** Abruptly, the lung findings change with a marked increase in the size and opacity. This is characteristic of pulmonary hemorrhage.

Pulmonary Lymphangiectasia

Pulmonary lymphangiectasia is a rare condition that, in the neonate, produces intractable respiratory distress, marked cyanosis, and, most often, rapid demise (1, 2). Survival beyond the neonatal period is rare. Pulmonary lymphangiectasia can occur as an isolated abnormality, but it also can be seen with generalized lymphangiectasia and in infants with certain congenital heart lesions (i.e., cases with severe pulmonary venous obstruction associated with lesions such as the hypoplastic left heart syndrome, total anomalous pulmonary venous return type III, and pulmonary vein atresia). This variability in presentation has prompted classifications of pulmonary lymphangiectasia into three groups: those infants with the isolated abnormality, those with associated congenital heart disease, and those with generalized lymphangiectasia (1, 3). It is the first two groups that one is concerned with in the neonatal period, for those infants with generalized lymphangiectasia show little in the way of clinical or roentgenographic neonatal pulmonary abnormality. Their major problem is often that of soft tissue tumors or intestinal lymphangiectasia with protein-losing enteropathy. Later on, however, pulmonary problems can develop.

In those infants in whom the abnormality is isolated or part of a syndrome such as Noonan's syndrome (4), the etiology is believed to lie in an early embryonic arrest of pulmonary lymphatic development and persistence of large dilated, obstructed lymphatic channels (5). In those cases in which congenital heart disease with severe pulmonary venous obstruction is present, it is believed that lymphatic dilatation and engorgement occur because of impaired lymph drainage, secondary to high pulmonary venous pressures. Pathologically, in cases of pulmonary lymphangiectasia, the lungs are extremely wet and show numerous overdistended, almost cystic, lymphatic channels scattered throughout the pulmonary parenchyma and subpleural spaces (5).

Roentgenographically, the conglomeration of distended lymphatics usually results in a congested, coarsely nodular, or somewhat reticular appearance to the lungs (Fig. 1.71). Overaeration is also usually present, and in the typical case,

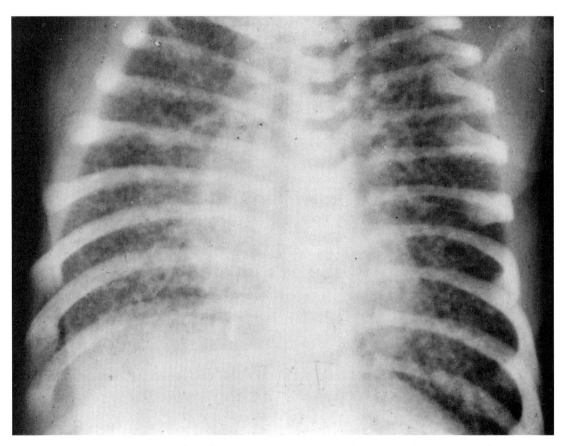

FIGURE 1.71. Pulmonary lymphangiectasia. Note bilateral reticulonodular pattern of congestion. Also note skin fold on the right. (Reproduced with permission from Singleton EB, Wagner ML. Radiologic atlas of pulmonary abnormalities in children. Philadelphia: Saunders, 1971; courtesy of Victor Mikity, M.D.).

there should be little difficulty in differentiating the coarsely nodular or reticular pattern from the fine granularity of surfactant deficiency disease. Pleural effusions also may be seen (6) and may be refractory. As such, the problem may provide a clue to the fact that pulmonary lymphangiectasia is the underlying cause of the effusions. The cystic changes of pulmonary lymphangioma also are readily demonstrable with high-resolution CT (7). Pulmonary angiomatosis can occasionally be mistaken for pulmonary lymphangiectasia, but since it is an extremely rare condition, this problem is unlikely to arise with any frequency. Pulmonary lymphangiectasia may also be familial (8). Generally, prognosis is poor if pulmonary lymphangiectasia is discovered in the neonatal period. However, if it presents later, survival has been documented, and clinical improvement seems to occur with time (9).

REFERENCES

1. Felman AH, Rhatigan RM, Pierson KK. Pulmonary lymphangiectasia: observations in 17 patients and proposed classification. AJR 1972;116:548–558.
2. Milovic I, Oluic D. Distress in a neonate. Pediatr Radiol 1992;22:156.
3. Noonan JA, Walters LR, Reeves JT. Congenital pulmonary lymphangiectasis. Am J Dis Child 1970;120:314–319.
4. Hernandez J, Stern AM, Rosenthal A. Pulmonary lymphangiectasis in Noonan syndrome. AJR 1980;1324:75–80.
5. Laurence KM. Congenital pulmonary cystic lymphangiectasis. J Clin Pathol 1959;12:62–69.
6. Hunter WS, Becroft DMO. Congenital pulmonary lymphangiectasis associated with pleural effusions. Arch Dis Child 1984;59:278–279.
7. Kim WS, Lee KS, Kim IL, et al. Cystic intrapulmonary lymphangioma: HRCT findings. Pediatr Radiol 1995;25:206–207.
8. Scott-Emuakpor AB, Warren ST, Kapur S, et al. Familial occurrence of congenital pulmonary lymphangiectasis. Am J Dis Child 1981;135:532–534.
9. Bouchard S, Di Lorenzo M, Youssef S, et al. Pulmonary lymphangiectasia revisited. J Pediatr Surg 2000;35:796–800.

Pulmonary Hypoplasia

A number of classifications of pulmonary hypoplasia are available (1–3), but, in essence, all reiterate that underdevelopment of the lungs can occur at different stages of intrauterine development and, in addition, that the final abnormality can range from total agenesis of both lungs to mild hypoplasia of the parenchyma of one lung only. Generally, patients with unilateral hypoplasia present with a somewhat different clinical picture than do those with bilateral disease, **and consequently, there is some reason to discuss pulmonary hypoplasia under these two broad categories.**

Bilateral pulmonary hypoplasia is quite variable in severity (1, 2). A rare form, usually lethal, is so-called "pulmonary alveolar-capillary dysgenesis" (3). In this condition,

TABLE 1.2. CLASSIFICATION OF BILATERAL PULMONARY HYPOPLASIA IN THE NEONATE

A. Extrathoracic Compression
1. Oligohydramnios with renal disease
   (a) Potter's syndrome
   (b) Bilateral cystic kidneys
   (c) Obstructive uropathy (posterior urethral valves, prune belly syndrome, neurogenic bladder, bilateral ureteropelvic junction, etc.)
2. Oligohydramnios without renal disease
   (a) Prolonged amniotic fluid leakage
   (b) Fetal development in amniotic-deficient uterine saccules, etc.
3. Chronically elevated diaphragm—no oligohydramnios
   (a) Large abdominal masses
   (b) Massive ascites
   (c) Membranous diaphragm

B. Thoracic Cage Compression
1. Thoracic dystrophies
   (a) Asphyxiating thoracic dystrophy
   (b) Achondrogenesis
   (c) Thanatophoric dwarfism
   (d) Severe achondroplasia
   (e) Congenital osteogenesis imperfecta
   (f) Ellis-van Creveld syndrome
   (g) Short-limb polydactyly syndrome
   (h) Metatrophic dwarfism, etc.
2. Muscular disease with "functional" compression
   (a) Myotonic dystrophy (?), arthrogryposis (?)
   (b) Amyotonia congenital (?)
   (c) Myasthenia gravis (?)
   (d) Decreased intrauterine breathing with "functional" compression (?)

C. Intrathoracic Compression
1. Diaphragmatic defects
   (a) Congenital diaphragmatic hernia
   (b) Agenesis of diaphragm
2. Excess pleural fluid
   (a) Chylohydrothorax
   (b) Fetal hydrops
3. Large intrathoracic tumor, cyst or heart

D. Primary Hypoplasia—No Cause of Compression Demonstrable

no alveoli or capillaries are present, only terminal airways develop, and ventilation along with gas diffusion are almost impossible to accomplish. In other cases, the problem usually is secondary to some form of intrauterine compression of the fetal thorax. Such compression is believed to inhibit the peripheral development of the lungs and, as such, result in parenchymal hypoplasia. Utilizing this basic concept, one can classify the condition in the following manner: (a) extrathoracic fetal compression, (b) thoracic cage compression of the fetal lung, (c) intrathoracic fetal compression of the lungs, and (d) primary pulmonary hypoplasia with no obvious cause of compression (Table 1.2).

The best-known cause of pulmonary hypoplasia secondary to **extrathoracic compression of the lungs** is Potter's syndrome (4). In this condition, renal agenesis leads to fetal anuria, maternal oligohydramnios, and subsequent compression of the fetal thorax and lungs by the uterus. Since its original description, however, it has become apparent that any urologic abnormality that predisposes to decreased urine output in the fetus can lead to the same phenomenon [i.e., obstructive uropathy, bilateral cystic disease (Fig. 1.72), prune belly syndrome, neurogenic bladder, etc.]. The lack of normal volumes of amniotic fluid in these cases is believed to predispose to direct uterine compression of the fetal thorax and thus to impaired peripheral pulmonary parenchymal development. In support of this hypothesis is the fact that similar hypoplasia can be seen with other causes of oligohydramnios not related to renal disease: namely, extrauterine pregnancy, pregnancy in an amniotic fluid-deficient, accessory saccule of a uterus, a deformed uterus, or a small amniotic sac for some other reason (5). Scoliosis of the spine and bending deformities of the ribs in these infants often attest to their cramped, compressed intrauterine environment (Fig. 1.73). Oligohydramnios also can result from premature rupture of the membranes and prolonged leakage of amniotic fluid (6).

External, extrathoracic compression of the fetal lungs also occurs in the absence of oligohydramnios. In these

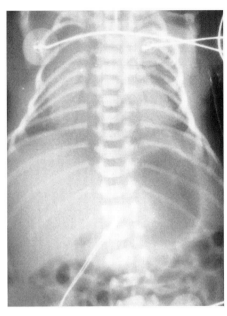

FIGURE 1.73. Hypoplastic lungs: oligohydramnios with leaking membranes. Note the small thorax in this patient with severely hypoplastic lungs secondary to leaking membranes in utero. Also note the deformed ribs.

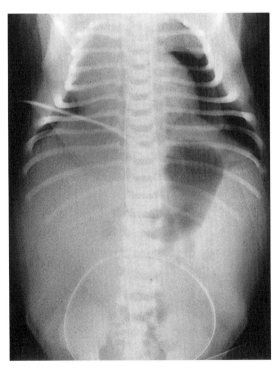

FIGURE 1.72. Hypoplastic lungs with oligohydramnios and polycystic kidneys. Note the grossly distended abdomen. Polycystic kidneys were present in this patient. Also note small lungs and a pneumothorax on the left. The thymus gland on the left is elevated off the cardiac silhouette and pushed into the apex of the left hemithorax. This attests to the presence of pneumomediastinum. A skin fold and small pneumothorax are present on the right.

cases, one usually is dealing with a large intraabdominal mass, massive ascites, a membranous diaphragm, or intrauterine phrenic nerve palsy (7). In all of these cases, persistent elevation of the diaphragm during fetal life is believed to cause chronic compression and underdevelopment of the lungs.

Hypoplasia secondary to **compression of the fetal lungs by the fetal thorax** also occurs in infants with restrictive bony dysplasias such as asphyxiating thoracic dystrophy (8), achondrogenesis, thanatophoric dwarfism, Ellis van Creveld syndrome, severe achondroplasia, the Pena-Shokeri syndrome (9, 10), and severe osteogenesis imperfecta. The degree of pulmonary hypoplasia in these infants often is severe, and stillbirth or death in the immediate postnatal period is not uncommon. It is the small, rigid thoracic cage that is believed to lead to restricted fetal respiratory movements in these infants, and this in turn to chronic compression of the lungs. Pulmonary hypoplasia secondary to "functional" compression of the lungs also exists in infants with muscular abnormalities such as amyotonia congenita, myotonic dystrophy, myasthenia gravis, arthrogryposis multiplex, and Werdnig-Hoffmann disease (11) (Fig. 1.74). As far as **intrathoracic compression of the fetal lungs** is concerned, the best-known example of this phenomenon is that which occurs with compression of the lungs secondary to congenital diaphragmatic hernia. Although one lung usually bears the brunt of the problem, both lungs are hypoplastic to one degree or another. Indeed, this is believed to be the major factor in the persisting high mor-

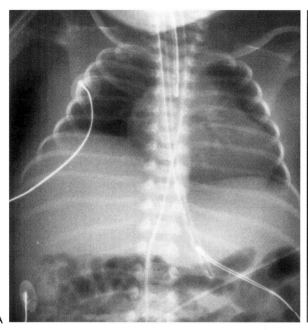
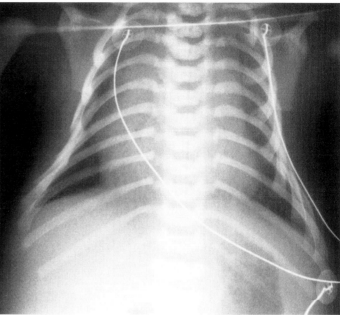

A B

FIGURE 1.74. Hypoplastic lung: chest wall dysfunction. A. Amyotonia congenita. Lung volumes are small and the diaphragm high in position. **B.** Baby with Down's syndrome demonstrating small, hypoplastic lungs and a bell-shaped chest.

bidity and mortality seen in this condition (12). A related condition, producing similar abnormalities, is the rare agenesis of the diaphragm.

In congenital diaphragmatic hernia, it has been demonstrated experimentally that pulmonary compression by the hernia must occur early in fetal life if pulmonary hypoplasia is to result (13). If the hernia develops in the third trimester or after birth, pulmonary hypoplasia does not occur. This is an important observation and almost certainly can be extrapolated to other causes of compressive pulmonary hypoplasia. In other words, no matter what the cause, compression of the lungs must occur early in fetal life for significant hypoplasia to develop.

Another cause of bilateral pulmonary hypoplasia resulting from intrathoracic compression of the lungs is bilateral fetal hydro-chylothorax (14). In this condition, fluid (chyle) accumulates in the fetal pleural space and causes pronounced compression of both lungs. These infants present with severe respiratory distress or absolute asphyxia, and unless the fluid is removed, rapid death is inevitable. However, even if the fluid is removed, the crisis is not over, for the small hypoplastic lungs do not expand to normal size immediately, and, indeed, if overinflated, refractory pneumothoraces result. ECMO therapy may be necessary in some of these infants.

A final cause of bilateral pulmonary hypoplasia resulting from intrathoracic compression of the lungs is the presence of a longstanding, compressive intrathoracic cyst, tumor, or even a very large heart (i.e., Epstein's anomaly, pulmonary

atresia type II). The latter may be more common than generally appreciated and should be included in this category of causes of bilateral pulmonary hypoplasia.

Infants with **primary pulmonary hypoplasia** (15, 16) often are difficult to diagnose, even though they show definite evidence of respiratory distress, tachypnea, mild to moderate cyanosis, and biochemical evidence of impaired gas exchange. The lungs, of course, are clear roentgenographically, and usually it is not noted at first that they also are small. Consequently, there is a tendency to assign another cause to the problem. However, after a number of chest roentgenograms are examined, one begins to note that the lungs are small on every study, and then the diagnosis of primary pulmonary hypoplasia can be suggested more confidently (Fig. 1.75). The etiology of primary pulmonary hypoplasia is unknown (2), and most cases are sporadic. However, a familial form has been described (17, 18).

Pathologically, the lungs of all infants with pulmonary hypoplasia show a decrease in size and weight and, histologically, a decrease in the number of alveoli (2, 19). The alveoli also often are immature but otherwise show no distinct abnormalities. The number of bronchioles and arterioles also is diminished, and there is proximal arrest of bronchial branching. Because of this, bronchioles near the pleural surface contain cartilage in their walls (Fig. 1.76). Ordinarily, of course, the terminal bronchioles do not contain cartilage in their walls. In addition, since the numbers of alveoli are diminished, the bronchioles lie close together

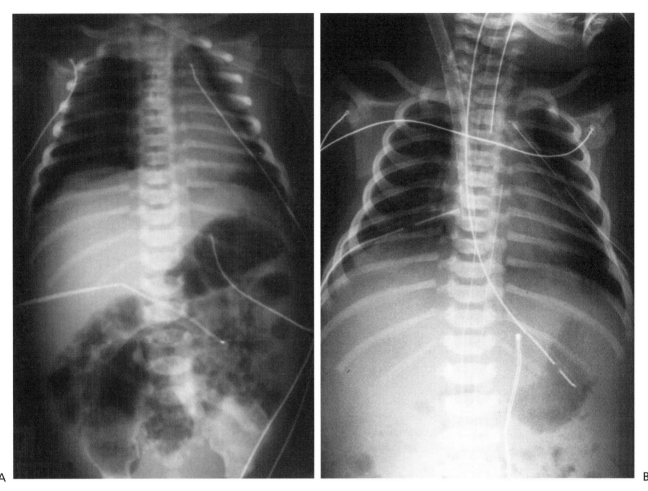

A   B

FIGURE 1.75. Primary bilateral pulmonary hypoplasia. A. This infant had immediate post-natal respiratory distress. The lungs are clear but small. Compare the size of the thorax to the overall size of the infant. Small, barely visible bilateral pneumothoraces are present. **B.** Later, the patient required extracorporeal membrane oxygenation therapy. Note bilateral chest tubes to decompress pneumothoraces. The lungs still are small.

and overcrowding is apparent (Fig. 1.76). The arterioles in these lungs often also show medial thickening, and this is believed to be an integral factor in the development of the commonly co-existent PFC syndrome.

Patients with pulmonary hypoplasia generally are prone to complications such as pneumomediastinum, pneumothorax, and pneumoperitoneum. Many times, these complications are the result of resuscitative measures, but just as often they are spontaneous in origin, resulting from the infant's own exuberant efforts to inflate the small lungs. It is interesting, however, that in those cases where the thoracic cage is rigid and acts as a splint (i.e., thoracic dystrophies, etc.) or where intrathoracic lesions such as a diaphragmatic hernia or bilateral hydro-chylothorax act as a cushion, these complications are much less common (3). It is only in those infants in whom the lungs become overin-

flated because there is nothing to inhibit their overinflation that these complications are common. Consequently, in diaphragmatic hernia and hydro-chylothorax, it is only after surgery or thoracentesis that pneumothorax occurs.

The ultimate prognosis in any infant with pulmonary hypoplasia is related to the degree of pulmonary underdevelopment. In those cases where hypoplasia is pronounced, death often ensues shortly after birth. On the other hand, in those infants in whom milder degrees of hypoplasia exist, nursing to survival is the rule. This is accomplished with conservative measures such as supportive oxygen and assisted ventilation, and many of these infants can be nursed over the critical period so as to allow their lungs to grow to the point where they can sustain life.

When **pulmonary hypoplasia is unilateral,** the clinical findings usually are considerably less severe than when the

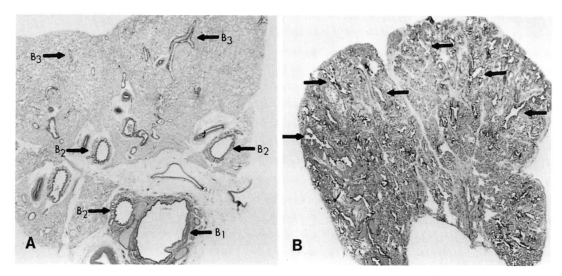

FIGURE 1.76. Pulmonary hypoplasia: histologic features. A. Normal lung demonstrating the progression of larger to smaller bronchi from the center of the lung toward the pleural surface. B, large central bronchus. Note cartilage around it. B₂ and B₃ represent progressively smaller bronchi as one travels to the pleural surface of the lung. Note the diminishing amount of parenchyma, resulting in a decrease of the distance between individual bronchi. **B.** Histologic material from infant demonstrated in Figure 1.75. First, note the crowded nature of the structures. Arrows point to the bronchioles equivalent to the B₂ stage of branching. Note how close to the pleural surface of the lung they occur, how little parenchyma is present in between, and that some contain cartilage in their walls. Bronchi this far out in the lungs should not contain cartilage.

disease is bilateral. Indeed, unilateral pulmonary hypoplasia often is unnoticed until accidentally discovered when the chest is examined for some other reason at a later time. It generally is a very benign condition. Indeed, in my experience, these lungs are not even susceptible to pulmonary infections any more than a perfectly normal lung. I believe the reason for this is that these lungs still can ventilate, and therefore there is no intrapulmonary air stasis, an important factor in the development of bacterial pulmonary infections. Associated pulmonary artery hypoplasia with decreased pulmonary blood flow co-exist in this condition, and some infants may show hemivertebra and ipsilateral rib or even upper extremity hypoplastic anomalies.

The roentgenographic findings in unilateral lung hypoplasia are rather typical in that the involved lung is smaller than the contralateral lung and the pulmonary blood flow diminished (Fig. 1.77). On inspiratory-expiratory views, these lungs will be seen to ventilate and thus change volume. This is important for the congenitally hypoplastic lung must be differentiated from the acquired hypoplastic lung of the Swyer-James syndrome (bronchiolitis obliterans). With these latter lungs, the obliterative bronchiolitis leads to air trapping and the lung does not significantly change size much during inspiration-expiration. Decreased pulmonary blood flow in congenital unilateral pulmonary hypoplasia can be confirmed with nuclear scintigraphy or arteriography.

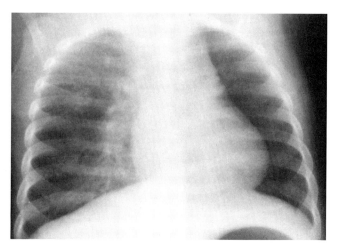

FIGURE 1.77. Pulmonary hypoplasia: unilateral. Hypoplasia of the left lung is characterized by increased lucency and smallness of the lung. In addition, note that the vascularity is compensatorily increased in the right lung because the left pulmonary artery also is hypoplastic and cannot accept its normal volume of blood.

REFERENCES

1. Minetto E, Galli E, Boglione G. Agenesia, aplasia, hypoplasia, pulmonare. Minerva Med 1958;49:4635.
2. Swischuk LE, Richardson CJ, Nichols MM, et al. Bilateral pulmonary hypoplasia in the neonate (a classification). AJR 1979; 133:1057–1063.
3. Newman B, Yunis E. Primary alveolar capillary dysplasia. Pediatr Radiol 1990;21:20–22.
4. Hislop A, Hey E, Reid L. The lungs in congenital bilateral renal agenesis and dysplasia. Arch Dis Child 1979;54:32–38.
5. Miller ME, Dunn PM, Smith DW. Uterine malformation and fetal deformation. J Pediatr 1979;94:387–390.
6. Thomas IT, Smith DW. Oligohydramnios, cause of the nonrenal features of Potter's syndrome, including pulmonary hypoplasia. J Pediatr 1974;84:811–814.
7. Goldstein JD, Reid LM. Pulmonary hypoplasia resulting from phrenic nerve agenesis and diaphragmatic amyoplasia. J Pediatr 1980;97:282.
8. Finegold MJ, Katzew H, Genieser NB, et al. Lung structure in thoracic dystrophy. Am J Dis Child 1971;122:153–159.
9. Moerman P, Fryns JP, Goddeeris P, et al. Multiple ankyloses, facial anomalies, and pulmonary hypoplasia associated with severe antenatal spinal muscular atrophy. J Pediatr 1983;103: 238–241.
10. Pena SDJ, Shokeri MHK. Syndrome of captodactyly, multiple ankylosis, facial anomalies and pulmonary hypoplasia: a lethal condition. J Pediatr 1974;85:373–375.
11. Cunningham M, Stocks J. Werdnig-Hoffmann disease; the effects of intrauterine onset on lung growth. Arch Dis Child 1978;53:921–925.
12. Boyden EA. The structure of compressed lungs in congenital diaphragmatic hernia. Am J Anat 1972;134:497–508.
13. Ohi R, Suzuki H, Kato T, et al. Development of the lung in fetal rabbits with experimental diaphragmatic hernia. J Pediatr Surg 1976;11:955–959.
14. Castillo R, Devoe L, Falls G, et al. Pleural effusions and pulmonary hypoplasia. Am J Obstet Gynecol 1987;157:1252–1255.
15. Langer R, Kaufmann HJ. Primary isolated bilateral pulmonary hypoplasia: a comparative study of radiologic findings and autopsy results. Pediatr Radiol 1986;16:175–179.
16. Swischuk LE, Richardson CJ, Nichols MM, et al. Primary pulmonary hypoplasia in the neonate. J Pediatr 1979;95:573–577.
17. Boylan P, Howe A, Gearty J, et al. Familial pulmonary hypoplasia. Br J Pediatr Surg 1978;13:179–180.
18. Green RAR, Shaw DG, Haworth SG. Familial pulmonary hypoplasia: plain film appearances with histopathological correlation. Pediatr Radiol 1999;29:455–458.
19. Askenazi SS, Pearlman M. Pulmonary hypoplasia: lung weight and radial alveolar count as a criteria of diagnosis. Arch Dis Child 1979;54:614.

Pulmonary Agenesis

Complete agenesis of the lungs is rare and, of course, incompatible with life (1–3). Unilateral pulmonary agenesis with ipsilateral absence of the pulmonary artery is more common, and when the problem occurs on the right, it is associated with a more serious prognosis, mostly because there is a greater propensity to kinking of the great arteries and veins with right-side agenesis. In addition, complex cardiac and venous abnormalities are more likely to co-exist. Tracheal compression by the normal aorta also can occur (4, 5).

Another interesting feature of unilateral pulmonary agenesis is that when the right lung is involved, the aortic arch usually is on the left, while if the left lung is involved, the arch lies on the right. In addition, as with unilateral pulmonary hypoplasia, it is not unusual to find tracheal, esophageal, spinal, and ipsilateral rib and upper extremity anomalies (4, 6, 7). Clinically, infants with unilateral agenesis can present with severe respiratory distress in the first few hours of life, but it is not uncommon for some to have no difficulty at all. In these latter cases, there appears to be an unusual degree of adaptability to the abnormal position of the mediastinum. On auscultation, mediastinal shift and hyperresonance of the contralateral hemithorax side are usually present. Roentgenographically, overdistention of the contralateral lung can be so marked that herniation of the lung across the mediastinum occurs. However, since no blood is delivered to the agenetic lung, the other lung, even though overdistended, shows increased blood flow (Fig. 1.78).

Isolated agenesis of a lobe or lobes is more common than total unilateral lung agenesis. This abnormality occurs more often on the right than on the left, and on the right usually involves the upper and middle lobes (Fig. 1.79, A and B). Characteristically, on frontal view, the involved hemithorax is smaller than normal and somewhat hazy. On lateral view (8), many of these patients demonstrate a characteristic retrosternal density (Fig. 1.79B). The tissue within this density was believed, for many years, to be due to alveolar and fatty tissue. However, more recently it has been demonstrated that the density represents the abnormal interface of the aerated left lung against the mediastinum. Other associated anomalies include accessory diaphragm, the scimitar syndrome, systemic arterial blood supply to the lungs from the aorta without true sequestration (pseudosequestration), and bronchopulmonary foregut anomalies with gastrointestinal tract communications (Fig. 1.79, D and E).

A peculiar configuration, in pulmonary agenesis, arises when the overdistended, contralateral lung is fluid filled. The problem can be especially perplexing if symptoms are minimal or nonexistent. This is exactly what occurred with the infant illustrated in Fig. 1.80, where the fluid in the contralateral normal lung eventually disappeared.

REFERENCES

1. DeBuse PJ, Morris G. Bilateral pulmonary agenesis, oesophageal atresia, and the first arch syndrome. Thorax 1972;28:526–528.
2. Markowitz RI, Frederick W, Rosenfield NS, et al. Single, mediastinal, unilobar lung—a rare form of subtotal pulmonary agenesis. Pediatr Radiol 1987;17:269–272.
3. Yahgmai I. Agenesis of the lung. AJR 1970;108:564–568.
4. Dohlemann C, Mantel K, Schneider K, et al. Deviated trachea in hypoplasia and aplasia of the right lung: airway obstruction and its release by aortopexy. J Pediatr Surg 1990;25:290–293.
5. McCormick TL, Kuhns LR. Tracheal compression by a normal aorta associated with right lung agenesis. Radiology 1979;130:659–660.
6. Hoffman MA, Superina R, Wesson DE. Unilateral pulmonary

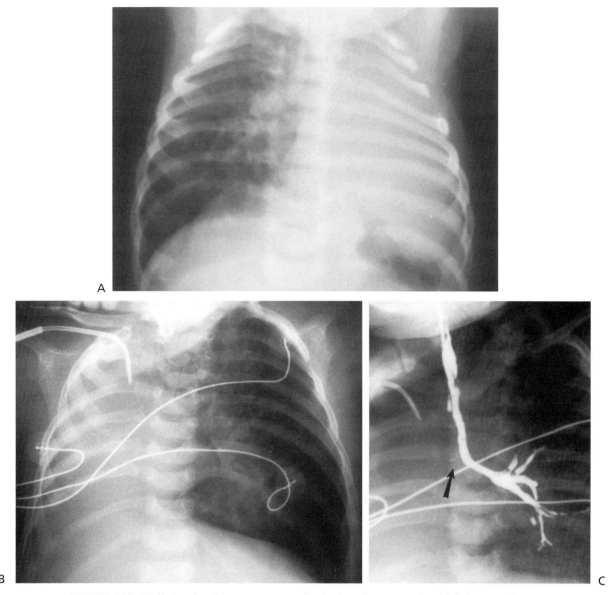

FIGURE 1.78. Unilateral pulmonary agenesis. A. Complete agenesis of left lung produces total shift of mediastinal structures into the left hemithorax and compensatory overdistension and hypervascularity of the right lung. However, note that the left hemithorax is only slightly smaller than the right. **B.** Right lung agenesis with similar findings. **C.** Bronchogram shows absence of the right main bronchus (arrow).

agenesis with esophageal atresia and distal tracheoesophageal fistula: report of two cases. J Pediatr Surg 1989;24:1084–1085.
7. Osborne J, Masel J, McCredie J. A spectrum of skeletal anomalies associated with pulmonary agenesis: possible neural crest injuries. Pediatr Radiol 1989;19:425–432.
8. Cremin BJ, Bass EM. Retrosternal density; a sign of pulmonary hypoplasia. Pediatr Radiol 1975;3:145–147.

Accessory Diaphragm

In this relatively rare condition, the extra diaphragm is fused anteriorly but duplicated posteriorly. As a result, it divides the affected hemithorax into two compartments (1, 2). This anomaly can occur on the left (3), but most often it is seen on the right. On the right, it frequently is associated with agenesis of the right upper and middle lobes of the right lung and its attendant anomalies (see previous section). The actual accessory diaphragm usually is discovered at surgery, as in most cases, plain film radiographic findings are those of unilateral pulmonary lung agenesis (see Fig. 1.79).

REFERENCES

1. Hart JC, Cohen IT, Ballantine TVN, et al. Accessory diaphragm in an infant. J Pediatr Surg 1981;16:947–949.
2. Ikeda T, Ishihara T, Yoshimatsu H, et al. Accessory diaphragm associated with congenital posterolateral diaphragmatic hernia,

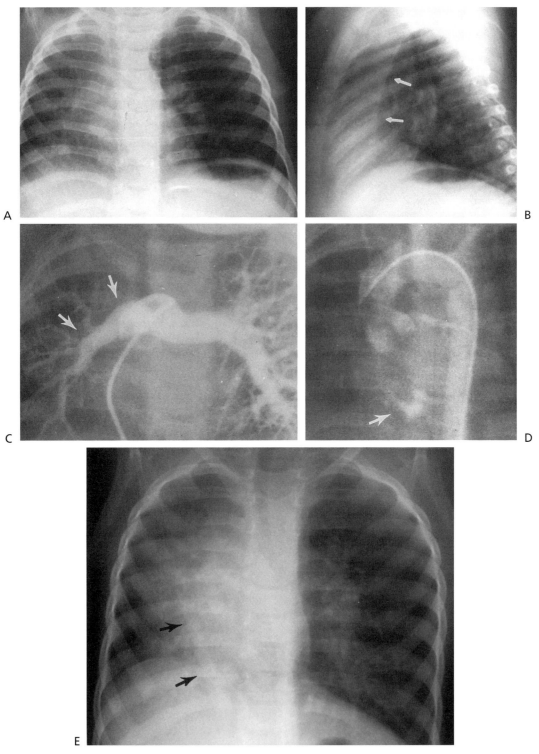

FIGURE 1.79. Right middle and upper lobe hypoplasia with associated anomalies. A. Note characteristic loss of volume on the right, semiopaqueness of the small, right hemithorax, and obliteration of the right cardiac border. **B.** Typical lateral view findings showing the retrosternal density (arrows) paralleling the chest wall. This represents the interface between the two lungs. In the past, it was believed to represent areolar and fatty tissue. **C.** Pulmonary arteriogram demonstrating a small, relatively branchless right pulmonary artery (arrows) supplying the hypoplastic right lung (lower lobe only). **D.** Aortogram demonstrating anomalous systemic blood supply (pseudosequestration) to a portion of the lower lobe on the right (arrow). **E. Scimitar syndrome.** Note the hypogenetic right lung and the abnormal draining vein (arrows), constituting the scimitar syndrome. The left lung is large, and the pulmonary artery is large.

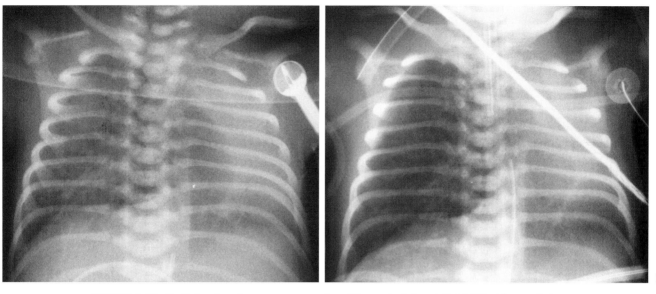

A   B

FIGURE 1.80. Unilateral pulmonary agenesis with contralateral fluid-filled lung. A. In this infant, note the large, fluid-filled right lung herniating across midline. The left hemithorax is small and opacified secondary to agenesis of the left upper lobe and lingula. **B.** Twenty-four hours later, fluid clears from the compensatorily enlarged right lung. Changes on the left remain about the same. This patient was basically asymptomatic.

aberrant systemic artery to the right lower lobe, and anomalous pulmonary vein. Review and report of a case. J Thorac Cardiovasc Surg 1972;64:18–25.
3. Kananoglu A, Tuncbilek E. Accessory diaphragm in the left side. Pediatr Radiol 1978;7:172–174.

Horseshoe Lung

Horseshoe lung is a rare anomaly of the lungs wherein a portion of the left lower lobe is ectopically located behind the heart and joined to the right lower lobe (1–5) (Fig.

1.81). The condition has many of the features seen with agenesis of the right and middle lobes, discussed previously, including vascular anomalies such as the scimitar syndrome (2–5). In addition, sequestration has been noted with horseshoe lung (2).

Radiographically, the chest findings resemble those of the hypogenetic right lung syndrome, with smallness and increased opacity of the right hemithorax (5). Pulmonary arteriography will demonstrate the abnormal arterial branch from the right pulmonary artery to the ectopic por-

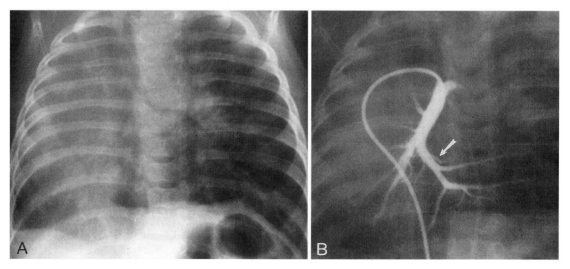

A   B

FIGURE 1.81. Horseshoe lung. A. Note the hypogenetic right lung with shift of the mediastinal structures to the right. There is minimal haziness in the left base. **B.** Pulmonary arteriogram demonstrates the aberrant left pulmonary artery branch (arrow) originating from the right pulmonary artery. (Reproduced with permission from Freedom RM, Burrows PE, Moes CAF. Horseshoe lung: report of five new cases. AJR 1986;146:211–215).

tion of the left lower lobe (Fig. 1.81). Most cases do not demonstrate communicating abnormal bronchi, but the condition known as "bridging bronchus" may be part of the spectrum of this abnormality. In bridging bronchus, there is no actual pulmonary tissue connecting the right and left lungs, but rather there is bronchial communication only.

On plain films, an additional useful finding in the detection of the horseshoe lung is a triangular-like density in the right lower lobe just adjacent to the spine, which represents the lateral extent of the isthmus of abnormal left lung tissue (1).

REFERENCES

1. Figa FH, Yoo SJ, Burrows PE, et al. Horseshoe lung: a case report with unusual bronchial and pleural anomalies and a proposed new classification. Pediatr Radiol 1993;23:44–47.
2. Frank JL, Poole CA, Rosas G. Horseshoe lung: clinical, pathologic features and a new plain film finding. AJR 1986;146:217–226.
3. Freedom RM, Burrows PE, Moes CAF. Horseshoe lung: report of five new cases. AJR 1986;146:211–215.
4. Takeda J, Kato N, Nakagawa T, et al. Horseshoe lung without respiratory distress. Pediatr Radiol 1990;20:604.
5. Hawass ND, Badawi MG, Al-Muzrakchi AM, et al. Horseshoe lung: differential diagnosis. Pediatr Radiol 1990;20:580–584.

Hyperviscosity or Polycythemia Syndrome

Polycythemia in the newborn infant is not an uncommon problem and has a variety of causes (1, 2). In some cases, it is due to placental or twin-to-twin transfusion or early clamping or milking of the cord. However, in other instances, it occurs as a primary phenomenon. Many of these infants exhibit respiratory distress, but not all demonstrate abnormal radiologic findings. Those who do, demonstrate cardiomegaly and vascular congestion (3, 4). In some cases, actual pulmonary edema develops, and fluffy infiltrates mimicking pneumonia can be seen. Pleural effusions also can be seen, and the lungs are hyperaerated. Cyanosis also can develop, and conservative measures such as phlebotomy produce dramatic results. Most patients recover and do well.

REFERENCES

1. Gross GP, Hathaway WE, McGaughey HR. Hyperviscosity in the neonate. J Pediatr 1973;82:1004–1012.
2. Wesenberg RL, Rumack CM, Lubchenco LO, et al. Thick blood syndrome. Radiology 1977;125:181–183.
3. O'Conner JF, Shapiro JH, Ingall D. Erythrocythemia as a cause of respiratory distress in the newborn; radiologic findings. Radiology 1968;90:333–335.
4. Saigal S, Wilson R, Usher R. Radiological findings in symptomatic neonatal plethora resulting from placental transfusion. Radiology 1977;125:185–188.

Persistent Fetal Circulation Syndrome (Pulmonary Hypertension)

Normally, the full-term infant has high pulmonary vascular resistance, and **the resultant phenomenon is termed "physiologic pulmonary hypertension."** However, in some cases, these pressures are extraordinarily high, and **the term "primary pulmonary hypertension" then is applied.** In such cases, if the ductus arteriosus is open, right-to-left ductal shunting of blood occurs, and thus there is persistence of the fetal circulatory pathway. This phenomenon then is referred to as the **"persistent fetal circulation (PFC) syndrome"** (1), and clinically, these patients present with respiratory distress and cyanosis. The condition may be primary or secondary to any number of hypoxia-inducing pulmonary or cardiac, congenital or acquired, conditions. In all of these cases, hypoxia is the cause of the problem for it induces pulmonary arteriolar vasoconstriction and elevation of pulmonary artery pressures (2–4).

Roentgenographically, in the primary form, the findings consist of clear lungs, decreased pulmonary vascularity, and right-side (right atrium and right ventricle) cardiomegaly (Fig. 1.82). Pathologically, patients with the PFC syndrome demonstrate thickening of the pulmonary arterioles. This, of course, is, to some degree, to be expected in the full-term infant, but in the PFC syndrome, the findings usually are more profound and do not regress. In addition, it also has been noted that some of these patients may show evidence of pulmonary microemboli (5, 6).

A rare cause of persistent pulmonary hypertension is so-called misalignment of pulmonary veins and alveolar capillary dysplasia (7–9). In this condition, there is congenital failure of formation and ingrowth of alveolar capillaries so that they do not make contact with the alveolar epithelium. There is associated medial muscular thickening of the pulmonary artery branches and hence resultant persistent pulmonary hypertension.

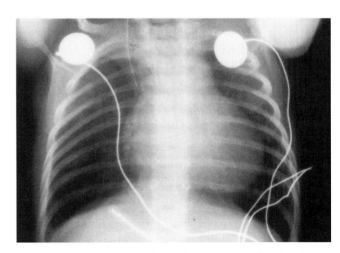

FIGURE 1.82. Pulmonary hypertension. Note the clear, hypovascularized lungs. The heart is enlarged with a right-side pattern.

Inhaled nitrous oxide, which leads to vasodilatation and improved oxygenation, has proved helpful in these patients. However, it has been noted that patients without associated pulmonary or cardiac problems are most likely to respond to this form of therapy (10–14). Eventually, refractory patients may require ECMO therapy.

REFERENCES

1. Gersony WM, Duc GV, Sinclair JC."PFC" syndrome (persistence of the fetal circulation). Circulation 1969;40:87.
2. Bauer CR, Tsipuras D, Fletcher BD. Syndrome of persistent pulmonary vascular obstruction of the newborn; roentgen findings. AJR 1974;120:285–290.
3. Merten DF, Goetzman BW, Wennberg RP. Persistent fetal circulation evolving clinical fetal circulation;evolving clinical and radiographic concept of pulmonary hypertension of the newborn. Pediatr Radiol 1977;6:74–80.
4. Silverstein EF, Ellis K, Casarella WJ, et al. Persistence of the fetal circulation; radiologic considerations. AJR 1977;128:781–788.
5. Levin DL, Weinberg AG, Perkin RM. Pulmonary microthrombi syndrome in newborn infants with unresponsive persistent pulmonary hypertension. J Pediatr 1983;102:299–303.
6. Morrow WR, Haas JE, Benjamin DR. Nonbacterial endocardial thrombosis in neonates; relationship to persistent fetal circulation. J Pediatr 1982;100:117–122.
7. Abdallah HI. Late presentation of misalignment of lung vessels with alveolar capillary dysplasia. Crit Care Med 1993;21: 628–630.
8. Boggs S, Harris MC, Hoffman DJ, et al. Misalignment of pulmonary veins with alveolar capillary dysplasia: affected siblings and variable phenotypic expression. J Pediatr 1994;124:125–128.
9. Chelliah BP, Brown D, Cohen M, et al. Alveolar capillary dysplasia—a cause of persistent pulmonary hypertension unresponsive to a second course of extracorporeal membrane oxygenation. Pediatrics 1995;96:1159–1161.
10. Barefield ES, Kattwinkel J, Dudell G, et al. Inhaled nitric oxide for the early treatment of persistent pulmonary hypertension of the term newborn: a randomized double-masked, placebo-controlled, dose response, multicenter study. Pediatrics 1998;101: 325–334.
11. Day RW, Lynch JM, White KS, et al. Acute response to inhaled nitric oxide in newborns with respiratory failure and pulmonary hypertension. Pediatrics 1996;98:698–705.
12. Goldman AP, Tasker RC, Haworth SG, et al. Four patterns of inhaled nitric oxide for persistent pulmonary hypertension of the newborn. Pediatrics 1996;98:706–713.
13. Kinsella JP, Truog WE, Walsh WF, et al. Randomized, multicenter traial of inhaled nitric oxide and high-frequency oscillatory ventilation in severe, persistent pulmonary hypertension of the newborn. J Pediatr 1997;131:55–62.
14. Nakagawa TA, Morris A, Gomez RJ, et al. Dose response to inhaled nitric oxide in pediatric patients wiuth pulmonary hypertension and acute respiratory distress syndrome. J Pediatr 1997; 131:63–69.

Thoracic Cage Dysfunction and Respiratory Distress

The bony thoracic cage or the muscles of respiration, including the diaphragm, if dysfunctional, can lead to severe respiratory distress. Muscular abnormalities include conditions such as myasthenia gravis, amyotonia congenita, myotonic dystrophy, Werdnig-Hoffmann disease, and other myopathies (1–5). All of these conditions can lead to severe hypoventilation and rapid death. In addition, the lungs in these patients are hypoplastic, and the roentgenograms usually show a small chest, generalized underaeration, and thin ribs. In the neonate, a picture similar to that seen with muscular disease can be seen with severe brain damage. In addition, in any of these infants, the chest cage may retain its original intrauterine bell-shaped configuration (see Fig. 1.74).

Severe deformity of the chest cage, usually consisting of shortening and hypoplasia or deformity of the ribs, can be seen with asphyxiating thoracic dystrophy, thanatophoric dwarfism, metatropic dwarfism, achondrogenesis, and other bony dysplasias such as osteogenesis imperfecta and hypophosphatasia. These bony abnormalities produce either a rigid or a flaccid thoracic cage, which leads to severe hypoventilation.

Therapeutic paralysis of infants on respiratory-assisted ventilation now is commonplace and may result in apparently underaerated lungs (6, 7). In addition, these patients demonstrate paucity of gas in the abdomen because they do not swallow air. At the same time, their soft tissues become edematous (6), probably owing to the lack of muscle activity resulting in stasis of lymph. Prolonged paralysis also can lead to muscle atrophy (7).

REFERENCES

1. Chassevent J, Sauvegrain J, Besson-Leaud M, et al. Myotonic dystrophy (Steinert's disease) in the neonate. Radiology 1978;127: 747–749.
2. Mellins RB, Hays AP, Gold AP, et al. Respiratory distress as the initial manifestation of Werdnig-Hoffmann disease. Pediatrics 1974;53:33–38.
3. Pearse RG, Howeler CJ. Neonatal form of dystrophia myotonica. Five cases in preterm babies and a review of earlier reports. Arch Dis Child 1979;54:331–338.
4. Conomy JP, Levinsohn M, Fanaroff A. Familial infantile myasthenia gravis; a cause of sudden death in young children. J Pediatr 1975;87:428–430.
5. Namba T, Brown SB, Grob D. Neonatal myasthenia gravis. Pediatrics 1970;45:488–504.
6. Kopecky K, Cohen M, Schreiner R. Therapeutic neuromuscular paralysis in neonates: characteristic radiographic features. AJR 1982;139:25–30.
7. Rutledge ML, Hawkins EP, Langston C. Skeletal muscle growth failure induced in premature infnats by prolonged pancuronium treatment. J Pediatr 1986;109:883–886.

SURGICALLY TREATED CAUSES OF RESPIRATORY DISTRESS

Diaphragmatic Abnormalities

A number of diaphragmatic abnormalities can lead to impaired respiratory function in neonates and infants. For the most part, these consist of phrenic nerve paralysis, diaphragmatic eventration, aplasia or hypoplasia of the diaphragm, and congenital diaphragmatic hernia.

Diaphragmatic Paralysis (Phrenic Nerve Injury)

Injury to the phrenic nerve with resultant elevation and fixation of a diaphragmatic leaflet can produce respiratory difficulty. This is especially significant if paradoxical leaflet motion is present. Such motion can be demonstrated with ultrasonography or fluoroscopy. **However, most times, paralysis is mild, paradoxical motion is not present, and symptoms are virtually absent.** Secondary paralysis of the diaphragmatic leaflets can occur with intracranial problems such as brainstem hemorrhage and posterior fossa anomalies and tumors.

In the neonate, paralysis of the diaphragmatic leaflet most often is believed to result from obstetric injury to the brachial plexus. Involvement of the right diaphragmatic leaflet is more common than the left, and frequently Erb's palsy is associated. Horner's syndrome also has been reported (1). Phrenic nerve injury also can be seen with chest tube and central line placement (2, 3) and thoracic surgery.

Roentgenographically, diaphragmatic paralysis can be suspected in any age group when the affected diaphragmatic leaflet is elevated and fixed (Fig. 1.83A). Fluoroscopic examination can demonstrate whether paradoxical move-

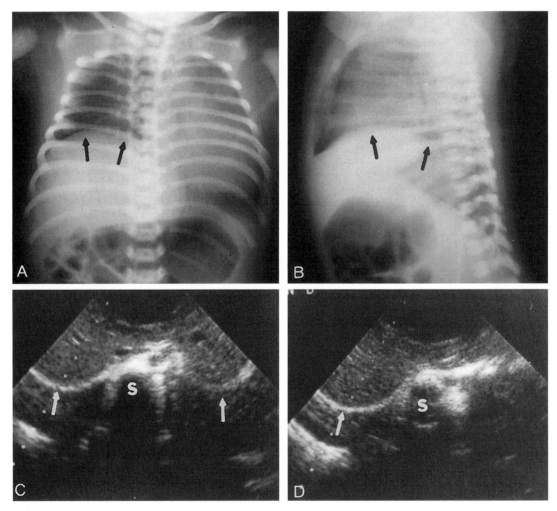

FIGURE 1.83. Diaphragmatic paralysis. A. Note the elevated right diaphragmatic leaflet (arrows). **B.** Lateral view demonstrates the characteristic smoothly domed and elevated diaphragmatic leaflet (arrows). **C. Ultrasound findings.** Expiratory phase demonstrates both the right and the left diaphragmatic leaflet (arrows) to be high in position and at the same level. **D.** With inspiration the left leaflet becomes flattened and moves downward while the right leaflet (arrow) remains domed and elevated. The right leaflet was paralyzed. Spine (S).

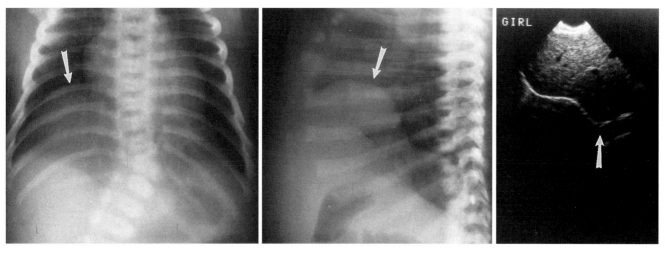

E,F

G

FIGURE 1.83. *Continued.* Diaphragmatic eventration. E. Note the elevated right diaphragmatic leaflet (arrow). This patient also had scoliosis secondary to vertebral anomalies. **F.** Lateral view demonstrates the characteristic localized bulge of an eventration (arrows). **G.** Longitudinal sonogram through the liver (L) demonstrates the hump (arrow) of the eventration.

ment of the involved leaflet is present. In neonates and young infants, ultrasonography now is often used to demonstrate diaphragmatic paralysis (Fig. 1.83, C and D).

The differential diagnosis of diaphragmatic leaflet elevation includes large diaphragmatic eventrations and enlargement of the liver with elevation of the right diaphragmatic leaflet. **However, in cases of phrenic nerve paralysis, the lower edge of the liver rises in proportion to the elevation of the diaphragmatic leaflet,** whereas with liver enlargement, the inferior edge of the liver is displaced downwardly.

Treatment of diaphragmatic paralysis is conservative, and many cases show spontaneous recovery. Continuous positive pressure ventilation is helpful in some infants, but when the problem is refractory, surgical intervention with plication of the diaphragm becomes necessary (4).

REFERENCES

1. Aldrich TK, Herman JH, Rochester DF. Bilateral diaphragmatic paralysis in the newborn infant. J Pediatr 1980;97:988–991.
2. Phillips AF, Rowe JC, Raye JR. Acute diaphragmatic paralysis after chest tube placement in a neonate. AJR 1981;136:824–825.
3. Nahum E, Ben Ari J, Schonfeld T, et al. Acute diaphragmatic paralysis caused by chest-tube trauma to phrenic nerve. Pediatr Radiol 2001;31:444–446.
4. Schwartz MZ, Filler RM. Plication of the diaphragm for symptomatic phrenic nerve paralysis. J Pediatr Surg 1978;13:259–263.

Eventration of the Diaphragm

Diaphragmatic eventration can occur unilaterally or bilaterally (1, 2). Roentgenographically, no matter what the age, a smooth bulge blending with the diaphragmatic leaflet is noted (Fig. 1.83, E–G). The abnormality represents a weakness in the diaphragm that allows upward herniation of the underlying organs such as the liver, kidney, spleen, and omentum. Usually, the condition is of no particular problem, but when the eventration is very large, or large and bilateral, respiratory distress can become a problem and surgical intervention may be required (3). Ultrasound is very effective in delineating any organs or other abdominal contents that may be seen in the eventration (Fig. 1.83F).

REFERENCES

1. Avnet NL. Roentgenologic features of congenital bilateral anterior diaphragmatic eventration. AJR 1962;88:743–750.
2. Paris F, Blasco E, Cantó A, et al. Diaphragmatic eventration in infants. Thorax 1973;28:66–72.
3. Tsugawa C, Kimura K, Nishijima E, et al. Diaphragmatic eventration in infants and children: is conservative treatment justified? J Pediatr Surg 1997;32:1643–1644.

Aplasia and Hypoplasia of the Diaphragm

Aplasia and hypoplasia of the diaphragm are extremely rare and can be unilateral or bilateral (1). This condition also can be familial and then is inherited as an autosomal recessive condition. When unilateral, the clinical and roentgenographic findings are similar to those of congenital diaphragmatic hernia.

REFERENCE

1. Tsang TM, Tam PKH, Dudley NE, et al. Diaphragmatic agenesis as a distinct clinical entity. J Pediatr Surg 1995;29:1439–1441.

Diaphragmatic Hernia

Congenital diaphragmatic hernia constitutes a major surgical emergency in the newborn, and the key to survival lies in the degree of underlying pulmonary hypoplasia. In terms of lung hypoplasia, as will be seen later, the degree of hypoplasia depends on whether herniation occurs early or late in intrauterine life.

Herniation of abdominal contents can occur through various portions of the diaphragm but most often occurs through the posterior foramina of Bochdalek, the old pleuroperitoneal canals. These are located just lateral to the spine, and, of the two sides, the left is much more common. Occasionally, bilateral hernias can be seen (1), and in some cases, the defect may be so large as to suggest complete absence of a hemidiaphragm. Hernias through the foramina of Morgagni are less commonly encountered (2, 3) and are not usually large enough to cause respiratory distress at birth or even later in life.

Clinically, infants with massive diaphragmatic hernias usually are in immediate respiratory distress. Symptoms are profound, and marked respiratory difficulty and cyanosis ensue. The hernia contents (intestine, stomach, spleen, liver, or omentum) fill the entire hemithorax and displace the mediastinal structures away from the affected side. As a result, the heart sounds are contralaterally displaced and the involved hemithorax dull to percussion. If the hernia is massive, the abdomen will be "empty" or scaphoid. Shortly, however, as the infant swallows more air, the herniated loops of intestine become distended and take up more space in the already crowded chest. Respiratory compromise becomes greater, and on auscultation, bowel sounds can be heard in the chest.

One cannot overstate the importance of obtaining a chest roentgenogram at the first sign of distress in these infants, as it usually permits accurate diagnosis. Of course, if the hernia is detected prenatally, the initial film does not represent such an emergency.

The classic roentgenographic appearance of a congenital diaphragmatic hernia is one in which the left hemithorax is filled with cyst-like structures (loops of bowel), the mediastinum is shifted to the right, and the abdomen is relatively void of gas (Fig. 1.84A). In some cases, a few loops of intestine can be seen in the abdomen, but more often, only the stomach remains visible. Interestingly enough, however, the stomach usually is in an abnormal location, often more central or lower than normal (Fig. 1.84C). The abnormal positioning of the stomach is helpful in differentiating congenital diaphragmatic hernia from those few cases of congenital cystic adenomatoid malformation where the cysts are large enough to mimic the air-filled intestinal loops. In congenital adenomatoid malformation of the lung, the stomach is normal in position and appearance.

In other cases, the stomach may be partially displaced into the chest, and in still other instances, it may be in the chest entirely and volved. In this regard, it has been demonstrated that when the stomach is in the chest, the prognosis is much poorer (4). Most likely, the problem here is that the stomach in the chest adds significantly to the compressive mass effect and leads to more hypoplasia of the lung. As far as abnormal abdominal positioning of the stomach is concerned, it probably is due to pulling on the stomach by the herniated intestine in association with a poorly fixed and underdeveloped mesentery.

If the chest roentgenogram is obtained before any air has entered the herniated bowel, it may be more difficult to diagnose the condition with accuracy (Fig. 1.84C). Similar difficulty arises when the liver alone is in the right hemithorax. In either case, the involved hemithorax is partially or totally opacified and mediastinal structures are shifted to the other side. For all one can say, one could be dealing with a large pleural fluid collection or a mass. However, in most of these cases, air soon enters the intestine and establishes the diagnosis. In other cases, the condition may be diagnosed by noting abnormal intrathoracic positioning of a nasogastric tube (5) (Fig. 1.84). If herniation occurs on the right, the intestine and liver, or liver alone, may fill the right hemithorax (Fig. 1.85). If the liver is in the chest, its silhouette will not be seen in the abdomen.

In spite of all the recent advances in the diagnosis and treatment of Bochdalek congenital diaphragmatic hernias, including ECMO therapy, the condition still remains high in terms of morbidity and mortality. Although some of these infants expire because of associated serious congenital heart or other anomalies, the main problem lies in the presence of pulmonary (lung) hypoplasia and the resultant PFC syndrome. Pulmonary hypoplasia results from longstanding intrauterine compression of the lungs by the hernia, and in this regard, infants with the largest and longest-standing hernias have the most hypoplastic lungs (Fig. 1.86) and are less

FIGURE 1.84. Left diaphragmatic hernia. A. Note numerous loops of air-filled intestine and the air-filled stomach (S) in the left hemithorax. There is marked contralateral shift of the mediastinal structures. The tip of the nasogastric tube is in the distal esophagus (arrow). **B.** Later, with the nasogastric tube now advanced into the stomach (arrow), note how the stomach has been decompressed and the intestines partially decompressed. There is much less mediastinal shift. Note paucity of gas in the abdomen. **C.** Another infant with an early film demonstrating an airless diaphragmatic hernia in the left hemithorax. Note the position of the stomach (S). There is marked contralateral shift of the mediastinal structures. **D.** A little later, some air is seen in the loops of intestine in the left hemithorax.

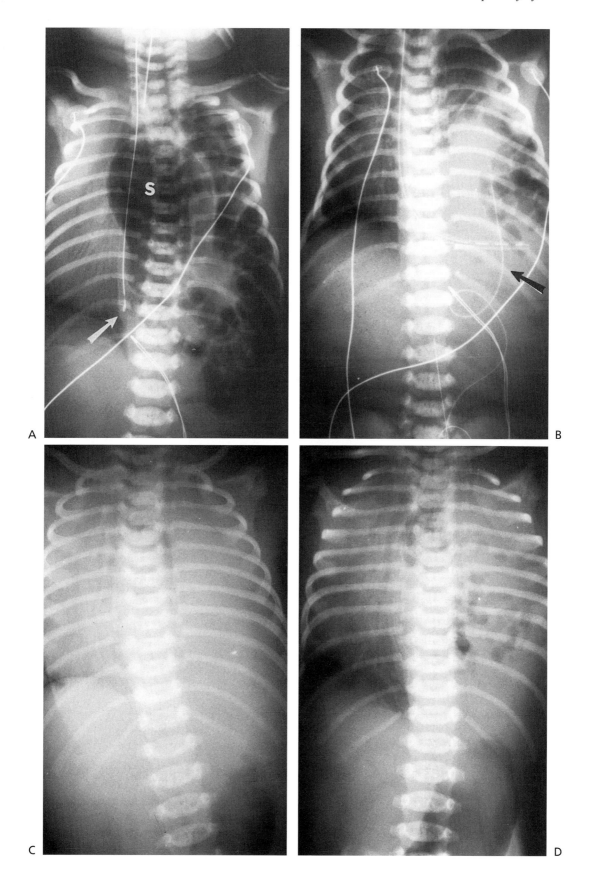

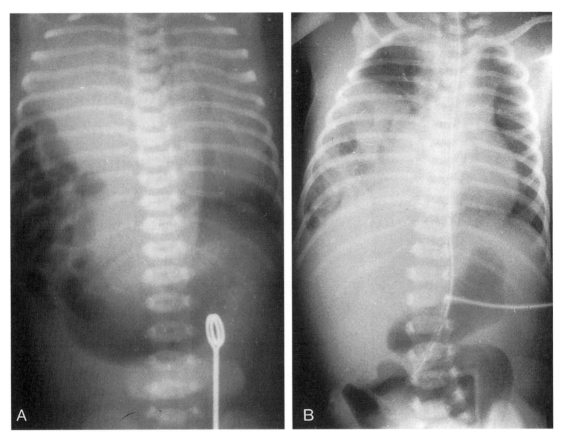

FIGURE 1.85. Right diaphragmatic hernia. A. The liver and intestines have been displaced into the right hemithorax. The central, air-filled structure in the abdomen is the stomach. Note its peculiar configuration and position. There is pronounced shift of the mediastinum to the left. **B.** Another patient with a right-side hernia with loops of intestine in the chest. However, herniation is not as massive as in **A** and thus the liver still remains in the abdomen.

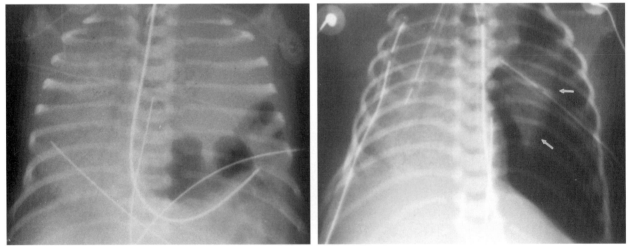

FIGURE 1.86. Diaphragmatic hernia with hypoplastic lungs. A. Note the typical appearance of a left diaphragmatic hernia. **B.** Postoperative film demonstrates a large iatrogenically produced pneumothorax and a small, hypoplastic nubbin of lung on the left (arrows).

likely to survive after birth. In all of these cases, compression by the hernia leads to retardation of normal alveolar growth, and it has been demonstrated experimentally that the hernia must be present early in fetal life for such hypoplasia to occur (6, 7). If a diaphragmatic hernia develops toward the end of pregnancy or after birth, pulmonary hypoplasia does not occur. In those early-onset cases of infants who survive, a demonstrably small lung on the involved side can persist for many years. This lung also usually is underperfused and, thus, roentgenographically small and hyperlucent. Regarding long-term follow-up, ventilatory impairment and lung dysfunction have been noted in older children and adults (8).

The PFC syndrome is a closely related and serious complication of the underlying pulmonary hypoplasia present in cases of congenital diaphragmatic hernia. It adds significantly, if not predominantly, to the morbidity of this condition because of resultant hypoxia-induced pulmonary arteriolar vasoconstriction, arteriolar muscular wall thickening, and hence persistent pulmonary hypertension. As a result, there is persistent right-to-left shunting across the patent ductus arteriosus and persistent cyanosis, that is, the PFC syndrome.

Complications of congenital diaphragmatic hernia include gastric volvulus, midgut volvulus, gastric or other intestinal perforation (9), compressive hypoplasia of the left ventricle with left-side hernias (10), and, on the right side, pleural effusions. The pleural effusions in these patients are believed due to lymphatic obstruction secondary to lymphatic compressive effects of the hernia.

Most congenital diaphragmatic hernias occur as isolated abnormalities, but in other cases, associated congenital heart disease, ipsilateral upper limb deformities, and other congenital anomalies of other systems co-exist. After surgical repair, gastroesophageal reflux can be a problem (11), and in some cases, the hernia may recur. In most cases, however, the hernia remains reduced, and immediately after reduction, the pleural space becomes filled with air and then fluid (Fig. 1.86). The initial presence of air, and then fluid, acts as a cushion to prevent the underlying hypoplastic lung from expanding too rapidly and rupturing. In those cases where hypoplasia is severe, the lung is slow to grow and expand, but in other less severe cases, the lung slowly enlarges and eventually occupies most of the hemithorax. However, in almost all cases, the ipsilateral lung eventually remains smaller than normal.

Small diaphragmatic hernias, mostly Bochdalek hernias, may go unnoticed and are discovered incidentally on chest films later in life. If the diagnosis is not obvious on the chest films, confirmation may be obtained with an upper gastrointestinal series, ultrasonography, or nuclear scintigraphy if the liver or spleen is suspected to be in the hernial sac.

Morgagni hernias are less common than Bochdalek hernias and, for the most part, are of no particular problem to the infant. Classically, Morgagni hernias present as unilateral,

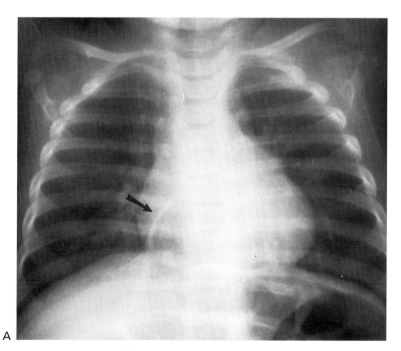
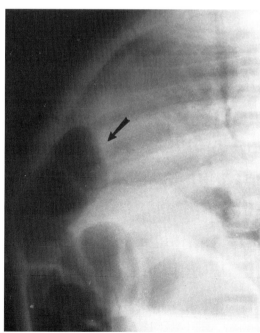

A   B

FIGURE 1.87. Morgagni hernia. A. Note a herniated loop of intestine just to the right of the spine (arrow). **B.** Lateral view showing herniation of intestine (arrow) through anterior defect.

medial and basal, masses containing a variety of abdominal organs but often air-filled loops of intestine (Fig. 1.87). Occasionally, they may be bilateral (1), and occasionally, they may produce significant respiratory distress (1).

Large, anterior, central diaphragmatic hernias, located just behind the sternum, can present very puzzling radiographic pictures. They may produce enlargement of the cardiac silhouette and bilateral bulges to either side of the lower mediastinum. However, more often, they produce nothing more than what appears to be rather marked cardiomegaly (Fig. 1.88). Ultrasound is of some use in these patients, but initial suspicion is based on familiarity with the phenomenon of central anterior herniations. Very often, these herniations occur into the pericardial cavity and are associated with pericardial effusions and serious cardiorespiratory compromise (12).

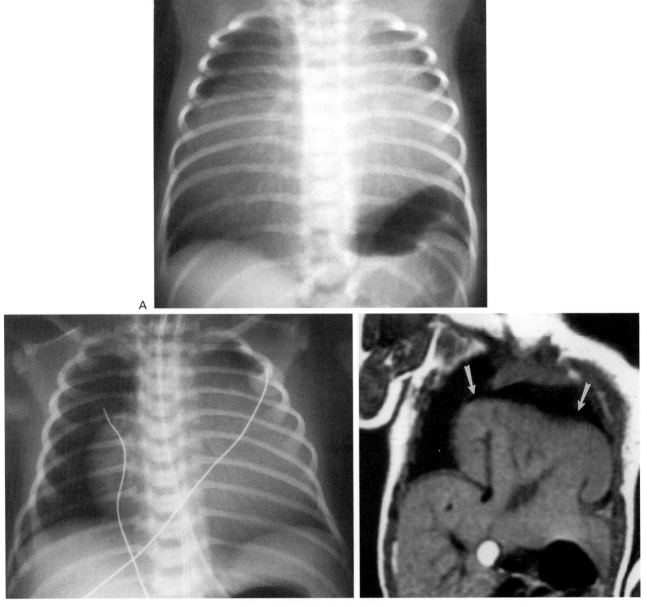

FIGURE 1.88. Central diaphragmatic hernia. A. Note the large cardiac silhouette caused by a large central diaphragmatic hernia. The hernial sac contained some liver, intestine, omentum, and the stomach. **B.** Another patient with less striking cardiac silhouette enlargement. **C.** Magnetic resonance study demonstrates the large central hernia (arrows), consisting primarily of liver.

REFERENCES

1. Furuta Y, Nakamura Y, Miyamoto K. Bilateral congenital posterolateral diaphragmatic hernia. J Pediatr Surg 1987;22:182–183.
2. Merten DF, Bowie JD, Kirks DR, et al. Anteromedial diaphragmatic defects in infancy: current approaches to diagnostic imaging. Radiology 1982;142:361–365.
3. Gross BR, D'Agostino C, Coren CV, et al. Prenatal and neonatal sonographic imaging of a central diaphragmatic hernia. Pediatr Radiol 1996;26:395–397.
4. Goodfellow T, Hyde I, Burge DM, et al. Congenital diaphragmatic hernia: the prognostic significance of the site of the stomach. Br J Radiol 1987;60:993–995.
5. Sakurai M, Donnelly LF, Klosterman LA, et al. Congenital diaphragmatic hernia in neonates: variations in umbilical catheter and enteric tube position. Radiology 2000;216:112–116.
6. Kent GM, Olley PM, Creighton RE, et al. Hemodynamic and pulmonary changes following surgical creation of a diaphragmatic hernia in fetal lambs. Surgery 1972;72:427–433.
7. Ohi R, Suzuki H, Kato T, et al. Development of the lung in fetal rabbits with experimental diaphragmatic hernia. J Pediatr Surg 1976;11:955–959.
8. Vanamo K, Rintala R, Sovijarvi A, et al. Long-term pulmonary sequelae in survivors of congenital diaphragmatic defects. J Pediatr Surg 1996;31:1096–1100.
9. Oshio T, Saito T, Sato Y. Gastric rupture associated with congenital diaphragmatic hernia. J Jpn Soc Pediatr Surg 1980;16:823–827.
10. Siebert JR, Haas JE, Beckwith JB. Left ventricular hypoplasia in congenital diaphragmatic hernia. J Pediatr Surg 1984;19:567–571.
11. Koot VCM, Bergmeijer JH, Bos AP, et al. Incidence and management of gastroesophageal reflux after repair of congenital diaphragmatic hernia. J Pediatr Surg 1993;28:48–52.
12. Stevens RL, Mathers A, Hollman AS, et al. An unusual hernia: congenital pericardial effusion associated with liver herniation into the pericardial sac. Pediatr Radiol 1996;26:791–793.

Delayed Diaphragmatic Hernia

Most of these patients initially are asymptomatic, but it has become increasingly apparent that late herniation of these previously occult Bochdalek hernias can be devastating (1–8). Indeed, these patients are prone to volvulus of the stomach and perforation of the stomach or other parts of the intestine. The clinical presentation can be very abrupt and confusing and consists of profound respiratory distress, vomiting, hematemesis, etc. Delayed herniation is believed due to an abrupt rise in intraabdominal pressures as might be seen with coughing, vomiting, or straining at stool. For the most part, the findings are not that different from intestinal herniation in the neonatal period, **but because one does not think of the diagnosis,** they can be misinterpreted for those of pneumonia (Fig. 1.89).

REFERENCES

1. Berman L, Stringer D, Ein SH, et al. The late-presenting pediatric Bochdalek hernia: a 20-year review. J Pediatr Surg 1988;23:735–739.
2. Byard RW, Bohn DJ, Wilson G, et al. Unsuspected diaphragmatic hernia: a potential cause of sudden and unexpected death in infancy and early childhood. J Pediatr Surg 1990;25:1166–1168.
3. Byard RW, Bourne AJ, Cockington RA. Fatal gastric perforation in a 4-year-old child with a late presenting congenital diaphragmatic hernia. Pediatr Surg Int 1991;6:44–46.
4. Brill PW, Gershwind ME, Krasna IH. Massive gastric enlargement with delayed presentation of congenital diaphragmatic hernia: report of three cases and review of the literature. J Pediatr Surg 1977;12:667–674.
5. Fotter R, Schimpt G, Sorantin E, et al. Delayed presentation of congenital diaphragmatic hernia. Pediatr Radiol 1992;22:187–191.
6. Manning PB, Murphy JP, Raynor SC, et al. Congenital diaphragmatic hernia presenting due to gastrointestinal complications. J Pediatr Surg 1992;27:1225–1228.
7. Swischuk LE. Vomiting blood for three days. Pediatr Emerg Care 1994;10:241–243.
8. Quah BS, Hashim I, Simpson H. Bochdalek diaphragmatic hernia presenting with acute gastric dilatation. J Pediatr Surg 1999;34:512–514.

Pneumothorax, Pneumomediastinum, and Interstitial Emphysema

Pneumothorax, pneumomediastinum, and interstitial emphysema are manifestations of terminal airway or alveolar overdistention and subsequent rupture of these structures. This can occur with (a) the infant's own forceful, initial respiratory efforts, (b) positive pressure assisted ventilation, (c) resuscitative measures, and (d) widespread or focal air trapping. Positive pressure assisted ventilation, however, still is the most common cause.

In all cases, when an alveolus or terminal airway ruptures, air escapes into the pulmonary interstitium and results in **PIE.** Air then dissects along the bronchovascular sheaths, in radiating fashion, to the outer periphery of the lung (1, 2). At any time, this air can decompress itself by passing directly into the mediastinum (through the hilus of the lung) or bursting through the visceral pleura into the pleural space. In the first case, pneumomediastinum is the result, while in the second, it is pneumothorax. When positive pressure ventilation is the cause of these complications, a continuous supply of air, under pressure, ensures that the interstitial "conduits," meandering along the bronchovascular sheaths, remain filled with air. These conduits were at first believed to be interstitial tunnels but now are believed to represent dilated lymphatics filled with air (3, 4). Just how air enters these lymphatics is not known, but there is reasonably good histologic evidence that the air, indeed, is intralymphatic.

The development of PIE in a lung is a serious problem, for the lung is severely splinted. To be sure, it is the "stiffest of stiff lungs" and does not fill or empty with respiration. In other words, it does not ventilate, and because of this, gas exchange cannot occur. Furthermore, since the air is under tension, pulmonary blood flow diminishes and aggravates the already compromised gas exchange in these infants.

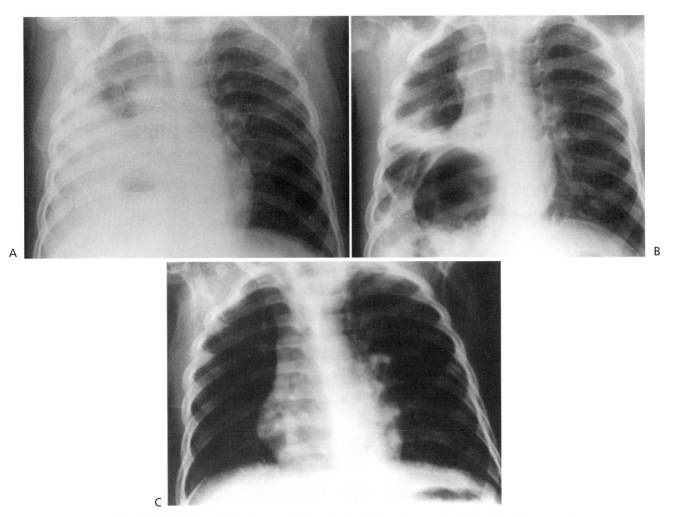

FIGURE 1.89. Delayed diaphragmatic hernia. A. The findings on the right first might suggest a cavitating pneumonia. **B.** Later, large bubbles are seen. **C.** Film in infancy on this patient is normal. Surgically proven diaphragmatic hernia.

Roentgenographically, the meandering collections of air tracking along the bronchovascular sheaths appear as tortuous air collections, radiating outward from the hilus of the lung, and measure from 2 to 3 mm in diameter (5). The findings are rather characteristic and histologically correlate well with the perivascular location of the air (Figs. 1.90 and 1.91). These air collections, or bubbles, termed "type II" bubbles (5), do not empty on expiration. Eventually, if the positive pressures that induced them are not lowered, the initially tortuous air bubbles become less tortuous and more cystic (Fig. 1.92). In some cases, this entire sequence of events is greatly accelerated (6), and the initially tortuous, meandering bubbles are rapidly replaced by large cystic pneumatoceles (6) in just a few hours. In other cases, findings can become localized to one

lobe or one lung and result in an acquired form of lobar emphysema (4). In the early years, these lungs were surgically removed, but later it was determined that they could be treated conservatively with decubitus positioning (afflicted side downward) or selective endobronchial intubation with occlusion of the involved bronchus. However, all of this is now very seldom required, but still an occasional case can be encountered (Fig. 1.93, A and B). Histologically, the distended air-filled lymphatics are quite prominent and, in addition, can be seen to be lined by reactive giant cells (Fig. 1.93C).

Once interstitial emphysema develops in a lung, one can expect to see complications such as pneumothorax, pneumomediastinum, pneumopericardium, pneumoperitoneum, and, terminally, massive gas embolism. It is not

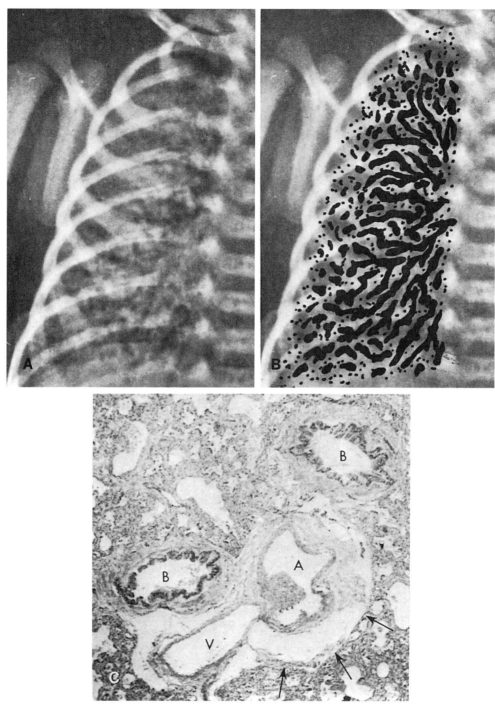

FIGURE 1.90. Pulmonary interstitial emphysema, type II bubble. A. Note the tortuous, meandering configuration of the bubbles of air in the interstitium. They radiate out from the hilus of the lung. **B.** Diagrammatic representation of the type II bubble. **C.** Histologic material demonstrating interstitial air (arrows) in a bronchovascular sheath. A, arteriole; V, venule; B, bronchiole. (Reproduced with permission from Swischuk LE. Bubbles in hyaline membrane disease; differentiation of three types. Radiology 1977;122: 417–426).

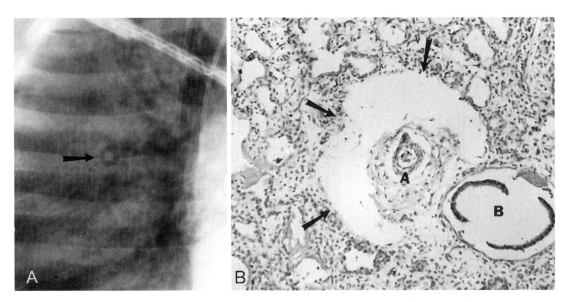

FIGURE 1.91. Pulmonary interstitial emphysema: perivascular location. A. In this patient with pulmonary interstitial emphysema, a target lesion is seen in the right midlung field (arrow). This configuration represents air surrounding the bronchovascular complex. **B.** Histologic material from another patient demonstrating air (arrows) surrounding an arteriole (A). The target-like configuration seen in **A** results from this type of air collection. B, adjacent bronchiole.

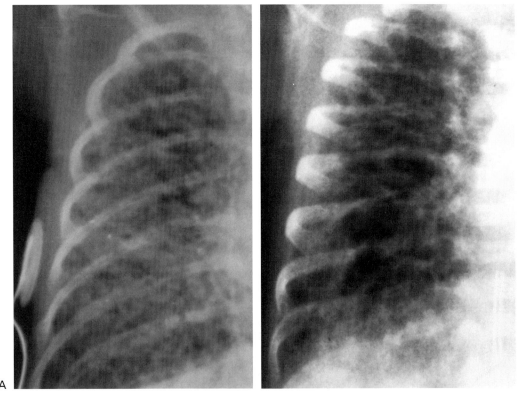

FIGURE 1.92. Pulmonary interstitial emphysema: varying bubble formation. A. In this patient, the bubbles basically still are tortuous. **B.** Another patient demonstrating much larger bubbles, which now are predominantly cyst-like.

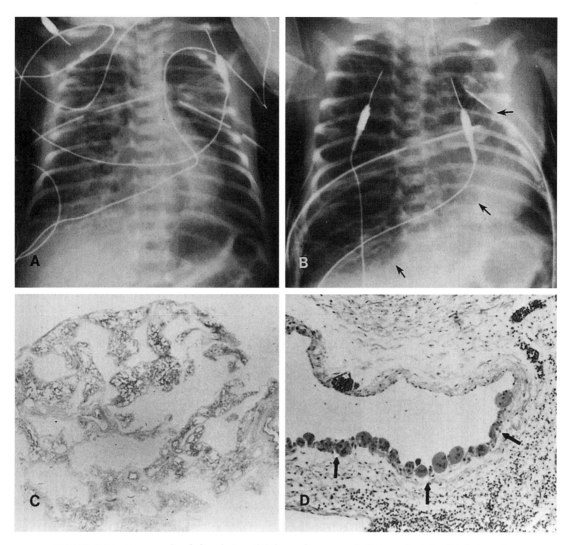

FIGURE 1.93. Progressive lobar interstitial emphysema. A. Note cystic interstitial air on the right. Bilateral chest tubes are in place for treatment of bilateral pneumothoraces. **B.** A few days later, there is marked overdistention of the right lung (arrows) with large pneumatocele formation. The mediastinal structure shows pronounced shift to the left. **C.** Histologic material from the removed right lung demonstrates large cystic spaces, eventually determined to be large, dilated lymphatics. **D.** High-power study of a dilated lymphatic. Note numerous giant cells (arrows) lining the lymphatic. These giant cells arise from the endothelium of the lymphatic and are presumed to be reactive to the air within.

known exactly how air enters the vascular system, but it is presumed that it does so through the pulmonary veins. The resultant findings often are striking (Fig. 1.94). When interstitial air reaches the pleural surface of the lung, subpleural blebs develop and can be quite large (6). These blebs, if symptomatic, can be catheter drained (7). When subpleural blebs, even ones quite small, burst, a **pneumothorax** develops. However, in most cases, the development of the bleb and subsequent pneumothorax is so rapid that there is no time to witness the entire sequence of events leading to the pneumothorax.

In terms of pneumothorax, large **pneumothoraces** can be diagnosed by transillumination, and actually, large pneumomediastinal air collections can be diagnosed in similar fashion. Lesser-volume pneumothoraces, however, are best detected roentgenographically. There is no problem with the radiographic identification of large pneumothoraces, and, when under tension, associated medial herniation of the pleural space across the anterior mediastinum occurs (8) (Fig. 1.95). Lesser-volume pneumothoraces are more difficult to identify, and, in this regard, one should be aware of all the potential locations for free air to collect. In

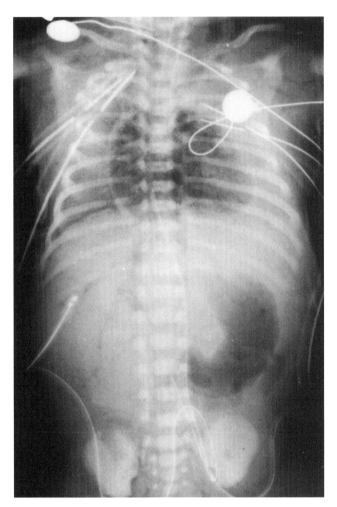

FIGURE 1.94. Air embolism with pulmonary interstitial emphysema. Note air within the heart itself. Also note air in the vessels leading to the upper extremities, in the liver, and in other parts of the body.

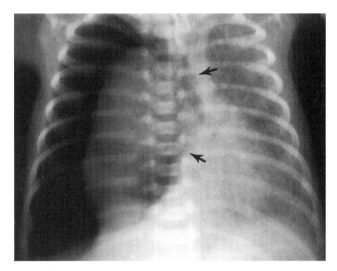

FIGURE 1.95. Tension pneumothorax. Note the large, right tension pneumothorax with herniation of the pleural space across the mediastinum (arrows). The underlying ipsilateral lung is compressed.

essence, air can cloak the lung in its entirety, but, most often, it does so less completely (Fig. 1.96). Knowledge of all of these areas of potential air collection is extremely helpful when a free lateral lung edge is not visualized (9).

When a pneumothorax collects medially (9, 10), the findings can be puzzling, but an important clue to the diagnosis of these pneumothoraces is the presence of increased sharpness of the ipsilateral mediastinal edge (Fig. 1.97). Another configuration of pneumothorax frequently missed is that seen with anterior air collections (9). In these cases, in the supine position, free air accumulates over the anterior surface of the lung and produces a hyperlucent, large hemithorax (Fig. 1.98). In addition, there is increased "sharpness" or "crispness" of the ipsilateral mediastinal edge, much as with medial pneumothoraces. Increased sharpness of the mediastinal edge results from the fact that

free air, rather than aerated lung tissue, abuts the mediastinum. In addition to these findings, the thymus gland frequently is compressed so as to form a bulging "pseudomass" (11) in the superior mediastinum (Fig. 1.98B).

When anterior pneumothoraces are bilateral, they present with a striking hyperlucent appearance to the entire chest and exceptional sharpness of the compressed mediastinal silhouette (Fig. 1.99A). In many of these cases, the compressed thymus gland appears as a superior mediastinal mass or the "figure 8" configuration of total anomalous pulmonary venous return (Fig. 1.99, B and C). Unless one is aware of these configurations, one will make a wrong diagnosis. Another helpful finding in these cases is visualization of the anterior junction line (12). The line is visible as a thin, opaque, mediastinal stripe, especially when the pneumothoraces are unequal and the larger one displaces the anterior junction line off midline (Fig. 1.100).

Confirmation of the presence of anterior or medial pneumothoraces can be accomplished with decubitus or cross-table lateral views (9, 10, 13). On the lateral view, the anterior location of the air layered over the lung often is clearly apparent (Fig. 1.101). It is important to appreciate the presence of these anterior pneumothoraces, for very often, when a chest tube is inserted for decompression, the tip of the chest tube lies posterior while the air is anterior (Fig. 1.101). In such cases, the pneumothorax will not clear unless the tube is repositioned or the patient's position is changed.

The causes of **pneumomediastinum** essentially are the same as those of pneumothorax. The condition, however, is

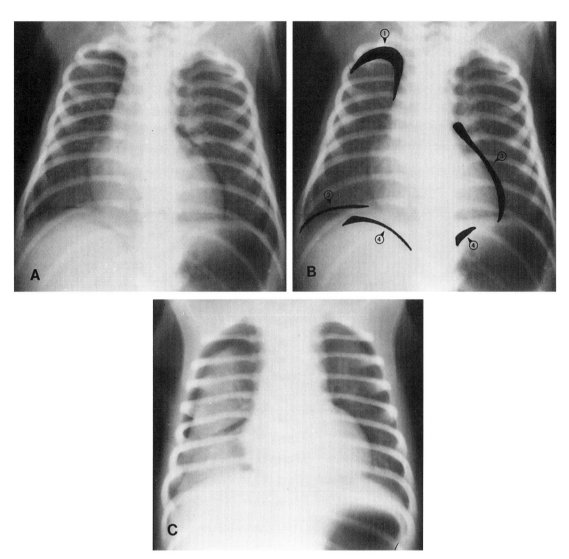

FIGURE 1.96. Pneumothorax: cloaking of the lung configurations. A. On first inspection, one might miss the fact that bilateral pneumothoraces are present. The radiolucency along the left cardiac border might be misinterpreted for a pneumopericardium. **B.** Diagrammatic representation of the sites of free air collection: (1) over the apex of the right lung, (2) over the anterior surface of the right diaphragmatic leaflet, (3) between the left lung and the heart (medial pneumothorax), and (4) deep, over the posterior aspects of the diaphragmatic leaflets. **C.** A little later, the pneumothoraces are much larger and more easily visualized. (Reproduced with permission from Swischuk LE. Two lesser known but useful signs of neonatal pneumothorax. AJR 1976;127:623–627).

less devastating and, for the most part, asymptomatic. Pneumomediastinal air also can track into the neck, and, indeed, air can extend over the entire chest wall. Nonetheless, even with large collections of air, there is surprisingly little respiratory difficulty. Every so often, an extremely large pneumomediastinal air collection, presumably under great tension, can produce respiratory distress, but this is very uncommon. Needle aspiration of the air may be required in these cases.

Roentgenographically, a wide variety of mediastinal free air configurations, sometimes quite bizarre, can be seen. Generally speaking, however, if one sees any peculiar air collection in the center of the chest outlining and/or elevating the lobes of the thymus gland, one should think of pneumomediastinum (Fig. 1.102). Outlining of the thymus gland is a most important finding and will differentiate pneumomediastinum from medial and anterior pneumothoraces where the thymus gland is compressed against, and not elevated

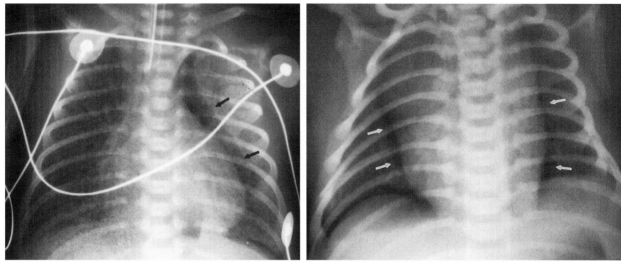

A   B

FIGURE 1.97. Medial pneumothorax. A. Note the large medial collection of free air (arrows) between the left lung and heart. Pulmonary interstitial emphysema is present throughout the right lung. **B.** Bilateral medial pneumothoraces produce a halo of free air around the heart. Some air also is present under the right lung.

from, the mediastinum. Confirmation of questionable pneumomediastinal air collections on the posteroanterior roentgenogram usually is readily accomplished with lateral views. On this view, an area of extreme hyperlucency in the superior retrosternal space almost always is seen.

When the thymus gland is outlined by air in the mediastinum, frequently it still looks like the thymus gland, except that the lobes are elevated (Fig. 1.103A), and the terms "angel wings" and "spinnaker sail" (14) have been suggested as descriptive terms for this phenomenon. However, when more air is present, the thymic lobes can be ele-

vated so far into the apices of the chest that they are misinterpreted for lobar atelectasis, consolidation, or apical pleural fluid (Fig. 1.103, B and C). At this point, one should recall that lobar pneumonias are uncommon in the newborn infant and that upper lobe atelectasis and apical effusions both are uncommon immediately after birth. When one appreciates these facts, one will arrive at the proper diagnosis. The thymus gland also can be so squeezed, flattened, and distorted by pneumomediastinal air that a bizarre "rocker-bottom thymus" configuration (Fig. 1.104B) has been described (15).

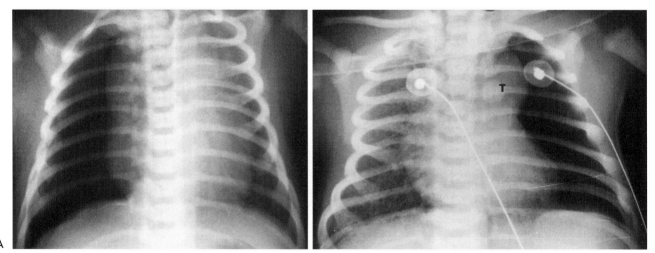

A   B

FIGURE 1.98. Anterior pneumothorax: large hyperlucent hemithorax sign. A. Note the slightly large but very hyperlucent right hemithorax. The ipsilateral mediastinal edge is sharp. **B.** In this infant, the left hemithorax is hyperlucent and the ipsilateral mediastinal edge very crisp. In addition, the thymus gland (T) is compressed so as to produce a pseudomass.

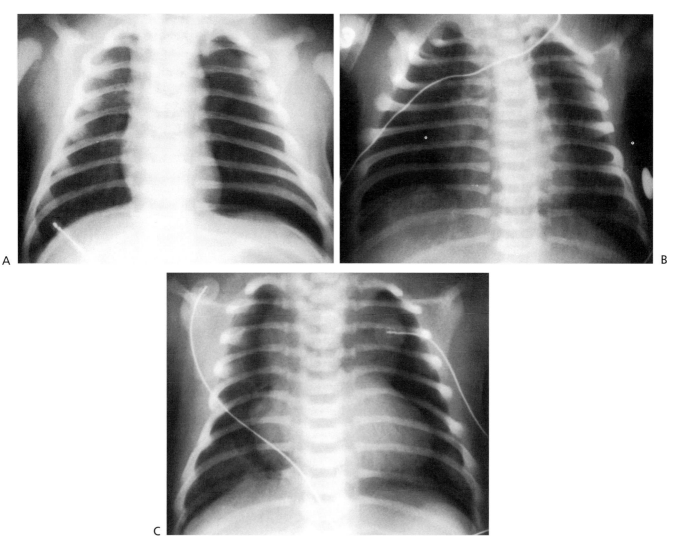

FIGURE 1.99. Bilateral anterior pneumothoraces. A. Note extreme hyperlucency of both lung fields. The mediastinal structures (thymus, heart) are compressed, and their edges are extremely sharp. **B.** After resolution of the pneumothoraces, the heart and thymus now appear normal. **C.** Another patient with bilateral pneumothoraces compressing the thymus gland and producing a pseudo-"snowman" or "figure 8" configuration.

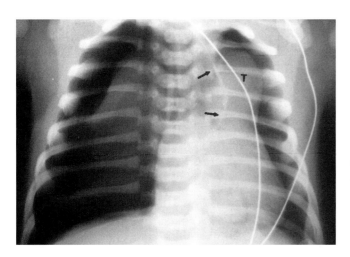

FIGURE 1.100. Bilateral pneumothoraces with anterior junction line. Note the massive pneumothorax on the right, compressing the right lung into a miniature of itself. Also note the anterior junction line (arrows) bulging across midline because of the distended pleural space on the right. The line is visible as a white line because air is present to either side of it. There also is an anterior pneumothorax on the left. Note the sharp mediastinal edge and that the thymus gland (T) is being compressed into a pseudomass configuration.

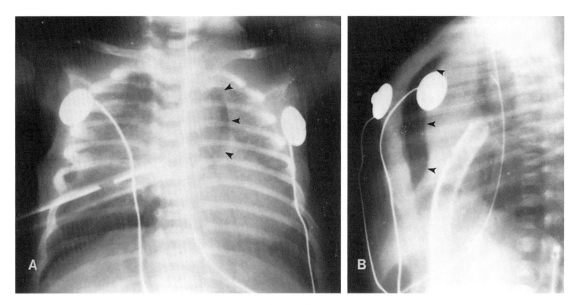

FIGURE 1.101. Anterior pneumothorax: faulty chest tube position. A. Note the chest tube in the right hemithorax. A large anterior pneumothorax is present. There is bulging of the pleural space across the mediastinum to the left side (arrows). **B.** Lateral view clearly shows the anterior pneumothorax (arrows) and the posterior position of the chest tube.

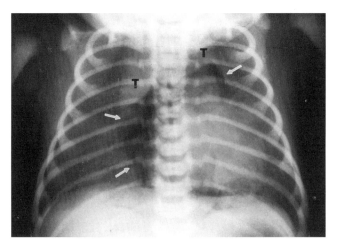

FIGURE 1.102. Pneumomediastinum. Note free air around the heart and great vessels (arrows), elevating both lobes of the thymus gland (T). Some air also is present along the inferior aspect of the heart.

FIGURE 1.104. Pneumomediastinum: other configurations. A. Note free air surrounding the heart in this older infant with adult respiratory distress syndrome. If this air represented that of pneumopericardium, **it would not outline the entire thymic lobe (T)** on the left. Air under the heart leads to the so-called "continuous diaphragm" sign (arrows). **B.** Peculiar-appearing "rocker-bottom thymus" (arrows) being compressed by pneumomediastinal air. This patient also had bilateral pneumothoraces. (**B** courtesy of M. Kogutt, M.D.).

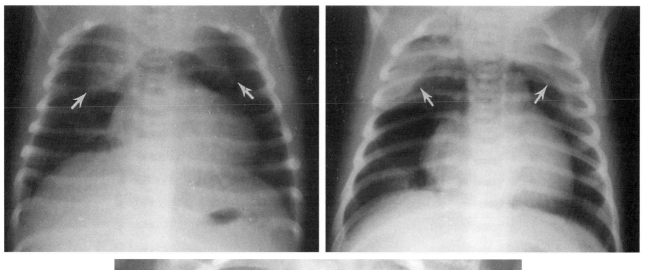

A

B

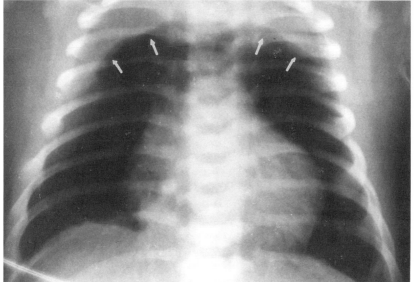

C

FIGURE 1.103. Pneumomediastinum: angel wing configuration. A. Note typical angel wing configuration of both thymic lobes (arrows) as they are elevated by free mediastinal air beneath them. **B.** Another patient with a large collection of air and more pronounced elevation of the thymic lobes (arrows). This patient also had bilateral anterior pneumothoraces. **C.** In still another infant, the thymic lobes (arrows) are pushed into the apices of the thorax.

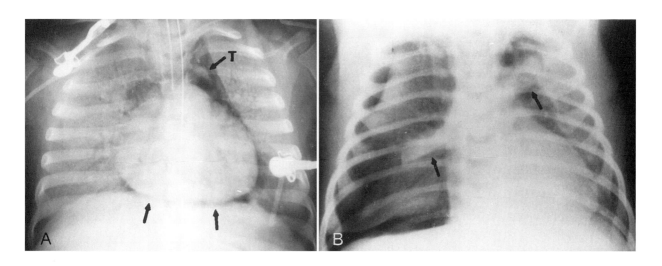

A

B

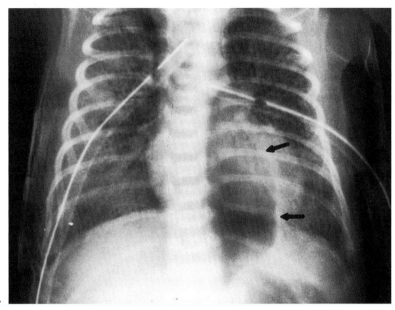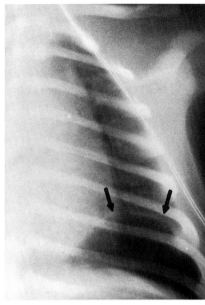

A

B

FIGURE 1.105. Pneumomediastinum: less common presentation. A. Note the central collection of pneumomediastinal air (arrows). This air is believed to lie in the infraazygos space. Bilateral chest tubes are in place for the treatment of bilateral pneumothoraces. Pulmonary interstitial emphysema also is present. **B.** Another patient with a similar collection of free air, but this time just to the left of the spine (arrows). This configuration is considered to represent air in the inferior pulmonary ligament. However, it must be noted that there is not universal agreement as to just where all of these air collections are located.

Other configurations of pneumomediastinum include air surrounding the heart and air outlining the inferior aspect of the heart (Fig. 1.04A). This latter finding often is referred to as the "continuous diaphragm sign" (16). Pneumomediastinal air surrounding the entire heart must be differentiated from pneumopericardium. With pneumopericardium, although the thymus gland may be elevated, it is not surrounded by air. With pneumomediastinum, the thymus gland usually is surrounded by air (Fig. 1.104A). Furthermore, with pneumopericardium, the pericardial sac itself often is visualized.

Mediastinal air can track into the subpleural space, that is, the space between the parietal pleura and diaphragm. This can result in a hyperlucent crescent of air, mimicking pneumothorax, just over the diaphragmatic leaflet (17) or, if localized, a pseudocyst configuration (Fig. 1.105B).

Mediastinal air, of course, also may track into the soft tissues of the neck and into the various ligaments in the mediastinum. Most commonly, the latter include the inferior pulmonary ligament (18), the infraazygos ligament (19), and the retrocardiac space (20) (Fig. 1.105A). There often is debate as to whether these latter collections are truly in the ligaments proposed, but, whatever, they usually require no specific therapy. In still other cases, air may pass from the mediastinum into the peritoneal cavity, and in such cases, while the volume of air in the mediastinum may be scant, the degree of pneumoperitoneum can be significant. It has been suggested that the air in these cases enters the peritoneal cavity through anterior retrosternal transdiaphragmatic communications between the thorax and abdomen. Such communications are normal and can account for either air or fluid traveling from the chest into the abdomen or vice versa.

REFERENCES

Pulmonary Interstitial Emphysema
1. Macklin MT, Macklin CC. Malignant interstitial emphysema of the lung and mediastinum as an important occult complication in many respiratory diseases and other conditions. Medicine 1944;23:281–358.
2. Ovenfors CO. Pulmonary interstitial emphysema; experimental roentgen diagnostic study. Acta Radiol [Suppl] 1964;224.
3. Boothroyd AE, Barson AJ. Pulmonary interstitial emphysema—a radiological and pathological correlation. Pediatr Radiol 1988;18:194–199.
4. Leonidas JC, Bhan K, McCauley RGK. Persistent localized pulmonary interstitial emphysema and lymphangiectasis: a causal relationship? Pediatrics 1979;64:165–171.
5. Swischuk LE. Bubbles in hyaline membrane disease. Radiology 1977;122:417–426.
6. deRoux SJ, Prendergast NC. Large sub-pleural air cysts: an extreme form of pulmonary interstitial emphysema. Pediatr Radiol 1998;28:981–983.
7. Kogutt MS, Lutrell CA, Puyau FA, et al. Decompression of pneumatocele in a neonate by percutaneous catheter placement. Pediatr Radiol 1999;29:488–489.
8. Fletcher BD. Medial herniation of the parietal pleura: a useful

sign of pneumothorax in supine neonates. AJR 1978;130: 469–472.

9. Swischuk LE. Two lesser known but useful signs of neonatal pneumothorax. AJR 1976;127:623–627.
10. Moskowitz PS, Griscom NT. The medial pneumothorax. Radiology 1976;120:143–147.
11. O'Keeffe FN, Swischuk LE, Stansberry SD. Mediastinal pseudomass caused by compression of the thymus in neonates with anterior pneumothorax. AJR 1991;156:145–148.
12. Markowitz RI. The anterior junction line: a radiographic sign of bilateral pneumothorax in neonates. Radiology 1988;167: 717–719.
13. Hoffer FA, Ablow RC. The cross-table lateral view in neonatal pneumothorax. AJR 1984;142:1283–1286.
14. Moseley JE. Loculated pneumomediastinum in the newborn: thymic "spinnaker sail" sign. Radiology 1960;75:788–790.
15. Kogutt MS. "Rocker-bottom thymus." A new sign of pneumomediastinum in the neonate. JAMA 1981;246:770–771.
16. Levin B. Continuous diaphragm sign: newly recognized sign of pneumomediastinum. Clin Radiol 1973;24:337–338.
17. Saezz F, Marco A, Martinez A, et al. Transient idiopathic subpleural cysts in the newborn: an observation in two patients. Pediatr Radiol 1985;15:249–250.
18. Volberg FM Jr, Everett CJ, Brill PW. Radiologic features of inferior pulmonary ligament air collections in neonates with respiratory distress. Radiology 1979;130:357–360.
19. Bowen A III, Quattromani FL. Infraazygos pneumomediastinum in the newborn. AJR 1980;135:1017–1021.
20. Rosenfeld DL, Cordell CE, Jadeja N. Retrocardiac pneumomediastinum: radiographic finding and clinical implications. Pediatrics 1990;85:92–97.

Pneumothorax and Pneumomediastinum with Pulmonary Hypoplasia

Pneumothorax and pneumomediastinum are common complications of pulmonary hypoplasia. Most often, such hypoplasia occurs with underlying renal disease (1–3), where intrauterine urine output is decreased and oligohydramnios results. Included are conditions such as renal agenesis (Potter's syndrome), renal cystic disease, prune belly syndrome, renal dysplastic disease, etc. With oligohydramnios, the normal cushioning effect of amniotic fluid is lost, and direct uterine compressive forces are transmitted to the thorax and abdomen of the fetus. Because of this, there is impairment of lung development, and, when the infant is born, the hypoplastic lungs are too small to provide adequate gas exchange. The infant, on its own, can overdistend these lungs and cause pneumothoraces to develop, but more often they are overdistended with resuscitative measures. Similar problems can arise with other pulmonary compressive problems such as congenital diaphragmatic hernia, bilateral hydro-chylothorax, restrictive thoracic dystrophies, and primary pulmonary hypoplasia. A more detailed discussion of pulmonary hypoplasia and its complications has been presented earlier in this chapter.

REFERENCES

1. Bashour BN, Balfe JW. Urinary tract anomalies in neonates with spontaneous pneumothorax and/or pneumomediastinum. Pediatrics [Suppl] 1977;59:1048–1049.
2. Renert WA, Berdon WE, Baker DH, et al. Obstructive urologic malformations of the fetus and infant: relation to neonatal pneumomediastinum and pneumothorax (air block). Radiology 1972; 105:97–105.
3. Wilkinson RH, Wheeler DB. Pneumothorax and renal disease in a newborn. Ann Radiol 1973;16:235–238.

Pneumothorax, Pneumomediastinum, and Interstitial Emphysema in Older Infants and Children

Generally, PIE is not seen in older infants and children unless they suffer from ARDS and are on ventilator-assisted therapy. Pneumomediastinum in children is most commonly seen with asthma, but it can also be seen with spasmodic coughing or Valsalva maneuvers for any other reason (1). Pneumomediastinal air also can track from the hypopharynx after perforating injuries (2). Pneumomediastinum and pneumothorax are seen after trauma to the chest, but pneumothorax is far less commonly seen in asthmatics than is pneumomediastinum. Both pneumomediastinum and pneumothorax can be seen with any condition that leads to acute or chronic air trapping, including foreign bodies.

Spontaneous pneumothorax is rather uncommon in infants and children and is generally the result of some underlying lung pathology (3). In older children, spontaneous pneumothorax tends to occur in males who are thin (4, 5). Very often, these patients suffer from subpleural apical blebs and the pneumothorax recurs. This has been our experience, and eventually these patients come to therapy in terms of surgical intervention, which is aimed at developing adhesions over the apex of the lung. Finally, small- and medium-size pneumothoraces can be treated conservatively (6) and, of course, are readily demonstrable with CT.

REFERENCES

1. Uva JL. Spontaneous pneumothoraces, pneumomediastinum, and pneumoperitoneum: consequence of smoking crack cocaine. Pediatr Emerg Care 1997;13:24–26.
2. McHugh TP. Pneumomediastinum following penetrating oral trauma. Pediatr Emerg Care 1997;13:211–213.
3. Alter SJ. Spontaneous pneumothorax in infants: a 10-year review. Pediatr Emerg Care 1997;13:401–403.
4. Poenaru D, Yazbeck S, Murphy S. Primary spontaneous pneumothorax in children. J Pediatr Surg 1994;29:1183–1185.
5. Wilcox DT, Glick PL, Karamanoukian HL, et al. Spontaneous pneumothorax: a single-institution, 12-year experience in patients under 16 years of age. J Pediatr Surg 1995;30:1452–1454.
6. Wolfman NT, Myers WS, Glauser SJ, et al. Validity of CT classification on management of occult pneumothorax: a prospective study. AJR 1998;171:1317–1320.

Congenital Lung Cysts

Congenital lung cysts are uncommon. Histologically, true congenital lung cysts contain smooth muscle and cartilage

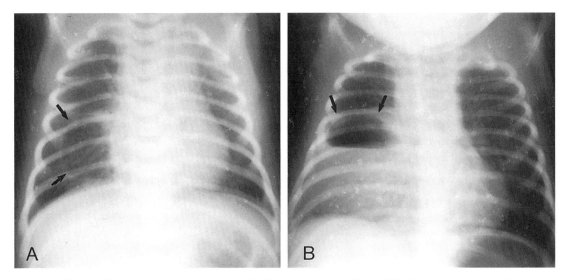

FIGURE 1.106. Congenital lung cyst. A. Newborn infant with air-filled lung cyst (arrows). **B.** One week later, the cyst nearly triples in size (arrows). This was due to a superimposed infection (note the air-fluid level).

in their wall. This finding is essential as the presence of columnar or squamocuboidal epithelium alone does not substantiate the diagnosis. Acquired lung cysts (pneumatoceles) can be similarly lined.

Occasionally, a cyst can undergo rapid enlargement and result in severe respiratory distress, but more often the problem is one of recurrent pulmonary infection (1). In those cases where rapid enlargement occurs, a ball-valve obstructive phenomenon at the point of communication with the normal airway is believed to exist. Such communications are common (2, 3), and with progressive air trapping, mediastinal shift and respiratory distress can reach severe proportions. Surgical removal of the involved lobe is usually required. Rhabdomyosarcoma arising within congenital pulmonary cysts also has been reported (4).

Single or multiple lung cysts occur most frequently in the lower lobes. They are usually thin walled, and, if fluid is present, an air-fluid level can be seen (Fig. 1.106). When an extremely large cyst is encountered, mediastinal shift may be seen, and the entire picture can mimic tension pneumothorax (4).

REFERENCES

1. Gwinn JL, Lee FA. Congenital pulmonary cysts. Am J Dis Child 1970;119:341–342.
2. Oestrich AE. Air fluid level detection in neonatal lung cyst identification. Pediatr Radiol 1973;1:244–245.
3. Reed JC, Sobonya RE. Congenital lung cyst. Radiology 1975;117:315–318.
4. Murphy JJ, Blair GK, Fraser GC, et al. Rhabdomyosarcoma arising within congenital pulmonary cysts: report of three cases. J Pediatr Surg 1992;27:1364–1367.

Cystic Adenomatoid Malformation

Cystic adenomatoid malformation is a relatively rare congenital lung abnormality (1, 2) that, however, can produce respiratory distress in the neonatal period. Occasionally, these infants are stillborn, and anasarca or fetal hydrops due to mechanical obstruction of venous return to the heart is seen. Polyhydramnios also can occur, and in the older infant, pulmonary infection may become a problem. In addition, complicating pneumothorax occasionally occurs (3).

Cystic adenomatoid malformation now can be identified prenatally with ultrasound. In terms of prenatal identification, some of these malformations have been seen to regress before birth (4, 5). In addition, it has been determined that polyhydramnios, anasarca, mediastinal shift, and the presence of a solid (type III) congenital adenomatoid malformation are associated with a poor postnatal prognosis (5).

Congenital cystic adenomatoid malformation is histologically diagnosed by the fact that the cysts contain clumps of cells showing definite adenomatous formation (2). The malformation has been classified into three types: type I demonstrating numerous relatively uniform air-filled cysts, type II demonstrating one dominant cyst with a background of smaller cysts, and type III, a solid lesion with numerous small cysts that are basically fluid filled (2). The latter tends to present in the neonatal period as a solid pulmonary mass (6, 7). However, since these cysts communicate with the airway, eventually the fluid is replaced by air, and the resultant air-filled bubbles progressively enlarge. The lesion usually is unilateral, although bilateral involvement occasionally can be seen. In some cases, blood supply can arise from the aorta, and confusion with bronchopulmonary foregut malformation and sequestration can occur.

Indeed, some overlap of all of these entities seems to exist (8).

Roentgenographically, the findings are quite variable and depend on the size and type of the lesion. With the type III abnormality, usually presenting in the neonatal period, initial findings, as previously noted, may suggest a solid pulmonary mass (Fig. 1.107A). In such cases, it may be difficult to differentiate the findings from those produced by other intrathoracic masses or pseudomasses such as the fluid-filled lung of lobar emphysema or bronchial atresia. In other instances, where air replaces the fluid, multiple bubbles of various sizes can be seen, and in some cases, the bub-

bles or cysts become quite large and mimic the pneumatoceles of a staphylococcal pneumonia or the air-filled intestinal loops of a congenital diaphragmatic hernia. However, as opposed to congenital diaphragmatic hernia, the abdominal gas pattern with congenital adenomatoid malformation is normal, and as far as staphylococcal pneumatoceles are concerned, this infection is uncommon in the immediate neonatal period. Finally, in a few cases, the cysts can become extremely large and so thin walled that they become difficult to detect as cysts. In such cases, the findings may at first suggest congenital lobar emphysema or a large pneumothorax. Examples of the various configura-

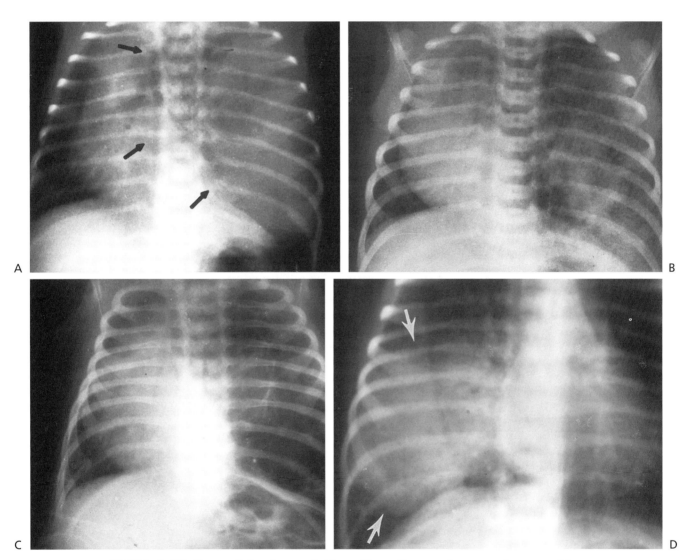

FIGURE 1.107. Congenital adenomatoid malformation: various roentgenographic appearances. A. Virtually airless adenomatoid malformation presenting as a large mass (arrows) in the left hemithorax. It is causing right-side displacement of the heart and trachea. **B.** Another patient with a less solid-appearing mass, which now also shows early cyst formation. **C.** In this patient, the air-filled cysts have become so large that the individual cyst walls are barely perceptible. Lobar emphysema or even a pneumothorax might erroneously be suggested. **D.** Smaller, airless malformation (arrows) on the right. (**B** courtesy of D. Kirks, M.D., and G. Shackelford, M.D.; **D** courtesy of Virgil Graves, M.D.).

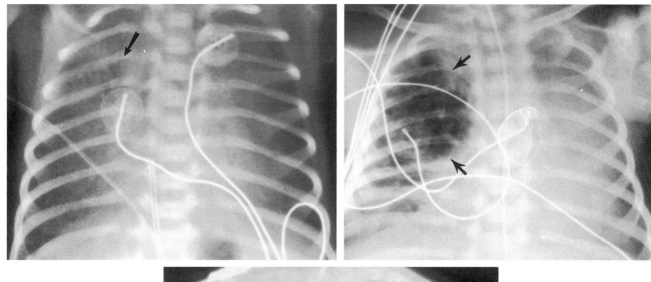

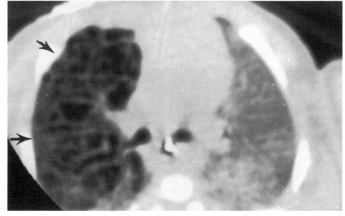

FIGURE 1.108. Cystic adenomatoid malformation: computed tomography findings. A. Note hazy/granular lungs secondary to surfactant deficiency disease. A small, tubular, air-filled structure (arrow) is seen in the right upper lobe. **B.** Later, a multicystic enlarging lesion (arrows) is seen in the right upper lobe. **C.** Computed tomography scan demonstrates the multiple air-filled cysts (arrows).

tions of congenital adenomatoid malformation are presented in Fig. 1.107.

In addition to plain films, congenital adenomatoid malformation can be evaluated with ultrasonography and CT (8) (Fig. 1.108). Ultrasonography is most rewarding in those cases where the lesion is fluid filled and solid appearing. In such cases, the lesion appears solid but does have internal echoes due to the cyst walls. CT findings merely reflect the plain film findings and consist of solid lung tissue interspersed with cystic structures containing both air and fluid.

Most patients with congenital adenomatoid malformation present with respiratory distress in the neonatal period or shortly thereafter. However, those with smaller lesions may present later (8), and in some of these patients, symptoms may take years to develop. The symptoms in these latter patients usually are those of pulmonary infection rather than respiratory compromise.

Finally, it should noted that there is overlap between congenital adenomatoid malformation and bronchopulmonary foregut malformation (9) and that some malformations may regress in utero (10).

REFERENCES

1. Fisher JE, Nelson SJ, Allen JE, et al. Congenital cystic adenomatoid malformation of the lung. Am J Dis Child 1982;136: 1071–1074.
2. Madewell JE, Stocker JT, Korsower JM. Cystic adenomatoid malformation of the lung; morphologic analysis. AJR 1975;124: 436–448.
3. Gaisie G, Oh KS. Spontaneous pneumothorax in cystic adenomatoid malformation. Pediatr Radiol 1983;13:281–283.
4. Fine C, Adzick NS, Doubilet PM. Decreasing size of a congenital cyst adenomatoid malformation in utero. J Ultrasound Med 1988;7:405–408.
5. Neilson IR, Russo P, Laberje J-M, et al. Congenital adenomatoid

malformation of the lung: current management and prognosis. J Pediatr Surg 1991;26:975–981.

6. Tucker TT, Smith WL, Smith JA. Fluid-filled cystic adenomatoid malformation. AJR 1977;129:323–325.

7. Wexler HA, Dapena MV. Congenital cystic adenomatoid malformation; a report of three unusual cases. Radiology 1978;126: 737–741.

8. Kim SS, Lee KS, Kim I-O, et al. Congenital cystic adenomatoid malformation of the lung: CT-pathologic correlation. AJR 1997; 168:47–53.

9. Cass DL, Crombleholme TM, Howell LJ, et al. Cystic lung lesions with systemic arterial blood supply: a hybrid of congenital cystic adenomatoid malformation and bronchopulmonary sequestration. J Pediatr Surg 1997;32:986–990.

10. vanLeeuwen K, Teitelbaum DH, Hirschl RB, et al. Prenatal diagnosis of congenital cystic adenomatoid malformation and its

postnatal presentation, surgical indications, and natural history. Ann J Pediatr Surg 1999;34:794–799.

Bronchopulmonary Foregut Malformation, Pulmonary Sequestration, and Accessory Lung

Embryologically, the entities of bronchopulmonary foregut malformation, pulmonary sequestration, and accessory lung are intertwined, and thus this will be the approach to these lesions in this section. They will be treated as the same lesion, and it should be noted that they can occur alone or be associated with other anomalies (1, 2). Generally, it is

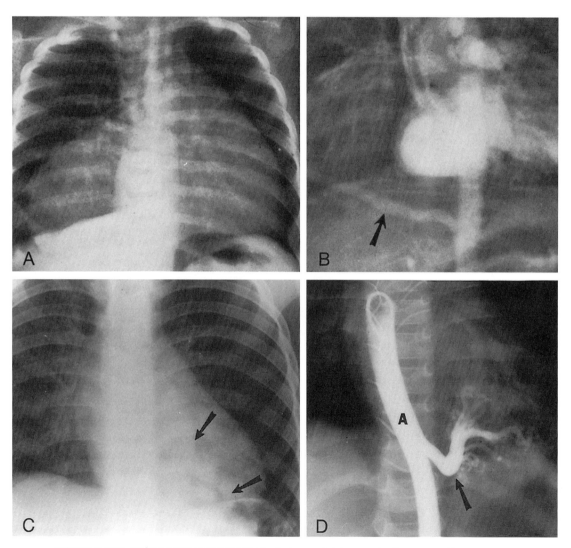

FIGURE 1.109. Pulmonary sequestration. A. Large right sequestration presenting as a mass in the right lung base. There is slight shift of the mediastinum to the opposite side. **B.** Aortogram showing aberrant vascular supply to the sequestrated lung from the aorta (arrow). **C.** Older patient with vague, nodular-appearing infiltrates behind the left side of the heart. **D.** Aortogram demonstrates the abnormal feeding vessel (arrow) arising from the aorta (A). (**A** and **B** reproduced with permission from Avery MA. The lung and its disorders in the newborn infant. Philadelphia: Saunders, 1968).

uncommon for neonatal infants with these abnormalities to present with difficulties in the neonatal period, but if these lesions are large, they can produce acute neonatal respiratory distress (1). They also can present acutely in older children (3, 4).

In the past, an intralobar-extralobar classification of sequestration usually was utilized, but since the lesion is so variable and since more and more it is being realized that gastroenteric communications and anomalies commonly co-exist (5–7), **the more encompassing term "bronchopulmonary foregut malformation" is more appropriate.** Even if one does not totally agree with this concept, it certainly is useful on a practical basis, and, indeed, many attempts at unifying congenital adenomatoid malformation, pulmonary sequestration, anomalous pulmonary venous return, and gastrointestinal anomalies also have been attempted (6–10).

Classically, pulmonary sequestrations are located in the lower lobes, and although bronchial and alveolar elements are seen within the malformation, there usually, but not always, is no connection with the bronchial tree (7). Arterial blood supply is from the lower thoracic or intraabdominal aorta, but it also can be derived from the upper mediastinum and neck (11). Venous return is directed into the pulmonary veins, systemic veins, or infradiaphragmatically into the portal vein (12). In the past, whether the sequestration was covered by the pleura of the normal lung or by its own pleura determined whether it was intra- or extralobar. If extralobar, it laid outside the pleura of the normal lung and venous drainage more often was to the systemic or portal veins. It is

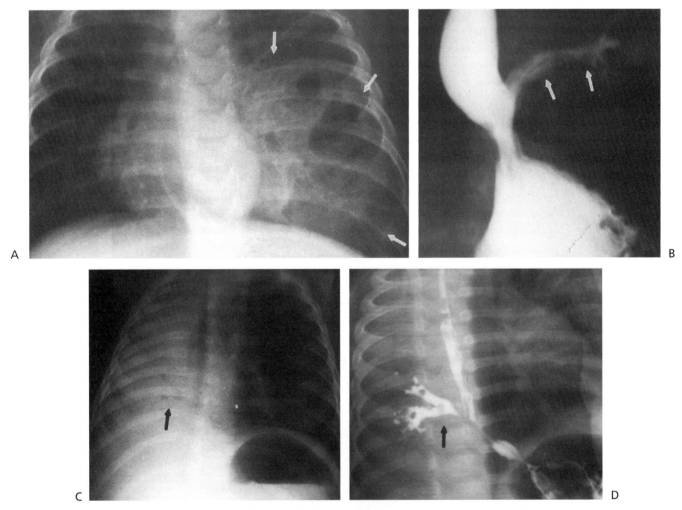

FIGURE 1.110. Bronchopulmonary foregut malformation. A. Note the mass on the left side (arrow). It is displacing the mediastinal structures to the right. Its margins are poorly defined, but two or three air-filled cysts are seen within it. **B.** Esophagram demonstrating communication (arrows) between the esophagus and malformation. **C.** This infant shows marked loss of volume on the right with compensatory emphysema of the left lung. A little air is seen in the base of the right lung (arrow). **D.** Esophagram shows a bronchoesophageal fistula (arrow). (**B** reproduced with permission from Graves VB, Dahl DD, Power HW. Congenital bronchopulmonary foregut malformations with anomalous pulmonary artery. Radiology 1975;114:423–424).

this form of sequestration that might be considered within the spectrum of so-called accessory lung. Sequestration also, but rarely, can occur in the upper lobe (13) and also can be found in the abdomen, mimicking a neuroblastoma (14–18). In addition, the opposite can occur where a neuroblastoma can be mistaken for sequestration (19).

Roentgenographically, the classic appearance of sequestration of the lung consists of a triangular or oval-shaped basal, posterior lung mass (Fig. 1.109). These masses usually are medial in position and can occur on the right or left, but left-side sequestrations are more common. Occasionally, bilateral sequestrations occur, and when a communication to the gastrointestinal tract is delineated, the term "bronchopulmonary foregut malformation" is preferred (Fig. 1.110).

Cystic changes are common, and because of this, the condition may be confused with congenital cystic adenomatoid malformation of the lung. Indeed, in some cases, cyst formation is so pronounced that congenital cystic adenomatoid malformation is one's first diagnosis. All of this is not so moot in that the two lesions can co-exist (20, 21).

In most cases, multiple cyst formation should suggest the diagnosis, but occasionally only one cavity exists and plain film or CT confusion with a simple lung cyst or abscess arises. After plain films, pulmonary sequestration customarily has been confirmed with aortography. But now, ultrasound, CT, and MRI can be employed (22–25). In most cases, MRI now is the definitive imaging modality, but the abnormal blood supply also is readily detected with ultrasonography utilizing color flow Doppler (Fig. 1.111).

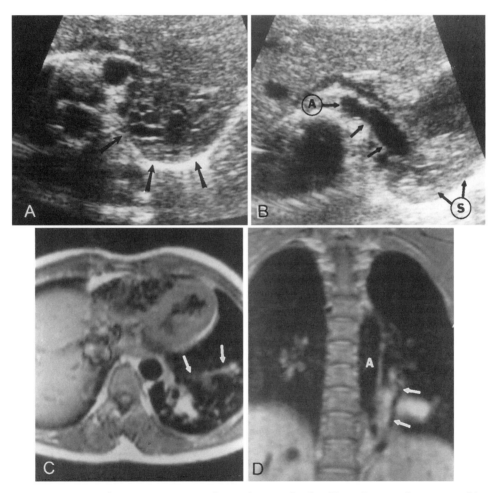

FIGURE 1.111. Pulmonary sequestration: other methods of imaging. A. Ultrasonographic demonstration of a cystic sequestration (arrows) in the left lung base. **B.** Another slice through the lesion demonstrates the aorta (A), large feeding vessel (arrows), and the sequestration (S). **C.** Axial magnetic resonance view in another patient with a cystic sequestration in the left base (arrows). **D.** The coronal image demonstrates the descending aorta (A) and the feeding vessel (arrows) of the sequestration. (**A** and **B** courtesy of C. Keith Hayden, Jr., M.D.).

Other features of pulmonary sequestrations include their occasional association and presentation with pleural effusions (26–28) (Fig. 1.112) and hydrops (29). Spontaneous hemorrhage into, or from, the sequestration (30) also can occur. Hemorrhage probably results from the arteriovenous fistula created by the abnormal systemic blood supply to the lesion. Pleural effusions are believed to result from obstruction of lymphatics (28), but torsion of the sequestration has been implicated as the cause in some cases (24). Arteriovenous shunting within a sequestration also can occur and may lead to cardiac failure (31, 32). Many times, these patients first are suspected of having cardiac disease, for the presence of the sequestration may not be readily apparent. These sequestrations, that is, those producing high-flow arteriovenous shunts, can be treated, nonsurgically, by interventional embolization (33).

As with all congenital lesions, now that prenatal sonography is so available, it has been witnessed that spontaneous involution of sequestrations can occur (34, 35).

"Pseudosequestration" is a term used to describe a lesion characterized by communication between an aberrant systemic artery and the pulmonary veins without evidence of sequestrated lung tissue (36–40). Generally, no mass is visible on plain films, and, indeed, no mass at all is present. Often, the abnormality is found incidentally during cardiac angiography or MR studies. In other cases, the abnormality may be seen in association with hypoplasia of the right lung, and in still other instances, it may present with features of a systemic arteriovenous malformation (Fig. 1.113). In the end, pseudosequestration may be nothing more than a variation of true sequestration, and to this end, **John et al. (9) have suggested that sequestration be con-**

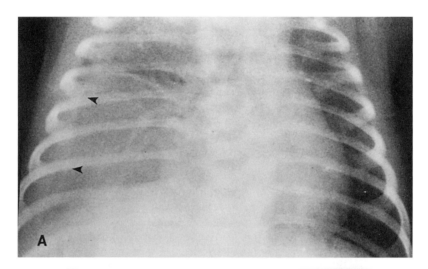

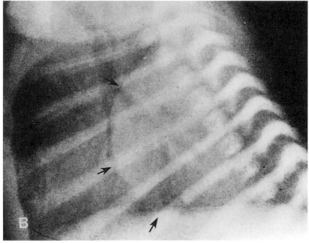

FIGURE 1.112. Pulmonary sequestration with pleural effusion. A. Note the pleural effusion on the right (arrows). Fluid also is layered along the posterior aspect of the right hemithorax and, on this supine view, is causing generalized haziness of the right lung field. A clear-cut mass is not defined. **B.** On lateral view, however, a clearly defined posterior mass is seen (arrows). This infant presented with respiratory distress. (Courtesy of Bill Schey, M.D.).

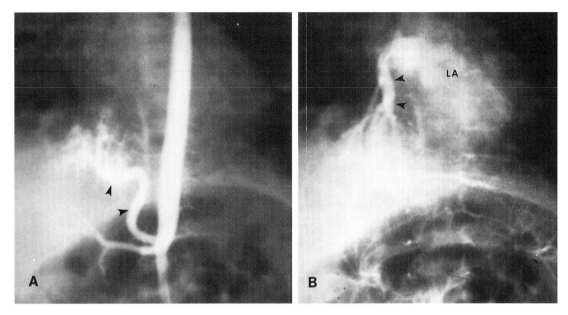

FIGURE 1.113. Pseudosequestration. A. Note the abnormal systemic artery (arrows) leading to the right lung base. **B.** Note the vein (arrows) draining into the left atrium (LA). The lung was normal, and no sequestration was found. (Reproduced with permission from Currarino G, Willis K, Miller W. Congenital fistula between an aberrant systemic artery and a pulmonary vein without sequestration. J Pediatr 1975;87:554–557).

sidered under three categories: (a) pulmonary parenchymal sequestration, (b) pulmonary arterial sequestration, and (c) both pulmonary parenchymal and arterial sequestration, the so-called "classic" form.

REFERENCES

1. Bratu I, Flageole H, Chen MF, et al. The multiple facets of pulmonary sequestration. J Pediatr Surg 2001;36:784–790.
2. Kim KW, Dim WS, Cheon J-E, et al. Complex bronchopulmonary foregut malformation: extralobar pulmonary sequestration associated with a duplication cyst of mixed bronchogenic and oesophageal type. Pediatr Radiol 2001;31:265–268.
3. Werthammer JW, Hatten HP Jr, Blake WB Jr. Upper thoracic extralobar pulmonary sequestration presenting with respiratory distress in a newborn. Pediatr Radiol 1980;9:116–117.
4. Spence LD, Ahmed S, Keohane C, et al. Acute presentation of cystic adenomatoid malformation of the lung in a 9-year-old child. Pediatr Radiol 1995;25:572–573.
5. Stanley P, Vachon L, Gilsanz V. Pulmonary sequestration with congenital gastroesophageal communication. Pediatr Radiol 1985;15:343–345.
6. Jamieson DH, Fisher RM. Communicating bronchopulmonary foregut malformation associated with esophageal atresia and tracheo-esophageal fistula. Pediatr Radiol 1993;23:557–558.
7. Leithiser RE Jr, Capitanio MA, Macpherson RI, et al. Communicating bronchopulmonary foregut malformations. AJR 1986;146:227–231.
8. Clements BS, Warner J. Pulmonary sequestration and related congenital bronchopulmonary vascular malformations: nomenclature and classification based on anatomical and embryological considerations. Thorax 1987;42:401–408.
9. John PR, Beasley SW, Mayne V. Pulmonary sequestration and related congenital disorders. Pediatr Radiol 1989;20:4–9.
10. Srikanth MS, Ford EG, Stanley P, et al. Communicating bronchopulmonary foregut malformations: classification and embryogenesis. J Pediatr Surg 1992;27:732–736.
11. Grigoryants V, Sargent SK, Shorter NA. Extralobar pulmonary sequestration receiving its arterial supply from the innominate artery. Pediatr Radiol 2000;30:696–698.
12. Kamata S, Sawai T, Nose K, et al. Extralobar pulmonary sequestration with a venous drainage to the portal vein: a case report. Pediatr Radiol 2000;30:492–494.
13. Hoeffel J-C, Bernard C. Pulmonary sequestration of the upper lobe in children. Radiology 1986;160:513–514.
14. Black MD, Bass J, Martin DJ, et al. Intraabdominal pulmonary sequestration. J Pediatr Surg 1991;26:1381–1383.
15. Chan YF, Oldfield R, Vogel S, et al. Pulmonary sequestration presenting as a prenatally detected suprarenal lesion in a neonate. J Pediatr Surg 2000;35:1367–1369.
16. Fenton LZ, Williams JL. Bronchopulmonary foregut malformation mimicking neuroblastoma. Pediatr Radiol 1996;26: 729–730.
17. Hernanz-Schulman M, Johnson JE, Holcomb GW III, et al. Retroperitoneal pulmonary sequestration: imaging findings, histopathologic correlation, and relationship to cystic adenomatoid malformation. AJR 1997;168:1277–1281.
18. Ross E, Chen MD, Lobe TE, et al. Infradiaphramatic extralobar pulmonary sequestration masquerading as an intra-abdominal, suprarenal mass. Pediatr Surg Int 1997;12:529–531.
19. Manson DE, Daneman A. Pitfalls in the sonographic diagnosis of juxta-diaphragmatic pulmonary sequestrations. Pediatr Radiol 2001;31:260–264.
20. Dibden LJ, Fischer JD, Zuberbuhler PC. Pulmonary sequestration and congenital cystic adenomatoid malformation in an infant. J Pediatr Surg 1986;21:731–733.
21. Morin C, Filiatrault D, Russo P. Pulmonary sequestration with

histologic changes of cystic adenomatoid malformation. Pediatr Radiol 1989;19:130–132.

22. Benya EC, Bulas DI, Selby DM, et al. Cystic sonographic appearance of extralobar pulmonary sequestration. Pediatr Radiol 1993;23:605–607.

23. Doyle AJ. Case report. Demonstration of blood supply to pulmonary sequestration by MR angiography. AJR 1992;158: 989–990.

24. Hernanz-Schulman M, Stein SM, Neblett WW, et al. Pulmonary sequestration: diagnosis with color Doppler sonography and a new theory of associated hydrothorax. Radiology 1991;180: 817–821.

25. Schlesinger AE, DiPietro MA, Statter MB, et al. Utility of sonography in the diagnosis of bronchopulmonary sequestration. J Pediatr Surg 1994;29:52–55.

26. Boyer J, Dozor A, Brudnicki A, et al. Extralobar pulmonary sequestration masquerading as a congenital pleural effusion. Pediatrics 1996;97:115–117.

27. Lucaya J, Garcia-Conesa JA, Bernado L. Pulmonary sequestration associated with unilateral pulmonary hypoplasia and massive pleural effusion. Pediatr Radiol 1984;14:228–229.

28. Vade A, Kramer LP. Extralobar pulmonary sequestration presenting as intractable pleural effusion. Pediatr Radiol 1989;19: 333–334.

29. Evans MG. Hydrops fetalis and pulmonary sequestration. J Pediatr Surg 1996;313:761–764.

30. Zumbro GL, Green DC, Brott W, et al. Pulmonary lung sequestration with spontaneous intrapleural hemorrhage. J Thorac Cardiovasc Surg 1874;68:673–674.

31. Fliegel CP, Rutishauser M, Gradel E. Pulmonary sequestrations with large blood flow, simulating and complicating congenital heart disease. Ann Radiol 1979;22:228–232.

32. Spinella PC, Strieper JJ, Callahan CW. Congestive heart failure in a neonate secondary to bilateral intralobar pulmonary sequestrations. Pediatrics 1998;101:120–124.

33. Takel K, Boyvat F, Varan B. Technical innovation. Coil embolization of pulmonary sequestration in two infants: a safe alternative to surgery. AJR 2000;175:993–995.

34. Garcia-Pena P, Lucaya J, Hendry GMA, et al. Spontaneous involution of pulmonary sequestration in children: a report of two cases and review of the literature. Pediatr Radiol 1998;28: 266–270.

35. Smulian JC, Guzman ER, Ranzini AC, et al. Color and duplex Doppler sonographic investigation of in utero spontaneous regression of pulmonary sequestration. J Ultrasound Med 1996; 15:789–792.

36. Currarino G, Willis K, Miller W. Congenital fistula between an aberrant systemic artery and a pulmonary vein without sequestration. J Pediatr 1975;87:554–557.

37. Kirks DR, Kane PE, Free EA, et al. Systemic arterial supply to normal basilar segments of the left lower lobe. AJR 1976;126: 817–821.

38. Macpherson RI, Whytehead L. Pseudo-sequestration. J Can Assoc Radiol 1977;28:17–25.

39. Miyake H, Hori Y, Takeoka H, et al. Systemic arterial supply to normal basal segments of the left lung: characteristic features on chest radiography and CT. AJR 1998;171:387–392.

40. Pernot C, Simon P, Hoeffel JC, et al. Systemic artery-pulmonary vein fistula without sequestration. Pediatr Radiol 1991;21: 158–159.

Congenital Lobar Emphysema

Congenital lobar emphysema is a common problem in the neonate and young infant, and although some infants are virtually asymptomatic, others can present with severe neonatal respiratory distress. In such cases, symptoms consist of tachypnea, grunting, retractions, and wheezing, and physical examination often reveals the presence of a hyperresonant hemithorax. Breath sounds are usually diminished over the involved lung, and the cardiac apex is shifted away from the involved side. In severe cases, treatment consists of emergency lobectomy, but if the infant is not in serious respiratory difficulty, no immediate treatment is necessary. At a later date, pulmonary infection, primarily viral bronchitis, may aggravate the problem (1). However, it also should be noted that some cases of congenital lobar emphysema have been known to remain relatively static and asymptomatic for years, and some even to resolve spontaneously (2, 3).

The upper lobes are most frequently involved, but it is not uncommon to have right middle lobe involvement. In fact, right middle lobe involvement may be as common as, or more so than, right upper lobe involvement. Overall, however, left upper lobe involvement is most common. Both lower lobe and multilobar involvement is extremely rare, accounting for less than 1% of cases (4).

Most cases of congenital lobar emphysema result from expiratory collapse of the bronchus secondary to segmental bronchial cartilage underdevelopment. The resultant loss of normal rigidity of the bronchus leads to redundancy and crinkling of the mucosa (Fig. 1.114), and this, together with the cartilage-deficient bronchial wall collapse, leads to a focal ball-valve mechanism of obstruction. This, of course, is what leads to air trapping in the involved lobe. Congenital lobar emphysema also has been documented with a tracheal bronchus (5) and in a mother and daughter (6).

Other causes of bronchial obstruction include congenital bronchial stenosis (7), intraluminal mucous plugs (8), and obstructing mediastinal cysts or tumors. In addition, a variety of vascular compressions, with or without underlying congenital heart disease, can produce bronchial obstruction and lobar emphysema (9–11). Lobar emphysema, on an acquired basis, also can occur in infants with BPD. Excess numbers of alveoli, or the so-called "polyalveolar lung," also have been described with some cases of congenital lobar emphysema (12).

In the usual case of congenital lobar emphysema, the roentgenographic findings are clear-cut. The affected lobe is overdistended and the mediastinum shifted to the contralateral side (Fig. 1.115). With upper lobe emphysema, secondary compression of the ipsilateral lower lobe is an important finding to look for. In addition, if emphysema is profound, herniation of the emphysematous upper lobe across the anterior superior mediastinum occurs. With right middle lobe emphysema, there is characteristic overaeration of the middle lobe and variable secondary compression of both the upper and the lower lobes (Fig. 1.115C). In these cases, there often is a tendency to pick the collapsed and opaque upper and lower lobes as being abnormal. However, this particular combination of atelectasis would be relatively

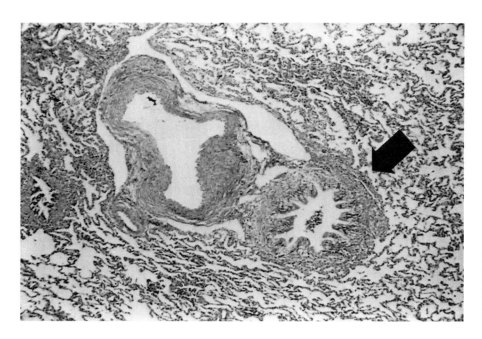

FIGURE 1.114. Congenital lobar emphysema: histologic features. Note the small collapsed bronchus (arrow), the crinkled nature of the mucosa, and absence of cartilage in the wall.

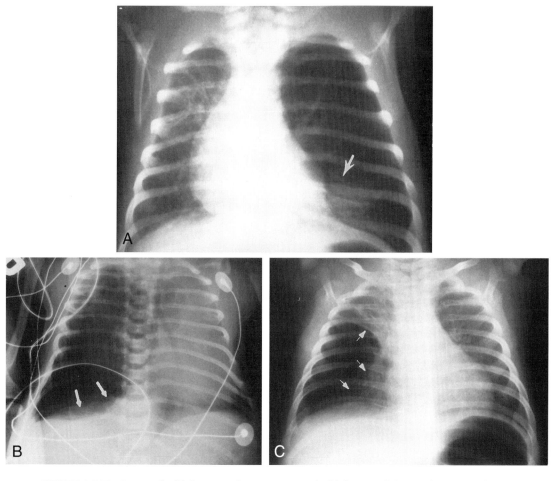

FIGURE 1.115. Congenital lobar emphysema. A. Typical left upper lobe emphysema with an overdistended left upper lobe and tell-tale atelectasis of the left lower lobe (arrow). There is mediastinal shift to the right. **B.** Right upper lobe emphysema with more pronounced overdistension of the involved lobe and marked compression of the right lower lobe (arrow). The overdistended right lung has herniated across the anterior mediastinum. **C. Right middle lobe emphysema.** Note the characteristic triangular radiolucency of the overinflated right middle lobe. It is causing compressive atelectasis of the right upper and lower lobes (arrows).

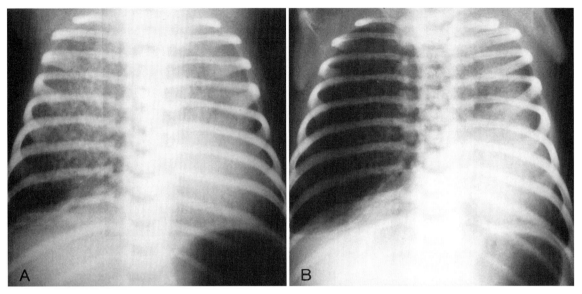

FIGURE 1.116. Opaque lung of lobar emphysema. A. The right lung is enlarged but somewhat opaque. There is pronounced mediastinal shift to the left. **B.** A few days later, the classic picture of congenital lobar emphysema of the right upper lobe has evolved. Note the collapsed right lower lobe, more left-side shift of the mediastinum, and striking hyperlucency of the overdistended right upper lobe. (Reproduced with permission from Fagan CJ, Swischuk LE. The opaque lung in lobar emphysema. AJR 1972;114:300–304).

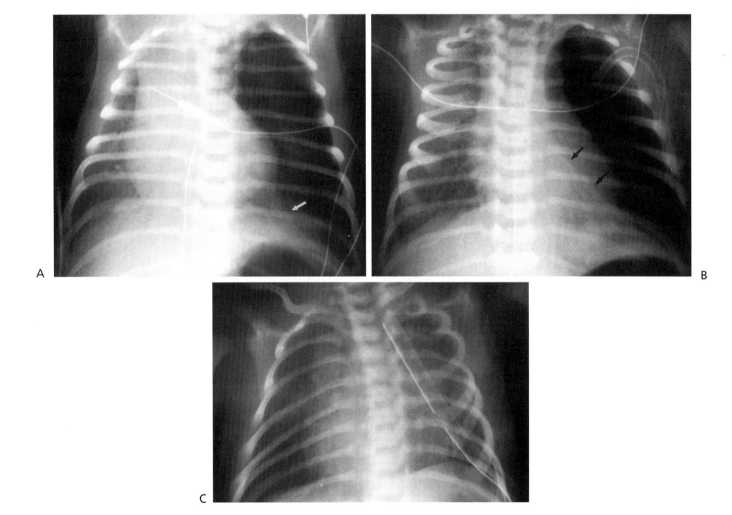

uncommon on a primary basis, and thus it is much more reasonable to suspect that the problem is obstructive emphysema of the right middle lobe with secondary compressive atelectasis of the other two lobes.

In some cases, the involved overdistended lungs may be opaque rather than hyperlucent (13–15). In these cases, obstruction is believed to occur early in intrauterine life, and fluid accumulates proximal to the obstruction. Because of this, the initial appearance of the lung is opaque (Fig. 1.116). Later on, as the fluid is cleared, the classic appearance of congenital lobar emphysema develops. Fluid from these lungs eventually is cleared by way of pulmonary lymphatics and veins (13). Indeed, dilated lymphatics traversing the emphysematous lung have been noted in some cases (16, 17), and this has brought up the added possibility of associated lymphatic obstruction. Actually, it is quite possible that the emphysematous lobe does cause some functional obstruction of the pulmonary lymphatics, for the inspiratory-expiratory excursion of a normal lobe is vital to the propulsion of fluid through the pulmonary lymphatics. In some cases of opaque fluid-filled lung in congenital lobar emphysema, the lung is so opaque that it mimics an intrathoracic mass.

Before leaving the topic of congenital lobar emphysema in infancy, it should be reemphasized that many apparent cases are transient and acquired and probably due to mucous plugs (8). Consequently, one should not rush into definitive therapy unless significant respiratory distress is present. In many such cases, findings dissipate with surprising rapidity. In addition, it should be noted that, in some instances, congenital lobar emphysema can present with a pneumothorax (Fig. 1.117). In these cases, the presence of the underlying emphysematous lobe may be missed on the first films. However, after the pneumothorax is treated, if it is noted that the lung remains overinflated, one should suspect the diagnosis.

REFERENCES

1. Newman B, Yunis E. Lobar emphysema associated with respiratory syncytial virus pneumonia. Pediatr Radiol 1995;25: 646–648.
2. Roghair GD. Nonoperative management of lobar emphysema: long-term follow-up. Radiology 1972;102:125–127.
3. Shannon DC, Todres ID, Moylan FMB. Infantile lobar hyperinflation; expectant treatment. Pediatrics 1977;59:1012–1018.
4. Hugosson C, Rabeeah A, Al-Rawaf A, et al. Congenital bilobar emphysema. Pediatr Radiol 1995;25:649–651.
5. Keller MS. Congenital lobar emphysema with tracheal bronchus. J Can Assoc Radiol 1983;34:306–307.
6. Wall MA, Eisenberg JD, Campbell JR. Congenital lobar emphysema in a mother and daughter. Pediatrics 1982;70:131–133.
7. Binstadt DH, Williams HJ, Jarvis CW. Bronchial stenosis and segmental emphysema in a neonate. J Can Assoc Radiol 1977; 28:297–299.
8. Talbert JL, Haller JA Jr. Obstructive lobar emphysema of the newborn infant; documentation of "mucous plug syndrome" with successful treatment by bronchotomy. J Thorac Cardiovasc Surg 1967;53:886–889.
9. Leape LL, Ching N, Holder TM. Lobar emphysema and patent ductus arteriosus. Pediatrics 1970;46:97–101.
10. Madan A, Parisi M, Wood BP. Radiological case of the month: absent pulmonic valve presenting with congenital lobar emphysema. Am J Dis Child 1992;146:113–114.
11. Sulayman R, Thilenius O, Replogle R, et al. Unilateral emphysema in total anomalous pulmonary venous return. J Pediatr 1975;87:433–435.
12. Tapper D, Schuster S, McBride J, et al. Polyalveolar lobe: anatomic and physiologic parameters and their relationship to congenital lobar emphysema. J Pediatr Surg 1980;15:931–937.
13. Fagan CJ, Swischuk LE. The opaque lung in lobar emphysema. AJR 1972;114:300–304.
14. Griscom NT, Harris GBC, Wohl MEB, et al. Fluid-filled lung due to airway obstruction in the newborn. Pediatrics 1969;43: 383–390.
15. Zumbro GL, Treasure RL, Geiger JP. Respiratory obstruction in the newborn associated with increased volume and opacification of the hemithorax. Ann Thorac Surg 1974;18:622–625.
16. Allen RP, Taylor RL, Requiam CW. Congenital emphysema with dilated septal lymphatics. Radiology 1966;86:929–932.

Chylothorax, Hydrothorax

Chylothorax is a relatively rare cause of respiratory distress in infants (1, 2), but its prompt recognition is most important, for treatment is simple and dramatic. The etiology of neonatal chylothorax is uncertain, although the most likely explanation lies in traumatic tear of the thoracic duct during delivery. It may not be so much that there is mechanical stretching or twisting of the duct but, rather, that temporary overdistension from elevation of central venous pressures during birth occurs. Another possible explanation is that leakage occurs through congenital defects in the thoracic duct (3). However, there is no conclusive evidence to support either theory. In addition, a case of fetal hydrothorax (chylothorax) has been documented secondary to pulmonary lymphatic hypoplasia (4).

FIGURE 1.117. Congenital lobar emphysema with pneumothorax. A. Note the large, anterior pneumothorax on the left, but, more importantly, note the tell-tale finding of compressive atelectasis of the left lower lobe (arrow). There also is pronounced shift of the mediastinal structures to the right. **B.** A chest tube has been inserted on the left, but the left upper lobe remains emphysematous. The compressed left lower lobe, again, also is seen (arrows). **C.** Postoperative radiograph demonstrates resolution of findings, but the left hemithorax and remaining lung are smaller than normal.

Chylothorax occurs most frequently on the right, but accumulations of chyle on the left are not uncommon. Occasionally, bilateral chylothorax can be seen (5). These fluid collections are readily demonstrable with ultrasound in utero. In addition, chylothorax, either unilateral or bilateral, secondary to superior vena caval thrombosis in infants also can occur (1, 5, 6). Thrombosis usually is secondary to the use of indwelling catheters. The problem can be severe, especially if fluid accumulations are bilateral, and then surgical intervention may be required. Roentgenographic findings in the usual case consist of opacification of one or the other side of the chest and contralateral shift of the mediastinum (Fig. 1.118A). In some cases, less fluid is seen and may collect along the base of the lung (subpulmonic effusion) or around the mediastinum. In those cases where the entire hemithorax is opacified, ultrasound is the best and easiest way to confirm the presence of pleural fluid (Fig. 1.118, B and C). There should be no confusion with atelectasis, for the problem is not one of volume loss. However, conditions such as neonatal empyema, opaque lung of congenital lobar emphysema, airless cystic adenomatoid malformation, or diaphragmatic hernia, and intrathoracic neoplasms can be a problem.

When fluid accumulations are bilateral, the infant presents with a totally opacified chest and restricted central aeration of small lungs (Fig. 1.119). Often, these patients also have fluid in the abdomen, and it may be that there is communication between the chest and abdomen through the various normally occurring foramina in the diaphragm. In addition, infants with bilateral fluid collections have associated bilateral pulmonary hypoplasia due to compression of the lungs in utero by the pleural fluid. This is an important aspect of the disease to appreciate, for even if the fluid is successfully removed, the lungs remain small and are prone to rupture (i.e., result in pneumothorax or pneumomediastinum). Because of all of this, respiratory distress may not completely resolve after the fluid is drained.

Treatment of chylothorax usually consists of thoracentesis, and even though multiple aspirations may be required (2), it is usually all the treatment that is necessary. It has been suggested that if three thoracenteses do not cure the problem, chest tube drainage of the thorax should be instigated (7). The condition also can be treated with a pleuroperitoneal shunt (8). All of this should be accompanied by cessation of oral feedings so as to decrease lymphatic flow through the gut. In addition, therapy with medium-chain triglycerides has been successful (9, 10). If fluid reaccumulates and does not respond to any of the foregoing therapeutic measures, surgery is indicated, and some form of pleural space obliterative procedure is performed.

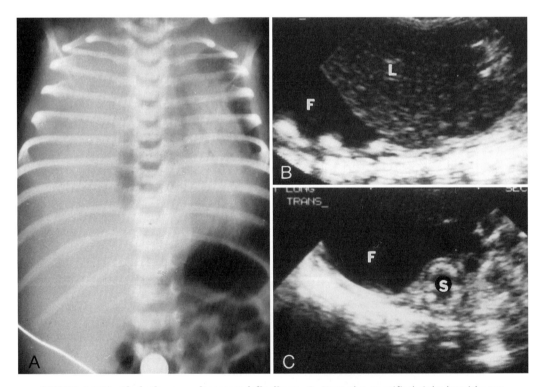

FIGURE 1.118. Chylothorax: ultrasound findings. A. Note the opacified right hemithorax. There is shift of the mediastinum to the right. **B.** Longitudinal sonogram demonstrates the liver (L) and sonolucent fluid (F) above the diaphragm. **C.** Transverse sonogram demonstrates fluid in the posterior pleural space (arrows). S, spine.

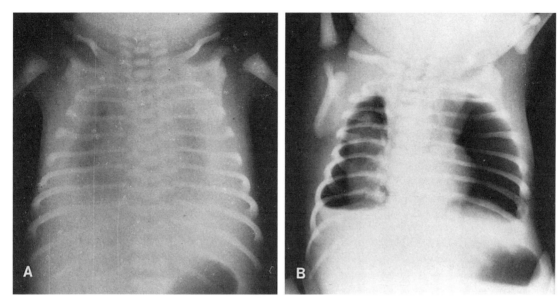

FIGURE 1.119. Bilateral hydro-chylothorax. A. Note the extensive collection of fluid on both sides of the chest. The small, aerated lungs produce a radiolucent halo around the poorly visible heart. **B. Post thoracentesis.** Note the bilateral, small, hypoplastic lungs. Bilateral pneumothoraces are present. (Courtesy of Brit Gay, M.D.).

Definitive diagnosis of chylothorax is made by studying the aspirated fluid. If the aspiration is performed after the infant begins to drink milk, the fluid is milky or chylous and fat globules are seen on microscopic examination. If the fluid is examined before the infant has been fed milk, the fluid is straw colored, for no fat is present. In such cases, the condition is often referred to as "hydrothorax."

Occasionally, chylothorax can result from thoracic duct tears secondary to known trauma to the chest or from thoracic duct obstruction with intrathoracic tumor (11). In other instances, chylothorax is secondary to iatrogenic injury to the thoracic duct during intrathoracic surgery.

Hydro-chylothorax also can be associated with hydro-chyloperitoneum where it is presumed that fluid crosses into the chest, or vice versa, through small, normally present diaphragmatic defects. In addition, pleural effusions (hydrothorax) commonly are encountered in fetal hydrops, and pleural effusions now are becoming a relatively common complication of hyperalimentation (12). In such cases, perforation of the vein with the catheter results in the hyperalimentation fluid being instilled into the thoracic cavity. The abnormal position of the catheter is the clue to the diagnosis in these cases.

REFERENCES

1. Vain NE, Xwarner OW, Cha CC. Neonatal chylothorax: a report and discussion of nine consecutive cases. J Pediatr Surg 1980; 15:261–265.
2. Van Aerde J, Campbell AN, Smyth JA, et al. Spontaneous hydrothorax in newborns. Am J Dis Child 1984;138:961–964.
3. McKendrie JB, Lindsay WK, Gearstein MC. Congenital defects of lymphatics in infancy. Pediatrics 1957;19:21–35.
4. Thibeault DW, Zalles C, Wickstrom E. Familial pulmonary lymphatic hypoplasia associated with fetal pleural effusions. J Pediatr 1995;127:979–983.
5. Kramer SS, Taylor GA, Garfinkel DJ, et al. Lethal chylothoraces due to superior vena caval thrombosis in infants. AJR 1981;137: 559–563.
6. Dhande V, Kattwinkel J, Alford B. Recurrent bilateral pleural effusions secondary to superior vena cava obstruction as complication of central venous catheterization. Pediatrics 1983;72: 109–113.
7. Brodman RF, Zavelson TM, Schiebler GL. Treatment of congenital chylothorax. J Pediatr 1974;85:516–517.
8. Engum SA, Rescorla FJ, West KW, et al. The use of pleuroperitoneal shunts in the management of persistent chylothorax in infants. J Pediatr Surg 1999;34:286–290.
9. Gershanik JJ, Jonsson HT Jr, Riopel DA, et al. Dietary management of neonatal chylothorax. Pediatrics 1974;53:400–403.
10. Kosloske AM, Martin LW, Schubert WK. Management of chylothorax in children by thoracentesis and medium-chain triglyceride feedings. J Pediatr Surg 1974;9:365–371.
11. Easa D, Balaraman V, Ash K, et al. Congenital chylothorax and mediastinal neuroblastoma. J Pediatr Surg 1991;26:96–98.
12. Knight L, Tobin J Jr, L'Heureux P. Hydrothorax; a complication of hyperalimentation with radiologic manifestations. Radiology 1974;111:693–695.

Hemothorax

This relatively uncommon cause of respiratory distress in the neonate is seen with hemorrhagic disease of the newborn (1). However, it can also be seen secondary to overt chest trauma, sustained either during birth or after postnatal resuscitation. Hemothorax also can be spontaneous or result from rupture of a ductal aneurysm. In the older infant and child, hemothorax usually is the result of chest trauma but also can be seen with aggressive germ cell intrathoracic tumors.

REFERENCE

1. Oppermann HC, Wille L. Hemothorax in the newborn. Pediatr Radiol 1980;9:129–134.

Tracheo- and Bronchomalacia

Tracheomalacia and bronchomalacia are difficult diagnostic problems. When focal, they can present with atelectasis or obstructive emphysema. Focal broncho- or tracheomalacia frequently occurs with lesions that compress the trachea in utero. Primarily, these include a variety of vascular anomalies and rings and the dilated proximal esophageal pouch of esophageal atresia. Indeed, many of these infants continue to have respiratory difficulties, including expiratory

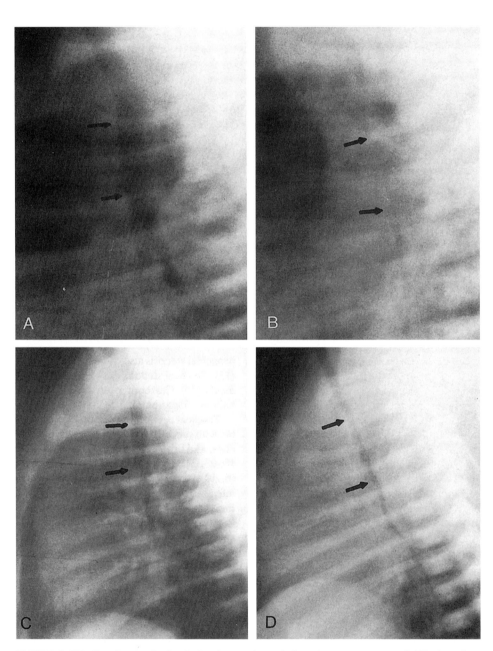

FIGURE 1.120. Tracheomalacia. A. Inspiratory lateral view demonstrates an air-filled trachea of normal diameter (arrows). **B.** With expiration, there is virtually no air remaining in the totally collapsed trachea (arrows). Similar findings were present on frontal view. This patient had expiratory stridor. **C. Pseudotracheomalacia.** Another patient with a normal trachea on inspiration (arrows). **D.** On expiration, the trachea shows marked collapse (arrows). This patient was asymptomatic.

wheezing and a barking cough, after the primary problem has been surgically corrected. In some of these cases, direct surgical repair of the trachea has been required. More recently, stenting of the abnormal portion of the trachea or bronchus has been accomplished (1, 2). Finally, it should be noted that acquired focal tracheomalacia is a frequent complication of endotracheal intubation and that in some cases focal tracheomalacia is of primary origin (3). In such cases, the problem may be persistent wheezing accompanied by other respiratory symptoms.

Generalized tracheomalacia is rather rare and is an expiratory problem. The abnormality is said to stem from the presence of extremely frail and underdeveloped tracheal cartilage (4). Because of this, adequate support for the tracheal wall is lacking, and exaggerated expiratory collapse of the entire trachea occurs (Fig. 1.120, A and B). There is associated air trapping and wheezing (4), and the condition also has been reported in association with polychondritis in a newborn infant (5). All in all, however, generalized tracheomalacia remains rare, and it is more common to see a hypercollapsible trachea in a normal infant with no respiratory distress or expiratory wheezing (Fig. 1.120, C and D).

REFERENCES

1. Filler RM, Forte V, Chait P. Tracheobronchial stenting for the treatment of airway obstruction. J Pediatr Surg 1998;33:304–311.
2. Tsugawa C, Nishijima E, Muraji T, et al. A shape memory airway stent for tracheobronchomalacia in children: an experimental and clinical study. J Pediatr Surg 1997;32:50–53.
3. Finder JD. Primary bronchomalacia in infants and children. J Pediatr 1997;130:59–66.
4. Levin SJ, Adler P, Scherer RA. Collapsible trachea (tracheomalacia); a non-allergic cause of wheezing in infancy. Ann Allergy 1964;22:20–25.
5. Johner CH, Szanto PA. Polychondritis in a newborn presenting as tracheomalacia. Ann Otol Rhinol Laryngol 1970;79:1114–1116.

Other Tracheobronchial Abnormalities

A number of generally less common tracheobronchial abnormalities may, on occasion, produce respiratory distress in the newborn or even later in life. One such anomaly is the so-called "tracheal bronchus." Most often occurring on the right, the aberrant bronchus arises above the normal right bronchus and supplies a portion of the right upper lobe. The anomaly may be asymptomatic but may also be the cause of repeated infections (1, 2). Almost always, there is a single anomalous bronchus, but double aberrant tracheal bronchi have been documented (1) and tracheal bronchus also has been seen on the left (3) and bilaterally (4). Radiographically, one might suspect the presence of the anomaly when repeated infections with chronic atelectasis are seen (Fig. 1.121). Short trachea with high carina is another uncommon tracheal abnormality (5, 6). In these cases, there often is left main stem bronchus compression by a ligamentous arteriosum because of the unusually high location of the left main bronchus.

Segmental congenital tracheal or bronchial stenosis or atresia is rare (7). Patients with bronchial stenosis or atresia may be asymptomatic in the newborn period, but in other cases, where stenosis is the problem, wheezing and obstructive emphysema may develop. With bronchial atresia, the obstructed lung may be fluid filled at birth and thus appear as a pulmonary mass (Fig. 1.122, B and C) (8). Later, as time passes, the fluid is replaced by air, but because the lung still is obstructed, the lobe becomes emphysematous. In addition, a central, oval, or fan-shaped density, representing inspissated mucus, just distal to the point of atresia, is clas-

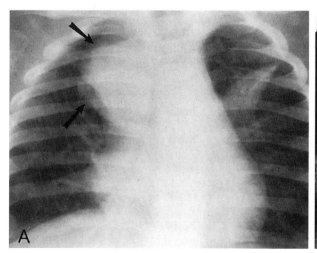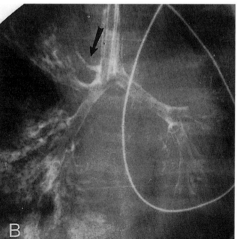

FIGURE 1.121. Right tracheal bronchus. A. Note the solid-appearing mass due to atelectasis of the right upper lobe (arrows). There also is an area of segmental atelectasis in the left upper lobe. This patient had recurrent pulmonary infections. **B.** Tracheogram demonstrates the right tracheal bronchus (arrow) and the collapsed right upper lobe.

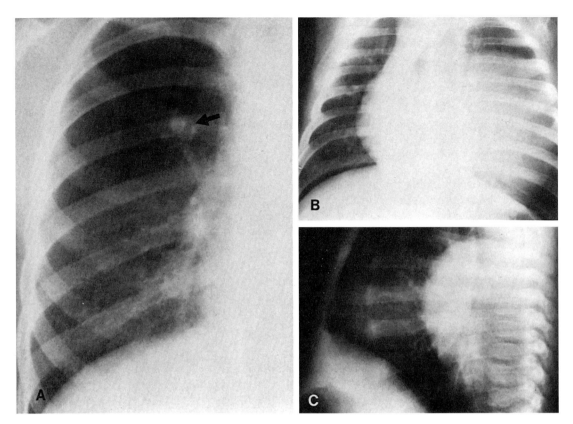

FIGURE 1.122. Bronchial atresia. A. Note hyperlucency of the right upper lobe and the central mucous impaction or mucocele (arrow). **B. Fluid-filled lung presenting as mass in neonate with bronchial atresia.** Note the mass-like configuration of fluid-filled lung on the left. Later on, as this fluid is cleared, the lung became emphysematous. **C.** Lateral view demonstrating that the involved portion of the left lower lobe is its superior segment. (**A** reproduced with permission from Genereux GP. Bronchial atresia: a rare cause of unilateral lung hypertranslucency. J Can Assoc Radiol 1971;22:71–82; **B** reproduced with permission from Rémy J, Ribet M, Pagniez B, et al. Segmental bronchial atresia; a study of three observations and a review of the literature. Ann Radiol 1973;16:615–628).

sic (Fig. 1.122A). The mucous collection often is referred to as a bronchocele or bronchial mucocele (8–10). Most often, the area of stenosis or atresia is segmental, and this also is true of congenital tracheal stenosis (Fig. 1.123A). Diffuse tracheal narrowing also can be seen with the storage diseases (11) (Fig. 1.23B).

Tracheal narrowing may be seen on plain films but is more vividly demonstrable with MRI, CT, and, less often, bronchography. Currently, helical or multislice CT with multiplanar and three-dimensional reconstruction, along with virtual bronchoscopy (Fig. 1.123C) are being used to demonstrate tracheal and bronchial narrowings (12–17).

Most cases of tracheobronchial stenosis are the result of simple underdevelopment of a segment of the airway, but an instance of stenosis due to esophageal remnants encircling the trachea also has been documented (18). Tracheal stenosis also can occur in the so-called "complete tracheal cartilaginous ring" syndrome (19). In these cases, the area of stenosis contains a complete cartilaginous ring, and the anomaly can be associated with an anomalous left pul-

monary artery, constituting the so-called "pulmonary ring-sling syndrome" (7, 19). Tracheobronchial stenosis also can be acquired after tracheal intubation and also can be seen with tracheoesophageal fistula (8). Currently, many of these cases can be treated with laser surgery and balloon dilatation (20–25).

Tracheal agenesis is extremely rare and generally incompatible with survival. It is usually associated with other major anomalies, and bronchoesophageal fistula is especially frequent (26, 27). **Bronchobiliary fistula** also is a rare anomaly, and respiratory distress, repeated respiratory infections, coughing, vomiting of bile, and failure to thrive can be the presenting symptoms. The fistula can be demonstrated with nuclear scintigraphy (28). **Bronchoesophageal fistula** also is a rare abnormality (29, 30), which can lead to chronic pulmonary problems. This fistula can be demonstrated with barium swallow or CT studies (30).

Tracheobronchomegaly is a rather uncommon condition consisting of marked dilatation of the tracheobronchial tree during inspiration (31). Generally considered to be due

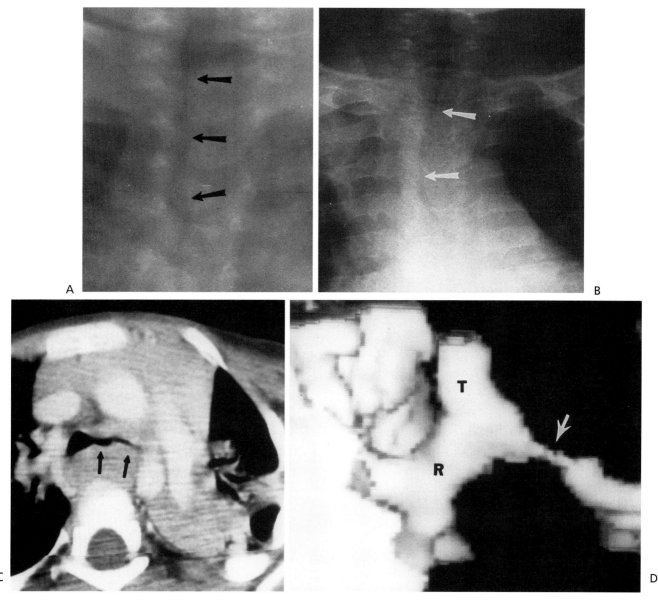

FIGURE 1.123. Tracheal stenosis. A. Note a long segment of narrowing of the tracheal air column (arrows). **B.** Tracheal stenosis (arrows) in Hurler's disease. **C. Bronchial stenosis: computed tomography findings.** Note stenosis (arrows) of the left bronchus. **D.** Three-dimensional study showing the stenotic area (arrow). T, trachea; R, right bronchus.

to an elastic tissue deficiency, similar cases with cartilage deficiency also have been described (32). The condition generally is considered to be congenital in origin.

REFERENCES

1. Iannaccone G, Capocaccia P, Colloridi V, et al. Double right tracheal bronchus. A case report in an infant. Pediatr Radiol 1983; 13:156–158.
2. McLaughlin FJ, Strieder DJ, Harris GBC, et al. Tracheal bronchus: association with respiratory morbidity in childhood. J Pediatr 1985;106:751–756.
3. Remy J, Smith M, Marache P, et al. Pathogenetic left "tracheal" bronchus: 4 cases and review of the literature. J Radiol Electrol Med Nucl 1977;58:621–630.
4. Cope R, Campbell JR, Wall M. Bilateral tracheal bronchi. J Pediatr Surg 1986;21:443–444.
5. Comerci SCD, Berdon WE, Levin TL, et al. Congenitally short trachea and high carina with left mainstem bronchus compression by the ligamentum arteriosum. Pediatr Radiol 1995;25:S194–S196.
6. Priester JA, de Vos GD, Waardenburg DA, et al. Congenitally short trachea with compression of the left mainstem bronchus: MRI findings. Pediatr Radiol 1998;28:342–343.
7. Benjamin B, Pitkin J, Cohen D. Congenital tracheal stenosis. Ann Otol Rhinol Laryngol 1981;90:364–371.
8. Remy J, Ribet M, Pagniez B, et al. Segmental bronchial atresia; a study of three observations and a review of the literature. Ann Radiol (Paris) 1973;16:615–628.

9. Genereux GP. Bronchial atresia; a rare cause of unilateral lung hypertranslucency. J Can Assoc Radiol 1971;22:71–82.

10. Tsuji S, Heki S, Kobara Y, et al. The syndrome of bronchial mucocele and regional hyperinflation of the lung; report of four cases. Chest 1971;64:444–447.

11. Peters ME, Arya S, Langer LO, et al. Narrow trachea in mucopolysaccharidoses. Pediatr Radiol 1985;15:225–228.

12. Konen E, Katz M, Rozeman J, et al. Original report. Virtual bronchoscopy in children: early clinical experience. AJR 1998; 171:1699–1702.

13. Lam WWM, Tam PKH, Chan F-L, et al. Esophageal atresia and tracheal stenosis: use of three-dimensional CT and virtual bronchoscopy in neonates, infants, and children. AJR 2000;174: 1009–1012.

14. Pumberger W, Metz V, Birnbacher R, et al. Tracheal agenesis: evaluation by helical computed tomography. Pediatr Radiol 2000;30:200–203.

15. Quint LE, Whyte RI, Kazerooni EA, et al. Stenosis of the central airways: evaluation by using helical CT with multiplanar reconstructions. Radiology 1995;194:871–877.

16. Toki A, Todani T, Watanabe Y, et al. Spiral computed tomography with 3-dimensional reconstruction for the diagnosis of tracheobronchial stenosis. Pediatr Surg Int 1997;12:334–336.

17. Manson D, Filler R, Gordon R. Tracheal growth in congenital tracheal stenosis. Pediatr Radiol 1996;26:427–430.

18. Lacasse JE, Reilly BJ, Mancer K. Segmental esophageal trachea: a potentially fatal type of tracheal stenosis. AJR 1980;134: 829–831.

19. Berdon WE, Baker DH, Wung J-T, et al. Complete cartilage ring tracheal stenosis associated with anomalous pulmonary artery: the ring-sling complex. Radiology 1984;152:57–64.

20. Bagwell CE, Talbert JL, Tepas JJ III. Balloon dilatation of long segment tracheal stenoses. J Pediatr Surg 1991;26:153–159.

21. Brown SB, Hedlund GL, Glasier CM, et al. Tracheobronchial stenosis in infants: successful balloon dilation therapy. Radiology 1987;164:475–478.

22. Jaffe RB. Balloon dilation of congenital and acquired stenosis of the trachea and bronchi. Radiology 1997;203:405–409.

23. Mateda K, Yasufuku M, Yamamoto T. New approach to the treatment of congenital tracheal stenosis: balloon tracheoplasty and expandable metallic stenting. J Pediatr Surg 2001;36: 1646–1649.

24. Morales L, Rovira J, Rottermann M, et al. Balloon dilatation of the lobar bronchi for symptomatic lobar bronchial stenosis. Pediatr Surg Int 1990;5:250–252.

25. Othersen HB Jr, Hebra A, Tagge EP. A new method of treatment for complete tracheal rings in an infant: endoscopic laser division and balloon dilation. J Pediatr Surg 2000;35:262–264.

26. Milstein JM, Lau M, Bickers RG. Tracheal agenesis in infants with Vater association. Am J Dis Child 1985;139:77–80.

27. Rovira J, Morales L, Rottermann M, et al. Agenesis of the trachea. J Pediatr Surg 1989;24:1126–1127.

28. Egrari S, Krishnamoorthy M, Yee CA, et al. Congenital bronchobiliary fistula: diagnosis and postoperative surveillance with HIDA scan. J Pediatr Surg 1996;31:785–786.

29. Wang CR, Tiu CM, Chou YH, et al. Congenital bronchoesophageal fistula in childhood. Case report and review of the literature. Pediatr Radiol 1993;23:158–159.

30. Kemp JL, Sullivan LM. Bronchoesophageal fistula in an 11-month-old-boy. Pediatr Radiol 1997;27:811–812.

31. Hunter TB, Kuhns LR, Roloff MA, et al. Tracheobronchiomegaly in an eighteen month old child. AJR 1975;123: 687–690.

32. Mitchell RE, Burgy RG. Congenital bronchiectasis due to deficiency of bronchial cartilage (Williams-Campbell syndrome). J Pediatr 1975;87:230–232.

MISCELLANEOUS NEONATAL CHEST PROBLEMS

Pulmonary Edema

Pulmonary edema is very common in premature infants, as seen with the LLS. Pulmonary edema also commonly results from a left-to-right shunt through a patent ductus arteriosus in premature infants and, in such cases, usually is associated with cardiomegaly. Less commonly, the left-to-right shunt may occur at the ventricular level, and, of course, other cardiac admixture conditions and left-side myocardial or obstructive problems also can lead to pulmonary edema. The most common left-side cardiac problems presenting in the neonate are the hypoplastic left heart syndrome, pulmonary vein atresia, and total anomalous pulmonary venous return type III. Very often, the pattern in the lungs of these latter patients is more reticular than hazy.

Pulmonary edema also can arise on a neurogenic basis when intracranial pressures are increased (1, 2). Most often, this occurs with intracranial hemorrhage in the premature infant, and the cause of such edema is unknown. However, it has been postulated that inappropriate antidiuretic hormone secretion occurs in these patients, but consideration also has been given to left-side cardiac dysfunction on a vagal basis.

In any of the foregoing cases, edema usually first accumulates in the interstitium of the lungs and leads to diffuse haziness of the lungs (Fig. 1.124). Some cases may show reticularity, but haziness is the predominant pattern. The differential diagnosis includes pneumonia and pulmonary hemorrhage. Pleural effusions, of course, may be associated.

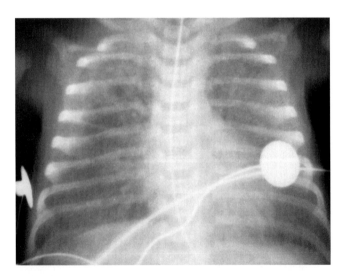

FIGURE 1.124. Pulmonary edema. Note diffusely hazy to opaque lungs due to pulmonary edema secondary to increased intracranial pressures resulting from an intracranial hemorrhage.

REFERENCES

1. Felman AH. Neurogenic pulmonary edema: observations in 6 patients. AJR 1971;112:393–396.
2. Milley JR, Nugent SK, Rogers MD. Neurogenic pulmonary edema in childhood. J Pediatr 1979;94:706–709.

Clear Chest Roentgenogram and Respiratory Distress

One often encounters an infant with severe respiratory difficulty and clear lungs. When the lungs also are overaerated, one should be familiar with the fact that infants with severe acidosis (renal disease, congenital adrenogenital syndrome, and severe dehydration) may, because of "overbreathing," show roentgenographic overaeration (Fig. 1.125).

Another group of infants with respiratory distress and clear lungs are those with hypoplastic lungs. In these cases, the lungs are persistently small but clear. The PFC syndrome also is present in these patients and is the most significant factor leading to their continued problems. The lungs also are clear in patients with apnea for a variety of reasons.

Extracorporeal Membrane Oxygenation

ECMO is now commonplace in the treatment of infants with severe compromising respiratory disease. Initially

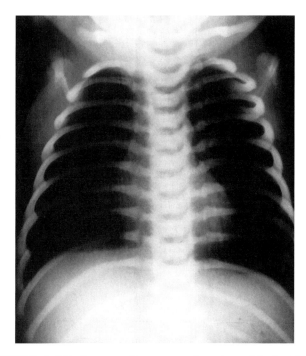

FIGURE 1.125. Overaeration secondary to acidosis. This newborn infant with profound metabolic acidosis shows pronounced overaeration with clear lungs.

designed for the infant with severe surfactant deficiency disease, it is now used more for infants with other severe pulmonary disease. The conditions are too numerous to list, but suffice it to say that infants who demonstrate cardiorespiratory failure to the point where death is inevitable now become candidates for ECMO therapy. In this regard, initially ECMO therapy was relegated to immature infants, but older infants and children now are commonly treated with ECMO therapy.

One's overall objective with ECMO therapy is to (a) circumvent the lungs, (b) let the lungs heal, and (c) protect the lungs from the effects of positive pressure ventilation therapy and oxygen toxicity. In other words, the lungs are placed to rest, almost as though they have been placed back in utero and the ECMO apparatus serves as the placenta. All of this has been very effective, and currently survival rates in patients on ECMO therapy are near 90% (1).

Classically, when an infant is placed on ECMO therapy, the lungs deflate and become opaque (Fig. 1.126), no matter what the underlying problem. Only minimal distending pressures are applied during the course of therapy, but as the patient begins to recover, the lungs are inflated a little more and finally normal aeration is restored. On the average, infants are kept on ECMO therapy for about 10 days, but some require significantly longer periods of time.

Prior to being placed on ECMO therapy, the infant is evaluated for the presence of intracranial bleeding and congenital heart disease that would be severe enough to preclude survival of the infant. From the radiologist's standpoint, it is the former with which one is most concerned, and in this regard, it has been demonstrated that grade I bleeds do not place the infant at risk for further bleeding while being anticoagulated for ECMO therapy. However, if problems such as periventricular leukomalacia or larger bleeds are present, the outlook is greatly compromised (2) and ECMO therapy is not initiated. Originally, only patients with normal intracranial ultrasound studies or those with grade I bleeds were placed on ECMO therapy, but more and more patients with grade II bleeds also are being placed on such therapy. Once placed on ECMO therapy, daily ultrasonographic examinations of the brain usually were obtained, although the need for this came to be questioned. Currently, we obtain daily studies for 5 days and thereafter only if clinically indicated for the detection of hemorrhagic complications. More recently, it has been suggested that negative pre- and 23-hour postultrasound studies should suffice and that repeated daily studies are not required. In this study (3), only 3% of infants with initially normal studies suffered bleeds at a later time.

Patients on ECMO therapy are anticoagulated, and because of this, the bleeds initially are hypoechoic (liquid) rather than echogenic (clotted). However, most of the bleeds we have seen in our institution have not been hypoechoic, but rather mixed or echogenic. In addition, there is a tendency for the bleeds to occur in the posterior fossa (4).

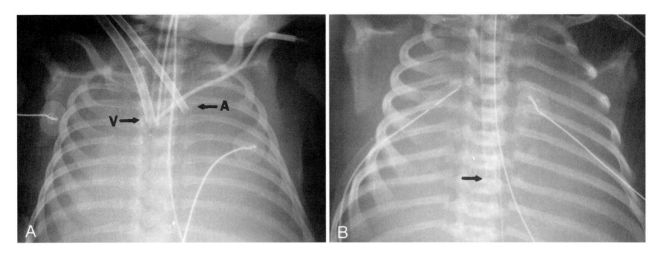

FIGURE 1.126. Extracorporeal membrane oxygenation therapy: cannula positions. A. Double cannula. Note the position of the venous (V) and atrial (A) cannulas. **B. Single cannula.** The tip of the single cannula rests in the right atrium (arrow).

Originally, because of permanently ligating the right jugular vein and common carotid artery after ECMO therapy, unilateral brain injury was feared and, in fact, documented. However, this has not turned out to be as great a problem as initially anticipated (5). The reason probably lies in the fact that there is good cross-circulation between the hemispheres. Attesting to this is that neurodevelopment in patients placed on ECMO is about the same as in those

patients not placed on ECMO (6, 7). In our institution, intracranial complications have been low (6).

When ECMO therapy was first utilized, two cannulas were used: one in the right jugular vein and the other in the right carotid artery. The tip of the arterial cannula usually lies just at the junction of the innominate artery and aortic arch, while the tip of the venous catheter lies at the junction of the superior vena cava and right atrium

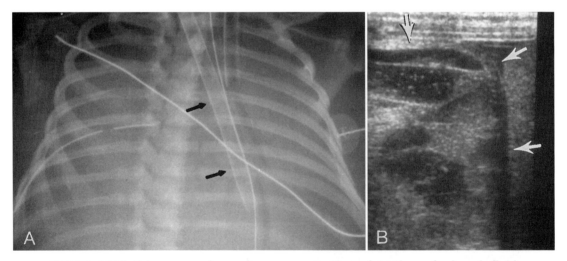

FIGURE 1.127. Extracorporeal membrane oxygenation: detection of pleural fluid (blood). A. Same patient as in Fig. 1.126B. Note, however, that on this film, the cannula has moved far to the left and that the endotracheal tube also is displaced. Although the patient is a little rotated, the degree of rotation would not account for such displacement. A chest tube is present on the right for a previous pneumothorax. The marked shift of the single cannula would suggest a space-occupying problem on the right, and this most likely would be a hemothorax. **B.** Ultrasonogram demonstrates a multiloculated hemothorax (arrows), with variable echogenicity of the numerous locules.

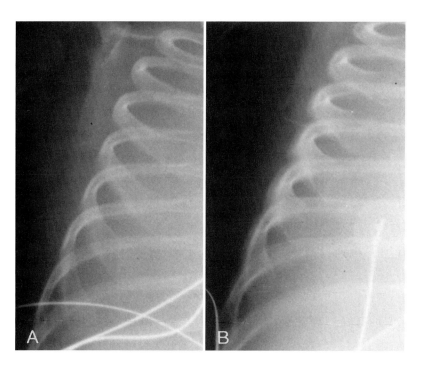

FIGURE 1.128. Extracorporeal membrane oxygenation therapy: periosteal new bone on ribs. A. Early in the course of extracorporeal membrane oxygenation therapy, the ribs appear normal. **B.** Days later, extensive periosteal new bone is seen on all the ribs.

(Fig. 1.126A). More recently, a venoveno single cannula has been advocated and has been shown to be as effective as the usual double-cannula setup (7, 8). In these cases, a single cannula is placed into the right atrium, approximately two-thirds down the length of the cavity (see Fig. 1.126B). Generally, these cannulas move very little as these patients are paralyzed, but they are checked daily for position. A good pictorial review of the various cannulas used is available in a communication by Gross et al. (9).

Complications of ECMO therapy primarily center around various hemorrhagic phenomenon. Although problems such as life-threatening pneumothorax (10) and pneumomediastinum can arise, most often problems center around bleeding into the pleural space or cardiac tamponade. The former is much more common (11, 12), but all of these complications must be recognized promptly. Of course, pneumothorax usually is readily detected, but blood in the pericardium or pleural space can be elusive. A clue to the fact that one or the other of these space-occupying problems has occurred consists of difficulty with aeration of the lungs on a clinical basis. Once this has occurred, one should look for the position of the cannulas or depression of the liver to signify that a unilateral space-occupying problem is occurring. Of course, if the problem is bilateral, one may never detect the abnormality on plain films. For this reason, ultrasound is invaluable and should be employed as soon as one of these com-

plications is suspected on a clinical basis (Fig. 1.127). Serous pericardial effusions also have been documented (13).

Other complications of ECMO therapy include benign cholestasis (14) secondary to associated total parental nutrition, and splenic enlargement. The latter is believed due to sequestration of damaged red blood cells and platelets. Fluid in the interhemispheric fissure also usually is seen in these patients, but volumes are small and interhemispheric fissure widths usually are no more than 4–5 mm (15). The problem is temporary and probably related to the fluid overload in these patients. Another interesting feature of ECMO therapy is periosteal reaction of the ribs (16, 17) in some of these infants (Fig. 1.128). This has been correlated with chest wall edema generally greater than 11 mm (16), and we have seen similar changes in the long bones.

REFERENCES

1. Moler FW, Custer JR, Barlett RH, et al. Extracorporeal life support for severe pediatric respiratory failure: an updated experience 1991–1993. J Pediatr 1994;124:875–880.
2. von Allmen D, Babcock D, Matsumoto J, et al. The predictive value of head ultrasound in the ECMO candidate. J Pediatr Surg 1992;27:36–39.
3. Heard ML, Clark RH, Pettignano P, et al. Daily cranial ultrasound during ECMO: a quality review cost analysis project. J Pediatr Surg 1997;32:1260.

4. Bulas DI, Taylor GA, Fitz CR, et al. Posterior fossa intracranial hemorrhage in infants treated with extracorporeal membrane oxygen: sonographic findings. AJR 1991;156:571–575.
5. Mondoza JC, Shearer LL, Cook LN. Lateralization of brain lesions following extracorporeal membrane oxygenation. Pediatrics 1991;88:1004–1009.
6. Griffin MP, Minifee PK, Landry SH, et al. Neurodevelopmental outcome in neonates after extracorporeal membrane oxygenation: cranial magnetic resonance imaging and ultrasonography correlation. J Pediatr Surg 1992;27:33–35.
7. Anderson HL III, Snedecor SM, Otsu T, et al. Multicenter comparison of conventional venoarterial access versus venovenous double-lumen catheter access in newborn infants undergoing extracorporeal membrane oxygenation. J Pediatr Surg 1993;28: 530–535.
8. Delius R, Anderson H III, Schumacher R, et al. Venovenous compares favorably with venoarterial access for extracorporeal membrane oxygenation in neonatal respiratory failure. J Thorac Cardiovasc Surg 1993;106:329–338.
9. Gross GW, McElwee DL, Baumgart S, et al. Bypass cannulas utilized in extracorporeal membrane oxygenation in neonates: radiographic findings. Pediatr Radiol 1995;25:337–340.
10. Zwischenberger JB, Bowers RM, Pickens GJ. Tension pneumothorax during extracorporeal membrane oxygenation. Ann Thorac Surg 1989;47:868–871.
11. Gross GW, Cullen J, Kornhauser MS, et al. Pictorial essay. Thoracic complications of extracorporeal membrane oxygenation: findings on chest radiographs and sonograms. AJR 1992;158: 353–358.
12. Zwischenberger JB, Cilley RE, Hirschl RB, et al. Life-threatening intrathoracic complications during treatment with extracorporeal membrane oxygenation. J Pediatr Surg 1988;23: 599–604.
13. Kurian MS, Reynolds ER, Humes RA, et al. Cardiac tamponade caused by serous pericardial effusion in patients on extracorporeal membrane. J Pediatr Surg 1999;34:1311–1314.
14. Shneider B, Maller E, VanMartger L, et al. Cholestasis in infants supported with extracorporeal membrane oxygenation. J Pediatr 1989;115:462–465.
15. Rubin DA, Gross GW, Ehrlich SM. Interhemispheric fissure width in neonates on ECMO. Pediatr Radiol 1990;21:12–15.
16. Feinstein KA, Fernbach SK. Periosteal reaction of the ribs in neonates treated with extracorporeal membrane oxygenation: prevalence and association with soft-tissue swelling. AJR 1993; 160:587–589.
17. Kogutt LM, Lovretich JO. Periosteal reaction of the long bones associated with extracorporeal membrane oxygenation: cause and effect? Pediatr Radiol 1999;29:797–798.

POSTNATAL PULMONARY INFECTIONS

Chest Roentgenograms in Febrile Infants

Chest roentgenograms often are obtained as part of a workup to determine the source of unexplained fever. Many times, the problem turns out to be sepsis or meningitis and the chest film is normal, and, indeed, it has been demonstrated that chest roentgenograms under these circumstances generally are unproductive unless respiratory tract symptoms also are present (1–3). However, it is difficult to put this type of philosophy into practice because of the fear of missing a serious pulmonary infection, and in this regard, it recently has been suggested that in patients with a leukocytosis and fever of 39°C or higher, empiric chest roentgenograms are in order if no other source for the fever is demonstrated (4). In spite of this, most of the roentgenograms in these patients will be normal. It is important to appreciate this, for otherwise there **will be a tendency to try to "squeeze something" out of a chest film that really is normal.**

REFERENCES

1. Bramson RT, Meyer TL, Silbiger ML, et al. The futility of the chest radiograph in the febrile infant without respiratory symptoms. Pediatrics 1993;92:524–526.
2. Crain EF, Bulas D, Bijur PE, et al. Is a chest radiograph necessary in the evaluation of every febrile infant less than 8 weeks of age? Pediatrics 1991;88:821–824.
3. Patterson RJ, Bisset GS III, Kirks DR, et al. Chest radiographs in the evaluation of the febrile infant. AJR 1990;155:833–835.
4. Bachur R, Perry H, Harper MB. Occult pneumonias: empiric chest radiographs in febrile children with leukocytosis. Ann Emerg Med 1999;33:166–173.

Imaging of Lower Respiratory Tract Infections

To this day, the chest radiograph is still the first and most important imaging study utilized in the evaluation of lower respiratory tract infections. In addition, it is becoming increasingly important that one can differentiate viral from bacterial infections (1). In interpreting the radiograph, it is important to appreciate that there is both inter- and intraobserver variation (2), and most often this deals with the misinterpretation of atelectasis, common with viral bronchitic infections, for pneumonia. **In other instances, especially along the right cardiac border and on lateral view in the retrocardiac space, clustering of bronchi, thickened by viral bronchitis, is misinterpreted for pneumonia (consolidations).** This is becoming less and less of a problem as imagers and other physicians become aware of these problems, but still errors in interpretation occur. On the other hand, there is almost universal agreement that all interpreters do well with the identification of bacterial consolidating pneumonias (2).

Other imaging modalities for the evaluation of lower respiratory tract infections in children include ultrasound and CT. The role of ultrasound is primarily that of detecting the presence of pleural fluid, either serous effusions or pyogenic empyemas. In this regard, it is very efficient and productive. CT is used primarily for evaluation of complications of pneumonia, and these, for the most part, include empyema and necrotizing pneumonia with abscess formation. CT generally is more informative than plain films once these complications occur (3) and almost invariably is necessary before radiologic or surgical intervention is contemplated. CT with both inspiratory and expiratory sequences also enables one to demonstrate occult areas of air trapping (4).

CT also plays a role in the evaluation of viral lower respiratory tract infections that involve the interstitium. There are numerous reports and dissertations on this subject (5–8), and all attest to the ability of CT to differentiate one condition from the other. However, my experience is that high-resolution CT plays a minimal role in the evaluation of acute lower respiratory tract infections and has limited diagnostic use in chronic problems as the patterns frequently overlap. It does, however, provide excellent data as far as the extent of disease is concerned.

REFERENCES

1. Donnelly LF. Review. Maximizing the usefulness of imaging in children with community-acquired pneumonia. AJR 1999;172: 505–512.
2. Davies HD, Wang EE-L, Manson D, et al. Reliability of the chest radiograph in the diagnosis of lower respiratory infections in young children. Pediatr Infect Dis J 1996;15:600–604.
3. Donnelly LF, Klosterman LA. The yield of CT of children who have complicated pneumonia and noncontributory chest radiography. AJR 1998;170:1627–1631.
4. Long FR, Castile RE. Technique and clinical applications of full-inflation and end-exhalation controlled ventilation chest CT in infants and young children. Pediatr Radiol 2001;31: 413–422.
5. Moon WD, Kim WS, Kim I-O, et al. Pictorial essay. Diffuse pulmonary disease in children: high-resolution CT findings. AJR 1996;167:1405–1408.
6. Oopley SI, Coren M, Nicholson AG, et al. Diagnostic accuracy of thin-section CT and chest radiography of pediatric interstitial lung disease. AJR 2000;174:549–554.
7. Ichikado K, Johkon T, Ikezoe J, et al. Acute interstitial pneumonia: high resolution CT findings correlated with pathology. AJR 1997;168:333–338.
8. Lynch DA, Hay T, Newell JDJ, et al. Pediatric diffuse lung disease: diagnosis and classification using high-resolution CT. AJR 1999;173:713–718.

Chest Roentgenograms and Wheezing

Classically, wheezing, especially expiratory wheezing, is seen with asthma, foreign bodies, cystic fibrosis, and viral, mycoplasma, or pertussis infections. All of these entities represent problems of the airway (tracheobronchial tree) and not the pulmonary parenchyma, and therefore, there is good reason for wheezing to be present. Wheezing is not characteristic of bacterial infections, for these infections are air space infections. This is an important point to appreciate for very often viral lower respiratory tract infections and/or asthma produce a good deal of atelectasis, both lobar and segmental, and then there is a tendency to misinterpret atelectasis for consolidation. In this regard, however, if wheezing is the predominant symptom, even in a febrile infant, atelectasis most likely is the problem. At the same time, it might be noted that wheezing in asthmatics is exaggerated with viral (1) and mycoplasma lower respiratory tract infections. Contrarily, when a bacterial infection is present in an asthmatic, wheezing is not exacerbated (2). Again, there is good reason for this to occur for, as previously noted, bacterial infections are alveolar space infections and not bronchial (airway) infections.

REFERENCES

1. Mitchell I, Inglis H, Simpson H. Viral infection in wheezy bronchitis and asthma in children. Arch Dis Child 1976; 51:707–711.
2. McIntosh K, Ellis EF, Hoffman LS, et al. The association of viral and bacterial respiratory infections with exacerbations of wheezing in young asthmatic children. J Pediatr 1973;82: 578–590.

Antibiotics in Lower Respiratory Tract Infections

There is no question that antibiotics are the answer to bacterial lower respiratory tract infections, but recently it has come to everyone's attention that antibiotics are inappropriately prescribed for children with colds, upper respiratory tract infections. and bronchitis (1). Obviously, this practice is to be discouraged for such practice in the past, has resulted in resistant streptococcal (pneumococcal) infection (*S. pneumoniae*). In this regard, we have seen more empyemas and more refractory empyemas in the last 3 years than we have seen in the last 15 years or so. For this reason alone, the judicious use of antibiotics in lower respiratory tract infections in children is paramount. In spite of this, however, there still is a tendency for patients who do not require antibiotics to receive them (2). **From the imaging standpoint, the main contribution to this dilemma is the accurate identification of atelectasis and parahilar peribronchial infiltration (Fig. 1.129).**

REFERENCES

1. Nyquist A-C, Gonzales R, Steinger JR, et al. Antibiotic prescribing for children with colds, upper respiratory tract infections, and bronchitis. JAMA 1998;279:875–877.

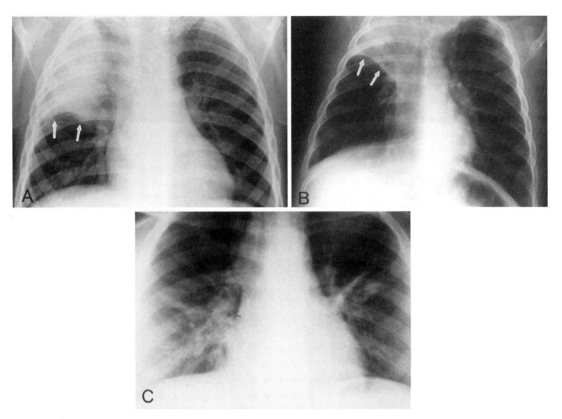

FIGURE 1.129. Consolidation versus atelectasis. A. Typical consolidation of the right upper lobe showing minimal elevation of the minor fissure, testifying to virtually no volume loss. **B.** Patient with viral bronchitis and classic atelectasis of the right upper lobe demonstrating marked elevation of the minor fissure. **C.** Asthmatic with viral bronchitis demonstrating extensive parahilar peribronchial infiltrates and bilateral streaky, wedge-like areas of segmental atelectasis.

2. Pichichero ME, Green JL, Francis AB, et al. Outcomes after judicious antibiotic use for respiratory tract infections seen in a private pediatric practice. Pediatrics 2000;105:753–759.

Bacterial Infections and Their Complications

Bacterial infections in patients beyond the neonatal period tend to present as homogeneous, lobar consolidations or fluffy (alveolar) infiltrates. For the most part, they are unilobar (Fig. 1.130) but can be multilobar (Fig. 1.131A). In any case, it is important to note that even with extensive consolidations, there is little or no lobar volume loss. Therefore,

confusion with atelectasis should not occur in most cases. In those cases where slight volume loss may be present, it is important to note that because consolidations begin in the periphery of the lobe, the peripheral density is more pronounced than the central density (Fig. 1.130C). With atelectasis, this constellation of findings usually is reversed, as there is more density centrally than peripherally. In a few cases, the infiltrate, rather than being a typical consolidation, assumes a more fluffy nodular pattern (Fig. 1.131B).

In infants younger than 2 years, the most commonly encountered organism, in the past, was *Haemophilus influenzae,* but this infection virtually has disappeared with current vaccination programs. Therefore, throughout the

FIGURE 1.131. Other patterns of bacterial pneumonia. A. Multilobar bacterial infection. Consolidations are present in the right upper and right lower lobes. The left lung is entirely clear. The minor fissure on the right shows minimal elevation. Overall, there is no significant volume loss of the right lung. **B. Nodular-appearing bacterial pneumonia.**

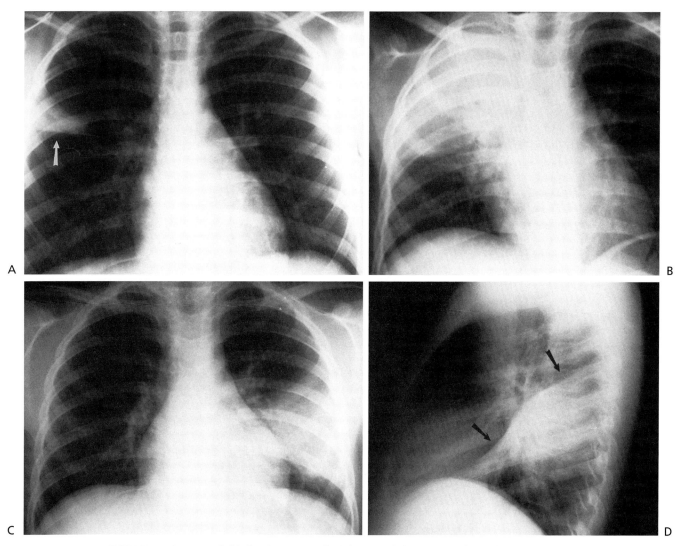

FIGURE 1.130. Bacterial infections. A. Early right upper lobe peripheral consolidation (arrow). Consolidations begin in the periphery of the lung and work inward. **B.** A well-developed right upper lobe consolidation. Note that there is no volume loss. **C.** Pneumonia in the left lower lobe. Note that there is no volume loss of the left lung. **D.** Lateral view also demonstrates that there virtually is no volume loss as the major fissure (arrows) is in near-normal position.

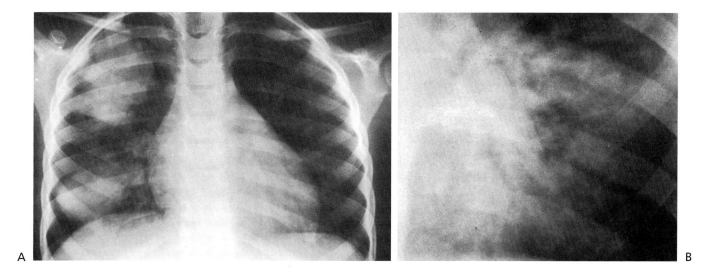

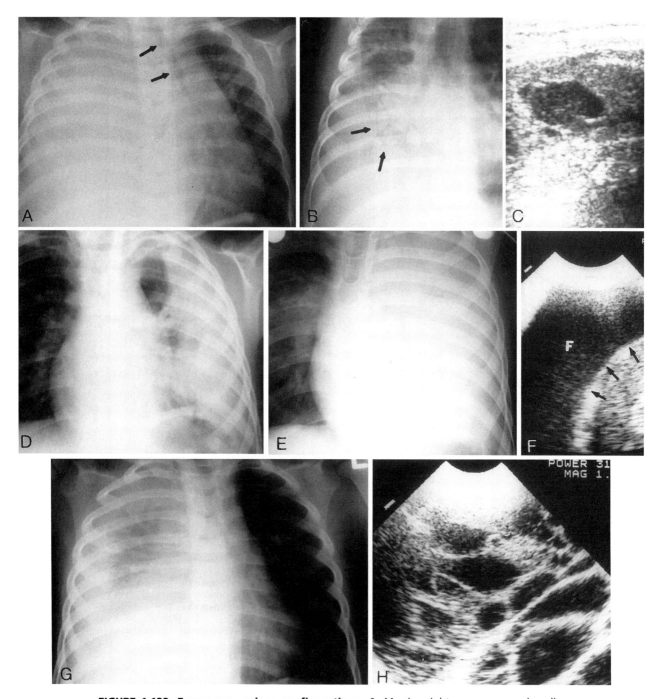

FIGURE 1.132. Empyema: various configurations. A. Massive right empyema causing displacement of the mediastinal structures. Note the position of the trachea (arrows). **B.** Smaller empyema in the right base extending up the lateral wall. This could be misinterpreted for a consolidation, but note that the air bronchograms (arrows) stop short of the periphery of the lung. This is a good finding to suggest that pleural fluid, and not simple consolidation, is present. **C.** Ultrasonogram demonstrates loculated pockets of fluid in the right pleural space. **D.** Another patient with an empyema developing along the left lateral wall. This configuration often is misinterpreted for pneumonia. Note that while the empyema is developing, the lung is being compressed centrally and that there is no volume loss or gain on the left side. **E.** Another patient with a large empyema on the left compressing the lung with air bronchograms centrally. Again, there is no mediastinal shift. **F.** Ultrasonogram in this patient demonstrates a large collection of fluid (F) above the left diaphragmatic leaflet (arrows). **G.** Another patient with a right empyema. **H.** Ultrasound demonstrates a multiloculated empyema.

pediatric age group, *Streptococcus (Diplococcus) pneumoniae* is now the most common causative organism. *Staphylococcus aureus* has not been a significant infection for two or three decades. Pleural effusions and frank empyema are common with bacterial pneumonia, and now, with resistant pneumococcal infections, more of a problem than they were 10 or 20 years ago. These empyemas definitely are more refractory to conservative therapeutic measures and, as with all empyemas, can develop very quickly, even over a period of hours. When empyema is accompanied by pneumothorax, the term "pyopneumothorax" is utilized, and this combination of findings has always been most common with staphylococcal infections.

Resolution of empyema can be quite slow, and this is especially true of staphylococcal and resistant pneumococcal infections. Even with vigorous therapy, tardy clearing is the rule, but eventually complete clearing usually occurs. There seldom is need for decortication even in this day and age of resistant infections. For this reason, one should not be overly concerned by lingering roentgenographic findings in the face of an otherwise clinically improving patient. In this regard, there is a tendency to obtain follow-up roentgenograms too frequently in these cases. As long as the patient is doing well clinically, one can space the follow-up roentgenographic studies quite far apart.

The volume of fluid present with empyema may be small or large, and when massive, mediastinal shift is obvious (Fig. 1.132A). Diagnosis in these cases is no real problem, but when the empyema is developing and there is no mediastinal shift, the findings can be a problem and usually are erroneously misinterpreted for total lung consolidation (Fig. 1.132D). The latter, however, is rare. Decubitus films are of no value in these cases for the hemithorax is so full of fluid that there is no room for shifting and layering to occur. However, the fluid is readily identified with ultrasound (Fig. 1.132, E and F). Decubitus films are useful in cases where less fluid is present, mostly to clearly delineate the volume of fluid present. Fluid collections identified ultrasonographically may be homogeneous or multiloculated (Fig. 1.132, F and H). The latter collections are more difficult to drain and may require fibrinolytic therapy (1). Empyema, unless multiloculated, is difficult to differentiate from simple pleural effusions on CT studies (2). However, CT studies generally are required before any therapeutic measure is considered, and in this regard, the video-assisted thoracoscopic surgical procedure is now a favored form of empyema drainage (3). In addition, intrapleural urokinase can be administered (4).

Pneumatoceles are another complication of bacterial pneumonia and result from the obstruction of a bronchus by the exudate produced by the infection. Many are subpleural blebs rather than intraparenchymal cystic structures, but, in any case, in the past, staphylococcal infections were the most likely to produce pneumatoceles. However, pneumatoceles can be seen with any bacterial lung infection.

Usually, pneumatoceles are of no particular consequence to the patient, but some can become very large and cause mediastinal shift and respiratory compromise (Fig. 1.133). Pneumatoceles usually are thin walled and eventually disappear, but some may become infected and demonstrate air-

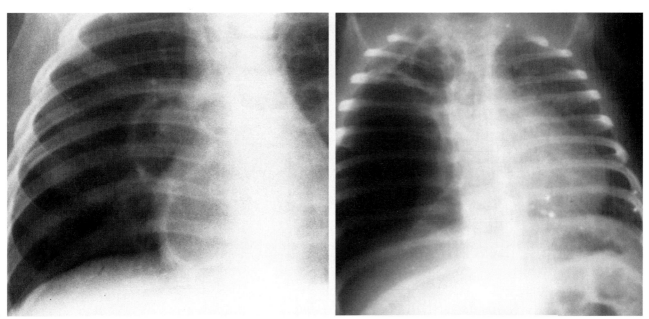

A   B

FIGURE 1.133. Pneumatoceles. A. Note two spherical pneumatoceles on the right (arrows). **B.** Large pneumatocele on the right.

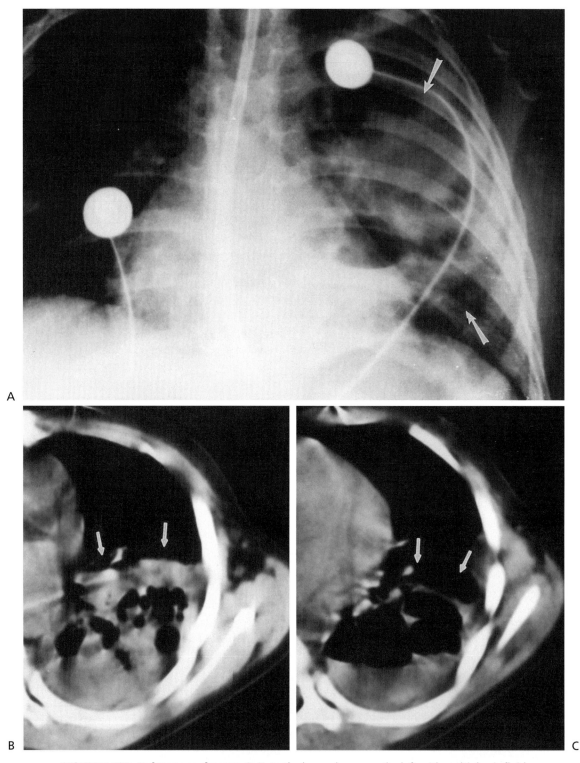

A

B

C

FIGURE 1.134. Pulmonary abscess. A. Note the large abscess on the left with multiple air-fluid levels. **B.** Computed tomography study shows numerous cavities in the abscess (arrows). **C.** At another level, a large cavity with an air-fluid level is seen (arrow).

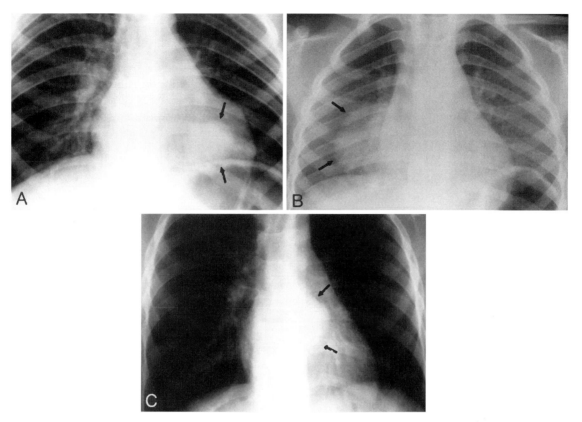

FIGURE 1.135. Round or mass-like pneumonias. A. Note the round, mass-like appearance of an early consolidation in the left lower lobe (arrows). **B.** Another patient with a mass-like configuration of an early consolidating pneumonia (arrows). **C.** Paraspinal mass-like pneumonia is seen on the left (arrows).

fluid levels. Infected pneumatoceles are difficult to differentiate from pulmonary abscess, but generally, pulmonary abscesses have thicker walls. Very seldom, a pneumatocele may rupture and produce a complicating pneumothorax.

Cavitary necrosis (5), leading to abscess formation, also can be a complication of bacterial pneumonia (Fig. 1.34). Many cases resolve without surgical intervention (5), but some can be refractory. CT studies usually are required for those cases where percutaneous (6, 7) or surgical drainage is to be accomplished. With CT, it has also been demonstrated that one can predict when cavitary necrosis might occur (8). This is accomplished on the basis of an area of decreased parenchymal enhancement on contrast CT studies.

Before I conclude the remarks on bacterial lung infections, it should be noted that some consolidations in their early phases may appear as round, parenchymal nodules or masses or mass-like lesions of the mediastinum (Fig. 1.135). One should not be misled by this appearance, for it is strictly fortuitous. If one were to examine these patients 12–24 hours later, a typical consolidation would be seen. **These consolidations are known as round or mass-like pneumonias** (9).

REFERENCES

1. Chen K-Y, Liaw Y-S, Wang H-C, et al. Sonographic septation: a useful prognostic indicator of acute thoracic empyema. J Ultrasound Med 2000;19:837–843.
2. Donnelly LF, Klosterman LA. CT appearance of parapneumonic effusions in children: findings are not specific for empyema. AJR 1997;169:179–182.
3. Doski JJ, Lou D, Hicks BA, et al. Management of parapneumonic collections in infants and children. J Pediatr Surg 2000;35:265–270.
4. Kornecki A, Silvan Y. Treatment of loculated pleural effusion with intrapleural urokinase in children. J Pediatr Surg 1997;32:1473–1475.
5. Donnelly LF, Klosterman LA. Cavitary necrosis complicating pneumonia in children: sequential findings on chest radiography. AJR 1998;171:253–256.
6. Ball WS Jr, Bisset GS III, Towbin RB. Percutaneous drainage of chest abscesses in children. Radiology 1989;171:431–434.
7. Lee SK, Morris RF, Cramer B. Percutaneous needle aspiration of neonatal lung abscesses. Pediatr Radiol 1991;21:254–257.
8. Donnelly LF, Klosterman LA. Pneumonia in children: decreased parenchymnal contrast enhancement—CT sign of intense illness and impending cavitary necrosis. Radiology 1997;205:817–820.
9. Rose RW, Ward BH. Spherical pneumonias in children simulating pulmonary and mediastinal masses. Radiology 1973;106:179–182.

Viral Infections

Viral infections generally are infections of the bronchi and peribronchial tissues (bronchitis) and thus produce changes different from those of intraalveolar bacterial infection (1–4). Even when the inflammatory process involves the parenchyma, it still generally involves the interstitium and not the alveolar space. **The most common pattern of infiltration is the so-called "parahilar peribronchial pattern."** This pattern results from thickening of the bronchial wall, both the mucosa and the peribronchial tissues. It leads to a classic pattern of radiating infiltrates that course outward from the hilar regions along the normal bronchovascular sheaths (Fig. 1.136). **In the past, the term "bronchopneumonia" also has often been used to describe these findings, but I believe it is a misleading term, for it suggests that a pneumonia is present, and yet there is no true pneumonia.** The problem in these patients is bronchitis-peribronchitis and not alveolar space disease (i.e.,

pneumonia), and therefore **"bronchopneumonia" seems an inappropriate, and confusing, term.** It probably is best that it not be used to describe the findings.

Parahilar peribronchial infiltrates, characteristic of viral lower respiratory tract infection, are generally very symmetric unless superimposed atelectasis is present. In addition, and most important with this pattern of infiltration, is that there is a central parahilar predominance. This results from the fact that the bronchi are closer together near the hilar regions and the resulting peribronchial edema becomes more confluent. In some cases, the central predominance is enhanced by the presence of hilar adenopathy. I have always underscored the fact that **the parahilar peribronchial infiltrative pattern is one that is bilateral, symmetric, and with a central predominance** (Fig. 1.136, A and C).

Organisms most often responsible for viral lower respiratory tract infections include respiratory syncytial virus, influenza and parainfluenza virus, adenovirus, and rhinovirus. Pleural effusions are rare, and occasionally other

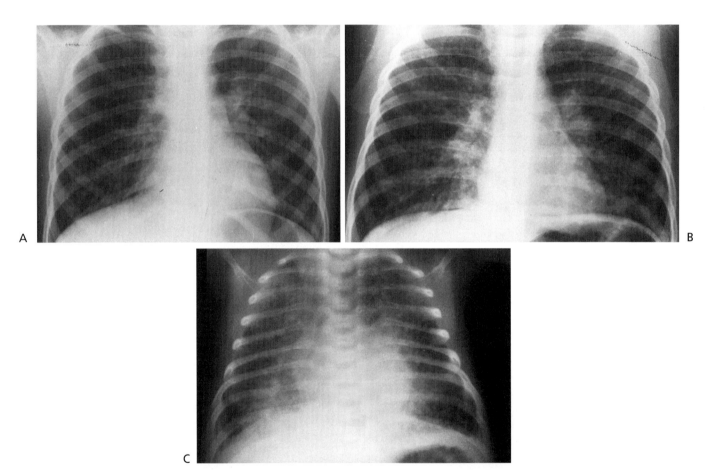

FIGURE 1.136. Spectrum of viral lower respiratory tract infection. A. Typical parahilar peribronchial infiltrates. **B.** More extensive central reticulonodularity and streakiness throughout both lungs. Hilar adenopathy is more pronounced. **C.** Very extensive parahilar peribronchial infiltration (interstitial) extending far into the parenchyma, leading to a more solid-appearing infiltrate. At this stage, however, the disease process still is interstitial, just more severe and extensive.

viral infections such as chickenpox, measles, and cytomegalic inclusion disease are encountered. The latter infection often occurs in immunocompromised individuals. Roentgenographically, it usually is not possible to distinguish one viral infection from another, but with adenoviral infection, there is a propensity for the disease process to be rather severe and result in an obliterative bronchiolitis with long-term respiratory sequelae (4, 5). These patients initially have the usual parahilar peribronchial inflammatory process common to viral infections, but the supervening necrotizing bronchitis leads to more extensive bronchial damage.

Bronchiolitis is a serious manifestation of viral lower respiratory tract infection occurring in infants in the first 2 years of life. The peak incidence is around 6 months, and the bronchial infection leads to such severe bronchospasm that these patients virtually cannot move air. **The problem is not so much toxicity or sepsis as an inability to move air.** Roentgenographically, overaeration of the lungs is the rule, and while many of these infants demonstrate typical parahilar peribronchial infiltrates (Fig. 1.137) with scattered areas of atelectasis, others, probably over 50%, demonstrate completely clear lungs. Almost exclusively the infection is due to respiratory syncytial virus, but other viruses, namely, influenza and adenovirus, can produce similar findings.

Although there are instances where both bacterial and viral infections co-exist, they are less common. In such cases, the viral infection precedes the bacterial infection, and after a week or so, a superimposed bacterial consolidation develops. In these cases, there is a change in the clinical picture, with abrupt onset of a more toxic-septic picture with high fevers (39–40°C), heralding the presence of the superimposed, more toxic bacterial infection. The consolidation usually is located in the periphery of the lung (Fig. 1.138) and, as such, can be differentiated from atelectasis, which tends to be more central.

One of the most common associated problems encountered with viral lower respiratory tract infection in children, especially young infants, is atelectasis, either lobar or segmental (1–3). Indeed, multiple areas of segmental and subsegmental atelectasis are the most problematic aspect of interpreting roentgenograms in infants and young children with viral lower respiratory tract infection. **They are no real problem for the patient but represent a serious pitfall for the interpreter of the roentgenogram, for very often they are misinterpreted for alveolar consolidations.**

The reason why atelectasis is so common in these patients, and not in older children and adults, is that the collateral air drift phenomenon in infants is not very effective (6, 7). Hypersecretion of mucus and bronchospasm lead to bronchial obstruction, and this usually results in atelectasis. In older children and adults, such atelectasis, via the collateral air drift phenomenon, disap-

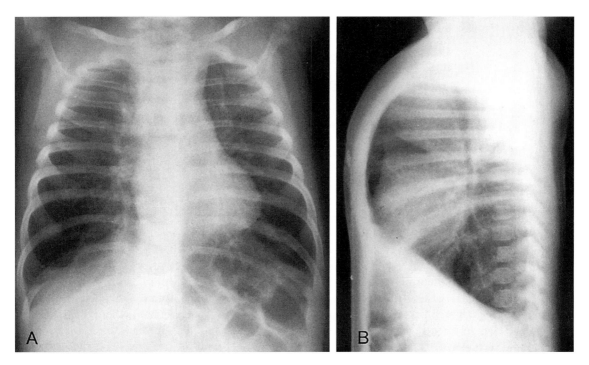

FIGURE 1.137. Bronchiolitis. A. Note markedly overaerated lungs and parahilar peribronchial infiltrates. **B.** Lateral view showing extensive overaeration of the lungs. Other cases may show simple overaeration and no infiltration whatsoever.

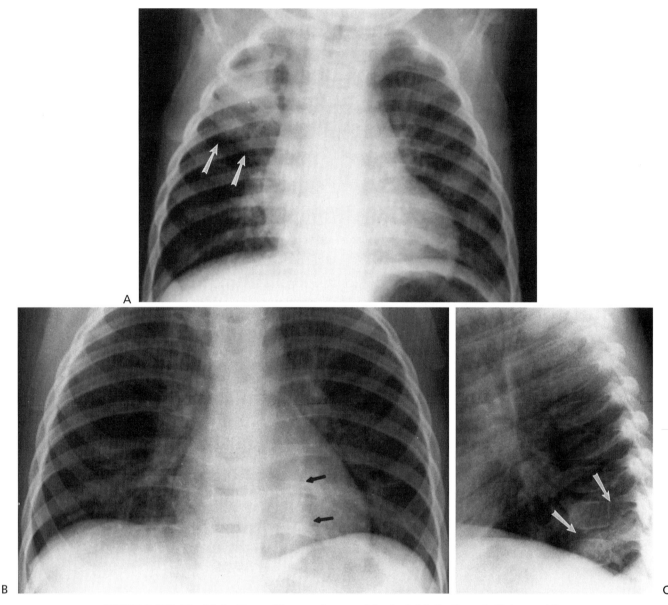

FIGURE 1.138. Viral infection with superimposed bacterial infection. A. Note parahilar peribronchial infiltrates and a consolidation (arrows) in the right upper lobe. **B.** Another infant with mild parahilar peribronchial infiltrates and some bilateral hilar adenopathy. A subtle pneumonia (arrows) is projected through the left side of the heart. **C.** Lateral view showing the posterior location of the pneumonia (arrows).

pears quickly, but in infants and young children, atelectasis persists. This being the case, there is a very good chance that atelectasis will be present on any given chest x-ray taken in these patients. **Unless one appreciates this, one will constantly call areas of atelectasis "lobar consolidations."** The key to the proper identification of atelectasis lies in the fact that there is significant lobar volume loss when a lobe is involved, and when subsegmental atelectasis is present, the infiltrates are not fluffy,

nodular, or hazy but rather angular, streaky, or wedge-like (Figs. 1.139 and 1.140).

When viruses involve the interstitium proper (i.e., interstitial pneumonitis), they produce reticulonodular or diffusely hazy infiltrates throughout both lung fields (Fig. 1.141). The former can be confused with the miliary infiltrates seen with tuberculosis, while the latter can be misinterpreted for total consolidation of both lungs. The latter, of course, would be most unusual, and thus when one

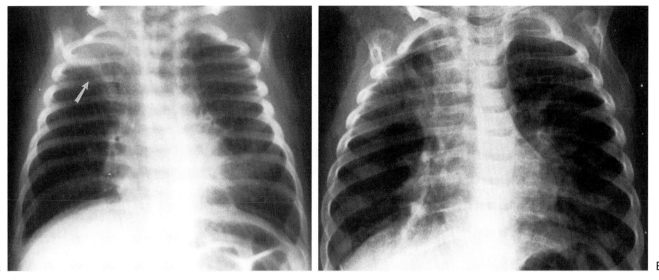

FIGURE 1.139. Viral lower respiratory tract infection with atelectasis. A. Note partial atelectasis of the right upper lobe (arrow) and bilateral parahilar peribronchial infiltrates. There is minimal atelectasis of the lingual and streaky atelectasis in the left lower lobe behind the heart. **B.** Bilateral parahilar peribronchial infiltrates with areas of wedge-like or streaky segmental atelectasis in the right upper and right lower lobes.

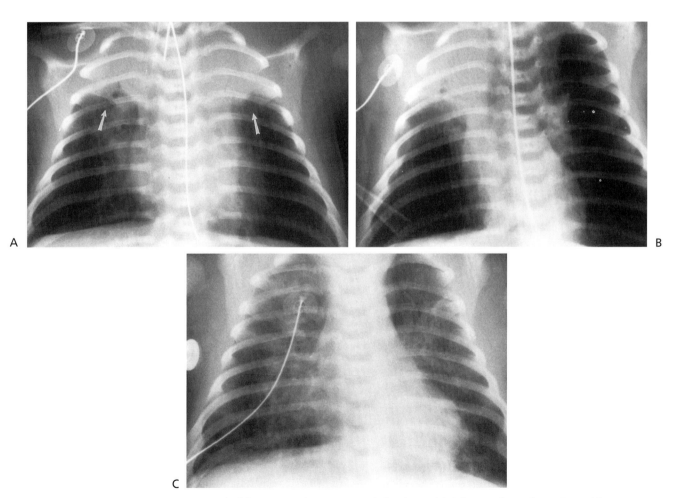

FIGURE 1.140. Viral lower respiratory tract infection with lobar atelectasis. A. Bronchiolitis with atelectasis. Note overall hyperinflation of the lungs and bilateral parahilar peribronchial infiltrates. Bilateral upper lobe atelectasis (arrows) easily could be misinterpreted for consolidating pneumonia. **B.** The next day, atelectasis on the left clears and there is midline shift of the mediastinum toward the right because of persistent right upper lobe atelectasis. **C.** Later, with both upper lobes reexpanded, only widespread parahilar peribronchial infiltrates and scattered segmental atelectatic areas are seen

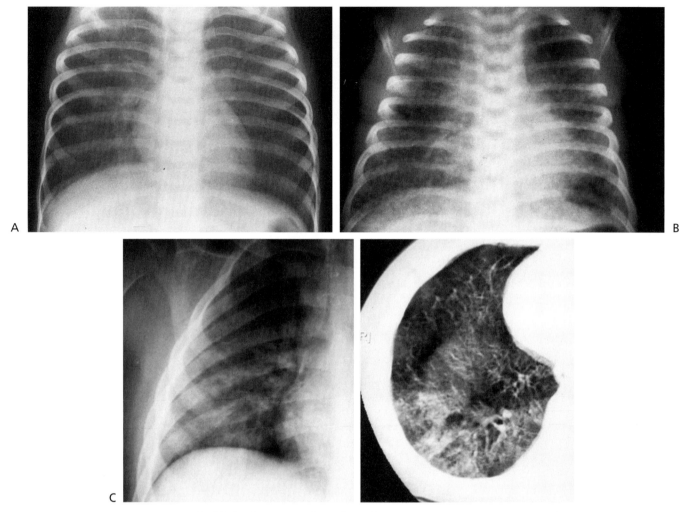

FIGURE 1.141. Viral infection: parenchymal involvement (interstitial pneumonitis). A. Diffuse, hazy lungs typical of interstitial pneumonitis. **B.** Diffuse haziness and reticulonodularity also characteristic of interstitial disease are present in this patient. **C.** In this patient, diffuse haziness and reticulonodularity are present in the right lung. **D.** High-resolution computed tomography (same patient) demonstrates diffuse ground-glass appearance, thickening of the interalveolar septum, and an area of pseudoconsolidation.

encounters bilateral, diffusely **hazy** lungs, even with visualization of air bronchograms, one should choose interstitial (viral) rather than intraalveolar (bacterial) disease. In many such cases, the hazy infiltrates are predominantly basal (see Fig. 1.142B). High-resolution CT can more vividly demonstrate these infiltrates (8–10) in that they produce the so-called "ground-glass" appearance of the lungs (Fig. 1.141D). Although not absolutely pathognomonic of interstitial pneumonitis, the ground-glass appearance is highly suggestive of the problem. This ground-glass appearance can be associated and intermingled with peribronchial inflammatory changes.

Rather than the lungs being diffusely hazy, only one lobe or the central parabilar region can become hazy or opaque.

This is not due to true consolidation but rather pseudoconsolidation caused by extensive inflammatory and edematous changes in the interstitium compressing the adjacent alveoli. The radiograph has no way of determining whether one is dealing with this type of pathophysiologic process or one where the alveoli are full of purulent exudates. Nonetheless, it is important to distinguish between consolidation and pseudoconsolidation. Pseudoconsolidation can involve one or more lobes (Fig. 1.142A) or just the bases of the lungs (Fig. 1.42B). In other cases, the original parahilar peribronchial pattern of infiltration leads to a more homogeneous and coalescent central and parahilar configuration (Fig. 1.142C). The bilateral symmetric and central location of these confluent infiltrates should provide the clue to the

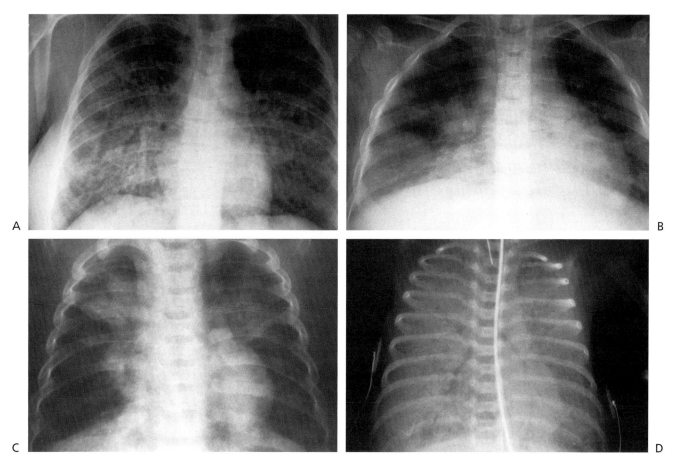

FIGURE 1.142. Viral interstitial parenchymal involvement: pseudoconsolidation. A. Varicella pneumonitis. Note the reticulonodular and hazy infiltrates. **B.** Bilateral basal pseudo-consolidations secondary to viral infection. **C.** Bilateral central coalescent density secondary to advanced interstitial involvement. **D.** Total lung opacification with air bronchograms, secondary to herpes pneumonitis.

fact that one is dealing with viral and not bacterial infection. Finally, the lungs can become almost totally opacified, not merely hazy but opaque, and the problem still is due to interstitial pneumonitis and not intraalveolar (air space) pneumonia (Fig. 1.42D). Adenoviral infections often are associated with a necrotizing bronchiolitis and hemmorhagic pneumonitis (11).

More recently, hantavirus also has been shown to produce early interstitial edema (12). However, in this infection and other viral infections with similar pathophysiologic virulence, a hemorrhagic component supervenes and the alveoli eventually become filled with edema fluid and blood. Bronchiolitis obliterans (13) is a rare complication of viral infection in children. There is a wide spectrum of pathologic change ranging from bronchiolar inflammation through peribronchiolar fibrosis and eventually complete cicatrization of the bronchiolar lumen (9). High-resolution CT is very helpful in demonstrating the presence of these findings for they may be somewhat subtle on plain films.

REFERENCES

1. Osborne D. Radiologic appearance of viral disease of the lower respiratory tract in infants and children. AJR 1978;13:29–33.
2. Khamapirad T, Glezen WP. Clinical and radiographic assessment of acute lower respiratory tract disease in infants and children. Semin Respir Infect 1987;2:130–144.
3. Swischuk LE, Hayden CK. Viral vs. bacterial pulmonary infections in children. (Is roentgenographic differentiation possible?) Pediatr Radiol 1986;16:278–284.
4. Wilden SR, Chonmaitree T, Swischuk LE. Roentgenographic features of common pediatric viral respiratory tract infections. Am J Dis Child 1988;142:43–46.
5. Gold R, Wilt JC, Adhikari PK, et al. Adenoviral pneumonia and its complications in infancy and childhood. J Can Assoc Radiol 1969;20:218–224.
6. Teper AM, Kofman CD, Maffey AF, et al. Lung function in infants with chronic pulmonary disease after severe adenoviral illness. J Pediatr 1999;134:730–733.
7. Griscom NT, Wohl MEB, Kirkpatrick JA Jr. Lower respiratory infections: how infants differ from adults. Radiol Clin North Am 1978;16:367–387.

8. Tal A, Maor E, Bar-Ziv J, et al. Fatal desquamative interstitial pneumonia in three infant siblings. J Pediatr 1984;104:873–876.
9. Hartman TE, Primack SL, Swensen SJ, et al. Desquamative interstitial pneumonia: thin-section CT findings in 22 patients. Radiology 1993;187:787–790.
10. Park JS, Lee KS, Kim JS, et al. Nonspecific interstitial pneumonia with fibrosis: radiographic and CT findings in seven patients. Radiology 1995;195:645–648.
11. Han BK, Son JA, Yoon H-K, et al. Original report. Epidemic adenoviral lower respiratory tract infection in pediatric patients: radiographic and clinical characteristics. AJR 1998;170:1077–1080.
12. Ketai LH, Williamson MR, Telepak RJ, et al. Hantavirus pulmonary syndrome: radiographic findings in 16 patients. Radiology 1994;191:665–668.
13. Chang AB, Masel JP, Masters B. Post-infectious bronchiolitis obliterans: clinical, radiological and pulmonary function sequelae. Pediatr Radiol 1998;28:23–29.

Follicular Bronchitis

Follicular bronchitis is an uncommon condition seen in children. It probably is of viral etiology and results in a chronic pulmonary problem characterized by lymphocytic infiltration around bronchi and interstitial lung reactive inflammatory changes (1). These often are best illustrated with high-resolution CT (2). Some cases may resolve spontaneously after 2 or 3 years (1). The radiographic findings in the early stages resemble those of viral parahilar peribronchial infiltrates. However, in this condition, these tend to persist, and there may be supervening areas of segmental and alveolar atelectasis. The peribronchial thickening, more vividly demonstrated with CT studies, can be associated with hilar adenopathy. Some suggest that a virus such as Epstein-Barr virus is responsible (1).

REFERENCES

1. Bramson RT, Cleveland R, Blickman JG, et al. Radiographic appearance of follicular bronchitis in children. AJR 1996;166:1447–1450.
2. Rettner P, Fotter R, Lindbichler F, et al. HRCT features in a 5-year-old child with follicular bronchiolitis. Pediatr Radiol 1997;27:877–879.

Mycoplasma pneumoniae Infection

Mycoplasma pneumoniae infections basically tend to produce roentgenographic findings similar to those produced by viruses (1, 2), and in this regard, the most common pattern of infiltration is that of bilateral parahilar peribronchial infiltrates. These infiltrates are virtually indistinguishable from those seen with viral lower respiratory tract infections and generally are seen in younger children and infants. There is another pattern, however, also quite common (2),

which is seen more in older children and adolescents. It consists of a predominantly unilobar reticular or reticulonodular infiltrate (Fig. 1.143). These predominantly unilobar infiltrates may be subtle, and clinically these patients usually present with a short-term (1–2 weeks) chronic cough and low-grade fever. It should be remembered that this pattern of unilobar, reticulonodular infiltrate also can be seen with viral infection, and in both cases, associated lobar or segmental atelectasis can be encountered, causing some problem with initial interpretation. The reason for this is that the superimposed atelectasis often sways one toward the direction of consolidation.

The similarity and overlap of radiographic findings seen with viral and mycoplasma infections is understandable since both infections involve the bronchi and pulmonary interstitium. Consolidations have been documented with *M. pneumoniae* infections, but they probably do not represent true alveolar air space consolidations. They probably represent the same **"pseudoconsolidation"** seen with viral disease wherein the interstitial disease process is so profound that the interstitium becomes very edematous and infiltrated and as such squeezes the air out of the alveoli. In addition, as with viral infections, these pseudoconsolidations tend to be more hazy than dense in their early stages (Fig. 1.144). True alveolar air space consolidations may be quite rare, or actually nonexistent, with *M. pneumoniae* infections. Obliterative bronchiolitis can be a complication of *M. pneumoniae* infections (3). This problem represents the end stage of severe bronchiolar inflammatory disease, and recently it has been demonstrated with high-resolution CT that the problem probably is more common than previously suspected (4).

REFERENCES

1. Guckel C, Benz-Bohm G, Widemann B. Mycoplasmal pneumonias in childhood: roentgen features, differential diagnosis, and review of the literatures. Pediatr Radiol 1989;19:499–503.
2. John SD, Ramanathan J, Swischuk LE. Spectrum of clinical and radiographic findings in pediatric mycoplasma pneumonia. Radiographics 2001;21:121–131.
3. Isles AF, Masel J, O'Duggy J. Obliterative bronchiolitis due to *Mycoplasma pneumoniae* infection in a child. Pediatr Radiol 1987;17:109–111.
4. Kim CK, Chung CY, Kim JS, et al. Late abnormal findings on high-resolution computed tomography after mycoplasma pneumonia. Pediatrics 2000;105:372–378.

Chlamydia Pneumonitis

Chlamydia pneumonitis (interstitial disease) characteristically occurs just after the newborn period (1, 2). The infecting organism, *Chlamydia trachomatis,* produces radiographic findings indistinguishable from those seen with

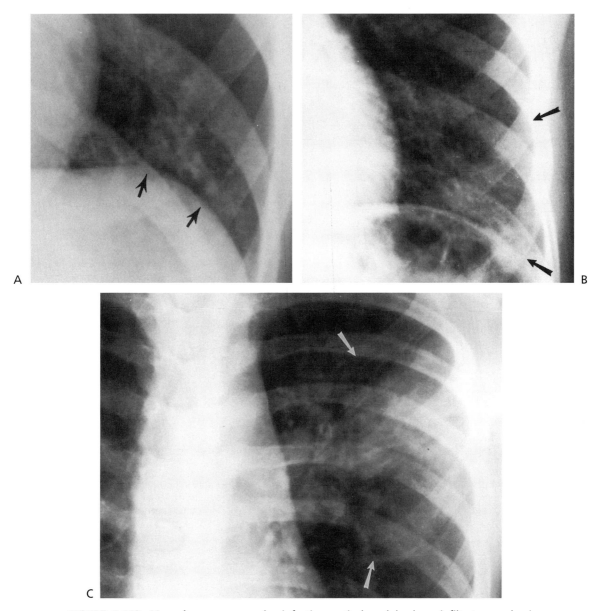

FIGURE 1.143. *Mycoplasma pneumoniae* infection: reticulonodular hazy infiltrates predominantly in one lobe. **A.** Note reticulonodular infiltrates in the left lower lobe (arrows). **B.** Another patient with more extensive reticularity (arrows) in the left lung base. **C.** In this patient, in the left upper lobe, reticulonodular infiltrates and bronchial wall thickening along with early diffuse parenchymal haziness are seen (arrows).

viral disease (i.e., parahilar peribronchial infiltrates with patches of segmental atelectasis) (1) (Fig. 1.145A). The clinical picture of moderate to severe respiratory distress and cough and marked eosinophilia should strongly suggest the diagnosis in a young infant. Febrile response often is minimal, but elevated IgG and IgM antibody titers usually are present. In the past, some of these cases were described as pertussoid eosinophilic pneumonitis, and understandably so, for the clinical and roentgenographic picture truly resembles that seen with pertussis.

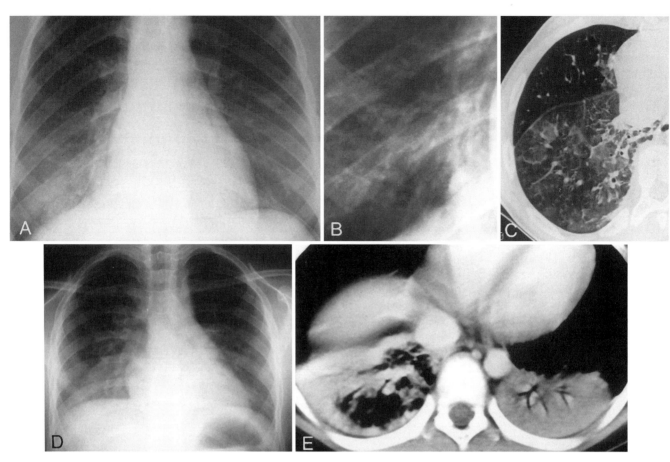

FIGURE 1.144. *Mycoplasma pneumoniae* infection: pseudoconsolidation. **A.** In this patient, note diffuse haziness in the right lower lobe, suggesting early pseudoconsolidation. **B.** Enlarged view of the right base shows diffuse haziness with some reticulonodularity, characteristic of interstitial disease. **C.** High-resolution computed tomography scan demonstrates ground-glass opacification typical of interstitial disease in the right lower lobe. Also note thickened bronchial walls. **D.** Another patient who presented with a high fever and demonstrates bilateral hazy basilar infiltrates suggesting pseudoconsolidation. **E.** Computed tomography scan demonstrates the bilateral lower lobe consolidations, with the one on the right showing some residual central aeration.

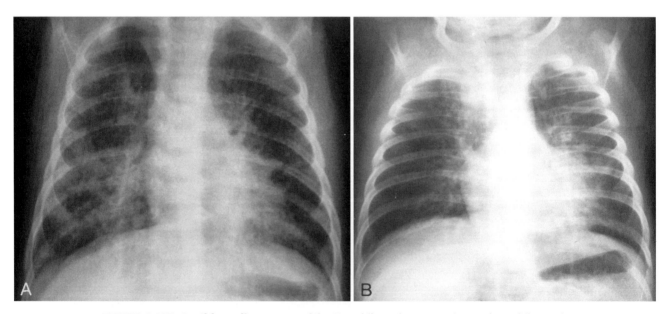

FIGURE 1.145. A. Chlamydia pneumonitis. Note bilateral overaeration and parahilar peribronchial infiltrates. **B. Pertussis.** Note extensive parahilar peribronchial infiltrates and bilateral overaeration. In both cases, the findings are virtually indistinguishable from those seen with viral lower respiratory tract infection.

REFERENCES

1. Attenburrow AA, Barker CM. Chlamydial pneumonia in the low birthweight neonate. Arch Dis Child 1985;60:1169–1172.
2. Radkowski MA, Kranzier JK, Beem MO, et al. Chlamydia pneumonia in infants: radiography in 125 cases. AJR 1981;137: 703–706.

Pertussis

Pertussis infection also resembles lower respiratory tract viral infection roentgenographically, and, indeed, it, too, is a bronchial, rather than an intraalveolar, infection. Clinically, the severe paroxysmal cough is the main clue to diagnosis. In most infants, chest findings consist of parahilar peribronchial infiltrates, with or without atelectasis (Fig. 1.145B). However, in one study, this pattern was present in only 25% of cases (1). The remaining cases showed clear but overdistended lungs, and this also has been our experience.

Because parahilar peribronchial infiltrates produce indistinctness of the mediastinal and cardiac edges, the term "shaggy heart" had, in the past, been utilized to describe the chest film (2). However, it should be noted that the commonest cause of the "shaggy heart" configuration is viral infection, after that mycoplasma infection, and then chlamydia and pertussis infections. Later on, if the initial pertussis infection goes unabated, much as with viral infections, the infant may develop a superimposed bacterial infection, producing consolidation, either lobar or widespread. However, currently, this complication seldom occurs.

REFERENCES

1. Bellamy EA, Johnston IDA, Wilson AG. The chest radiograph in whooping cough. Clin Radiol 1987;38:39–43.
2. Barnhard HJ, Kniker WT. Roentgenologic findings in pertussis. With particular emphasis on the "shaggy heart" sign. AJR 1960; 84:445–450.

Pneumocystis carinii Pneumonia (Plasma Cell Pneumonia)

Pneumocystis carinii pneumonia is caused by the organism *P. carinii,* a protozoan. It is an uncommon infection in the full-term neonate but occurs with greater frequency in premature infants or immunologically suppressed patients (1). The most common roentgenographic manifestation is that of hazy interstitial infiltrates of the lungs (2). Overaeration, emphysema, and absence of hilar lymph node enlargement also are clues to the diagnosis (Fig. 1.146). Less commonly, the infiltrate can appear more nodular, consolidative, or even as a solitary nodule (3).

REFERENCES

1. Stagno S, Pifer LL, Hughes WT, et al. *Pneumocystis carinii* pneumonitis in young immunocompetent infants. Pediatrics 1980;66:56–62.
2. Capitanio MA, Kirkpatrick JA Jr. *Pneumocystis carinii* pneumonia. AJR 1966;97:174–180.
3. Bier S, Halton K, Krivisky B, et al. *Pneumocystis carinii* pneumonia presenting as a single pulmonary nodule. Pediatr Radiol 1986; 16:59–60.

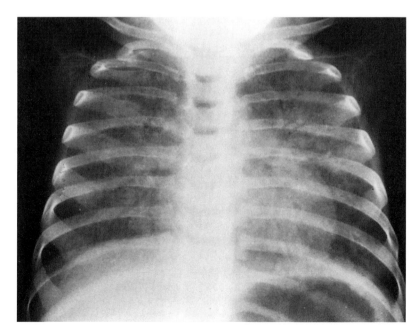

FIGURE 1.146. *Pneumocystis carinii* pneumonia. Note the generalized, hazy pattern of interstitial infiltration. Adenopathy is not prominent. More rarely, the infiltrates can appear nodular and fluffy.

Tuberculosis

Congenital tuberculosis, that is, infection of the fetus or unborn infant, is uncommon in America (1–3). In most such cases, the infection is acquired transplacentally, and the primary complex lodges in the liver and adjacent lymph nodes rather than in the lungs. Less commonly, the infant may swallow infected amniotic fluid and develop intestinal and mesenteric tuberculosis. Pulmonary findings in patients with congenital tuberculosis are variable and may not become apparent until 2 or 3 weeks after birth. Usually, widespread infiltrates, often nodular or fluffy, are seen, but miliary infiltrates also have been described (3).

In those infants in whom the infection is acquired after birth, pulmonary findings also are variable, and occasionally one may be fortunate enough to demonstrate the peripheral Ghon lesion (Fig. 1.147). In these cases, the inhalation of the organism from another infected individual is how the infection is acquired. In recent years, primary tuberculosis in children has seen a resurgence (4).

The roentgenographic findings of primary tuberculosis in the infant and older child are different from those seen in the immediate neonatal period. In this regard, **the radiographic hallmark of primary postnatal tuberculous infection of the lungs is unilateral, hilar, or paratracheal adenopathy, with or without associated atelectasis of the involved lung.** Bilateral adenopathy also can occur (5, 6), but unilateral adenopathy is more common, and in any case, it very often is accompanied by atelectasis (Fig. 1.148A). In these cases, while occasionally atelectasis may be secondary to compression of the bronchus by the enlarged lymph nodes (7), much more often it is due to endobronchial granulomatous disease causing obstruction. Hilar adenopathy often is more easily assessed on the lateral chest film (8) (Fig. 1.148B).

Obstructive emphysema also can be seen with primary tuberculosis but is much less frequent than atelectasis. Occasionally, consolidation of the lung also can occur (Fig. 1.149A), and once the infection erodes into the bloodstream, hematogenous spread leads to miliary tuberculosis (Fig. 1.149B). In older children, miliary tuberculosis is more classic in that very fine dots are seen scattered throughout the lung, almost blending into a diffuse haze. However, in infants, the nodules usually are larger and the resultant pattern is more reticulonodular than military (9, 10). Cavitary primary tuberculosis also occurs but is not common (11), and actually the cavities most likely represent pneumatoceles rather than true necrotic cavities (Fig. 1.49, C and D). Pleural effusions also can occur with primary tuberculosis (12).

Finally, it might be noted that some infants with pulmonary tuberculosis present with a surprisingly silent respiratory picture. Rather, they may present with signs and symptoms of meningitis. These patients may have a near-normal chest film and a negative skin test (6, 9), **and the findings of meningitis may so dominate the picture that tuberculosis, as a cause for the meningitis, is not considered until the chest film is obtained.**

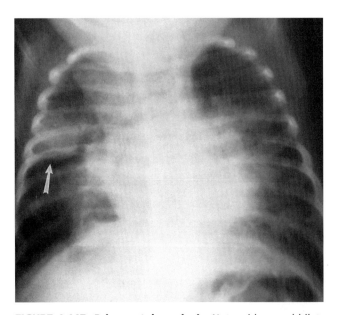

FIGURE 1.147. Primary tuberculosis. Note widespread bilateral parahilar infiltrates, right hilar adenopathy, and a peripheral Ghon lesion (arrows) in this 1-month-old infant who contracted tuberculosis from his mother. The triangular density in the right upper lobe probably represents atelectasis of the right upper lobe.

REFERENCES

1. Hageman J, Shulman S, Schreiber M, et al. Congenital tuberculosis: critical reappraisal of clinical findings and diagnostic procedures. Pediatrics 1980;66:980–984.
2. Myers JP, Perlstein PH, Light I J, et al. Tuberculosis in pregnancy with fatal congenital infection. Pediatrics 1981;67:89–94.
3. Stallworth JR, Brasfield DM, Tiller RE. Congenital miliary tuberculosis. Am J Dis Child 1980;134:320–321.
4. Amodio J, Abramson S, Berdon W. Primary pulmonary tuberculosis in infancy: a resurgent disease in the urban United States. Pediatr Radiol 1986;16:185–189.
5. Stansberry SD. Tuberculosis in infants and children. J Thorac Imag 1990;5:17–27.
6. Leung AN, Muller NL, Pineda PR, et al. Primary tuberculosis in childhood: radiographic manifestations. Radiology 1992;18:287–291.
7. Pereira KD, Mitchell RB, Eyen TP, et al. Tuberculous lymphadenopathy masquerading as a bronchial foreign body. Pediatr Emerg Care 1997;13:329–330.
8. Smuts NA, Beyers N, Gie RP, et al. Value of the lateral chest radiograph in tuberculosis in children. Pediatr Radiol 1994;24:478–480.
9. Hussey G, Ghisholm T, Kibel M. Miliary tuberculosis in children: a review of 94 cases. Pediatr Infect Dis J 1991;10:832–836.
10. Jamieson DHJ, Cremin BJ. High resolution CT of the lungs in

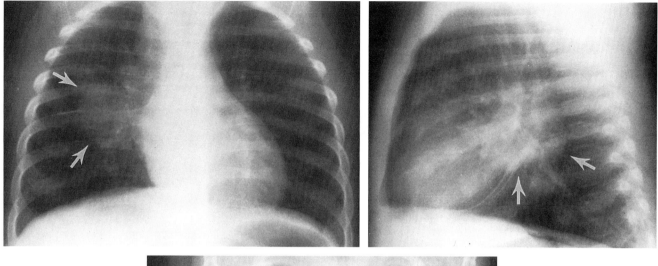

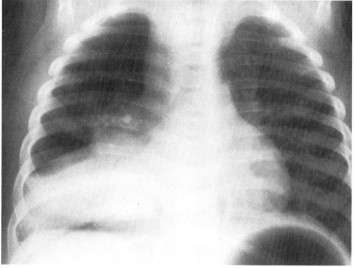

FIGURE 1.148. Tuberculosis with adenopathy. A. Note extensive right hilar and paratracheal adenopathy (arrows). **B.** Lateral view demonstrates the typical central location of the hilar adenopathy (arrows). **C.** Later, the patient develops atelectasis of the right middle and lower lobes. There is compensatory overinflation of the right upper lobe.

acute disseminated tuberculosis and a pediatric radiology perspective of the term "miliary." Pediatr Radiol 1993;23:380–383.

11. Weizman Z, Shvil Y, Ayalon A. Primary cavitary tuberculosis in an infant. Chest 1980;77:578.

12. Moon WK, Kim WS, Kim I-O, et al. Complicated pleural tuberculosis in children: CT evaluation. Pediatr Radiol 1999;29: 153–154.

Atypical Tuberculosis

Atypical tuberculosis is caused by *Mycobacterium tuberculosis*-related mycobacteria. Generally, the pulmonary changes are the same as those of ordinary tuberculosis, but there is less of a tendency to develop complications such as miliary or widespread bronchial spread. Most often, the findings consist of unilateral hilar or paratracheal adenopathy and atelectasis.

Fungal Infection

Fungal pulmonary infection in neonates is quite rare. However, neonatal candidiasis can be seen in premature infants with indwelling catheters associated with prolonged debilitating disease. The radiographic findings in any fungal infection are nonspecific and may consist of consolidations, parenchymal nodules, and fluffy or miliary infiltrates (1–4). Hilar and paratracheal adenopathy also frequently are

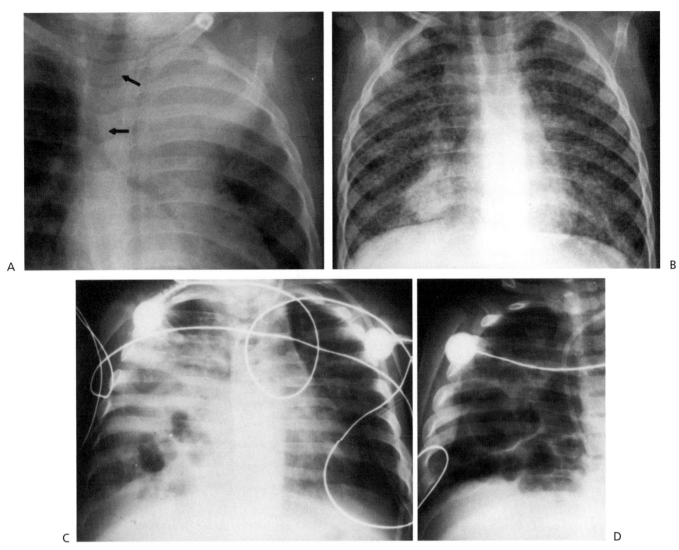

FIGURE 1.149. Tuberculosis: other manifestations. A. Left upper lobe consolidation. Note deviation of the trachea to the right, indicating the presence of paratracheal adenopathy. **B. Miliary tuberculosis.** Note extensive, fine nodules throughout both lungs. In addition, there is some right paratracheal adenopathy and a peripheral Ghon lesion in the right base. **C.** Another patient with cavities in a consolidated lung. **D.** With recovery, these cavities are seen to be pneumatoceles.

encountered, and in this regard, the findings mimic those of tuberculosis (Fig. 1.150). Associated pleural effusions also may be seen, and chest wall involvement can occur, especially with actinomycosis.

Allergic pulmonary aspergillosis is not as common in children as it is in adults. It can be seen in asthmatics, immunologically compromised patients, and patients with cystic fibrosis (5–7). The findings consist of nodular densities in the lungs, often "Y" shaped as they conform to the fungal-mucous plugs in the branching tracheobronchial tree. When the disease becomes invasive, parenchymal destruction is seen, and pneumothorax and pneumomediastinum can complicate the picture (6). In addition, systemic arterialization of an involved lobe can lead to so-called "pseudosequestration" (5).

Finally, a word is in order regarding acute histoplasmic inhalation. The disease process in these patients differs from the usual case of fungal pulmonary infection. Very often, these patients have just cleaned a chicken coop and inhaled the dust from the debris. There is a massive inhalation and inoculation of the histoplasmosis organism, and a diffuse inflammatory response in the lungs results in diffuse, fluffy infiltrates. **The history is key to diagnosis in these patients.**

REFERENCES

1. Alkrinawi S, Reed MH, Pasterkamp H. Pulmonary blastomycosis in children: findings on chest radiographs. AJR 1995;165: 651–654.

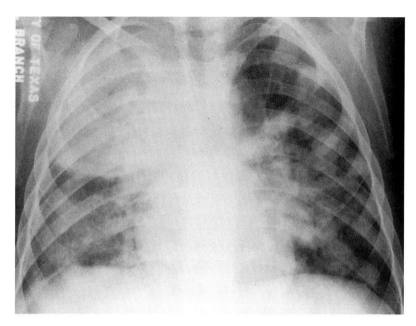

FIGURE 1.150. Actinomycosis. Note consolidation in the right upper lobe and numerous nodular infiltrates scattered throughout both lungs. All of these findings are typical of alveolar infiltrates seen with any fungal infection.

2. John SD, Swischuk LE. Fungus infections of the chest in infants and children. J Thorac Imag 1992;7:91–98.
3. Kim OH, Yang HR, Bahk YW. Pulmonary nocardiosis manifested as miliary nodules in a neonate—a case report. Pediatr Radiol 1992;22:229–230.
4. Chusid MJ, Sty JR, Wells RG. Pulmonary aspergillosis appearing as chronic nodular disease in chronic granulomatous disease. Pediatr Radiol 1988;18:232–234.
5. Matsuzono Y, Togashi T, Narita M, et al. Pulmonary aspergillosis and pseudosequestration of the lung in chronic granulomatous disease. Pediatr Radiol 1995;25:201–203.
6. Serrano-Gonzalez A, Merino-Arribas JM, Ruiz-Lopez MJ, et al. Invasive pulmonary aspergillosis with pneumopericardium and pneumothorax. Pediatr Radiol 1992;22:601–602.
7. Taccone A, Occhi M, Garaventa A, et al. CT of invasive pulmonary aspergillosis in children with cancer. Pediatr Radiol 1993; 23:177–180.

Syphilitic Pneumonitis

The roentgenographic findings of luetic infection in the lungs of the neonate or young infant are nonspecific and consist of reticulonodular or hazy-appearing lungs due to interstitial pneumonitis (1). The roentgenographic diagnosis most often depends on identification of typical osseous lesions (Fig. 1.151). In terms of the pneumonitis present in

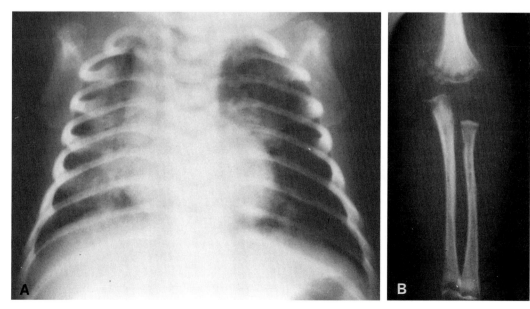

FIGURE 1.151. Pneumonia alba in congenital lues. A. Note nonspecific infiltrates throughout both lungs of this 2-month-old infant who presented with the nephrotic syndrome. **B.** Typical osseous lesions of congenital lues.

these patients, because of the pale, pink lungs, the problem often is referred to as "pneumonia alba."

REFERENCE

1. Pieper CH, van Gelderen WFC, Smith J, et al. Chest radiographs of neonates with respiratory failure caused by congenital syphilis. Pediatr Radiol 1995;25:198–200.

OTHER PULMONARY ABNORMALITIES

Cystic Fibrosis

Cystic fibrosis, inherited as an autosomal recessive trait, is a devastatingly progressive disease without cure. The main problem in patients suffering from it is the production of abnormally thick secretions by a variety of organs of the body. Usually, it is the lungs that receive most attention, but in the neonate, the most common manifestation is low small bowel obstruction secondary to meconium ileus. Cystic fibrosis is a disease primarily of the white race; it also can occur in blacks, but much less commonly (1, 2). Furthermore, the disease can show considerable variation in terms of severity, and currently patients are surviving longer because of more effective supportive therapy (3).

As far as the pulmonary findings in cystic fibrosis are concerned, it might be noted that infants with cystic fibrosis often first present with recurrent and refractory bronchiolitis. Thick mucous secretions aggravate the viral infection, producing the bronchiolitis, and widespread air trapping

results. Consequently, the lungs are overaerated, and, as with viral infections, areas of lobar and segmental atelectasis are common (Fig. 1.152A).

In terms of the roentgenographic chest findings in cystic fibrosis, it should be appreciated that lung consolidations are not particularly common. These patients develop all sorts of changes related to bronchial (airway) disease, but classic consolidations are uncommon. Later, as repeated infections take their toll, chronic atelectasis, fibrosis, and bronchiectasis result (Fig. 1.152B). In addition to these problems, as the chronic infection becomes more deeply embedded, its need for a greater blood supply leads to parasitization of the systemic blood flow to the lungs. In other words, collaterals from the hypertrophied bronchial arteries connect at their peripheries with the pulmonary vasculature, and when these communications become large enough, arteriovenous fistula formation and hemoptysis result. Refractory pneumothoraces also can be a problem in these patients (4).

High-resolution CT is now available for evaluation of these patients (5–7). However, it has been determined that for mapping of lung pathology in these patients, the CT study is not as effective as is single-photon emission perfusion nuclear scintigraphy. In addition, the chest film still is the main imaging modality with which these patients are initially and continuously evaluated. CT should be used when complications arise and is especially beneficial in the mapping of bronchiectasis.

In addition to the pulmonary problems, because thick, exocrine secretions are a generalized problem in these patients, other organ systems sooner or later become

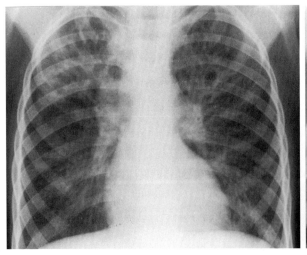
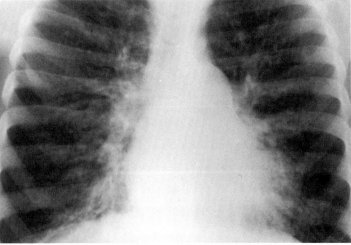

A   B

FIGURE 1.152. Cystic fibrosis. A. Extensive changes in an older child, consisting of chronic, streaky parahilar peribronchial infiltration, hilar adenopathy, and bronchiectatic changes especially evident in the upper lobes. **B.** Another patient with typical chronic parahilar peribronchial infiltrates and thickening of the bronchial walls (i.e., bronchial cuffing and railroad tracking). In addition, note that the pulmonary artery (arrow) is prominent and that the heart is enlarged. These findings are due to pulmonary hypertension as this patient also had cor pulmonale.

involved, for example, sinusitis (8), nasal polyps, and in the gastrointestinal tract meconium ileus equivalent in older children, fatty liver, cholestasis, gallstones, cholecystitis, and biliary cirrhosis. Recurrent pancreatitis also becomes a problem, and the pancreas slowly undergoes atrophy with resultant pancreatic insufficiency, malabsorption, and, in some cases, diabetes mellitus. Calcifications of the pancreas also occur. An interesting manifestation is aspermia due to blockage of the vas deferens or actual atrophy of this structure early in infancy (9).

Numerous radiographic classifications, both plain film and CT motivated, are available for the categorization of the severity of cystic fibrosis (10–12).

REFERENCES

1. McColley SA, Rosenstein BJ, Cutting GR. Differences in expression of cystic fibrosis in blacks and whites. Am J Dis Child 1991; 145:94–97.
2. Hamoch A, Fitz-Simmons SC, Macek M Jr, et al. Comparison of the clinical manifestations of cystic fibrosis in black and white patients. J Pediatr 1998;132:255–259.
3. FitzSimmons SC. The changing epidemiology of cystic fibrosis. J Pediatr 1993;122:1–9.
4. McLaughlin FJ, Matthews WJ, Strieder DJ, et al. Pneumothorax in cystic fibrosis: management and outcome. J Pediatr 1982;100: 863–869.
5. Brody AS, Molina PL, Klein JS, et al. High-resolution computed tomography of the chest in children with cystic fibrosis: support for use as an outcome surrogate. Pediatr Radiol 1999;29: 731–735.
6. Santamaria F, Grillo G, Guidi G, et al. Cystic fibrosis: when should high-resolution computed tomography of the chest be obtained? Pediatrics 1998;101:908–913.
7. Donnelly LF, Gelfand MJ, Brody AS, et al. Comparison between morphologic changes seen on high-resolution CT and regional pulmonary perfusion seen on SPECT in patients with cystic fibrosis. Pediatr Radiol 1997;27:920–925.
8. Wiatrak BJ, Myer CM III, Cotton RT. Cystic fibrosis presenting with sinus disease in children. Am J Dis Child 1993;147: 258–260.
9. Auguiano A, Oates RD, Amos JA, et al. Congenital bilateral absence of the vas deferens: a primarily genital form of cystic fibrosis. JAMA 1992;267:1794–1797.
10. Bhalla M, Turcios N, Aponte V, et al. Cystic fibrosis: scoring system with thin-section CT. Radiology 1991;179:783–788.
11. Meerman GJ, Dankert-Roelse J, Martijn A, et al. A comparison of the Schwachman, Chrispin-Norman and Brasfield methods for scoring the chest radiographs of patients with cystic fibrosis. Pediatr Radiol 1985;15:98–101.
12. Weatherly MR, Palmer CGS, Peters ME, et al. Wisconsin cystic fibrosis chest radiograph scoring system. Pediatrics 1993;91: 488–495.

Asthma

Asthma is not a problem of very young infants, although children who become asthmatics often present with repeated episodes of bronchiolitis or viral lower respiratory tract infection in the first year or two of life. Nonetheless, most asthmatics are not clearly declared (except by their grandmothers, who usually know what is going on) until after the age of 2 years.

Roentgenographically, the most common findings are overaeration and parahilar peribronchial infiltrates, virtually indistinguishable from those seen with viral lower respiratory tract infection (Fig. 1.153). In addition, much as with viral infection, these patients develop areas of segmental and lobar atelectasis, which frequently are misinter-

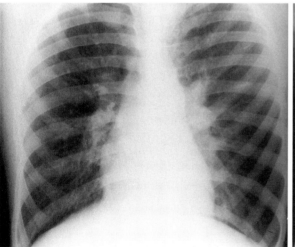
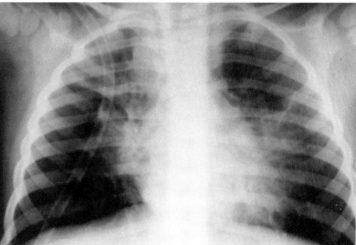

A B

FIGURE 1.153. Asthma. A. Note typical overaeration, parahilar peribronchial radiating infiltrates, and hilar prominence. **B.** Another patient with a superimposed viral infection leading to more extensive parahilar peribronchial infiltrates and bilateral areas of scattered wedge-like segmental atelectasis.

preted for bacterial consolidations. However, it should be noted that patients with asthma are not particularly susceptible to bacterial infections. Viral and mycoplasma lower respiratory tract infections are the problem for they play havoc with the already compromised respiratory tract of asthmatics (1–3). Complications of asthma include pneumomediastinum and pneumothorax, but pneumomediastinum is more common by far. Transient pulmonary hypertension due to the obstructive emphysema present can lead to prominence of the pulmonary artery, but this complication is not considered a significant problem.

Very often, in asthmatics, the baseline chest film appears exactly the same as the film of a patient with viral parahilar peribronchial infiltrates. Indeed, when asthmatics acquire a superimposed viral infection, it is difficult to tell the two patterns apart. Because the problem is bronchitic (airway) rather than alveolar (air space), patients with asthma have the same propensity to develop atelectasis as do those patients with viral bronchitis. There also is the same propensity to misinterpret the areas of atelectasis for areas of consolidation. When bacterial consolidation occurs in an asthmatic, it occurs as a separate entity, and the clinical picture is quite different. Bacterial consolidations do not cause exacerbation of the patient's asthma (1). Viral and mycoplasma infections, on the other hand, do cause exacerbation of asthma (1–3).

It is debatable as to just how important it is to obtain chest radiographs with asthma exacerbation. In this regard, it recently has been suggested that chest radiographs be obtained only when barotrauma (pneumothorax, pneumomediastinum) is suspected or persistent high fever or localized physical findings are present (4). We are currently studying this aspect of asthma and lower respiratory tract infection, and our preliminary results suggest that patients who are wheezing and have a low-grade fever probably do not require chest radiographs. **They will be normal or show potentially confusing atelectasis along with parahilar peribronchial infiltrates.** On the other hand, infants with high fever could have a superimposed bacterial infection. In this regard, even though it is very uncommon to have a bacterial infection result in exacerbation of asthma, one cannot afford not to obtain a chest radiograph. At the same time, however, it should be appreciated that the likelihood of discovering a consolidating pneumonia is low, but that the likelihood of discovering atelectasis, which could be confused with pneumonia, is high.

REFERENCES

1. McIntosh K, Ellis EF, Hoffman LS, et al. The association of viral and bacterial respiratory infections with exacerbations of wheezing in young asthmatic children. J Pediatr 1973;82:578–590.
2. Minor TE, Dick EC, DeMeo AN, et al. Viruses as precipitants of asthmatic attacks in children. JAMA 1974;227:292–298.
3. Mitchell I, Inglis H, Simpson H. Viral infection in wheezy bronchitis and asthma in children. Arch Dis Child 1976;51:707–711.
4. Faiqa Q. Management of children with acute asthma in the emergency department. Pediatr Emerg Care 1999;15:206–213.

Aspiration Pneumonia

Aspiration pneumonia is common in young infants, and usually the aspirate is gastric contents or oropharyngeal secretions. Infants with esophageal atresia, tracheoesophageal fistula, pharyngeal incoordination, vascular rings, familial dysautonomia (Riley-Day syndrome), and high gastrointestinal obstruction are especially prone to aspirate.

In cases where aspiration is massive, bilateral fluffy infiltrates are seen. In infants, if aspiration is related to the supine or recumbent-oblique position in which infants frequently are fed, right upper lobe atelectasis may be seen and be the predominant finding. When aspiration becomes a chronic problem, pulmonary fibrosis ensues, and chronic parahilar peribronchial streaky infiltrates similar to those seen with viral bronchitis and asthma develop.

Aspiration also occurs when hydrocarbons are accidentally ingested. These substances, because they destroy surfactant (1), play havoc with the respiratory tract. Usually, the changes are most profound in the lung bases (lower lobes) medially (Fig. 1.154, A and B). However, the first film often shows little or no change, but within 24 hours, infiltrates develop. These result from areas of focal atelectasis and, if severe enough, hemorrhage and edema. Pneumatoceles also may develop during the recovery phase (2, 3). Hydrocarbons with the least viscosity are the most injurious. Among these is red furniture polish, which contains mineral seal oil (1).

Aspiration of lipoid materials is less common (4, 5), but I have encountered a case wherein mineral oil was ill advisedly administered to a constipated infant whose basic problem was Hirschsprung's disease (Fig. 1.154D). The infiltrates with lipid aspiration often are very dense centrally and in the lung bases. Histologically, a dense, reactive lymphocytosis has been noted (5).

Massive aspiration of acidic gastric contents can lead to extensive pulmonary edema (Fig. 1.154C) and lung destruction. The term "Mendelson's syndrome" is applied to this condition (6). An unusual form of aspiration is that of massive baby powder aspiration. This can cause severe respiratory distress and pulmonary edema (7). Similarly, sand aspiration can cause severe respiratory compromise (8), and finally occult aspiration can be detected with a radionuclide sialogram (9, 10).

REFERENCES

1. Giamonna ST. Effects of furniture polish on pulmonary surfactant. Am J Dis Child 1967;113:6:658–663.

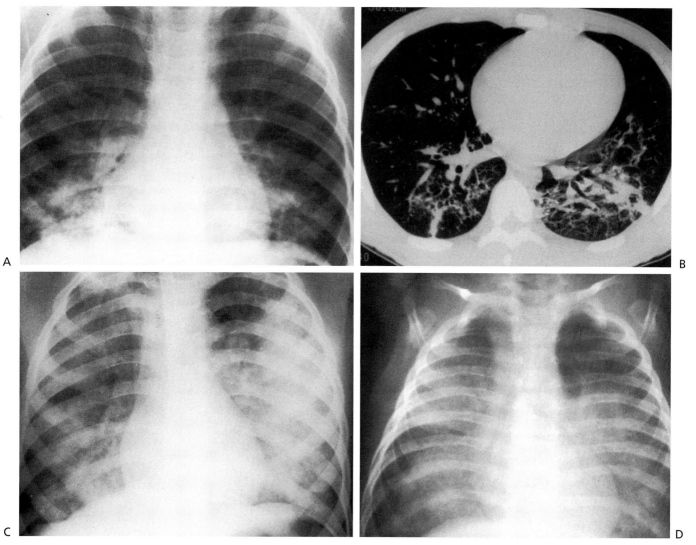

FIGURE 1.154. Aspiration pneumonia. A. Typical basal distribution of patchy, nodular infiltrates seen in hydrocarbon aspiration. **B.** Another patient whose computed tomography study demonstrates the typical posterior dependent location of the infiltrates. **C.** Massive aspiration with pulmonary edema producing bilaterally opaque lungs. This is termed **"Mendelson's syndrome"** and is due to aspiration of acid gastric contents. **D.** Diffuse, hazy infiltrates secondary to lipid aspiration.

2. Bergeson PS, Hales SW, Lustgarten MD, et al. Pneumatoceles following hydrocarbon ingestion. Am J Dis Child 1975;129: 49–54.

3. Harris VJ, Brown R. Pneumatoceles as a complication of chemical pneumonia after hydrocarbon ingestion. AJR 1975;125: 531–537.

4. de Oliveira GA, Del Caro SR, Lamego CMB, et al. Radiographic plain film and CT findings in lipoid pneumonia in infants following aspiration of mineral oil used in the treatment of partial small bowel obstruction by *Ascaris lumbridoides.* Pediatr Radiol 1985;15:157–160.

5. Hugosson CO, Riff EJ, Moore CCM, et al. Lipoid pneumonia in infants: a radiological-pathological study. Pediatr Radiol 1991; 21:193–197.

6. Esquirol E, Bruneton JN, Larroque CH, et al. Mendelson's syndrome; a radiological study. Ann Radiol 1974;17:523–530.

7. Motampsu K, Adachi H, Uno T. Two infant deaths after inhaling baby powder. Chest 1979;75:448–450.

8. Choy IO, Idowu O. Sand aspiration: a case report. J Pediatr Surg 1996;31:1448–1450.

9. Heyman S, Respondek M. Detection of pulmonary aspiration in children by radionuclide "salivagram." J Nucl Med 1989;30: 697–699.

10. Bar-Sever Z, Connolly LP, Treves ST. The radionuclide salivagram in children with pulmonary disease and a high risk of aspiration. Pediatr Radiol 1995;25:S180–S183.

Airway Foreign Bodies

Airway foreign bodies, if opaque, are readily identified on chest films. Generally, in the past, it was considered that most foreign bodies in children passed into the right bronchus, but over the years, it has been demonstrated that the incidence of right and left foreign bodies is about equal (1–3). If the foreign body lodges in the larynx, the problem usually is quite acute, and films generally are not obtained prior to its removal. Tracheal foreign bodies also are rather uncommon, and in these patients, inspiratory chest films may show inadequate distention of the lungs and paradoxical dilatation of the heart (4). Another unusual manifestation of foreign body aspiration is that which occurs when numerous small fragments are inhaled deep into the airway. Respiratory distress is severe, and the patients behave just as do those infants with viral bronchiolitis or severe emphysema (5). There is very little to see on the roentgenogram except overaerated lungs.

More commonly, the foreign body lodges in a major bronchus and most often causes obstructive emphysema (Fig. 1.155, A and B). This is readily detected on chest

films, but if in doubt, one should obtain inspiratory-expiratory sequences (Fig. 1.155, C and D). This is most important for the inspiratory film may be normal in up to 25–33% of cases (6, 7). In other cases, one may obtain decubitus films whereupon, with the involved side down, the overdistended lung will not collapse (8). However, most often this is not required, as inspiratory-expiratory films suffice. If, however, further documentation is required in questionable cases, fluoroscopy is in order. In addition, in some cases, the location of the foreign body in a bronchus can be ascertained by noting the interrupted air-filled bronchus, as the interrupted bronchus sign (9).

It might also be noted that, in some cases, a foreign body may produce atelectasis (6) rather than emphysema (Fig. 1.156, A and B). Such atelectasis may be acute but more often is chronic and may be associated with pneumonia (Fig. 1.156C), empyema, or even abscess formation. Longstanding foreign bodies usually present as chronic pulmonary infec-

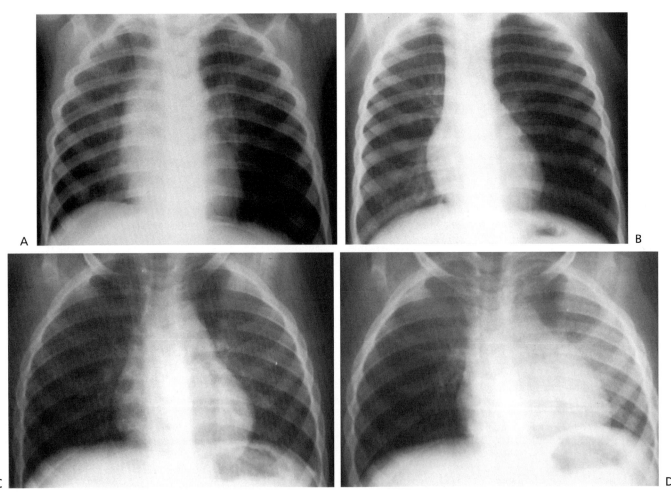

FIGURE 1.155. Airway foreign bodies. A. Classic left endobronchial foreign body. Note the markedly overdistended, hyperlucent left lung causing shift of the mediastinum to the right. **B. Less pronounced findings.** Note slight enlargement and hyperlucency of the left lung. **C. Subtle changes.** The right lung is only slightly larger and darker than the left lung. **D.** Expiratory view clearly shows air trapping in the right lung. The left lung empties normally.

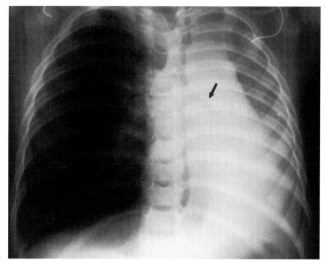
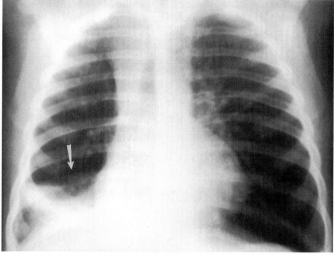
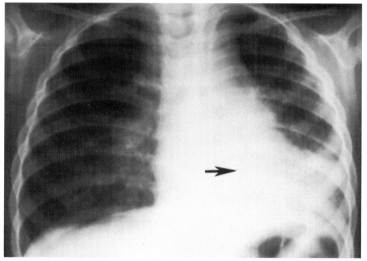

A

B

C

FIGURE 1.156. Foreign body: atelectasis and pneumonia. A. Total atelectasis of the left lung with overaeration of the right lung. Note cut-off of the air column of the left bronchus (arrow). **B.** Chronic atelectasis of the right lower lobe (arrow) due to a tack in the right bronchus. **C. Pneumonia with volume loss.** Note left lower lobe pneumonia and volume loss due to superimposed atelectasis, secondary to a chronic foreign body. The mediastinum is shifted to the left (arrow). With acute pneumonia, atelectasis (volume loss) is not a feature.

tions. This tends to occur with less irritating foreign bodies (i.e., plastic, chicken bones, seeds, etc.). Oily foreign bodies such as peanuts or popcorn produce a more severe bronchial mucosal reaction and bring the patient in sooner. One of the reasons that less irritating foreign bodies may become chronic is that, as can occur with all foreign bodies, **once the initial coughing episode is over, the patients may be surprisingly asymptomatic.** Pneumothorax and pneumomediastinum are rare complications of airway foreign bodies (10, 11).

REFERENCES

1. Blazer S, Naveh Y, Friedman A. Foreign body in the airway: review of 200 cases. Am J Dis Child 1980;134:68–71.

2. Cleveland RH. Symmetry of bronchial angles in children. Radiology 1979;133:89–93.

3. Linegar AG, van Oppel UO, Hegemann S, et al. Tracheobronchial foreign bodies: experience at Red Cross Children's Hospital. S Afr Med J 1992;82:164–167.

4. Capitanio MA, Kirkpatrick JA. Obstructions of the upper airway in children as reflected on the chest radiograph. Radiology 1973; 107:159–161.

5. Swischuk LE. Acute respiratory distress with cyanosis. Pediatr Emerg Care 1987;3:209–210.

6. Laks Y, Barzilay Z. Foreign body aspiration in childhood. Pediatr Emerg Care 1988;4:102–106.

7. Svedstrom E, Puhakka H, Kero P. How accurate is chest radiography in the diagnosis of tracheobronchial foreign bodies in children? Pediatr Radiol 1989;19:520–522.

8. Capitanio MA, Kirkpatrick JA. The lateral decubitus film, an aid in determining air-trapping in children. Radiology 1972;103: 460–462.

9. Lim-Dunham JE, Yousefzadeh DK. The interrupted bronchus: a fluoroscopic sign of bronchial foreign body in infants and children. AJR 1999;173:969–972.

10. Burton EM, Riggs W Jr, Kaufman RA, et al. Pneumomediastinum caused by foreign body aspiration in children. Pediatr Radiol 1989;20:45–47.

11. Saoji R, Ramchandra C, D'Cruz AJ. Subcutaneous emphysema: an unusual presentation of foreign body in the airway. J Pediatr Surg 1995;30:860–862.

α₁-ANTITRYPSIN DEFICIENCY

α_1-Antitrypsin deficiency is not a common problem in infancy but later on can produce overaeration mimicking bronchiolitis or cystic fibrosis (1). In infants, liver parenchymal disease most often first brings the patient to the attention of the physician.

REFERENCE

1. Talamo RC, Levison H, Lynch MJ, et al. Symptomatic pulmonary emphysema in childhood associated with hereditary A₁ antitrypsin and elastase inhibitor deficiency. J Pediatr 1971;79:20–26.

Cutis Laxa

Cutis laxa is an uncommon condition where there is generalized elastic tissue deficiency throughout the body. In the lungs, lack of this elastic tissue in the tracheobronchial tree results in collapse of the airway during expiration and thus widespread overaeration (1–3). In addition, lung cysts can be encountered. These cysts are transient and probably represent pneumatoceles rather than true cysts (4, 5). This would be in keeping with the obstructive emphysema seen in these patients.

REFERENCES

1. Lally JF, Gohel VK, Dalinka MK, et al. The roentgenographic manifestations of cutis laxa (generalized elastolysis). Radiology 1974;113:605–606.

2. Meine F, Grossman H, Forman W, et al. The radiographic findings in congenital cutis laxa. Radiology 1974;113:687–690.

3. Merten DF, Rooney R. Progressive pulmonary emphysema associated with congenital generalized elastolysis (cutis laxa). Radiology 1974;113:691–692.

4. Baumer JH, Hankey S. Transient pulmonary cysts in an infant with the Ehlers-Danlos syndrome. Br J Radiol 1980;53:598–599.

5. Herman TE, Mcalister WH. Cavitary pulmonary lesions in type IV Ehlers-Danlos syndrome. Pediatr Radiol 1994;24:263–265.

Milk Allergy (Heiner's Syndrome)

Heiner's syndrome results in chronic coughing, dyspnea, wheezing, and recurrent episodes of allergic pneumonia (1).

In addition, iron deficiency anemia is present. Diagnosis depends on recognizing the clinical and roentgenographic findings and demonstrating circulating milk antibodies. The roentgenographic findings are not specific (2, 3) and consist of recurrent pulmonary infiltrates that tend to wax and wane. Clearing usually occurs with the withdrawal of milk from the infant's diet.

In some of the cases originally reported by Heiner et al. (1) and in some more recently reported cases (4), pulmonary hemosiderosis also was present. It has been considered, therefore, that a relationship between this syndrome and idiopathic pulmonary hemosiderosis might exist. However, no conclusive evidence for such an association is available.

REFERENCES

1. Heiner DC, Sears JW, Knicker WT. Multiple precipitins to cow's milk in chronic respiratory disease. A syndrome involving poor growth, gastrointestinal symptoms, evidence of allergy, iron deficiency anemia, and pulmonary hemosiderosis. Am J Dis Child 1962;103:634–654.

2. Chang CH, Wittig HJ. Heiner's syndrome. Radiology 1969;92:507–508.

3. Diner WC, Knicker WT, Heiner DC. Roentgenologic manifestations in the lungs in milk allergy. Radiology 1961;77:564–572.

4. Boat TE, Polmar SH, Whitman V, et al. Hyperreactivity to cow milk in young children with pulmonary hemosiderosis and cor pulmonale secondary to nasopharyngeal obstruction. J Pediatr 1975;87:23–29.

Idiopathic Pulmonary Hemosiderosis

Although idiopathic pulmonary hemosiderosis usually affects children over the age of 1 year (1), infants as young as 10 months (2) have been reported. In the acute phase, marked respiratory distress, cyanosis, and hemoptysis are present. Hemoptysis is a most important feature of the disease but, unfortunately, is not always present in very young infants. Hypochromic anemia is also present and, in some cases, may be the presenting problem. The disease is progressive and usually fatal, and after many bouts of hemorrhage, the lungs show interstitial fibrosis and widespread hemosiderin deposits. Pulmonary hypertension with cor pulmonale usually eventually develops. Steroid therapy has been temporarily effective in some cases.

Roentgenographically, the findings are nonspecific, but when taken in context with the clinical findings, they should suggest the diagnosis. Small hemorrhages into the lungs manifest as patchy areas of alveolar infiltration, and during acute attacks, infiltration may be extensive (Fig. 1.157, A and B). Remissions are common, and with clinical remission, there is usually roentgenographic clearing. Because of the nonspecificity of the pulmonary infiltrates, one may, at first, believe them to be inflammatory or allergic. Eventually, with repeated bouts of bleeding into the

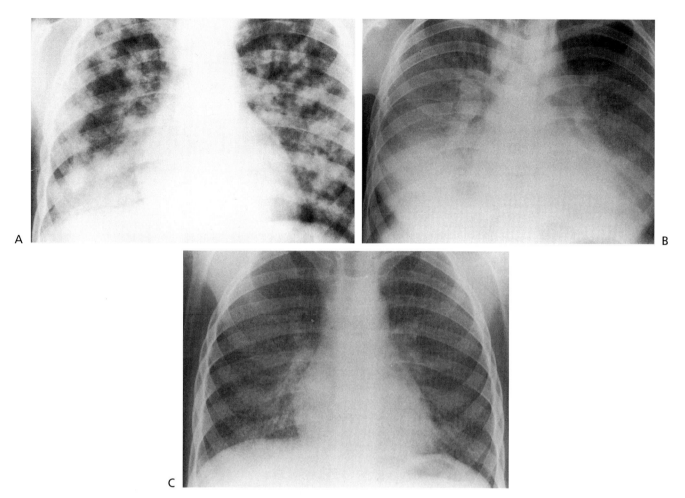

FIGURE 1.157. Pulmonary hemosiderosis. A. Acute phase demonstrating multiple fluffy alveolar infiltrates due to bleeding into the parenchyma. **B.** Another patient with acute bleeding into the lung, resulting in near-total opacification of both lungs. Some pleural fluid is present on the right, along the lateral chest wall, and in the minor fissure. Pleural fluid is also present on the left. **C.** Pulmonary fibrosis in another patient, resulting in miliary infiltrates producing haziness of the lungs.

lung, pulmonary fibrosis is seen, and then one may see diffuse haziness of the lungs or even a diffuse miliary or reticulonodular infiltrate (Fig. 1.157C).

REFERENCES

1. Foulon E, Nogues C, Joron F, et al. Idiopathic pulmonary hemosiderosis in children; two cases. Ann Pediatr 1974;21:145–160.
2. Repetto G, Lisboa C, Emparanza E, et al. Idiopathic pulmonary hemosiderosis; clinical, radiologic and respiratory function studies. Pediatrics 1967;40:24–32.

Pulmonary Fibrosis (Fibrosing Alveolitis and Hamman-Rich Syndrome)

Pulmonary fibrosis is not common in childhood but does occur (1). Clinically, there is progressive respiratory insufficiency, and roentgenographically, diffuse interstitial fibrosis causes increasing haziness of the lung fields. A familial form of pulmonary fibrosis also has been described (2). Pulmonary fibrosis (fibrosing alveolitis) also can be seen with viral pneumonitis, idiopathic pulmonary hemosiderosis (late stages), and as the aftermath of lung injuries secondary to drugs, intoxicant inhalants, and chronic pulmonary edema.

REFERENCES

1. Hewitt CJ, Hull D, Keeling JW. Fibrosing alveolitis in infancy and childhood. Arch Dis Child 1977;52:22–37.
2. Nezelof C, Brieu A, Beal G, et al. Familial pulmonary fibrosis; two cases. Ann Pediatr 1974;21:135–144.

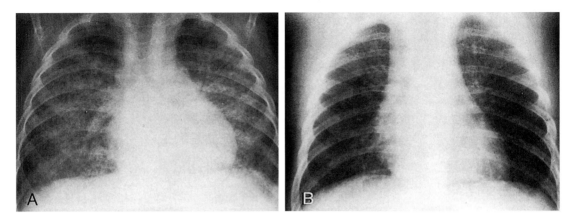

FIGURE 1.158. Reticuloendotheliosis. A. Note numerous reticulonodular infiltrates in this infant with Letterer-Siwe disease. **B.** In this patient, hilar adenopathy and some streaky parahilar infiltrates are present.

Reticuloendothelioses and Histiocytoses of the Lung

The reticuloendothelioses, or Langerhans' cell histiocytoses, that most commonly involve the lung in young infants are the nonlipid Letterer-Siwe disease and Hand-Schüller-Christian disease (cholesterol storage disease). Less commonly, eosinophilic granuloma can produce pulmonary infiltration, but, no matter what the underlying condition, pulmonary involvement in infants under 4–6 months of age is uncommon (1). Roentgenographically, the pattern often consists of symmetric bilateral reticulonodular infiltrates (Fig.1.158A), hilar and paratracheal lymphadenopathy, and, in some cases, honeycombing or cystic change of the lungs (2, 3). Similar interstitial infiltrates can be seen in the severe infantile forms of Gaucher's disease and Niemann-Pick disease. Other patients may show hilar adenopathy (Fig. 1.158B).

REFERENCES

1. Vade A, Hayani A, Pierce K. Congenital histiocytosis X. Pediatr Radiol 1993;23:181–182.
2. Carlson RA, Hattery RB, O'Connell EJ, et al. Pulmonary involvement by histiocytosis X in the pediatric age group. Mayo Clin Proc 1976;51:542–547.
3. Moore A, Godwin JD, Muller NL, et al. Pulmonary histiocytosis X: comparison of radiographic and CT findings. Radiology 1989;172:249–254.

Sarcoidosis

Sarcoidosis in young infants is very uncommon. In fact, young infants are more apt to present with one of its other nonpulmonary manifestations such as arthritis, uveitis, or renal disease (1). In older children, pulmonary manifestations are not particularly different from those seen in young adults and consist of hilar or paratracheal adenopathy (Fig. 1.159), fluffy alveolar infiltrates, or variable interstitial infiltration (2).

REFERENCES

1. Hetherington S. Sarcoidosis in young children. Am J Dis Child 1982;136:13–15.
2. Harris RO, Spock A. Childhood sarcoidosis: pulmonary infiltrates as an early sign in a very young child. Clin Pediatr 1978;17: 119–121.

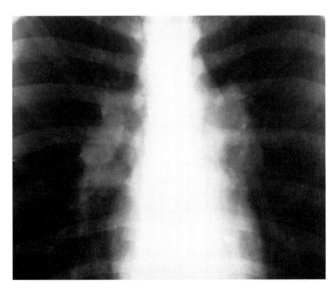

FIGURE 1.159. Sarcoidosis. Note clear lungs but bilateral hilar adenopathy.

Pulmonary Alveolar Proteinosis (Surfactant B Deficiency)

Pulmonary alveolar proteinosis can be seen in children, infants, and even neonates (1, 2). The abnormality arises from the degeneration of abnormally enlarged alveolar pneumocytes (3). These cells (type II pneumocytes) accumulate proteinaceous matter within them and eventually, as they disintegrate, deposit it into the pulmonary interstitium and alveolar space (3, 4). Eventually, pulmonary fibrosis results (3). Unlike some cases reported in adults, pulmonary alveolar proteinosis is usually a fatal disease in young infants. It is also termed "surfactant B deficiency disease" (5–7).

The roentgenographic findings usually consist of bilateral radiating parahilar infiltrates (8) (Fig. 1.160). Although they can appear finely nodular, they can also coalesce and bear a striking resemblance to the typical butterfly configuration of pulmonary edema. In other cases, the soft, fluffy infiltrates extend far into the periphery of the lungs. On CT imaging, one sees a diffuse ground-glass appearance to the parenchyma and prominent interlobular septa (9).

REFERENCES

1. Mahut B, Delacourt C, Scheinmann P, et al. Pulmonary alveolar proteinosis: experience with eight pediatric cases and a review. Pediatrics 1996;97:117–122.
2. Schumacher RE, Marrogi AJ, Heidelberger KP. Pulmonary alveolar proteinosis in a newborn. Pediatr Pulmonol 1989;7:178–182.
3. Farrell PM, Gilbert EF, Zimmerman JJ, et al. Familial lung disease associated with proliferation and desquamation of type II pneumonocytes. Am J Dis Child 1986;140:262–266.
4. Albafouille V, Sayegh N, De Coudenhove S, et al. CT scan patterns of pulmonary alveolar proteinosis in children. Pediatr Radiol 1999;29:147–152.
5. Ballard PL, Nogee LM, Beers MF, et al. Partial deficiency of surfactant protein B in an infant with chronic lung disease. Pediatrics 1995;96:1046–1052.
6. deMello DE, Nogee LM, Heyman S. Molecular and phenotypic variability in the congenital alveolar proteinosis syndrome associated with inherited surfactant protein B deficiency. J Pediatr 1994;125:43–50.
7. Nogee LM, Garnier G, Dietz HC, et al. A mutation in the surfactant protein B gene responsible for fatal neonatal respiratory disease in multiple kindreds. J Clin Invest 1994;93:1860–1863.
8. Herman TE, Nogee LM, McAlister WH, et al. Surfactant protein B deficiency: radiographic manifestations. Pediatr Radiol 1993;23:373–375.
9. Newman B, Kuhn JP, Kramer SS, et al. Congenital surfactant protein B deficiency—emphasis on imaging. Pediatr Radiol 2001;31:327–331.

Protozoan Disease

Protozoan lung disease is not particularly common in children unless the child lives in an endemic area. The lungs can be involved with visceral larva migrans, and involvement can be severe (1). Generally, the infiltrates are nonspecific but often widespread (2). The organism *Strongyloidies stercoralis,* a nematode, also may involve the lung, producing nonspecific infiltrates, but this time often more lobar than widespread. Associated findings may be seen in the gastrointestinal tract. Pulmonary paragonimiasis can produce consolidations with abscess formation simulating ordinary lung abscesses (3). The condition is caused by the parasite *Paragonimus westereni,* an organism present in freshwater crabs and crayfish.

Finally, echinococcal involvement of the lung is quite common in Alaska and the Canadian Northwest. The dis-

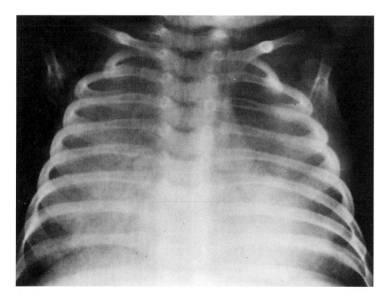

FIGURE 1.160. Pulmonary alveolar proteinosis. Ten-week-old infant with extensive bilateral pulmonary infiltration. Note that the costophrenic angles are spared and that infiltration is most pronounced centrally. (Reproduced with permission from Singleton EB, Wagner MI. Radiologic atlas of pulmonary abnormalities in children. Philadelphia: Saunders, 1971).

ease is caused by the tapeworm *Echinococcus granulosus,* whose definitive host is the dog or wolf. The pulmonary parenchyma is involved in the form of a cyst of one type or another. Most commonly, the cysts are fluid filled and consist of two layers: the exocyst and endocystic layers. Daughter cysts develop from the inner layer and may protrude into the fluid-filled cystic cavity. The cyst may rupture into a bronchus, and then an air-filled cyst with an air-fluid level may be seen. Rupture may also occur between the two layers of the cyst, permitting air to outline the two layers in a variety of crescent-shaped configurations.

The most severe form is the pastoral form. In Alaska and the Canadian Northwest, the sylvatic form of the disease is endemic and produces less severe clinical findings (4).

REFERENCES

1. Beshear JR, Hendley JO. Severe pulmonary involvement in visceral larva migrans. Am J Dis Child 1973;125:599–600.
2. Woodring JH, Halfhill H II, Reed JC. Review. Pulmonary strongyloidiasis: clinical and imaging features. AJR 1994;162:537–542.
3. Moon WK, Kim WS, Im J-G, et al. Pulmonary paragonimiasis simulating lung abscess in a 9-year-old: CT findings. Pediatr Radiol 1993;23:626–627.
4. Lamy AL, Cameron BH, LeBlanc JG, et al. Giant hydatid lung cysts in the Canadian Northwest: outcome of conservative treatment in three children. J Pediatr Surg 1993;28:1140–1143.

Idiopathic Pulmonary Alveolar Microlithiasis

Idiopathic pulmonary alveolar microlithiasis is uncommon in children (1, 2), and its etiology is unknown. It is autosomal recessive in derivation and more common in females (3). A case associated with lymphocytic interstitial pneumonitis has been documented (4), but generally pulmonary alveolar microlithiasis usually is an unexpected finding on chest roentgenograms. Most patients are asymptomatic. Roentgenographically, the findings consist of small punctate calcifications scattered throughout the parenchyma of the lungs, demonstrable both on plain films (1, 2) and on high-resolution CT (3).

REFERENCES

1. Volle E, Kaufmann HJ. Pulmonary alveolar microlithiasis in pediatric patients—review of the world literature and two new observations. Pediatr Radiol 1987;17:439–442.
2. Schmidt H, Lorcher U, Kitz R, et al. Pulmonary alveolar microlithiasis in children. Pediatr Radiol 1996;26:33–36.
3. Helbich TH, Wojnarovsky C, Wunderbaldinger P, et al. Case report. Pulmonary alveolar microlithiasis in children: radiographic and high-resolution CT findings. AJR 1997;168:63–65.
4. Ratjen FA, Schoenfeld B, Weisemann HG. Pulmonary alveolar microlithiasis and lymphocytic interstitial pneumonitis in a ten-year-old girl. Eur Respir J 1992;5:1283–1285.

Wegener's Granulomatosis

Wegener's granulomatosis is an uncommon condition in childhood (1). The findings are the same as those in adults (1, 2). They consist of midline facial granulomas involving the paranasal sinuses and nose. In the chest, the findings are those of multiple pulmonary nodules, some of which may cavitate.

REFERENCES

1. McHugh K, Manson D, Eberhard BA, et al. Wegener's granulomatosis in childhood. Pediatr Radiol 1991;21:552–555.
2. Wadsworth DT, Siegel MJ, Day DL. Wegener's granulomatosis in children: chest radiographic manifestations. AJR 1994;163:901–904.

Immunologic Deficiency and Chest Disease

There are a great number of congenital and acquired immunologic deficiency states that predispose the patient to numerous and repeated pulmonary infections. Infections of other organ systems also are common, but as far as the chest is concerned, the radiologist's most important role lies in detecting the degree of pulmonary involvement in any given case and whether any complications have arisen. In this regard, it has been shown that in patients with clear chest films, high-resolution CT is very useful in detecting subtle infiltrates (1). Nonetheless, organ-specific interpretation of the roentgenogram is not always possible. However, certain subgroupings can be made, and these are determined by the basic immunologic defect present and whether the patients are more susceptible to regular or opportunistic infections. Furthermore, while certain conditions are more prone to viral infections, others are more prone to bacterial or fungal infections.

In terms of the various immunologic defects encountered, one can consider the problems as being due to either T-cell or B-cell lymphocyte deficiency. The T cells are produced in the thymus gland and provide cell-mediated immunity. B cells are found in the bone marrow, lymph nodes, and spleen and are responsible for humoral immunity. B lymphocytes mature into plasma cells and are the ones responsible for producing a variety of immunoglobulins. Finally, there are phagocytic cells: both macrophages and neutrophils. These cells engulf and destroy bacteria and then produce antigens that trigger B lymphocytes into producing immunoglobulins. Deficiency of any of these cells, either alone or in combination, leads to the various disease entities encountered.

A group of patients frequently considered, along with patients with the immunodeficiency syndromes, are those with the **dysmotile cilia syndrome.** In these patients, a variety of defects of the cilia can be encountered, and the result is deficient mucociliary cleansing of mucus and topical debris from the airways (2, 3). These patients suffer from recurrent bacterial infections, not only in the lungs but also the sinuses, upper airway, and ears. For the most part, the infections do not appear different from those seen in healthy patients with similar infections except that the chronicity present does take its toll. Frequently, the dysmotile cilia syndrome is associated with situs inversus, and then the term **Kartagener's syndrome** is employed.

Bacterial infections also are the main problem in patients with **chronic granulomatous disease** (neutrophil dysfunction) of childhood, but fungal infections also can be a problem. Again, the resulting roentgenographic findings of consolidations, abscesses, empyemas, etc., are no different from those seen in normal patients. These patients also are very prone to developing hepatic abscesses, and the organism most responsible for all of these infections is *Staphylococcus aureus.* This bacterium is catalase positive, and the abnormal neutrophils cannot phagocytize and kill the bacteria. On the other hand, they can fend off catalase-negative organisms such as *Streptococcus pneumoniae* and *Haemophilus influenzae.* Chronic granulomatous disease occurs in both sexes, but most cases occur in males and are X linked in their transmission.

The rare **Cediak-Higashi syndrome,** an autosomal recessive condition characterized by oculocutaneous albinism and neurologic cerebellar abnormalities, also is associated with abnormal neutrophil function. However, as opposed to patients with granulomatous disease, these patients also have difficulty dealing with coagulase-negative organisms.

Congenital agammaglobulinemia is an X-linked recessive condition where absence of normal B lymphocytes results in deficient immunoglobulins and humoral immunity. While T-cell immunity is normal, the lack of immunoglobulin production makes these patients very susceptible to ordinary bacterial infections.

Another condition where humoral (B-cell) immunodeficiency is present is **hypergammaglobulinemia E** or the **Job syndrome** (4, 5). These patients suffer from eczema-like lesions and also are prone to infections due to *S. aureus.* One of the unique features of this condition is that the patients tend to develop large pneumatoceles in association with their staphylococcal pulmonary infections.

In summary, patients with the foregoing immunologic deficiency problems tend to develop bacterial infections in the lungs and other organs throughout the body. Problems stem from ciliary abnormalities, neutrophil dysfunction, or B-lymphocyte deficiency. In the lungs, there is a great propensity for pulmonary abscesses, empyemas, and bronchiectasis to develop.

In those conditions where **T-lymphocyte deficiency occurs, viral infections are more the problem.** Not only are these patients susceptible to ordinary viral infections, but they also are susceptible to other more opportunistic viruses. This is the main problem in the **DiGeorge syndrome,** which is characterized by absence of the thymus and parathyroid glands along with congenital heart anomalies such as persistent truncus arteriosus. A similar immunologic deficiency also occurs in the **cartilage-hair hypoplasia** (McKusick metaphyseal dysostosis) syndrome, where the patients also suffer from pancreatic insufficiency and neutropenia. Finally, there are a large group of abnormalities where combined immunodeficiency is the problem. These include **severe combined immune deficiency,** which usually is X-linked recessive in its inheritance. It can be associated with absence of adenosine deaminase in the red blood cells and thus also has been referred to as **adenosine deaminase deficiency syndrome.** Patients with the **Wiskott-Aldrich syndrome** also have combined immune deficiency and have problems with severe eczema and thrombocytopenia. Similarly, in the ataxia-telangiectasia syndrome characterized by cerebellar ataxia and ocular and cutaneous telangiectasia, a combined immune deficiency problem exists. Of course, the most notorious of the combined immune deficiency states is **HIV infection.**

In children with **HIV-acquired immunodeficiency,** the infection is acquired transplacentally from the mother or in later life through transfusion or intravenous drug use. Because of the combined nature of the immunodeficiency in all these patients, they are susceptible not only to ordinary bacterial, viral, and fungal infections but also to less virulent or frankly opportunistic organisms such as *Pneumocystis carinii* (6), tuberculosis, atypical tuberculosis, Epstein-Barr virus (7), herpes virus, and cytomegalic inclusion virus. These patients also tend to have a pronounced lymphocytic response in the lungs, leading to so-called "**lymphoid interstitial pneumonia**" (8). The aggregates of lymphocytes can be seen throughout the interstitium or as collections (nodules) around small bronchi. They probably represent a form of delayed response to an infection with which the host is having difficulty dealing.

Although bacterial and fungal infections in these patients tend to present much as they do in ordinary individuals, they also tend to be more widespread. Viral infections often present with diffuse, interstitial infection in the form of diffuse haziness or reticulonodularity (Fig. 1.161) of the lungs (8–10). Reticulonodular infiltrates also can be seen with military tuberculosis. Diffusely hazy lungs can be seen with *P. carinii* infection (9–12). Chronic bronchitis also leads to parahilar peribronchial infiltrates, but lobar consolidations are rather uncommon. Indeed, what might at first appear to be a consolidation is actually a pseudo-consolidation due to alveolar compressive atelectasis secondary to extensive interstitial inflammation and edema (Fig. 1.162).

Some patients may develop "bronchiolitis obliterans organizing pneumonia," or the so-called "BOOP." For the most part, this is a histologic diagnosis but can be suspected with high-resolution CT. Pathologically, the problem lies in

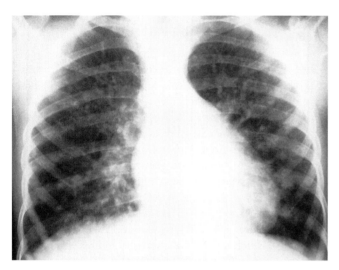

FIGURE 1.161. Immunodeficiency: reticulonodular infiltrates. Note extensive reticulonodular infiltrates in this patient due to a combination of cytomegalic inclusion and lymphocytic interstitial pneumonitis.

a necrotizing bronchiolitis with subsequent bronchiolar obliteration and adjacent parenchymal interstitial disease (13).

Thymic enlargement can occur and may simply be due to hyperplasia (14), but multicystic enlargement of the thymus also occurs (12, 15, 16). It is suggested that in these patients, abnormal immune regulation leads to follicular hyperplasia and then cystic degeneration (16). If thymic enlargement is due to multicystic involvement, no biopsy is

necessary, but if thymic enlargement is not due to multicystic disease, biopsy is in order (15).

Finally, it should be noted that **bony changes** can be seen with certain immunologic deficiency states. Severe demineralization and osteoporosis have been documented with the hypergammaglobulinemia E syndrome (17), but more important is that a variety of metaphyseal dysostoses (chondrodystrophies) can be seen in association with immunodeficiency. These include the cartilage-hair hypoplasia (McKusick metaphyseal dysostosis), metaphyseal dysostosis thymolymphopenia, and Schwachman-Diamond syndrome. In addition, it should be recalled that certain individuals with trisomy 21 also have immune deficiency states. For the most part, all of these are combined immune deficiency problems.

REFERENCES

1. Heussel CP, Kauczor H-U, Heussel G, et al. Early detection of pneumonia in febrile neutropenic patients: use of thin-section CT. AJR 1997;169:1347–1353.
2. Goldman AS, Schochet SS Jr, Howell JT. The discovery of defects in respiratory cilia in the immotile cilia syndrome. J Pediatr 1980;96:244–247.
3. Nadel HR, Stringer DA, Levison H, et al. The immotile cilia syndrome: radiological manifestations. Radiology 1985;154:651–656.
4. Dreskin SC, Goldsmith PK, Gallin JI. Immunoglobulins in the hyperimmunoglobulin E and recurrent infection (Job's) syndrome. Deficiency of anti-*Staphylococcus aureus* immunoglobulin. Am J Clin Invest 1985;75:26–34.
5. Fitch SJ, Magill HL, Herrod HF, et al. Hyperimmunoglobuline-

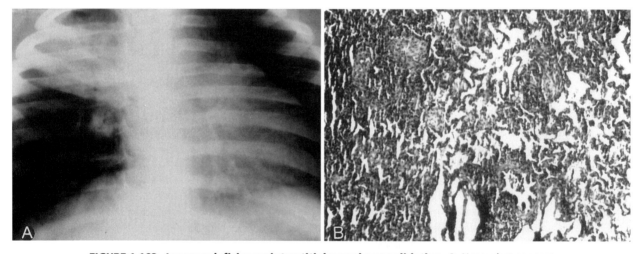

FIGURE 1.162. Immunodeficiency: interstitial pseudoconsolidation. A. Note what appears to be a consolidation in the right upper lobe. **B.** Histologic material demonstrates extensive interstitial infiltration but no significant intraalveolar (air space) disease. The alveoli on the left side of the preparation are compressed and atelectatic. In some areas, the interstitial infiltrate is beginning to assume a nodular configuration. (Reproduced with permission from Marquis JR, Berman CZ, DiCarlo F, et al. Radiographic patterns of PLH/LIP in HIV positive children. Pediatr Radiol 1993;23:328–330).

mia E syndrome: pulmonary imaging considerations. Pediatr Radiol 1986;16:285–288.

6. Glatman-Freedman A, Ewig JM, Dobroszycki J, et al. Simultaneous *Pneumocystis carinii* and pneumococcal pneumonia in human immunodeficiency virus-infected children. J Pediatr 1998;132:169–171.

7. Katz BZ, Berkman AB, Shapiro ED. Serologic evidence of active Epstein-Barr virus infection in Epstein-Barr virus associated lymphoproliferative disorders of children with acquired immunodeficiency syndrome. J Pediatr 1992;120:228–232.

8. Marquis JR, Berman CZ, DiCarlo F, et al. Radiographic patterns of PLH/LIP in HIV positive children. Pediatr Radiol 1993;23:328–330.

9. Suster B, Akerman M, Orenstein M, et al. Pulmonary manifestation of AIDS: review of 106 episodes. Radiology 1986;161: 87–93.

10. Naidich DP, Garay SM, Leitman BS, et al. Radiographic manifestations of pulmonary disease in the acquired immunodeficiency syndrome (AIDS). Semin Roentgenol 1987;22:14–30.

11. Sivit CJ, Miller CR, Rakusan TA, et al. Spectrum of chest radiographic abnormalities in children with AIDS and *Pneumocystis carinii* pneumonia. Pediatr Radiol 1995;25:389–392.

12. Marks MJ, Haney PJ, McDermott MP, et al. Thoracic disease in children with AIDS. Radiographics 1996;16:1349–1362.

13. Helton KJ, Kuhn JP, Fletcher BD, et al. Bronchiolitis obliterans organizing pneumonia (BOOP) in children with malignant disease. Pediatr Radiol 1992;22:270–274.

14. Mercado-Deane M-G, Sabio H, Burton EM, et al. Case report. Cystic thymic hyperplasia in a child with HIV infection: imaging findings. AJR 1996;166:171–172.

15. Avila NA, Mueller BU, Carrasquillo JA, et al. Multilocular thymic cysts: imaging features in children with immunodeficiency virus infection. Radiology 1996;201:130–134.

16. Kontny HU, Sleasman JW, Kingma DW, et al. Multilocular thymic cysts in children with human immunodeficiency virus infection: clinical and pathologic aspects. J Pediatr 1997;131: 264–270.

17. Kirchner SG, Sivit CJ, Wright PF. Hyperimmunoglobulinemia E syndrome: association with osteoporosis and recurrent fractures. Radiology 1985;156:362.

Adult Respiratory Distress Syndrome

The main problem in the acquired respiratory distress syndrome (ARDS) is hypoperfusion of the lungs (1, 2). The condition initially was termed "shocked lung," but whatever terminology one wishes to choose, the initial impact on the hypoperfused lung is decreased surfactant production with capillary damage and increased capillary wall permeability (1–5). The latter problem leads to widespread pulmonary edema, and the entire picture is similar to that seen in the LLS of immature infants. Indeed, surfactant therapy has been attempted in some of these patients (4). The whole problem usually is further aggravated when these patients are placed on ventilator therapy where high oxygen concentrations lead to oxygen toxicity and further damage to the capillaries.

In any given case, the lungs first become hazy (interstitial edema) and then more opaque (alveolar spill) (Fig. 1.163). When this occurs, these patients become refractory to conservative therapeutic measures, and ventilator assis-

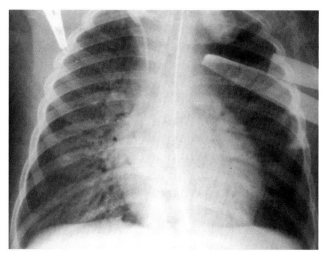

FIGURE 1.163. Acquired respiratory distress syndrome. Note the extensive and diffuse pattern of interstitial edema in this patient, who suffered severe burns and marked hypovolemia.

tance is then required. This results in barotrauma and the usual associated complications, namely, PIE, pneumothorax, and pneumomediastinum. Eventually, fibrosis occurs, blebs develop, and uneven pattern of aeration of the parenchyma occurs. The findings are very reminiscent of those seen with BPD in immature infants with chronic lung disease. Pulmonary hypertension also can occur and is believed to result from thrombosis of the smaller, peripheral pulmonary vessels during the acute phase of the injury.

REFERENCES

1. Lyrene RK, Truog WE. Adult respiratory distress syndrome in a pediatric intensive care unit: predisposing conditions, clinical course, and outcome. Pediatrics 1982;67:790–794.

2. Royall JA, Levin DL. Adult respiratory distress syndrome in pediatric patients. I. Clinical aspects, pathophysiology, pathology, and mechanisms of lung injury. J Pediatr 1988;112:169–180.

3. Greene R. Adult respiratory distress syndrome: acute alveolar damage. Radiology 1987;163:57–66.

4. Tortorolo L, Chiaretti A, Piastra M, et al. Surfactant treatment in a pediatric burn patient with respiratory failure. Pediatr Emerg Care 1999;15:410–411.

5. Pfenninger J, Gerber A, Tshappeler H, et al. Adult respiratory distress syndrome in children. J Pediatr 1982;101:352–357.

Pulmonary Embolism and Infarction

Pulmonary embolism in childhood is not particularly common, but any condition including the presence of indwelling catheters, which predisposes to thromboembolic disease, can result in pulmonary embolism. In the pediatric age group, pulmonary infarction is common in the acute chest syndrome of sickle cell disease (see next section). Pul-

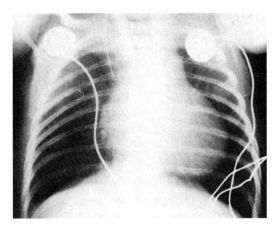

FIGURE 1.164. Pulmonary embolism with pulmonary hypertension. Note cardiomegaly with right ventricular hypertrophy, diminished pulmonary vascularity, and prominence of the pulmonary artery. The latter finding is a manifestation of pulmonary hypertension secondary to multiple small pulmonary emboli.

monary embolism secondary to intravenous fat infusion or fat embolism complicating long bone fractures is rare.

Roentgenographically, pulmonary infarction appears, more or less, as a consolidation with or without pleural effusion. Occasionally, if the infiltrate is wedge shaped and peripheral, one can suggest the diagnosis of infarction, but usually one can offer it only as part of a differential diagnosis. With widespread small vessel pulmonary emboli, cardiomegaly with right ventricular hypertrophy, prominence of the pulmonary artery, and diminution of the pulmonary vasculature is seen (Fig. 1.164). Ventilation-perfusion lung scans are more definitive in identifying perfusion defects in the light of normal ventilation. These are especially useful with massive lobar or unilateral embolism. On plain films, in some of these patients, the lobe or lung involved will appear hyperlucent due to oligemia.

Identifying pulmonary emboli in the past was accomplished with standard arteriography, but now digital arteriography can be performed and has been shown to be less invasive and equally as effective (1, 2). In addition, MR angiography with gadolinium enhancement has been shown to be useful (3).

REFERENCES

1. Hagspiel KD, Polak JF, Grassi CJ, et al. Pulmonary embolism: comparison of cut-film and digital pulmonary angiography. Radiology 1998;207:139–145.
2. Johnson MS, Stine SB, Shah H, et al. Possible pulmonary embolus: evaluation with digital subtraction versus cut-film angiography—prospective study in 80 patients. Radiology 1998;207: 131–138.
3. Meaney JFM, Weg JG, Chenevert TL, et al. Diagnosis of pulmonary embolism with magnetic resonance angiography. N Engl J Med 1997;336:1422–1427.

Acute Chest Syndrome in Sickle Cell Disease

Patients with sickle cell disease are well known to have an increased incidence of pneumonia or pneumonitis due to *Streptococcus pneumoniae* or *Mycoplasma pneumoniae* as part of the acute chest syndrome. However, it is becoming increasingly apparent that many episodes of chest pain leading to lung consolidation are secondary to venoocclusive disease (1, 2). Microvascular occlusion of the arterioles leads to pulmonary microembolism and pulmonary infarction. The resultant radiographic findings may be indistinguishable from those of bacterial consolidation, except that the resulting consolidations, when due to infarction alone, develop very rapidly. In this regard, it may be that even in those cases where consolidation is due to infection, the primary insult is infarction. This whole problem has not been resolved, but it has been demonstrated that 87% of cases of acute chest syndrome do not demonstrate an infectious etiology (2). In addition, the acute left chest syndrome is usually less severe in children than in adults (3).

REFERENCES

1. Bhala M, Abboud MR, McLoud TC, et al. Acute chest syndrome in sickle cell disease: CT evidence of microvascular occlusion. Radiology 1993;187:45–49.
2. Martin L, Buonoma C. Acute chest syndrome of sickle cell disease: radiographic and clinical analysis of 70 cases. Pediatr Radiol 1997;27:637–641.
3. Vichinsky EP, Styles LA, Colangelo LH, et al. Acute chest syndrome in sickle cell disease: clinical presentation and course. Blood 1997;89:1787–1792.

Chest Tube Complications

Any time tubes are introduced into the chest, complications can result, and most common is a misplaced endotracheal tube, occluding one or another of the bronchi, resulting in atelectasis of the lung. In addition, endotracheal and endoesophageal tubes can perforate the trachea or esophagus and result in refractory pneumothorax or pneumomediastinum (1–3). Similarly, intravenous tubes used for total parenteral hyperalimentation can perforate the superior vena cava and result in a hydro- or hemothorax (4, 5). Indwelling catheters in the vein and heart can also predispose to thromboembolic phenomenon. In addition, damage to the phrenic nerve can occur with intrathoracic tubes and result in paralysis of the diaphragm.

Endotracheal tubes also can be inadvertently placed into the esophagus. Such misplacement may elude the observer if the tube is so positioned that it is difficult to determine that it is out of the trachea and in the esophagus. In such cases, one may have to rely on other clues such as excessive esophageal air, marked gastric distension, or a peculiar position of a tube (Fig. 1.165). Other abnormal tube placements are also demonstrated in Fig. 1.165.

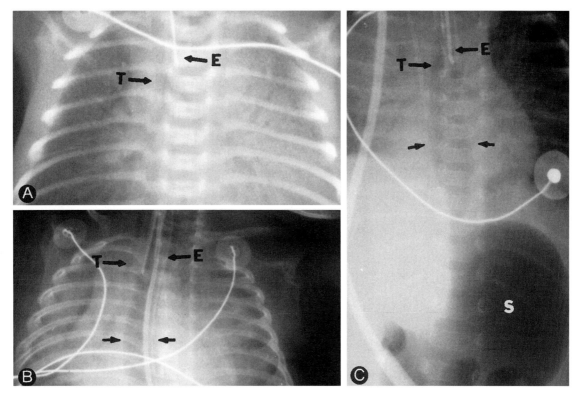

FIGURE 1.165. Malpositioning of endotracheal tube. A. There is air in the trachea (T), but the endotracheal tube (E) is outside the trachea and in the esophagus. **B.** In this patient, an endotracheal tube (E) in the esophagus results in marked distention of the esophagus with air (arrows). T, trachea. **C.** Another patient in whom not only is the air-filled esophagus distended, but so is the stomach (S). The endotracheal tube (E) is outside the trachea (T).

REFERENCES

1. Amodio JB, Berdon WE, Abramson SJ, et al. Retrocardiac pneumomediastinum in association with tracheal and esophageal perforations. Pediatr Radiol 1986;16:380–383.
2. Purohit DM, Lorenzo RL, Smith CD, et al. Bronchial laceration in a newborn with persistent posterior pneumomediastinum. J Pediatr Surg 1985;20:82–85.
3. Strife JL, Smith P, Dunbar JS, et al. Chest tube perforation of the lung in premature infants: radiographic recognition. AJR 1983; 141:73–75.
4. Bellini F, Beluffi G, Principi N. Total intravenous hyperalimentation (TIH) complications in childhood: a radiological survey. Pediatr Radiol 1984;14:6–10.
5. Krasna IH, Krause T. Life-threatening fluid extravasation of central venous catheters. J Pediatr Surg 1991;26:1346–1348.

Bronchial Fistulas

Bronchial fistulas can communicate with the pleural space or the esophagus. Congenital bronchoesophageal fistula occurs in the bronchopulmonary foregut malformation complex of conditions, but on an acquired basis, it usually is seen after pulmonary infections (1). Bronchopleural fistulas also occur after iatrogenic perforation of the tracheobronchial tree (2). They also can occur after blunt trauma to the chest.

Roentgenographically, a bronchopleural fistula can be suspected when there is chronic reaccumulation of fluid and air in the pleural space.

REFERENCES

1. Lucaya J, Sole S, Badosa J, et al. Bronchial perforation and bronchoesophageal fistulas: tuberculous origin in children. AJR 1980; 135:525–528.
2. Grosfeld JL, Lemons JL, Ballantine TVN, et al. Emergency thoracotomy for acquired bronchopleural fistula in the premature infant with respiratory distress. J Pediatr Surg 1980;15:416–421.

Swyer-James Lung

The Swyer-James lung is an acquired hypoplastic lung (1–4). Most often, the problem is an obliterative viral bronchiolitis, frequently secondary to adenoviral infection (2). However, any infection that leads to an obliterative bronchiolitis can produce the syndrome. In essence, the small peripheral bronchioles are damaged and scarred, leading to narrowed lumina and faulty aeration of the lung. Secondarily, there is decreased blood flow to the lung, and the lung therefore becomes hyperlucent.

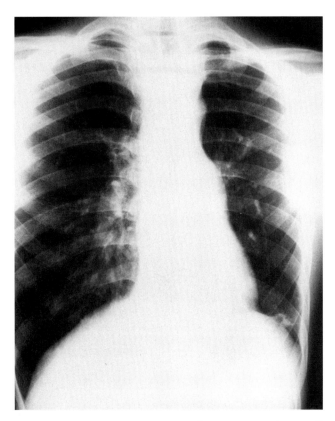

FIGURE 1.166. Swyer-James syndrome. Note the small hyperlucent left lung. It is clear, but the compensatorily overdistended right lung is larger and demonstrates relatively more blood flow than the left lung.

The Swyer-James lung originally was described as a clear, small, hyperlucent lung that did not change its size on expiration-inspiration (4), but the lung also can demonstrate diffuse reticulonodularity secondary to interstitial fibrosis (Fig. 1.166). The differential diagnosis for this type of lung is pulmonary vein atresia with repeated bouts of pulmonary infarction and edema, leading to pulmonary underdevelopment and interstitial fibrosis.

REFERENCES

1. Kogutt MS, Swischuk LE, Goldblum R. Swyer-James syndrome (unilateral hyperlucent lung) in children. Am J Dis Child 1973; 125:614–618.
2. MacPherson RI, Cumming GR, Chernick V. Unilateral hyperlucent lung; a complication of viral pneumonia. J Can Assoc Radiol 1969;20:225–231.
3. Moore ADA, Godwin JD, Dietrich PA, et al. Swyer-James syndrome: CT findings in eight patients. AJR 1992;158:1211–1215.
4. Swyer P, James C. Case of unilateral pulmonary emphysema. Thorax 1953;8:133–136.

Collagen Vascular Disease

For the most part, collagen vascular diseases consist of lupus erythematosus, dermatomyositis, rheumatoid arthritis, and periarteritis nervosa. The latter tends to produce coronary artery and other systemic artery aneurysms, while the former three do not. Dermatomyositis produces extensive soft tissue calcification, and rheumatoid arthritis, of course, presents primarily as joint inflammation. As for pulmonary changes, any of these conditions can lead to interstitial pulmonary infiltrates or pulmonary nodules, but they are most common with lupus erythematosus and periarteritis nodosa. Interstitial consolidation of the lung due to edema secondary to the vasculitis seen in these conditions also can be encountered, but most often it is seen in systemic lupus erythematosus. Almost all of these findings are nonspecific but, in the proper clinical context, can be quite suspicious (1). There is a tendency for these infiltrates to develop in the lung bases, and CT, for the demonstration of fibrosis, has been determined to be important, especially in symptomatic patients whose lungs remain clear on plain films (2).

REFERENCES

1. Nodorra RL, Landing BH. Pulmonary lesions in childhood onset systemic lupus erythematosus: analysis of 26 cases, and summary of literature. Pediatr Pathol 1987;7:1–18.
2. Seely JM, Jones LT, Wallace C, et al. Systemic sclerosis: using high-resolution CT to detect lung disease in children. AJR 1998;170: 691–697.

Henoch-Schönlein Purpura

Henoch-Schönlein purpura manifests primarily in a cutaneous hemorrhagic rash but also commonly involves the gastrointestinal tract and even the kidneys. It is less well known that it also can involve the lungs, leading to interstitial hemorrhage and pulmonary edema (1, 2). The findings are no different from any other cause of interstitial pulmonary edema.

REFERENCES

1. Chaussain M, de Boissieu D, Kalifa G, et al. Impairment of lung diffusion capacity in Schönlein-Henoch purpura. J Pediatr 1992; 121:12–16.
2. Olson JC, Kelly KJ, Pan CG, et al. Pulmonary disease with hemorrhage in Henoch-Schönlein purpura. Pediatrics 1992;89: 1177–1181.

Pulmonary Edema

The causes of pulmonary edema are numerous, and in the early stages, chest films show variable increase in prominence and fuzziness of the bronchovascular markings (Fig. 1.167A). The reason for this is that at this stage, edema fluid still is predominately interstitial. In other cases, diffuse haziness is seen (Fig. 1.67, B and C), but sooner or later, enough fluid oozes out of the interstitium so as to begin

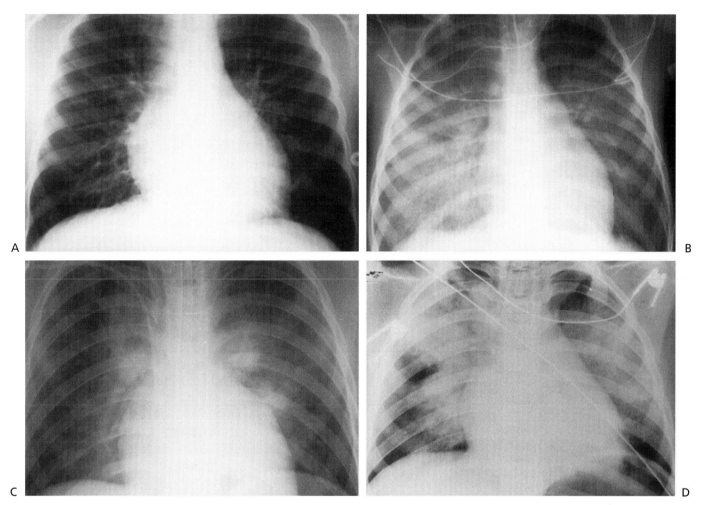

FIGURE 1.167. Pulmonary edema. A. Parahilar radiating reticulonodular infiltrates in a patient with renal failure secondary to glomerulonephritis. The superior vena cava is prominent, and there is slight cardiomegaly. **B.** Hazy pattern of interstitial pulmonary edema in a patient with acutely increased intracranial pressure. **C.** Diffuse interstitial emphysema resulting from fluid overload. **D.** Typical butterfly distribution of alveolar pulmonary edema in a patient who suffered an intracranial bleed from a ruptured aneurysm (neurogenic pulmonary edema).

seeping into the alveolar spaces. At this point, pulmonary edema can present with its typical butterfly (parahilar) distribution (Fig. 1.67D).

Pulmonary edema can result from any cause of obstruction to, or failure of, the left side of the heart but also can be seen with any type of fluid overload. In this regard, one of the most common fluid overload problems in children leading to pulmonary edema in the past was acute glomerulonephritis (1) (Fig. 1.167A). The roentgenographic findings may be profound and, as such, mimic those of myocarditis with cardiac failure. However, once the fluid overload problem is corrected, they resolve. The problem now is not as common because of the prevalent use of antibiotics to treat the original streptococcal infection.

Pulmonary edema also can result from increased intracranial pressure (i.e., neurogenic pulmonary edema), hot air or toxic fume inhalation, aerosol spray inhalation,

near drowning, and renal failure. The development of edema in most of these cases is straightforward, but it is poorly understood in those cases where it develops from increased intracranial pressure. It has been suggested that these latter patients develop pulmonary edema because of vagal-induced left-side cardiac dysfunction.

Pulmonary edema also is a key feature of the ARDS and can be seen as a complication of upper airway obstruction (2). In the latter cases, edema can occur during the obstruction or after it has been relieved. The etiology of edema associated with airway obstruction is incompletely understood (2).

REFERENCES

1. Macpherson RI, Banerjee AJ. Acute glomerulonephritis; a chest film diagnosis? J Can Assoc Radiol 1974;25:58–64.

2. Oudjhane K, Bowen A, Oh KS, et al. Pulmonary edema complicating upper airway obstruction in infants and children. Can Assoc Radiol J 1992;43:278–282.

Goodpasture's Syndrome

Goodpasture's syndrome is seldom encountered in childhood. The condition classically presents with a combination of renal and pulmonary findings. There is a hypersensitivity reaction involving the basement membranes of the glomerular and the alveolar capillaries. As a result, bleeding into the interstitium and then into the alveolar space of the lungs occurs. The infiltrative pattern resembles that of pulmonary edema. Either the renal or the pulmonary problems can precede each other, and the pulmonary changes can be rapidly progressive. However, the condition is usually one of young adulthood and not of children.

Eosinophilic (Allergic) Pneumonia

Allergic, or acute eosinophilic, pneumonia usually presents with fluffy infiltrates that tend to come and go (1, 2). The diagnosis usually is suspected when a previously healthy child develops respiratory distress and has many eosinophils in the bronchoalveolar lavage fluid (1). Radiographic findings are nonspecific and merely suggest fluffy or consolidative infiltrates. Pleural effusion may be seen (2).

REFERENCES

1. Alp H, Daum RS, Abrahams C, et al. Acute eosinophilic pneumonia: a cause of reversible, severe, noninfectious respiratory failure. J Pediatr 1998;132:540–543.
2. Cheon JE, Lee KS, Jung GS, et al. Original report. Acute eosinophilic pneumonia: radiographic and CT findings in six patients. AJR 1996;167:1195–1199.

Pleural Fluid

A small amount of pleural fluid commonly is present in normal children (1), leading to slight blunting of the costophrenic angle. Apart from this, however, pleural fluid usually indicates an underlying disease process of the lungs or pleura, and most often one is dealing with bacterial pneumonia. However, other infections, except for viral infections, also can produce pleural effusions. In addition, pleural effusions can be seen with renal disease such as glomerulonephritis and the nephrotic syndrome and with collagen vascular diseases. Furthermore, any time generalized body fluid overload or pulmonary edema occurs, for any reason, pleural fluid frequently accompanies the problem.

In early stages, pleural fluid may present more as mere thickening of the various pleural fissures, but later it assumes its more characteristic configuration along the chest wall (Fig. 1.168, A and B). Smaller amounts are easily detected with

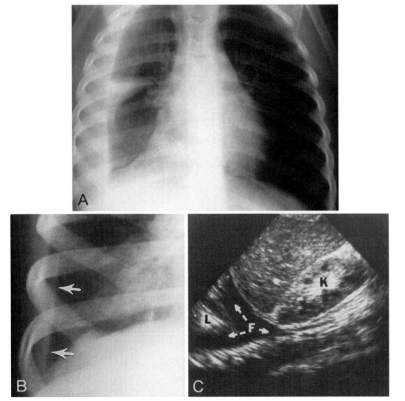

FIGURE 1.168. Pleural fluid. A. Typical pleural effusion on the right extending into the minor fissure. **B.** Another patient with a small, but typical, pleural effusion along the right lateral chest wall (arrows). **C.** Ultrasonography confirms the presence of the fluid (arrows). The liver is seen above the kidney (K). L, compressed lung.

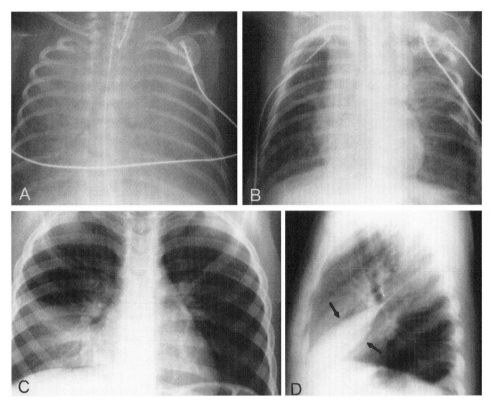

FIGURE 1.169. Pleural fluid: other configurations. A. This patient appears to have bilateral lung consolidations. However, it is pleural fluid layering along the posterior wall of the chest, on supine positioning, that produces the increase in density. **B.** After removal of the fluid (note bilateral chest tubes), one can see that the lungs actually were clear. **C.** Another patient with a density in the right lung base that might at first suggest an infiltrate. **D.** Lateral view clearly demonstrates a characteristic spindle-shaped pleural effusion (arrows) located in the major fissure.

ultrasound (Fig. 1.168C). When pleural fluid accumulations are massive, there is complete opacification of the involved hemithorax and contralateral shift of the mediastinum. Of course, bilateral pleural effusions also can occur and are common in the neonate as chylo-hydrothorax.

A few peculiarities about pleural fluid collections include layering along the posterior wall of the chest in the supine position. In such cases, the findings may erroneously suggest total consolidation of the lung (Fig. 1.169, A and B). In other cases, as pleural fluid accumulates in the various fissures, a pseudotumor appearance can result (Fig. 1.169, C and D). Very often, the oval or spindle-shaped configuration of the fluid collection is the clue to proper diagnosis. Because these collections tend to disappear on their own, they have been called "vanishing tumors."

Subpulmonic effusions are common in children. They occur most often with the nephrotic syndrome but also can be seen with lymphoma in the chest or abdomen. Of course, they are not limited to these conditions but merely are most common with them. The fluid is free flowing but accumulates along the lung base between the diaphragmatic leaflet and the lung. This creates the erroneous impression that one or both diaphragmatic leaflets are elevated (Fig. 1.170).

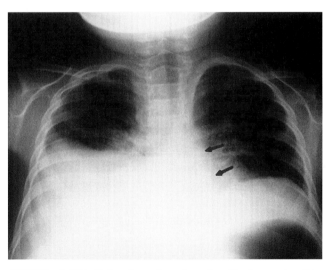

FIGURE 1.170. Subpulmonic pleural effusions. In this patient with nephrotic syndrome, note what would at first appear to be elevated diaphragmatic leaflets. This appearance is caused by bilateral basal pleural effusions, and the squared-off appearance of the leaflets is suggestive of fluid. Also note pleural fluid extending along the paraspinal gutter on the left (arrows).

However, the leaflets often have a somewhat laterally squared configuration, and associated fluid in the paraspinal gutter frequently is seen. In addition, there is loss of gradation of gray behind the involved leaflet. In other words, the leaflet becomes abruptly opaque. Once one becomes familiar with these findings, it is not so difficult to identify that subpulmonic pleural effusions, rather than elevated diaphragmatic leaflets, are present (Fig. 1.70).

REFERENCE

1. Ecklof O, Torngren A. Pleural fluid in healthy children. Acta Radiol 1971;11:346–349.

Bronchiectasis

Bronchiectasis is not exceptionally common in children but, as in any age group, can result from any longstanding pulmonary infection or foreign body. It also is a common feature of chronic pulmonary problems such as cystic fibrosis and the various immunologic deficiency syndromes. Radiographically, the findings can be seen on plain chest films where they consist of saccular or tubular dilatations of air-filled bronchi. These findings as well as those in less pronounced cases are best demonstrated with high-resolution CT (1, 2). CT also is more accurate in defining the distribution of bronchiectasis, an important consideration in those patients for whom surgical intervention is contemplated.

REFERENCES

1. Herman M, Michalkova K, Kopriva F. High-resolution CT in the assessment of bronchiectasis in children. Pediatr Radiol 1993;23:376–379.
2. Kornreich L, Horev G, Ziv N, et al. Bronchiectasis in children: assessment by CT. Pediatr Radiol 1993;23:120–123.

Castleman's Disease

Castleman's disease is not common in children. It is manifest primarily by the presence of large, intrathoracic lymph nodes (1, 2). The etiology of the condition is unknown, and there apparently are two types. The localized type has a better prognosis, while the more diffuse intrathoracic form has a poorer prognosis.

REFERENCES

1. Johkoh T, Mullr ND, Ichikado K, et al. Intrathoracic multicentric Castleman disease: CT findings in 12 patients. Radiology 1998;209:477–481.
2. McAdams HP, Rosado-de-Christenson M, Fishback NF, et al. Castleman disease of the thorax: radiologic features with clinical and histopathologic correlation. Radiology 1998;209:221–228.

Lung Transplantation

Lung transplantation can be performed on either one lung or both lungs and accompanied by transplantation of the heart. A detailed dissertation on lung transplantation is beyond the scope of this book, but the procedure is definitely becoming more common. Unfortunately, complications in the realms of both rejection and infection are commonplace, and roentgenographically usually it is difficult to differentiate one from the other. The main problem is that the findings of rejection often resemble those of opportunistic infections such as cytomegalovirus or *Pneumocystis carinii* infection. These patients, of course, because they are immunosuppressed, are prone to develop a wide variety of pulmonary infections, much as do those patients with primary immunologic deficiencies. In the end, the chest film is used primarily as an indicator of the presence of clinically suspected pulmonary complications, and most often bronchial lavage or transbronchial biopsy is required for final diagnosis (1, 2). CT also is helpful in identifying the complications associated with lung transplantation (3).

REFERENCES

1. Medina LS, Siegel MJ, Bejarano PA, et al. Pediatric lung transplantation: radiographic-histopathologic correlation. Radiology 1993;187:807–810.
2. Medina LS, Siegel MJ, Glazer HS, et al. Diagnosis of pulmonary complications associated with lung transplantation in children: value of CT vs. histopathologic studies. AJR 1994;162:969–974.
3. Medina LS, Siegel MJ. CT of complications in pediatric lung transplantation. Radiographics 1994;14:1341–1349.

Chest Trauma

Chest trauma most commonly occurs with motor vehicle accidents but also can be seen with the battered child syndrome and other forms of trauma. The findings are generally much the same as in adults, and I have dealt with these in another publication (1).

In terms of what can be seen, one can see traumatic diaphragmatic hernias (2), tracheobronchial ruptures (3, 4), pneumothorax, pneumomediastinum, mediastinal hematoma, rib fractures, vertebral fractures, pulmonary contusions, pulmonary hematomas, intercostal hernias (5), and posttraumatic pneumatoceles (6, 7). The latter can be confused with traumatic diaphragmatic hernias (6).

Problems with the thymus are not encountered in adults but frequently are encountered in infants and even children. In supine position, the normal thymus gland can make the superior mediastinum appear very wide, to the point of suggesting a mediastinal hematoma secondary to aortic injury. In these cases, it is most important to look for the position of the trachea or of endotracheal and endoesophageal tubes, if they are present (they usually are). If there is no displacement of the trachea or the esophagus, or the tubes within them, that is, to the right, and there is no apical cap over the left lung apex (blood), then most likely one is dealing with a normal thymus and not a hematoma.

REFERENCES

1. Swischuk LE. Emergency imaging of the acutely ill or injured child. 4th ed. Philadelphia: Lippincott Williams & Wilkins, 2000:95–104.
2. Koplewitz BZ, Ramos C, Manson DE, et al. Traumatic diaphragmatic injuries in infants and children, imaging findings. Pediatr Radiol 2000;30:471–479.
3. Becmeur F, Donoto L, Horta-Geraud P, et al. Rupture of the airways after blunt chest trauma in two children. Eur J Pediatr Surg 2000;10:133–135.
4. Slimane MAA, Becmeur F, Aubert D, et al. Tracheobronchial ruptures from blunt thoracic trauma in children. J Pediatr Surg 1999;34:1847–1850.
5. Min S, Gow KW, Blair GK. Traumatic intercostal hernia: presentation and diagnostic workup. J Pediatr Surg 1999;34:1544–1545.
6. Allbery AM, Swischuk LE, John SD. Posttraumatic pneumatoceles mimicking diaphragmatic hernia. Emerg Radiol 1997;4: 94–96.
7. Fagan CJ, Swischuk LE. Traumatic pneumatoceles in children. Radiology 1976;120:18.

Chest Pain in Children

It is well known that chest pain in children most often is musculoskeletal or the result of anxiety (1). It is generally believed that it is uncommon for it to be secondary to cardiac disease. It can, of course, be associated with pulmonary disease such as pneumonia, pleurisy, etc., but central chest pain generally is not associated with cardiac disease in the ordinary setting. Recently, however, it has been demonstrated that in the emergency room setting, 15% of children with chest pain did, in fact, have associated cardiac disease (2).

REFERENCES

1. Swischuk LE. Emergency imaging of the acutely ill or injured child. 4th ed. Philadelphia: Lippincott Williams & Wilkins, 2000: 114.
2. Zavaras-Angelidou KA, Weinhouse E, Nelson DB. Review of 180 episodes of chest pain in 134 children. Pediatr Emerg Care 1992;8:819.

CHEST MASSES

Chest masses of various types are not uncommon in infants and children, but they are less common in newborns. In addition, these masses often are rather silent and reach enormous size before they are detected. However, if they are critically located in the chest, they may present earlier with respiratory distress, stridor, or dysphagia. In still other cases, recurrent pneumonia or bleeding may be a problem. Overall, the chest film is the most sensitive study in detecting chest masses, be they in the mediastinum, lungs, or chest wall. Data available on plain films include size and location of the mass, calcifications within the mass, chest wall involvement, and tracheal deviation. In some cases, the diagnosis is clearly apparent from an analysis of these findings alone, but in other cases, further investigation to specifically outline the perimeters of the tumor is in order, and this usually consists of CT or MRI (1). Nuclear scintigraphy is used primarily for lesions suspected of being thyroid in origin or in the determination of whether suspected gastroenteric cysts contain gastric mucosa. Ultrasonography is useful only if the lesion abuts the chest wall.

Mediastinal Masses

In older children, the most common mediastinal mass is that due to adenopathy resulting from lymphoma. Thereafter, and in all ages, various neurogenic tumors and cysts make up the majority of mediastinal masses in childhood. In children as in adults, mediastinal masses are considered on the basis of their location in the mediastinum (i.e., anterior, middle, and posterior).

Posterior mediastinal lesions usually are neurogenic in origin and primarily consist of neuroblastoma, neurenteric cysts, and intrathoracic meningocele. Middle mediastinal lesions consist mainly of enlarged lymph nodes (inflammatory or tumoral) or developmental cysts of some type (i.e., bronchogenic or duplication cysts). In the anterior mediastinum, tumors usually are teratomas, dermoids, thymomas, cystic hygromas, lymphomas, or some thyroid tumor or cyst.

Posterior Mediastinal Tumors

As has been noted, posterior mediastinal tumors, for the most part, are neurogenic in origin. When they become large, they may extend into the middle mediastinum and, in addition, may arise in the neck and extend into the chest. Tumor types encountered include neuroblastoma, ganglioneuroma, and neurofibroma, but the **neuroblastoma-ganglioneuroma** complex is most common, accounting for 90% of cases (2). Most frequently, these tumors occur in the upper one-third to one-half of the posterior mediastinum and, in some cases, can be so large as to be associated with respiratory distress (3) and Horner's syndrome (4). On the other hand, 50% of these tumors are discovered incidentally (2), attesting to the generally acknowledged more favorable prognosis for primary intrathoracic neuroblastoma (5), especially if discovered under 1 year of age (2).

Roentgenographically, with neuroblastoma, a variably sized, often lobulated posterior mediastinal mass is seen. Usually, it is not as round or oval as a benign cyst, and displacement of the trachea and esophagus and adjacent lung is common (Fig. 1.171). Calcification, usually irregular or granular, often also is present, but the calcifications are not as discrete or well formed as in a teratoma or dermoid. Furthermore, they are more commonly seen in older children with the more benign ganglioneuroma. In these latter cases and, indeed, in all cases, diagnostically important associated rib erosion is frequently present and may be associated with spreading of the ribs (Fig. 1.171). Although the diagnosis usually is secured on plain films (6), CT or MRI now usually is employed to define the tumor's exact borders and to determine whether there is any intraspinal extension (i.e., the so-called "dumbbell" tumor) (7). In the pediatric age group, a "dumbbell" tumor usually is a neuroblastoma or ganglioneuroma and not a neurofibroma. With these dumbbell tumors, in addition to rib erosion, there may be intervertebral fora-

men enlargement, pedicular flattening, posterior vertebral scalloping, spinal canal widening, and localized kyphosis or scoliosis. It is most important to recognize the presence of such extensions before definitive therapy of the tumor is contemplated. MRI is best for determining the presence of intraspinal extension (Fig. 1.172) and generally is favored over CT (2). Most neuroblastomas are solid, but occasionally cystic neuroblastomas can be encountered (7).

Neurofibroma is rare in children and, when encountered, produces changes similar to those seen in older children or adults, that is, a posterior mediastinal mass and associated intervertebral foramen enlargement. Plexiform mediastinal neurofibromas produce a more diffuse mass effect (8). Rarely, one may encounter posterior mediastinal teratomas (9), hemangiomas (10, 11), cystic hygromas (12), and juvenile fibromas (13).

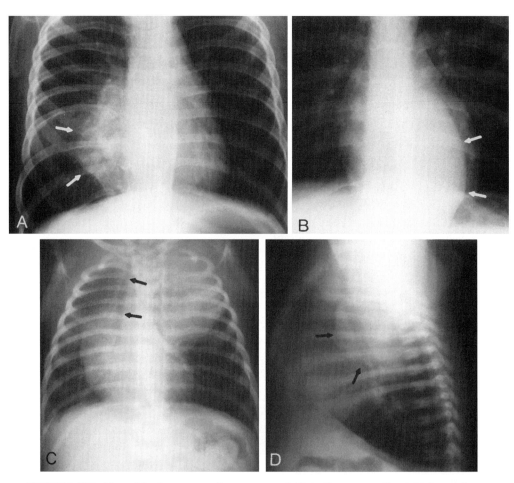

FIGURE 1.171. Neuroblastoma-ganglioneuroma. A. Note the mass on the right (arrows) containing calcification and causing erosion of the ribs. This was a ganglio-neuroblastoma in an infant. **B.** Older child with a smooth mass, located behind the heart (arrows). This was a ganglioneuroma in an older child. **C.** Large mass (neuroblastoma) projected over the left upper lung field displacing the trachea (arrows) and mediastinal structures to the right. Supraclavicular extension was present clinically. Also note thinning of the posterior aspect of the second rib on the left. **D.** Lateral view shows typical posterior location of the neuroblastoma (arrows).

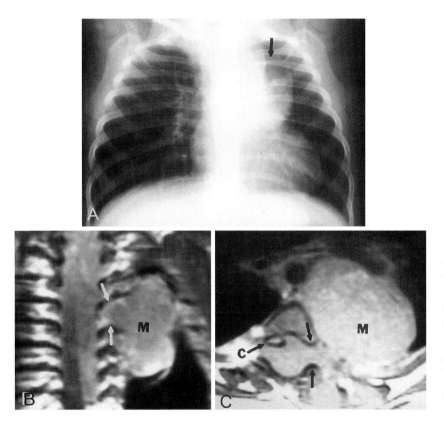

FIGURE 1.172. Dumbbell neuroblastoma. A. Note the large lobulated posterior mediastinal mass producing erosion and displacement of the third rib on the left (arrow). **B.** Coronal T1-weighted magnetic resonance study demonstrates the large paraspinal mass (M) with extension into the intravertebral foramina (arrows). **C.** Axial image demonstrates the same mass (M) with evidence of extension in dumbbell fashion into the spinal canal (arrows). The spinal cord (C) is displaced and compressed. (Courtesy of C. Keith Hayden, Jr., M.D.).

Middle Mediastinal Masses

Most tumors occurring in the middle mediastinum arise from the lymph nodes. Lesions involving the thymus gland can become so large that they may extend into the middle mediastinum, and the same can occur with large posterior mediastinal lesions. Lymphoma is probably the most common tumor occurring in the medial mediastinum and results from enlargement of the hilar and paratracheal lymph nodes. The findings are those of a mass of endless configurations (Figs. 1.173 and 1.174). Lymphomas can demonstrate calcification after therapy, and residual lymphoma tissue does not always require further imaging (14). This often is a problem because the residual mass is difficult to identify as being either end fibrosis or residual tumor. Positron emission tomography scanning is useful in making this distinction.

Anterior Mediastinal Tumors

In the anterior mediastinum of infants and children, one most often encounters **dermoids, teratomas,** and **germ cell tumors.** Often, these are now considered together under the single term "germ cell tumor." However, there still is some use to separate the two because the term "germ cell tumor" usually denotes a tumor that is growing more rapidly and has a greater malignant potential. Tumors of the thyroid are less common (discussed in Chapter 2), and thymomas, along with thymolipomas, have been discussed earlier in this chapter.

As far as teratomas are concerned, they frequently attain considerable size before producing symptoms. When large, their posterior limits can extend into the middle mediastinum, and some can extend into the neck. Fifty percent of these tumors occur in neonates, and malignancy is more common when the tumor presents in older children (15).

Histologically, dermoids are said to contain only ectodermal elements, but it is believed that if all dermoids were more closely examined, cells arising from the other two dermal layers would frequently be found. True mediastinal dermoids are probably rare. Teratomas contain elements of all three dermal layers and can be either cystic or solid. If gastric mucosa is present, hemoptysis can be a problem (16). Hemoptysis also can be a problem if the tumor bleeds and forms pleural adhesions. In these cases, systemic-to-pulmonary artery communications lead to pulmonary hemorrhage (17).

Roentgenographically, teratomatous tumors produce posterior and lateral displacement of the trachea and esophagus. This single fact allows one to differentiate them from normal thymus, for the **completely** normal thymus does not displace the airway. In addition, however, if irregular calcifications or formed skeletal structures are present, the diagnosis is assured (Fig. 1.175, A and B), even if obscured by an associated pleural effusion. CT and MRI are excellent in demonstrating

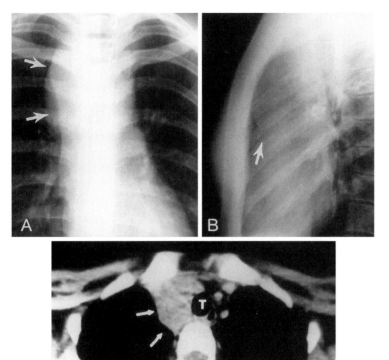

FIGURE 1.173. Lymphoma. A. Note right paratracheal widening due to lymphoma (arrows). **B.** Lateral view clearly places the lesion in the anterior mediastinum (arrow). **C.** Axial computed tomography image demonstrates the relatively small mass in the right paratracheal region (arrows). T, trachea.

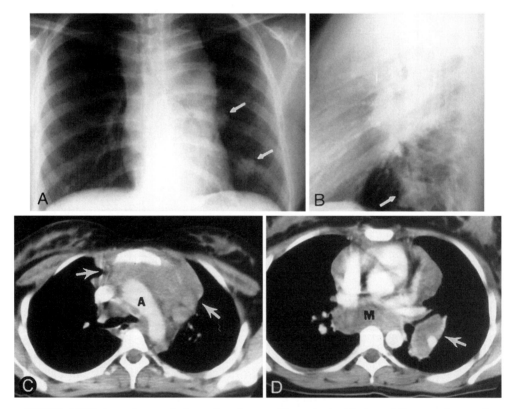

FIGURE 1.174. Lymphoma. A. Large lymphoma with marked widening of the superior mediastinum. Also note fullness in the left hilar region and two lung nodules (arrows). **B.** Lateral view demonstrating the anterior mediastinal mass and the hilar adenopathy. The lower, larger pulmonary nodule also is visible (arrow). **C.** Computed tomography at the level of the aortic arch (A) demonstrates the large, anterior mediastinal mass (arrows). **D.** A lower cut demonstrates the posterior extension of the mass (M) and left hilar adenopathy (arrow). The left pulmonary artery (P) is encased by the adenopathy. A, descending aorta.

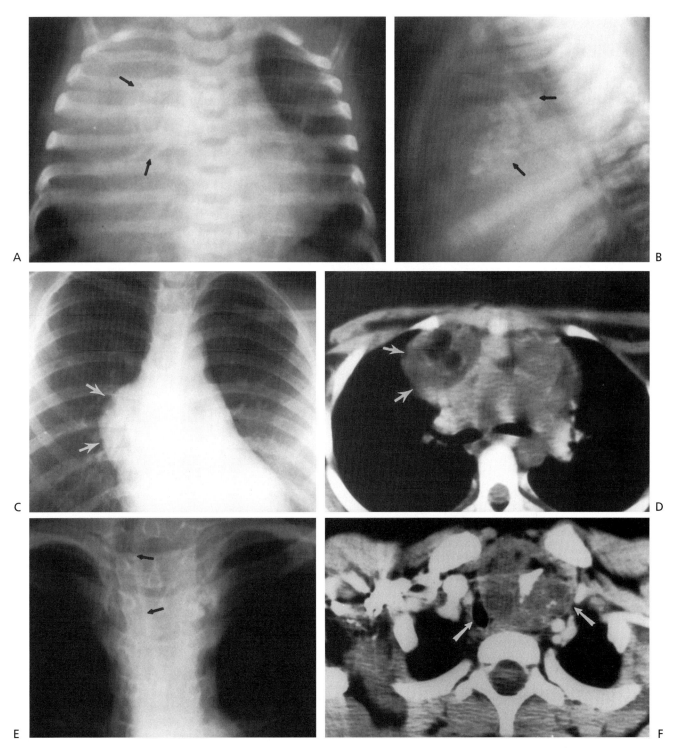

FIGURE 1.175. Teratoma: anterior mediastinum. A. Note the large mass with central calcifications (arrows) displacing the trachea to the left. **B.** Lateral view demonstrates the anterior mediastinal position of the mass (arrows) and calcifications. **C.** Another patient with a small teratoma (arrows). **D.** Computed tomography study demonstrates the anterior mass (arrows) consisting of solid tissue, fluid-filled cyst, and fat collections. **E.** Another patient with a high anterior mediastinal mass causing deviation of the trachea (arrows). Note calcification within the mass. **F.** Computed tomography in this patient demonstrates typical mixed findings (arrows) of a teratoma.

the heterogeneous nature of these lesions (Figs. 1.175 and 1.176). Ultrasound is not as useful because the lesions often are quite large, but still it can detect the multitissue aspect of the tumor. An interesting feature identified with ultrasound is floating fatty spherules in the cysts of cystic teratomas (17, 18). Most often, teratomas are located in the anterior mediastinum, but occasionally a posterior mediastinal location is encountered (19) (Figs. 1.176 and 1.177). With teratomas, one often clearly will see the presence of fluid-filled cysts, nonspecific soft tissue, fatty tissue, and calcification. With germ cell tumors, the heterogenicity of the tumor is not as marked (Fig. 1.178). In fact, calcification is not common. But since these tumors are quite vascular, bleeding into and around the tumor can be a significant problem (Fig. 1.179). In some cases, mediastinal teratomas may be located within the pericardium, and then cardiac enlargement may initially be suggested. Intrapericardial teratomas can produce extensive pericardial effusions and severe respiratory distress.

Other tumors occurring in the anterior mediastinum include yolk cell tumors (20) and cystic hygromas, the latter of which can mimic teratomas in some cases (see next section).

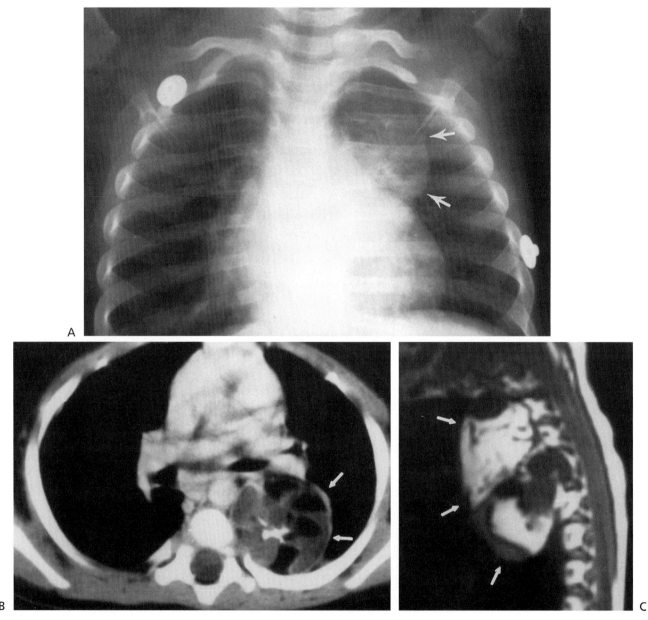

FIGURE 1.176. Teratoma: posterior mediastinum. A. Note mass on the left (arrows). **B.** Computed tomography demonstrates the typical cystic, fat, and calcific components of a teratoma (arrows). **C.** Magnetic resonance image demonstrating the fatty content of the mass (arrows).

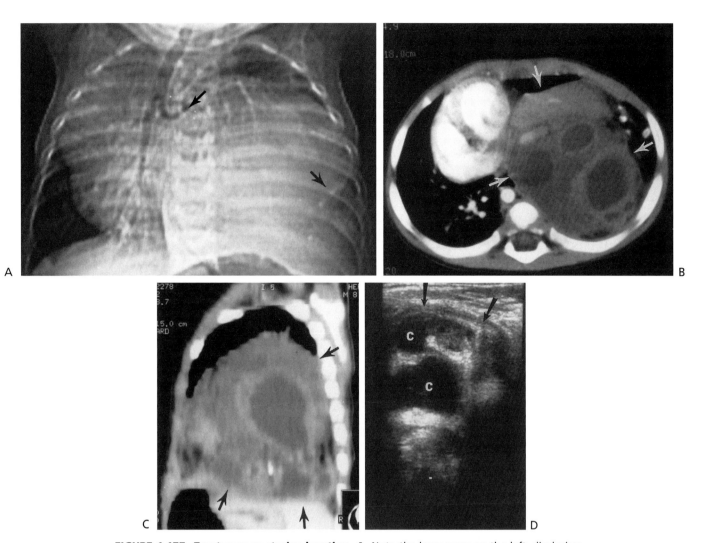

FIGURE 1.177. Teratoma: posterior location. A. Note the large mass on the left, displacing the mediastinum to the right. Note the cut-off of the left bronchus (upper arrow) and calcifications (lower arrow). **B.** Axial computed tomography study demonstrates the large mass (arrows) consisting of mixed tissue including fat and calcium. The heart is displaced to the left. **C.** Sagittal reconstructed computed tomography study demonstrates the mass (arrows). **D.** Ultrasound study demonstrates the fluid-filled cysts (C) and echogenic fat.

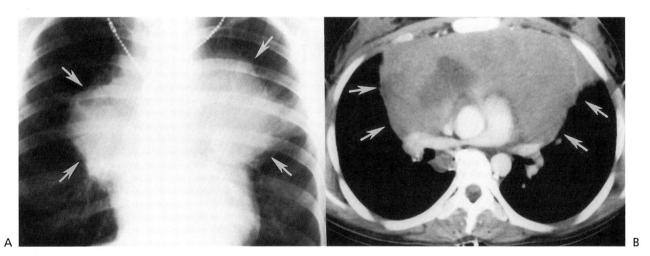

FIGURE 1.178. Germ cell tumor. A. Note the large mediastinal mass (arrows). **B.** Computed tomography demonstrates the anterior location of the mass (arrows), which contains areas of hypodensity due to the presence of fatty tissue (arrows).

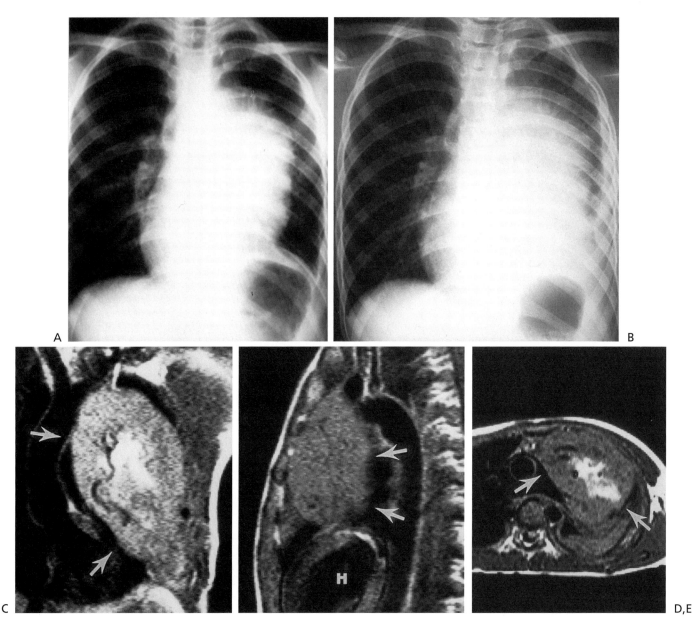

FIGURE 1.179. Aggressive teratoma (germ cell tumor). A. Note the large anterior mediastinal mass and small left pleural effusion. **B.** One day later, the mass increased in size owing to hemorrhage, and more pleural fluid developed. **C.** Coronal T1-weighted magnetic resonance image demonstrates the large medium-signal mass (arrows), with central high signal due to blood. Also note the tortuous supplying blood vessel. **D.** Lateral view demonstrates the anterior location of the tumor (arrows). H, heart. **E.** Axial view demonstrates the mass (arrows) with central bleeding (high signal) and numerous flow voids due to feeding blood vessels. The left lung is compressed posteriorly.

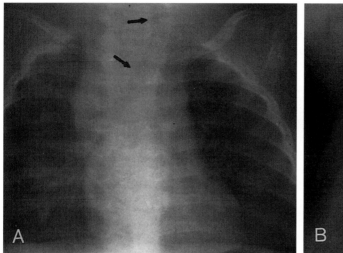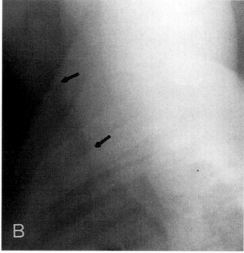

FIGURE 1.180. Cystic hygroma. A. Note right superior mediastinal widening (outer arrows) extending into the neck. Also note displacement of the trachea to the left. **B.** Lateral view demonstrates anterior displacement of the trachea (arrows).

Other Mediastinal Tumors

In addition to the tumors already mentioned, one also may encounter lesions such as lipomas (21), lipoblastoma (22), mediastinal lipomatosis (23, 24), lipomatosis secondary to steroid therapy, mesothelioma, hemangioma, and cystic hygromas. Cystic hygroma is the most common of the tumors just mentioned and most often arises in the neck. However, occasionally the tumor can arise primarily in the mediastinum (24–27) and can occur in the anterior, posterior, and middle mediastinal compartments (12, 20, 25–27). When cystic hygromas are large, they can produce tracheal and esophageal displacement (Fig. 1.180), for even though these tumors are rather soft, they still can compress adjacent structures. Cystic hygromas tend to extend over large areas and insinuate themselves between various surrounding structures. For this reason, they are difficult to remove surgically, and in this regard, MRI has proved of considerable value in delineating the precise location and extent of these tumors. Cystic hygromas, on ultrasonography, have a characteristic multiloculated appearance, as do they on both CT and MRI, and in longstanding cases may show calcifications secondary to presumed infection or hemorrhage (Fig. 1.181). In such cases, very often one first considers teratoma to be the diagnosis (28). Hemangiomas generally are more heterogeneously echogenic on ultrasound and show high signal on MRI. Indeed, these tumors stay very bright on the second echo of the T2 imaging sequence. Color flow Doppler also is useful in detecting hemangiomas as very frequently increased blood flow is seen in the tumor. This does not occur with cystic hygromas. Cystic hygromas also can be associated with lytic, cystic skeletal lesions (27).

REFERENCES

1. Daldrup HE, Link TM, Worlet K, et al. Pictorial essay. MR imaging of thoracic tumors in pediatric patients. AJR 1998;170: 1639–1644.
2. Saenz NC, Schnitzer JJ, Eraklis AE, et al. Posterior mediastinal masses. J Pediatr Surg 1993;28:172–176.
3. Illescas FL, Williams RL. Neonatal neuroblastoma presenting with respiratory distress. J Can Assoc Radiol 1984;35: 310–312.
4. Jaffe N, Cassady R, Filler RM, et al. Heterochromia and Horner syndrome associated with cervical and mediastinal neuroblastoma. J Pediatr 1975;87:75–77.
5. Adams GA, Schochat SJ, Smith E, et al. Thoracic neuroblastoma: a pediatric oncology group. J Pediatr Surg 1993;28:372–378.
6. Slovis TL, Meza MP, Cushing B, et al. Thoracic neuroblastoma: what is the best imaging modality for evaluating extent of disease? Pediatr Radiol 1997;27:273–275.
7. Fagan CJ, Swischuk LE. Dumbbell neuroblastoma or ganglioneuroma of the spinal canal. AJR 1968;102:453–460.
8. Chalmers AH, Armstrong P. Plexiform mediastinal neurofibromas. A report of two cases. Br J Radiol 1977;591:215–217.
9. Karl SR, Dunn J. Posterior mediastinal teratomas. J Pediatr Surg 1985;20:508–510.
10. Fowler CL, Bloss RS. Hemangioma of a thoracic sympathetic ganglion mimicking a neuroblastoma. Pediatr Radiol 1994;24:1 48–149.
11. Herman TE, McAlister WH, Dehner LP. Posterior mediastinal capillary hemangioma with extradural extension resembling neuroblastoma. Pediatr Radiol 1999;29:517–519.
12. Curley SA, Ablin DS, Kosloske AM. Giant cystic hygroma of the posterior mediastinum. J Pediatr Surg 1989;24:398–400.
13. Ko S-F, Ng S-H, Hsiao C-C, et al. Juvenile fibromatosis of the posterior mediastinum with intraspinal extension. AJNR 1996; 17:522–524.
14. Brisse H, Pacquement H, Burdairon E, et al. Outcome of residual mediastinal masses of thoracic lymphomas in children: impact on managemnt and radiological follow-up strategy. Pediatr Radiol 1998;28:444–450.

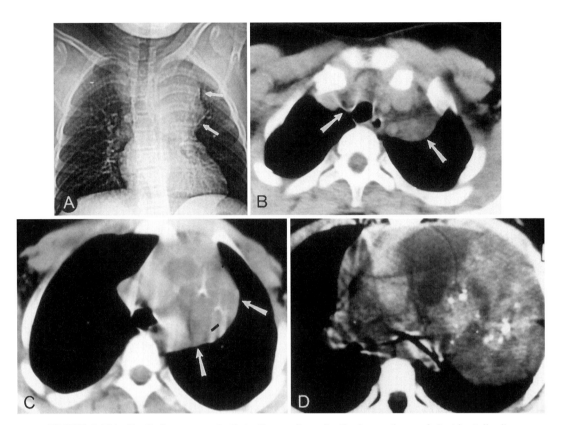

FIGURE 1.181. Cystic hygroma. A. Note the small mediastinal mass (arrows), incidentally discovered in this patient. It is located in the anterior mediastinum. **B.** Computed tomography demonstrating the anterior location of the mass (arrows), which is somewhat inhomogeneous and seems to be surrounding the vessels. **C.** Slightly lower cut demonstrates calcifications within the mass (arrows). **D. Another case.** Large cystic hygroma mimicking a teratoma with marked heterogenicity of the parenchyma and scattered calcifications. In both these patients, it is believed that hemorrhage and/or infection may have resulted in the calcifications. Both lesions initially were considered to be teratomas. (**D** courtesy of Jean Claude Hoeffel, M.D.).

15. Laakhoo K, Boyle M, Drake DP. Mediastinal teratomas: review of 15 pediatric cases. J Pediatr Surg 1993;28:1161–1164.

16. Hayden CK Jr, Swischuk LE, Schwartz MZ, et al. Systemic-pulmonary shunting and hemoptysis in a benign intrathoracic teratoma. Pediatr Radiol 1984;14:52–54.

17. Shih J-Y, Wang H-C, Chang Y-L, et al. Echogenic floating spherules as a sonographic sign of cystic teratoma of mediastinum: correlation with CT and pathologic findings. J Ultrasound Med 1996;15:603–605.

18. Hession PR, Simpson W. Case report: mobile fatty globules in benign cystic teratoma of the mediastinum. Br J Radiol 1996;69:186–188.

19. Solsona-Narbon B, Sanchez-Paris O, Bernal-Sprekelsen JC, et al. Hourglass thoracic lipoma of infancy: case report and review of the literature. J Pediatr Surg 1997;32:785–786.

20. Uchiyama M, Iwafuchi M, Matsuda Y, et al. Mediastinal yolk sac tumor in a young girl: case report and review of the literature. J Pediatr Surg 1996;31:1318–1321.

21. Federici S, Cuoghi D, Sciutti R. Benign mediastinal lipoblastoma in a 14-month-old infant. Pediatr Radiol 1992;22:150–151.

22. Shukla LW, Katz JA, Wagner ML. Mediastinal lipomatosis: a complication of high dose steroid therapy in children. Pediatr Radiol 1988;19:57–58.

23. Irgau I, McNicholas KW. Mediastinal lipoblastoma involving the left innominate vein and the left phrenic nerve. J Pediatr Surg 1998;33:1540–1542.

24. Agartan C, Olguner M, Mirac Akgur F, et al. A case of mediastinal cystic hygroma whose only symptom was hoarseness. J Pediatr Surg 1998;33:642–643.

25. Perkes EA, Haller JO, Kassner EG, et al. Mediastinal cystic hygroma in infants; two cases with no extension into the neck. Clin Pediatr 1979;18:168–170.

26. Wright CC, Cohen DM, Vegunta RK, et al. Intrathoracic cystic hygroma: a report of three cases. J Pediatr Surg 1996;31:1430–1432.

27. Gupta AK, Berry M, Raghav B, et al. Mediastinal and skeletal lymphangiomas in a child. Pediatr Radiol 1991;21:129.

28. Swischuk LE, Hoeffel J-C, John SD. Primary intrathoracic lymphangioma masquerading as teratoma. Pediatr Radiol 1996;26:827–829.

INTRATHORACIC CYSTS

The most commonly encountered cyst in the chest is the **bronchogenic cyst.** Many occur around the carina, upper trachea, or along the bronchi (1), but some can be infradiaphragmatic (2). Symptoms may be striking or entirely absent, depending on the position and size of the cyst. The most common symptomatic location is around the carina. In addition, small cysts around the upper trachea and lower esophagus can grow without necessarily compromising the airway and are often discovered as incidental findings. Most bronchogenic cysts are fluid filled and do not connect with the tracheobronchial tree. In some cases, when the cyst becomes infected, enlargement is rapid. Respiratory distress, of course, can be profound in these infants. Roentgenographically, these cysts appear as smooth, round, or oval masses in the chest (Fig. 1.182). In a few cases, the cysts can be multiple (3), and when the cyst compresses a pulmonary blood vessel, localized stenosis can result (4).

Neurenteric or enteric cysts (gastrointestinal duplication) are commonly located in the posterior mediastinum. Since they have their origin in faulty separation of the gastrointestinal tract from the primitive neural crest, they occasionally connect with the spinal canal, and enterogenous cysts can co-exist (5). The connection may be through a demonstrable sinus tract or merely by means of a fibrous band. Vertebral anomalies and anterior vertebral body defects are commonly associated (Fig. 1.183), and because of this, the main differential diagnosis is intrathoracic meningocele. Cord compression can occur in these patients (6), and occasionally a neurenteric cyst can extend, in dumbbell fashion, below the diaphragm and be both intraabdominal and intrathoracic (7).

Other enteric cysts have no residual communication with the spinal canal and often are located more in the middle mediastinum, close to the esophagus. These cysts frequently are referred to as "gastrointestinal duplication cysts." They infrequently connect with the gastrointestinal

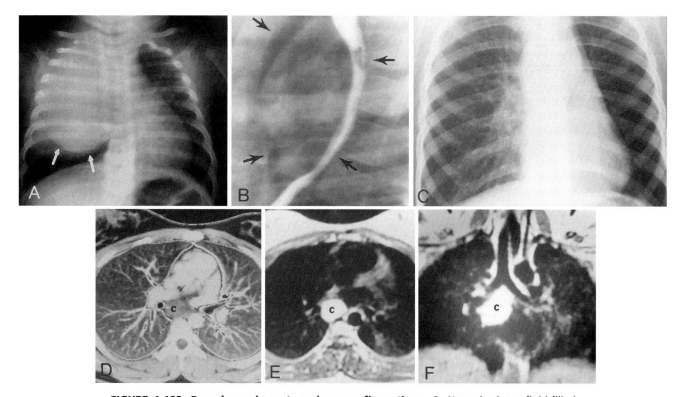

FIGURE 1.182. Bronchogenic cyst: various configurations. A. Note the large fluid-filled bronchogenic cyst (arrows) in this infant with respiratory distress. **B.** Another patient with a bronchogenic cyst displacing the trachea anteriorly and the barium-filled esophagus posteriorly (arrows). **C.** Same patient, demonstrating hypoplasia of the left lung secondary to compression of the pulmonary artery by the bronchogenic cyst. **D.** Small subcarinal bronchogenic cyst (C) in another patient, demonstrated on computed tomography. **E.** Same finding (C) is seen on this axial proton density magnetic resonance image. **F.** Coronal view demonstrates the subcarinal location of the cyst (C). High signal indicates dense proteinaceous content.

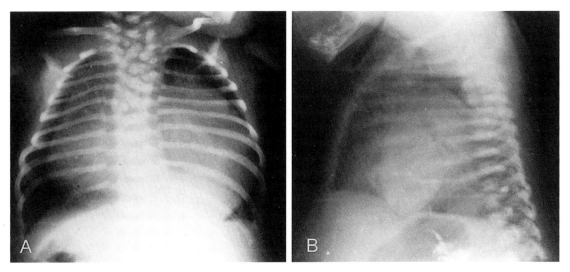

FIGURE 1.183. Neurenteric cyst. A. There is a large mass in the superior mediastinum in this infant. It is blending with the cardiac and thymic silhouettes and overall is causing marked enlargement of these structures. However, note the characteristic vertebral anomalies. **B.** Lateral view demonstrates the posterior location of this mass. Also note forward displacement of the trachea. (Courtesy of S. Rubin, M.D.).

tract and, on roentgenographic examination, appear as round or oval masses, displacing the esophagus and other adjacent structures (Fig. 1.184). Roentgenographic differentiation from bronchogenic cysts is difficult.

Histologically, neurenteric or enteric cysts are lined with esophageal, gastric, or intestinal epithelium, and the cyst wall contains layers of smooth muscle with interspersed myenteric plexuses. When gastric mucosa lines the cyst, peptic ulceration is more than a passing compli-

cation, and erosion into the lung parenchyma, bronchus, or esophagus can occur. Indeed, these patients can present with significant hemorrhages, even to the point of exsanguination and death. In most instances, bleeding is the result of ulceration of a cyst containing gastric mucosa. This gastric mucosa can be identified with nuclear scintigraphy using technetium-99m studies. Intrathoracic cysts, of any type are readily demonstrable with CT and MRI (Fig. 1.185).

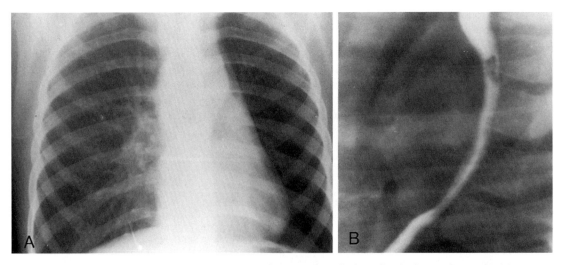

FIGURE 1.184. Duplication cyst. A. Note the smooth-walled mediastinal mass (arrows). This was incidentally discovered in this older boy who had nonrelated syncopal episodes. **B.** Lateral view demonstrates characteristic displacement of the trachea and esophagus, clearly placing the mass in the middle mediastinum. Surgically proven duplication cyst.

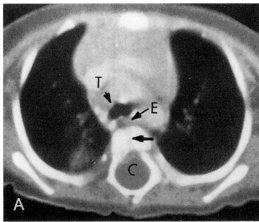

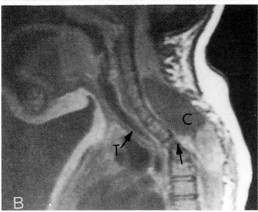

FIGURE 1.185. Neurenteric cyst: computed tomography and magnetic resonance findings. A. This unusual cyst fills the entire thoracic spinal canal (C). Note the connection, through the vertebral body (arrow), between the cyst and the esophagus (E) and trachea (T) anteriorly. **B.** T1-weighted magnetic resonance image demonstrates the large intraspinal cyst (C) and the anterior communication (arrow). Note that the trachea (T) and the esophagus are tethered to the spine. (Reproduced with permission from Kantrowitz LR, Pais MJ, Burnett K, et al. Intraspinal neuroenteric cyst containing gastric mucosa: CT and MRI findings. Pediatr Radiol 1986;16:324).

REFERENCES

1. DuMontier C, Grauiss ER, Siberstein MJ, et al. Bronchogenic cysts in children. Clin Radiol 1985;36:431–361.
2. Rozenblit A, Igbal A, Kaleya R, et al. Case report: intradiaphragmatic bronchogenic cyst. Clin Radiol 1998;53:918–920.
3. Agha FP, Master K, Kaplan S, et al. Multiple bronchogenic cysts in the mediastinum. Br J Radiol 1975;48:54–57.
4. Harris M, Woo-Ming MO, Miller CG. Acquired pulmonary stenosis due to compression by a bronchogenic cyst. Thorax 1973;28:394–398.
5. Kincaid PK, Stanley P, Kovanlikaya A, et al. Coexistent neuroenteric cyst and enterogenous cyst. Further support for a common embryologic error. Pediatr Radiol 1999;29:539–541.
6. Piramoon AM, Abbassioun K. Mediastinal enterogenic cyst with spinal cord compression. J Pediatr Surg 1974;9:543–545.
7. Snodgrass JJ. Transdiaphragmatic duplication of the alimentary tract. AJR 1953;69:42–53.

MISCELLANEOUS MEDIASTINAL LESIONS

Suppurative mediastinitis or actual abscess formation as a cause of respiratory distress in young infants has been reported (1, 2). Overall, however, the problem is rare and usually due to perforation of the esophagus. Such perforation may be iatrogenic or spontaneous. The former is more common. Both suppurative mediastinitis and mediastinal hemorrhage lead to widening of the superior mediastinum and, in many cases, associated pleural effusions. Pancreatic pseudocysts extending into the chest, accumulation of mediastinal fat in patients on steroid therapy, and anomalous vessels such as a persistent left superior vena cava, total anomalous pulmonary venous return, etc., round out the less common causes of mediastinal widening.

REFERENCES

1. Feldman R, Gromisch DS. Acute suppurative mediastinitis. Am J Dis Child 1971;121:79–81.
2. Fields JM, Schwartz DS, Gosche J, et al. Idiopathic bilateral anterior mediastinal abscesses. Pediatr Radiol 1997;27:596–597.

INTRAPULMONARY MASSES AND NODULES

Pulmonary nodules are not nearly as common in childhood as in adulthood, and most often a solitary nodule, calcified or otherwise, is a granuloma. Occasionally, calcification also can be encountered in a hamartoma, and most often they assume the typical "popcorn" calcification of cartilage (Fig. 1.186A). Rarely, malignant degeneration can occur in a hamartoma (1). One also can encounter peripheral nodules due to bronchogenic cysts, but these are rather uncommon, and it is even more uncommon for them to calcify (Fig. 1.186B). Most often, bronchogenic cysts lie closer to the mediastinum and are uncalcified.

Multiple nodules, of course, are seen with metastatic disease (Fig. 1.186C) but also are seen with fungal disease, Wegner's granulomatosis, juvenile papillomatosis, multiple hemangiomatosis (Fig. 1.186D), multiple septic emboli (abscesses), and the collagen vascular diseases. Those nodules most prone to cavitation are the ones seen with Wegner's granulomatosis, juvenile papillomatosis, collagen vascular disease, and septic emboli. Occasionally, cavitation also is seen with metastatic nodules, and, in addition, metastatic nodules often are of variable size and quite discrete. Inflammatory nodules tend to be more even in size and have slightly fuzzier margins. Metastases from osteogenic sarcoma frequently show calcification due to ossified bone.

Primary pulmonary or pleural tumors are very rare in childhood, and perhaps the one most often reported is the pulmonary blastoma or pleuroblastoma (2–6). Mesothe-

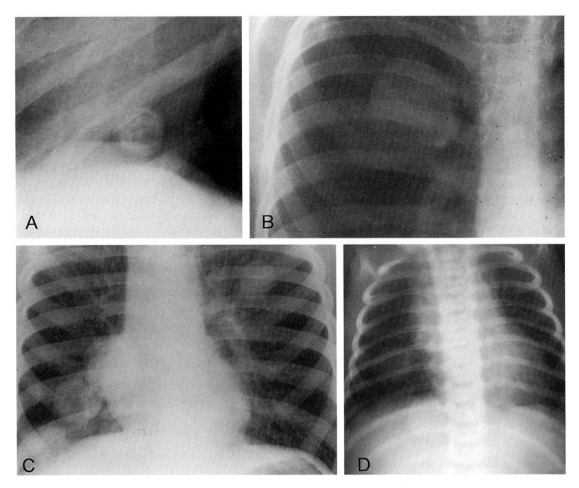

FIGURE 1.186. Pulmonary nodules. A. Calcified nodule, an incidental hamartoma. **B.** Peripheral calcification in a bronchogenic cyst. **C.** Numerous discretely outlined nodules due to metastatic disease from a peripheral hemangiopericytoma. **D.** Note two faintly visible masses in the lower right lung. The lower one is partially obscured by the diaphragm and liver. These were hemangiomas in the lung. The patient also had hemangiomas over the body. (**B** courtesy of C. J. Fagan, M.D.).

lioma is extremely rare but can present as a very large mass (Fig. 1.187A). Pulmonary blastoma or pleural blastoma can present as a solitary nodule or a very large mass that can be bilateral and cystic (5, 6). The findings are usually vividly demonstrable with CT (Fig. 1.187B). The tumor probably arises from primitive mesenchymal pulmonary blastoma and is capable of producing metastases (5). Squamous cell carcinoma of the lung is extremely rare in children (7) but, in addition to being primary, also can be seen in cases of juvenile papillomatosis with bronchial seeding. Lymphoma of the lung is extremely rare (Fig. 1.187C).

Other rare tumors documented in infancy and childhood include bronchoalveolar carcinoma (8), pulmonary leiomyosarcoma (9), rhabdomyosarcoma (10, 11), and fibrosarcoma. Endobronchial lesions are rare but include bronchial adenoma (12), bronchial carcinoid (13, 14), mucoepidermoid carcinoma (13, 15), and bronchial adenoma (12). Endobronchial lesions tend to present more with atelectasis and infection rather than as pulmonary masses.

A pulmonary varix or an arteriovenous malformation also may produce a nodule in the lungs, and often feeding vessels can be identified on plain films. However, these vessels can be seen with greater clarity with contrast-enhanced CT. If they touch the chest wall, they also can be evaluated with color flow Doppler (16). Pulmonary nodules can be seen with hemangiomas of the lung. Calcified pulmonary nodules can be seen on a metastatic basis with chronic renal failure (17) and in older children with metastatic osteosarcoma, old granulomatous disease, and, as has been noted earlier, hamartomas.

Finally, one should appreciate that an early consolidating pneumonia may present as a nodule in the lung and that occasionally old, incompletely resolved pulmonary infections can leave a residual reactive nodule or so-called "pseudotumor" (18, 19). These pseudotumors consist of fibroblasts, histiocytes, and plasma cells, and hence the term "plasma cell granuloma" (20, 21) also is used to describe them.

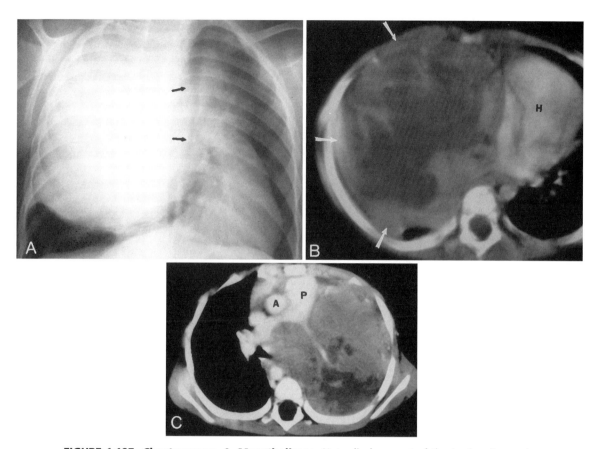

FIGURE 1.187. Chest masses. A. Mesothelioma. Note displacement of the trachea (arrows) and mediastinum to the left by the large mass occupying most of the right hemithorax. **B. Pulmonary blastoma.** Axial computed tomography image demonstrates a heterogeneous mass (arrows) occupying the entire right hemithorax and displacing the heart (H) to the left. **C. Lymphoma of lung.** Note the heterogeneous and nonspecific nature of the mass in the left hemithorax. A, aorta; P, pulmonary artery. (**B** reproduced with permission from Senac MO Jr, Wood BP, Isaacs H, et al. Pulmonary blastoma: a rare childhood malignancy. Radiology 1991;179:743–746; **C** courtesy of C. Keith Hayden, Jr., M.D.).

REFERENCES

1. Hedlund GL, Bisset GS III, Bove KE. Malignant neoplasms arising in cystic hamartomas of the lung in childhood. Radiology 1989;173:77–79.
2. Kovanlikaya A, Pirnar T, Olgun N. Pulmonary blastoma: a rare case of childhood malignancy. Pediatr Radiol 1992;22:155.
3. Cappuccino H, Heleotis T, Krumerman M. Pulmonary blastoma as a unique cause of fatal respiratory distress in a newborn. J Pediatr Surg 1995;30:886–888.
4. Priest JT, McDermott MB, Bhatia S, et al. Pleuropulmonary blastoma. A clinicopathologic study of 50 cases. Cancer 1997;80: 147–161.
5. Picaud J-C, Levrey H, Bouivier R, et al. Bilateral cystic pleuropulmonary blastoma in early infancy. J Pediatr 2000;136: 834–836.
6. Tagge EP, Mulvihill D, Chandler JC, et al. Childhood pleuropulmonary blastoma: caution against nonoperative management of congenital lung cysts. J Pediatr Surg 1996;31:187–190.
7. Shelley BE, Lorenzo RL. Primary squamous cell carcinoma of the lung in childhood. Pediatr Radiol 1983;13:92–94.
8. Ohye RG, Cohen DM, Caldwell S, et al. Pediatric bronchioloalveolar carcinoma: a favorable pediatric malignancy? J Pediatr Surg 1998;33:730–732.
9. Beluffi G, Bertolotti P, Mietta A, et al. Primary leiomyosarcoma of the lung in a girl. Pediatr Radiol 1986;16:240–244.
10. Hancock BJ, DiLorenzo M, Youssef S, et al. Childhood primary pulmonary neoplasms. J Pediatr Surg 1993;28:1133–1136.
11. Noda T, Todani T, Watanabe Y, et al. Alveolar rhabdomyosarcoma of the lung in a child. J Pediatr Surg 1995;30:1607–1608.
12. Wildburger R, Hollwarth ME. Bronchoadenoma in childhood. Pediatr Surg Int 1989;4:373–380.
13. Bellah RD, Mahboubi S, Berdon WE. Malignant endobronchial lesions of adolescence. Pediatr Radiol 1992;22:563–567.
14. Spunt SL, Pratt CB, Rao BN, et al. Childhood carcinoid tumors: the St. Jude Children's Research Hospital experience. J Pediatr Surg 2000;35:1282–1286.
15. Tsuchiya H, Nagashima K, Ohashi S, et al. Childhood bronchial mucoepidermoid tumors. J Pediatr Surg 1998;33:1586–1587.
16. Kuo P-H, Yuan A, Yang P-C, et al. Diagnosis of pulmonary arteriovenous malformation with color Doppler ultrasonography. J Ultrasound Med 1995;14:53–56.
17. Beerman PJ, Crowe JE, Sumner TE, et al. Radiological case of the month—metastatic pulmonary calcification from chronic renal failure. Am J Dis Child 1983;137:1119–1120.

18. Hadimeri U, Hadimeri H, Resjo M. Inflammatory pseudotumor of the lung. A case report. Pediatr Radiol 1993;23:624–625.
19. Kim I, Kim WS, Yeon KM, et al. Inflammatory pseudotumor of the lung manifesting as a posterior mediastinal mass. Pediatr Radiol 1992;22:467–468.
20. Laufer L, Cohen Z, Mares AJ, et al. Pulmonary plasma-cell gran-uloma. Pediatr Radiol 1990;20:289–290.
21. Mas Estelles F, Andres V, Vallcanera A, et al. Plasma cell granu-loma of the lung in childhood: atypical radiologic findings and association with hypertrophic osteoarthropathy. Pediatr Radiol 1995;25:369–372.

CHEST WALL MASSES

Chest wall masses in children usually are secondary to car-tilaginous or mesenchymal hamartomas of the ribs (1–4). These tumors often are very large. They can be bilateral and cause considerable rib deformity and destruction (Fig. 1.188). Indeed, they may at first appear malignant, although most are benign and can be treated conservatively (5). In addition, an aneurysmal bone cyst has been docu-mented as arising within one of these tumors (6).

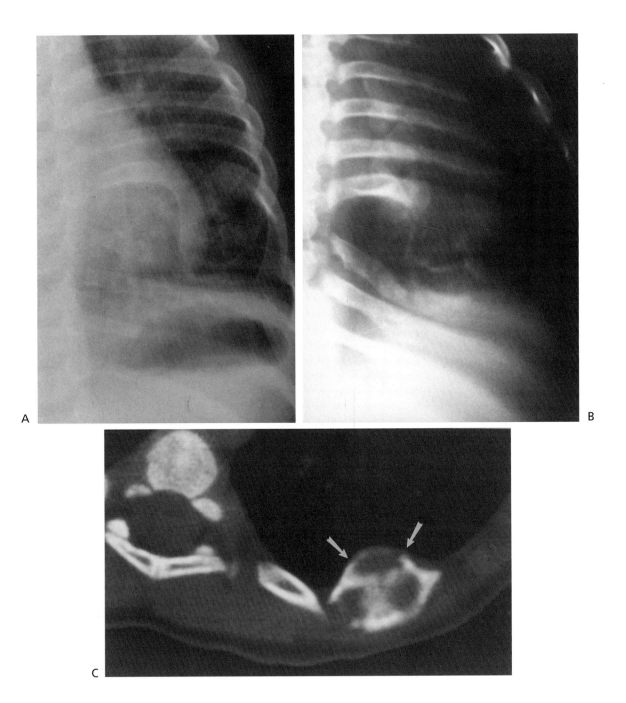

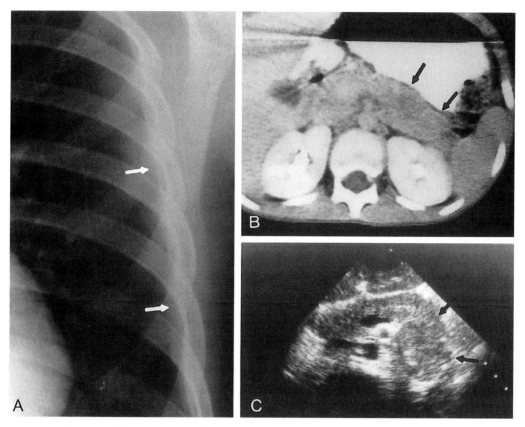

FIGURE 1.189. Metastatic neuroblastoma. A. Note pleural thickening (arrows) in this patient who presented with diffuse bone pain. The findings are secondary to neuroblastoma metastases to the ribs. **B.** Computed tomography in the same patient demonstrates a retroperitoneal neuroblastoma (arrows). It is difficult to separate it from the pancreas. **C.** Ultrasound study in the same patient demonstrates the same mass (arrows).

Pleural thickening can be a manifestation of bone marrow infiltration of the ribs with leukemia (7), lymphoma, or metastatic neuroblastoma (Fig. 1.189). This may be the first roentgenographic clue to the presence of one of these round cell infiltrating malignancies.

Other chest wall tumors include lipomas, hemangiomas, lymphangiomas, teratomas, sarcomas, osteoid osteomas (8), and desmoids (9). In addition, one not uncommonly can encounter Ewing's sarcoma or primitive neuroectodermal tumor and Askin tumors (all probably the same tumor) throughout childhood (10–15). However, these tumors tend to present in older children and often produce massive lysis of the ribs (Fig. 1.190). Associated pleural effusions are common, and on ultrasound, the findings are nonspecific. CT with three-dimensional reconstruction is very helpful in demonstrating the topography of these tumors (16).

FIGURE 1.188. Mesenchymoma of rib. A. Note the deformed ribs on the left. **B.** The deformed ribs are displaced by the cartilaginous mass. **C.** Computed tomography study demonstrates the expanded mixed nature of the tumor (arrows). (Courtesy of J. C. Hoeffel, M.D.).

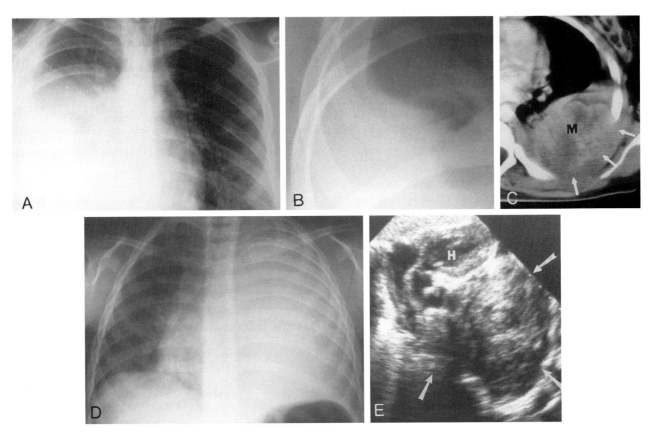

FIGURE 1.190. Ewing's sarcoma. A. Note the right pleural effusion and absent (destroyed) rib. **B.** Focused view of the destroyed rib. **C.** Computed tomography demonstrates the large, heterogeneous mass (M) associated with rib destruction (arrows). **D. Askin (primitive neuroectodermal) tumor.** The left hemithorax is completely opacified secondary to a large tumor and some pleural fluid. **E.** Ultrasonography demonstrates the heterogeneous nature of the tumor (arrows). H, displaced heart.

REFERENCES

1. Gwyther SJ, Hall CM. Mesenchymal hamartoma of the chest wall in infancy. Clin Radiol 1991;43:24–25.
2. Andiran F, Ciftci AO, Senocak ME, et al. Chest wall hamartoma: an alarming chest lesion with a benign course. J Pediatr Surg 1998;33:727–729.
3. Oakley RH, Carty H, Cudmore RE. Multiple benign mesenchymoma of the chest wall. Pediatr Radiol 1985;15:58–60.
4. Schlesinger AE, Smith MB, Genez BM, et al. Chest wall mesenchymoma (hamartoma) in infancy: CT and MR findings. Pediatr Radiol 1989;19:212–213.
5. Cameron D, Ong TH, Borzi P. Conservative management of the mesenchymal hamartomas of the chest wall. J Pediatr Surg 2001;36:1346–1349.
6. Balci P, Obuz F, Gore O, et al. Aneurysmal bone cyst secondary to infantile cartilaginous hamartoma of rib. Pediatr Radiol 1997;27:767–769.
7. Siegel MJ, Shackelford GD, McAlister WH. Pleural thickening: an unusual feature of childhood leukemia. Radiology 1981;138:367–369.
8. Hoeffel JC, Lascombes P, Delgoffe C, et al. Osteoid osteoma of the rib: a case report. J Pediatr Surg 1993;28:741–743.
9. Okamura H, Marayama S, Murakami J, et al. CT manifestations of pediatric intrathoracic desmoid tumors. Pediatr Radiol 1995;25:S202–S204.
10. Dang NC, Siegel SE, Philips JD. Malignant chest wall tumours in children and young adults. J Pediatr Surg 1999;34:1773–1778.
11. Pineschi A, Cavallaro S, Bardini T, et al. Askin's tumor in children: a report of two cases. Pediatr Surg Int 1992;7:73–75.
12. Saenz NC, Hass DJ, Meyers P, et al. Pediatric chest wall Ewing's sarcoma. J Pediatr Surg 2000;35:550–555.
13. Sallustio G, Pirronti T, Lasorella A, et al. Diagnostic imaging of primitive neuroectodermal tumour of the chest wall (Askin tumour). Pediatr Radiol 1998;28:697–702.
14. Shamberger RC, Tarbell NJ, Perez-Atayde AR, et al. Malignant small round cell tumor (Ewing's-PNET) of the chest wall in children. J Pediatr Surg 1994;29:179–185.
15. Winer-Muram HT, Kauffman WM, Gronemeyer SA, et al. Primitive neuroectodermal tumors of the chest wall (Askin tumors): CT and MR findings. AJR 1993;161:265–268.
16. Donnelly LF. Pictorial essay. Use of three-dimensional reconstructed helical CT images in the recognition and communications of chest wall anomalies in children. AJR 2001;177:441–445.

Diaphragmatic Tumors

Diaphragmatic tumors in children are rare. Among those encountered, one can see primitive neuroectodermal tumors and rhabdomyosarcoma (1, 2). These tumors can present with what at first might appear to be an elevated diaphragmatic leaflet (1), while in others, a pleural effusion may at first obscure the tumor (2).

REFERENCES

1. Gupta AK, Mitra DK, Berry M. Primary embryonal rhabdomyosarcoma of the diaphragm in a child: case report. Pediatr Radiol 1999;29:823–825.
2. Smerdely MS, Raymond G, Fisher KL, et al. Primitive neuroectodermal tumor of the diaphragm: case report. Pediatr Radiol 2000; 30:702–704.

MISCELLANEOUS CHEST WALL PROBLEMS

Tietze's Syndrome

Tietze's syndrome consists of acute costochondritis. Often, the patient will present with pain or a painful mass along a costochondral junction. The diagnosis should be accomplished clinically (1). The typical physical findings (i.e., pain, mass) usually require no further imaging studies. Indeed, if a chest film is obtained, it will be normal (1).

REFERENCE

1. Mukamel M, Kornreich L, Horev G, et al. Tietze's syndrome in children and infants. J Pediatr 1997;131:774–775.

Pectus Carinatum and Pectus Excavatum

Pectus carinatum is commonly seen with congenital heart disease and often is associated with sternal fusion (Fig. 1.191A). Pectus excavatum produces a very narrow chest on lateral view and on frontal view a characteristic downward slanting of the anterior ribs and more horizontal positioning of the posterior ribs (Fig. 1.191B). In addition, the heart is shifted to the left, and the right paraspinal structures become a little more prominent and may erroneously suggest an infiltrate (Fig. 1.191C). Pectus excavatum can be demonstrated with CT scans, and this is of value in pre- and postoperative assessment (1).

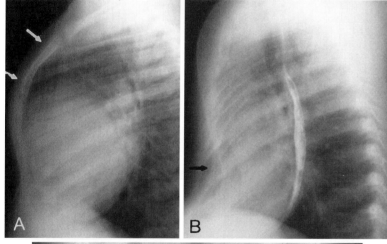

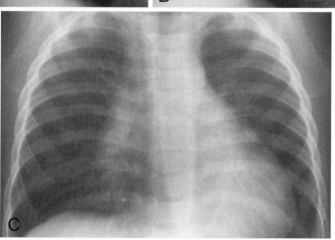

FIGURE 1.191. Pectus abnormalities. A. Pectus carinatum. The sternum bulges anteriorly (arrows) and has prematurely fused in this patient with over-aerated lungs and underlying congenital heart disease. **B. Pectus excavatum.** Lateral view demonstrates the typical depression of the sternum (arrow). **C.** Frontal view demonstrates apparent shift of the mediastinum to the left, increased pulmonary markings in the right lower paraspinal region, horizontal positioning of the posterior ribs, and downward slanting of the anterior ribs.

REFERENCE

1. Chuang J-H, Wan Y-L. Evaluation of pectus excavatum with repeated CT scans. Pediatr Radiol 1995;25:654–656.

BREAST DISEASE

Breast disease in childhood and adolescence is not nearly as common as in adulthood. On the other hand, breast infections, abscesses, and tumors can be encountered (1, 2). Most malignant tumors are metastatic in origin (1), and the most common benign tumor is a fibroadenoma. However, breast cancer (3) and other tumors such as rhabdomyosarcoma (1, 4) and lymphoma (1) also can be encountered.

The evaluation of breast abnormalities in childhood centers around ultrasonography (5) and not mammography. Mammography, in fact, is to be discouraged except for very select cases. Breast abscesses usually show a clearly hypoechoic center (Fig. 1.192A) with an inflammatory rim showing hyperemia on color flow Doppler studies, and in some cases, scattered debris may be seen with the abscess (Fig. 1.192B). Simple cysts are smooth walled and hypoechoic (Fig. 1.192C) but are not particularly common. Fibroadenomas are echogenic but relatively hypoechoic as compared with the adjacent adipose and glandular tissue (Fig. 1.192D). Simple gynecomastia also can be evaluated with ultrasonography whereupon an overabundance of normal tissue will be seen.

REFERENCES

1. Boothroyd A, Carty H. Breast masses in childhood and adolescence. A presentation of 17 cases and a review of the literature. Pediatr Radiol 1994;24:81–84.
2. Rogers DA, Lobe TE, Roa BN, et al. Breast malignancy in children. J Pediatr Surg 1994;29:48–51.
3. Murphy JJ, Morzaria S, Gow KW, et al. Breast cancer in a 6-year-old child. J Pediatr Surg 2000;35:765–767.
4. Herrera LJ, Lugo-Vicente H. Primary embryonal rhabdomyosarcoma of the breast in an adolescent female: a case report. J Pediatr Surg 1998;33:1582–1584.
5. Garcia CK, Espinoza A, Dinamarca V, et al. Breast US in children and adolescents. Radiographics 2000;20:1605–1612.

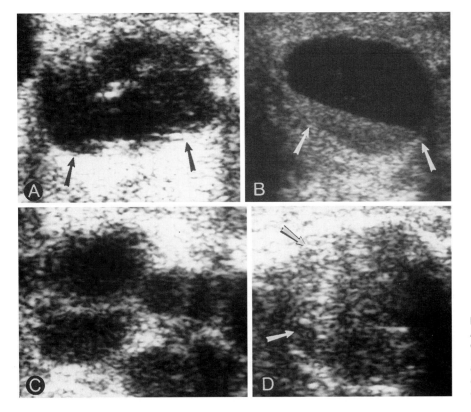

FIGURE 1.192. Breast abnormalities. A. Breast abscess (arrows) with a hypoechoic fluid-filled center. **B.** Another breast abscess (arrows) with echogenic debris layering along its base. **C.** Numerous hypoechoic fluid-filled cysts. **D.** Echogenic fibroadenoma (arrows).

NASAL PASSAGES, MANDIBLE, AND UPPER AIRWAY

Air in the nose, pharynx, larynx, and upper trachea provides a natural contrast medium that proves most useful in the assessment of the soft tissues of the neck. These tissues are best assessed on the lateral roentgenogram, obtained during inspiration, with the neck partially extended. If the neck is flexed or if the infant is crying (expiration), the airway buckles forward and the prevertebral soft tissues become more prominent, suggesting a mass (Fig. 2.1). Buckling of the airway has been suggested to be the result of upward crowding of the prevertebral soft tissues by the jamming effect of the thymus being pushed into the thoracic inlet during expiration (1). However, this can be avoided if the

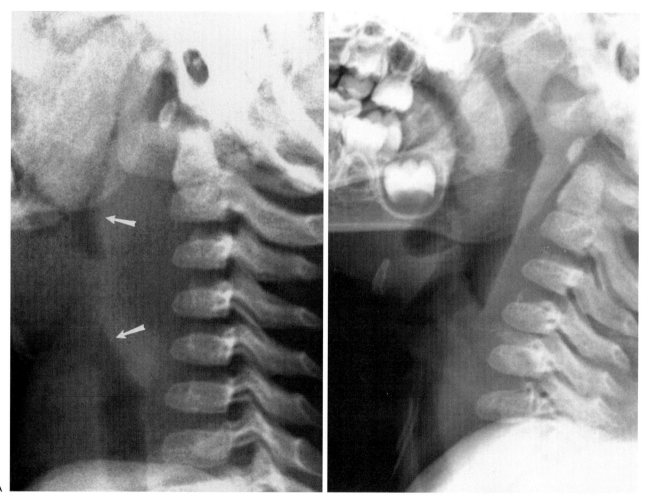

A   B

FIGURE 2.1. Normal airway buckling. A. Note exaggerated anterior buckling of the airway, producing the appearance of a retropharyngeal mass (arrows). Such a configuration is commonly seen with forward flexion of the neck and during expiration. **B.** With deep inspiration and with extension of the neck the airway is normal.

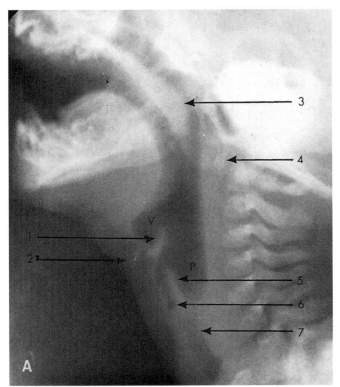

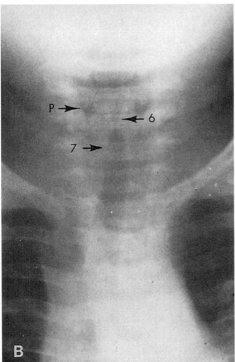

examination is properly performed (Fig. 2.1B), whereupon one can clearly identify the entire airway and surrounding soft tissues (Fig. 2.2A). In many cases, the same structures also are visible on frontal projection (Fig. 2.2B), but it is the lateral view that is most uniformly informative. It is for this reason that the plain film study of the airway, especially the lateral view, still is the most important and productive imaging study in the assessment of stridor and other upper airway problems (2). Computed tomography (CT) and magnetic resonance imaging (MRI) are used in specific instances, but initial impressions usually are accomplished on clinical and plain film findings.

As far as the retropharyngeal soft tissues are concerned, undue thickening should alert one to the presence of a retropharyngeal mass or inflammatory process, but it should be remembered that this area is proportionately thicker in newborn and young infants than in older children because the vertebral bodies are not yet fully ossified. Unfortunately, it is difficult to outline precise prevertebral soft tissue measurements, but it has been generally accepted that in infants, with the neck fully extended, the soft tissue space from C1 to C4 is equal to one-half of the width of the vertebral body. Later on, as the infant grows older, the vertebral bodies become larger and wider, and prevertebral soft tissues become correspondingly less prominent. Below the

FIGURE 2.2. Normal airway. A. Lateral view with neck in extension shows normal cervical spine, normal prevertebral soft tissue thickness, and normal airway. 1, epiglottis; 2, hyoid bone; 3, soft palate and uvula; 4, anterior arch of C1; 5, aryepiglottic folds; 6, air in ventricle of glottis. False cords are just above the ventricle, and true cords are just below. 7, subglottic portion of trachea; V, valleculae; P, pyriform sinuses. Note the normal step-off of the posterior pharyngeal and tracheal walls. **B.** Frontal view.

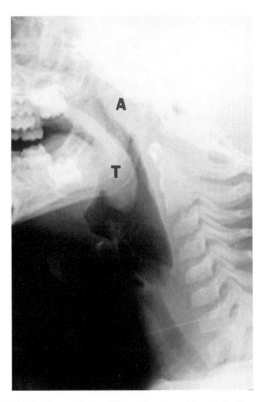

FIGURE 2.3. Normal tonsils and adenoids. Note the prominent tonsils (T) and adenoids (A) in this 3-year-old child.

TABLE 2.1. NORMAL NASOPHARYNGEAL LYMPHOID TISSUE

		Thickness of Soft Tissue		
Age	No. of Infants	0.0 cm	0.5 cm or less	Over 0.5 cm
1 day to 1 month	36	36	0	0
1–3 months	76	36	39	1
3–6 months	47	7	25	15
6–12 months	56	0	16	40
12–24 months	42	0	3	39

Source: From Capitanio MA, Kirkpatrick JA. Nasopharyngeal lymphoid tissue. Roentgen observations in 257 children two years of age or less. Radiology 1970;96:389–391, with permission of the Radiological Society of North America, Inc.

level of C4, that is, below the level of the larynx, the soft tissue space normally doubles in width. The resulting step-off between the posterior pharyngeal and tracheal walls is probably the most important thing to note. On a well-positioned film, if the step-off is lost, one should suspect retropharyngeal pathology.

Nasopharyngeal adenoidal tissue is sparse in the newborn, but as the infant grows older, it becomes more abundant (Fig. 2.3). For specific measurements of the adenoids, one is referred to Table 2.1.

REFERENCES

1. Mandell GA, Bellah RD, Boulden MEC, et al. Cervical trachea: dynamics in response to herniation of the normal thymus. Radiology 1993;186:383–386.
2. John SD, Swischuk LE. Stridor and upper airway obstruction in infants and children. Radiographics 1992;12:625–643.

ABNORMALITIES OF THE NASAL PASSAGES

Choanal Atresia

Choanal atresia, a congenital obstruction of the nasal passages, can be either membranous or bony (1). When it is bilateral, severe respiratory distress develops, and, in fact, until the infant learns to mouth-breathe, the mouth may have to be held open mechanically. Feeding also can be a problem. When choanal atresia is unilateral, it poses less of a problem and frequently passes unnoticed until the infant is older.

Plain film roentgenographic changes are absent, but in the past, contrast studies of the nasal passages were helpful. These now have been replaced by CT (2), where detailed delineation of the abnormal anatomy is possible. CT identifies both the membranous and the bony forms of the condition (Fig. 2.4). Slovis et al. (2) have indicated that in bony atresia, the vomer (midline bone) is thickened and also that there is inward thickening of the lateral nasal bony wall

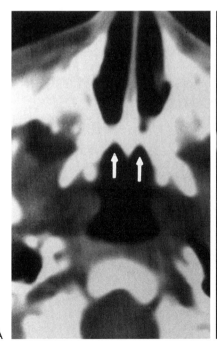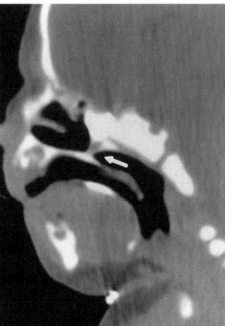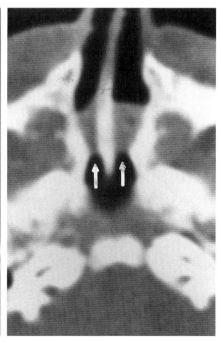

A

B,C

FIGURE 2.4. Choanal atresia: computed tomography findings. A. Bony choanal atresia. Note bony obstruction of both nares (arrows). In addition, note that the vomer, the bone in between, is thickened. **B. Membranous choanal atresia.** On this sagittal reconstructed view, note the discrete membrane (arrow). **C.** In this patient with membranous choanal atresia (arrows), fluid has accumulated distal to the obstructing membranes. Also note that the vomer is only slightly thickened.

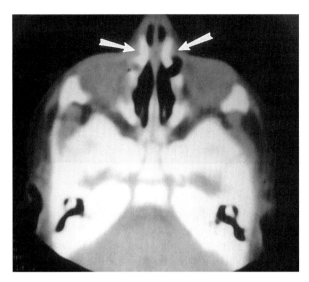

FIGURE 2.5. Inlet or pyriform aperture stenosis, anterior choanal atresia. Note the anterior location of the choanal stenosis (arrows) in this infant. (Reproduced with permission from Ey EH, Han BK, Towbin RB, et al. Bony inlet stenosis as a cause of nasal airway obstruction. Radiology 1988;168:477–479).

(Fig. 2.4A). The membrane in membranous obstructions may be thin, and in addition, there is less thickening of the lateral nasal wall and vomer (Fig. 2.4B). The precise location of the obstructing membrane or bone can be further delineated with sagittal reconstruction views (Fig. 2.4B). Associated mucoid impaction can appear as an intranasal mass (3) and on fluid collections may suggest that an obstructing membrane is thicker than it really is (Fig. 2.4C). To remedy this, it has been suggested that the nasal passages be thoroughly cleaned and that topical decongestants be applied before CT examination is undertaken (2).

The vast majority of congenital stenoses or frank obstructions of the nasal passages occur posteriorly, in the form of

posterior choanal stenosis or atresia. Rarely, somewhat similar stenoses can be encountered anteriorly and have been termed "inlet" (4), or congenital, nasal piriform aperture stenosis (5–7). This abnormality also is best demonstrated with CT (Fig. 2.5), where it has been suggested that a width of less than 11 mm through the aperture be considered abnormal (6). These patients have been demonstrated to have associated abnormalities consisting of absence of the anterior pituitary gland and abnormal dentition (6).

REFERENCES

1. Stahl RS, Jurkiewicz MJ. Congenital posterior choanal atresia. Pediatrics 1985;76:429–436.
2. Slovis TL, Renfro B, Watts FB, et al. Choanal atresia: precise CT evaluation. Radiology 1985;155:345–348.
3. Kleinmann P, Winchester PP. Pseudotumor of the nasal fossa secondary to mucoid impaction in choanal atresia. Pediatr Radiol 1975;4:47–48.
4. Ey EH, Han BK, Towbin RB, et al. Bony inlet stenosis as a cause of nasal airway obstruction. Radiology 1988;168:477–479.
5. Bignault A, Castillo M. Congenital nasal piriform aperture stenosis. AJNR 1994;15:877–878.
6. Belden CJ, Mancuso AA, Schmalfuss IM. CT features of congenital nasal piriform aperture stenosis: initial experience. Radiology 1999;213:495–501.
7. Beregszaszi M, Leger J, Gaerl C, et al. Nasal piriform aperture stenosis and absence of the anterior pituitary gland: report of two cases. J Pediatr 1996;128:858–861.

Nasal Polyps

Nasal polyps are not particularly common in children. Occasionally so-called "allergic polyps" are encountered, and occasionally recurrent bouts of allergy and infection lead to chronic hypertrophic polypoid rhinosinusitis. However, most commonly when nasal polyps are encountered in children, the underlying problem is cystic fibrosis. In any of

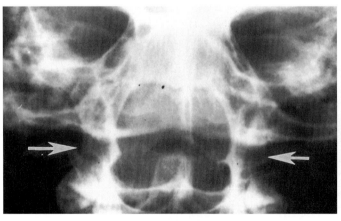
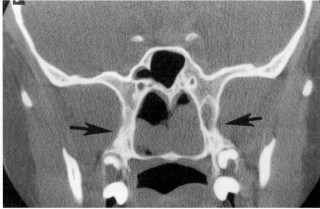

FIGURE 2.6. Nasal polyps. A. Note widening of the nasal passages (arrows) in this patient with polyposis secondary to cystic fibrosis. **B.** Another patient demonstrating similar findings on a computed tomography scan (arrows). (**A** courtesy of J. Arndt, M.D.).

these cases, if the polyps are massive and chronic, they can completely fill the nose, extend into the nasopharynx, and even widen the nose. If clearer definition of polyps is required, CT examination is useful (Fig. 2.6).

Antrochoanal polyps are peculiar lesions of older children and young adults (1–3). These benign polyps are of unknown etiology but probably not inflammatory or allergic in origin. They most commonly arise from the maxillary sinuses but also can arise from the sphenoid and ethmoid sinus cavities (4–7). In any case, they may fill the nasal cavity or plunge back into the oropharynx. As such, they can present as a pharyngeal mass (Fig. 2.7). In addition, the

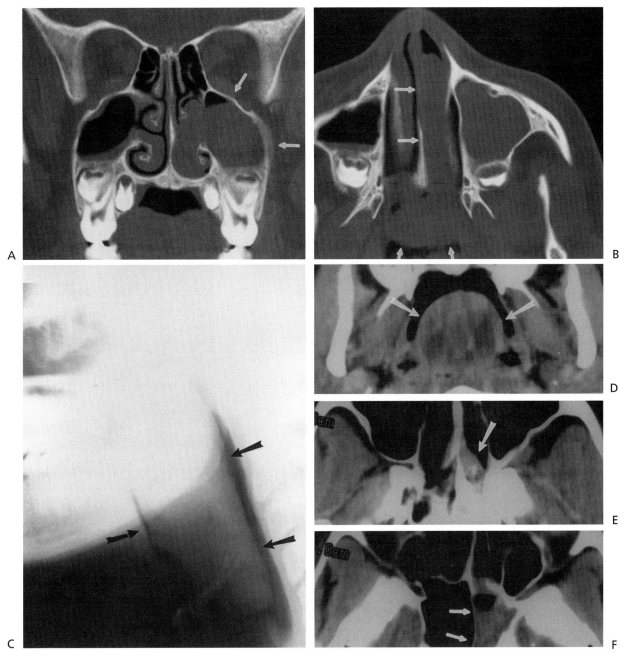

FIGURE 2.7. Antrochoanal polyp. A. Antrochoanal polyp producing opacification of the left maxillary sinus and nasal passage (arrows). **B.** Axial view demonstrates the extent of the polyp in the nasal passage and the pharynx (arrows). **C. Another patient.** Note the large mass (polyp) in the nasopharynx (arrows). **D.** Axial computed tomography (CT) study demonstrates the hypodense mass (arrows) in the pharynx. **E.** On this axial CT view, the stalk of the polyp (arrow) is seen within the nasal passage. Note that the maxillary sinuses are clear. **F.** A higher CT cut demonstrates the obliterated left sphenoid sinus cavity. This polyp arose from the sphenoid sinus. (Reproduced with permission from Swischuk LE, Hendrick EP. Antrochoanal polyp originating from sphenoid sinus causing acute dysphagia. Emerg Radiol 2000;7:358–360).

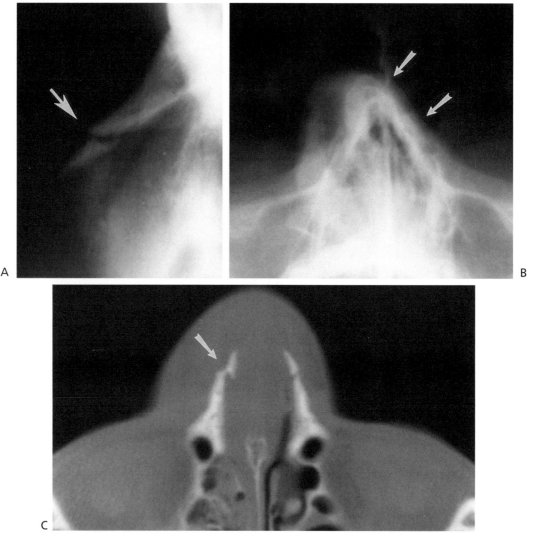

FIGURE 2.8. Nasal fractures. A. Comminuted nasal fracture (arrow). **B.** Water's view demonstrates nasal deformity (arrows) and deviation of the septum. **C.** Another patient with a minimally displaced nasal fracture (arrow) seen on an axial computed tomography view. There also are swelling of the soft tissues and slight deviation of the nose.

involved sinus, usually the ipsilateral maxillary sinus, is opacified (Fig. 2.7, A and B). Ultimately, it is the CT study that more clearly demonstrates the polyp and its site of origin (Fig. 2.7). Antrochoanal polyps can produce secondary symptoms such as sleep apnea (8) and dysphagia (6). Finally, it should be noted that the so-called "hairy" polyp can be encountered in the newborn (9).

REFERENCES

1. Min Y-G, Chung JW, Shin J-S, et al. Histologic structure of antrochoanal polyps. Acta Otolaryngol 1995;115:543–547.
2. Rashid A-MH, Soosay G, Morgan D. Unusual presentation of a nasal antrochoanal polyp. Br J Clin Pract 1994;48:108–109.
3. Sharma HS, Daud ARA. Antrochoanal polyp—a rare paediatric emergency. Int J Pediatr Otorhinolaryngol 1997;41:65–70.
4. Crampette L, Mondain M, Rombaux PH. Sphenochoanal polyp in children; diagnosis and treatment. Rhinology 1995;33:43–45.
5. Weissman JL, Tabor EK, Curtin HD. Sphenochoanal polyps: evaluation with CT and MR imaging. Radiology 1991;178:145–148.
6. Lopatin A, Bykova V, Piskunov G. Choanal polyps: one entity, one surgical approach? Rhinology 1997;35:79–83.
7. Swischuk LE, Hendrick EP. Antrochoanal polyp originating from sphenoid sinus causing acute dysphagia. Emerg Radiol 2000;7:358–360.
8. Rodgers GK, Chan KH, Dahl RE. Antral choanal polyp presenting as obstructive sleep apnea syndrome. Arch Otolaryngol Head Neck Surg 1991;117:914–916.
9. Kelly A, Bough ID Jr, Luft JD, et al. Hairy polyp of the oropharynx: case report and literature review. J Pediatr Surg 1996;31:704–705.

Nasal Foreign Bodies

Foreign bodies in the nose are common in childhood and, if embedded deeply in the nasal passages, may remain occult and lead to chronic infection. If these foreign bodies are radiopaque, they are easily identified, but if nonopaque, they may remain undetected even with more sophisticated imaging.

Nasal Trauma

Nasal trauma is common in infants but most of the time does not lead to underlying bony injury. However, fractures can occur transversely across the nasal bone or longitudinally in the septal portion of the bone. What is most important is to determine whether septal deviation has occurred, and this is best accomplished on the Water's view or with CT (Fig. 2.8). It is important not to misinterpret the normal nasociliary groove and frontonasal suture for fractures.

Nasal Tumors and Cysts

Nasal tumors and cysts are not particularly common, and as far as cysts are concerned, dermoid cysts are probably the most common (1). Most often, they are midline, round, and best demonstrated with CT or MRI (2) (Fig. 2.9, A and B). Patients with nasal dermoids also may demonstrate hypertelorism, and the findings should be differentiated from those seen with nasal encephalocele and congenital dermal sinus. In both the latter instances, there is communication with the subarachnoid space of the brain, while with a dermoid cyst, no such communication exists. Nasal encephaloceles are discussed in Chapter 6.

Nasal tumors generally are uncommon in childhood, but include nasal gliomas (1), teratomas, fibrous histiocytomas (2), osteomas, olfactory neuroblastomas (3), rhinolithiasis (4), and hemangiomas. Nasal gliomas present with a progressively enlarging mass over the bridge of the nose. Hypertelorism and localized bony erosion can be seen, and some of these tumors may communicate intracranially. Teratomas can be identified by the presence of extensive calcification, and osteomas, of course, are very dense and radiopaque (Fig. 2.9C). All of these lesions finally are imaged with CT and/or MRI.

REFERENCES

1. Barkovich AJ, Vandermarck P, Edwards MSB, et al. Congenital nasal masses: CT and MR imaging features in 16 cases. AJR 1991;156:587–598.

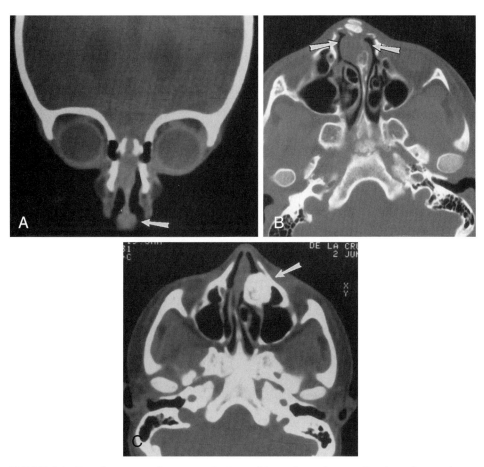

FIGURE 2.9. Nasal cysts and tumors. A. Dermoid cyst (arrow) extending into the nasal passage. Note the bony defect through the floor of the skull in the interorbital region. **B.** Another patient with a dermoid (arrows) causing a deformity of the septum. **C.** Dense osteoma (arrow) in another patient.

2. Shearer WT, Schreiner RL, Ward SP, et al. Benign nasal tumor appearing as neonatal respiratory distress; first reported case of nasopharyngeal fibrous histiocytoma. Am J Dis Child 1973; 126:238–241.

3. Ferlito A, Micheau C. Infantile olfactory neuroblastoma: a clinicopathological study with review of the literature. J Otorhinolaryngol 1971;41:40—45.

4. Royal SA, Gardner RE. Rhinolithiasis: an unusual pediatric nasal mass. Pediatr Radiol 1998;28:54–5.

ABNORMALITIES OF THE TONGUE

A large tongue can be seen with acute glossitis (1) and primary tumors such as rhabdomyosarcoma (2), lymphangioma (3), and hemangioma. Enlargement also can be seen with cretinism and the Beckwith-Wiedemann syndrome. A small tongue is less common and often is associated with a small mandible. An absent tongue can be seen as part of the aglossia-adactylia syndrome (4). Finally, glossoptosis (posterior dropping of the tongue) can lead to sleep apnea and can be documented fluoroscopically during sleep (5).

REFERENCES

1. Stoddard JJ, Deshpande JK. Acute glossitis and bacteremia caused by Streptococcus pneumoniae: case report and review. Am J Dis Child 1991;145:598–599.

2. Liebert PS, Stool SE. Rhabdomyosarcoma of the tongue in an infant. Results of combined radiation and chemotherapy. Ann Surg 1973;178:621.

3. Lobitz B, Lang T. Lymphangioma of the tongue. Pediatr Emerg Care 1995;11:1983–1185.

4. Johnson GF, Robinow M. Aglossia-adactylia. Radiology 1978; 128:127–132.

5. Donnelly LF Strife JL, Myer CM III. Glossoptosis (posterior displacement of the tongue during sleep): a frequent cause of sleep apnea in pediatric patients referred for dynamic sleep fluoroscopy. AJR 2000;175:1557–1559.

ABNORMALITIES OF THE SALIVARY GLANDS

Infections of the salivary glands usually are viral and most often are caused by the mumps virus. Suppurative infections usually result from bacterial infection. Some children also have chronic recurrent swelling of the salivary glands of unknown etiology, but presumed to be of autoimmune origin (1). Sjögren's syndrome, also an autoimmune-mediated disease, is uncommonly documented in children, as are salivary gland stones. The stones may be visualized on plain films, CT, or with ultrasound and can be located in the ducts or in the glands themselves. In the past, the ducts themselves were visualized by way of contrast sialography, but this has been replaced by MR sialography (2) (Fig 2.10D).

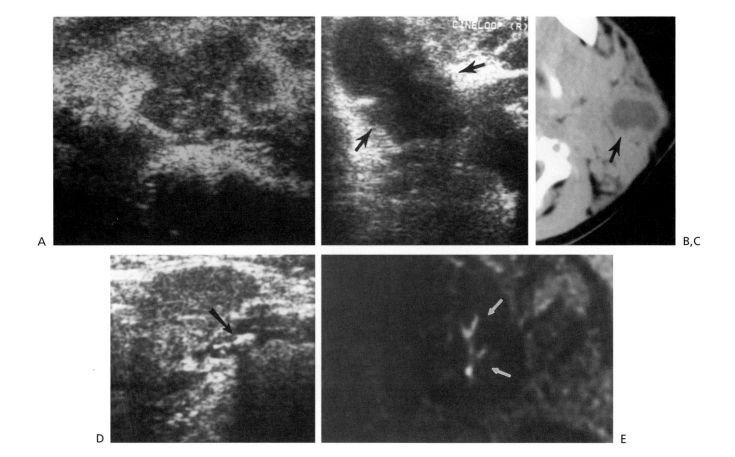

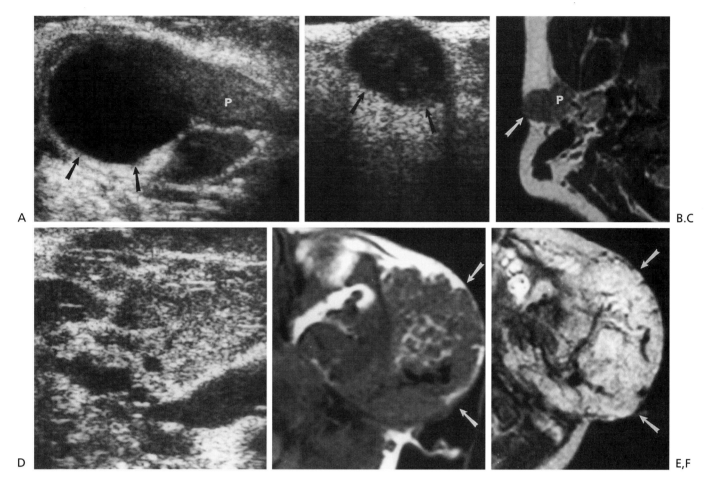

FIGURE 2.11. Salivary gland tumors and cysts. A. Note, on this ultrasound study, the hypoechoic parotid cyst (arrows) within the parotid (P) gland. **B. Hypoechoic fibroma (arrow) of parotid gland. C.** Fast spin echo axial magnetic resonance (MR) study demonstrates the low signal fibroma (arrow). Note the residual parotid gland (P) just to the side. **D. Parotid hemangioma: ultrasound study.** Note the heterogeneous echotexture and the numerous hypoechoic flow voids. **E.** T1-weighted MR study demonstrates the large medium-signal mass (arrows). Scattered high-signal fat is seen within the lesion, and in addition, flow void reflecting the vascularity of the lesion is seen. **F.** Fast spin echo axial MR study demonstrates the relatively high-signal tumor (arrows) with numerous tortuous flow voids representing vessels.

Generally, lesions of the salivary glands now are first investigated with ultrasound (3, 4) and then CT or MR. Ultrasound can detect stones, abscesses, and intraglandular lymphoid tissue (Fig. 2.10, A–E). The latter, first believed to be seen only in human immunodeficiency virus-positive patients (5, 6), is now known also to occur in other patients. Ultrasonographically, infected salivary glands show a nonspecific pattern of echogenicity of the enlarged gland (Fig. 2.10A). If suppuration occurs, a central hypoechoic collection of pus can be seen (Fig. 2.10B).

Salivary gland stones usually are the result of chronic infection but also can be seen with cystic fibrosis. Tumors of the salivary glands in childhood, be they primary or secondary, are uncommon but include mixed tumors, carcinomas (7), embryonomas (8), teratomas (9), lipomas (10), mucoepidermoid tumors, and hemangiomas (11). For the most part, it is difficult to histologically type the tumor on the basis of the features seen on any given imaging modality (Fig. 2.11), except for hemangiomas. Hemangiomas produce coarse echogenicity on ultrasound and markedly

FIGURE 2.10. Salivary gland inflammation. A. Parotid gland. Note the echogenic background of the parenchyma and three hypoechoic areas representing intraglandular lymphoid tissue. **B.** Hypoechoic abscess (arrows) in another patient. **C.** Computed tomography demonstrates the same hypodense abscess (arrow). **D. Sialectasis with stone.** On this ultrasound study, note the echogenic stone (arrow) in the dilated duct. **E. Magnetic resonance sialography.** Note high signal in the dilated intraglandular ducts (arrows). This patient suffered from chronic recurrent salivary gland infection.

increased signal on T2-weighted MR images. In addition, with both studies, one can identify feeding vessels and internal blood flow. This is especially well documented with color flow Doppler.

REFERENCES

1. Wilson WR, Eavey RD, Lang DW. Recurrent parotitis during childhood. Clin Pediatr 1980;19:235–236.
2. Becker M, Marchal F, Becker CD, et al. Sialolithiasis and salivary ductal stenosis: diagnostic accuracy of MR sialography with a three-dimensional extended-phase conjugate-symmetry rapid spin-echo sequence. Radiology 2000;217:347–358.
3. Seibert RW, Seibert JJ. High-resolution ultrasonography of the parotid gland in children. Part II. Pediatr Radiol 1988;19:13–18.
4. Garcia CJ, Flores PA, Arce JD, et al. Ultrasonography in the study of salivary gland lesions in children. Pediatr Radiol 1998;28:418–425.
5. Goddart D, Francois A, Ninane J, et al. Parotid gland abnormality found in children seropositive for the human immunodeficiency virus (HIV). Pediatr Radiol 1990;20:355–357.
6. Soberman N, Leonidas JC, Berdon WE, et al. Parotid enlargement in children seropositive for human immunodeficiency virus: imaging findings. AJR 1991;157:553–556.
7. Rogers DA, Ral BN, Bowman L, et al. Primary malignancy of the salivary gland in children. J Pediatr Surg 1994;29:44–47.
8. Som PM, Brandwein M, Silvers AR, et al. Sialoblastoma (embryoma): MR findings of a rare pediatric salivary gland tumor. AJNR 1997;18:847–850.
9. Rose PE, Howard ER. Congenital teratoma of the submandibular gland. J Pediatr Surg 1982;17:414–416.
10. Holland AJA, Hay GSB, Brennan BA. Parotid lipomatosis. J Pediatr Surg 1996;31:1422–1423.
11. Hebert G, Ouimet-Oliva D, Ladouceur J. Vascular tumors of the salivary glands in children. AJR 1975;123:815–819.

ABNORMALITIES OF THE MANDIBLE

Hypoplasia of the Mandible (Micrognathia)

Hypoplasia of the mandible can involve the entire mandible or just one side. When unilateral underdevelopment is pre-

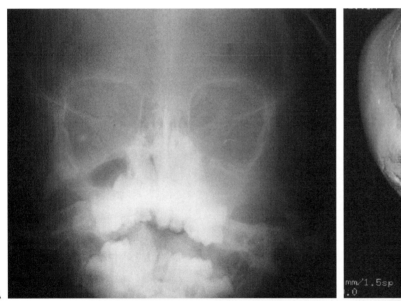

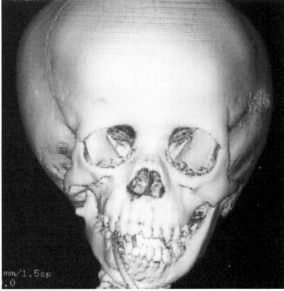

A

B

C

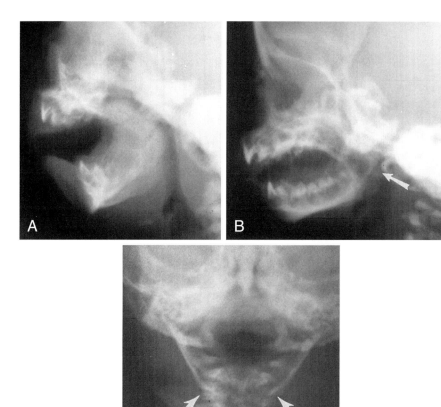

FIGURE 2.13. Mandibular underdevelopment: small mandible. A. Note the small mandible in this patient with Pierre-Robin syndrome. The mandible is recessed into the airway, and airway compromise results. **B.** Another patient with generalized mandibular hypoplasia but, more specifically, hypoplasia of the rami (arrow). **C.** Note pointed, small mandible (arrows) in this patient with aglossia.

sent, the condition frequently is referred to as "hemifacial microsomia." In such cases, associated temporomandibular joint hypoplasia, facial hypoplasia, and congenital hearing defects can be seen (1). The imaging findings are straightforward and especially well demonstrated with three-dimensional reconstructed CT studies (Fig. 2.12).

Generalized hypoplasia of the mandible frequently is seen as part of the "first arch" syndromes (e.g., Pierre Robin syndrome, Goldenhar's syndrome, Weyers' mandibulofacial dysostosis, and Treacher Collins mandibulofacial dysostosis). It is also often seen in the trisomy 17–18 and 13–15 and cri-du-chat syndromes. In all cases, there is mandibular underbiting and recessing of the mandible and tongue into the oropharynx (Fig. 2.13A). This often leads to severe airway compromise and marked respiratory distress. Cor pul-

monale with pulmonary edema (secondary to chronic upper airway obstruction) also can result.

As the infant grows older, the mandible usually becomes larger, more normal in position, and less prone to produce airway obstruction. Nonetheless, in the early days and weeks of life, mandibular hypoplasia and its associated posterior displacement of the tongue can produce profound respiratory distress, especially if the infant is kept in a recumbent position. Therefore, these infants should be kept in the prone position, and in severe cases, prolonged nasoesophageal intubation is required.

Another variation of mandibular hypoplasia includes isolated hypoplasia of the mandibular rami. In these cases, the body of the mandible is relatively normal, but the rami short (Fig. 2.13B). Still another variation is smallness of the

FIGURE 2.12. Hemifacial microsomia. A. Plain film, Water's view, demonstrates the underdevelopment of the right side of the face. **B.** Reconstructed three-dimensional computed tomography study demonstrates the same findings. **C.** Note absence of the middle and outer ear on the right side (arrows).

mandible with a pointed symphysis menti, a deformity usually seen with aglossia (Fig. 2.13C).

REFERENCE

1. Cavo JW Jr, Pratt LL, Alonso WA. First branchial cleft syndromes and associated congenital hearing loss. Laryngoscope 1976;86: 739–745.

Inflammatory Lesions of the Mandible

Osteomyelitis of the mandible is rarely encountered in the young infant, but later may be seen in association with chronic tooth infection or as a focus of hematogenous osteomyelitis. Although most often osteomyelitis is due to a pyogenic organism, it also can be seen with actinomycosis or other fungal disease. Whatever the cause, the roentgenographic findings are about the same, for there is mandibular destruction, and when the disease is chronic, reactive hyperostosis occurs. A paramandibular mass also may be present and often is best demonstrated with CT or MRI scanning (Fig. 2.14).

In the past, one of the most common inflammatory conditions to involve the mandible of a young infant was infantile cortical hyperostosis. This condition is discussed in more detail in the chapter on bone disease, but the mandible frequently was involved and, indeed, the presenting problem. Usually, there is considerable swelling of the jaw, and roentgenographically, the characteristic findings are those of periosteal new bone deposition along the mandible (Fig. 2.15). This disease, however, now is virtually nonexistent, suggesting that it may have been due to some infectious process, perhaps a viral infection.

The findings should not be confused with reactive periostitis secondary to cellulitis and lymphadenitis of the submandibular lymph glands (1). This condition, usually occurring in older infants and children, has periosteal new bone appear a week or so after the lymph node inflammation begins. The underlying bone is completely normal.

REFERENCE

1. Suydan MJ, Mikity VG. Cellulitis with underlying inflammatory periostitis of the mandible. AJR 1969;56:133–135.

Trauma to the Mandible

For the most part, mandibular fractures are sustained with forceful injuries to the chin, and not mere tumbles. In some cases, only transient problems with temporomandibular joint movement occur, but in other instances, one can encounter a variety of hairline to frankly displaced or

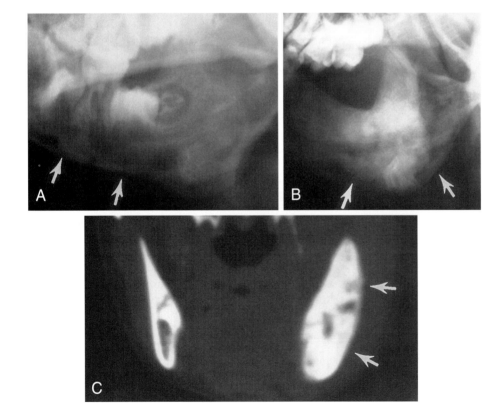

FIGURE 2.14. Osteomyelitis. A. Note multiple areas of destruction in the ramus of the mandible (arrows). **B.** Chronic osteomyelitis in another patient demonstrating hyperostosis and absence of teeth (arrows). **C.** Computed tomography demonstrating the thickened hyperostotic right mandibular ramus (arrows).

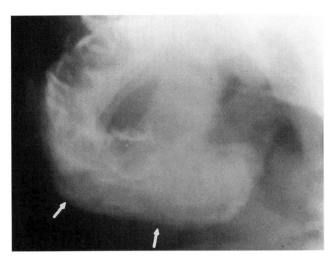

FIGURE 2.15. Caffey's disease (infantile cortical hyperostosis) of the mandible. Note homogeneous, thick periosteal new bone deposition (arrows) on the mandible.

angled fractures of the mandible. Because the mandible is a ring-like bone, fractures in more than one place tend to occur. CT is best for demonstrating mandibular fractures, although Panorex (Gendex) studies also are useful.

It should be noted that bending fractures of the mandibular condyles also may be seen in infants and young children and, indeed, are common (1) (Fig. 2.16). These fractures are easily overlooked (2) and usually are the result of falling on the chin (3).

REFERENCES

1. Ahrendt D, Swischuk LE, Hayden CK Jr. Incomplete (bending?) fractures of the mandibular condyle in children. Pediatr Radiol 1984;14:140–141.

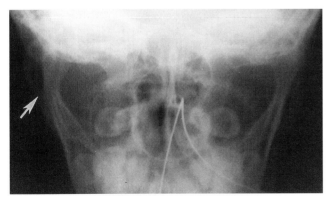

FIGURE 2.16. Bending fracture of mandible. Note the bending fracture of the right mandibular ramus (arrow).

2. Myall RWT, Sandor GKB, Gregory CEB. Are you overlooking fractures of the mandibular condyle? Pediatrics 1987;79:639–641.
3. Hurt TL, Fisher B, Peterson BM, et al. Mandibular fractures in association with chin trauma in pediatric patients. Pediatr Emerg Care 1988;4:121–123.

Temporomandibular Joint

The temporomandibular joint now usually is best assessed with MRI where open and closed views are obtained, but the joints also can be assessed with CT and sagittal reconstruction. In childhood, one may see congenital hypoplasia of the mandible and condyle (see Fig. 2.11B), and while most times the finding is isolated, it also may be associated with some of the syndromes producing generalized mandibular hypoplasia noted in the previous section. Temporomandibular joint dislocation can occur with trauma to the chin, and dislocation also can occur secondary to exaggerated opening of the mouth, as can occur with vomiting (1). The temporomandibular joint also can be involved in rheumatoid arthritis, but joint space narrowing secondary to cartilage destruction is seen with advanced disease only. MR is useful in evaluating the temporomandibular joints in rheumatoid arthritis (2).

REFERENCES

1. Whiteman PJ, Pradel EC. Bilateral temporomandibular joint dislocation in a 10-month-old infant after vomiting. Pediatr Emerg Care 2000;16:418–419.
2. Kuseler A, Pedersen TK, Herlin T, et al. Contrast enhanced magnetic resonance imaging as a method to diagnose early inflammatory changes in the temporomandibular joint in children with juvenile chronic arthritis. J Rheumatol 1998;25:1406–1412.

Tumors and Cysts of the Mandible

Tumors of the mandible are rather uncommon (1) and are extremely rare in the newborn infant. In older children, one may encounter ossifying and nonossifying fibromas, cementomas, ameloblastomas, and fibrous dysplasia. Ossifying fibromas and cementomas usually are unilocular, with distinct margins. They are often seen to contain variable amounts of calcifications within them. Ameloblastomas may produce multilocular, expanding cystic lesions that may be difficult to differentiate from other cystic abnormalities of the mandible.

Fibrous dysplasia may involve the mandible as part of generalized fibrous dysplasia but more often appears as a solitary finding. In the mandible, it usually produces a multiloculated cystic lesion and may be unilateral or bilateral (Fig. 2.17A). It tends to be familial, and in such cases, bilateral involvement leads to the term "cherubism" (1, 2).

As far as cysts of the mandible are concerned, the two most commonly occurring ones in childhood are dentigerous cysts and the so-called "reparative" or "giant cell granu-

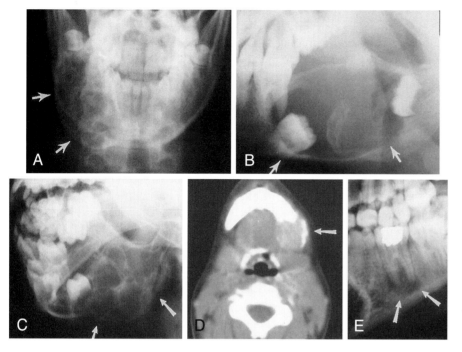

FIGURE 2.17. Mandibular tumors. A. Fibrous dysplasia. Note typical, bubbly, expanded appearance of fibrous dysplasia (arrows). **B. Dentigerous cyst.** Note typical unilocular thin-walled dentigerous cyst (arrows) with ectopic tooth. **C.** Reparative granuloma. Typical multiloculated appearance of a large reparative granuloma. **D.** Computed tomography study in another patient with a reparative granuloma demonstrates the expansile nature of the lesion (arrow). **E. Radicular cyst.** Note the radiolucent cyst (arrows) around the root of the tooth.

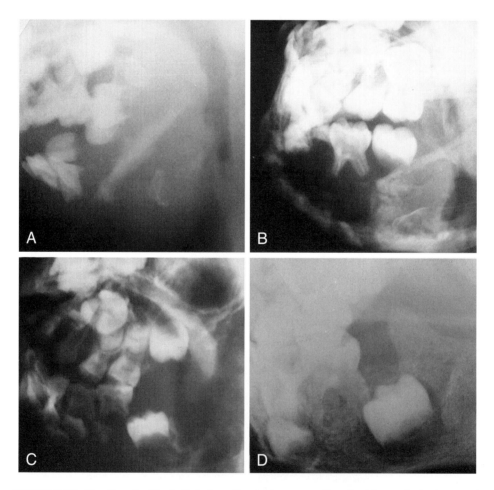

FIGURE 2.18. Floating teeth. A. Note how the teeth seem to float in this massively destroyed mandible in a patient with histiocytosis X. **B.** Less pronounced findings in another patient. **C.** Similar findings in a patient with metastatic neuroblastoma. **D.** Another patient with metastatic neuroblastoma demonstrating mottled destruction of the mandible and early bone dissolution around the wisdom tooth. (**D** courtesy of C. Keith Hayden, Jr., M.D.)

loma" (3, 4). Odontogenic, primordial cysts are rare and develop in the tooth bud before the crown is formed. Dentigerous cysts are much more common and usually present with swelling of the mandible. They demonstrate a typical unilocular appearance with a displaced, ectopic, and tilted tooth in their periphery (Fig. 2.17B). The margins of the cyst are well defined but can be very thin, and occasionally the roots of the involved tooth may be eroded. Dentigerous cysts may be unilateral or bilateral and are common manifestations of the basal cell nevus syndrome.

Reparative granulomas are a peculiarity of childhood, and their roentgenographic appearance is that of either a unilocular or, more often, a multilocular cystic lesion (Fig. 2.17, C and D). Although originally believed to be developmental, they probably represent a reaction to trauma or inflammatory insult to the mandible. Generally, the lesion is well circumscribed and involves the posterior body and ramus of the mandible.

Finally, a note regarding the so-called "radicular cyst" of the mandible is in order. This is not a true cyst but rather an apical root abscess seen with carious teeth in older children. These lesions seldom become very large, are intimately related to a root tip, and usually are associated with surrounding demineralization and indistinctness of the cyst wall (Fig. 2.17E). The tooth root may be partially resorbed, and caries may be seen on its surface.

Destruction of the mandible also can be seen with leukemia, lymphoma, metastatic disease, (usually neuroblastoma), and histiocytosis X. Histiocytosis X often leads to a very homogeneous and complete destruction of the mandible, leaving the teeth to appear to be floating in a liquid matrix (Fig. 2.18, A and B). This has led to the term "floating teeth sign," but while very suggestive of histiocytosis X, the sign can be seen with other causes of bony destruction such as metastases to the mandible (Fig. 2.18, C and D) or leukemia.

REFERENCES

1. Kozlowski K, Masel J, Sprague P, et al. Mandibular and paramandibular tumors in children. Report of 16 cases. Pediatr Radiol 1981;11:183–192.
2. Cornelius EA, McClendon JL. Cherubism—hereditary fibrous dysplasia of the jaws. AJR 1969;106:136–140.
3. Waldron CA, Shafer WG. The central giant-cell reparative granuloma of the jaws: an analysis of 38 cases. Am J Clin Pathol 1966;45:437–447.
4. Bodner L, Bar-Ziv J. Radiographic features of central giant cell granuloma of the jaws in children. Pediatr Radiol 1996;26:148–151.

Dental Abnormalities

In the normal newborn infant, unerupted teeth with well-calcified crowns are present in the mandible and maxilla. In fact, the appearance of the enamel crown of the first and second molars can be used to determine ges-

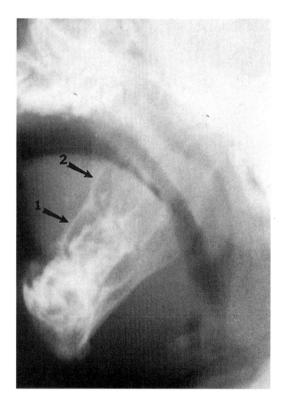

FIGURE 2.19. Determination of neonatal age from mandible. Since the mandible is frequently seen on chest films of the neonate, it is relatively easy to define the degree of calcification of the deciduous molars. The first molar (arrow 1) does not usually appear calcified before 33–34 weeks of gestation, whereas the second molar (arrow 2) does not usually appear calcified until 36–37 weeks of age.

tational age (1). The roots of the various teeth are usually poorly defined, but the enamel cap and surrounding dental sac (radiolucent space around the tooth) are readily identified (Fig. 2.19).

Underdevelopment or total absence of the teeth can occur with conditions such as the aglossia-adactylia syndrome, cleidocranial dysostosis, pyknodysostosis, ectodermal dysplasia (anhidrotic type), and the otopalatodigital syndrome. The most commonly appreciated of these conditions is ectodermal dysplasia, and the findings can be seen at birth (Fig. 2.20A).

Premature neonatal teeth are even rarer but can be seen with conditions such as the Ellis-van Creveld syndrome, the Hallermann-Streiff syndrome, the adrenogenital syndrome, and the pachyonychia congenita syndrome. In addition, occasionally premature teeth may appear in normal neonates, on both a sporadic (2) and a familial (3) basis. We have also seen premature eruption of natal teeth in an infant whom we believed to have Noonan's syndrome (Fig. 2.20B). Odontogenesis imperfecta is the term applied to the generally underdeveloped and dysplastic teeth seen with osteogenesis imperfecta.

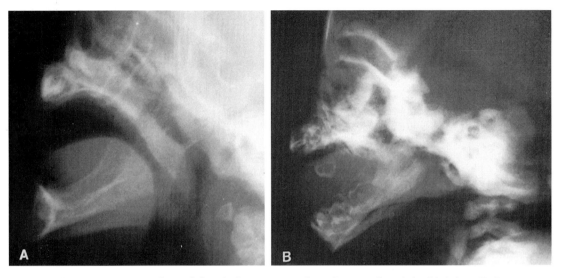

FIGURE 2.20. A. Ectodermal dysplasia. Note complete absence of teeth in this infant. **B.** Premature natal teeth in Noonan's syndrome. Note the prematurely erupted teeth in this patient with suspected Noonan's syndrome. This male infant also demonstrated webbing of the neck and lymphedema.

REFERENCES

1. Kuhns LR, Sherman MP, Poznanski AK. Determination of neonatal maturation on the chest radiography. Radiology 1972;102:597–603.
2. King NM, Lee AMP. Prematurely erupted teeth in newborn infants. J Pediatr 1989;114:807–809.
3. Sibert JR, Porteous JR. Erupted teeth in the newborn; 6 members in a family. Arch Dis Child 1974;49:492–493.

NECK MASSES

Neck masses are common in infants and children, and one's best initial imaging modality is ultrasound. Ultrasound can very quickly determine whether the mass is cystic or solid, and thereafter MRI provides excellent soft tissue resolution and geography for location of the mass. Little else in the way of imaging often is required, but if it is, we favor MRI over CT. If the mass is related to the thyroid gland, one also should perform nuclear scintigraphy.

In terms of masses that turn out to be cysts, the two most common are the midline thyroglossal duct cyst and the laterally located branchial cleft cyst. Thyroglossal duct cysts may be associated with ectopically located thyroid tissue, best detected with nuclear scintigraphy. In this regard, if nuclear scintigraphy identifies a normal thyroid gland, one can confidently exclude ectopic thyroid tissue (1). Thyroglossal duct cysts and sinuses usually are midline and represent remnants or rests of the thyroglossal duct. Branchial cleft cysts and their sinus tracts tend to occur off midline, and most arise from the branchial cleft pouches (2, 3). They occur in the anterior neck. Other cysts in the neck are uncommon (Fig. 2.21E), and some tumors, both benign and malignant, may have a cystic component. In addition, thymic cysts can occur in the neck (4, 5). Ultrasonographically, both thyroglossal duct and branchial cleft cysts usually are well demarcated as round or oval, hypoechoic structures (Fig. 2.21). If bleeding or infection occurs, debris will be seen within the cysts (Fig. 2.21D), and overall the findings can be quite variable (6). Both branchial cleft and thyroglossal duct cysts may calcify, but this is rare.

Inflammatory masses consist of inflamed lymph nodes, suppurative lymph nodes, or frank soft tissue abscesses. In addition, the various salivary glands, but most often the parotid gland, can become infected and enlarged. Ultrasound, again, is the best initial imaging modality with which to detect enlarged lymph nodes. They are relatively hypoechoic and of uniform texture and show increased blood flow with color flow Doppler (7) (Fig. 2.22). When suppuration occurs, the involved node, or a portion thereof, becomes more hypoechoic, in whole or in part (Fig. 2.23). CT and MRI generally are not required for evaluation of inflammatory adenopathy in the neck, but abscesses may require these modalities to delineate their precise location. Abscesses, of course, have a variable picture ultrasonographically, depending on the amount of debris present within the abscess (Fig. 2.22). On CT and MR, an enhancing rim usually is seen with contrast administration.

Malignant tumors of the neck, other than lymphoma, are relatively uncommon. As far as lymphoma is concerned, both Hodgkin's and non-Hodgkin's lymphoma may be encountered. These tumors, as do all malignant tumors, present primarily as firm to hard masses and are clearly demonstrable with CT or MR scanning. On MR scanning,

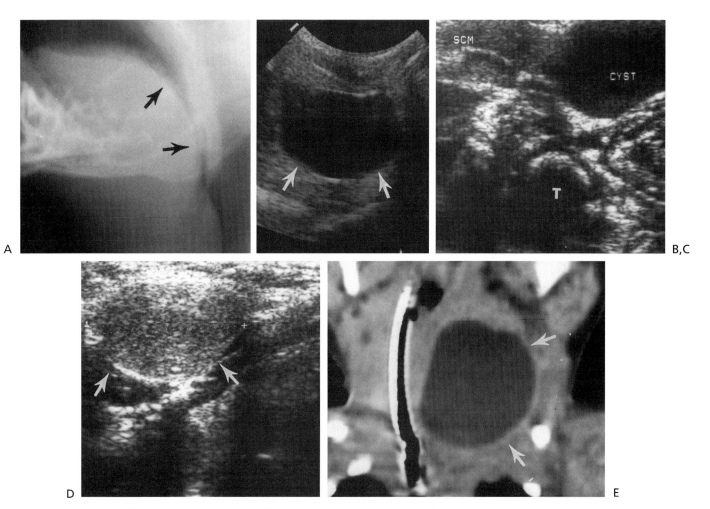

FIGURE 2.21. Cysts. A. Thyroglossal duct cyst (arrows) encroaching upon the airway. **B.** Same patient whose midsagittal sonogram demonstrates the anechoic cyst (arrows). **C.** Sonogram in another patient demonstrating a bronchial cleft cyst (cyst) off midline. T, trachea; SCM, stern-ocleidomastoid muscle. **D.** Another branchial cleft cyst (arrows), which is echogenic because of debris due to bleeding. **E. Duplication cyst.** Note the large cyst (arrows) compressing the airway.

they generally show variable increase in signal on T1- and T2-weighted images (Fig. 2.24A), but on CT, they are rather nonspecific in their appearance. On ultrasonography, lymphoma lymph nodes appear relatively hypoechoic (Fig. 2.24B) and also may demonstrate increased blood flow with color flow Doppler (7). In some cases, many enlarged nodes may be clustered (Fig. 2.24C). In addition, we have found that patients with sclerosing Hodgkin's disease demonstrate more echogenicity in the enlarged nodes than do patients with other forms of lymphoma (Fig. 2.24D). A rare cause of lymph node enlargement is so-called "sinus histiocytosis" (8). This benign condition can be confused with lymphoma, but on histologic examination, the lymph nodes show characteristically dilated sinusoidal spaces containing foamy histiocytes and multinucleated giant cells. The etiology of the condition is unknown, and there is no specific treatment.

Other malignancies encountered in the neck include rhabdomyosarcoma (9), neurofibroma, fibrosarcoma, malignant vascular tumors, salivary gland tumors, and teratomas (10–12). On ultrasonography, all are echogenic, but the pattern is nonspecific. CT and MR studies usually are required for final definition, but MR studies provide more discrete soft tissue delineation (11). Vascular tumors may show their feeding or draining vessels on CT, MR, and ultrasound.

Neuroblastoma may be metastatic or primary in the neck. The primary form is less malignant than when it is intraabdominal (12). It may, as does neuroblastoma elsewhere, show calcification, and on ultrasound, increased blood flow may be seen. There may be involvement of the skull and intracranial contents (13), but even in these cases (Fig. 2.25), the tumor is less aggressive and malignant than neuroblastoma arising in the abdomen or even the chest.

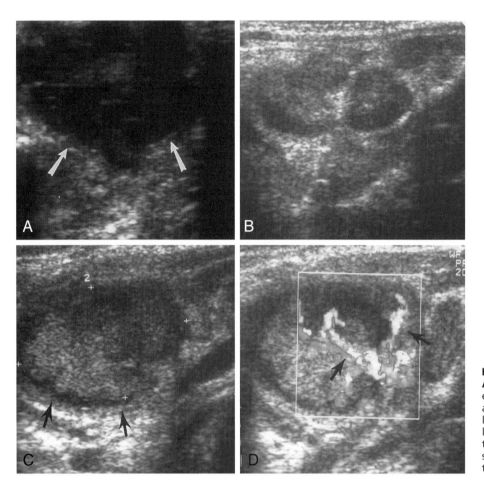

FIGURE 2.22. Inflammatory masses. A. Large abscess (arrows) with some echogenic debris. **B.** Inflammatory adenopathy with numerous enlarged lymph nodes. **C.** A larger, inflamed lymph node (arrows) in another location. **D.** Color flow Doppler demonstrates increased blood flow (arrows) to the large inflamed node.

As far as benign tumors are concerned, the most common is cystic hygroma. These tumors represent congenital malformations of the cervical lymph sac, and the greatest problem they pose is their tendency to extend into adjacent soft tissues by way of soft, finger-like extensions. Sonographically, cystic hygromas usually appear hypoechoic and multicystic or multiseptate (Fig. 2.26). If bleeding occurs into the tumor, echogenicity of the involved cyst is seen (Fig. 2.27). Bleeding may be massive and lead to rapid enlargement of the tumor and significant respiratory distress. Lymphangiomas also can become infected and enlarge precipitously.

Sonography is useful in first identifying and categorizing the cystic hygroma, but MRI is best in defining its geographic limits. With this latter modality, T1-weighted images show medium signal unless bleeding has occurred. If bleeding has occurred, signal is increased. On T2-weighted images, signal in uncomplicated tumors increases (Fig. 2.27C), and when bleeding occurs, signal is variable depending on the age of the bleed (Fig. 2.27D). These findings, together with the ultrasonographic features, should confidently secure the diagnosis.

Hemangiomas of the neck are a little less common and may or may not co-exist with subglottic hemangiomas. Most often, they are separate but, because of their size, may compress the airway. Hemangiomas, as opposed to cystic hygromas, characteristically produce rather homogeneous ultrasonographic echogenicity with varying numbers of hypoechoic sinusoids. If the lesion is primarily a capillary hemangioma, echogenicity is more uniform and sinusoids less prominent (Fig. 2.28). In addition, draining and feeding vessels can be identified in many cases, and on MRI, hemangiomas characteristically produce markedly increased signal intensity on T2-weighted images (Fig. 2.28). The large blood vessels also are clearly identified as low-signal structures (flow void). Color flow Doppler is especially valuable in demonstrating these vessels. However, blood flow to hemangiomas is variable, and in some cases it may be exuberant, while in others it may be barely detectable. Most hemangiomas are treated with steroids, and the natural history is for these tumors to slowly regress.

Another neck mass encountered in infants is the one associated with the sternocleidomastoid muscle abnormal-

(text continues on page 193)

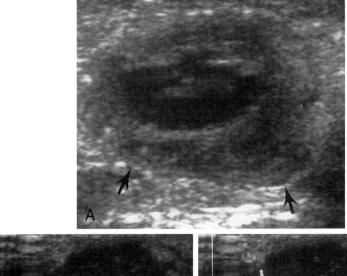

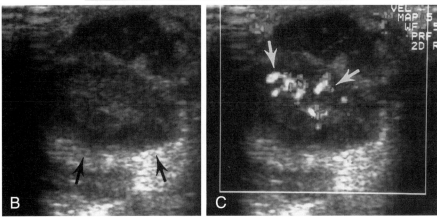

FIGURE 2.23. Suppurative adenopathy. A. Large inflamed lymph node (arrows) with center of liquefaction resulting from suppuration. **B.** Another patient with a large inflamed lymph node (arrows), above which is an area of anechoic suppuration. **C.** Color flow Doppler demonstrates increased blood flow (arrows) to the lymph node but no blood flow to the area of suppuration.

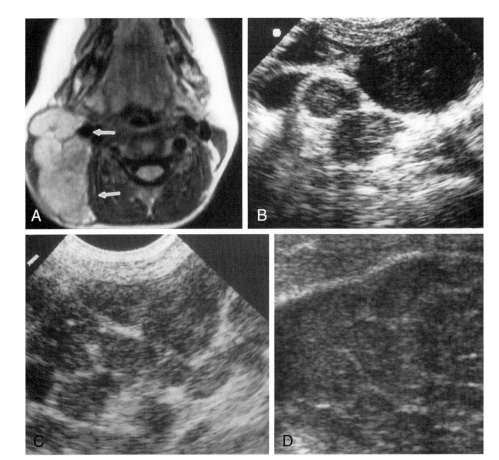

FIGURE 2.24. Lymphoma. A. Proton density magnetic resonance image demonstrates numerous enlarged lymph nodes (arrows) resulting from lymphoma. **B.** Ultrasonogram in another patient demonstrates hypoechoic to moderately echoic enlarged lymph nodes. **C.** Another patient with clustering of moderately echogenic lymph nodes. **D.** More confluent mass somewhat more echogenic in sclerosing Hodgkin's lymphoma.

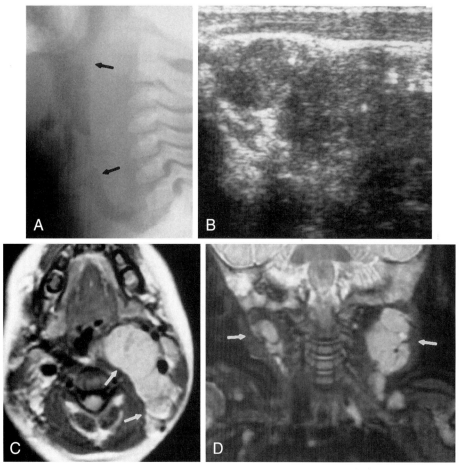

FIGURE 2.25. Cervical neuroblastoma. A. Note the retropharyngeal mass (arrows) with barely visible central punctate calcification. **B.** Ultrasound study demonstrates the solid lobulated nature of the mass with heterogeneous echogenicity and echogenic foci of calcification. **C.** Axial proton density magnetic resonance image demonstrates the large mass on the left (arrows). A smaller mass is present around the jugular vein on the right. **D.** Coronal view demonstrates the bilateral tumor masses (arrows). On the left, some lymph nodes also are seen in the supraclavicular region.

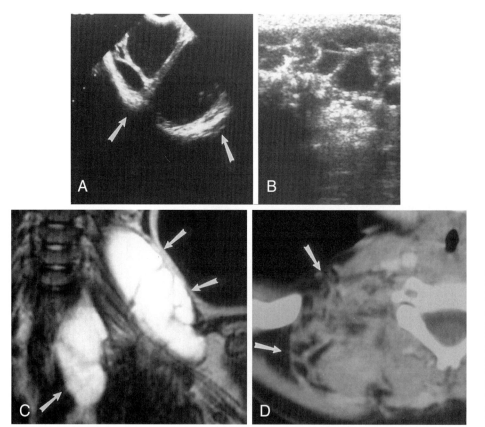

FIGURE 2.26. Cystic hygroma. A. Note large sonolucent cystic structures on ultrasound (arrows). **B.** Another patient with smaller similar sonolucent cystic structures. **C.** In this patient, a proton density magnetic resonance image demonstrates multicystic high-signal structures in the neck (arrows) insinuating between the muscles. **D.** Computed tomography study in another patient demonstrates the multiple fluid-filled cysts (arrows).

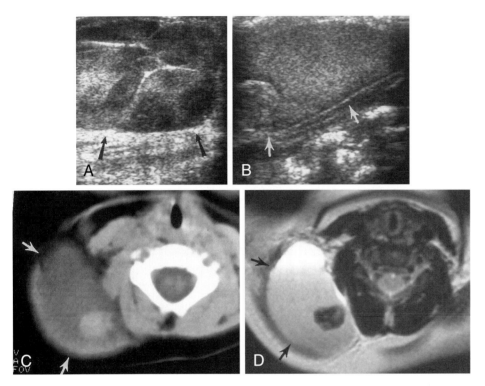

FIGURE 2.27. Cystic hygroma with bleeding. A. Ultrasonogram demonstrates a multicystic structure (arrows) with echogenic debris secondary to bleeding. **B.** Another patient with an echogenic solitary cyst (arrows) and an echogenic blood clot. **C.** Computed tomography demonstrates the cystic structure (arrows) with a blood clot. **D.** Proton density magnetic resonance image demonstrates the cystic structure (arrows) with variable signal and a low-signal old blood clot.

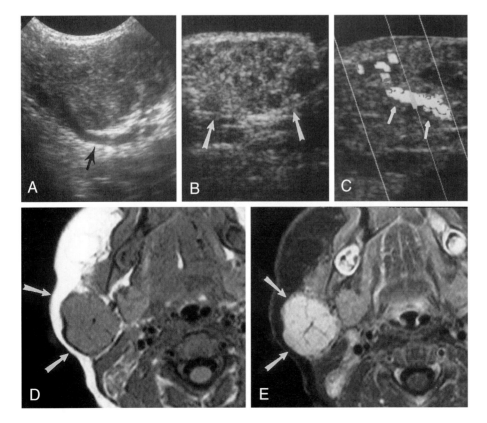

Figure 2.28. Hemangioma. A. Note typical coarse echogenic pattern of a hemangioma with a feeding vessel (arrow). **B.** Another hemangioma (arrows) with coarse echogenicity and numerous anechoic sinusoids. **C.** Color flow Doppler demonstrates increased blood flow to the lesion (arrows). **D.** T1-weighted image demonstrating characteristic density of a hemangioma. Flow voids represent feeding vessels. **E.** T2-weighted image, first echo, demonstrates high signal intensity of the lesion (arrows) and flow voids resulting from the feeding vessels. (**A–C** courtesy of C. Keith Hayden, Jr., M.D.; **D** and **E** courtesy of Frank Crnkovich, M.D.).

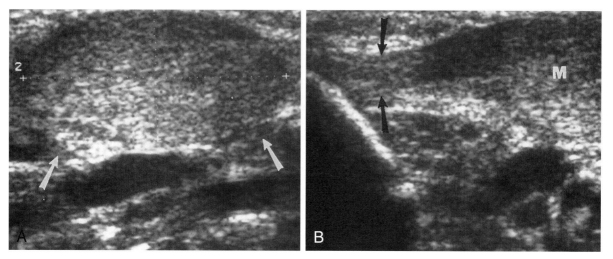

FIGURE 2.29. Sternocleidomastoid muscle mass. A. Note the echogenic oval, bulging mass (arrows). **B.** Another image shows blending of the mass (M) with the normal muscle (arrows).

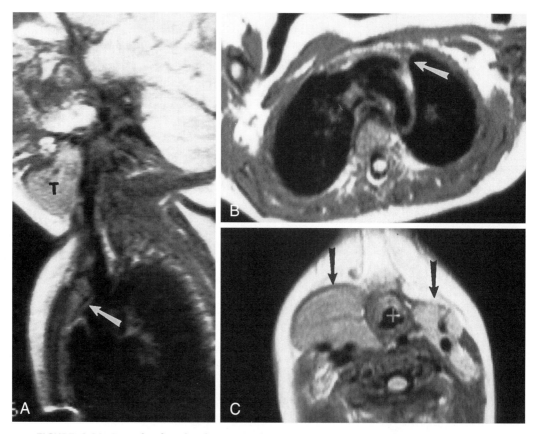

FIGURE 2.30. Ectopic thymic tissue. A. Sagittal T1-weighted magnetic resonance study demonstrates ectopic thymic tissue (T) in the neck and no thymic tissue in the chest (arrow). **B.** Axial T1-weighted magnetic resonance image through the chest demonstrates absence of normal thymic tissue (arrow). **C.** Axial tomogram through the lower neck demonstrates bilateral ectopic thymic tissue (arrows).

ity known as fibromatosis colli. The problem here is a fibrotic tumor of the muscle resulting in torticollis (wry neck). The tumor usually is firm to hard and on ultrasonography can be slightly hypoechoic to echogenic (14). Its location in the belly of the sternocleidomastoid muscle is diagnostic and readily demonstrable with ultrasonography (Fig. 2.29) as it is with CT or MR (15), but ultrasonography usually suffices. The etiology of the condition is unknown, but with physiotherapy, the muscle mass and wry neck deformity usually disappear over a period of time.

Another unusual mass encountered in the neck is ectopic thymic tissue. Most often, the finding comes as a surprise after biopsy (Fig. 2.30). In such cases, there is lack of normal descent of thymic tissue into the neck, but in addition, there may be accessory islands of such tissue present.

REFERENCES

1. Lim-Dunham JE, Feinstein KA, Yousefzadeh DK, et al. Sonographic demonstration of a normal thyroid gland excludes ectopic thyroid in patients with thyroglossal duct cyst. AJR 1995;164:1489–1491.
2. Chin AC, Radhakrishnan J, Slatton D, et al. Congenital cysts of the third and fourth pharyngeal pouches or pyriform sinus cysts. J Pediatr Surg 2000;35:1252–1255.
3. Mahomed A, Youngson G. Congenital lateral cervical cysts of infancy. J Pediatr Surg 1998;33:1413–1415.
4. Lyons TJ, Dickson JAS, Variend S. Cervical thymic cysts. J Pediatr Surg 1989;24:241–243.
5. Cure J, Tagge EP, Richardson MS, et al. MR of cystic aberrant cervical thymus. AJNR 1995;16:1124–1127.
6. Wadsworth DT, Siegel MJ. Thyroglossal duct cysts: variability of sonographic findings. AJR 1995;163:1475–1478.
7. Swischuk LE, Desai PB, John SD. Exuberant blood flow in enlarged lymph nodes: findings on color flow Doppler. Pediatr Radiol 1992;22:419–421.
8. Puczynski MS, Demos TC, Suarez CR. Sinus histiocytosis with massive lymphadenopathy: skeletal involvement. Pediatr Radiol 1985;15:259–261.
9. Yousem DM, Lexa FJ, Bilaniuk LT, et al. Rhabdomyosarcomas in the head and neck: MR imaging evaluation. Radiology 1990;177:683–686.
10. Elmasalme F, Giacomantonio M, Clarke KD, et al. Congenital cervical teratoma in neonates. Case report and review. Eur J Pediatr Sur 2000;10:252–257.
11. Green JS, Dickinson FL, Rickett A, et al. MRI in the assessment of a newborn with cervical teratoma. Pediatr Radiol 1998;28:709–710.
12. Saing H, Lau WF, Chan YF, et al. Parapharyngeal teratoma in the newborn. J Pediatr Surg 1995;29:1524–1527
13. Goldberg RM, Keller IA, Schonfeld SM, et al. Intracranial route of a cervical neuroblastoma through skull base foramina. Pediatr Radiol 1996;26:715–716.
14. Crawford SC, Harnsberger HR, Johnson L, et al. Fibromatosis colli of infancy: CT and sonographic findings. AJR 1988;151:1183–1184.
15. Bedi DG, John SD, Swischuk LE. Fibromatosis colli of infancy: variability of sonographic appearance. J Clin Ultrasound 1998;26:345–348.

ABNORMALITIES OF THE PHARYNX

Tonsils and Adenoids

In the newborn infant, and in the first few weeks of life, the tonsils and adenoids are not very large (Fig. 2.31A). Thereafter, there is an increase in bulk of both these collections of lymphoid tissue, but maximum growth occurs between 3 and 5 years (1). After this time, even though the pharynx enlarges, lymphoid tissue bulk remains rather stable and at all times is clearly visible on regular lateral views of the neck (Fig. 2.31), CT scans, and MR images. On MR studies, normal lymphoid tissue usually shows increased signal on T2-weighted images (Fig. 2.32).

In some children, when the tonsils and adenoids become large (Fig. 2.33A), upper airway obstruction may result. This may lead to snoring and inspiratory obstruction, and, in some cases, cor pulmonale (2). The latter problem is more likely to occur in young infants, for, as has been noted earlier, growth of the adenoidal and tonsillar tissue is out of proportion to growth of the airway. As a consequence, increased bulk is more of a problem, and cor pulmonale in these patients is believed to be secondary to chronic hypoxia and acidosis. These factors lead to pulmonary arterial spasm, hypertrophy of the media, and subsequent pulmonary hypertension (Fig. 2.33).

If the adenoids are absent or their bulk markedly diminished, one should look for a cause. Of course, one merely might be dealing with a patient who has had an adenoidectomy; but in the absence of such a history, sparse adenoidal tissue should suggest hypogammaglobulinemia, agammaglobulinemia, or the ataxia-telangiectasia syndrome (3). Tonsillar tumors are rare, but teratomas can occur in the neonate (4,5), and we have encountered one fibroma (Fig. 2.34A) in the neonate. Tonsillar abscesses are more common and are best identified with CT (Fig 2.34B).

REFERENCES

1. Jeans WD, Fernando DCJ, Maw AR, et al. A longitudinal study of the growth of the nasopharynx and its contents in normal children. Br J Radiol 1981;54:117–121.
2. Macartney FJ, Panday J, Scott O. Cor pulmonale as a result of chronic nasopharyngeal obstruction due to hypertrophied tonsils and adenoids. Arch Dis Child 1969;44:585–592.
3. Ozonoff MB. Ataxia-telangiectasia: chronic pneumonia, sinusitis, and adenoidal hypoplasia. AJR 1974;120:297–299.
4. Shah BL, Vasan U, Raye JR. Teratoma of the tonsil in a premature infant. Am J Dis Child 1979;133:79–80.
5. Valente A, Grant C, Orr JD, et al. Neonatal tonsillar teratoma. J Pediatr Surg 1988;23:364–366.

Uvulitis

The uvula can become inflamed or frankly infected (1, 2). In such cases, it enlarges and the enlargement can be seen

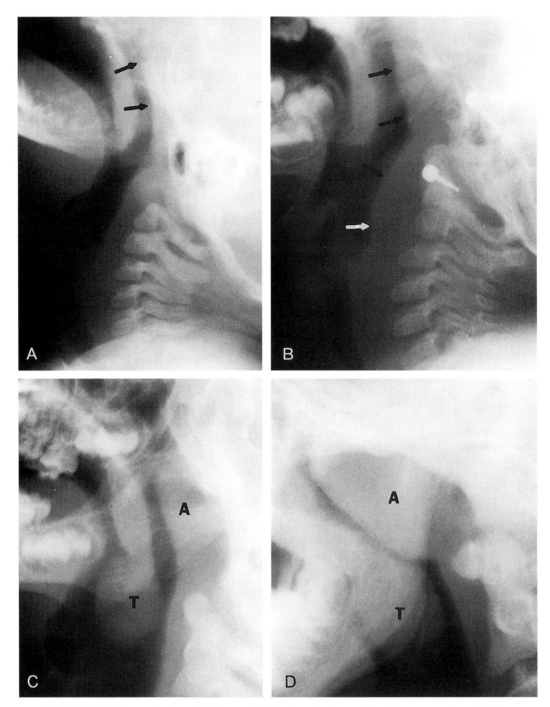

FIGURE 2.31. Normal adenoidal tissue. A. Infant under 3 months. Note sparse adenoidal tissue (arrows). **B.** Older infant. Note abundant adenoidal tissue extending into the retropharynx (arrows). **C.** Young child demonstrating prominent adenoids (A) and palatine tonsils (T). **D.** Older child demonstrating very prominent adenoids (A) and palatine tonsils (T).

FIGURE 2.34. Tonsillar masses. A. Fibroma of tonsil. Note the mass (arrows) in the hypopharynx of this 3-day-old infant with respiratory distress and stridor from birth. Pathologically proven fibroma of tonsil. **B. Tonsillar abscess.** Note the hypodense abscess (arrows).

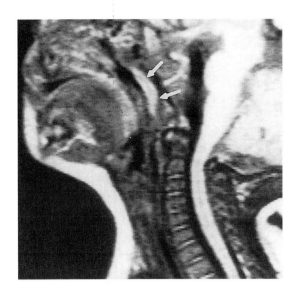

FIGURE 2.32. Normal adenoidal tissue: magnetic resonance imaging. In this infant, on a T2-weighted image, note increase signal in the thin strip of adenoidal tissue (arrows).

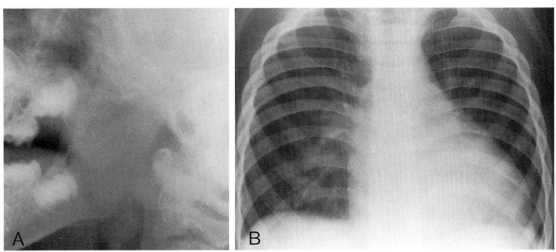

FIGURE 2.33. Large tonsils and adenoids with cor pulmonale. A. Note large adenoids virtually obliterating the nasopharynx. **B.** Chest film demonstrates cardiomegaly.

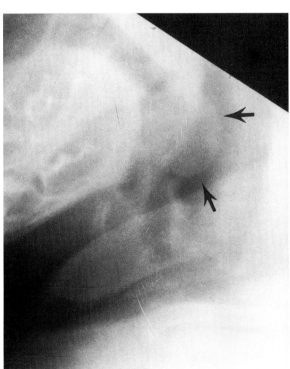

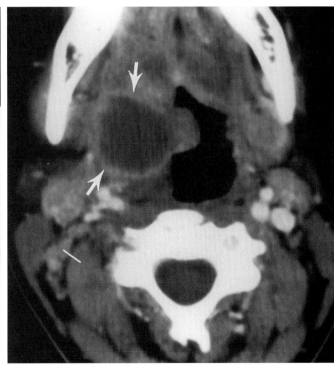

A

B

on lateral views of the neck. It can also enlarge with angioneurotic edema and with hot air inhalation or hot fluid ingestion. The condition usually does not require any form of imaging, but if a lateral view of the neck is obtained, the swollen uvula will be seen.

REFERENCES

1. Aquino V, Terndrup TE. Uvulitis in three children: etiology and respiratory distress. Pediatr Emerg Care 1992;8:206–208.
2. Brook I. Uvulitis caused by anaerobic bacteria. Pediatr Emerg Care 1997;13:221.

Retropharyngeal Abscess, Tumor, and Soft Tissue Thickening

Thickening of the soft tissues in the retropharyngeal region may be the result of tumor growth, inflammation-infection, frank retropharyngeal abscess, or edema. The most common cause in children is inflammation, most often bacterial adenitis, which may or may not go on to abscess formation. Abscesses also can occur secondary to perforation of the hypopharynx. In the newborn, such perforation usually is iatrogenic, but later it usually is the result of trauma, either accidental or part of the battered child syndrome (1). In any of these cases, gas may be seen to accumulate in the retropharyngeal area, and with infection, when such gas is seen, an abscess can be suggested with confidence. However, if only thickening is present, an abscess may or may not also be present, and, in fact, usually is not. Ultrasonography or CT scanning are of assistance in determining whether an abscess or just inflammation is the problem. With retropharyngeal infection, the initial problem is inflammatory adenopathy, which then may go on to suppuration and actual abscess formation. When this occurs, it is important to evaluate the airway for compression, and this usually is best performed with plain films and CT scanning.

Other plain film findings in cases of retropharyngeal inflammation consist of straightening of the normal curve of the spine and smooth, forward displacement and compression of the airway (Fig. 2.35). In those cases where the findings are minimal, one may use a barium swallow to delineate the soft tissues with greater clarity. If neck spasm is profound, there may be such forward flexion of the upper cervical spine that pathologic dislocation at the C1-dens or C2–3 levels is erroneously suggested. Ultrasound and CT both can demonstrate the presence of adenopathy or suppuration with abscess formation (Fig. 2.36), but CT may be misleading as often it is difficult to completely differentiate confluent adenopathy from an abscess.

Associated vasospasm of both the artery and the vein frequently is seen (Fig. 2.36) and can lead to thrombosis of the

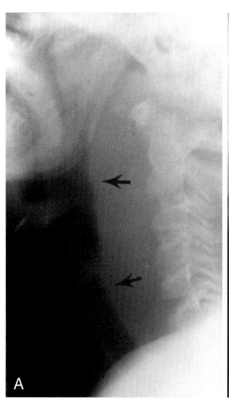
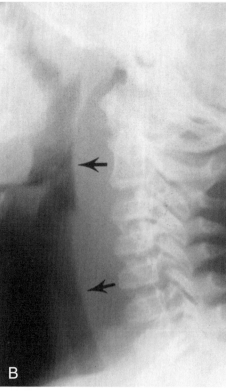

FIGURE 2.35. Retropharyngeal abscess-inflammation. A. Note characteristic anterior displacement of the hypopharynx and trachea (arrows) in a smooth curving fashion. **B.** Another patient with less pronounced thickening of the retropharyngeal soft tissues producing less displacement of the airway. However, note that the posterior wall of the pharynx and trachea form a continuous smooth line (arrows). This is important, as it signifies a retropharyngeal mass or mass-like problem.

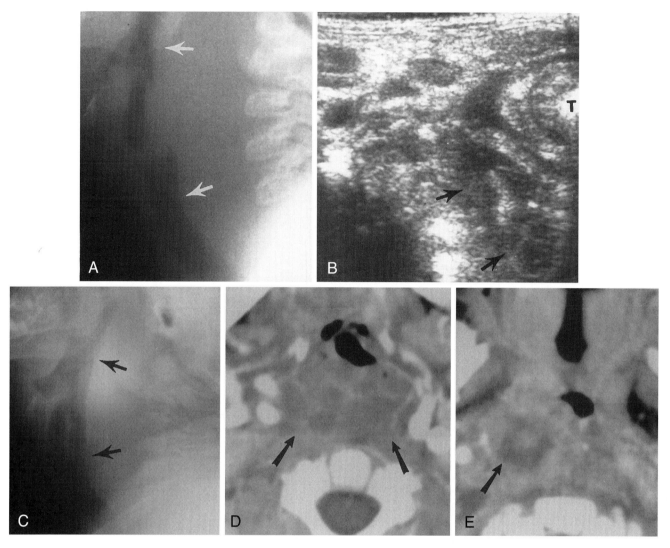

FIGURE 2.36. Retropharyngeal abscess. A. Note marked anterior displacement of the airway (arrows). **B.** Ultrasonogram demonstrates a few hypoechoic lymph nodes, just lateral to the trachea (T). Posterior to the trachea is an area suggesting an abscess (arrows). **C.** Another patient with characteristic anterior displacement of the airway (arrows). **D.** Axial computed tomography demonstrates numerous hypodense lymph nodes (arrows) in the retropharyngeal area. **E.** A slightly lower slice demonstrates an area suggesting an abscess (arrow).

jugular vein and so-called "Lemierre's syndrome" (2,3). In addition, the disease process can extend into the mediastinum to produce a necrotizing mediastinitis (4, 5) (Fig. 2.37).

The most common tumor to occur in the retropharyngeal region is cystic hygroma. This tumor has been discussed earlier, but it should be noted that it is not at all uncommon for it to arise in the neck and extend into the retropharynx. Other masses encountered in the retropharyngeal area include goitrous thyroid tissue and a variety of retropharyngeal tumors such as teratoma, neurofibroma, and primary or secondary neuroblastoma. The findings in any of these lesions are nonspecific, and one usually cannot differentiate one lesion from another on the basis of plain films alone. Neuroblastoma can show calcification and seems to have a much better prognosis when it is primary in the neck (6).

Lymphadenopathy (other than that resulting from inflammation) also can produce retropharyngeal thickening and may be seen with histiocytosis X, the leukemia-lymphoma group of diseases, and metastatic disease. Thickening of the retropharyngeal space also may be seen with trauma to the cervical spine, where the finding is the result of bleeding into the soft tissues. In addition, retropharyngeal edema may be seen with allergic (angioneurotic) edema and thrombosis of the superior vena cava (7), where, in addition to retropharyngeal soft tissue thickening, one also sees the full-blown superior vena caval syndrome (i.e.,

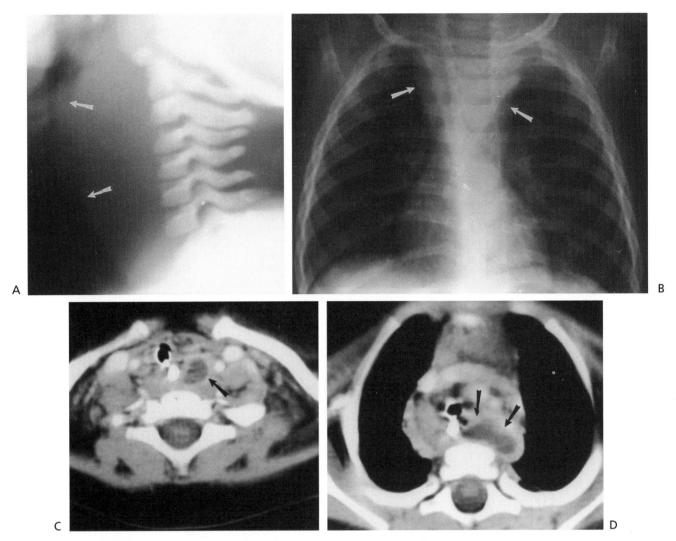

FIGURE 2.37. Retropharyngeal abscess extending into chest. A. Note marked anterior displacement of the airway (arrows). **B.** Chest film shows superior mediastinal widening (arrows). **C.** Axial computed tomography study through the neck shows an abscess (arrow). **D.** Lower axial slice through the chest shows the mediastinal extension of the abscess (arrows).

edema of the neck and cyanosis of the head). Myxedematous thickening of the retropharyngeal tissues in young infants with hypothyroidism also has been described (8) and is not an uncommon manifestation of the disease in the neonate and young infant.

REFERENCES

1. McDowell HP, Fielding DW. Traumatic perforation of the hypopharynx—an unusual form of abuse. Arch Dis Child 1984;59: 888–889.
2. Barker J, Winer-Muram HT, Grey SW. Lemierre syndrome. South Med J 1996;89:1021–1023.
3. De Sena S, Rosenfeld DL, Santos S, et al. Jugular thrombophlebitis complicating bacterial pharyngitis (Lemierre's syndrome). Pediatr Radiol 1996;26:141–144.
4. Kono T, Kohno A, Kuwashima S, et al. CT findings of descending necrotising mediastinitis via the carotid space ("Lincoln Highway"). Pediatr Radiol 2001;31:84–86.
5. Smith JK, Armato DM, Specter BB, et al. Danger space infection: infection of the neck leading to descending necrotizing mediastinitis. Emerg Radiol 1999;6:129–132.
6. Abramson SJ, Berdon WE, Ruzal-Shapiro C, et al. Cervical neuroblastoma in eleven infants—a tumor with favorable prognosis. Clinical and radiologic (US, CT, MRI) findings. Pediatr Radiol 1993;23:253–257.
7. Hayden CK Jr, Swischuk LE. Retropharyngeal edema, airway obstruction and caval thrombosis. AJR 1982;138:757–758.
8. Grunebaum M, Moskowitz G. The retropharyngeal soft tissues in young infants with hypothyroidism. AJR 1970;108:543–545.

Tumors and Cysts in and around the Pharynx

Tumors in this area of the upper airway are rather uncommon but, at the same time, varied. In this regard, one may

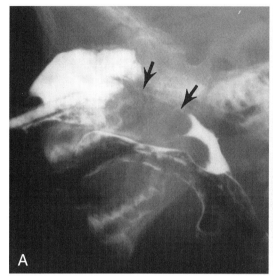
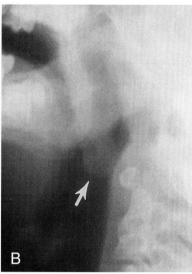

FIGURE 2.38. Nasopharyngeal teratoma. A. Note the teratoma (arrows) outlined by contrast material. **B. Hairy polyp.** Note the polypoid lesion dangling into the hypopharynx (arrow). (**A** reproduced with permission from Frech RS, McAlister WH. Teratoma of the nasopharynx producing depression in the posterior hard palate. J Can Assoc Radiol 1969;20:204–205).

encounter lesions such as dermoid, teratoma (1, 2), neuroblastoma, neurofibroma, hemangioma , choristoma (3), hamartoma (4), and a variety of foregut, thymic, thyroglossal, and lingual cysts. In the neonate, one can also encounter the so-called "hairy polyp." In general, on plain films, these lesions appear as nonspecific masses encroaching upon, or actually protruding into, the pharyngeal air column (Fig. 2.38). However, in most cases, contrast studies, CT, or MRI is required for complete delineation. Clinically, respiratory distress, dysphagia, and stridor are the usual presenting symptoms, but if the tumor is large enough, asphyxia may result.

In the older child, the two most important pharyngeal tumors are the juvenile nasopharyngeal angiofibroma and lymphoepithelioma. Nasopharyngeal angiofibroma, however, is much more common and characteristically is seen in the preadolescent male, where presenting symptoms usually consist of epistaxis and sinusitis. Angiographically, the appearance of these tumors is rather characteristic, consisting of dilated, nodular vessels with a hypertrophied, internal maxillary artery supplier. Occasionally, however, blood supply also may be derived from the internal carotid system or even the vertebral arteries. Embolization often is performed preoperatively, as this tends to stem the hypervascularity. Surgical resection is the treatment of choice, but if there is intracranial extension, radiation may be required. CT and MR (5) identify these tumors clearly, including visualization of the signal void resulting from feeding and draining blood vessels (Fig. 2.39). Characteristically, hemangiomas have very high signal on T2-weighted images, which persists on the second echo, and finally, it might be noted that some hemangiomas are confined to the pterygoid region (6), while others can present as nasal masses (Fig. 2.40). Under such circumstances, one might

not think of hemangioma as the diagnosis and suggest some other tumor.

Lymphoepithelioma, as opposed to the juvenile angiofibroma, is a malignant tumor and, in essence, is an undifferentiated epidermoid carcinoma arising from Waldeyer's ring. It too occurs in older children and usually presents with tender cervical adenopathy resulting from metastatic disease. The tumor may spread throughout the body, but does so at a later stage. It must be differentiated from juvenile angiofibroma, and currently this is best accomplished with MRI, for the T2-weighted features characteristic of angiofibromas will be absent. The lesion simply appears as a solid mass with moderately increased T2 signal. This tumor also can be demonstrated with CT, but the findings are nonspecific (Fig. 2.41). Other masses that might be encountered in the nasopharynx include basal encephaloceles, chordomas, and rhabdomyosarcomas. These are discussed in Chapter 6.

REFERENCES

1. Alter AD, Cove JK. Congenital nasopharyngeal teratoma: report of a case and review of the literature. J Pediatr Surg 1987;22: 179–181.
2. Jawad AJ, Khattak A, Al-Rabeeah a, et al. Congenital nasopharyngeal teratoma in newborn: case report and review of the literature. Z Kinderchir 1990;45:375–378.
3. Johnson JF. Oropharyngeal choristoma in a newborn. Br J Radiol 1980;53:1007–1009.
4. Cook K, DiPietro MA, Bogdasarian RS. An elusive nasopharyngeal hamartoma in a neonate. Pediatr Radiol 1988;18:351–352.
5. Lloyd GAS, Phelps PD. Juvenile angiofibroma: imaging by magnetic resonance, CT and conventional techniques. Clin Otolaryngol 1986;11:247–259.
6. Seo CS, Han MH, Chang KH, et al. Angiofibroma confined to

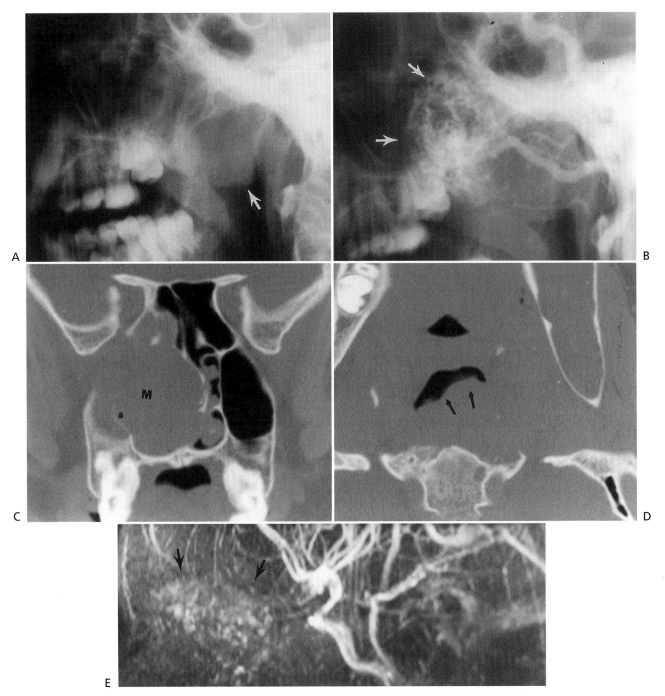

FIGURE 2.39. Angiofibroma. A. Note the nasopharyngeal mass (arrows). **B.** Arteriogram demonstrates the leash of abnormal vessels (arrow). **C.** Another patient with a large angiofibroma producing a mass (M) that fills and expands the maxillary sinus. **D.** Axial computed tomography study demonstrates the nasopharyngeal extension of the mass (arrow). **E.** Magnetic resonance angiography study demonstrates the abnormal vascularity of the tumor (arrows).

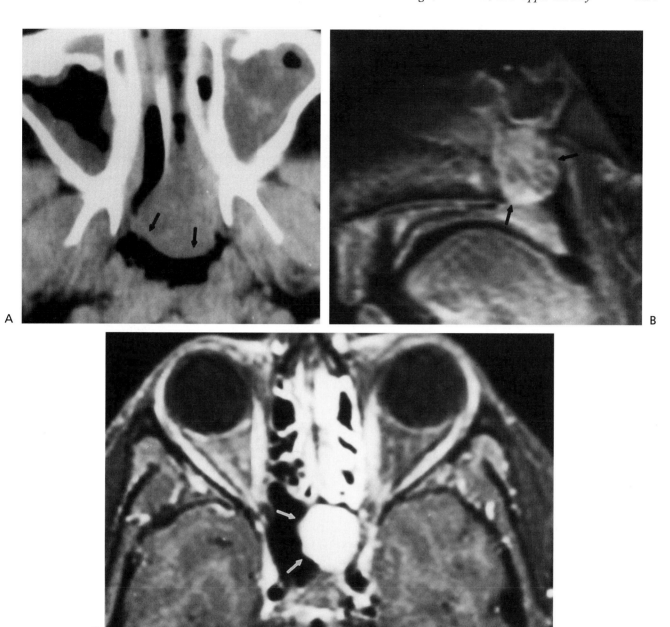

FIGURE 2.40. Angiofibroma: nasal passage extension. A. Axial computed tomography study demonstrates a mass (arrows) extending into the left nasal passage. **B.** Sagittal magnetic resonance study with contrast enhancement demonstrates the mass (arrows) in the juxtanasal position. **C.** Arteriogram demonstrates the abnormal leash of vessels (arrows) within the tumor.

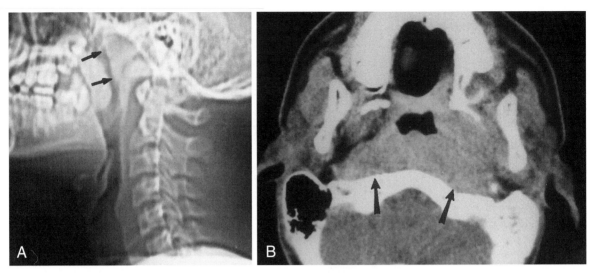

FIGURE 2.41. Lymphoepithelioma. A. Note slight prominence of the nasopharyngeal soft tissues (arrows). This patient presented with a left neck mass. **B.** A computed tomography study demonstrates the large tumor mass (arrows) with slightly more tumor bulk on the left.

the pterygoid muscle region: CT and MR demonstration. AJNR 1996;17:374–376.

Pharyngeal Incoordination (Cricopharyngeal Achalasia)

Pharyngeal incoordination is a relatively common problem in the neonate but, for the most part, is transient (1). How-

ever, a more permanent form can be seen in conjunction with cerebellar injury, Chiari malformations (2), other neurologic or neuromuscular disease, and familial dysautonomia or the Riley-Day syndrome.

In all cases, there is failure of cricopharyngeal and upper esophageal sphincter relaxation, hypertrophy of the cricopharyngeus muscle, and massive reflux of barium into the nasal passages (Fig. 2.42). In addition, spillover of barium into the trachea also usually occurs. Posterior indenta-

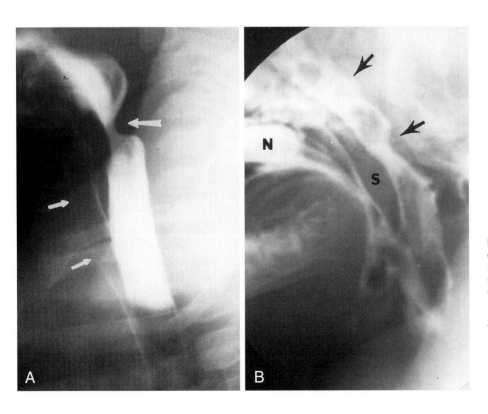

FIGURE 2.42. Pharyngeal incoordination. A. Lateral view showing pronounced spasm of cricopharyngeus muscle (large arrow). Note that constriction is circumferential, but most pronounced posteriorly. Also note some spillover of barium into the trachea (small arrows). **B.** Same infant during swallowing shows pronounced regurgitation of barium into the nasopharynx and posterior nasal passages (arrows). S, soft palate and uvula; N, nipple.

tion of the upper esophagus by the cricopharyngeus muscle (Fig. 2.42) is variable and not always pronounced.

Clinically, these patients demonstrate difficulty in feeding, regurgitation of food into the nose, and repeated aspirations. Esophageal obstruction can be profound (3), and in some cases, it may become necessary to nonsurgically dilate the muscle (4) or perform a sphincterotomy (5). A feeding gastrostomy also may be required, but most infants do not have this much difficulty. In most cases, as the infant matures, the degree of incoordination slowly diminishes and eventually disappears. The problem probably represents nothing more than transient immaturity of the swallowing mechanism.

REFERENCES

1. Reichert TJ, Bluestone CD, Stool SE, et al. Congenital cricopharyngeal achalasia. Ann Otol Rhinol Laryngol 1977;86:603–610.
2. Putnam PE, Orenstein SR, Pang D, et al. Cricopharyngeal dysfunction associated with Chiari malformations. Pediatrics 1992;89:871–876.
3. Bergman AB, Lewicki AM. Complete esophageal obstruction from cricopharyngeal achalasia. Radiology 1977;123:289–290.
4. Mihailovic T, Perisic VN. Balloon dilatation of cricopharyngeal achalasia. Pediatr Radiol 1992;22:522–524.
5. Salih SA, Aubert D, Valioulis I, et al. Cricopharyngeal achalasia—a cause of major dysphagia in a newborn. Eur J Pediatr Surg 1999;9:406–408.

Velopalatine Incompetence

The radiographic evaluation of function of the soft palate in patients with speech problems is an important part of their overall evaluation and, for the most part, is accomplished with videotaped fluoroscopy. The patient pronounces and executes various letters, phrases, and sentences (1), and the function of the palate is observed during these procedures. Basically, one documents upward and posterior movement of the palate on lateral view and closure of the lateral pharyngeal walls on submentovertex or basal views.

Normally, with phonation, the soft palate moves upward and posteriorly in a brisk fashion. It assumes a high, right angle configuration as it apposes the posterior pharyngeal wall, usually against the adenoidal tissue mass (Fig. 2.43, A and B). With velopalatine incompetence, the soft palate

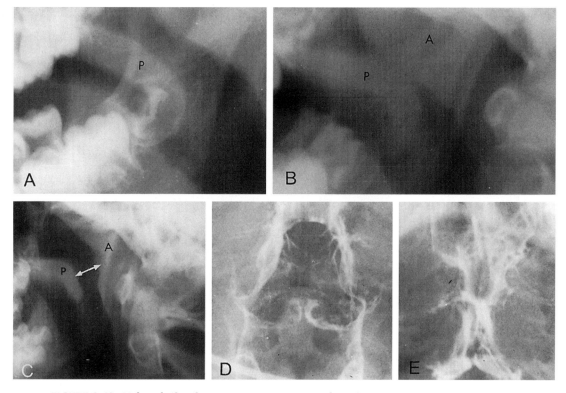

FIGURE 2.43. Velopalatine incompetence. A. Normal resting. Note size, position, and configuration of the soft palate and uvula (P). **B. Normal phonation.** There is elevation of the soft palate (P) resulting in an acute right angle configuration and its apposition against the adenoids (A). **C. Abnormal soft palate.** Note that the soft palate (P) is underdeveloped and that, with phonation, there is lack of apposition against the adenoids (A). An air gap (arrows) results. Also note that bending of the soft palate is somewhat short of the normal right angle. **D.** Another patient demonstrating lack of apposition of the lateral pharyngeal walls with the letter "E." **E.** This same patient with the letter "S," however, shows good apposition of the lateral walls toward center.

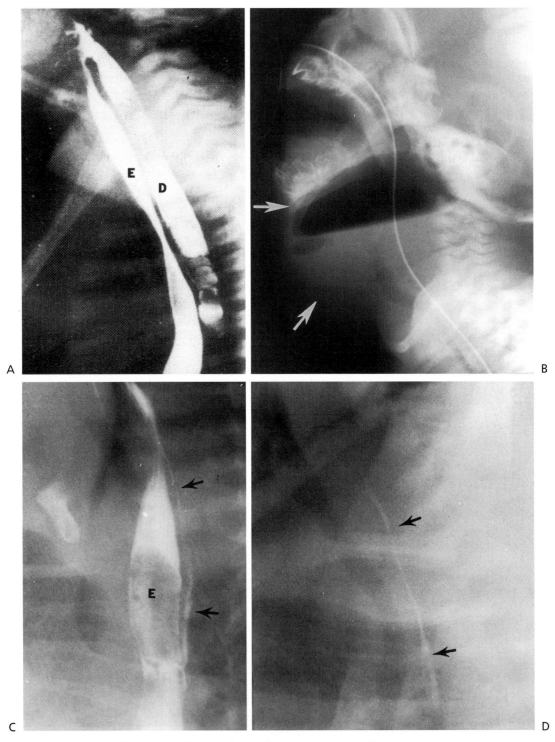

FIGURE 2.44. Pharyngeal diverticula. A. Congenital diverticulum. Note the long congenital posterior pharyngeal diverticulum (D) extending far into the chest. Anterior to it is the normal esophagus (E). **B.** Large congenital diverticulum with an air-fluid level (arrows). **C. Iatrogenic diverticulum.** Note the thin sinus-like tract (arrows) posterior to the esophagus (E). This was a diverticulum. **D.** Weeks later, residual barium is seen in the diverticulum (arrows.) (**A** reproduced with permission from MacKellar A, Kennedy JC. Congenital diverticulum of the pharynx simulating esophageal atresia. J Pediatr Surg 1972;7:408–411).

does not reach the posterior wall but falls short, and the result is an air gap (Fig. 2.43C). Often, in an attempt to close the gap, there is a compensatory bulge of the posterior pharyngeal wall, the so-called "Passavant's ridge." This ridge is a compensatory mechanism aimed at closing the air gap and not present in all patients.

On basal or frontal views, the lateral pharyngeal walls in normal patients come together briskly and meet in midline. With velopalatine incompetence, there is failure of such central apposition of the lateral walls (Fig. 2.43, D and E). Visualization of the pharyngeal walls on the basal view is facilitated by the introduction of barium into the nasopharynx. This usually is accomplished with a tube placed through the nose. Ultrasonography also has been used to assess lateral wall movement (2).

Study of velopalatine incompetence is a little more detailed than just outlined, and numerous other vocal maneuvers can be performed, but if one is involved in the investigation of these patients, one soon becomes acquainted with all the details. Otherwise, the resume here should serve as a brief introduction to the subject.

REFERENCES

1. Barr LL, Hayden CK Jr, Hill LC, et al. Pictorial essay. Radiographic evaluation of velopharyngeal incompetence in childhood. AJR 1989;153:811–814.
2. Hawkins CF, Swisher WE. Evaluation of a real-time ultrasound scanner in assessing lateral pharyngeal wall motion during speech. Cleft Palate J 1978;15:161–166.

Sleep Apnea

Sleep apnea is best investigated with fluoroscopy (1), but ultrasonography (2) and MRI (3) also have been used. Basically, during sleep in the normal patient, there is very little movement of the soft tissues of the hypopharynx and tongue. However, in patients with sleep apnea, during inspiration, the hypopharynx collapses, resulting in posterior displacement of the tongue and anterior movement of the posterior pharyngeal wall. Together these movements cause closure of the airway.

REFERENCES

1. Fernbach SK, Brouilette RT, Riggs TW, et al. Radiologic evaluation of adenoids and tonsils in children with obstructive sleep apnea: plain films and fluoroscopy. Pediatr Radiol 1983;13:258–265.
2. Marsh RR, Potsic WP, Pasquariello PS. Reliability of sleep sonography in detecting upper airway obstruction in children. Int J Pediatr Otorhinolaryngol 1989;18:1–8.
3. Suto Y, Matsu T, Kato T, et al. Evaluation of the pharyngeal airway in patients with sleep apnea: value of ultrafast MR imaging. AJR 1993;160:311–314.

Pharyngeal Diverticula

Pharyngeal diverticula are uncommon (1) and many times are identified only after barium swallow (Fig. 2.44). Occasionally, however, they may be seen as air-filled structures on neck films (1). There are two types of pharyngeal diverticula: congenital and acquired. The latter may now be more common and are believed to result from iatrogenic perforation of the pharynx, above the cricopharyngeus muscle, during intubation (2). Most often seen in the neonate, they may be indistinguishable from congenital diverticula. Zenker's diverticula also can occur in childhood but are rare. Consequently, any time one encounters a pharyngeal diverticulum in an infant, one should first consider an iatrogenic etiology.

An interesting feature regarding these acquired diverticula is that whereas in the older child, pharyngeal perforation often results in mediastinitis, in the neonate the perforation remains remarkably silent. Indeed, the first findings may suggest obstruction secondary to esophageal atresia (3, 4). These diverticula often lie posterior to the esophagus but in other cases may be positioned to one side or the other of this structure (Fig. 2.44).

REFERENCES

1. Burge D, Middleton A. Persistent pharyngeal pouch derivatives in the neonate. J Pediatr Surg 1983;18:230–234.
2. Lucaya J, Herrera M, Salcedo S. Traumatic pharyngeal pseudodiverticulum in neonates and infants. Two case reports and review of the literature. Pediatr Radiol 1979;8:65–69.
3. MacKellar A, Kennedy JC. Congenital diverticulum of the pharynx simulating esophageal atresia. J Pediatr Surg 1972;7:408–411.
4. Heller RM, Kirchner SG, O'Neill JA. Perforation of the pharynx in the newborn: a new look-alike for esophageal atresia. AJR 1977;129:335–337.

ABNORMALITIES OF THE LARYNX AND UPPER TRACHEA

Laryngomalacia

Laryngomalacia (congenital flaccid larynx) is the most common abnormality of the larynx in the neonate. Symptoms most often appear shortly after the neonatal period and consist primarily of inspiratory stridor. Variable degrees of intercostal and substernal retractions occur, but the cry usually is normal. This latter point is of value in differentiating these infants from those with laryngeal tumors and vocal cord paralysis. In addition, laryngomalacia is the only cause of infantile stridor that worsens at rest. Although not invariably so (1), the stridor usually improves with activity and crying. The condition usually is sporadic, but familial laryngomalacia also has been documented (2), and, of course, the problem can last into early infancy.

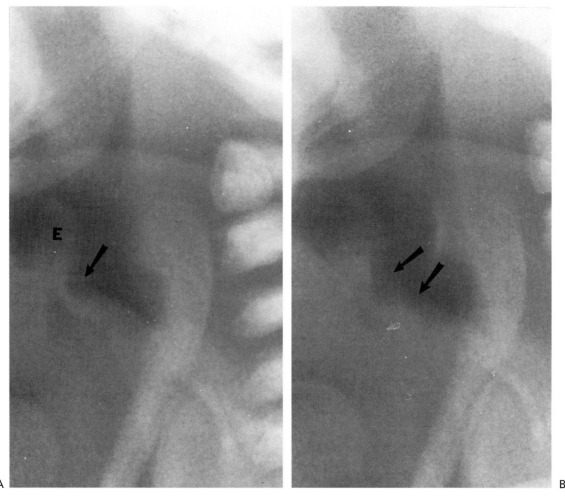

A

B

FIGURE 2.45. Laryngomalacia. A. Early inspiratory phase. Note the position of the epiglottis (E). It is just beginning to bend backward, and the aryepiglottic folds just below it are beginning to buckle forward (arrow). **B.** Moments later, the entire larynx collapses (arrows) and causes obstruction.

Other causes of congenital stridor must be excluded before the diagnosis of congenital flaccid larynx or laryngomalacia is made, for other laryngeal abnormalities such as webs, stenoses, cysts, and tumors can present with a similar clinical picture. In the usual case, however, with laryngomalacia, during inspiration, the larynx tends to collapse upon itself. The prognosis is usually good, and with time, stridor lessens. By the age of 1 year, it usually completely disappears. However, in some cases, stridor can persist for up to 5 years (2), but this is rather uncommon. In addition, long-term studies have shown that some residual laryngeal flaccidity can persist, but with no real clinical compromise (3).

Roentgenographically, on inspiration, one sees hypopharyngeal overdistention, anteroinferior collapse of the aryepiglottic folds, downward and backward bending of the floppy epiglottis, and paradoxical narrowing of the subglottic portion of the trachea (Fig. 2.45). Although one can see these findings on regular lateral views of the neck obtained

during inspiration, the findings often are best assessed with fluoroscopy.

REFERENCES

1. McSwiney PF, Cavanagh NPC, Languth P. Outcome in congenital stridor (laryngomalacia). Arch Dis Child 1977;52:215–218.
2. Shulman JB, Hollister DW, Thibeault DW, et al. Familial laryngomalacia; a case report. Laryngoscope 1976;86:84–91.
3. Macfarlane PI, Olinsky A, Phelan PD. Proximal airway function 8 to 16 years after laryngomalacia: follow-up using flow-volume loop studies. J Pediatr 1985;107:216–218.

Laryngotracheoesophageal Cleft (Persistent Esophagotrachea)

Laryngotracheoesophageal cleft can vary from simple posterior laryngeal clefting to persistence of a common tube

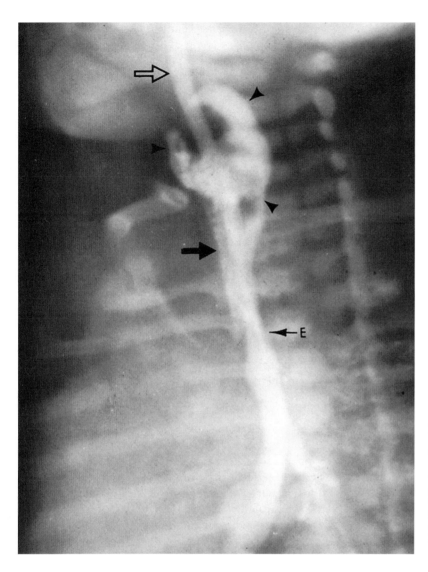

FIGURE 2.46. Laryngotracheoesophageal cleft. Barium passes freely from the upper esophagus, through the wide communication (small arrows), into the trachea (large filled arrow). The nasogastric tube (large open arrow) extends into the midesophagus (E). (Reproduced with permission from Felman AH, Talbert JL. Laryngotracheoesophageal cleft. Description of a combined laryngoscopic and roentgenographic diagnostic technique and report of two patients. Radiology 1972;103:641–644).

comprised of the trachea and esophagus (1). The posterior clefting of the larynx results from failure of fusion of the posterior cricoid cartilage. In the more extensive persistent esophagotrachea, there is complete lack of separation of the trachea from the esophagus, for the septum, which normally separates these structures, fails to develop.

Clinically, infants with a simple posterior laryngeal cleft present with an abnormal cry or mutism. They also may have difficulty with swallowing, as there is a tendency to aspirate food into the larynx. With more severe clefting and the development of a common tracheoesophageal tube, symptoms resembling those seen in infants with esophageal atresia or tracheoesophageal fistula are present. There is excessive accumulation of secretions and marked difficulty with swallowing. Aspiration is usually pronounced and respiratory distress marked. Mutism, because of the extensive laryngeal abnormality, is the rule. In such cases, the roentgenographic examination reveals massive aspiration into the trachea (Fig. 2.46), and on plain lateral chest and

neck roentgenograms, it is often difficult to separate the tracheal air column from that of the esophagus.

REFERENCE

1. Fuzesi K, Young DG. Congenital laryngotracheoesophageal cleft. J Pediatr Surg 1976;11:933–937.

Inflammatory Lesions of the Larynx and Upper Trachea (Epiglottitis and Croup)

Epiglottitis and croup (laryngotracheobronchitis) are the most common inflammatory conditions of the larynx and upper trachea in childhood. Although occasionally one can encounter fungal and monilial infections in this area (1), epiglottitis almost always, in the past, was due to *Haemophilus influenzae* bacterial infection and croup to viral infection. However, viral epiglottitis also can occur (2)

Croup tends to occur in younger infants (under 2 years of age), while epiglottitis is seen in older children (3–5 years or older). However, epiglottitis also occasionally can be seen in young infants (3). Clinically, croup presents primarily with inspiratory stridor and a "barking" cough and often is associated with other findings of an upper respiratory tract infection. Epiglottitis usually presents more as a swallowing problem with drooling. However, respiratory distress also can be significant, and other causes of epiglottitis besides acute bacterial (*Staphylococcus aureus* and *H. influenzae*) epiglottitis include allergic epiglottitis, thermal epiglottitis (4–6), epiglottic edema resulting from radiation therapy, and epiglottic infiltration with sarcoidosis (7).

Roentgenographically, the findings of epiglottitis are rather typical. They consist of thickening of the epiglottis and aryepiglottic folds. It is important that one identify both epiglottic and aryepiglottic fold thickening, for pseudothickening of the epiglottis occurs with the so-called "omega epiglottis." The epiglottis in these children has prominent lateral flaps, and when examined on lateral view, the flaps overlie the epiglottis and erroneously suggest thickening (Fig. 2.47). This is most important to appreciate, for in true epiglottitis, both the epiglottis and the aryepiglottic folds are thickened (Fig. 2.48). However, it is important to know where to measure the aryepiglottic folds. In this regard, it has been shown (8) that measuring them through their middle portions or just behind the epiglottis is required. They should not be measured at their base, as the base normally tends to be somewhat wide and there is too much overlap with normal.

The location of the inflammation in epiglottitis has led to the alternate term "supraglottitis," but it should be noted that in some more severe cases, edema also can extend into the subglottic region and mimic the steeple sign of croup on frontal view (9). However, on lateral view, although there is variable distension of the hypopharynx, the subglottic portion of the trachea usually is normal in diameter. It is only on frontal view that confusion with croup occurs.

With croup, the typical lateral view roentgenographic findings during inspiration are those of pronounced hypopharyngeal overdistension, indistinctness and thickening of the vocal cords, prominence of the laryngeal ventricle, and subglottic tracheal narrowing (Fig. 2.49) (10). The latter finding is not specific for it merely is the result of paradoxical collapse of the subglottic trachea secondary to decreased subglottic intratracheal pressures. This phenomenon occurs with any cause of glottic or paraglottic obstruction and can be demonstrated to be nonfixed on expiratory views (Fig. 2.49B). However, this is not true in all cases, for in bacterial (membranous) croup, the narrowing often is more fixed or an actual membrane may be seen (Fig. 2.50). Narrowing is the result of extensive inflammation and edema in this area. This form of croup also has been referred to as bacterial tracheitis (11, 12). The problem often is more severe than with ordinary viral croup, and many of these patients require endotracheal intubation. In addition, the membranes produced in and around the larynx may be mistaken for those seen with diphtheria. Croup also can be allergic in etiology, especially in older children.

On frontal view, and often visible on routine chest films, slit-like narrowing of the glottis is seen (Fig. 2.49C). This has been termed the "steeple" or "funnel" sign and, although not pathognomonic, is highly suspicious for croup. The finding, however, also can be seen in some cases of epiglottitis and regularly with vocal cord paralysis, subglottic laryngeal webs, and vocal cord thickening resulting

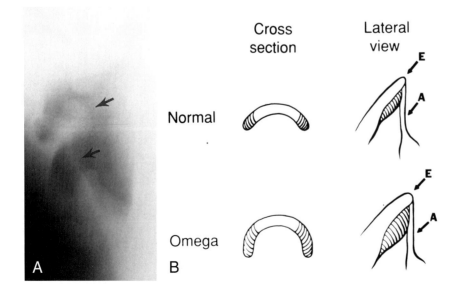

FIGURE 2.47. Omega epiglottis. A. Note the apparently thick and swollen epiglottis (upper arrow). The aryepiglottic folds (lower arrow), however, are thin. **B.** Diagrammatic representation of the omega epiglottis. Note the size and prominence of the lateral flap (shaded areas) as they appeared in cross-section and on lateral view. E, epiglottis; A, aryepiglottic folds.

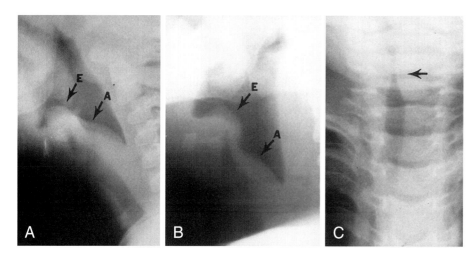

FIGURE 2.48. Epiglottitis. A. Classic epiglottitis with a thickened epiglottis (E) and aryepiglottic fold (A). **B.** Another patient with milder changes, but still the epiglottis (E) and aryepiglottic folds (A) are thickened. **C.** In this patient, on frontal view, the glottic-subglottic area is narrowed to produce the steeple sign (arrow) more characteristic of croup.

from any type of cord edema or infiltration. In those instances where the inspiratory effort is not very deep, hypopharyngeal overdistension may not be striking, and the only finding may be indistinctness and thickening of the vocal cords (Fig. 2.51). It is in these cases that the narrow-ing of the glottic and subglottic regions seen on frontal view is most valuable. This narrowing is the result of spasm and edema of the cords and persists during both inspiration and expiration. Indeed, it is so persistent that it usually is ran-domly seen on associated chest films.

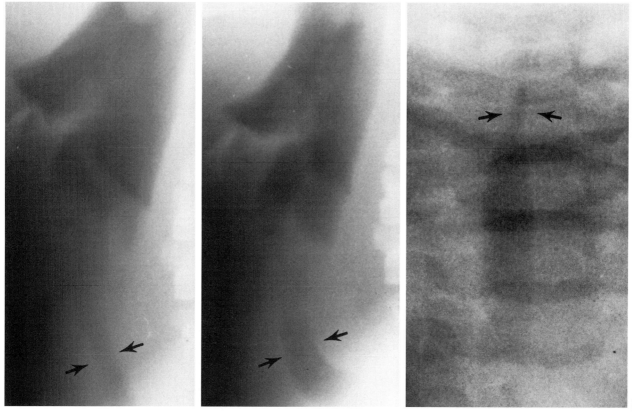

A   B,C

FIGURE 2.49. Croup. A. With deep inspiration, the hypopharynx overdistends and paradoxical narrowing of the subglottic portion of the trachea occurs (arrows). Also note indistinctness of the vocal cord region. The epiglottis is normal. **B.** With expiration, the subglottic portion of the tra-chea (arrows) is seen to be of normal diameter. **C.** Frontal view demonstrates the classic steeple sign (arrow) of croup.

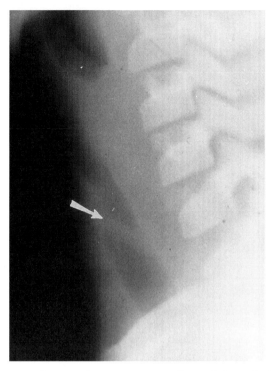

FIGURE 2.50. Membranous croup (bacterial tracheitis). Note narrowing of the subglottic portion of the trachea, but in addition note the membrane (arrow) traversing the trachea.

REFERENCES

1. Balsam D, Sorran D, Barax CH. *Candida* epiglottis presenting as stridor in a child with HIV infection. Pediatr Radiol 1992;22: 235–236.

2. Grattan-Smith T, Forer M, Kilham H, et al. Viral supraglottitis. J Pediatr 1987;110:434–435.
3. Brilli RG, Benzing G III, Cotcamp DH. Epiglottitis in infants less than two years of age. Pediatr Emerg Care 1989;5:16–21.
4. Herman TE, McAlister WH. Epiglottic enlargement: two unusual causes. Pediatr Radiol 1991;21:139–140.
5. Harjacek M, Kornberg AE, Yates EW, et al. Thermal epiglottitis after swallowing hot tea. Pediatr Emerg Care 1992;8:342–344.
6. Kulick RM, Selbst SM, Baker MD, et al. Thermal epiglottitis after swallowing hot beverages. Pediatrics 1988;81:441–444.
7. McHugh K, deSilva M, Kiham HA. Epiglottic enlargement secondary to laryngeal sarcoidosis. Pediatr Radiol 1993;23:71.
8. John SD, Swischuk LE, Hayden CK Jr, et al. Aryepiglottic fold width in patients with epiglottitis: where should measurements be obtained? Radiology 1994;190:123–125.
9. Shackelford GD, Siegel MJ, McAlister WH. Subglottic edema in acute epiglottitis in children. AJR 1978;131:603–605.
10. Currarino G, Williams B. Lateral inspiration and expiration radiographs of the neck in children with laryngotracheitis (croup). Radiology 1982;145:365–366.
11. Denneny JC III, Handler SD. Membranous laryngotracheobronchitis. Pediatrics 1982;70:705–707.
12. Henry RL, Mellis CM, Benjamin B. Pseudomembranous croup. Arch Dis Child 1983;58:180–183.

Subglottic Stenosis

Prior to the commonplace intubation of infants in intensive care nurseries, the most common cause of subglottic stenosis of the trachea, by far, was congenital. However, most cases now are iatrogenic, and although in a few instances the findings are identical to those seen in congenital subglottic stenosis, more often one sees stenosis resulting from membranes, irregular tracheal narrowings, or granulomas (Fig. 2.52, C and D). In congenital subglottic stenosis, the characteristic finding consists of circumferential, smooth

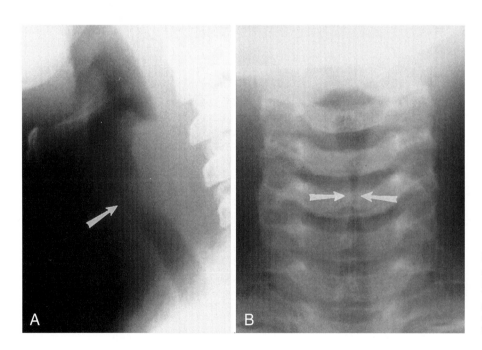

FIGURE 2.51. Croup: other changes. A. On this lateral view with only minimal inspiration, the only abnormal finding is indistinctness of the vocal cords (arrow). **B.** Frontal view, however, demonstrates the typical steeple sign (arrows).

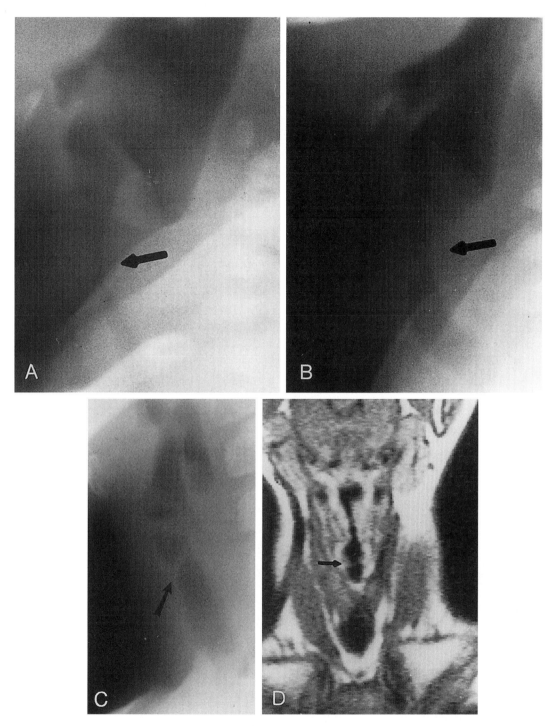

FIGURE 2.52. Subglottic stenosis. A. Inspiratory phase. Note marked overdistention of the hypopharynx and pronounced narrowing of the subglottic portion of the trachea (arrow). **B. Expiratory film.** Note that the degree of narrowing of the subglottic portion of the trachea (arrow) has changed very little. Also note that the trachea below it is more distended (obstructed) than on the inspiratory film. **C. Iatrogenic subglottic stenosis.** Note membranous subglottic stenosis (arrow) in an infant who was intubated for a long period of time. **D.** Another case of an iatrogenic web (arrow) demonstrated with magnetic resonance imaging.

narrowing of the immediate subglottic portion of the trachea (1). This narrowing persists during both inspiration and expiration (Fig. 2.52, A and B) and in this way can be differentiated from the inspiratory subglottic narrowing seen in most cases of croup. With croup, since inspiratory narrowing usually is paradoxical, during expiration, it either disappears completely or diminishes markedly. If the narrowing remains about the same on inspiration and expiration, congenital subglottic stenosis should be one's diagnosis. The only significant differential diagnosis in the immediate neonatal period is that of subglottic hemangioma, and the differentiation can be made with ease for subglottic hemangiomas usually present with eccentric subglottic mass-like narrowing.

Patients with subglottic stenosis present with inspiratory and expiratory stridor, although the inspiratory component frequently predominates. The findings usually are aggravated by viral croup, and overall there is a marked tendency for the problem in these patients to mimic the findings of croup, not only roentgenographically but also clinically. However, since most of these patients demonstrate stridor from birth, one can lessen the consideration of ordinary croup.

REFERENCE

1. John SD, Swischuk LE. Stridor and upper airway obstruction in infants and children. Radiographics 1992;12:625–643.

Atresia, Stenosis, and Laryngeal Web

Atresia, stenosis, and laryngeal web are rather uncommon abnormalities, but they can be immediately life threatening, and so prompt recognition and subsequent tracheostomy may be required. Laryngeal atresia or stenosis often is primary but also can occur with esophageal atresia and tracheoesophageal fistula (1). Laryngeal stenosis may be glottic, supraglottic, or infraglottic and may be membranous (web) or cartilaginous (2). Roentgenographically, with laryngeal webs, the findings mimic those of croup or vocal cord paralysis and consist of fixation of the cords and paradoxical subglottic narrowing of the trachea on inspiration (Fig. 2.53). Glottic stenosis also can be acquired, and CT and MR are useful in its delineation (Fig. 2.54).

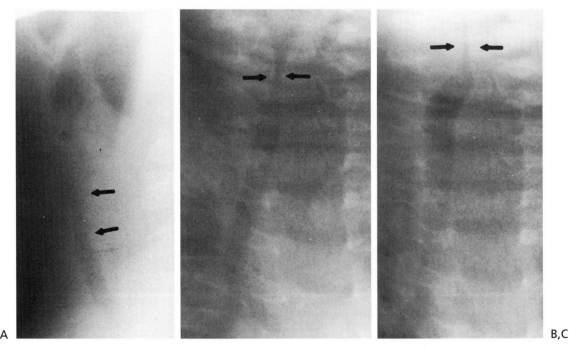

A   B,C

FIGURE 2.53. Laryngeal web: subglottic stenosis. A. Lateral view demonstrates hypopharyngeal overdistention, a normal epiglottis and aryepiglottic folds, some indistinctness of the vocal cords, and narrowing of the subglottic portion of the trachea (arrows). The findings are virtually indistinguishable from those of croup. **B.** Frontal view demonstrates fixed cords (arrows). This was an inspiratory view, and the findings are indistinguishable from those of vocal cord paralysis. **C.** Expiratory view demonstrates overdistention of the trachea secondary to fixed, glottic obstruction. Buckling of the trachea to the right is normal.

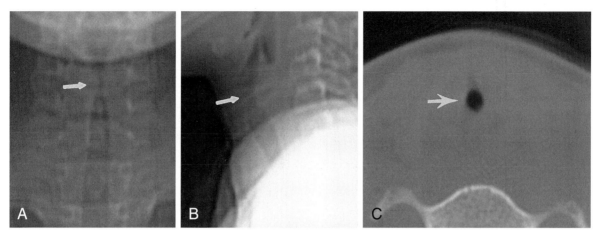

FIGURE 2.54. Glottic stenosis: acquired. A. Note narrowing of the glottis (arrow). **B.** Lateral view during expiration (note overdistension of the trachea) demonstrates fixed narrowing in the region of the glottis (arrow). **C.** Computed tomography demonstrates an extremely narrow glottic lumen (arrow).

REFERENCES

1. Sayre JW, Hall EG. Anomalies of the larynx associated with tracheo-esophageal fistula. Pediatrics 1954;13:150–154.
2. Benjamin B. Congenital laryngeal webs. Ann Otol Rhinol Laryngol 1983;92:317–326.

Vocal Cord Paralysis

Vocal cord paralysis in the neonate is not uncommon. It can be central (1) and related to brainstem injury resulting from perinatal anoxia, the Arnold-Chiari malformation, cerebellar agenesis, or posterior fossa meningoceles. However, birth injury and anoxic damage to the brainstem probably are the most common causes in the neonate.

Vocal cord paralysis is readily demonstrated with plain films and fluoroscopic examination of the larynx. On lateral view, indistinctness of the vocal cords, loss of definition of the ventricle, and, on deep inspiration, paradoxical collapse of the subglottic portion of the trachea are seen. The findings mimic those of croup, but the frontal view will pinpoint the problem as being in the vocal cords, for they show little variation in position during resting and phonation, and when both cords are involved, a narrow, slit-like glottic air passage is seen (Fig. 2.55). If only one cord is paralyzed, it will fail to reach the midline on phonation and to relax completely with quiet breathing. Unilateral vocal cord paralysis also can result from stretching of the recurrent laryngeal nerve during birth or by vascular rings or masses in the chest. In addition, it also can be seen after iatrogenic injury of the nerve. Usual imaging of vocal cord paralysis, as previously mentioned, entails fluoroscopy. However, ultrasound (2, 3) also has been used, for it is easy to detect cord motion with this modality (Fig. 2.56).

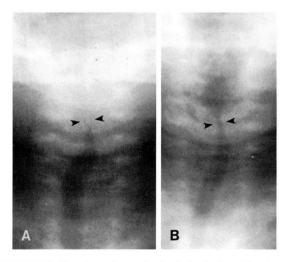

FIGURE 2.55. Vocal cord paralysis. A. Expiratory film demonstrating complete meeting of the cords in the midline (arrows). **B.** Inspiratory film shows little motion of the cords. A narrow slit-like column of air is seen in the glottis (arrows). Normally, the cords would have fallen away from the midline and the glottic air column would be just slightly narrower than the tracheal air column.

REFERENCES

1. Ross DA, Ward PH. Central vocal cord paralysis and paresis presenting as laryngeal stridor in children. Laryngoscope 1990;100:10–13.
2. Garel C, Contencin P, Polonovski JM, et al. Laryngeal ultrasonography in infants and children: a new way of investigating. Normal

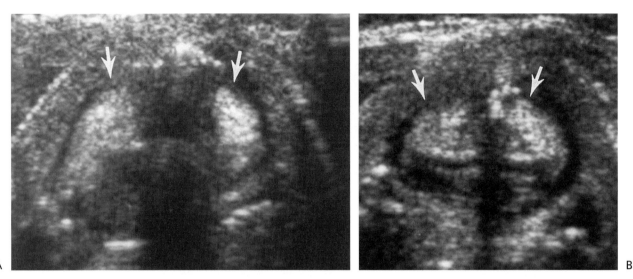

FIGURE 2.56. Normal vocal cord motion: ultrasound. A. On inspiration, the vocal cords (arrows) move apart. **B.** On phonation, they come together (arrows).

and pathological findings. Int J Pediatr Otorhinolaryngol 1992; 23:107–115.
3. Garel C, Hassan M, Legrand I, et al. Laryngeal ultrasonography in infants and children: pathological findings. Pediatr Radiol 1991; 21:164–167.

Laryngocele

Laryngoceles are quite uncommon in childhood, and especially in infancy (1). In adults, they often are the result of occupations that require build-up of high pressures in the upper airway (i.e., singing, wind instrument playing, etc.). The etiology of laryngoceles in infants is unknown but probably is congenital. Laryngoceles may protrude inward and bulge into the airway or outward and produce lateral neck masses. These masses may be fluid or air filled, and the latter occasionally can be demonstrated radiographically. Often, they are associated with hoarseness, but some may be asymptomatic. They also can be vividly demonstrated with CT or MRI.

REFERENCE

1. Walpita PR. Laryngocele in an infant. J Pediatr Surg 1975;10: 843–844.

Laryngeal Asthma

In the peculiar condition of laryngeal asthma, there is paradoxical vocal cord closure on inspiration, and the findings are very confusing during fluoroscopic examination. What happens is that during inspiration, these patients close their glottis, whereas normal individuals would open their glottis (i.e., vocal cords). It is not certain as to whether this is an organic or emotional problem (1), but once recognized, the condition can be diagnosed with confidence.

REFERENCE

1. Shao W, Chung T, Berdon WE, et al. Fluoroscopic diagnosis of laryngeal asthma (paradoxical vocal cord motion). AJR 1995;165: 1229–1231.

Upper Esophageal Foreign Body and Stridor

Upper esophageal foreign bodies generally produce dysphagia, but in many infants, the foreign body may become lodged in the upper esophagus and lead to stridor (1–5). **These infants quickly circumvent their swallowing difficulties and switch to a liquid diet. So smooth is this transition that often it goes unnoticed by the parent.** Thereafter, paraesophageal edema develops and compresses the upper trachea. This can occur within a day or two after the foreign body becomes lodged in the upper esophagus, and the stridor produced usually misleads the physician into thinking that an airway problem, rather than an esophageal problem, is present. If the foreign body is opaque, it can be seen on plain films of the neck and chest (Fig. 2.57), but if it is nonopaque, the diagnosis can be much more elusive, and barium swallow may be required for final verification (4).

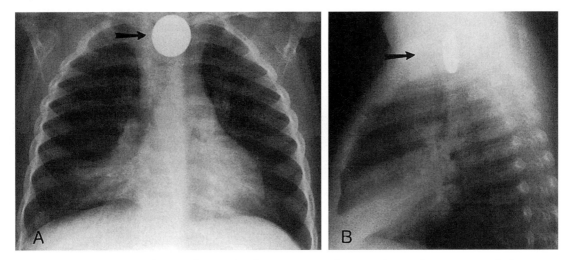

FIGURE 2.57. Esophageal foreign body causing respiratory obstruction. A. Note coin in the esophagus (arrow). **B.** Lateral view demonstrates some narrowing of the trachea anterior to the embedded coin (arrow). This patient presented with chronic cough and stridor, and not so much with dysphagia.

REFERENCES

1. Beer S, Avidan G, Viure E, et al. A foreign body in the oesophagus as a cause of respiratory distress. Pediatr Radiol 1982;12:41–42.
2. Jeffers RG, Weir MR, Wehunt WD, et al. Pull-tab the foreign body sleeper. J Pediatr 1978;92:1023–1024.
3. Schidlow DV, Palmer J, Balsara RK, et al. Chronic stridor and anterior cervical "mass" secondary to an esophageal foreign body. Am J Dis Child 1981;135:869–870.
4. Smith PC, Swischuk LE, Fagan CJ. An elusive and often unsuspected cause of stridor or pneumonia (the esophageal foreign body). AJR 1974;122:80–89.
5. Spitz L, Hirsig J. Prolonged foreign body impaction in the oesophagus. Arch Dis Child 1982;57:551–553.

Laryngeal and Upper Tracheal Tumors and Cysts

Generally, laryngeal tumors and cysts are rare in the neonate and young infant, but when they occur, they can produce considerable respiratory distress. Since many of these lesions involve the vocal cords, the infant will have a hoarse or altered cry in addition to findings such as stridor and cyanosis.

With laryngeal cysts (1, 2), a mass of varying size, encroaching upon the airway, will be visualized. Many of these cysts are located within the aryepiglottic folds (Fig. 2.58). If they are inadequately visualized on plain films, CT or MRI may be used for further delineation. Subglottic cysts also have been identified after chronic airway intubation (3), and their eccentricity may mimic the findings of subglottic hemangioma.

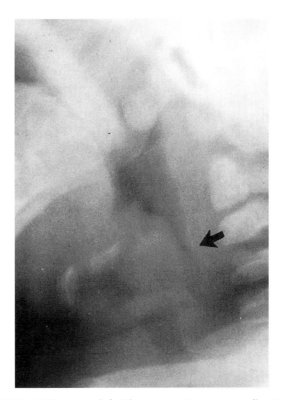

FIGURE 2.58. Aryepiglottic cyst. Note mass distorting aryepiglottic fold and filling the hypopharynx (arrow). (Reproduced with permission from Dunbar JS. Upper respiratory tract obstruction in infants and children; Caldwell lecture. AJR 1970;109:227–246).

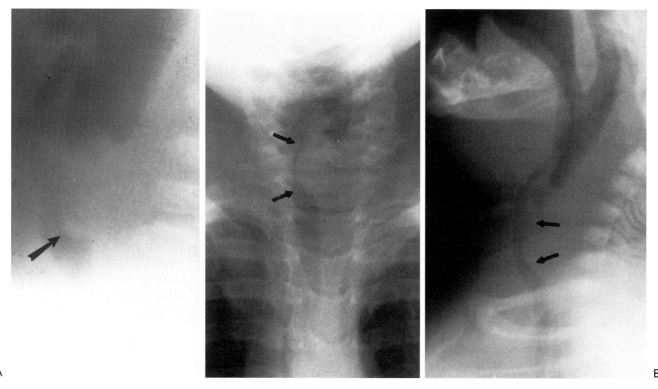

A

B,C

FIGURE 2.59. Subglottic hemangioma. A. Note the characteristic posterior subglottic mass (arrow). **B.** Another patient with a typical lateral subglottic mass (arrows). **C.** A more unusual circumferential hemangioma producing long segment narrowing of the trachea (arrows).

In terms of tumors of the larynx in infants, subglottic hemangioma is most common. These tumors occur directly below the glottis and most often are posterior or lateral in position. Roentgenographically, they present as relatively small, eccentric, rounded masses encroaching upon the airway, just below the glottis (Fig. 2.59, A and B). The finding is virtually pathognomonic, for it is uncommon to encounter other tumors in this area.

Hemangiomas tend to regress on their own or with the aid of steroid therapy, but the process is long and arduous. On the other hand, they can become large and then will require some form of surgical removal, usually in the form of laser or cryotherapy. In addition, while it is classic for subglottic hemangiomas to be eccentric, they also can be circumferential (4), producing findings similar to those of congenital subglottic stenosis. In some cases, the area of stenosis can be quite long (Fig. 2.59C). These hemangiomas also can be detected with MR (5), where they produce high signal on T2-weighted images.

In the older child, the most common tumor is the vocal cord papilloma. Often readily visible on plain films (Fig. 2.60), these tumors usually present in males with insidious hoarseness or voice alteration. Stridor also may be present, and the nodular masses on the vocal cords are characteristic. They can be visualized with greater clarity on CT examination, but generally plain films and direct laryngoscopy suffice.

Vocal cord papillomas are believed to be warts and most likely are of viral (human papilloma) origin (5) contracted from the mother at birth. They tend to regress on their own toward adolescence, but most often they produce so much respiratory difficulty that one cannot wait until that time. Consequently, some form of surgical therapy is required. Unfortunately, in the past, once surgical removal was attempted, there was seeding of these warts into the lower respiratory tract, resulting in chronic pulmonary nodules, some of which cavitate (Fig. 2.60C) (6, 7). This now is less of a problem with current surgical procedures such as cryosurgery or laser surgery. A rare complication in such patients is the development of squamous cell carcinoma from the lung (8) (Fig. 2.60C). Other tumors of the larynx, although rare, include chordoma (9) and neurofibromas (10).

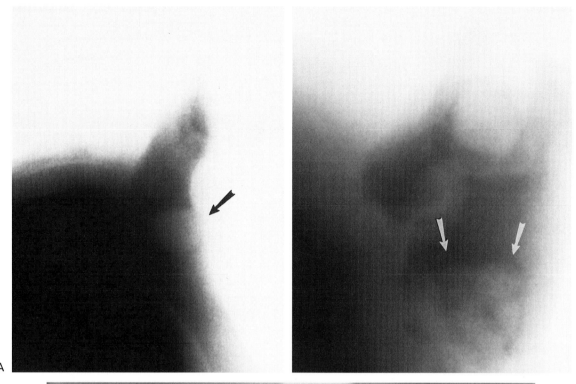

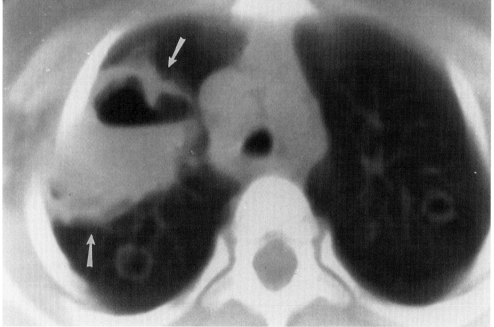

FIGURE 2.60. Juvenile papillomatosis. A. Typical nodule (arrow) on the vocal cords. **B.** In this patient, a large lobulated nodule (arrows) is seen in the hypopharynx. **C.** Cavitating, metastatic squamous cell carcinoma (arrows) in another patient with longstanding papillomatosis. Also note other cavitating nodules on both sides.

REFERENCES

1. Conway EE Jr, Bye MR, Wirtshafter K, et al. Epiglottic cyst: an unusual cause of stridor in an infant. Pediatr Emerg Care 1991; 7:85–86.
2. Shita L, Rypens F, Hassid S, et al. Sonographic demonstration of a congenital laryngeal cyst. J Ultrasound Med 1999;18:665–667.
3. Holinger LD, Torium DM, Anandappa EC. Subglottic cysts and asymmetrical subglottic narrowing on neck radiograph. Pediatr Radiol 1988;18:306–308.
4. Cooper M, Slovis TL, Madgy DN, et al. Congenital subglottic hemangioma: frequency of symmetric narrowing on frontal radiographs of the neck. AJR 1992;159:1269–1271.
5. Boyle WF, Riggs JL, Oshino LS. Electron microscopic identification of papovavirus in laryngeal papilloma. Laryngoscope 1973; 93:1102–1108.
6. Fagan CJ, Swischuk LE. Juvenile laryngeal papillomatosis with spread to the lung. Am J Dis Child 1972;123:139–140.
7. Kramer SS, Wehunt WD, Stocker JT, et al. Pulmonary manifestations of juvenile laryngotracheal papillomatosis. AJR 1985; 144:687–694.
8. Chaput M, Ninane J, Gosseye S, et al. Juvenile laryngeal papillomatosis and epidermoid carcinoma. J Pediatr 1989;114: 269–272.
9. Gundlach P, Radke C, Waldschmidt J. Congenital chondroma of the larynx: an unusual cause of connatal stridor. Z Kinderchir 1990;45:182–184.
10. Masip MJ, Esteban E, Alberto C, et al. Laryngeal involvement in pediatric neurofibromatosis: a case report and review of the literature. Pediatr Radiol 1996;26:488–492.

Cartilaginous Laryngeal and Tracheal Abnormalities

It is uncommon to encounter a newborn or young infant with a true cartilaginous dysplasia of the larynx, but it is certainly not unheard of. In this regard, Capitanio and Kirkpatrick (1) described localized hyperplasia of the cricoid cartilage leading to subglottic compression and respiratory distress in an infant with apparent metatropic dwarfism. Otherwise, calcification of the laryngeal and tracheal cartilages usually is idiopathic (Fig. 2.61) and rarely associated with respiratory distress (2). Even in these latter cases, it is unclear as to whether one can justifiably associate stridor with the calcifications, and, indeed, the calcifications may be incidental (3). The calcifications themselves are unexplained, and in most reported cases, stridor eventually disappears.

Calcification of the larynx or trachea also can be seen in idiopathic hypercalcemia (4) and in chondrodystrophia cal-

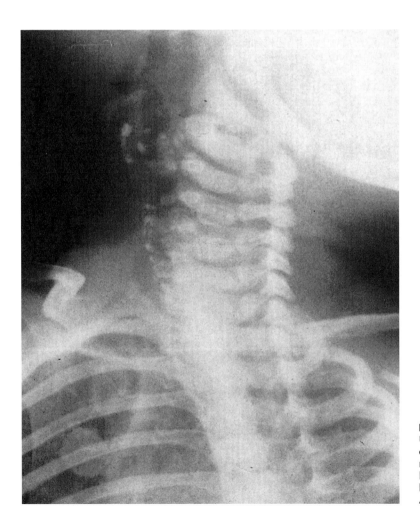

FIGURE 2.61. Calcified trachea and larynx. Unusual calcifications of the laryngeal and tracheal cartilages. This rare problem can be associated with respiratory distress in the neonate. (Same case published by Russo PE, Coin CG. Calcification of the hyoid, thyroid, and tracheal cartilages in infancy. AJR 1958;80:440–442).

cificans congenita (5). In these cases, of course, other manifestations of the respective diseases will be noted throughout the skeleton. In isolated laryngeal and tracheal cartilage calcification, the skeleton is normal. Finally, in a recent study of laryngeal and tracheal calcifications associated with chondrodysplasia punctata, long-term follow-up showed undergrowth and stenosis of the trachea (5). However, the findings did not compromise overall growth of these patients, although there was a certain predisposition to lower respiratory tract infections. For a resume of laryngeal cartilage calcification, one can be referred to the publication by Santos (6).

REFERENCES

1. Capitanio MA, Kirkpatrick JA Jr. Upper respiratory tract obstruction in infants and children. Radiol Clin North Am 1968;6: 265–277.
2. Goldbloom RB, Dunbar JS. Calcification of cartilage in the trachea and larynx in infancy associated with congenital stridor. Pediatrics 1960;26:669–673.
3. Marchal G, Baert AL, van der Hauwaert L. Calcification of larynx and trachea in infancy. Br J Radiol 1974;47:896–897.
4. Shiers JA, Neuhauser EBD, Bowman JR. Idiopathic hypercalcemia. AJR 1957;78:19–29.
5. Kaufmann HJ, Mahboubi S, Spackman TJ, et al. Tracheal stenosis as a complication of chondrodysplasia punctata. Ann Radiol 1976; 19:203–209.
6. Santos JMG. Laryngotracheobronchial cartilage calcification in children. A case report and review of the literature. Pediatr Radiol 1991;21:377–378.

PULMONARY EDEMA AND UPPER AIRWAY OBSTRUCTION

Pulmonary edema is a known complicating factor in upper airway obstruction in infants and children. It can occur during the obstruction or after the obstruction has been relieved (1–6). It is not known exactly why pulmonary edema should develop in such cases, but it has been suggested that capillary damage secondary to hypoxia leads to increased permeability and the development of pulmonary edema (2, 4). At any rate, one should be aware of this phenomenon so as not to misinterpret the findings for some other problem.

REFERENCES

1. Galvis AG. Pulmonary edema complication: relief of upper airway obstruction. Am J Emerg Med 1987;5:294–297.
2. Iszak E. Pulmonary edema due to acute upper airway obstruction for aspirated foreign body. Pediatr Emerg Care 1986;2:235–237.
3. Kanter RK, Watchko JF. Pulmonary edema associated with upper airway obstruction. Am J Dis Child 1984;138:356–358.
4. Oudjhane K, Bowen A, Oh KS, et al. Pulmonary edema complicating upper airway obstruction in infants and children. Can Assoc Radiol J 1992;43:278–282.
5. Rivera M, Hadlock FP, O'Meara ME. Pulmonary edema secondary to acute epiglottitis. AJR 1979;132:991–992.
6. Travis KW, Todres ID, Shannon DC. Pulmonary edema associated with croup and epiglottitis. Pediatrics 1977;59:695–698.

THYROID AND PARATHYROID GLANDS

Parathyroid disease in childhood is rather uncommon, and imaging usually centers around initial sonography and thereafter CT or MRI. Diseases of the thyroid gland are more common, and the gland also is readily amenable to imaging with ultrasound, CT, or MRI.

Normal Thyroid Gland

The normal thyroid gland is readily identified with ultrasonography, CT, and MRI but most often is first imaged ultrasonographically. Both lobes are similar in size and shape (oval), and the isthmus also can be identified. On ultrasound, the normal gland has a very homogeneous pattern of echogenicity (Fig. 2.62).

Developmental Abnormalities

Agenesis of the thyroid gland is one of the more common causes of cretinism, but in the newborn, hypothyroidism probably is more commonly caused by (a) a nonfunctioning thyroid gland or (b) a gland suppressed by maternal antithyroid medication. Initial imaging of the thyroid gland in hypothyroidism usually is accomplished with ultrasound wherein the size and texture of the gland are easily evaluated. In this regard, most of these glands, although smaller than normal (1), usually have a normal echotexture. However, if the gland is entirely absent, no thyroid tissue is detected in its usual place. Under these circumstances, one should look for ectopic thyroid tissue, usually taking the form of a sublingual thyroid gland. These sublingual collections of thyroid tissue can be identified with ultrasound, but their presence often is finally confirmed with nuclear scintigraphy (Fig. 2.63). In this regard, however, although ectopic thyroid tissue usually occurs in the sublingual region, it can be found at any point between the base of the tongue and the diaphragm.

Parenchymal Disease and Goiter

Goiter is a nonspecific term that merely indicates that the thyroid gland is enlarged. Many causes for enlargement exist, but the more common include thyrotoxicosis (Graves' disease), lymphocytic thyroiditis (Hashimoto's disease), and nonspecific multinodular goiter. Almost invariably, all of these lesions now are first imaged with ultrasound.

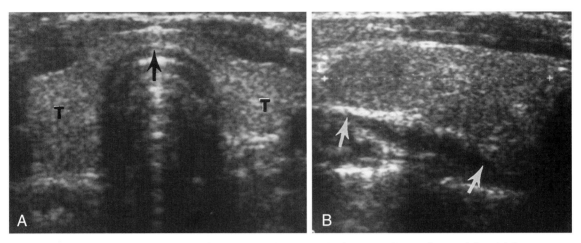

FIGURE 2.62. Normal thyroid: ultrasound. A. Note the fine granularity of normal thyroid tissue throughout both thyroid lobes (T). Arrow denotes isthmus. **B.** Longitudinal view demonstrates the shape and fine granularity of normal thyroid tissue (arrows).

In thyrotoxicosis, the thyroid gland is enlarged and shows echogenicity similar to that of a normal gland. With lymphoid thyroiditis (Hashimoto's disease), the findings are variable, but generally the gland shows nonspecific variation of echogenicity (Fig. 2.64). In some cases, actual echogenic nodules may be seen, but most often there is a basic stroma of coarse echogenicity interspersed with small hypoechoic areas (2). Grading of the degree of change has been attempted (3), but generally cannot be applied on a practical basis. The reason for this is that when a thyroid gland responds to decreased thyroxin production for any reason, it usually shows rebound hypertrophy in a nonuniform pattern. In other words, erratic hypertrophic nodules arise, and the end result is a multinodular goiter with no specificity.

Suppurative bacterial thyroiditis is rare in children, but it has been reported in association with pyriform sinus fistulas (4, 5). The pyriform sinus is thought to be an embryonic remnant of either the third or the fourth pharyngeal pouches, and infections through the fistula are believed to cause secondary infections of the thyroid gland. Abscesses of the thyroid gland appear just as abscesses do in any other part of the body. Basically, they are hypoechoic through their center, but if debris is present, echogenicity is seen.

Cysts and Tumors of the Thyroid Gland

Simple cysts of the thyroid are rare and usually are the result of cystic degeneration of a benign adenoma. In this regard,

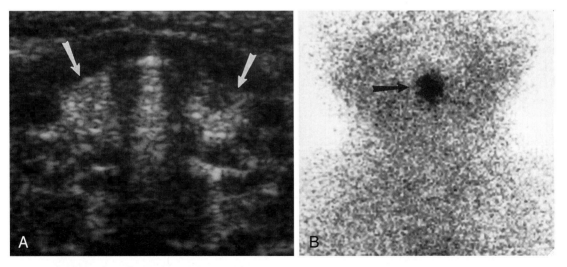

FIGURE 2.63. Sublingual thyroid. A. Ultrasonogram demonstrates abnormal echogenicity in the areas where the thyroid gland would ordinarily be located. **B.** Nuclear scintigraphy demonstrates a sublingual thyroid.

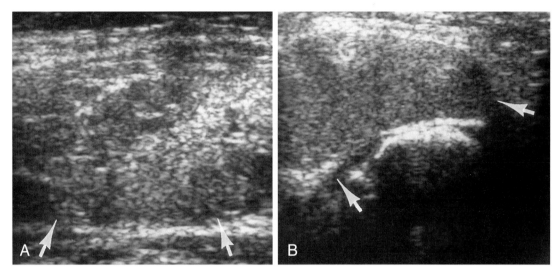

FIGURE 2.64. Thyroiditis. A. Hashimoto's thyroiditis. Note the coarse, echogenic heterogeneous texture of the thyroid gland (arrows). **B.** Another patient in cross-section demonstrating lesser changes, but still the echotexture of the thyroid gland (arrows) is more coarse than normal.

the most common benign nodule in the thyroid gland of children is the follicular adenoma. It usually is hypoechoic, and most of these nodules also demonstrate a sonolucent halo surrounding the lesion (Fig. 2.65), but the finding is not entirely pathognomonic (6). In addition, and as has been noted, adenomas very frequently undergo necrosis and cystic degeneration.

Malignant tumors of the thyroid gland in children are not particularly common, and in terms of the imaging feature of carcinoma of the thyroid gland, the appearance is about the same as that in adults. In this regard, if a cold nodule is detected on nuclear scintigraphy, it may or may not be malignant, but if the nodule is active or hot, it is benign. The incidence of malignancy in solitary nodules of the thyroid gland ranges from 17% to 57%, depending on the series reviewed (6). Follicular papilloma of the thymus gland deserves special attention, for while low in malignancy, it may spread to regional lymph nodes and even the lungs. Treatment with ^{131}I is successful, and in spite of extensive pulmonary disease, pulmonary function remains relatively normal.

Thyroglossal Duct Cysts

Thyroglossal duct cysts are common in childhood. They occur in the midline and thus can be differentiated from laterally placed branchial cleft cysts. These cysts usually are well

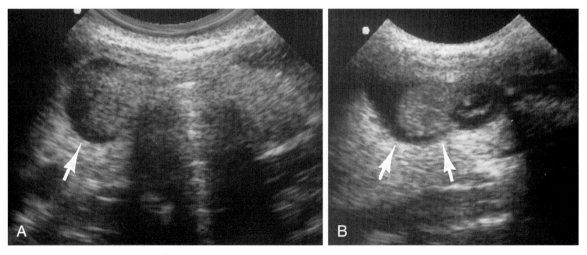

FIGURE 2.65. Thyroid adenoma. A. Note the echogenic nodule in the left thymic lobe. Some fluid surrounds the nodule (arrow). **B.** Sagittal view demonstrates the same findings (arrows).

defined sonographically and may be hypoechoic (fluid filled) or show echogenicity resulting from infection, bleeding, etc. (see Fig. 2.21). If a thyroglossal duct fistula is present, it can be injected with contrast material, and when a fistula is present, repeated thyroid gland infections are not uncommon.

The Parathyroid Gland

Parathyroid abnormalities in childhood are rare, but one can encounter cysts (7) and adenomas (8). Cysts appear just as cysts do anywhere in the body, and adenomas usually are echogenic and homogeneous. Parathyroid tumors also can be detected with MRI and with nuclear scintigraphy using ^{99m}Tc-sestamibi.

REFERENCES

1. Ueda D, Mitamura R, Suzuki N, et al. Sonographic imaging of the thyroid gland in congenital hypothyroidism. Pediatr Radiol 1992; 22:102–105.
2. Mache CJ, Schwingshandl J, Riccabona M, et al. Ultrasound and MRI findings in a case of childhood amyloid goiter. Pediatr Radiol 1993;23:565–566.
3. Ivarsson SA, Ericsson U-B, Fredriksson B, et al. Ultrasonic imaging in the differential diagnosis of diffuse thyroid disorders in children. Am J Dis Child 1989;143:1369–1372.
4. Hatabu H, Kasagi K, Yamamoto K, et al. Acute suppurative thyroiditis associated with piriform sinus fistula: sonographic findings. AJR 1990;155:845–847.
5. Lucaya J, Berdon WE, Enriquez G, et al. Congenital pyriform sinus fistula: a cause of acute left-sided suppurative thyroiditis and neck abscess in children. Pediatr Radiol 1990;21:27–29.
6. Hung W, Anderson KD, Chandra RS, et al. Solitary thyroid nodules in 71 children and adolescents. J Pediatr Surg 1992;27: 1407–1409.
7. Entwistle JWC, Pierce CV, Johnson DE, et al. Parathyroid cysts: report of the sixth youngest pediatric case. J Pediatr Surg 1994;29: 1528–1529.
8. Rai M, Agrawal JK, Sasikumar V, et al. Familial childhood parathyroid adenoma. J Pediatr Surg 1994;29:1530–1531.

3

CARDIOVASCULAR SYSTEM

Cardiac problems in neonates and infants usually are congenital in origin, while in older children, acquired heart disease is more the problem. In all groups, imaging modalities used for the investigation of heart disease in children include plain films, magnetic resonance imaging (MRI) (1, 2), computed tomography (CT), and cineradiography. However, even in this sophisticated age of imaging, the plain film still is the first imaging study obtained and still is useful (3). Thereafter, ultrasonography usually is performed, but this generally is performed by cardiologists and not radiologists.

REFERENCES

1. Bisset GS III. Magnetic resonance imaging of congenital heart disease in the pediatric patient. Radiol Clin North Am 1991;29: 279–291.
2. Fellows KE, Weinberg PM, Baffa JM, et al. Evaluation of congenital heart disease with MR imaging: current and coming attractions. AJR 1992;159:925–931.
3. Swenson JM, Fischer DR, Miller SA, et al. Are chest radiographs and electrocardiograms still valuable in evaluating new pediatric patients with heart murmurs or chest pain? Pediatrics 1997;99:1–3.

NORMAL HEART AND VARIATIONS

There is little difference in evaluating the heart of an older child from that of an adult, but in infancy, because of the overlying thymus gland, the individual great vessels are more difficult to identify and analyze. Cardiac measurements for the determination of cardiac size have the same pitfalls in children as in adults, and it generally is accepted by imagers that these measurements are of questionable value. There simply is too much overlap with normal for them to be useful, and for this reason, they generally are not used by experienced imagers.

It also has been demonstrated that cardiac size differs very little during systole and diastole in newborn infants (1). This is different from the situation in older children and adults where the difference may be substantial and is a well-known radiologic phenomenon. It also should be noted that in otherwise apparently healthy newborn infants, transient cardiac enlargement is not uncommon. There are many reasons why the heart might enlarge in these babies, including placental-to-fetal transfusion, excessive cord stripping, hypoglycemia, hypocalcemia, and myocardial schemia secondary to hypoxia. All of these entities are discussed later in this chapter, but **it should be noted here that not every large heart in the neonate stays large and, indeed, not every one is significantly pathologic.** This is different from the problem in the older child where cardiomegaly generally indicates underlying cardiac or pericardial disease.

Normal variations commonly encountered in children include prominence of the superior vena cava (2), normal visualization of the left atrial silhouette on frontal views (3), and the ductus bump in neonates (4). Prominence of the superior vena cava produces unilateral widening of the mediastinum on the right. This finding often is indistinguishable from that seen with a normal thymus gland, but it might be noted that with either of these causes of right-side mediastinal widening, there is no displacement of the trachea. This is important, for with true mediastinal masses (i.e., cysts or tumors), tracheal displacement occurs.

Visualization of the normal right edge of the left atrium, through the cardiac silhouette on frontal view, is a common normal finding in infants and children (Fig. 3.1A). It should not be confused with the enlarged double silhouette seen with an enlarged left atrium. With the latter, the left atrial edge is seen further to the right and somewhat lower (Fig. 3.1B) than the position occupied by the normal left atrium.

The ductus bump is a finding limited to newborn infants and is seen in the region of the aortic knob (Fig. 3.2). It represents the dilated ductal infundibulum of the closing ductus and disappears as the infant grows older. It is not seen beyond the neonatal period, and consequently, if one sees a similar bulge in an older infant, one should suspect a ductus arteriosus aneurysm. This is especially true if the bulge shows progressive enlargement.

Finally, another normal finding is calcification of the ligamentum arteriosum (5) typically located between the aortic knob and pulmonary artery (Fig. 3.3).

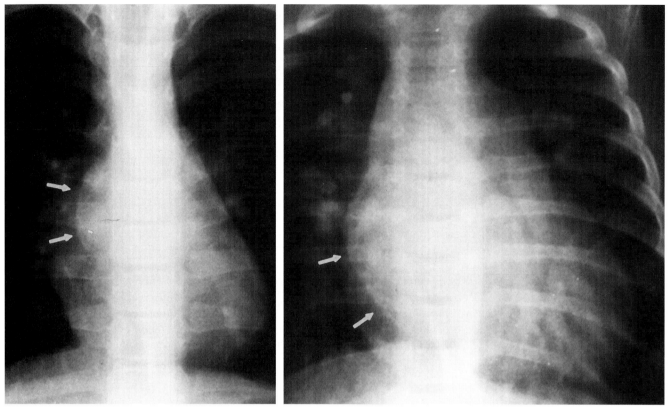

A   B

FIGURE 3.1. Left atrial silhouette, normal and abnormal. A. Normal left atrial silhouette (arrows). **B.** Abnormal left atrial silhouette (arrows) in a patient with an enlarged left atrium associated with a ventricular septal defect.

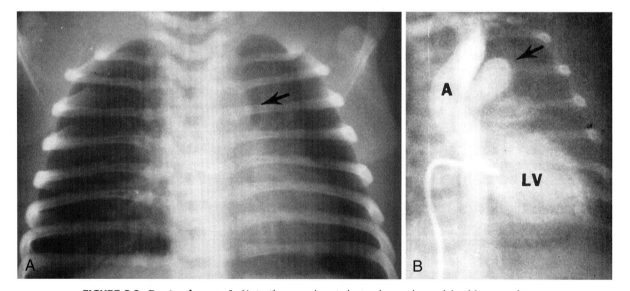

FIGURE 3.2. Ductus bump. A. Note the prominent ductus bump (arrow) in this normal newborn infant. **B.** Aortogram in another infant demonstrates a large ductal remnant or bump (arrow). A, aorta; LV, left ventricle.

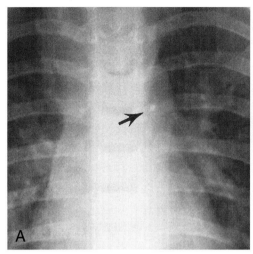
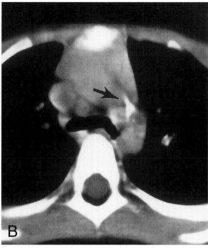

FIGURE 3.3. Calcification of ligamentum arteriosum. A. Note typical punctate calcification (arrow) of the ligamentum arteriosum. **B.** Computed tomography study demonstrating the same finding (arrow). (Reproduced with permission from Bisceglia M, Donaldson JS. Calcification of ligamentum arteriosum in children; a normal finding on CT. AJR 1991;156:351–352).

REFERENCES

1. Burnard ED, James LS. The cardiac silhouette in newborn infants: a cinematographic study of the normal range. Pediatrics 1961;27:713–725.
2. Heil BJ, Felman AH, Talbert JL, et al. Idiopathic dilatation of the superior vena cava. J Pediatr Surg 1978;13:193.
3. Rosario-Medina W, Strife JL, Dunbar S. Normal left atrium: appearance in children on frontal chest radiographs. Radiology 1986;161:345–346.
4. Berdon WE, Baker DH, James LS. The ductus bump (a transient physiologic mass in chest roentgenograms of newborn infants). AJR 1965;95:91–98.
5. Bisceglia M, Donaldson JS. Calcification of the ligamentum arteriosum in children: a normal finding. AJR 1991;156:351–352.

NORMAL ROENTGENOGRAPHIC ANATOMY

It is not possible to completely assess all cardiac chambers on any one projection, so in the past, multiple roentgenographic views were employed. The frontal projection, however, was, and still is, the most valuable. It provides most of the vital information on a single view (i.e., cardiomegaly, state of the vasculature, configuration of the great vessels, etc.) (Fig. 3.4).

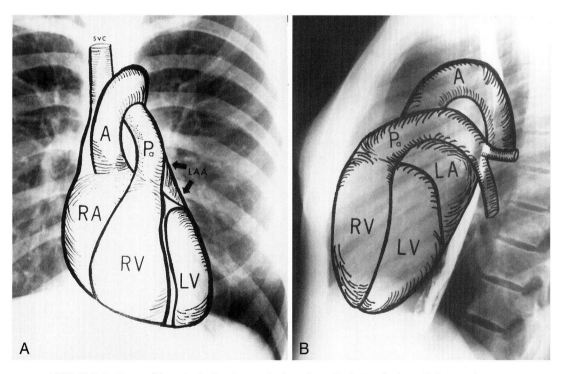

FIGURE 3.4. Normal heart. A. Posteroanterior view. B. Lateral view. SVC, superior vena cava; A, aorta; Pa, pulmonary artery; LA, left atrium; RA, right atrium; LAA, left atrial appendage; LV, left ventricle; RV, right ventricle.

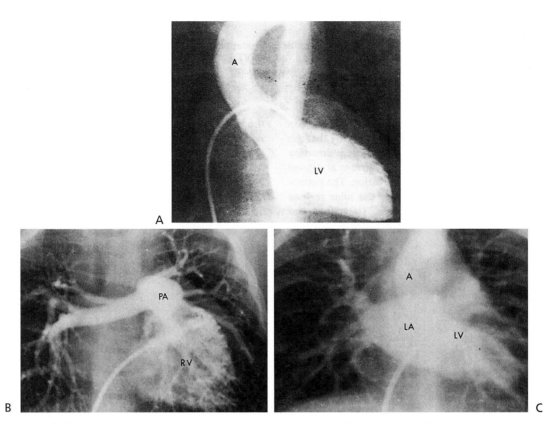

FIGURE 3.5. Normal cardioangiogram: frontal view. A. Note the aorta (A) and smooth-walled left ventricle (LV). The aortic valve is not clearly visualized. The right border of the left ventricle demarcates the closed mitral valve. **B.** View of another patient demonstrates the pulmonary artery (PA) and characteristically trabeculated right ventricle (RV). Note the course and configuration of the pulmonary artery branches. **C.** Drainage film in the same patient demonstrates the more horizontal orientation of the pulmonary veins draining into the left atrium (LA). Subsequent filling of the left ventricle (LV) and the aorta (A) is seen.

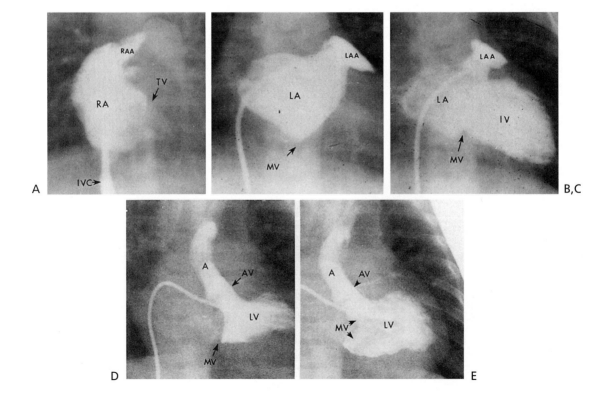

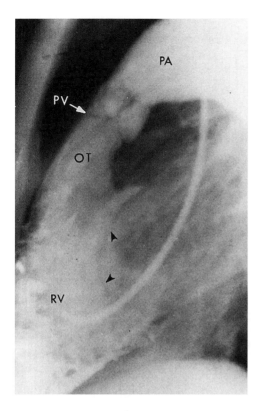

FIGURE 3.7. Normal cardioangiogram: lateral view. Note the right ventricle (RV), right outflow tract (OT), cusps of the pulmonary valve (PV), and the pulmonary artery (PA). Also note the thin curved radiolucency of the bulging tricuspid valve (arrowheads).

ANGIOCARDIOGRAPHIC ANATOMY

Frontal, lateral, and both oblique projections are the standard angiocardiographic views. The views obtained in any given case are selected according to the lesion or lesions suspected. On standard frontal views, all four chambers of the heart can, depending on the site of injection, be identified (Figs. 3.5 and 3.6). The right ventricle usually is identified by its more midline position and by its being much more trabeculated than the left ventricle. The left ventricle lies to the left and, of course, gives rise to the aorta. The right atrium is rather crescent shaped, while the left atrium, lying somewhat more medially, is more oval. The lateral view is used primarily for identification of the right ventricle and great vessels (Fig. 3.7). The right ventricle and pulmonary artery are anterior, while the left ventricle and aorta are posterior. On the left anterooblique view, perhaps the most used view, the left atrium, left ventricle, intraventricular septum, right ventricle, and both the aorta and the pulmonary artery can be evaluated (Fig. 3.8). The mitral and tricuspid valves also can be seen on the left anterooblique view.

FIGURE 3.6. Normal cardioangiogram: frontal view. A. Note the characteristic configuration of the right atrium (RA) and right atrial appendage (RAA). TV, tricuspid valve; IVC, inferior vena cava. **B.** The left atrium (LA), which was injected with contrast medium through the catheter that had passed through the foramen ovale, is visualized. LAA, left atrial appendage. Note the location of the closed mitral valve (MV). **C.** View in another patient demonstrates the left atrium (LA), left atrial appendage (LAA), and the smooth-walled left ventricle (LV). Note the location of the mitral valve (MV). **D.** View of still another patient demonstrates filling of the left ventricle (LV) and aorta (A) and the aortic valve (AV) in between these two structures. Note the closed mitral valve (MV). **E.** Later view in the same patient demonstrates the aorta (A), thin curved aortic valve (AV), left ventricle (LV), and the now-opened mitral valve (MV).

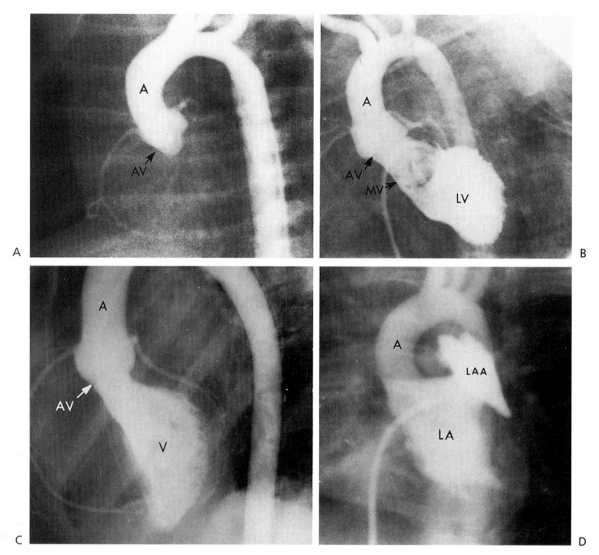

FIGURE 3.8. Normal cardioangiogram: left anterooblique views. A. Supravalvular aortic injection demonstrates the aorta (A) and all three cusps of the aortic valve (AV). Also note the right and left coronary arteries. **B.** View in another patient demonstrates the aorta (A), aortic valve (AV), and left ventricle (LV). The round radiolucency just below the aortic valve is the open mitral valve (MV). **C.** View of another patient demonstrates the left ventricle (V), aortic valve (AV), bulging sinuses of Valsalva above, ascending aorta (A), and the right and left coronary arteries. The straight edge anterior to the contrast-filled left ventricle demarcates the interventricular septum. **D.** Injection into the left atrium (LA) demonstrates the left atrial appendage (LAA) and the aorta (A).

MAGNETIC RESONANCE IMAGING ANATOMY

MRI is extremely useful in delineating the cardiac chambers, great vessels, and various cardiac valves. The reason for this is that moving blood is vividly depicted, since with movement, there is lack of signal generation and blood appears black. Consequently, a natural contrast medium is available, and in those cases where delineation of the anatomy is of prime consideration, MRI is very useful.

The views obtained with MRI generally correspond to those used for cardioangiography. Of course, with the infinite number of slices and angles available with MRI, many more images can be produced (Figs. 3.9–3.12).

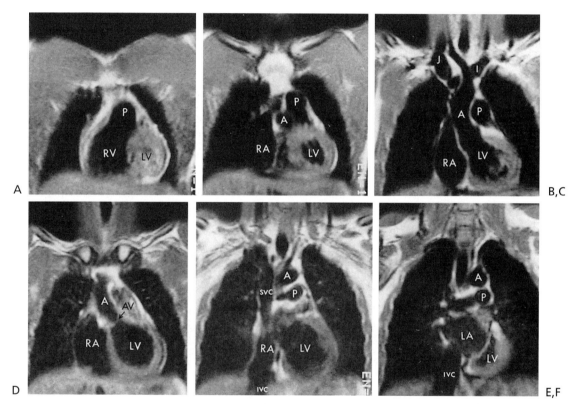

FIGURE 3.9. Normal magnetic resonance images: coronal sections. A. Anterior slice demonstrates the anterior wall of the left ventricle (LV), the cavity of the right ventricle (RV), and the pulmonary artery (P). **B.** Slightly more posterior cut demonstrates the left ventricular cavity (LV), right atrium (RA), pulmonary artery (P), and the root of the aorta (A). **C.** A still more posterior cut demonstrates the right atrium (RA) and the left ventricle (LV), giving rise to the aorta (A) and innominate artery, which heads up to the right. P, pulmonary artery; I, innominate vein; J, jugular vein. **D.** Anterior coronal slice of another patient demonstrates the right atrium (RA), left ventricle (LV), aortic valve (AV), and aorta (A). **E.** A slightly more posterior cut again demonstrates the left ventricle (LV), right atrium (RA), both the superior (SVC) and inferior (IVC) venae cavae, and aorta (A), giving rise to the left common carotid artery and the pulmonary artery (P). **F.** Posteriormost cut demonstrates the left atrium (LA) and left ventricle (LV). The crescent-shaped density between the two structures represents the wall of the left atrium. Also note the inferior vena cava (IVC), aorta (A), and pulmonary artery (P). The right pulmonary artery arises from the main pulmonary artery and crosses the mediastinum just above the left atrium.

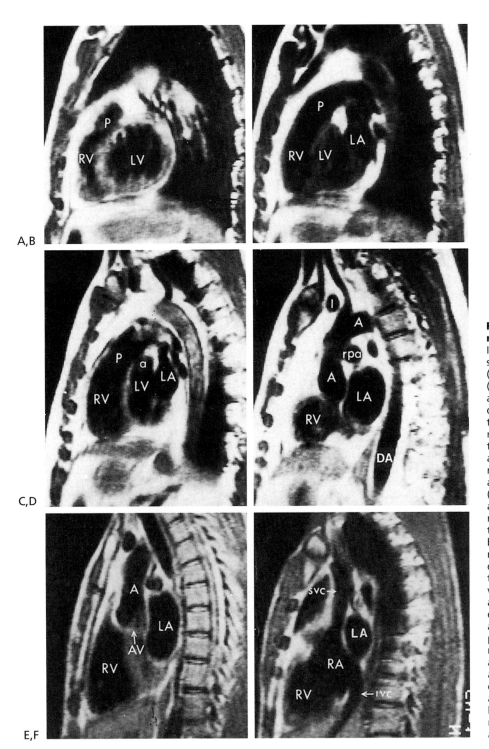

FIGURE 3.10. Normal magnetic resonance images: sagittal sections. A. Image well to the left of the spine demonstrates the posteriorly located left ventricle (LV) and anteriorly located right ventricle (RV). Also note the root of the pulmonary artery (P). **B.** Slightly more medial cut demonstrates the right ventricle (RV) and the pulmonary artery (P) arising from the right ventricle (RV). Note the position of the left ventricle (LV) and that the left atrium (LA) now is visualized. **C.** Still more medially, one can see the left ventricle (LV) and the proximal portion of the aortic root (a). Note the left atrium (LA) and, once again, the right ventricle (RV) and pulmonary artery (P). The descending aorta is the gray tubular structure (flow artifact) behind the heart. **D.** Another slice more medial and just to the left of the spine demonstrates what is left of the right ventricle (RV). The left ventricle is no longer visualized, but the aorta is seen in both its ascending and transverse portions (A). DA, descending aorta; rpa, right pulmonary artery; I, innominate vein. **E.** Another patient: midsagittal cut. Note the anterior right ventricle (RV), the aortic valve (AV), and the ascending aorta (A). LA, left atrium. **F.** Cut to the right of the spine demonstrates the right ventricle (RV), right atrium (RA), and left atrium (LA). Note both the superior vena cava (svc) and inferior vena cava (ivc) entering the right atrium.

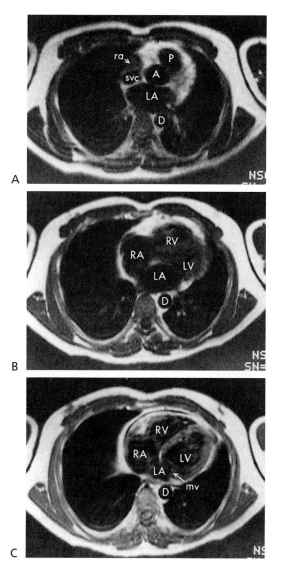

FIGURE 3.11. **Normal magnetic resonance scans: axial views. A.** Note the pulmonary artery (P) and the root of the aorta (A) on this cut through the top of the heart. Also note the posteriorly located left atrium (LA). The superior vena cava (svc) is seen just posterior to the right atrium (ra). D, descending aorta. **B.** Slightly lower cut demonstrates the left atrium (LA), right atrium (RA), left ventricle (LV), and right ventricle (RV). D, descending aorta. **C.** A still lower cut demonstrates the right atrium (RA), the very bottom of the left atrium (LA), and the mitral valve (mv) between the left atrium and the left ventricle (LV). RV, right ventricle; D, descending aorta.

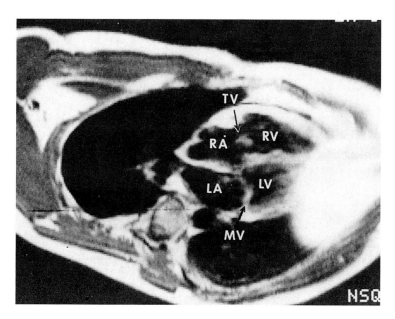

FIGURE 3.12. **Normal magnetic resonance image: oblique axial view.** Note all four chambers of the heart and the atrioventricular valves between them. LV, left ventricle; RV, right ventricle; RA, right atrium; LA, left atrium; TV, tricuspid valve; MV, mitral valve.

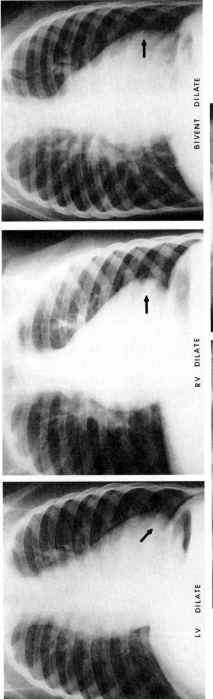

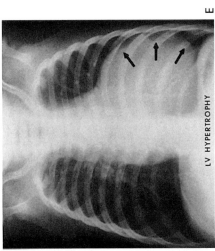

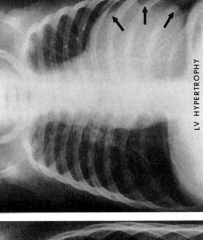

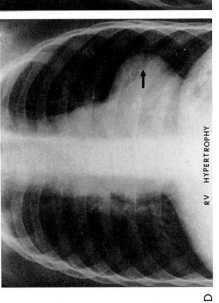

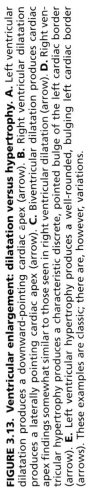

A   LV DILATE

RV DILATE   BIVENT DILATE   B,C

D   RV HYPERTROPHY

LV HYPERTROPHY   E

FIGURE 3.13. Ventricular enlargement: dilatation versus hypertrophy. A. Left ventricular dilatation produces a downward-pointing cardiac apex (arrow). **B.** Right ventricular dilatation produces a laterally pointing cardiac apex (arrow). **C.** Biventricular dilatation produces cardiac apex findings somewhat similar to those seen in right ventricular dilatation (arrow). **D.** Right ventricular hypertrophy produces a characteristic discrete, pointed bulge of the left cardiac border (arrow). **E.** Left ventricular hypertrophy produces a well-rounded, bulging left cardiac border (arrows). These examples are classic; there are, however, variations.

PHYSIOLOGIC CONSIDERATIONS IN CONGENITAL HEART DISEASE

Systolic (Pressure) and Diastolic (Volume) Ventricular Overloading

The concepts of systolic and diastolic overloading of the ventricles are important to the understanding of congenital heart disease and especially to the understanding of the effects on the ventricles. Diastolic overloading occurs in patients with lesions that produce a left-to-right shunt or valvular insufficiency. In such patients, the altered hemodynamics require that the involved chamber receive an extra volume of blood during diastole. This results in early ventricular dilatation and enlargement, findings that are readily appreciated roentgenographically. Of course, some reactive hypertrophy also must occur, but dilatation predominates and is what is seen on the x-ray (Fig. 3.13).

Systolic overloading results when a valvular or vascular lesion produces obstruction to the normal flow of blood through the heart. This occurs with such lesions as aortic stenosis, pulmonary stenosis, and coarctation of the aorta. The ventricles respond to systolic overloading with concentric hypertrophy rather than dilatation; thus, there is little or no chamber enlargement. Consequently, often there is little in the way of roentgenographic abnormality, and in many cases, the roentgenogram may appear to be entirely normal. Eventually, however, the specific patterns of right and left ventricular hypertrophy evolve (Fig. 3.13).

Postnatal Pulmonary Vascular and Right Ventricular Involution

The phenomena of postnatal pulmonary vascular and right ventricular involution are important to the understanding of certain congenital heart lesions, especially those associated with left-to-right shunts. These phenomena occur because in the fetus, the pulmonary arteriolar walls are thicker than normal and resistance to pulmonary blood flow is increased. As a result, pulmonary artery pressures are greater than normal and the right ventricle hypertrophies. Thickening of the arteriolar walls is primarily the result of hypertrophy of the media, and the entire problem is believed to represent a reaction of the pulmonary arterioles to the relatively hypoxic state of the fetus during the third trimester of pregnancy. There is some support for this concept in that full-term infants almost always develop this vascular pattern, while premature infants usually do not.

The presence of this "physiologic" pulmonary hypertension after birth significantly inhibits the flow of blood through the lungs. Consequently, if a potential left-to-right shunt is present, it will not become manifest until later. It usually takes days, or even weeks, for left-to-right shunting to occur and allow these infants to flood their lungs with blood. This entire phenomenon is referred to as "involution of the pulmonary vasculature" and is the usual sequence of events in the normal neonate. However, if it fails to occur, pulmonary vascular resistance remains high, and the result is "primary pulmonary hypertension." This leads to the so-called "persistent fetal circulation syndrome" where right-to-left ductal shunting results. These patients are cyanotic and therefore often first thought to have significant structural cyanotic heart disease.

BASIC PULMONARY VASCULAR PATTERNS

Increased Pulmonary Vascularity

Increased pulmonary vascularity resulting from active congestion is seen with left-to-right shunts (i.e., atrial septal defect, ventricular septal defect, patent ductus arteriosus, etc.) and in admixture lesions, where there is preferential blood flow into the lower-pressure pulmonary circulation (i.e., transposition of the great vessels, persistent truncus arteriosus, single ventricle, etc.). In all instances, however, it is the increased volume of blood flowing through the pulmonary vessels that leads to vascular congestion. Pulmonary vascular congestion or engorgement involves both arteries and veins and is uniform throughout both upper and lower lobes. However, usually only the arteries are seen on plain films. Perhaps this is because their walls are thicker, but whatever the reason, the veins are never clearly visualized. The individual arteries are dilated and tortuous (Fig. 3.14A) and extend further than usual into the periphery of the lungs. Their walls, however, are still relatively distinct.

Generally, roentgenographically detectable engorgement of the pulmonary arteries with underlying left-to-right shunts does not occur until right ventricular output is more than twice left ventricular output; indeed, in more precise terms, this does not occur until the ratio of cardiac output is about 2.5:1 in favor of the right ventricle. When the shunt reaches this level, the pulmonary vessels become visibly, but not strikingly, dilated. This assessment, for the most part, is subjective, but Coussement and Gooding (1) presented material that enables a more objective assessment. In their study of normal children, they compared the diameter of the right descending pulmonary artery with the diameter of the trachea and found them to be nearly the same, differing at most by only 2 mm. In patients with significant left-to-right shunts (i.e., more than 2.5:1), they found that the diameter of the right descending pulmonary artery always was greater than the diameter of the trachea. These observations are readily duplicated and are objective, but on a practical basis, most settle for a simple subjective evaluation.

Passive congestion occurs whenever there is pulmonary venous hypertension, and pulmonary venous hypertension results from left-side obstructive lesions or left-side myocardial dysfunction. In either case, left-side failure leads to dilation of pulmonary veins and the transudation of fluid into the perivascular tissues. **In other words, pulmonary inter-**

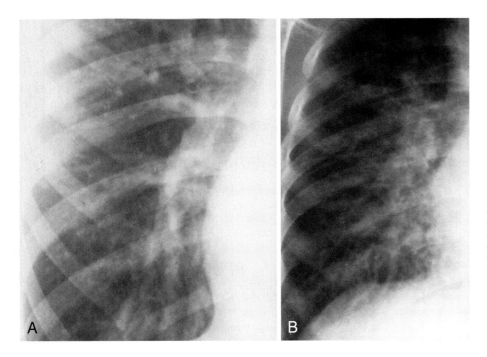

FIGURE 3.14. Increased pulmonary vascularity. A. Active congestion. The individual vessels dilate, extend further into the periphery than usual, yet retain relatively distinct walls. **B. With passive congestion,** the problem is increased pressure in the pulmonary venous system with transudation of fluid into the interstitial space, resulting in indistinct, fuzzy-appearing vessels. The pulmonary artery branches are not dilated as they are in **A.**

stitial edema develops, and because of this, the individual vessels lose their normal sharpness and become hazy and indistinct on plain films (Fig. 3.14B). In severe cases, frank alveolar pulmonary edema and pleural effusions can be seen, and in almost all cases, the changes are more pronounced in the parahilar regions. As opposed to active congestion, the pulmonary artery branches do not dilate and enlarge.

In the neonate, certain lesions produce pronounced passive congestion where the lungs appear hazy, granular, or reticular and the findings mimic pulmonary disease, including surfactant deficiency (hyaline membrane) disease (Fig.

3.15A). In other cases, a very reticular pattern of congestion results, and the findings mimic those of primary pulmonary lymphangiectasia (Fig. 3.15B). For the most part, lesions producing this picture include total anomalous pulmonary venous return below the diaphragm (type III), pulmonary vein atresia, and the hypoplastic left heart syndrome.

Decreased Pulmonary Vascularity

Decreased pulmonary vascularity reflects diminished pulmonary blood flow, and the finding is seen with right out-

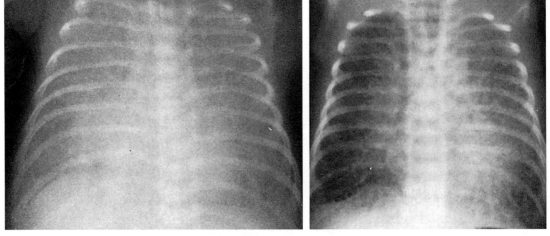

FIGURE 3.15. Passive congestion: high-grade venous obstruction in neonates. A. Note the hazy-appearing lungs in this infant with total anomalous pulmonary venous return below the diaphragm. This finding is typical of interstitial pulmonary edema. **B.** Another patient with hypoplastic left heart syndrome and a typical reticulonodular pattern.

flow tract-obstructing lesions associated with a right-to-left shunt. Because of the shunt, blood is diverted from the right side of the heart to the left, and because of this, less blood flows through the lungs. In addition, the shunt results in cyanosis, and lesions showing this combination of findings include tetralogy of Fallot, hypoplastic right heart syndrome, severe pulmonary stenosis with right-to-left atrial shunt (trilogy of Fallot), and Ebstein's anomaly. When pulmonary blood flow is diminished, the lungs demonstrate a generalized hyperlucency (pulmonary oligemia), and the blood vessels appear thin and stringy (Fig. 3.16). Indeed, it is difficult to identify a normal-caliber pulmonary artery branch. This all is more evident when compared with normal pulmonary blood vessels (Fig. 3.4A).

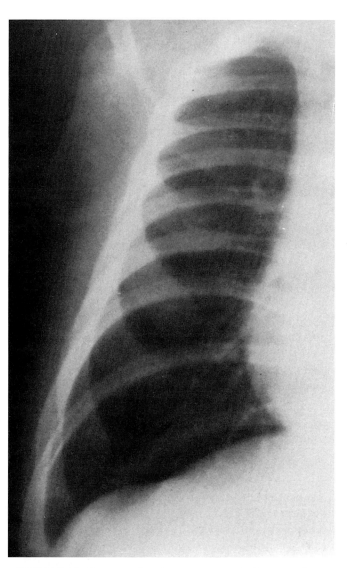

FIGURE 3.16. Decreased pulmonary vascularity: tetralogy of Fallot. Note characteristically thin and stringy pulmonary artery branches. It is difficult to identify a normal-caliber vessel.

Unequal Pulmonary Blood Flow

Unequal pulmonary blood flow is a valuable adjunctive roentgenographic finding in the assessment of congenital heart disease and occurs most often in tetralogy of Fallot, persistent truncus arteriosus, and pulmonary valve stenosis. In tetralogy of Fallot, it is the left lung that usually shows diminished blood flow, while in persistent truncus arteriosus, either lung or just one lobe of a lung (Fig. 3.17) can manifest this finding. In pulmonary valve stenosis, the flow of blood through the stenotic valve preferentially enters the left pulmonary artery. As a result, the left pulmonary artery enlarges and vascularity through the left lung is slightly increased. This latter finding is readily demonstrable with nuclear scintigraphy but is difficult to detect on plain films, especially in infants and children. In adults, the discrepancy may be more readily detectable.

Pulmonary Hypertension with Increased Pulmonary Blood Flow

Pulmonary hypertension most often is associated with a longstanding left-to-right shunt or intracardiac mixing lesion. The pulmonary artery changes result from the constant delivery of excessive volumes of blood to the lungs. To protect the lungs from this excessive flow of blood, the peripheral pulmonary arterioles constrict, first resulting in transient pulmonary hypertension and eventually, with muscular hypertrophy of the media, permanent pulmonary hypertension (Eisenmenger's physiology). This results in diminution of peripheral pulmonary blood flow and prominence of the main pulmonary artery and proximal right and left pulmonary artery branches. At first, these findings are subtle (Fig. 3.18A), but eventually the main pulmonary artery and the right and left pulmonary artery branches become more dilated, and indeed aneurysmal (Fig. 3.18B). At this stage, the findings must be differentiated from those of bilateral hilar adenopathy. In extremely longstanding cases, the dilated proximal pulmonary arteries can develop calcifications within their walls (Fig. 3.18C).

Heart Size

Barring variations resulting from shallow inspiratory efforts, an increase in heart size indicates underlying cardiac disease. On the other hand, a normal cardiac silhouette does not necessarily exclude underlying pathology. A truly small heart (microcardia) is probably not seen with congenital heart disease and is, for the most part, acquired. In my estimation, cardiothoracic ratio measurements are of little value; there is no substitute for experience, and with experience, even minimal degrees of cardiac enlargement can be detected by inspection alone.

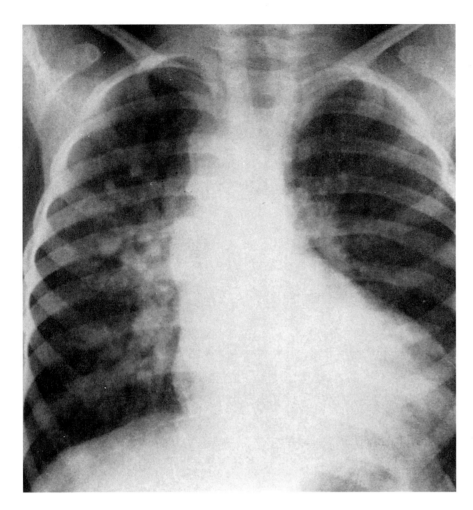

FIGURE 3.17. Unequal pulmonary vascularity. Note marked discrepancy of blood flow between the two lungs. There is much more blood flowing to the right lung. Patient with persistent truncus arteriosus.

SPECIFIC CHAMBER ENLARGEMENT

Generally, cardiac chambers enlarge for one of two reasons: Either they must accept more blood than normal, or they must pump against an obstructive lesion at their outlet. Enlargement resulting from the chamber's acceptance of increased volumes of blood occurs with left-to-right shunts, intracardiac mixing lesions, anomalous drainage of pulmonary veins to the right side of the heart, and insufficient valves. Obstruction to the outflow of blood from a cardiac chamber results from atresia or stenosis of the output valve, subvalvular obstructing lesions of the ventricle such as diaphragms or muscular hyperplasia, and stenosing lesions of the aorta or pulmonary artery distal to their valves. In addition, it should be recalled that, with obstruction to the flow of blood from a cardiac chamber, the atria and ventricles behave differently. Generally, the atria dilate and enlarge soon and rapidly, while ventricles, because they are pumping chambers, respond to obstruction with hypertro-

phy rather than with dilatation. This is important, for overall when ventricular hypertrophy is present, cardiomegaly is not pronounced, and thus as long as hypertrophy is the dominant or sole problem, cardiomegaly is subtle. However, when the involved ventricle decompensates and dilates, radiographic evidence of cardiomegaly becomes more visible (see Fig. 3.13).

Right Atrium

Roentgenographically, right atrial enlargement often is difficult to assess, since mild enlargement is not always clearly apparent. On the other hand, when the right atrium is markedly enlarged, there is no real problem. In this regard, the most useful information is available on the **posteroanterior view.** On this view, moderate to marked right atrial enlargement produces bulging or prominence of the right cardiac border extending high into the region of the right pulmonary artery (Fig. 3.19).

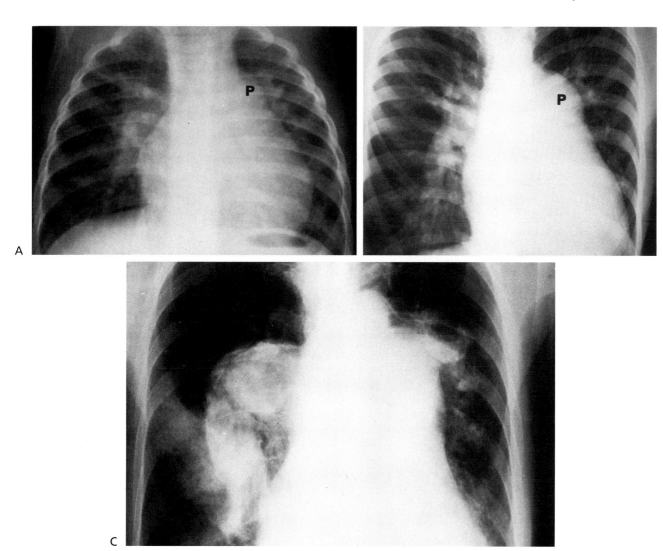

FIGURE 3.18. Pulmonary hypertension. A. Note cardiomegaly with a prominent main pulmonary artery (P) and left and right pulmonary artery branches. **B.** More advanced changes with a much more prominent and enlarged pulmonary artery (P) and central pulmonary artery branches. In contrast, the peripheral pulmonary artery branches show an abrupt diminution in caliber. **C.** Adult with pulmonary hypertension and calcified pulmonary arteries. In this patient with an atrial septal defect, the aneurysmally dilated main pulmonary artery and its branches have calcified.

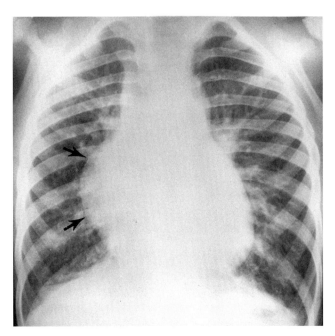

FIGURE 3.19. Right atrial enlargement: posteroanterior view. There is marked bulging of the lower half of the right cardiac border (arrows) extending high into the right hilar region.

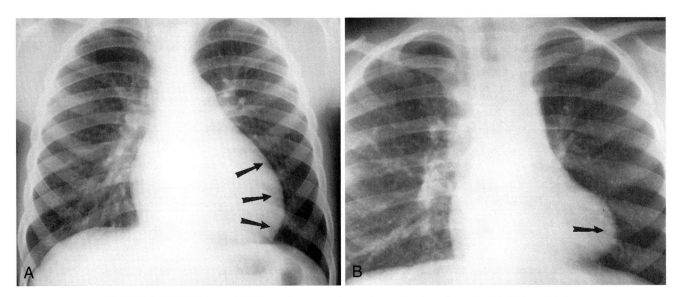

FIGURE 3.20. Right ventricular enlargement: posteroanterior view. A. Dilatation. Note marked bulging of the left cardiac border and lateral displacement of the cardiac apex (arrows). There is slight straightening of the left cardiac border. Atrial septal defect. **B. Hypertrophy.** Note pronounced elevation of cardiac apex (arrow) and lack of cardiac enlargement. Tetralogy of Fallot.

Right Ventricle

The roentgenographic assessment of right ventricular enlargement **on the posteroanterior view** depends on the fact that as the right ventricle dilates, a clockwise rotation of the heart ensues. This results in upward displacement and lateral pointing of the roentgenographic cardiac apex and slight straightening of the left cardiac border (Fig. 3.20A). With right ventricular hypertrophy, enlargement is less pronounced, but apical uptilting and lateral pointing are more pronounced (Fig. 3.20B). The picture is quite different from that seen with right ventricular dilatation.

Left Atrium

Left atrial enlargement on frontal view is not as clearly manifest in infants and children with congenital heart disease as it is in older children and adults with acquired disease such as mitral stenosis. However, in some instances, enlargement of the left atrium can be seen on frontal view as a double density through the right side of the cardiac silhouette (Fig. 3.21A). This density should not be confused with a similar double density frequently seen in normal young infants and children (see Fig. 3.1A). The latter density represents the edge of the normal left atrium and is located higher than when true left atrial enlargement is present. In addition, as opposed to adults with left atrial enlargement, widening of the carina is not easy to see in infants. Indeed, it actually does not occur very often. Another manifestation of left atrial enlargement is seen on lateral views of the chest and consists of posterior displacement of the left main bronchus (Fig. 3.21B).

Left Ventricle

Enlargement (dilatation) of the left ventricle can be appreciated on the posteroanterior view, and added information may be available on the lateral view. On the **posteroanterior view,** as the left ventricle dilates, a counterclockwise rotation of the heart occurs. This rotation, directly opposite that which occurs with right ventricular dilatation, produces downward displacement and pointing of the roentgenographic cardiac apex. In addition, there is slight accentuation of the normal concavity of the left cardiac border. As a result, the cardiac silhouette has a "droopy" or "saggy" appearance (Fig. 3.22A). The lateral view is useful only in assessment of marked left ventricular enlargement (dilatation). In these cases, bulging of the inferior portion of the posterior cardiac silhouette is seen (Fig. 3.22B).

Changes associated with left ventricular hypertrophy are more subtle, and the detection of even marked hypertrophy is often elusive. Hypertrophy of the left ventricle produces increased, but not marked, enlargement of the heart. Rather, it produces relatively subtle "roundness" or "bulging" of the left cardiac border (Fig. 3.22C). This "well-rounded" or "firm" appearance of the left cardiac border is different from the "sagging" or "drooping" cardiac configuration produced by left ventricular dilatation. In fact, it more resembles right or biventricular dilatation.

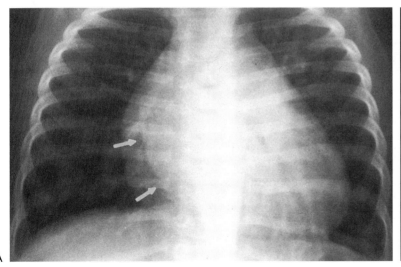 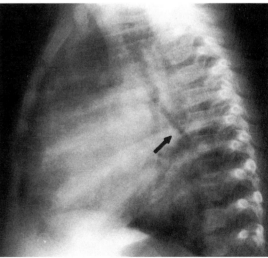

A ‎ B

FIGURE 3.21. Left atrial enlargement. A. In this patient with a large ventricular septal defect and biventricular enlargement, note the enlarged left atrium presenting as a double silhouette (arrows) through the right side of the heart. **B.** Left atrial enlargement: lateral view. Note characteristic posterior displacement of the left main bronchus (arrow) by an enlarged left atrium.

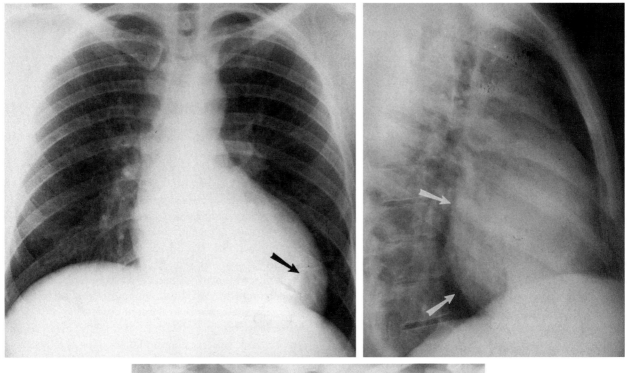

A

B

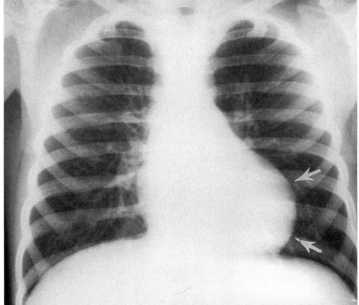

C

FIGURE 3.22. Left ventricular enlargement. A. Left ventricular dilatation: posteroanterior view. Note the pronounced "drooping" or "sagging" of the cardiac apex (arrow) and increased concavity of the left cardiac border. Also note the enlarged aorta in this patient with aortic insufficiency. **B. Lateral view.** There is posterior bulging of the lower half of the cardiac silhouette (arrows). Aortic insufficiency. **C. Left ventricular hypertrophy: posteroanterior view.** Note the well-rounded or firm appearance of the left cardiac border (arrows).

ANCILLARY FINDINGS

Rib Notching

Bilateral rib notching is a valuable ancillary finding in the diagnosis of coarctation of the aorta. Unilateral rib notching can be seen in patients on whom a Blalock-Taussig anastomotic procedure has been performed and, occasionally, in patients with thoracotomies performed early in life for right outflow track-obstructing lesions. In such patients, it is believed that subsequent pleural adhesions facilitate the development of intercostal artery-to-pulmonary artery collateral communications. In time, these dilated intercostal arteries cause rib notching.

Bone Changes

In congenital heart disease, some bone changes are congenital, while others are acquired. Perhaps the best-known congenital abnormality seen in congenital heart disease is hypoplasia of the upper extremity, specifically of the radius and thumb. This is the characteristic bony abnormality seen in the Holt-Oram syndrome, a syndrome in which congenital heart disease, such as atrial or ventricular septal defect

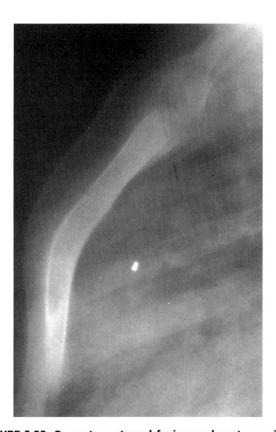

FIGURE 3.23. Premature sternal fusion and pectus carinatum. Note the bulging sternum in this patient with cyanotic heart disease and cardiomegaly. The anterior bulging results in a pectus carinatum deformity. Also note that almost all of the sternal segments have fused prematurely.

or pulmonary stenosis, is associated with radial ray hypoplasia.

Premature sternal fusion, with associated pectus carinatum (pigeon breast) deformity, is a relatively common bony abnormality seen in congenital heart disease (Fig. 3.23). The abnormality most often is seen with severe cyanotic heart disease, which results in marked cardiomegaly. In many of these cases, the sternum is shorter than normal, and perhaps more than premature sternal fusion, the sternum shows diminished segmentation. Scoliosis of the spine also is a commonly associated bony abnormality with congenital heart disease.

Bone changes resulting from the polycythemia associated with cyanotic heart disease include pulmonary osteoarthropathy and medullary cavity changes reflecting bone marrow hypertrophy. Bone marrow hypertrophy involves the erythroid elements primarily and can lead to thickening and spiculation of the diploë of the skull, widening of the medullary bone space, and trabecular atrophy in the long bones. In very extensive cases, the changes can mimic those of Cooley's anemia.

Intracardiac, Vascular, and Valvular Calcifications

In congenital heart disease, intracardiac, vascular, and valvular calcifications are relatively rare. However, they occasionally are encountered in the older patient with aortic stenosis, coarctation of the aorta (1), patent ductus arteriosus (2), and pulmonary stenosis (3). In addition, patients with longstanding pulmonary hypertension, usually associated with atrial septal defects, eventually can develop calcification within the dilated pulmonary arteries. In some of these patients, findings can be striking and are quite pathognomonic (see Fig. 3.18C).

AERATION DISTURBANCES

Focal Disturbances

Focal aeration disturbances in patients with congenital heart lesions usually result from the compressive effects of abnormally enlarged arteries, veins, or cardiac chambers. Overall, one can see either focal hyperinflation (obstructive emphysema) or focal hypoinflation (atelectasis). Left lower lobe atelectasis (Fig. 3.24) commonly is seen in those lesions producing marked enlargement of the left side of the heart, and for the most part, these lesions include ventricular septal defect, patent ductus arteriosus, and left-side cardiomyopathy such as endocardial fibroelastosis.

Generalized Overaeration

Generalized overaeration is a common phenomenon in children with congenital heart lesions. It can occur with

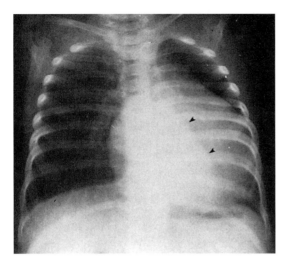

FIGURE 3.24. Left lower lobe atelectasis with left-side enlargement. Note the characteristic triangular configuration of the collapsed left lower lobe (arrowheads) seen behind the enlarged heart. This patient had endocardial fibroelastosis with marked left ventricular dilatation.

both increased pulmonary blood flow (4) and decreased pulmonary blood flow. In either case, overaeration is a reflection of compensatory overbreathing and, as such, represents a normal homeostatic response to decreased oxygen levels in the blood. In many of these cases, overaeration is profound (Fig. 3.25). In left-to-right shunts, the distended pulmonary arteries and veins lead to stiffness or decreased compliance of the lungs, and the lungs tend not to deflate as easily.

REFERENCES

Basic Pulmonary Vascular Problems
1. Flynn PJ, Kattus AA. Coarctation of aorta with proximal aortic dilatation and calcific atheromatous degeneration corrected by endarterectomy. J Thorac Cardiovasc Surg 1959;38:369–373.
2. Pochaczevsky R, Dunst ME. Coexistent pulmonary artery and aortic arch calcification; its significance and association with patent ductus arteriosus. AJR 1972;116:141–145.
3. Dinsmore RE, Sanders CA, Harthorne JW, et al. Calcification of congenitally stenotic pulmonary valve. Radiology 1966;87:429–436.
4. Markowitz RI, Johnson KM, Weinstein EM. Hyperinflation of the lungs in infants with large left-to-right shunts. Invest Radiol 1988; 23:354–358.

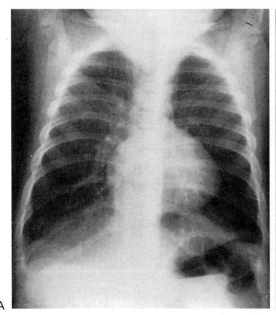
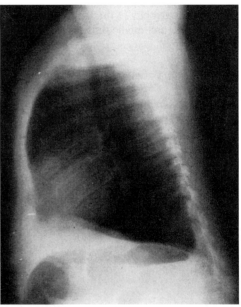

A   B

FIGURE 3.25. Generalized overaeration with congenital heart disease. A. Note the marked degree of overaeration of both lungs in this patient with an endocardial cushion defect and pulmonary atresia. **B.** Lateral view demonstrates findings virtually indistinguishable from those seen with obstructive emphysema. Such overaeration is common in patients with congenital heart lesions in whom oxygenation is impaired. In cases where vascularity is decreased, overaeration is secondary to compensatory overbreathing as a result of hypoxia. Overaeration also can be seen with underlying left-to-right shunts where the increased blood flow through the lungs splints them and reduces pulmonary compliance. The lungs tend to be stiff and do not collapse easily.

THE LEFT-TO-RIGHT SHUNTS

The left-to-right shunts include atrial septal defect, patent ductus arteriosus, aortopulmonary window, rupture of a sinus of Valsalva, partial anomalous pulmonary venous return, and coronary artery fistula (Table 3.1). All of these lesions have in common a large pulmonary artery with increased pulmonary blood flow leading to prominence of the pulmonary artery branches. Specific chamber enlargement depends on the site of the shunt. If the shunt occurs at the level of the great vessels (i.e., patent ductus arteriosus), a pure left-side (left ventricle and left atrium) pattern of enlargement results. If it occurs at the ventricular level, depending on the size of the shunt, there will be either predominant left-side enlargement or bilateral ventricular enlargement. The latter tends to occur with larger shunts, for shunting occurs both during systole and during diastole. If the defect is located at the atrial level, the right atrium and right ventricle undergo enlargement, and the left side of the heart is not involved in the resultant abnormal hemodynamics. In all cases of left-to-right shunt, however, if the shunt is not corrected in time, pulmonary hypertension develops.

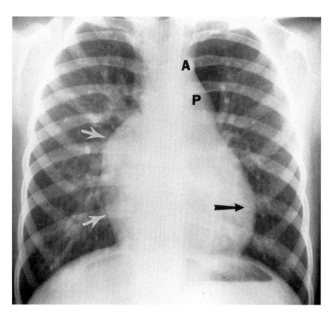

FIGURE 3.26. Atrial septal defect: posteroanterior view. Note the prominent right atrium (arrows), increased pulmonary vascularity, and large pulmonary artery (PA). The aorta (A) is diminutive. The right ventricle is slightly dilated, and the cardiac apex points laterally (arrow).

Atrial Septal Defect

Atrial septal defect occurs in two forms: primum and secundum defects. The secundum defect results from the absence of, or a defect in, the flap of tissue derived from the septum primum, which covers and closes the foramen ovale. The resulting shunt leads to the delivery of increased volumes of blood to the right atrium, during both systole and diastole. This causes volume overloading and enlargement of the right atrium and subsequently the right ventricle (Fig. 3.26). Thereafter, there is enlargement of the pulmonary artery and engorgement of the pulmonary vasculature. The aorta is small in atrial septal defect, because the left-to-right

shunt occurs below the level of the great vessels. This leads to left-to-right shunting of blood before it is delivered to the aorta. As a result, less than normal volumes of blood are handled by the aorta, and it becomes smaller than normal. Angiocardiography is not usually necessary for the diagnosis of a secundum atrial septal defect. However, with the angled four-chamber view, atrial septal defects usually are demonstrable after injection of contrast material into the right superior pulmonary vein (Fig. 3.27A). Atrial septal defects most often now are diagnosed with ultrasound, and in the usual case, no further imaging is required prior to surgery.

Ostium primum defects are low defects resulting from maldevelopment of the primitive endocardial cushions. Both the intraatrial and the intraventricular septa are defective, resulting in a low atrial septal defect (Fig. 3.27B) and a high ventricular septal defect. Associated is a cleft, deformed mitral valve, and mitral regurgitation. Depending on the particular combination of these abnormalities, a wide spectrum of abnormalities is seen, but generally the entire complex of abnormalities is classified either as partial or as complete. The partial form has (a) two discrete atrioventricular valves; (b) a low ostium primum atrial septal defect; (c) an abnormal, often insufficient mitral valve with a cleft in the anterior leaflet; and (d) a ventricular septal defect of variable size and hemodynamic significance. A cleft in the tricuspid valve also may be present.

The complete form of the endocardial cushion defect complex has a common atrioventricular valve, usually with five leaflets. This results from contiguous clefting of the

TABLE 3.1. INCREASED PULMONARY VASCULARITY WITHOUT CYANOSIS

Active congestion (left-to-right shunts)
  ASD (except AV communis)
  VSD
  Left ventricle-to-right atrium shunt
  PDA
  Miscellaneous
    AP window
    Ruptured aortic sinus aneurysm
    Coronary artery fistula
    Partial anomalous pulmonary venous return
Passive congestion (failing heart with left-side obstructing or
  myocardial dysfunction lesions)[a]

ASD, atrial septal defect; AV, aortic valve; VSD, ventricular septal defect; PDA, patent ductus arteriosus; AP, aortopulmonary.
[a]See Table 3.4.

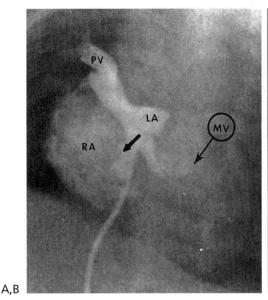
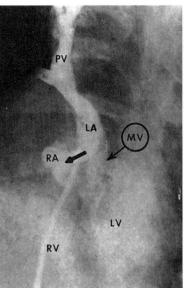

A,B

FIGURE 3.27. Atrial septal defect: angiocardiographic findings. A. Angled four-chamber view demonstrates contrast passing from the left atrium (LA) to the right atrium (RA) through the intraatrial septal defect (arrow). This is a low secundum defect. MV, region of mitral valve; PV, pulmonary vein. B. View of another patient demonstrates a low primum defect (arrow). LA, left atrium; LV, left ventricle; MV, region of mitral valve; PV, pulmonary vein; RA, right atrium; RV, right ventricle.

atrioventricular valves. There also is juxtapositioning of low atrial and high ventricular septal defects, and as a result, a large common communication involving all four cardiac chambers is created. For this reason, patients with the full-blown complex of abnormalities show considerable cardiomegaly. Cardiomegaly usually is oval, with a prominent right atrium (Fig. 3.28).

Angiocardiographically, in the complete defect, left ventricular injections in the posteroanterior projection lead to characteristic findings. During diastole, there is deep excursion of the abnormal anterior mitral valve leaflet into the left ventricle, resulting in apparent elongation of the left

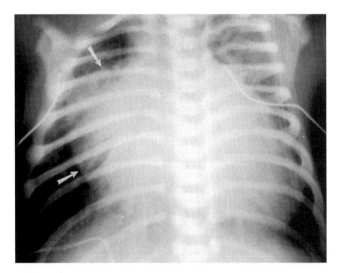

FIGURE 3.28. **Atrioventricular** communis. Note marked right atrial (arrows) and right ventricular enlargement. The heart is oval shaped, and the vascularity is increased. Some failure is present.

ventricular outflow tract and the so-called "gooseneck" deformity (Fig. 3.29). In systole, the deformed mitral valve may appear bilobed, irregular, or scalloped (Fig. 3.29). Left-to-right atrial shunting, after regurgitation of contrast material into the left atrium, also is seen (Fig. 3.29C). MRI also can vividly demonstrate the findings (Fig. 3.30).

Ventricular Septal Defect

Ventricular septal defect is a very common congenital heart abnormality and is found either in isolated form or in association with other abnormalities. The remarks in this section pertain to the isolated defect: either membranous (high) or muscular (low). The natural history for small to medium membranous, but not muscular, defects is spontaneous closure, a phenomenon different from that seen with atrial septal defects.

The hemodynamics and resultant pattern of chamber enlargement in ventricular septal defect depend on the size of the defect. In all cases, however, the excessive blood flow through the lungs leads to active pulmonary vascular engorgement and increased pulmonary venous return to the left side of the heart. Consequently, there is diastolic (volume) overloading and enlargement of the left atrium and left ventricle (Fig. 3.31A). With larger defects, however, there is ready decompression of blood from the left to the right ventricle during both systole and diastole, and as a result, both chambers enlarge. This leads to a pattern of biventricular dilatation or enlargement (Fig. 3.31B). This does not occur with small defects for there is very little shunting during diastole. In addition, of course, because of the increased pulmonary blood flow in these individuals, pulmonary vascular disease with pulmonary hypertension is a frequent and early complication.

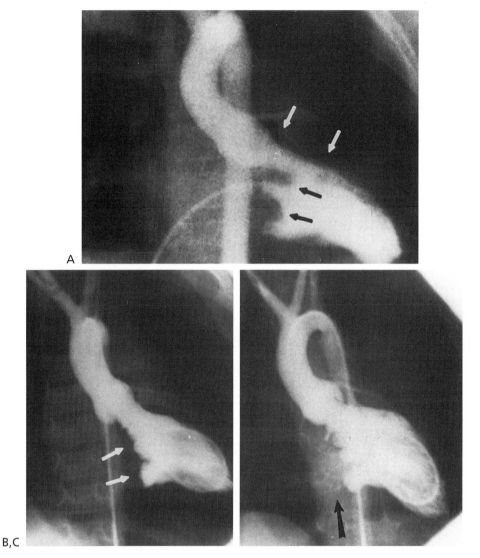

A

B,C

FIGURE 3.29. Endocardial cushion defect: angiographic findings. A. Note typical elongated outflow tract (white arrows), leading to the gooseneck deformity. Also note the bilobed appearance of the deformed mitral valve (black arrows). **B.** Similar view in another patient demonstrates a typical deformed mitral valve (arrows). **C.** Later, in early systole, initial mitral regurgitation (arrow) is seen.

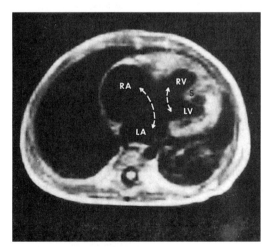

FIGURE 3.30. Magnetic resonance imaging of atrioventricular canal: transaxial view. Note the large high ventricular septal defect and low atrial septal defect (arrows) communicating, respectively, between the right (RV) and left (LV) ventricles and the right (RA) and left (LA) atria. Also note the intraventricular septum (S). (Courtesy of R. M. Peshock, M.D.).

Left atrial enlargement in ventricular septal defect, although occasionally seen on frontal view (see Fig. 3.1B), most often is best seen on the lateral chest film. On this view, one looks for displacement of the left main bronchus posteriorly (Fig. 3.31C). In addition to these findings, the aorta is small, for much as in atrial septal defect, shunting occurs below the great vessel level. As a result, blood is shunted away from the systemic circulation before it reaches the aorta, and the aorta is reactively small. In addition, because of the increased high-pressure pulmonary blood flow in these individuals, pulmonary vascular disease with pulmonary hypertension is a frequent and early complication.

Angiocardiographically, ventricular septal defects are best demonstrated on the left anterooblique view, with injection into the left ventricle. Most often, the catheter is passed from the right side of the heart, through the foramen

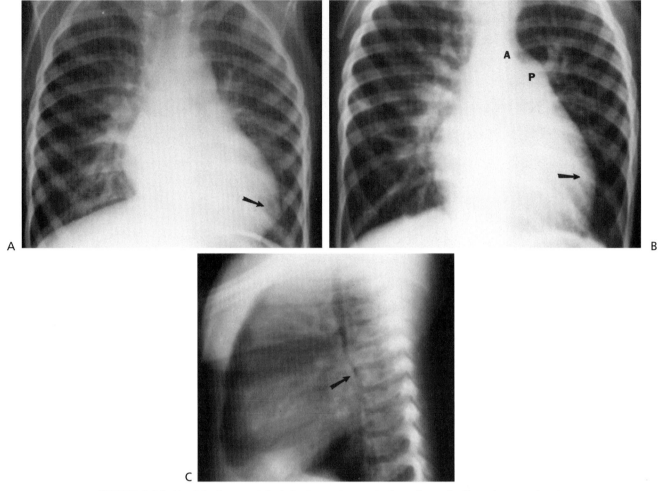

FIGURE 3.31. Ventricular septal defect: posteroanterior view. A. Note increased pulmonary vascularity and moderate cardiomegaly. Left ventricular dilatation produces "dipping" or "sagging" of the roentgenographic apex, which points downward (arrow). The enlarged pulmonary artery is hidden in the superior mediastinum by normal thymic tissue. **B.** Biventricular enlargement with a large shunt. The apex (arrow) points laterally. The heart is more oval in shape. The pulmonary artery (P) is large, but the aorta (A) is small. **C.** Lateral view. Note that the heart is enlarged and that the left main bronchus is posteriorly displaced (arrow).

ovale, into the left atrium, and then down into the left ventricle (Fig. 3.32, A–C). MRI also can demonstrate ventricular septal defects (Fig. 3.32, D and E) but, in general, has not replaced angiocardiography and ultrasonography.

Patent Ductus Arteriosus

When the ductus arteriosus fails to close, a communication between the great vessels persists, and while this communication is essential in the fetus, its persistence after birth results in a left-to-right shunt. The shunt functions in both systole and diastole, and the resultant extra blood volume circulated through the lungs is returned to the left atrium and then the left ventricle, causing these chambers to

enlarge (Fig. 3.33). The right side of the heart is totally excluded from the hemodynamics of uncomplicated patent ductus arteriosus, and the aorta, as opposed to being small as in atrial and ventricular septal defects, is normal in size or enlarged. The reason for this is that in patent ductus arteriosis, the shunt occurs at the great vessel level. Longstanding shunts lead to pulmonary hypertension, but as opposed to atrial and ventricular septal defects, both the pulmonary artery and the aorta enlarge in patent ductus arteriosus.

Patent ductus arteriosus also is a common problem in the premature infant. Ordinarily in the full-term infant, the originally patent ductus arteriosus closes within a few hours or days after birth. However, in the premature infant, where hypoxic pulmonary disease is commonplace,

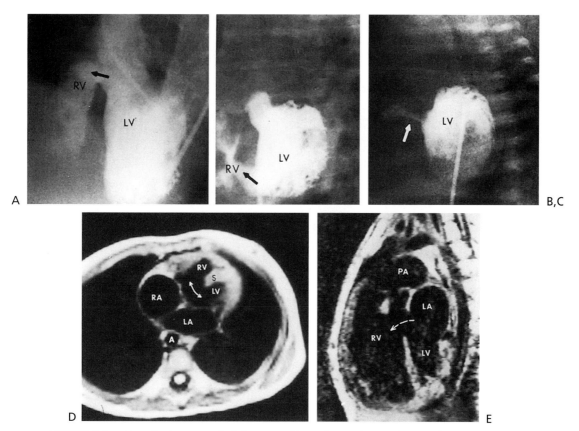

FIGURE 3.32. Ventricular septal defect: cardioangiographic and magnetic resonance findings. A. Large high ventricular septal defect in the membranous septum (arrow). LV, left ventricle; RV, right ventricle. **B.** Large low defect in the muscular septum (arrow). LV, left ventricle; RV, right ventricle. **C.** Small muscular defect (arrow) from the left ventricle (LV) to the right ventricle. **D.** Magnetic resonance image, axial view, demonstrating a large ventricular septal defect (arrow). S, interventricular septum; LA, left atrium; LV, left ventricle; RA, right atrium; RV, right ventricle; A, aorta. **E.** Parasagittal view of another patient with a high ventricular septal defect (arrow) in the interventricular septum. LV, left ventricle; RV, right ventricle; LA, left atrium; PA, pulmonary artery. (**D** courtesy of R. M. Peshock, M.D.).

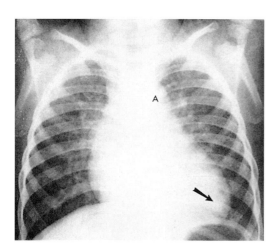

FIGURE 3.33. Patent ductus arteriosus: posteroanterior view. The pulmonary vascularity is engorged. There is cardiomegaly, and the roentgenographic cardiac apex shows pronounced downward dipping (arrow) resulting from left ventricular dilatation. Also note the enlarged aortic knob (A).

the ductus, being very sensitive to hypoxia, remains open. This is important, for the premature infant does not have the luxury of the presence of physiologic pulmonary hypertension as exists in the full-term infant. For this reason, pulmonary pressures in the pulmonary vascular bed remain lower than those in the systemic circulation, and left-to-right shunting occurs. This leads to cardiac failure, cardiac enlargement, and passive pulmonary vascular congestion (Fig. 3.34).

Angiocardiographically, patent ductus arteriosus is readily demonstrable with injection into the aorta, just around the level of the ductus. The ductus usually is best visualized in the left anterooblique and lateral positions (Fig. 3.35). Patency of the ductus arteriosus also can be documented with ultrasound and commonly is detected in this manner. Coil occlusion (1) of the ductus is now commonly accomplished.

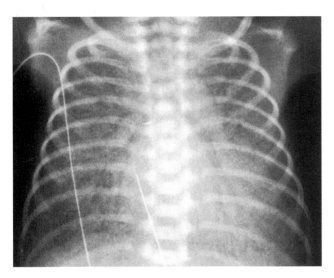

FIGURE 3.34. Patent ductus arteriosus in premature infants. Note nonspecific cardiomegaly and extensive pulmonary edema secondary to passive congestion.

Left Ventricular-to-Right Atrial Shunt

A left ventricular-to-right atrial shunt is a rare congenital heart anomaly resulting from a communication between the left ventricle and the right atrium. The defect involves either the tricuspid valve annulus or the right atrium just above it. In the first type, the septal leaflet of the tricuspid valve usually is cleft, and the valve itself frequently is insufficient. The radiographic findings usually resemble those of an atrial, rather than a ventricular septal defect.

Aortopulmonary Window

Hemodynamically and roentgenographically, aortopulmonary window manifests much the same as patent ductus

arteriosus. It is much rarer, however, and the specific anomaly consists of a communication between the pulmonary artery and the aorta, just above their valves. The lesion results from a failure of complete septation of the primitive truncus arteriosus. Roentgenographically, left ventricular and left atrial enlargement, pulmonary artery dilatation, increased pulmonary vascularity, and a prominent aorta are seen. Cardioangiographically, the window is best visualized on left anterooblique or lateral views.

Ruptured Aneurysm of Sinus of Valsalva

A ruptured aneurysm of the sinus of Valsalva is a relatively uncommon condition that results from a deficiency in the supporting structure of the aortic valve cusps. The result is aneurysmal bulging of the aortic sinuses and, in some cases, rupture of these structures. Most often, it is the right (anterior) aortic sinus that is affected, and rupture is into the outflow tract of the right ventricle.

Roentgenographically, the findings consist of pulmonary vascular congestion, dilatation of the pulmonary artery, and right ventricular enlargement. Angiographically, abnormal bulging of the involved aortic sinus is seen, and when a shunt occurs, contrast material is seen to be shunted to the right ventricle from the aorta.

Coronary Artery Fistula

In coronary artery fistula, the most common anatomic arrangement consists of one of the coronary arteries communicating with a cardiac chamber or pulmonary artery. In this regard, the right coronary artery is affected most often, and the communication most commonly is to the right ventricle, right atrium, coronary sinus, or pulmonary artery. In any of these cases, since there is a communication between the coronary artery (systemic circulation) and a right-side cardiac chamber or great vessel, a left-to-right

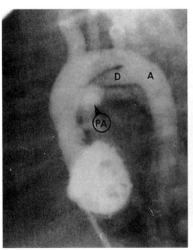
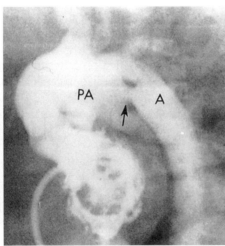

A,B

FIGURE 3.35. Patent ductus arteriosus: cardioangiographic findings. A. Note the moderately long ductus (D) between the descending aorta (A) and the pulmonary artery (PA). **B.** View of another patient with a short ductus (arrow). Note the aorta (A) and large, dilated pulmonary artery (PA).

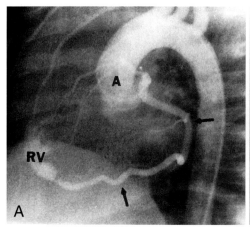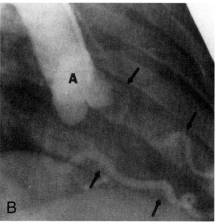

FIGURE 3.36. Coronary artery fistula. A. The left coronary artery (arrows) is dilated and communicates with the right ventricle (RV). A, aorta. **B.** View of the same patient demonstrates that both right and left coronary arteries (arrows) are involved and dilated. A, aorta.

shunt results. Aberrant left coronary artery is another form of coronary artery fistula. In these cases, the left coronary artery arises from the pulmonary artery and fills retrogradely from the right coronary artery.

Roentgenographically, in coronary artery fistula, the shunt produces pulmonary vascular engorgement and pulmonary artery dilatation. The chambers receiving blood from the coronary vessel show specific enlargement; thus, if the right ventricle is affected, it alone enlarges, while if the right atrium is affected, both the right atrium and the right ventricle enlarge. A definitive diagnosis usually is accomplished with angiocardiography (Fig. 3.36), but ultrasonography also can detect the lesion.

Partial Anomalous Pulmonary Venous Return

Partial anomalous pulmonary venous return occurs in isolated form or more often in association with atrial septal defect. The clinical and roentgenographic findings are virtually indistinguishable from those of isolated atrial septal defect, and in most circumstances, the anomaly is discovered during ultrasonography or cardiac catheterization.

REFERENCE

1. Rothman A, Lucas VW, Sklansky MS, et al. Percutaneous coil occlusion of patent ductus arteriosis. J Pediatr 1997;130:447–454.

INTRA- AND EXTRACARDIAC MIXING LESIONS WITH CYANOSIS

Intra- and extracardiac mixing lesions with cyanosis (Table 3.2) include total anomalous pulmonary venous return, the transposition complexes, persistent truncus arteriosus, and single ventricle. All of these patients demonstrate cyanosis.

Total Anomalous Pulmonary Venous Return

Embryologically, total anomalous pulmonary venous return results from the persistent connection of the pulmonary veins to the right side of the heart, that is, the right atrium, coronary sinus, or systemic vein. Normally, of course, they would empty into the left atrium, but in total anomalous pulmonary venous return, because of abnormal development of the common pulmonary vein, the pulmonary veins unite to form a single vessel posterior to the heart, which then joins the right-side circulation. Because of the variable site of insertion of the pulmonary veins into the right heart, some categorization is required, and the classification originally proposed by Darling et al. (1) is the one most often referred to. These authors grouped the lesions into four types. In the type I (50–55%) and type II (30%) lesions,

TABLE 3.2. INCREASED PULMONARY VASCULARITY WITH CYANOSIS

Active congestion
  Total anomalous pulmonary venous return, types I and II
  Persistent truncus arteriosus
  Pseudotruncus arteriosus type I (old truncus type IV), some cases
  Complete endocardial cushion defect (AV communis)
  Transpositions with no pulmonary stenosis
    Complete transposition of the great vessels
    Incomplete transposition (Taussig-Bing anomaly—DORV type II)
    Double-outlet right ventricle (DORV type I)
  Single (common) ventricle with no pulmonary stenosis
  Tricuspid atresia with transposition and no pulmonary stenosis
Passive congestion (pulmonary venous obstruction)
  Total anomalous pulmonary venous return, type III
  Pulmonary vein atresia

AV, aortic valve.

venous return is supradiaphragmatic. These types are the most common. In the type III anomaly, there is infradiaphragmatic insertion of the anomalous pulmonary vein, and the type IV anomaly is a mixture of the first three types (Fig. 3.37). In the type I anomaly, the common pulmonary vein most often joins the so-called "vertical vein" on the left (persistent left superior vena cava) and then the azygos vein on the right. In the type II anomaly, the common pulmonary vein usually drains into the right atrium by way of the coronary sinus. In the type III anomaly, the abnormal vein travels with the esophagus, through the diaphragm, and inserts into a systemic abdominal vein, most frequently the portal vein.

Hemodynamically in the type I and II anomalies, a large "functional" left-to-right shunt is present, for blood is delivered from the lungs to the right atrium, completely bypassing the left atrium. It is then delivered to the right ventricle and exits through the pulmonary artery. As a result, the right atrium and right ventricle enlarge, the pulmonary artery dilates, and the pulmonary vasculature engorges. Thereafter, the blood, on reaching the right atrium, is shunted back to the left atrium through an atrial septal defect or a persistently patent foramen ovale. This is an obligatory, cyanosis-producing, right-to-left shunt and is absolutely necessary for survival. Without it, no blood would reach the left side of the heart, and there would be no perfusion of the systemic circulation. In the type III anomaly, the same functional left-to-right and obligatory right-to-left shunts are present, but marked pulmonary venous obstruction complicates the picture. As a result, the left-to-right shunt is attenuated for it is believed that there is impedance of blood flow through the long, thin anomalous common pulmonary vein inserting into the portal vein.

The presence of the aforementioned pulmonary venous impedence in the type III anomaly drastically reduces pulmonary blood flow, and actually, it is almost obliterated. As a result, right-side pressure overloading and cardiac enlargement are absent, and the problem is shifted to the left side of the circulation; the result is pulmonary venous hypertension and pulmonary edema. Occasionally, this occurs with the other types of total anomalous pulmonary venous return, but most often it is seen with type III. In regard to the former situation, the problem can arise with the type I ("snowman") anomaly, when the vertical vein is compressed

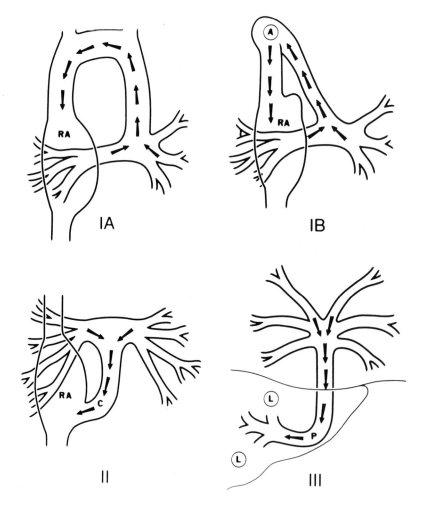

FIGURE 3.37. Total anomalous pulmonary venous return classification. Type I. Drainage into the right atrium (RA) occurs through the supracardiac veins, either the superior vena cava (IA) or the azygos vein (IB). **Type II.** Drainage is to the right atrium (RA) or coronary sinus (C). **Type III.** Drainage occurs infradiaphragmatically into a systemic, most often the portal, vein (P). L, liver. **Type IV.** Type IV anomalies represent a mixture of the preceding types.

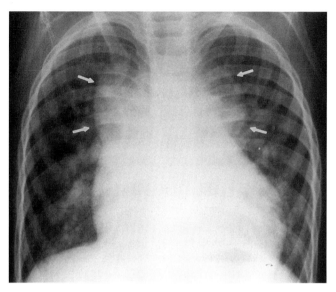

FIGURE 3.38. Total anomalous pulmonary venous return: type I. Frontal view demonstrates the "snowman" or "figure 8" heart. Note right atrial and right ventricular dilatation and enlargement. Superior mediastinal widening (arrows) results from the large inverted U-shaped vein. The pulmonary vascularity is engorged, but the large pulmonary artery is hidden in the superior mediastinal silhouette.

by the pulmonary artery and left bronchus, resulting in a so-called "pulmonary vise syndrome" (2, 3).

Roentgenographically, the changes in total anomalous pulmonary venous return are varied and depend on the specific type of venous connection. The most characteristic and

diagnostic plain film configuration in the type I anomaly group is that of the so-called "snowman" or "figure 8" heart (Fig. 3.38). In this anomaly, the pulmonary veins join to form a common vessel just behind the left atrium. This common vein then joins the vertical vein (persistent left superior vena cava), and this vein then joins the innominate vein, which travels across the mediastinum and empties into the superior vena cava. The resultant connections form an inverted U-shaped vessel (Fig. 3.39). It is this inverted U-shaped vessel that accounts for the upper portion of the snowman.

In young infants, this U-shaped vessel still is small and thus not clearly visible on plain films. Indeed, if one believes that the vessel is visible in a young infant, even with an enlarged heart and increased pulmonary vascularity, one should ask, **"Could I be dealing with a large thymus and some other left-to-right shunt?" The answer to this question almost always will be "Yes" since a large ventricular septal defect with a large thymus gland represents the most common circumstance wherein a snowman heart is erroneously suggested (Fig. 3.40).**

In other patients in the type I group, when the pulmonary veins drain into the azygos vein, localized bulging of the azygos vein can be seen (Fig. 3.41). Angiocardiographically, with retrograde injection into the pulmonary veins, the abnormal anatomy is explicitly delineated (Fig. 3.42).

In the type II anomaly, the abnormal confluent pulmonary veins enter the right atrium or, more usually, the coronary sinus. The cardiac configuration, although abnor-

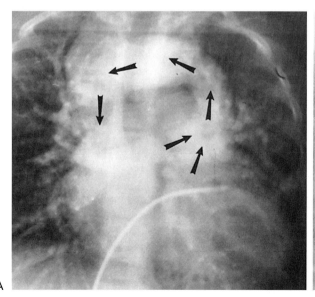 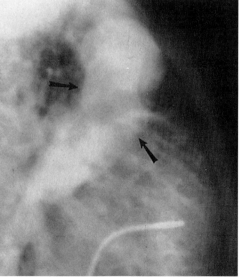

A   B

FIGURE 3.39. Total anomalous pulmonary venous return type I with "snowman" heart: cardioangiogram. A. Frontal view demonstrates that all of the pulmonary veins drain into the inverted U-shaped vessel, which eventually empties into the superior vena cava (arrows). **B.** Lateral view demonstrates the large abnormal vein anterior to the trachea (arrows).

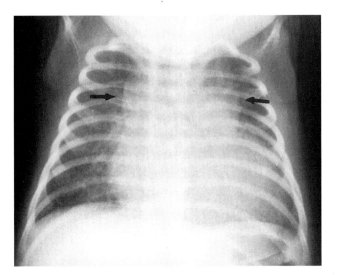

FIGURE 3.40. Large thymus versus "figure 8" or "snowman" heart. The heart is enlarged in this patient because of an underlying ventricular septal defect. However, the large thymus (arrows) gives the cardiac silhouette an overall configuration virtually indistinguishable from the figure 8 or snowman heart of type I total anomalous pulmonary venous return.

mal, is less specific than with the snowman heart. Usually, these patients present with diffuse cardiomegaly with suggestion of right atrial and right ventricular predominance (Fig. 3.43). Angiocardiographically, in the type II anomaly with direct injection into the pulmonary veins, the abnormal drainage pattern is clearly identified (Fig. 3.44).

Roentgenographic findings in the type III anomaly (infradiaphragmatic insertion) are distinctly different from

those in the other types. Because of severe pulmonary venous obstruction, instead of the pulmonary vessels being dilated and engorged (active congestion), only interstitial pulmonary edema (passive congestion) is seen (Fig. 3.45A). Angiocardiographically, the abnormal descending vein is readily identified and most often enters the portal vein (Fig. 3.45D). MRI (Fig. 3.46) and three-dimensional reconstruction CT angiograms also are useful in demonstrating the anatomy of the various forms of total anomalous pulmonary venous return (4, 5). These studies are especially useful in the older patient.

A final interesting feature of total anomalous pulmonary venous return occurs in those patients with the type III anomaly (infradiaphragmatic). Because of the high degree of obstruction, varicosed venous connections to the gastrointestinal tract can result in gastrointestinal hemorrhage (6, 7).

Pulmonary Vein Atresia

Atresia of the pulmonary veins can be unilateral or bilateral. If bilateral, the plain film findings and underlying hemodynamics are virtually indistinguishable from those seen in total anomalous pulmonary venous return type III. This is because there is similar total obstruction to pulmonary venous drainage. Clinically, of course, these patients also are in severe respiratory distress and are very cyanotic. Cyanosis results from right-to-left shunting through an atrial septal defect or persistent foramen ovale. Cardioangiographically, the findings differ from those of patients with total anomalous pulmonary venous return type III in that no abnormal subdiaphragmatic pulmonary vein is seen. The problem, however, is rare.

With unilateral pulmonary vein atresia, symptoms are not as pronounced; in fact, it may take some time before the actual diagnosis is established. This occurs because, while venous drainage to one lung is totally obstructed, circulation through the other lung is normal. When the two lungs are considered together, the resultant hemodynamics and clinical picture are less abnormal than when both lungs have obstructed pulmonary venous return. Roentgenographically (8, 9), the involved lung often is reticulated (chronic interstitial edema), small (Fig. 3.47), and prone to recurrent infections. Clinically, hemoptysis also can be a presenting feature (1).

Persistent Truncus Arteriosus

Persistent truncus arteriosus, a relatively uncommon anomaly, results from failure of division of the common truncus arteriosus into the aorta and pulmonary artery. Consequently, a single vessel drains both ventricles and supplies the systemic, pulmonary, and coronary circulations. Most patients with this anomaly have a high ventricular septal defect. Various attempts to classify persistent truncus arte-

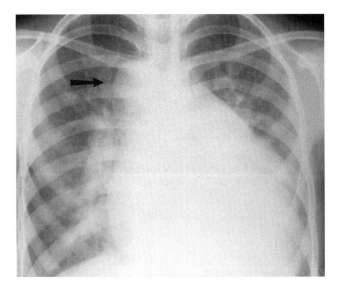

FIGURE 3.41. Total anomalous pulmonary venous return type I: azygos vein. Note marked cardiomegaly, vascular congestion, and the large dilated azygos vein in the right paratracheal region (arrow).

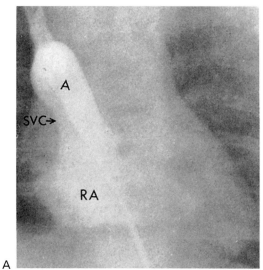

A

FIGURE 3.42. Total anomalous pulmonary venous return type I: azygos vein. A. The catheter is in the azygos vein (A), which drains into the superior vena cava (SVC). RA, right atrium. **B.** The catheter has been advanced into the right lower pulmonary vein (arrows). Note how this vein communicates with the previously delineated azygos vein. **C.** Still another injection demonstrates both right and left lower pulmonary veins (arrows) coming to a confluence just at the catheter tip. They drain into the azygos vein, as delineated in **A.**

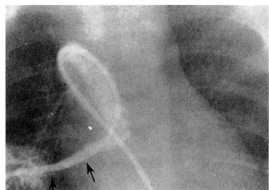

B

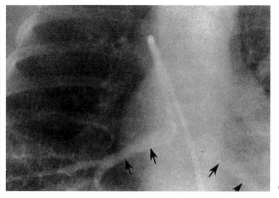

C

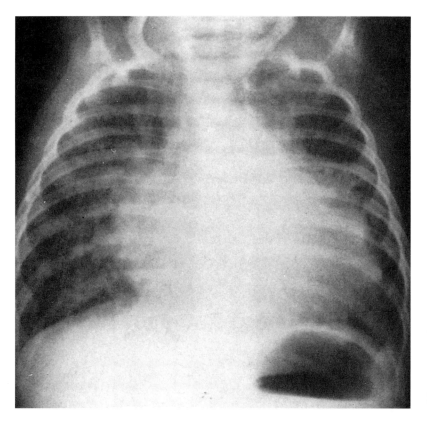

FIGURE 3.43. Total anomalous pulmonary venous return type II: posteroanterior view. Note marked vascular engorgement and cardiomegaly. The large pulmonary artery is hidden in the superior mediastinum. Right atrial enlargement is striking, and lateral displacement of the cardiac apex indicates right ventricular dilatation. The aorta is diminutive.

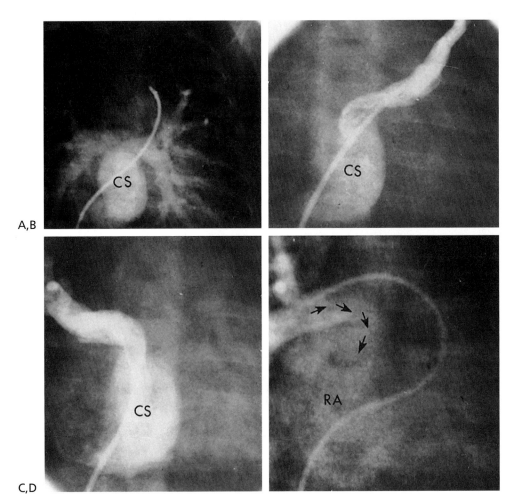

FIGURE 3.44. Total anomalous pulmonary venous return type II: cardioangiogram. A. Note the pulmonary veins draining into the coronary sinus (CS). **B.** View of same patient with selective injection into left superior pulmonary vein draining into the coronary sinus (CS). **C.** This view shows similar findings, after another injection from the right side. CS, coronary sinus. **D.** View of another patient with anomalous pulmonary venous drainage (arrows) into the right atrium (RA).

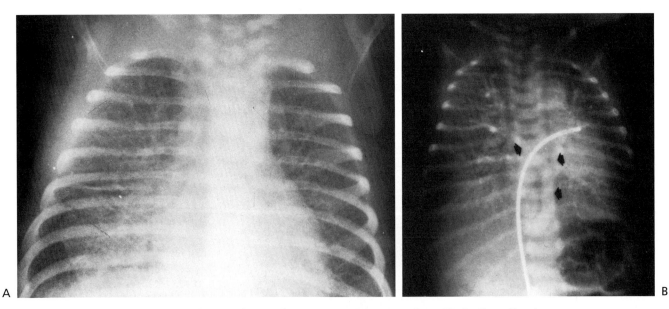

FIGURE 3.45. Total anomalous pulmonary venous return type III. A. Chest film demonstrates typical fine reticular vascularity characteristic of passive congestion resulting in interstitial pulmonary edema. Note the absence of cardiomegaly. **B.** Cardioangiogram demonstrates the anomalous pulmonary vein (arrows) descending below the diaphragm and inserting into the portal vein. (Courtesy of R. I. MacPherson, M.D.).

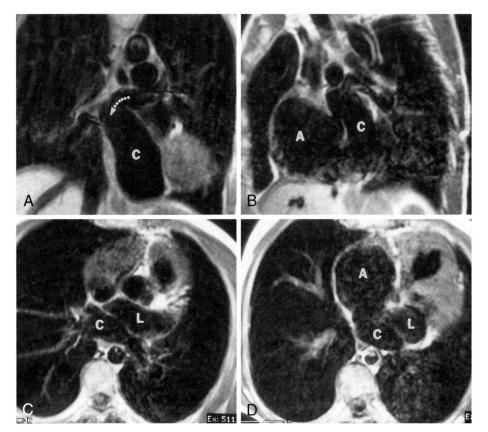

FIGURE 3.46. Type II total anomalous pulmonary venous return: magnetic resonance imaging findings. A. In this adult, note the large coronary sinus (C) and draining into it the left pulmonary vein (arrow). **B.** Left anterooblique view demonstrates the large coronary sinus (C) and large right atrium (A). **C.** Axial view demonstrates the posterior position of the coronary sinus (C) with the pulmonary vein draining toward it. The left atrium (L) is anterior. **D.** A slightly lower slice demonstrates the coronary sinus (C) and large right atrium (A). L, left atrium.

riosus have been suggested, but that of Collett and Edwards (10), based on the site of pulmonary artery origin, is still the one most often referred to. This classification is summarized in Fig. 3.48.

Hemodynamically, in all forms of persistent truncus arteriosus, the truncus drains both ventricles and overrides the interventricular septum. Blood is delivered to the truncus under systemic pressures, and thus, a good portion of the blood is preferentially directed into the lower-pressure pulmonary artery. This creates a systemic-to-pulmonary (left-to-right) shunt, and the pulmonary vascularity engorges. The extra blood is then returned to the left side of

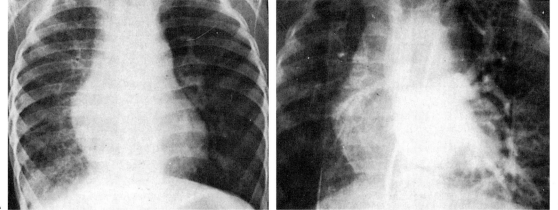

FIGURE 3.47. Unilateral pulmonary vein atresia. A. Note the hazy reticular appearance of the right lung resulting from chronic interstitial pulmonary edema secondary to high-grade pulmonary venous obstruction associated with unilateral right-side pulmonary vein atresia. **B.** Late-phase angiogram shows absence of the right pulmonary veins. The vessels visible in the right lung are thin pulmonary artery branches demonstrating characteristic prolonged opacification.

PERSISTENT TRUNCUS ARTERIOSUS AND RELATED CONDITIONS
Sites of Origin of the Pulmonary Artery or Arteries

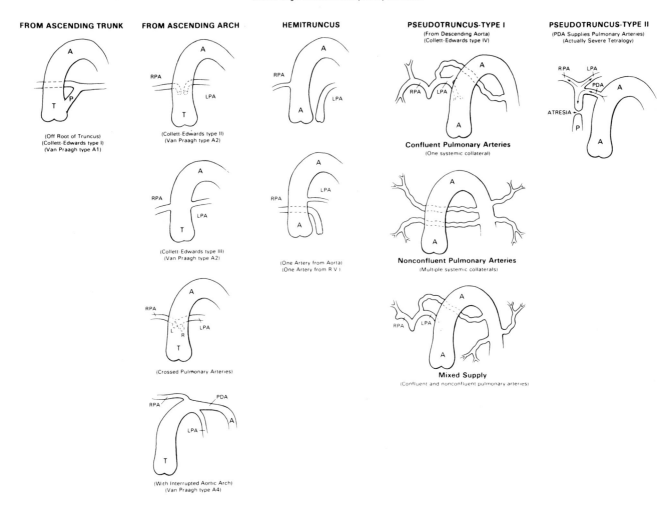

FIGURE 3.48. Persistent truncus arteriosus: classification. These diagrammatic representations include most of the forms of persistent truncus arteriosus. In pseudotruncus arteriosus type I (old truncus arteriosus type IV), pulmonary blood flow is derived through bizarre systemic collaterals. In pseudotruncus arteriosus type II (severe tetralogy of Fallot), pulmonary blood flow is derived primarily through a patent ductus arteriosus. Infants with an associated interrupted aortic arch (type A4) present with findings suggestive of the hypoplastic left heart syndrome. In hemitruncus arteriosus, one of the pulmonary arteries arises from the truncus (aorta), while the other arises from its normal position off the right ventricle. In the latter and, indeed, in all forms of persistent truncus arteriosus, it is not uncommon for one or the other of the pulmonary arteries to be hypoplastic or atretic.

the heart, and both the left atrium and the left ventricle dilate and enlarge. Right ventricular hypertrophy also is present and, in many cases, dominates the picture. It occurs because the right ventricle works against systemic pressures.

Roentgenographically, in most cases of persistent truncus arteriosus, the heart is significantly enlarged, but because of the complexity of the lesion, no chamber predominates and overall the cardiac configuration usually is oval. In addition, in all cases other than in the type I anomaly, the pulmonary artery is misplaced and its site is concave. The aorta (truncus), on the other hand, is enlarged

and frequently right sided (30–35% of cases) (Fig. 3.49). In the type II and III anomalies, the abnormal vessels are readily demonstrated with CT or ordinary angiography (Fig. 3.50) or with MRI (Fig. 3.51).

Type I persistent truncus arteriosus differs from the other types of persistent truncus arteriosus in that the main pulmonary artery arises from a "near"-normal position. Because of this, it is visible on plain films and, indeed, usually is enlarged. In addition, these patients usually demonstrate a different cardiac contour, reflecting considerable left-side chamber preponderance with a definitely down-

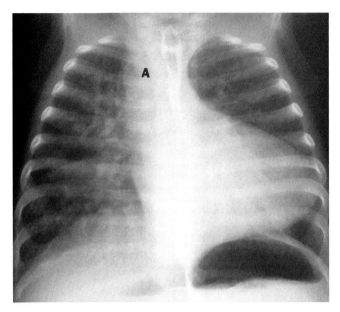

FIGURE 3.49. Persistent truncus arteriosus. Note increased pulmonary vascularity, which in this case is a little more prominent on the right than on the left. The aorta (A) is on the right side and enlarged. The heart is enlarged and oval.

ward-dipping cardiac apex (Fig. 3.52). Angiography and MRI (Fig. 3.53) clearly demonstrate the underlying pathology in these patients.

Classification of the old type IV persistent truncus arteriosus of Collett and Edwards (10) always has been controversial, and over the years, there has been a distinct trend to separate this form of truncus arteriosus from the other forms. Consequently, it now often is identified by the term "pulmonary agenesis or atresia with ventricular septal defect and systemic collaterals." The reason for this is that the type IV anomaly probably does not represent a problem of abnormal septation of the truncus. Rather, it most likely results from pulmonary conal agenesis, and because of this, the pulmonary blood supply is derived from the descending aorta. This is accomplished via collateral vessels that usually are bizarre and tortuous and not at all reminiscent of normal pulmonary arteries, at least in their proximal portions. More distally, they connect with normal-appearing intrapulmonary artery branches, but proximally, they appear bizarre. **However, all of this notwithstanding, the condition still is most commonly referred to as type IV truncus arteriosus.**

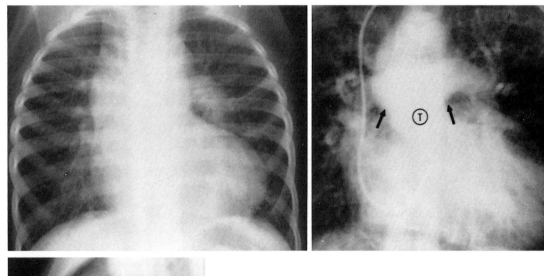

FIGURE 3.50. Persistent truncus arteriosus type II. A. Note pulmonary vascular congestion, concavity of the main pulmonary artery segment, and enlargement and slight elevation of the left main pulmonary artery. The aorta (truncus) is enlarged but, in this case, is on the left. The heart is oval. **B.** Angiogram demonstrates the common origin of the pulmonary arteries (arrows) from the ascending portion of the persistent truncus arteriosus (T). **C.** Lateral view demonstrates the posterior origin of the common pulmonary artery (arrow) from the posterior wall of the ascending truncus (T).

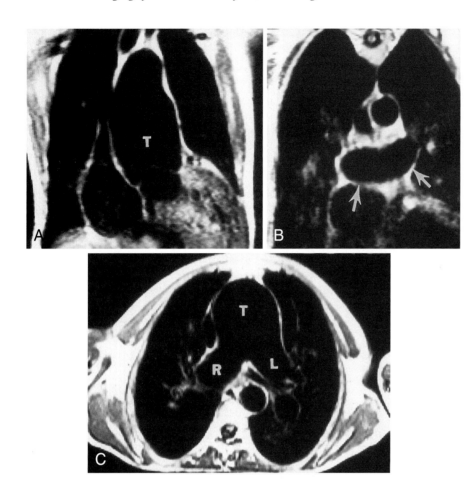

FIGURE 3.51. Truncus type II: magnetic resonance imaging findings. A. Coronal view demonstrating large ascending truncus (T). **B.** Slightly more posterior slice demonstrates the origin of the pulmonary arteries (arrows). **C.** Axial view demonstrates the right (R) and left (L) pulmonary arteries originating from the posterior wall of the truncus (T).

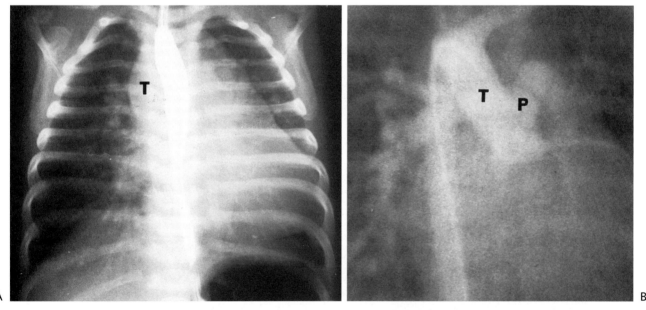

FIGURE 3.52. Persistent truncus arteriosus type I. A. Note cardiomegaly and downward dipping of the roentgenographic cardiac apex, suggesting left ventricular dilatation. The truncus (T) is on the right and enlarged. The pulmonary artery is difficult to identify, but there is an unusual sloping flatness to the upper left cardiac border. **B.** Aortogram demonstrates the right-side truncus (T) and the pulmonary artery trunk (P) arising in the typical type I truncus arteriosus position. Note how the left branch of the pulmonary artery contributes to straightening of the upper left cardiac border.

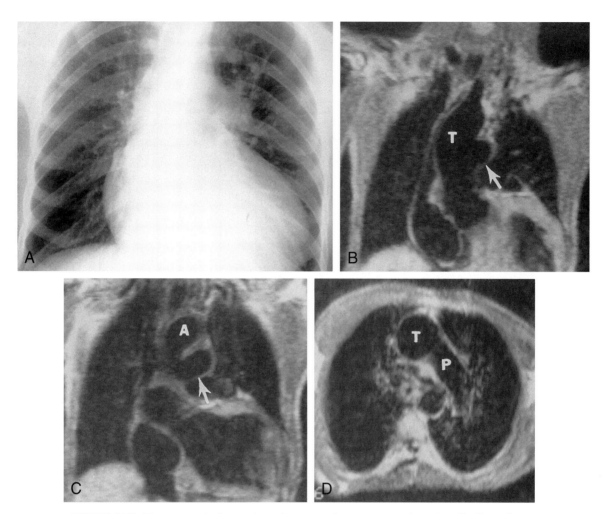

FIGURE 3.53. Truncus arteriosus type I: magnetic resonance imaging findings in an older patient. A. Note oval cardiomegaly, prominent pulmonary vascularity, a prominent aorta, and fullness in the region of the pulmonary artery. **B.** Coronal magnetic resonance image demonstrates the dilated truncus (T) and the pulmonary artery (arrow) as it originates from the base of the truncus. **C.** Slightly more posterior cut demonstrates the truncus forming the aortic arch (A) and the clearly separated pulmonary artery (arrow). **D.** Axial view demonstrates the large dilated truncus (T) and, originating from it, the pulmonary artery (P).

In the past, the collateral vessels in the type IV anomaly usually were referred to as "bronchial artery collaterals," but they are more properly referred to as "primitive, nonspecific, systemic collaterals." Indeed, these bizarre vessels can arise from as high as the brachiocephalic arteries and as low as the infradiaphragmatic portion of the aorta. In addition, they can be large or small, and because of this, the pulmonary vascularity can be markedly engorged (active congestion) or greatly attenuated (diminished vascularity). However, whichever the pattern, it usually is present from birth and does not change. On plain films, in patients with type IV persistent truncus arteriosus, the findings resemble those of tetralogy of Fallot except that there is more cardiac enlargement (Fig. 3.54A).

Final diagnosis in patients with this form of persistent truncus arteriosus usually is accomplished with aortography, and in this regard, a variety of systemic-to-pulmonary artery communications have been demonstrated. Overall, however, these patients have been classified into one of three groups: (a) those with confluent pulmonary arteries, (b) those with nonconfluent pulmonary arteries, and (c) those with a mixed pulmonary artery pattern. Those patients with confluent pulmonary arteries are more amenable to surgical correction by way of a conduit from the right ventricle to the pulmonary artery. The variations of these two basic pulmonary artery configurations are endless (Fig. 3.54, B–D), and in addition, the pulmonary artery on one side or the other commonly is atretic or

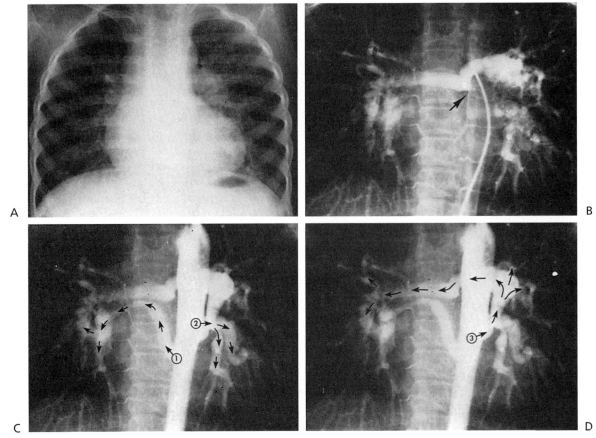

FIGURE 3.54. Pseudotruncus arteriosus type IV: patterns of pulmonary blood flow. A. Note typical oval cardiomegaly and a large, slightly elevated left pulmonary artery. In addition, there is a little more blood flowing to the left lung than to the right. **B.** The main pulmonary artery (arrow) is atretic, and the right and left pulmonary arteries are confluent. These structures have filled in retrograde fashion by way of systemic collaterals as seen in **C** and **D. C.** Earlier-phase aortogram. Route 1: systemic collateral arising from the aorta and supplying the right lower lobe. Route 2: systemic collateral arising from the descending aorta and supplying the left lower lobe. **D.** Same aortogram as in **C.** Route 3: systemic collateral arising from the descending aorta and supplying the left upper lobe and, in retrograde fashion, the confluent pulmonary arteries and the branches to the right upper lobe.

hypoplastic. The findings also are demonstrable with MRI (Fig. 3.55).

The final condition to be discussed under the broad umbrella of persistent truncus arteriosus is the so-called "hemitruncus arteriosus" (Fig. 3.56). In this condition, one of the pulmonary arteries arises from the ascending aorta, while the other arises from the right ventricle in normal fashion. The pulmonary artery arising from the ascending aorta is believed to result from abnormal septation of the primitive truncus, and because of this, the term "hemitruncus arteriosus" has been applied to the condition. Most often, the abnormal pulmonary artery is the right, and thus the condition also is referred to as "right pulmonary artery arising from the ascending aorta." Blood flow to the involved lung may be accentuated or diminished, depend-

ing on whether the systemic communication from the aorta is large or small. Hemodynamically, this anomaly differs from true persistent truncus arteriosus in that there is no misdirection of venous blood into the aorta, and thus no cyanosis.

The Transposition Complexes

The transposition complexes include simple transposition of the great vessels and the double-outlet right ventricle complexes. In addition, congenitally corrected transposition and single ventricle are considered.

There are several approaches to the classification of these abnormalities, but the one summarized in Fig. 3.57 has been helpful for me. It focuses on the relative positions of

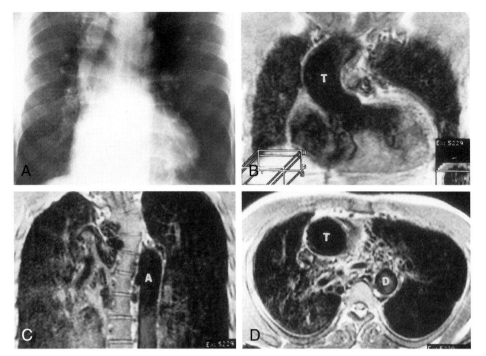

FIGURE 3.55. Persistent truncus arteriosus type IV: magnetic resonance imaging findings. A. In this adult with typical oval cardiomegaly, a large dilated truncus and a concave pulmonary artery segment also are seen. **B.** Coronal magnetic resonance image demonstrates the large truncus (T). There is no pulmonary artery. **C.** More posterior coronal cut demonstrates the descending aorta (A) and extensive collaterals especially visible on the right. **D.** Axial view demonstrating the truncus (T), descending aorta (D), no pulmonary artery, and numerous tortuous collateral vessels throughout the mediastinum.

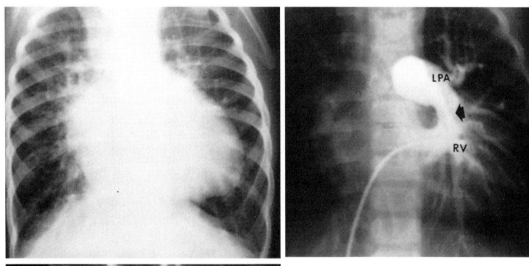

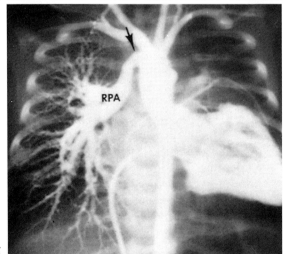

FIGURE 3.56. Hemitruncus (right pulmonary artery from ascending aorta). A. Note oval cardiomegaly, overaeration, and vascular congestion in the right lung. The vascularity is not engorged in the left lung (compare the outer thirds of the lung fields on both sides). **B.** Right ventriculogram demonstrates the right ventricle (RV), right outflow tract (arrow), and left pulmonary artery (LPA). No right pulmonary artery is identified. **C.** Aortogram demonstrates a single systemic arterial communication (arrow) between the aorta and right pulmonary artery (RPA). This communication creates a left-to-right shunt through the right lung and explains why the right lung shows engorged vascularity. Loosely, this abnormality could be considered a form of persistent truncus arteriosus, although it should be remembered that a ventricular septal defect usually is absent in these patients.

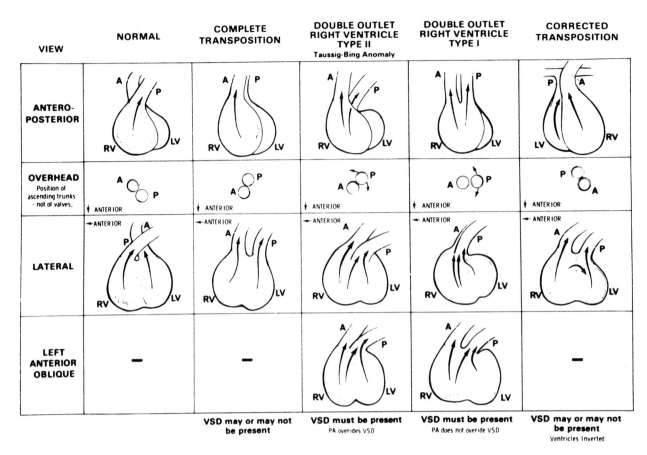

VIEW	NORMAL	COMPLETE TRANSPOSITION	DOUBLE OUTLET RIGHT VENTRICLE TYPE II Taussig-Bing Anomaly	DOUBLE OUTLET RIGHT VENTRICLE TYPE I	CORRECTED TRANSPOSITION
ANTERO-POSTERIOR					
OVERHEAD Position of ascending trunks - not of valves.					
LATERAL					
LEFT ANTERIOR OBLIQUE	—	—			—
	VSD may or may not be present	VSD may or may not be present	VSD must be present PA overides VSD	VSD must be present PA does not overide VSD	VSD may or may not be present Ventricles Inverted

FIGURE 3.57. Transposition and double-outlet complexes: great vessel configurations.
Diagrammatic representation of "classic" great vessel relationships in various transposition and double-outlet complexes. Variations, however, are to be expected, especially in the double-outlet right ventricle group. Very often, one must examine these infants in the left anterooblique position (cardioangiogram) to delineate more clearly the relative position of the pulmonary artery, interventricular septum, and ventricular septal defect. In type II double-outlet right ventricle (Taussig-Bing anomaly), the pulmonary artery overrides the ventricular septal defect, while in the type I anomaly, it does not.

the aorta and pulmonary artery and considers simple or complete transposition and the two types of incomplete transposition or the so-called "double-outlet right ventricle abnormalities." It also includes congenitally corrected transposition. The reason I have found it helpful to consider all of these lesions in the group is that the aorta is transposed in all. In other words, it assumes an abnormal anterior position and drains the right ventricle. The pulmonary artery is more variable in position from one condition to the other.

In simple (complete) transposition, the anteroposterior relationship of the great vessels is reversed, but the aorta remains in normal position from side to side, and thus the term "D-transposition," or dextro-transposition, is used to describe the anomaly. Generally, the pulmonary artery lies directly behind the aorta in this form of transposition. In terms of the "double-outlet right ventricle" abnormalities,

both great vessels receive blood from the right ventricle. However, while the aorta always arises solely from the right ventricle, the pulmonary artery may arise from the right ventricle alone or from both ventricles. In the latter instance, the pulmonary artery overrides a high ventricular septal defect, and the abnormality constitutes the Taussig-Bing or "double-outlet right ventricle type II" anomaly.

In complete or simple transposition of the great vessels, in the first few days of life, heart size and pulmonary vascularity usually are normal. This is because the high pulmonary vascular resistance in the neonate prevents flooding of the lungs and thus protects the heart from diastolic ventricular overloading and enlargement. Thereafter, however, if the condition is not corrected, pulmonary blood flow increases, cardiomegaly becomes apparent, and all chambers dilate. Pulmonary vascular congestion is both active

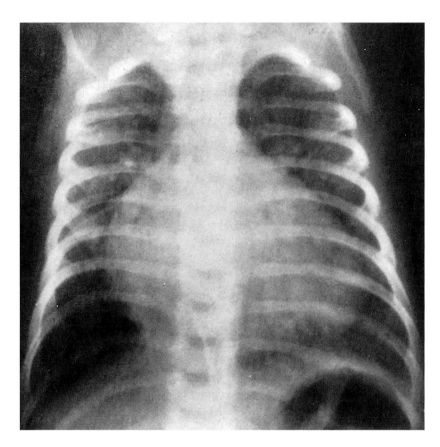

FIGURE 3.58. Transposition of great vessels: posteroanterior view. Note the large oval heart and congested lung fields. The apex of the heart tends to slope slightly downward. The base of the cardiac silhouette is narrow. This is the "egg-shaped" heart.

and passive, and it is difficult to separate one from the other. The specific cardiac configuration is oval or egg shaped (Fig. 3.58). In addition, narrowness of the pedicle, due to the anteroposterior positioning of the aorta and pulmonary artery, is present. This finding is further accentuated by the absence of thymic tissue due to stress atrophy. This latter phenomenon is not totally peculiar to transposition of the great vessels and occurs with other severe congenital heart lesions, but its resultant appearance is accentuated in transposition of the great vessels by their anteroposterior lineup.

The cardioangiographic findings in simple transposition are best seen on lateral or left anterooblique views (Fig. 3.59). Characteristically, the aortic valve is higher in position than when the aorta is normal and drains the left ventricle. The aorta, of course, also is anterior. The presence of an associated ductus arteriosus or ventricular septal defect also is readily determined. If these communications are inadequate, a balloon septostomy or a Raskind procedure is performed (Fig. 3.60). The altered anatomy in transposition of the great vessels also can be demonstrated with MRI where the anterior aorta and posterior pulmonary artery are clearly visualized (Fig. 3.61).

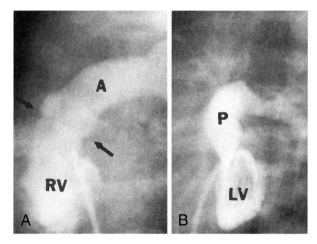

FIGURE 3.59. Transposition of the great vessels: angiocardiographic findings. A. Injection into the right ventricle (RV) demonstrates the anteriorly placed aorta (A). The aortic valve (arrows) is higher in position than usual. There is no communicating ventricular septal defect or patent ductus arteriosus. **B.** Injection into the left ventricle (LV) demonstrates the pulmonary artery (P), which is located posterior to the aorta.

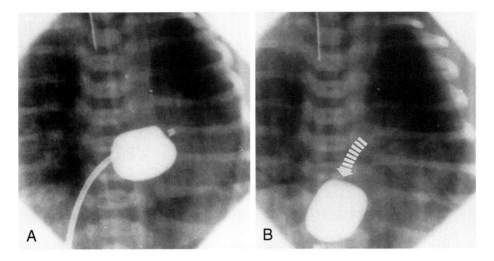

FIGURE 3.60. Raskind procedure. A. Note the position of the contrast-filled balloon in the left atrium. **B.** With pulling, the balloon passes through the foramen ovale (arrow) deep into the right atrium. In so doing, the foramen ovale is dilated and enlarged.

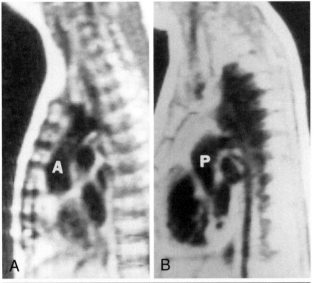

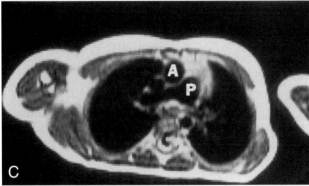

FIGURE 3.61. Transposition: magnetic resonance imaging and ultrasound findings. A. Sagittal magnetic resonance imaging study demonstrates the anterior aorta (A). **B.** Another sagittal slice demonstrates the posteriorly placed pulmonary artery (P) originating from the left ventricle. **C.** Axial view demonstrates the anterior position of the aorta (A) and posterior position of the pulmonary artery (P).

Double-Outlet Right Ventricle

In double-outlet right ventricle, the aorta is transposed and anterior, but the pulmonary artery may arise from the right ventricle entirely or from both the left and the right ventricles as it overrides a high ventricular septal defect (Taussig-Bing anomaly). The cardiac configuration, in any case, is usually oval, and the mediastinum is wider than in simple transposition because the aorta and pulmonary artery do not lie directly behind one another (Fig. 3.62). Angiocardiographically, distinction between simple and the double-outlet right ventricle complexes is made on the basis of the left anterooblique view findings. On this view, the intraventricular septum is seen on edge, and the imager can determine whether the pulmonary artery overrides the ventricular septal defect (Fig. 3.63). In simple double-outlet right ventricle, the pulmonary artery lies totally anterior to the defect and septum, while in the Taussig-Bing anomaly, the pulmonary artery overrides the ventricular septal defect and accepts blood from both ventricles. MRI also can be used to define the anatomy of these lesions (11).

"Congenitally Corrected" Transposition of Great Vessels

As has been noted earlier, in congenitally corrected transposition of the great vessels, the great vessels are transposed, but, in addition, the great vessels and ventricles are inverted (Fig. 3.64). Inversion of the great vessels places the aorta on the left, or in the so-called "L-transposition location." Hemodynamically, this results in a "normal" circulation. In other words, blood returning from the lungs is delivered to the left atrium, then to the anatomic right ventricle, and finally out the aorta. On the other side, blood from the systemic circulation is returned to the right atrium, then to the

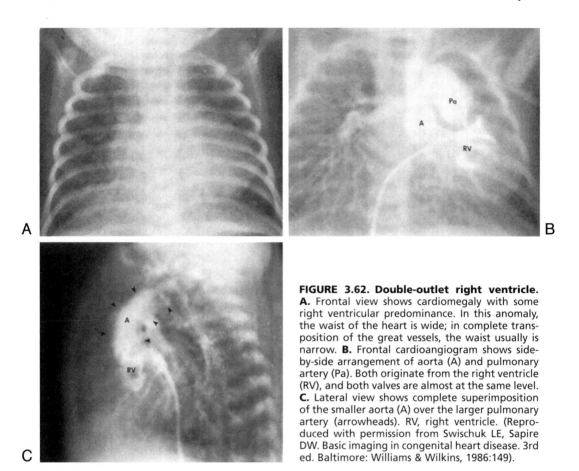

FIGURE 3.62. Double-outlet right ventricle. A. Frontal view shows cardiomegaly with some right ventricular predominance. In this anomaly, the waist of the heart is wide; in complete transposition of the great vessels, the waist usually is narrow. **B.** Frontal cardioangiogram shows side-by-side arrangement of aorta (A) and pulmonary artery (Pa). Both originate from the right ventricle (RV), and both valves are almost at the same level. **C.** Lateral view shows complete superimposition of the smaller aorta (A) over the larger pulmonary artery (arrowheads). RV, right ventricle. (Reproduced with permission from Swischuk LE, Sapire DW. Basic imaging in congenital heart disease. 3rd ed. Baltimore: Williams & Wilkins, 1986:149).

anatomic left ventricle, and finally out the pulmonary artery. Even though these ventricles are discordant in their anatomic connections with the atria and great vessels, functionally they deliver blood to the appropriate circulation. In other words, even though the ventricle delivering blood to

the aorta is the anatomic right ventricle, it receives blood from the left atrium and functions as the left ventricle. The same occurs in reverse with the anatomic left ventricle, which functions as the right ventricle and delivers blood to the pulmonary artery.

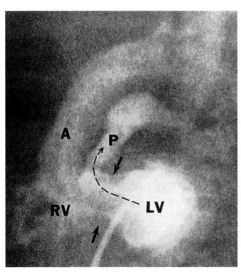
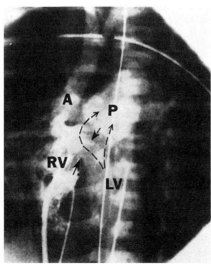

FIGURE 3.63. Double-outlet right ventricle: cardioangiographic differentiation. A. Double-outlet right ventricle type I. The slightly stenotic pulmonary artery (P) lies totally on the right ventricular side of the ventricular septal defect (arrows). For blood to pass into the pulmonary artery from the left ventricle, it must cross the ventricular septal defect (dotted arrow pathway). A, aorta; LV, left ventricle; RV, right ventricle. **B.** Double-outlet right ventricle type II (Taussig-Bing anomaly). The large pulmonary artery (P) overrides the ventricular septal defect (arrows). Blood from the left ventricle (LV) may enter the pulmonary artery directly from the left ventricle or, after it has crossed into the right ventricle, through the ventricular septal defect (dotted arrow pathways). A, aorta; RV, right ventricle.

NORMAL   CORRECTED TRANSPOSITION

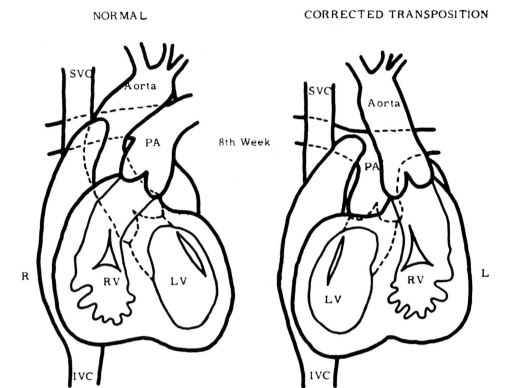

FIGURE 3.64. Corrected transposition. Note the position of the aorta and right ventricle (RV). The outflow tract of the right ventricle and the base of the aorta produce the bulge seen on the posteroanterior roentgenogram. IVC, inferior vena cava; LV, left ventricle; PA, pulmonary artery; SVC, superior vena cava. (Reproduced with permission from Ellis K et al. Congenitally corrected transposition of the great vessels. Radiology 1962;79:35–50).

Patients with this anomaly are acyanotic, and many are completely asymptomatic. Those who are symptomatic usually have some other congenital heart defect such as a ventricular septal defect or pulmonary stenosis. In later life, however, even those with an apparently normal heart can develop conduction defects and atrioventricular valve insufficiency.

Roentgenographically, if there is no shunt, the pulmonary vasculature is normal and the heart is not enlarged. On the other hand, in some cases, the posteroanterior roentgenogram reveals an abnormal, almost squared-off, bulge along the upper left cardiac border (Fig. 3.65A). This bulge may be the only clue to the underlying problem and represents the inverted aorta arising from the concomitantly inverted right ventricle (Fig. 3.65, B and C). Once recognized, this finding should alert one to the possibility of congenitally corrected transposition of the great vessels.

Single Ventricle

The term "single ventricle" most often refers to the situation in which one ventricle is large and the other is rudimentary (12). This anomaly essentially can be regarded as taking one of three forms: (a) underdevelopment of the right ventricle (most common), (b) underdevelopment of the left ventricle (next most common), and (c) an undifferentiated ventricle with no development of the intraventricular septum (rare). In addition, transposition of the great vessels, either simple or congenitally corrected, frequently is present. However, since only a single ventricle exists, this fact is of little hemodynamic or clinical significance. Of more importance is the presence or absence of pulmonic stenosis or atresia, for if they are present, some surgical procedure will be required to improve blood flow. Roentgenographically, it is difficult to identify a characteristic plain film pattern for single ventricle. Usually, one sees nonspecific cardiomegaly and vascular congestion. However, the abnormality can be identified cardioangiographically and with MRI (Fig. 3.66).

REFERENCES

1. Darling RC, Rothney WB, Craig JM. Total pulmonary venous drainage into the right side of the heart: report of 17 autopsied cases not associated with other major cardiovascular anomalies. Lab Invest 1957;6:44–65.

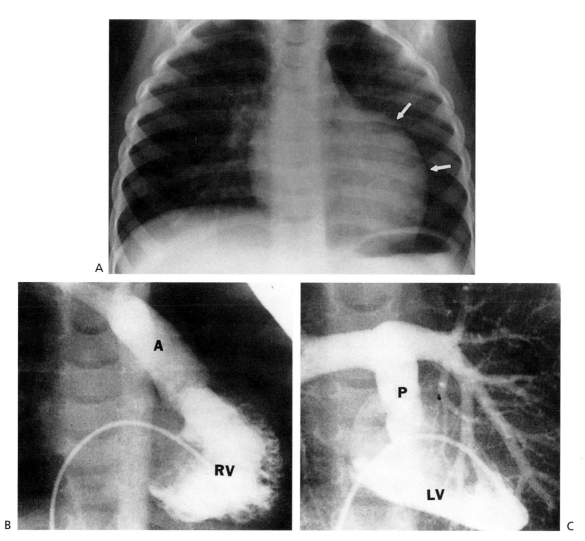

FIGURE 3.65. "Congenitally corrected" transposition of great vessels. A. Plain film demonstrates cardiomegaly with a very prominent left cardiac border and upper left hump (arrows). Note also that while the descending aorta is identified to the left of the trachea, delineation of the aortic knob and pulmonary artery is not possible. The reason for this is that they are inverted. **B.** Injection into the right ventricle (RV) shows its inverted position and the inverted aorta (A) draining it. The problem is referred to as "L-transposition." **C.** The left ventricle (LV), identified by its smooth wall, gives rise to the inverted pulmonary artery (P). The aorta and pulmonary artery also are transposed, in that the pulmonary artery is more posterior and drains the left ventricle, while the aorta is anterior and drains the right ventricle.

2. Casta A, Sappire DW, Swischuk LE. True congenital aneurysm of the septum primum not associated with obstructive right-or left-sided lesions: identified by two-dimensional echocardiography and angiography in a newborn. Pediatr Cardiol 1983;4:159–162.

3. Patton WL, Momenah T, Gooding CA, et al. The vascular vise causing TAPVR type I to radiographically mimic TAPVR type III. Pediatr Radiol 1999;29:323–326.

4. Elias-Jones AC, Cordner SV. Infra-diaphragmatic total anomalous pulmonary venous drainage presenting with rectal bleeding. Arch Dis Child 1983;58:637–639.

5. King DR, Marchildon MB. Gastrointestinal hemorrhage; an unusual complication of total anomalous pulmonary venous drainage. J Thorac Cardiovasc Surg 1977;73:316–318.

6. Kastler B, Livolsi A, Germain P, et al. Contribution of MRI in supracardiac total anomalous pulmonary venous drainage. Pediatr Radiol 1992;22:262–263.

7. Kim TH, Kim YM, Suh CH, et al. Helical CT angiography and three-dimensional reconstruction of total anomalous pulmonary venous connections in neonates and infants. AJR 2000;175:1381–1386.

8. Swischuk LE, L'Heureux P. Unilateral pulmonary vein atresia: hemoptysis, infection and reticular lung. AJR 1980;135:667–672.

9. Heyneman LE, Nolan RL, Harrison JK, et al. Original report. Congenital unilateral pulmonary vein atresia radiologic findings in three adult patients. AJR 2001;177:681–685.

10. Collett RW, Edwards JE. Persistent truncus arteriosus: a classification according to anatomic types. Surg Clin North Am 152:149.

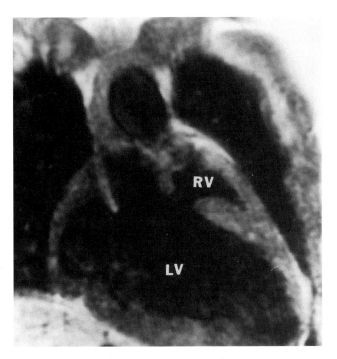

FIGURE 3.66. Single ventricle: magnetic resonance imaging. A. Axial image through the upper portion of the heart demonstrates the normal-size left ventricle (LV) and rudimentary right ventricle (RV).

11. Akins EW, Martin TD, Alexander JA, et al. Case report. MR imaging of double-outlet right ventricle. AJR 1989;152: 128–130.
12. Swischuk LE. Single ventricle. Semin Roentgenol 1985;20: 130–133.

DECREASED PULMONARY VASCULARITY

A pattern of decreased pulmonary vascularity denotes diminished pulmonary blood flow and usually is seen in patients with right outflow tract obstruction and an associated right-to-left shunt (Table 3.3). With right outflow tract obstruction, the obstructive lesion can be located anywhere from the tricuspid valve to the peripheral pulmonary artery branches. This results in elevation of right-side cardiac pressures and, if an intracardiac communication is present, a right-to-left shunt. Clinically, this results in cyanosis and, roentgenographically, reduced pulmonary blood flow and decreased pulmonary vascularity.

Tetralogy of Fallot

Tetralogy of Fallot is the most common cause of cyanotic congenital heart disease beyond the first 30 days of life. The developmental defect is rather complex and involves the interventricular septum, right outflow tract (right ventricular infundibulum), pulmonary artery, and aorta. Specifically, the anomaly consists of a high ventricular septal

TABLE 3.3. DECREASED PULMONARY VASCULARITY

Right outflow tract obstruction (with right-to-left shunt and cyanosis)
    Tetralogy of Fallot
        Pseudotruncus arteriosus type II (severe tetralogy of Fallot)
    Hypoplastic right heart syndrome
        Tricuspid atresia
        Pulmonary atresia
        Tricuspid stenosis
        Isolated hypoplasia of right ventricle
    Ebstein's anomaly
    Uhl's disease
    Trilogy of Fallot (pulmonary stenosis with intact ventricular septum and right-to-left atrial shunt)
    Various transpositions with pulmonary stenosis or atresia
    Single (common) ventricle with pulmonary stenosis or atresia
    Tricuspid or pulmonary insufficiency with right-to-left shunt
Absent or hypoplastic pulmonary artery or branches
    Pseudotruncus arteriosus type I (old truncus type IV), some cases
    Unilateral absent pulmonary artery (unilateral decreased vascularity)

defect, some form of pulmonary stenosis, and associated septal overriding by the aorta. Other abnormalities of the pulmonary artery or its branches also frequently are present and include peripheral pulmonary artery coarctations, unilateral absence or hypoplasia of a pulmonary artery (usually the left), and absence of the pulmonary valve.

Hemodynamically, the critical component of tetralogy of Fallot is pulmonary stenosis. It results in right ventricular hypertrophy and ultimately regulates the degree of right-to-left shunting and aortic overriding. In other words, with severe stenosis, right-to-left shunting and aortic overriding are marked, while with mild stenosis, shunting is decreased and overriding is minimal. Overriding is probably related more to aortic size than to actual displacement of the interventricular septum. For example, in patients with severe pulmonary stenosis, right ventricular obstruction is so great that almost all the blood from both ventricles is delivered out the aorta. As a result, the aorta shows marked enlargement and greater "overriding." The reverse is true in patients with mild pulmonary stenosis (i.e., "pink tetralogy of Fallot"), where the radiographic findings are basically normal.

In the more severe cases of tetralogy of Fallot, the pulmonary vascular pattern is distinctly diminished and the pulmonary artery silhouette shallow or concave (Fig. 3.67A). Because the right ventricle hypertrophies and does not dilate, overall cardiac size usually is normal or even "small." However, right ventricular hypertrophy causes the cardiac apex to be displaced laterally and upwardly, resulting in the classic "coeur en sabot" configuration (Fig. 3.67A). In other cases, however, findings may resemble pulmonary atresia more than tetralogy of Fallot (Fig. 3.67B).

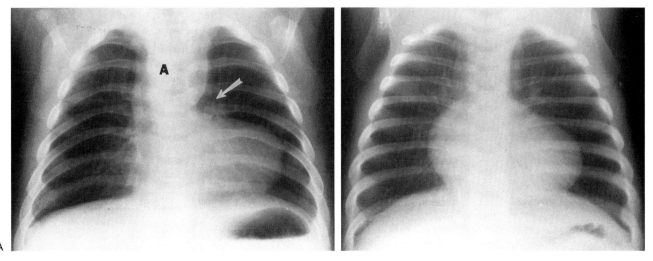

FIGURE 3.67. Tetralogy of Fallot: various configurations. A. Classic findings consist of decreased pulmonary vascularity, a very concave pulmonary artery segment (arrow), a prominent right-sided aorta (A), and a typical "coeur en sabot" heart, reflective of right ventricular hypertrophy. **B.** Posteroanterior view of another infant with markedly decreased pulmonary vascularity and oval heart. The findings resemble those of pulmonary atresia. The pulmonary artery is concave, while the aorta is on the left and not particularly large.

The size and side of the aorta are important in the assessment of tetralogy of Fallot. A right-side aorta is variably estimated to be present in 20–30% of cases and is useful in differentiating tetralogy of Fallot from other congenital heart lesions producing diminished pulmonary vascularity. A right-side aorta occurs in less than 5% of other conditions, except for persistent truncus arteriosus, where it is seen in approximately 33% of cases.

The right-side aorta produces fullness in the right paratracheal region, emptiness in the left paratracheal region (where the aorta normally should lie), and often a slanted paraspinal line on the right (Fig. 3.68A). This results from

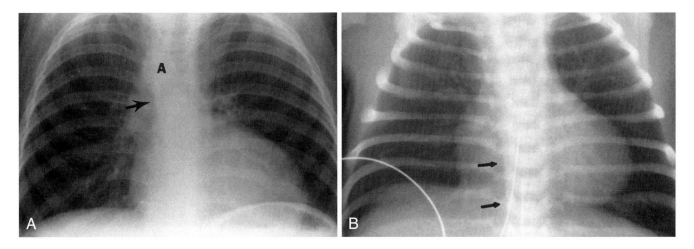

FIGURE 3.68. Tetralogy of Fallot: right-side aorta. A. Note the right side aortic knob (A) and the slanted right oblique paraspinal stripe (arrow). Other findings include right ventricular hypertrophy, slight cardiomegaly, concavity of the main pulmonary artery segment, and decreased pulmonary vascularity. **B.** Another patient with relatively normal vascularity, some suggestion of right ventricular hypertrophy (although the film is lordotic), fullness in the right paratracheal region without actual visualization of the right aortic arch and trachea, and finally, the most important clue, the slanted line (lower arrow) of the right-side aorta descending on the right (arrows).

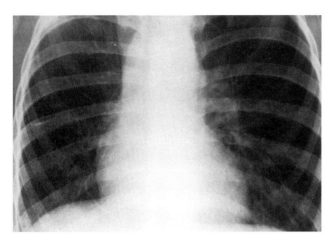

FIGURE 3.69. Tetralogy of Fallot: unequal pulmonary blood flow. There is decreased blood flow to both lungs, but there is virtually no blood flow to the right lung and the right lung also is smaller because it is hypoplastic.

the right-side aorta descending just to the right of the spine. Later, the aorta tends to cross midline and may descend on the left, but in the thoracic region, the right-side slanted paravertebral stripe is an important plain film finding (Fig. 3.68B). It usually is accentuated with rotation to the right.

Unequal pulmonary blood flow also frequently is present in patients with tetralogy of Fallot; most commonly, it is the left pulmonary artery that is hypoplastic or absent. However, diminished pulmonary vascularity also can occur on the right, as seen in Fig. 3.69. **Another abnormality that can occur with tetralogy of Fallot is absence of the pulmonary valve.** These patients demonstrate larger hearts

than do regular tetralogy of Fallot patients, but still a tetralogy-like cardiac silhouette usually is retained (Fig. 3.70). However, the most reliable finding in these patients is marked dilatation of the main, right, and left pulmonary arteries. In some cases, dilatation is aneurysmal and causes bronchial obstruction (1, 2), while in other cases, the left pulmonary artery may be absent, and only right hilar prominence is seen.

Cases of tetralogy of Fallot where pulmonary valve atresia is present often are referred to as cases of "pseudotruncus arteriosus." The term "pseudotruncus arteriosus" came into use because the overall pattern of blood flow in these patients was similar to that seen in true persistent truncus arteriosus. In other words, a single vessel delivers blood to all three circulations (i.e., systemic, coronary, and pulmonary). Anatomically, however, the lesions are different, but the plain film findings may be indistinguishable. In pseudotruncus arteriosus, the main communication between the aorta and the atretic pulmonary valves is via the patent ductus arteriosus (Fig. 3.71), which can be quite large and tortuous in some cases. The abnormal systemic connecting vessels seen in persistent truncus arteriosus type IV are not present in these cases.

Over a period of time, tetralogy of Fallot patients with high-grade pulmonary stenosis or pulmonary atresia derive some of their pulmonary blood from the bronchial arteries. The resultant enlarged bronchial arteries are seldom visible on plain films, since it is only after many years that these vessels hypertrophy to the point where they can be detected on plain films. In this day and age, this is uncommon. When present, these collaterals usually are detected with aortography. Angiocardiographically, the diagnosis of tetralogy is rather straightforward. On either the frontal,

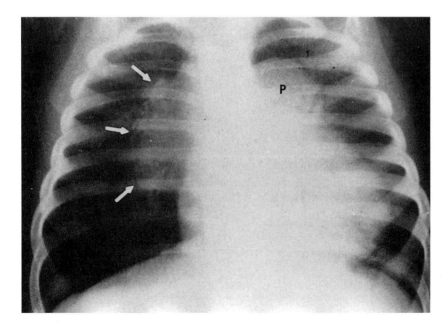

FIGURE 3.70. Tetralogy of Fallot with absent pulmonary valve. Note cardiomegaly with right ventricular hypertrophy and a very large, mass-like main pulmonary artery (P) and right pulmonary artery (arrows). The left pulmonary artery also is enlarged but is hidden behind the main pulmonary artery. Note also that the vascularity distal to the dilated proximal pulmonary arteries is decreased. This appearance is typical of tetralogy of Fallot with absence of the pulmonary valve.

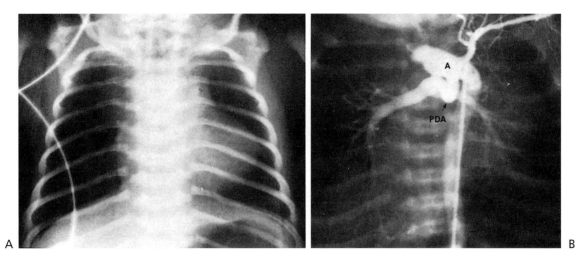

FIGURE 3.71. Pseudotruncus arteriosus: tetralogy of Fallot with pulmonary atresia and patent ductus arteriosus. A. Note the typical "coeur en sabot" appearance of the heart in this infant with tetralogy of Fallot. The vascularity is decreased, but the aorta is difficult to define. This patient was markedly cyanotic. **B. Frontal aortogram.** Note the aorta (A) and the patent ductus arteriosus (PDA). The patent ductus arteriosus is supplying the pulmonary arteries. Note that there are no visible systemic collaterals.

the lateral, or the left anterooblique projections, infundibular stenosis and pulmonary valve stenosis are readily identified (Fig. 3.72). In most cases, the entire pulmonary arterial tree is hypoplastic, and peripheral coarctations may co-exist. In other instances, one of the pulmonary arteries may be totally absent or very atretic. MRI also demonstrates

the abnormalities seen in tetralogy of Fallot but generally is used in older patients in whom, for one reason or another, cardioangiography cannot be performed (Fig. 3.73). Postoperatively, in tetralogy of Fallot, after placement of an infundibular patch, the patch may dilate and eventually calcify (Fig. 3.74).

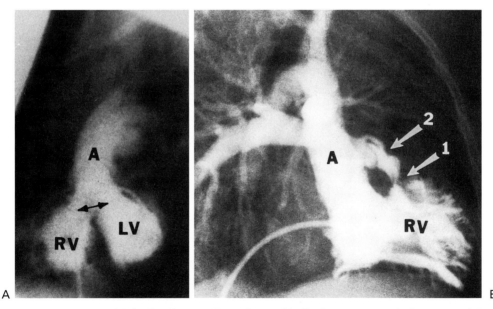

FIGURE 3.72. Tetralogy of Fallot: cardioangiographic findings. A. Note the large aorta (A) overriding the ventricular septal defect (arrow). The septum is the radiolucent wedge between right ventricle (RV) and the left ventricle (LV). **B.** Right anterooblique view demonstrates infundibular stenosis (1) and some thickening of the stenotic pulmonary valve (2). The aorta (A) is on the right. RV, right ventricle.

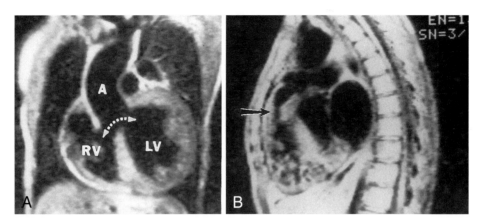

FIGURE 3.73. Tetralogy of Fallot: magnetic resonance imaging findings. A. Left anterooblique view demonstrates the large aorta (A), overriding the ventricular septal defect (arrows). LV, left ventricle; RV, right ventricle. **B.** Lateral view demonstrates the infundibular stenosis (arrow).

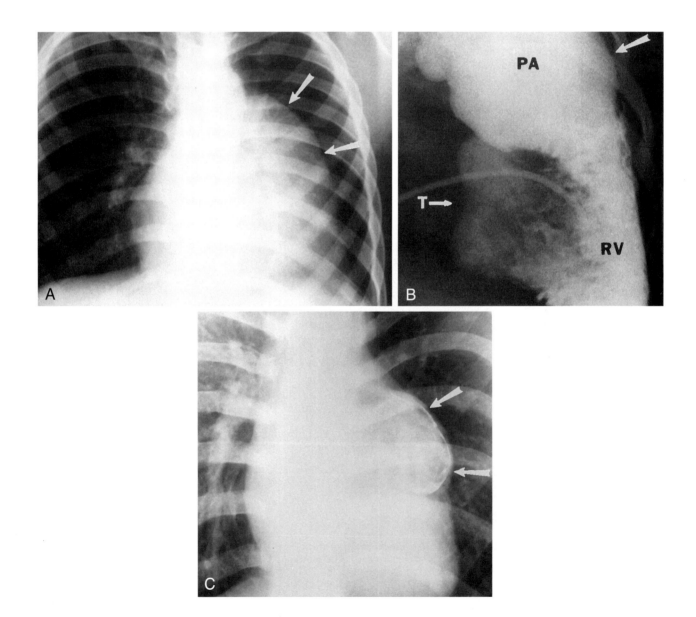

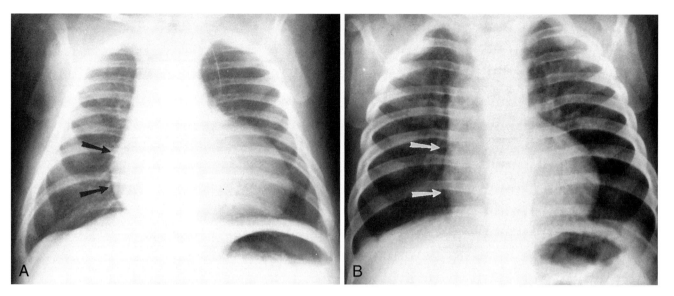

FIGURE 3.75. Tricuspid atresia: variable configurations. A. In this patient, there is oval cardiomegaly. The vascularity is diminished, and the pulmonary artery segment is concave. There is some right atrial fullness (arrows). **B.** In this patient, because the atrial septal defect is large, the right atrial region is flat (arrows).

Hypoplastic Right Heart Syndrome

A wide variety of conditions compose the hypoplastic right heart syndrome. These include tricuspid atresia and stenosis, pulmonary atresia, and isolated hypoplasia of the right ventricle. All have in common a small right ventricle, a large left atrium and ventricle, varying degrees of right atrial enlargement, and right-to-left atrial shunting. The latter, of course, is responsible for the cyanosis seen in these patients.

Tricuspid Atresia and Stenosis

In tricuspid atresia, the tricuspid valve is atretic or stenotic and the right ventricle hypoplastic. The pulmonary artery also is underdeveloped, and pulmonary stenosis may be present. Transposition of the great vessels also may be present.

In such cases, pulmonary stenosis usually is absent, and as a result, blood flow to the lungs is increased rather than decreased.

Roentgenographically, decreased pulmonary vascularity and a flat or concave pulmonary artery are seen. The heart usually is enlarged, and if the decompressing atrial septal defect is small, right atrial enlargement is present (Fig. 3.75A). On the other hand, if the atrial septal defect is large, right atrial enlargement is minimal or absent (Fig. 3.75B). Angiocardiography clearly demonstrates the enlarged right atrium, the atretic tricuspid valve, right-to-left atrial shunting, and hypoplasia of the right ventricle (Fig. 3.76). Tricuspid stenosis is rarer than tricuspid atresia but, for practical purposes, can be considered functionally and roentgenographically similar. The difference is anatomic, in that a smaller than normal tricuspid orifice is still present.

FIGURE 3.74. Tetralogy of Fallot: postoperative dilated patch. A. Note the characteristic bump over the upper left cardiac border (arrows). **B.** Cardioangiogram demonstrates the right ventricle (RV) and the enormously dilated pulmonary artery (PA), which leads to the bump (arrow) seen in **A.** T, tricuspid valve. **C.** Another patient with a longstanding aneurysmally dilated patch showing peripheral curvilinear calcification (arrows).

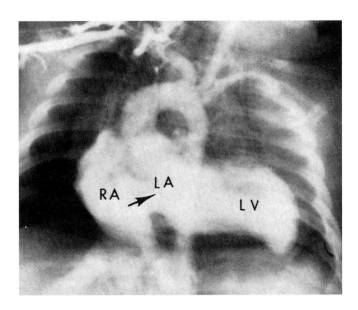

FIGURE 3.76. Tricuspid atresia: angiocardiogram. There is shunting (arrow) from the right atrium (RA) to the left atrium (LA). Filling of the large left ventricle (LV) is seen, but there is no filling of the right ventricle (i.e., triangular radiolucent space or right ventricular window along the inferior margin of the heart).

Pulmonary Atresia

In most cases of pulmonary atresia, a small hypoplastic right ventricle and tricuspid valve are present. Hemodynamically, right ventricular pressures are exceedingly high, and shunting from right to left occurs at the atrial level. In addition, variable degrees of tricuspid insufficiency are present, and because of this, there are two types of pulmonary atresia: types I and II. The type I anomaly constitutes those cases where the right ventricle is severely hypoplastic and the tricuspid valve is virtually atretic. In such cases, there is no significant tricuspid regurgitation and no right atrial enlargement. In the type II anomaly, the right ventricle is more developed and the tricuspid valve more patent. As a result, gross tricuspid insufficiency can occur, and the result is marked enlargement of the right atrium. In both types of pulmonary atresia, the intraventricular septum is intact, and therefore the condition often is referred to as "pulmonary atresia with an intact intraventricular septum." In addition, in both types, since the pulmonary valve is atretic, postnatal patency of the ductus arteriosus is critical. It is through the ductus that blood is delivered to the pulmonary circulation, and thus once the ductus closes, the infant's condition rapidly deteriorates. Prostaglandin therapy can maintain ductal patency until surgery is performed.

Roentgenographically, all cases of pulmonary atresia show decreased pulmonary vascularity and a shallow or concave pulmonary artery. Cardiac enlargement is variable, but there usually is significant right atrial and right ventricular enlargement. In the type II anomaly, the one often presenting in the neonatal period, the heart is very large as there is gross tricuspid insufficiency. The findings are indistinguishable from those of Ebstein's anomaly (Fig. 3.77). In these cases, there is a significant residual right ventricular

cavity remaining, and therefore, regurgitation can occur into the right atrium. In the type I anomaly, the right ventricle is very small, and there is virtually no tricuspid valve present. Therefore, tricuspid regurgitation does not occur, and the heart is not enlarged. However, right atrial predominance still is present (Fig. 3.78).

Hypoplasia of the Right Ventricle

Hypoplasia of the right ventricle is a rare variation of the hypoplastic right heart syndrome, and in most cases, plain film findings mimic those of tricuspid or pulmonary atresia. Angiocardiography shows a small bulbous or spherical right ventricle. MRI also can demonstrate the virtually lumenless right ventricular muscle mass (Fig. 3.79). Tricuspid stenosis frequently is associated with hypoplasia of the right ventricle, but the pulmonary valve is open.

Ebstein's Anomaly

Ebstein's anomaly consists of downward displacement of the septal and, frequently, the posterior leaflet of the tricuspid valve. As a result, a variable portion of the right ventricle is functionally and anatomically incorporated into the right atrium. In severe cases, only a small portion of the right ventricle remains as the true muscular right ventricle. The atrialized portion of the right ventricle has a very thin wall, and even though it contracts with the muscular portion, contraction is so feeble and ineffective that it contributes little to right ventricular emptying. Therefore, the large atrialized portion of the right ventricle can be thought of as a large venous reservoir impeding the flow of blood from the right atrium to the right ventricle.

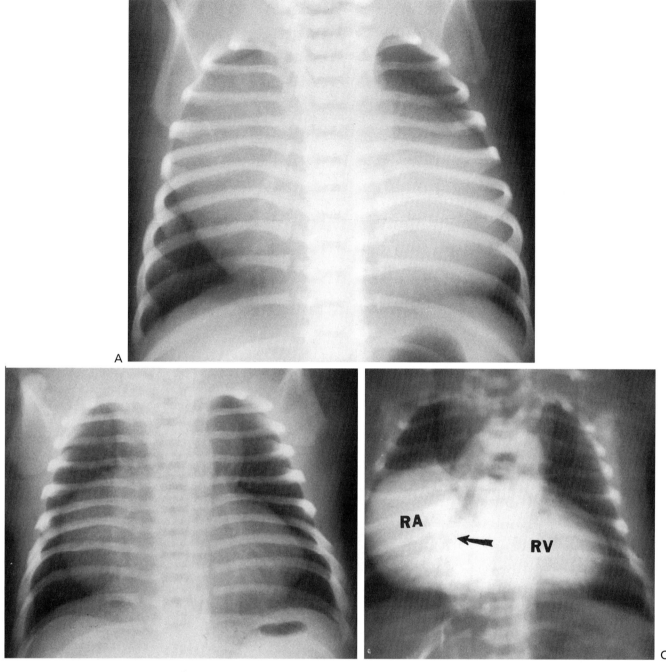

FIGURE 3.77. Pulmonary atresia with intact ventricular septum type II. A. Note aneurysmal dilatation of the right atrium. Cardiomegaly is enormous. A similar cardiac configuration can be seen in Ebstein's anomaly but in pulmonary atresia is seen only in the type II form. **B.** Another patient showing decreased pulmonary vascularity, a concave pulmonary artery segment, and marked oval cardiomegaly with marked right atrial enlargement. **C.** Angiogram demonstrates the large right ventricle (RV), regurgitation of contrast material through the insufficient tricuspid valve (arrow), and the large right atrium (RA).

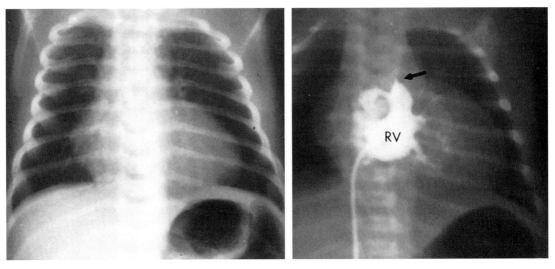

FIGURE 3.78. Pulmonary atresia type I. A. Note typical oval cardiomegaly, moderately bulging right atrium, decreased pulmonary vascularity, and a concave pulmonary artery segment. **B.** Cardioangiogram demonstrates the typical findings of a small, markedly trabeculated right ventricle (RV), with numerous intramural sinusoids and atretic pulmonary valve (arrow).

Roentgenographically, the findings are variable and depend on the severity of the lesion. However, pulmonary vascularity is decreased in most patients. In some patients, usually those surviving into adulthood, the findings may be minimal or near normal. In others, with more significant anatomic disturbance, cardiomegaly resulting from right atrial and right ventricular dilatation is present (Fig. 3.80A). In newborn infants, severe disease is the rule, and car-

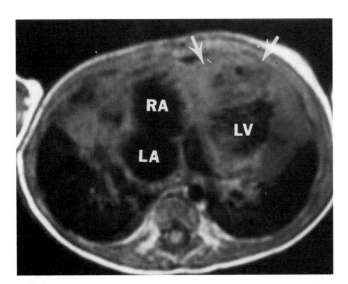

FIGURE 3.79. Hypoplasia of right ventricle: magnetic resonance imaging findings. Magnetic resonance imaging, axial view, demonstrates the left ventricle (LV), left atrium (LA), right atrium (RA), but no cavity for the right ventricle. Only rudimentary small channels are seen within the central muscle mass (arrows).

diomegaly is profound, duplicating the findings seen in cases of pulmonary atresia type II (Fig. 3.80B). In long-standing cases, a bulge resulting from the elevated "residual" right ventricle is seen along the upper left cardiac border. This bulge has resulted in the so-called "squared" or "boxed" cardiac appearance demonstrated in Fig. 3.80C. Angiocardiographically, one sees stagnation of the circulation so that the entire heart seems to be opacified (Fig. 3.81). MRI also is useful in demonstrating this abnormality (3).

Uhl's Disease

Uhl's disease is a rare condition that can present in early infancy and whose findings are similar to those of Ebstein's anomaly. Anatomically, there is focal or complete absence of the right ventricular myocardium, and the right ventricle becomes a thin-walled, fibroelastic bag (4). It contracts poorly and impedes the emptying of blood from the right side of the heart. Tricuspid insufficiency also is present, and cyanosis results from a right-to-left atrial shunt.

Pulmonary Stenosis

Congenital pulmonary stenosis is a common anomaly and may be found in isolated form or in combination with other abnormalities. This section deals primarily with isolated pulmonary stenosis, where the pulmonary valve itself is affected. The valve cusps fuse to form a diaphragm with an orifice of variable size, and the valve leaflets are variably thickened and dysplastic. Many cases of valvular pulmonary

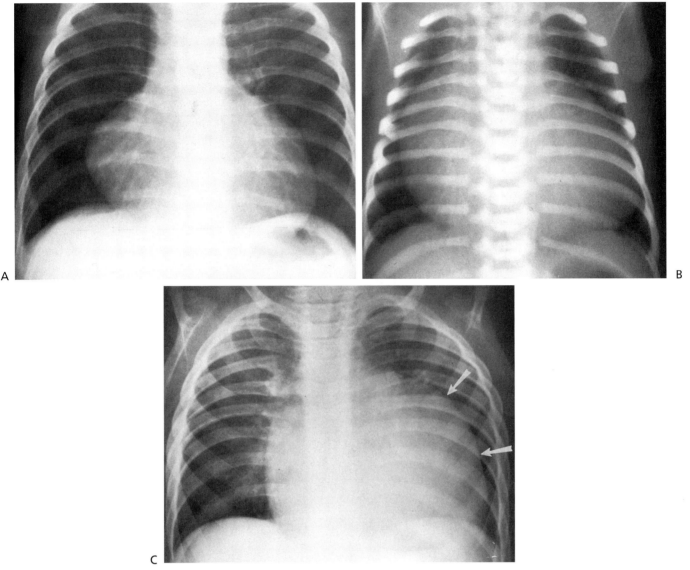

A

B

C

FIGURE 3.80. Ebstein's anomaly: posteroanterior view. A. Note the markedly diminished pulmonary vasculature and a flat pulmonary artery segment. There is marked right atrial enlargement (bulging on the right). The left cardiac border also is prominent. The configuration is not unlike that seen with pulmonary or tricuspid atresia. **B.** View of another patient with marked cardiomegaly and enormous enlargement of the right atrium. The enlarged right atrium could be misinterpreted for a large thymus gland or even a cardiac tumor. This cardiac configuration also can be seen with pulmonary atresia type II. **C.** View of another older patient with pronounced cardiomegaly, less bulging of the right atrium, and a more definite hump along the left upper cardiac border (arrows). This configuration leads to the so-called "squared" or "boxed heart."

stenosis demonstrate normal pulmonary vascularity, but if stenosis is associated with a right-to-left shunt (trilogy of Fallot), decreased vascularity is seen. These cases, of course, are in the minority, for most cases of valvular pulmonary stenosis are associated with normal pulmonary vascularity. However, I have seen cases of severe pulmonary stenosis without an underlying atrial defect where the vascularity appeared decreased.

Hemodynamically, in all cases, obstruction at, near, or distal to the pulmonary valve results in systolic overloading and hypertrophy of the right ventricle and its infundibulum. The degree of hypertrophy parallels the severity of stenosis, and in addition, in cases of pure valvular stenosis, the pulmonary artery just distal to the stenotic valve dilates (poststenotic dilatation). This dilatation is not seen with infundibular (subvalvular) or supravalvular stenoses.

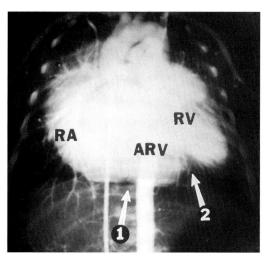

FIGURE 3.81. Ebstein's anomaly: angiographic findings. Cardioangiogram demonstrates filling of the entire heart with delineation of the right atrium (RA), atrialized right ventricle (ARV), and residual right ventricle (RV). These are separated by the tricuspid valve annulus (1) and the displaced septal and posterior leaflets of the tricuspid valve (2).

Roentgenographically, in mild cases of pulmonary valvular stenosis, there may be little or no abnormality seen. One may see only slight prominence of the pulmonary artery (Fig. 3.82). In more severely afflicted individuals, the pulmonary artery and left pulmonary artery branch show marked enlargement (Fig. 3.83). However, the heart still usually is normal. Poststenotic dilatation is the result of the high-pressure jet of blood decompressing itself in the postvalvular portion of the main pulmonary artery. This phenomenon often extends into the left main pulmonary artery, which then also dilates, but this finding is not always visible on plain films of infants and children.

Poststenotic dilatation of the pulmonary artery caused by stenosis of the pulmonary valve must be differentiated from idiopathic dilatation of the pulmonary artery. This latter finding is a common finding in adolescents and young adults, especially young females. In infants and children, however, it is not prevalent, and thus, when one sees a prominent pulmonary artery in a young infant, he or she should suspect some other problem besides idiopathic dilatation.

With cardioangiography, as noted earlier, poststenotic dilatation of the pulmonary artery along with doming of the pulmonary valve are readily identified. The findings are characteristic, and in some cases, the pulmonary valve leaflet may appear thickened. All of these findings are demonstrated in Fig. 3.84.

Pulmonary Stenosis with Intact Ventricular Septum and Right-to-Left Atrial Shunt (Trilogy of Fallot)

Patients with pulmonary stenosis and an intact ventricular septum mandate the presence of a right-to-left, cyanosis-producing atrial shunt and thus differ from the usual

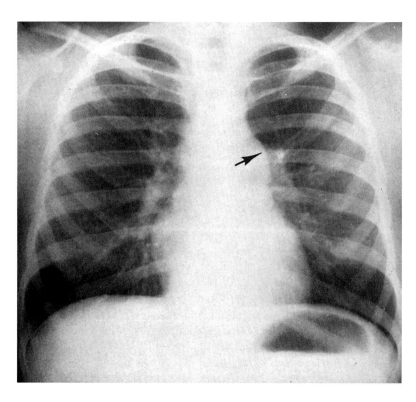

FIGURE 3.82. Mild pulmonary stenosis: posteroanterior view. The pulmonary vascularity and cardiac configuration are normal. There is slight prominence of the main and left pulmonary arteries resulting from mild poststenotic dilatation (arrow).

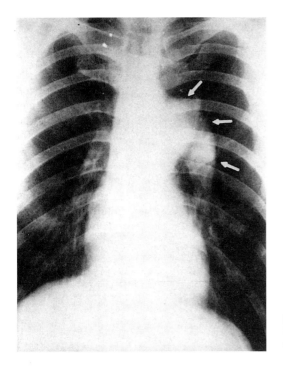

FIGURE 3.83. Pulmonary stenosis: large left pulmonary artery. Note the large main pulmonary artery and the large, slightly elevated left pulmonary artery (arrows).

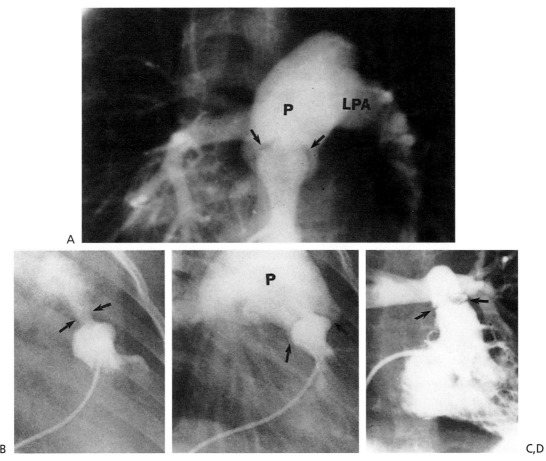

FIGURE 3.84. Valvular pulmonary stenosis: angiocardiographic findings. A. Note the typical domed stenotic pulmonary valve (arrows). There is marked poststenotic dilatation of the main pulmonary artery (P) and the left branch (LPA). **B.** View in another patient, in the right anterooblique position, demonstrates the characteristic jet (arrows) through the domed stenotic pulmonary valve. **C.** View of the same patient, a little later, demonstrates the domed stenotic valve (arrows). Note marked dilatation of the pulmonary artery (P) and its branches. There is a mild degree of secondary infundibular stenosis in this patient. **D.** Slightly thickened, dysplastic pulmonary valve (arrows) in another patient with pulmonary valve stenosis.

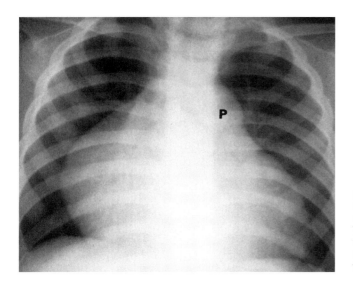

FIGURE 3.85. Pulmonary stenosis with intact ventricular septum and right-to-left atrial shunt: trilogy of Fallot. Note enormous right atrial and moderate right ventricular dilatation. The pulmonary artery (P) shows marked poststenotic dilatation, while the pulmonary vascularity is decreased. Except for the pulmonary artery dilatation, the cardiac configuration is not unlike that seen in pulmonary atresia or Ebstein's anomaly.

patient with pulmonary valve stenosis. Cyanosis results from right-to-left shunting through a patent foramen ovale or true atrial septal defect and from the markedly elevated right-side cardiac pressures induced by the stenotic pulmonary valve. Roentgenographically, since a right-to-left shunt is present, the pulmonary vascularity is diminished, and because of associated atrial regurgitation, the right atrium is enlarged (Fig. 3.85).

Supravalvular Pulmonary Stenosis

The most common form of supravalvular pulmonary stenosis is that which is manifest by multiple peripheral pulmonary artery coarctations. These coarctations usually are best demonstrated with pulmonary angiography, since plain films most often are normal in these patients. Peripheral stenoses also occur in the arteriohepatic dysplasia or Allegiles syndrome.

Insufficiency of Right-Side Cardiac Valves

As an isolated anomaly, congenital tricuspid insufficiency is an extremely rare condition. However, it can result in severe, early heart failure in the neonate. More frequently, of course, tricuspid insufficiency is found in association with conditions such as Ebstein's anomaly, pulmonary atresia type II, and trilogy of Fallot. Tricuspid insufficiency results in marked dilatation of the right atrium and right ventricle and, if associated with a right-to-left shunt, in variably diminished pulmonary vascularity. If, however, there is no such shunt, the pulmonary vascularity is normal.

REFERENCES

1. Kurlander GJ. Bronchial obstruction from aneurysm of the pulmonary artery associated with absence of the pulmonary valve. Lancet 1965;85:129–132.
2. Owens CM, Rees P, Elliot M, et al. Plain chest radiographic changes of the absent pulmonary valve syndrome. Br J Radiol 1994;67: 248–251.
3. Chli YH, Park JH, Choe YH, et al. Pictorial essay. MR imaging of Ebstein's anomaly of the tricuspid valve. AJR 1994;163:539–544.
4. Zuberbuhler JR, Blank E. Hypoplasia of right ventricular myocardium (Uhl's disease). AJR 1970;110:491–496.

LEFT-SIDE OBSTRUCTION

The group of patients with left-side obstruction are those who, in spite of having serious cardiac lesions, characteristically show normal pulmonary vascular patterns for years. Basically, these patients have left-side valvular or vascular obstructing lesions that result in systolic (pressure) overloading of the left ventricle (Table 3.4). This type of cardiac overload is notoriously well tolerated by the patient, and consequently, these patients can carry on for many years without showing evidence of heart failure. Eventually, however, the left ventricle decompensates, and passive pulmonary congestion (edema) results. Lesions included under this category of anomalies are aortic stenosis, mitral stenosis, coarctation of the aorta, hyperplastic left heart syndrome, interrupted aortic arch, and cor triatriatum.

Aortic Stenosis

Aortic stenosis usually is valvular but also may be subvalvular or supravalvular. Subvalvular stenosis may take the form of a band or, more usually, a thin diaphragm located some 5–10 mm below the aortic valve. Another subgroup of these patients consists of those patients with idiopathic hypertrophy of the left ventricle and interventricular septum. Patients who have supravalvular aortic stenosis are believed

TABLE 3.4. NORMAL PULMONARY VASCULARITY (UNLESS THERE IS FAILURE OR A RIGHT-TO-LEFT SHUNT IS PRESENT)

Left-side valvular or vascular lesions (normal vascularity until failure occurs; then passive congestion)

    Aortic stenosis—valvular[a]
        —subvalvular[a]
        —supravalvular[a]
    Coarctation of the aorta—with no VSD or PDA[a]
                      —with VSD or PDA[b]
    Interrupted aortic arch[b]
    Hypoplastic left heart syndrome[c]
    Mitral stenosis[b]
    Mitral insufficiency[b]
    Aortic insufficiency[b]
    Cor triatriatum[b]

Left-side endomyocardial lesions (normal vascularity until failure occurs; then passive congestion)

    Endocardial fibroelastosis[b]
    Aberrant left coronary artery[b]
    Cardiomyopathy[b]

Right-side valvular or vascular lesions (normal vascularity unless a right-to-left shunt is present; then decreased[d])

    Pulmonary stenosis
    Pulmonary insufficiency
    Tricuspid insufficiency

VSD, ventricular septal defect; PDA, patent ductus arteriosus.
[a]Left-side failure usually develops late in childhood.
[b]Left-side failure usually develops early in infancy (i.e., after the first week of life).
[c]Left-side failure usually develops in the first few days of life (under 1 week).
[d]See Table 4.3.

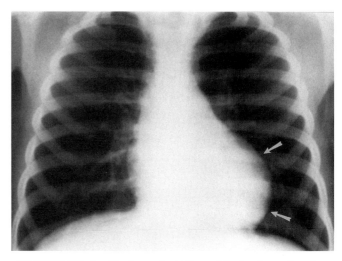

FIGURE 3.86. Aortic stenosis: left ventricular hypertrophy. Note the well-rounded bulging left cardiac border (arrows). This is characteristic of left ventricular hypertrophy. The aorta, in this patient, appears relatively normal.

to constitute a distinct syndrome, consisting of supravalvular aortic stenosis, other systemic and pulmonary vessel stenoses, mental retardation, and a peculiar, although distinctive, elfin facial appearance. All of these characteristics are believed to represent the sequelae of, or at least to be associated with, the infantile hypercalcemia (Williams) syndrome (1).

Hemodynamically, the basic abnormality in all types of aortic stenosis is obstruction to the flow of blood from the left ventricle. This obstruction results in systolic overloading and hypertrophy of the left ventricle and, in severe cases, enlargement of the left atrium. **Clinically, symptomatology is variable, but it generally is late in onset.** This does not mean that significant left outflow tract obstruction is absent in early life; rather, it reiterates the fact that the left side of the heart is able to tolerate considerable degrees of systolic overloading before decompensating.

Roentgenographically, **abnormal findings frequently are minimal or even absent.** The pulmonary vascularity is neither increased nor decreased, and the heart is of normal size. However, with time and with more severe lesions, left ventricular hypertrophy becomes more obvious (1). On the posteroanterior view, this results in increased convexity or prominence of the left cardiac border and a "firm" or "well-rounded" appearance to the left side of the heart (Fig. 3.86).

Prominence of the ascending aorta in patients with valvular aortic stenosis is another subtle, but extremely valuable, roentgenographic finding. It represents poststenotic dilatation and is best appreciated on the posteroanterior roentgenogram (Fig. 3.87). The aortic knob also may become prominent. Prominence of the ascending aorta results from the jet phenomenon associated with valvular stenosis. The constant hammering by the jet causes the aortic wall to dilate. This is vividly demonstrated angiographically where characteristic systolic doming of the valve and the jet of blood (contrast material) are seen (Fig. 3.88). Some of these features also can be seen with MRI (Fig. 3.89). The valve also may be thickened or dysplastic and, in some cases, bicuspid (Fig. 3.90) rather than tricuspid. The latter is commonly associated with coarctation of the aorta.

Poststenotic dilatation of the ascending aorta is absent in most cases of subvalvular and supravalvular aortic stenosis. Only occasionally will poststenotic dilatation of the aorta be seen in subvalvular stenosis, and in these cases, the obstructing lesion will be a subvalvular diaphragm. What occurs is that the jet through the diaphragm is directed through the center of the stenotic valvular orifice. Otherwise, there is no reason for the aorta to dilate in any form of subvalvular aortic stenosis. Consequently, although many of these cases show profound left ventricular hypertrophy, the aorta remains normal in size (Fig. 3.91A). In some cases, hypertrophy of the left ventricle is so pronounced that it produces a shoulder or bump along the upper left cardiac border.

Angiocardiographically, both forms of subvalvular aortic stenosis are readily demonstrable. When a membrane is seen cardioangiographically, it produces a radiolucent line in the opacified subaortic portion of the left ventricle (Fig. 3.91B). With hypertrophic subvalvular aortic stenosis, the

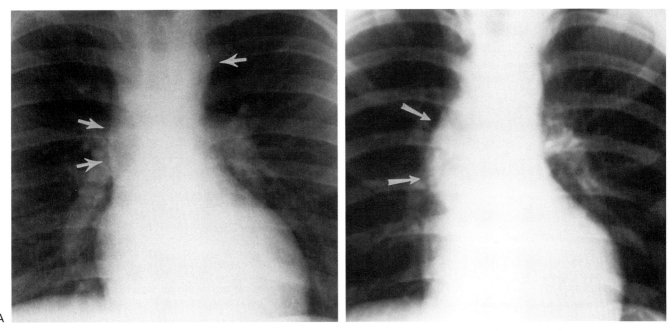

A

B

FIGURE 3.87. Aortic stenosis; prominence of the ascending aorta. A. In this patient, the ascending aorta and aortic knobs (arrows) are slightly prominent. There is mild left ventricular hypertrophy. **B.** In this patient, the ascending aorta (arrows) is much more prominent.

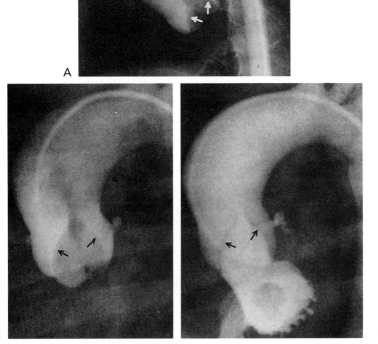

A

B,C

FIGURE 3.88. Valvular aortic stenosis: cardioangiography. A. Left anterooblique view, with injection into the aorta above the valve, demonstrates poststenotic dilatation of the ascending aorta and the stenotic domed aortic valve (arrows). Note also the radiolucent jet of unopacified blood passing through the valve into the ascending aorta, causing it to dilate. **B.** View of another patient with doming of the aortic valve (arrows) and a radiolucent jet. Note also dilatation of the ascending aorta. **C.** View of the same patient with injection below the aortic valve demonstrates the thin but domed valve (arrows).

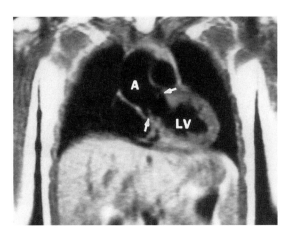

FIGURE 3.89. Aortic stenosis: magnetic resonance imaging. Note the dilated ascending aorta (A) and hypertrophied left ventricle (LV). The domed aortic valve leaflets are just visible (arrows).

typical findings consist of a funnel-shaped left ventricular cavity resulting from marked thickening of the interventricular septum and left ventricular myocardium (Fig. 3.91C).

In supravalvular aortic stenosis, since the supravalvular portion of the aorta is underdeveloped and stenotic, the aortic knob frequently is smaller than normal (Fig. 3.92A). Angiocardiographically, variable hypoplasia and often a fusiform constriction above the aortic valve are seen (Fig.

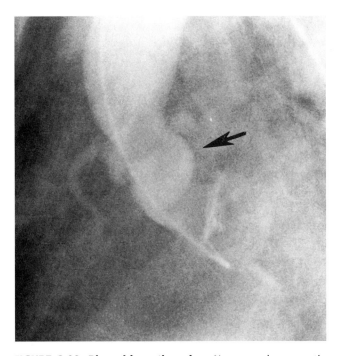

FIGURE 3.90. Bicuspid aortic valve. Note one large aortic valve cusp (arrow), with a smaller cusp seen opposite it. This is typical of a bicuspid aortic valve.

3.92B). MRI also can be employed to demonstrate some of the foregoing abnormalities.

Aortic Insufficiency

Isolated congenital aortic insufficiency is an extremely rare lesion, but when it is present, marked dilatation and enlargement of the left ventricle and ascending aorta occur. Both structures dilate and enlarge as a result of volume overloading. Specifically, the left ventricle is overloaded in diastole and the aorta in systole. This exemplifies a phenomenon seen with all insufficient valves; that is, the chamber proximal and distal to the involved valve shows dilatation and enlargement. In effect, in a to-and-fro manner, an excessive volume of blood is regurgitated into the proximal chamber and then propelled back into the distal chamber. Roentgenographically, left ventricular dilatation and aortic enlargement are best appreciated on the posteroanterior roentgenogram (Fig. 3.93A), and angiocardiographically, aortic insufficiency is demonstrated with supravalvular aortic injections of contrast material (Fig. 3.93B) in the left anterooblique position.

Coarctation of the Aorta

There are two types of coarctation of the aorta, but the most frequently encountered type is the juxtaductal variety. In this type, previously known as the adult type, the area of coarctation is located at, or just distal to, the left subclavian artery and ductus arteriosus and usually is short and discrete. In the rarer second type, the area of narrowing lies proximal to the ductus arteriosus, somewhere between it and the left subclavian artery. This type is referred to as "preductal," "isthmic," or "infantile coarctation" and, in contrast to the juxtaductal variety, usually consists of a long segment of narrowing. In addition, a ventricular septal defect often is present, and a patent ductus arteriosus always is present. Blood is delivered to the descending aorta from the pulmonary artery through the latter structure.

Hemodynamically, in the juxtaductal variety, aortic narrowing results in systolic overloading and hypertrophy of the left ventricle. Prestenotic and poststenotic dilatation of the aorta occurs, and there is progressive development of a collateral circulation. The usual arteries affected include the intercostal (usually T4 through T8), internal mammary, and those around the scapula. Development of a collateral circulation is important, for it supplies blood to the systemic circulation below the level of coarctation. In other cases, even more collaterals develop in the mediastinum, and the resulting leash of vessels can be very extensive and impressive.

In the preductal or isthmic type, the hemodynamics are somewhat different. Left ventricular systolic overloading is still a prominent feature, but since a ventricular septal defect often also is present, an associated left-to-right shunt

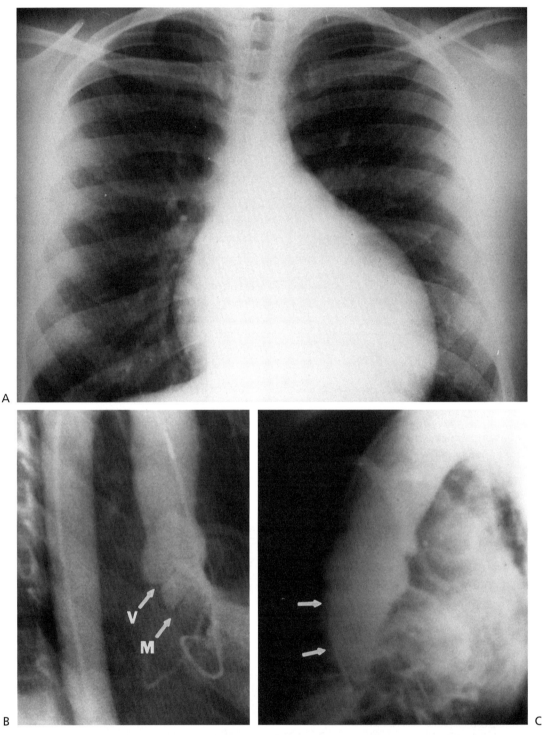

FIGURE 3.91. Subvalvular aortic stenosis. A. Note marked left ventricular hypertrophy caus-ing a well-rounded, prominently bulging left cardiac border. However, as opposed to valvular aortic stenosis, the ascending aorta and the aortic knob are not enlarged. In fact, the aorta may be a little small. The pulmonary vasculature is normal. **B.** Membranous stenosis. Note the thin membrane (M) below the normal aortic valve cusps (V). **C.** Typical cone-shaped left ventricular cavity (arrows) in subvalvular muscular hypertrophy.

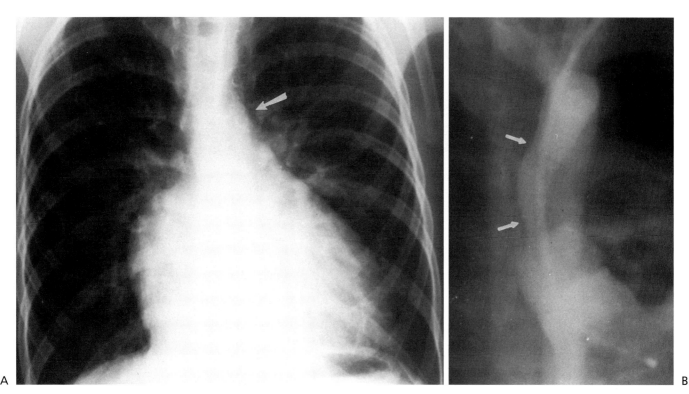

FIGURE 3.92. Supravalvular aortic stenosis. A. Note the small aortic knob (arrow). Not all patients with supravalvular aortic stenosis demonstrate this finding, but many do. In addition, note that the heart is enlarged. This patient had an associated atrial septal defect and peripheral pulmonary artery coarctations. **B.** Angiogram demonstrates marked narrowing of the supravalvular portion of the aorta (arrows). The aortic valve (V) is located about an inch below the narrowed portion of the aorta.

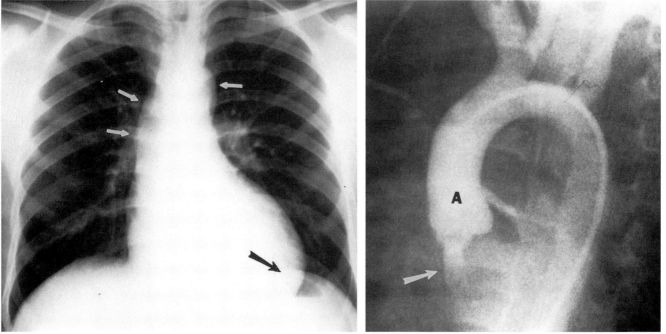

FIGURE 3.93. Aortic insufficiency. A. Posteroanterior view in older patient, with left ventricular dilatation causing the cardiac apex to point downward (black arrow). Also note prominence of the ascending aorta and aortic knob (white arrows). **B.** Supravalvular aortic injection in same patient shows regurgitation of contrast material into the left ventricle (arrow). A, aorta.

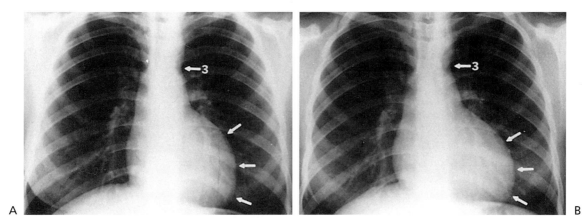

FIGURE 3.94. Coarctation of aorta: juxtaductal type. A. Note the well-rounded appearance of the left cardiac border resulting from left ventricular hypertrophy (lower arrows). The pulmonary vascularity is normal, and there is minimal suggestion of a figure 3 sign (upper arrow). **B.** Another patient with similar findings but with more pronounced fullness of the left cardiac border (lower arrows). Upper arrow indicates the presence of a figure 3 sign.

develops and, together with the obstructing coarctation, leads to marked overloading of the heart and cardiomegaly along with congestion. A collateral circulation is not so critical in these patients, since blood is delivered to the descending aorta through the patent ductus arteriosus.

However, since this blood is unoxygenated, the lower half of the body is cyanotic.

Early congestive heart failure also occurs in infants with juxtaductal coarctation of the aorta when it is associated with either a ventricular septal defect or a patent ductus

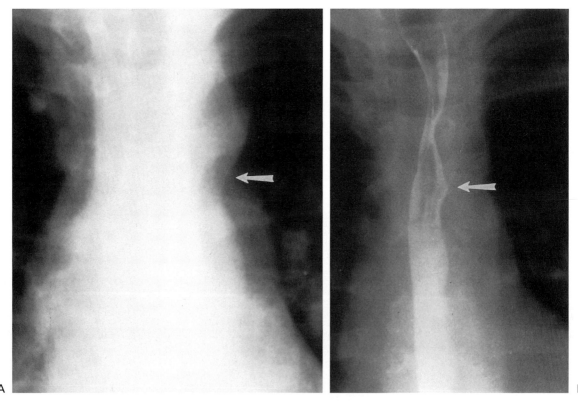

FIGURE 3.95. Coarctation of aorta. A. "Figure 3" sign. Arrow indicates the center of the "3." The upper bulge represents prestenotic dilatation, while the lower bulge represents poststenotic dilatation. **B. "Figure E" sign.** Arrow indicates the middle of the "E." The curve above represents prestenotic dilatation, while the curve below represents poststenotic dilatation.

arteriosus. In such cases, left-to-right shunting through either of these communications results in an added overload (volume) on the left side of the heart. It is this added overload that is the cause of early failure in these patients, and in this regard, the problem is similar to that in infantile coarctation of the aorta.

Roentgenographically, cardiac findings in patients with juxtaductal coarctation of the aorta are similar to those in patients with aortic stenosis. In early and in mild cases, the findings are normal or barely noticeable. Eventually, however, some bulging or prominence of the left cardiac border becomes apparent, and the well-rounded appearance of left ventricular hypertrophy is seen (Fig. 3.94). Definite pre- and poststenotic dilatation of the aorta is not present in all patients, but when present produces a figure 3 sign on the posteroanterior roentgenogram (Figs. 3.94 and 3.95) and a reverse figure 3, or a figure E, sign on the barium esopha-

gram (Fig. 3.95B). The proximal bulge represents dilatation of the proximal aorta and base of the left subclavian artery, while the distal bulge represents poststenotic dilatation of the aorta.

Other findings, commonly seen in coarctation of the aorta, are a prominent descending aorta and rib notching. Widening of the descending aorta is due to more extensive poststenotic dilatation (Fig. 3.96). Rib notching, usually involving the posterior fourth to eighth ribs, while frequently present in older patients (Fig. 3.97), is uncommonly seen in patients under the age of 4 or 5, since this length of time is required to produce pressure erosion by the progressively dilating and pulsating collateral vessels. Retrosternal notching (dilated mammary artery) also is occasionally seen in these patients, as is scapular notching. It also has been noted that, after surgical correction of coarctation of the aorta, rib notching can regress (2).

The roentgenographic findings in infants with the infantile type of coarctation and juxtaductal coarctation associ-

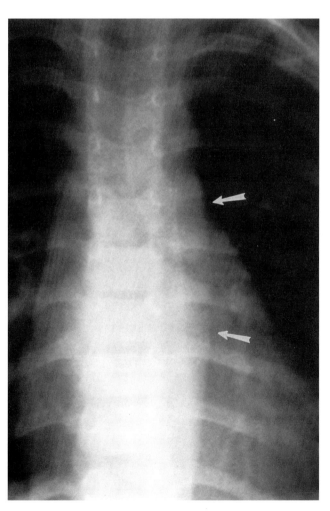

FIGURE 3.96. Coarctation of aorta: juxtaductal type with prominent descending aorta. Note prominent descending aorta (arrows).

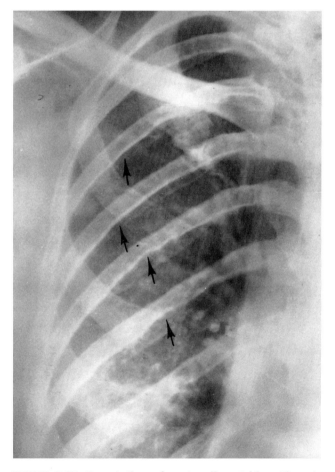

FIGURE 3.97. Coarctation of aorta: rib notching. There is notching of the posterior fourth to eighth ribs (arrows). Notches are also seen at sites other than those indicated by the arrows.

ated with left-to-right shunting through a ventricular septal defect or a patent ductus arteriosus are different from those seen in juxtaductal coarctation without a left-to-right shunt. As opposed to the findings in these latter patients, nonspecific oval cardiac enlargement, rather than left ventricular hypertrophy, is seen. Passive congestion due to car-

diac failure is present, and overall the findings resemble those of the hypoplastic left heart syndrome.

Angiocardiographically, in coarctation of the aorta, the findings consist of demonstration of the area of narrowing, collateral circulation, and the frequently associated and often stenotic bicuspid aortic valve. In juxtaductal coarcta-

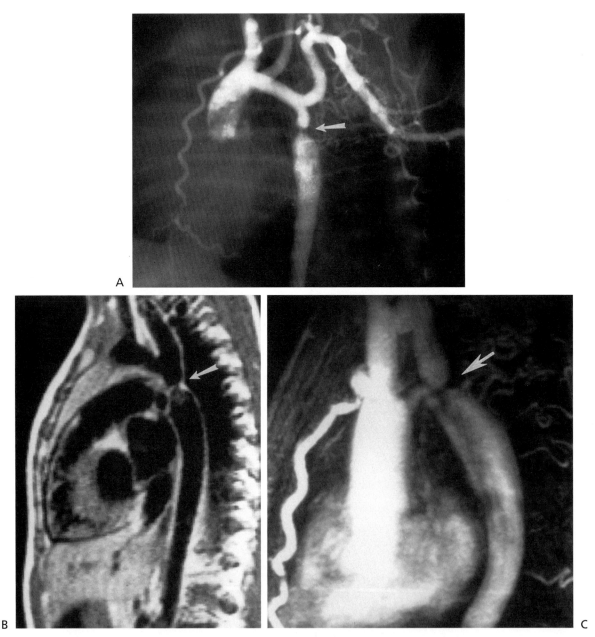

FIGURE 3.98. Coarctation of the aorta. A. Cardioangiography. Note the discrete area of severe coarctation (arrow), just distal to the large and prominent left subclavian artery. The aortic arch is hypoplastic, and collaterals have already been established. Note specifically the tortuous internal mammary coursing in front of the aortic arch. **B. Magnetic resonance imaging.** Left anterooblique view demonstrates discrete stenosis (arrow) of the aorta. The aortic arch proximally is a little hypoplastic, and the left subclavian artery, just above the coarctation, is large and dilated. Note poststenotic dilatation of the descending aorta, similar to that seen in **A. C. Magnetic resonance angiography.** Note the area of coarctation (arrow), the hypoplastic arch proximal to this area, and a large internal mammary artery coursing tortuously behind the sternum.

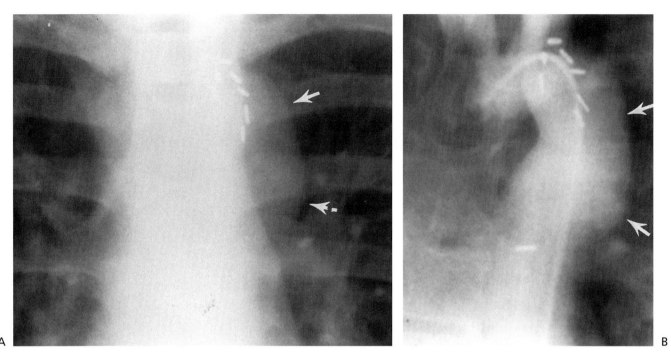

FIGURE 3.99. Coarctation of the aorta: postangioplasty patch dilatation. A. Note the bulge (arrows) of the patch angioplasty. Telltale metal clips are seen in the area. **B.** Aortogram demonstrates the dilated patch (arrows). Usually, these focal dilatations are of no particular consequence.

tion, the area of narrowing is relatively discrete (Fig. 3.98A) and usually best visualized in the left anterooblique position. Collateral circulation is variable, and the bicuspid aortic valve is identified by visualization of only two cusps, one being overlarge (see Fig. 3.90). MRI and MR angiography (3, 4), however, now are the modalities of choice for demonstrating coarctation, for they vividly demonstrate the lesion in all planes, but most clearly in the left anterooblique plane (Fig. 3.98, B and C). Postoperatively, if the coarctation is repaired with a patch, the patch may dilate and produce a mediastinal bump (5) (Fig. 3.99).

In preductal or isthmic coarctation, there is pronounced narrowing of the aortic arch, proximal to the ductal region. This lesion closely resembles interrupted aortic arch, discussed in the next section. Hypoplasia of the preductal portion of the aorta also occurs with juxtaductal coarctation (Fig. 3.98A), but to a lesser degree.

Pseudocoarctation of Aorta

In pseudocoarctation of the aorta, the aortic arch is tortuous, dilated, and kinked, and in many cases, plain film findings suggest true coarctation (Fig. 3.100). However, since no pressure gradient across the area of kinking is noted, the term "pseudocoarctation" is applied to the condition (6). Clues to its proper diagnosis lie in the facts that the figure 3 sign often is extremely well demarcated and that the aortic knob is higher in position than in true coarctation of the aorta. However, these differences are subjective, and generally the condition is not definitely diagnosed until cardiac catheterization and aortography, CT angiography, or MRI is performed (Fig. 3.100).

Interrupted Aortic Arch

Congenital interruption of the aortic arch is an uncommon lesion (7) and usually presents with symptoms similar to those of preductal or isthmic coarctation of the aorta. Anatomically, a variable length of aortic arch is absent or atretic, and blood is delivered to the descending aorta through a patent ductus arteriosus. The area of atretic aortic arch can be located distal to the left subclavian artery, distal to the left common carotid artery, or between the left common carotid and innominate arteries. Roentgenographically, the plain film findings are difficult to differentiate from coarctation of the aorta presenting in infancy and the hypoplastic left heart syndrome. Cardiomegaly is rather nonspecific, and vascular congestion is mixed; that is, both active and passive but most often the passive component predominates (Fig. 3.101A). In addition, the pulmonary artery often is large and higher in position than is expected (Fig. 3.101A). Cardioangiography can demonstrate the exact site of interruption (Fig. 3.101B), the large pulmonary artery, the mandatory shunting ductus (2), and, in some cases, a congenital subclavian steal syndrome (Fig. 3.101, C and D).

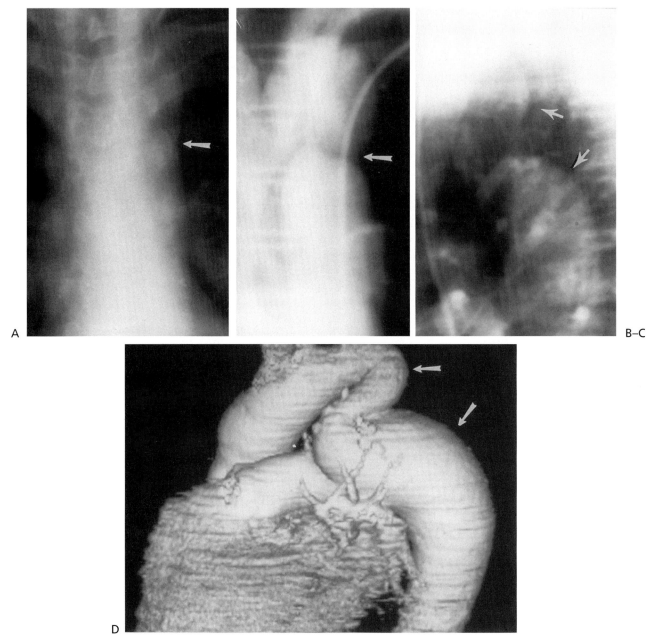

FIGURE 3.100. Pseudocoarctation (kinking) of the aorta. A. Frontal view demonstrates an unusually prominent figure 3 sign (arrow) and a large aortic knob, which is higher in position than normal. **B.** Aortogram demonstrating the same findings. **C.** Oblique aortogram demonstrates the large tortuous aorta and typical kinking (arrows). **D.** Three-dimensional computed tomography in another patient demonstrates the tortuous aorta (arrows).

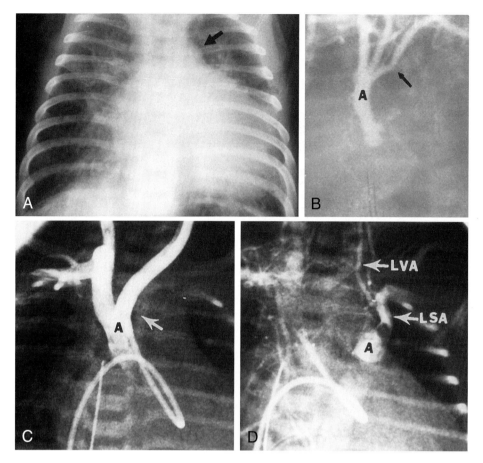

FIGURE 3.101. Interrupted aortic arch. A. Plain film demonstrates marked, nonspecific cardiomegaly and profound congestive heart failure. Note the prominent pulmonary artery (arrow), which is somewhat high in position. **B.** Another patient whose aortogram demonstrates the ascending aorta (A) and interruption of the hypoplastic arch just at the takeoff (arrow) of the subclavian artery. The innominate and left common carotid arteries are present. **C.** Another patient with interruption (arrow) just distal to the left common carotid artery. A, aortic arch. The innominate artery also is present. **D.** Same patient, later phase, demonstrates retrograde filling of the left subclavian artery (LSA) via the left vertebral artery (LVA), constituting a congenital subclavian steal syndrome. A, descending aorta.

Hypoplastic Left Heart Syndrome

The hypoplastic left heart syndrome encompasses a variety of cardiac lesions, all of which have in common some degree of underdevelopment of the left side of the heart (8). In the most marked cases, severe stenosis or atresia of the aortic and mitral valves is present, and the left atrium, left ventricle, and ascending aorta show marked underdevelopment. In other cases, only the aortic valve is atretic. In these cases, the left ventricle still is small and thickened, but the left atrium may be normal or enlarged. Premature closure of the foramen ovale (9) is a condition producing severe findings similar to the hypoplastic left heart syndrome.

Hemodynamically, all cases show severe impairment of blood flow from the left side of the heart, which also is underdeveloped. Such underdevelopment predisposes to shunting of blood from the left to the right atrium through a persistent atrial septal defect. The blood then passes to the right ventricle and out an enlarged pulmonary artery. Blood reaches the aorta through a patent ductus arteriosus; thus,

this structure is extremely important for the maintenance of the systemic circulation.

Symptoms in the hypoplastic left heart syndrome manifest early, and often there is congestive heart failure in the immediate neonatal period. In fact, the hypoplastic left heart syndrome probably is the most common cause of congestive heart failure in the first day or two of life. In addition, because of systemic hypoperfusion, these patients also are mildly cyanotic or ashen gray and, as such, tend to mimic infants with neonatal sepsis. This should not be a surprise, for infants with sepsis also are underprofused owing to the presence of septic shock.

Roentgenographically, the findings are variable, and in the early hours of life, many of these infants show a normal heart and normal pulmonary vascularity. However, within a few hours, and certainly by the end of a day or two, cardiomegaly and vascular congestion become apparent. Often, the heart is oval (Fig. 3.102A), a configuration that results from a combination of right atrial and right ventricular enlargement. In some cases, right atrial enlargement can be pronounced (Fig. 3.102B). The underdeveloped

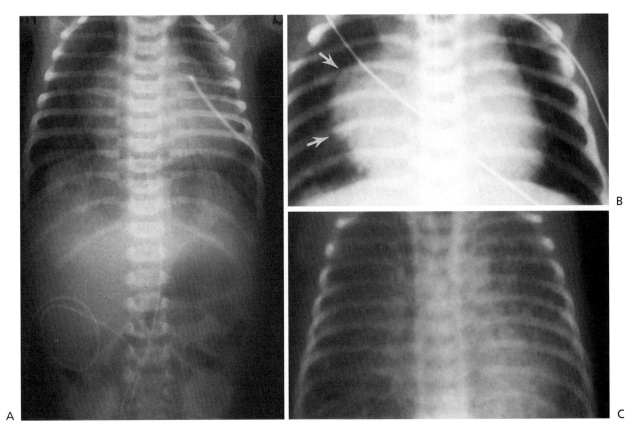

FIGURE 3.102. Hypoplastic left heart syndrome: plain film findings. A. Note nonspecific cardiomegaly and considerable passive congestion of the lungs. Also note that the liver is enlarged. **B.** In this infant, some passive congestion is present along with cardiomegaly, but the right atrium (arrows) is quite prominent. **C.** In this patient, note the extremely dense, reticular lungs consistent with passive congestion and pronounced pulmonary edema. The heart is slightly enlarged.

aorta is small or virtually nonexistent (atretic), but often this is difficult to determine from plain films alone. The pattern of pulmonary vascular congestion in these patients is passive, and in other cases, dilatation of the small pulmonary veins and lymphatics results in a very wet, reticular appearance of the lungs (Fig. 3.102, C and D).

In the hypoplastic left heart syndrome, ultrasonography and cardioangiography can identify the specific valves and chambers affected. On cardioangiography, with injection into the left atrium via the foramen ovale, the examiner can see the atretic mitral valve (Fig. 3.103A). Similarly, retrograde injection into the aortic arch can demonstrate a small aorta and aortic atresia (Fig. 3.103B). In addition, on pulmonary artery injection, the usually rather large patent ductus arteriosus, passing from the pulmonary artery to the aorta, can be identified (Fig. 3.103C). Congenital mitral stenosis can be considered under the broad umbrella of the hypoplastic left heart syndrome. It is, however, an uncommon lesion, and its clini-

cal and roentgenographic findings are similar to those of acquired mitral stenosis.

Congenital Mitral Insufficiency

As an isolated anomaly, congenital mitral insufficiency is an extremely rare lesion (7). When it is encountered, there are marked left atrial and left ventricular enlargement and passive congestion of the pulmonary vascularity. Angiocardiography and ultrasound demonstrate dilatation of the left ventricle and regurgitation of contrast material through a dilated mitral annulus into the large left atrium.

Insufficiency of the mitral valve also occurs with **mitral valve prolapse.** Prolapse of the posterior, anterior, or both leaflets of the mitral valve occurs as a congenital heredofamilial lesion. Most frequently, it is seen in young females, but it also is seen in patients with Marfan's syndrome.

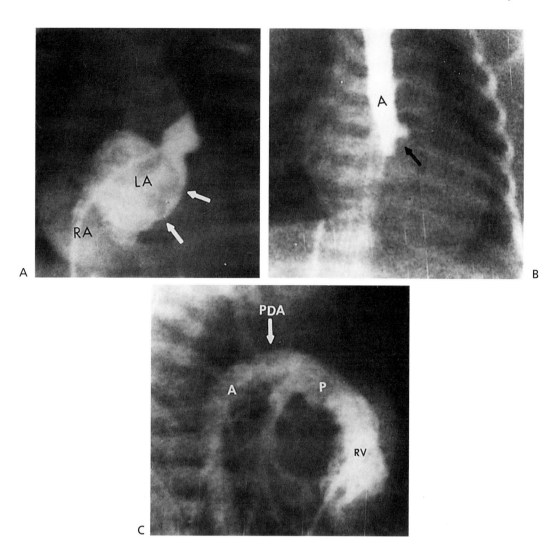

FIGURE 3.103. Hypoplastic left heart syndrome: cardioangiographic findings. A. Mitral atresia with atretic mitral valve (arrows). Contrast material has not passed to the left ventricle. The catheter has passed into the left atrium (LA) through the foramen ovale. RA, right atrium. **B.** Retrograde injection into the ascending aorta (A) of another patient demonstrates the dimple (arrow) of the atretic aortic valve. **C.** Lateral view in the same patient demonstrates the right ventricle (RV), pulmonary artery (P), and patent ductus arteriosus (PDA) communicating with the descending aorta (A).

Cor Triatriatum

Cor triatriatum is a rare anomaly with **abnormal hemodynamics similar to those of congenital mitral stenosis.** The difference is anatomic, in that an extra chamber is present proximal to the left atrium. Embryologically, it represents persistence of the common pulmonary vein and into it drain the normal pulmonary veins. Blood then passes to the true left atrium, but its flow is obstructed by a perforated membrane separating the left atrium from this chamber (10). Symptoms are similar to those of congenital mitral stenosis, and roentgenographically, the

main difference is absence of left atrial enlargement. In addition, passive congestion may be profound (Fig. 3.104, A and B). The membrane itself can be demonstrated angiocardiographically (Fig. 3.104C) or with ultrasound (Fig. 3.104D).

Aberrant or Anomalous Left Coronary Artery

In aberrant or anomalous left coronary artery, which is a relatively rare condition, the left coronary artery arises from

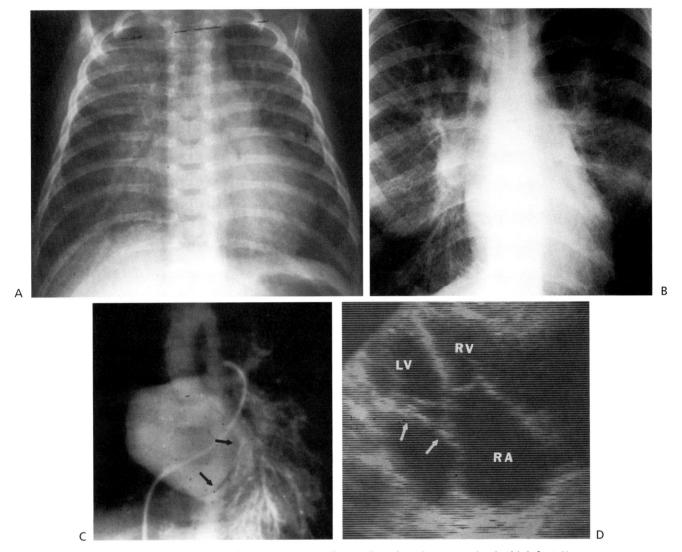

FIGURE 3.104. Cor triatriatum. A. Note cardiomegaly and passive congestion in this infant. No specific identifying features are seen. **B.** In this 15-year-old boy, the heart is normal, but there is extensive passive congestion of the lungs. **C.** Cardioangiogram in another patient demonstrates the typical prevalvular membrane (arrows) in the left atrium. **D. Ultrasonogram of cor triatriatum.** Note the membrane (M) just proximal to the mitral valve. LV, left ventricle; RV, right ventricle; RA, right atrium.

the pulmonary artery. Hemodynamically, the changes are dependent on whether a collateral circulation between the coronary arteries is established. In the initial stages, collateral circulation usually is minimal, no significant left-to-right shunt is present, and the presentation is early in infancy with congestive heart failure (Fig. 3.105A) and electrocardiographic abnormalities suggesting anterolateral myocardial schemia or infarction. Later, however, if a greater collateral circulation is established, a significant left-to-right shunt develops, and a pattern of active pulmonary vascular congestion becomes superimposed. In effect, these

patients have a coronary artery fistula, and angiocardiography usually is required to substantiate the diagnosis (Fig. 3.104, B and C). Ultrasound also can demonstrate the fistula.

REFERENCES

1. Beuren AJ, Schulze C, Eberle P, et al. The syndrome of supravalvular aortic stenosis, peripheral pulmonary stenosis, mental retardation and similar facial appearance. Am J Cardiol 1964;13:471–483.

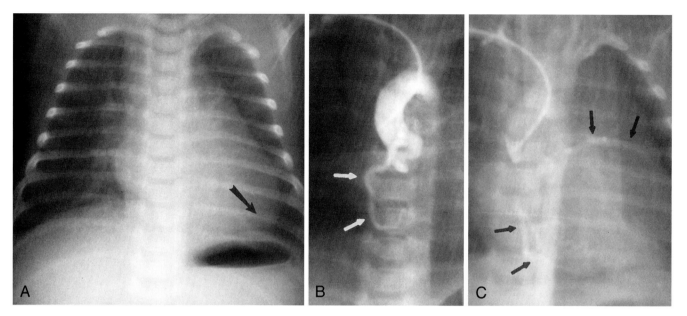

FIGURE 3.105. Aberrant left coronary artery. A. Note passive congestion, cardiomegaly, and a downward-dipping cardiac apex (arrow) signifying the presence of left ventricular dilatation. **B.** Early-phase aortogram demonstrates a large tortuous right coronary artery (arrows). **C.** Later film demonstrates further filling of the distal branches of the right coronary artery (lower arrows). The left coronary artery (upper arrows) arises aberrantly from the pulmonary artery (i.e., the low-pressure circulation) and fills in retrograde fashion from the right coronary artery, which arises normally from the high-pressure systemic circulation. In this way, a left-to-right shunt results.

2. Gooding CA, Glickman MG, Suydam MJ. Fate of rib notching after correction of aortic coarctation. AJR 1969;106: 21–23.

3. Nyman R, Hallberg M, Sunnegardh J, et al. Magnetic resonance imaging and angiography for the assessment of coarctation of the aorta. Acta Radiol 1989;30:481–485.

4. von Schulthess CK, Higashino SM, Higgins SS, et al. Coarctation of the aorta: MR imaging. Radiology 1986;158: 469–474.

5. Swischuk LE, Alexander A, Hayden CK, et al. Postoperative lumps and bumps in congenital heart disease: their significance. Perspect Radiol 1990;3:45–52.

6. Hoeffel JC, Henry M, Mentgre B, et al. Pseudocoarctation or congenital kinking of the aorta: radiologic considerations. Am Heart J 1975;89:428–436.

7. Neye-Bock S, Fellows KE. Aortic arch interruption in infancy: radio- and angiographic features. AJR 1980;135:1005–1010.

8. Deely WJ, Ehlers KH, Levin AR, et al. Hypoplastic left heart syndrome: anatomic, physiologic and therapeutic considerations. Am J Dis Child 1971;121:168–175.

9. Naeye RL, Blanc WA. Prenatal narrowing or closure of the foramen ovale. Circulation 1964;30:736–742.

10. Mortensson W. Radiologic diagnosis of cor triatriatum in infants. Pediatr Radiol 1973;1:92–95.

CARDIAC MALPOSITIONS

Dextrocardia, Dextroversion, and Mesoversion

Dextrocardia, as discussed here, deals with primary cardiac malposition rather than dextroposition of the heart resulting from some mediastinal shifting thoracic abnormality. Dextrocardia is a complex subject, and a simplified approach is presented in Table 3.5. In the assessment of type of dextrocardia, it is of extreme importance to determine abdominal situs, that is, whether it is situs inversus or situs solitus. This usually is readily appreciated on the posteroanterior roentgenogram and, once determined, allows further differentiation of the various types of cardiac malposition.

The most common type of dextrocardia is so-called "mirror image dextrocardia." In these cases, the cardiac apex points to the right, and there is complete inversion of the cardiac chambers. In other words, the left atrium and ventricle become right sided, and the right atrium

TABLE 3.5. CARDIAC MALPOSITIONS

GENERAL RULES:

1. Right atrium is usually on the same side as the liver.
2. Right atrium usually receives blood from the inferior vena cava.
3. Right atrium is usually opposite the gastric bubble.
4. Left atrium is usually opposite the liver.
5. Right ventricle is markedly trabeculated and has an infundibulum.
6. Left ventricle is smooth walled and has no infundibulum.
7. Ventricular inversion means anatomic right ventricle becomes left sided and anatomic left ventricle becomes right sided.

8. (a) The primitive tubular heart can bend to the right (D-loop—Fig. A1) or, more rarely, to the left (L-loop—Fig. A2). With D-loop bending, the ventricles are not inverted, while with L-loop bending, they are inverted.

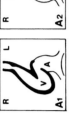

   (b) If bending is to the same side as the liver and right atrium, it is termed concordant, while if it is opposite, it is termed discordant.
   (c) In situs solitus, D-loop bending is concordant (i.e., normal heart), while L-loop bending is discordant (i.e., corrected transposition).
   (d) In situs inversus, D-loop bending is discordant, while L-loop bending is concordant.
   (e) Great vessel transposition, usually congenitally corrected, is present with discordant D- or L-loops.

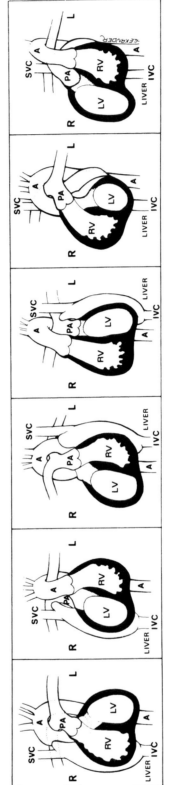

| | NORMAL | CORRECTED TRANSPOSITION | SITUS INVERSUS (Dextrocardia) | | SITUS SOLITUS (Dextroversion) | |
			COMMON FORM (Mirror Image)	LESS COMMON FORM	COMMON FORM	LESS COMMON FORM
	CONCORDANT D-LOOP	DISCORDANT L-LOOP	CONCORDANT L-LOOP	DISCORDANT D-LOOP	CONCORDANT D-LOOP	DISCORDANT L-LOOP
	Situs solitus	Situs solitus	(Type IIA)	(Type IIB)	(Type IA)	(Type IB)
	Ventricles not inverted	Ventricles inverted	Ventricles inverted	Ventricles not inverted	Ventricles not inverted	Ventricles inverted
	Great vessels not transposed	Great vessels transposed	Great vessels not transposed	Great vessels transposed	Great vessels usually not transposed	Great vessels transposed

ASPLENIA and POLYSPLENIA SYNDROMES:

Cardiac malposition often present. Situs often indeterminate. Liver midline. Stomach bubble variable. Complex cardiac anomalies.

V, ventricle; A, aorta; SVC, superior vena cava; PA, pulmonary artery; RV, right ventricle; LV, left ventricle; IVC, inferior vena cava.

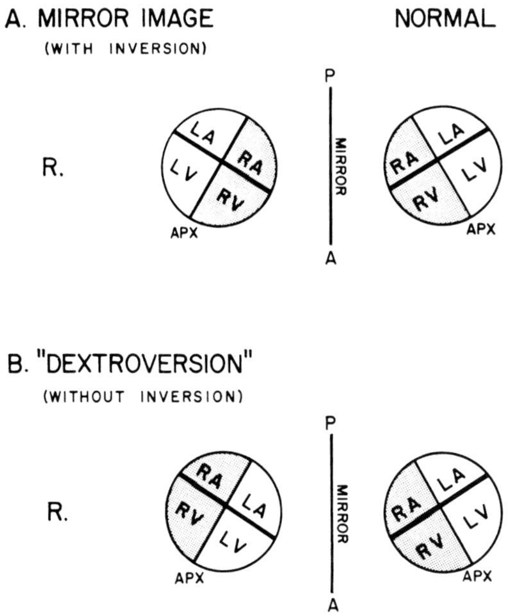

A. MIRROR IMAGE   NORMAL
(WITH INVERSION)

R.

B. "DEXTROVERSION"
(WITHOUT INVERSION)

R.

FIGURE 3.106. Dextropositions. A. Mirror image dextrocardia. There is inversion of the cardiac chambers: That is, the left ventricle (LV) is on the right, and the right ventricle (RV) in on the left. However, the left ventricle is still posterior, while the right ventricle is anterior. APX, apex; LA, left atrium; RA, right atrium. **B.** In dextroversion, there is no chamber inversion, but marked right-sided rotation of the heart places the right chambers posterior. APX, apex; LA, left atrium; LV, left ventricle; RA, right atrium; RV, right ventricle. (Reproduced with permission from Nadas AS. Pediatric cardiology. 2nd ed. Philadelphia: Saunders, 1964).

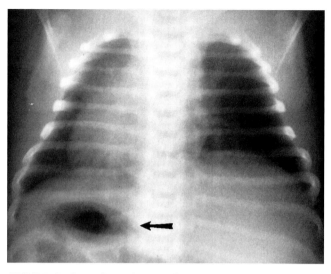

FIGURE 3.107. Mirror image dextrocardia. Note that the entire heart lies to the right of the spine. The gastric bubble (arrow) also is on the right, and the liver is on the left.

and ventricle become left sided (Fig. 3.106A). Normal anteroposterior chamber relationships, however, are preserved. Situs inversus is always present, but generally, there is no increased incidence of congenital heart disease (Fig. 3.107).

The next most common type of cardiac dextroposition is referred to as "dextroversion." For the sake of simplicity, this condition can be thought of as extreme right-sided rotation of the heart. As a result, the cardiac chambers lose their normal anteroposterior relationships, but chamber inversion does not occur. In other words, the right atrium and ventricle, as they rotate to the right, become more posterior but remain on the right, while the left atrium and ventricle become anterior but remain on the left (Fig. 3.106B). Situs inversus may or may not be present (Fig. 3.108), but associated cyanotic congenital heart disease is common. Other cases of cardiac malposition come under the category of mesocardia, perhaps more properly termed "mesoversion." In these cases, the heart lies halfway between normal levoposition and abnormal dextroposition and can be consid-

ered incompletely dextroverted. In other words, there is only partial right-sided rotation of the heart; consequently, the apex, instead of pointing to the right, points anteriorly (Fig. 3.109).

Finally, there are the somewhat related asplenia (Ivemark) and polysplenia syndromes, which usually present in the neonatal period. Serious and complicated congenital heart lesions are the rule, including problems such as pulmonary atresia, transposition of the great vessels, total anomalous pulmonary venous return, single ventricle, and aortic atresia. Systemic venous abnormalities such as persistent left superior vena cava and azygos continuation of the inferior vena cava are common, especially in the polysplenia syndrome. In terms of localization of the spleen in these patients, it may be difficult to determine whether the spleen is truly absent or multiple, and in this regard, nuclear scintigraphy and ultrasonography are helpful.

Numerous other visceral abnormalities exist in these patients, but only a few are noted here. The liver often is midline or near midline, the stomach midline and small (microgastria), and the intestines malrotated. In addition, the lungs are abnormally lobated, and in asplenia, both lungs usually have three lobes and result in bilateral right lungs. In polysplenia, bilateral bilobed or left lungs occur. Howell-Jolly bodies are seen in the peripheral red blood cells of infants with asplenia (1) and occasionally in patients with polysplenia. Finally, biliary atresia (2), horseshoe adrenal gland (3), polycystic kidneys (4), Kartagener's syn-

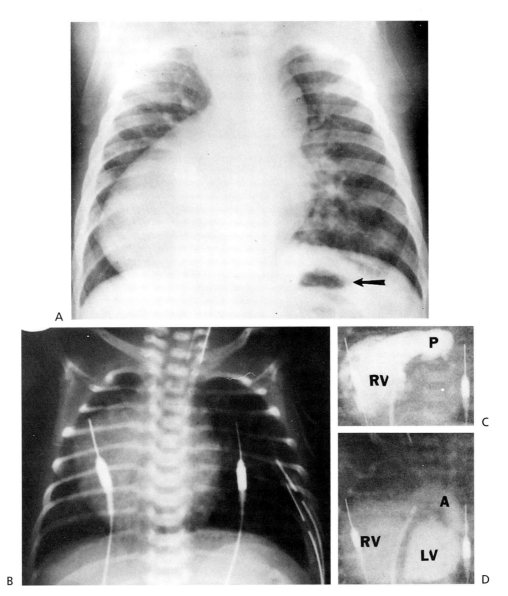

FIGURE 3.108. Dextroversion. A. In this patient, the cardiac apex points to the right, while the gastric bubble is on the left: situs solitus (arrow). The cardiac configuration is bizarre, and complex cyanotic congenital heart disease was present. The patient was cyanotic. **B.** Another patient with dextroversion and typical plain film findings. **C.** Cardioangiogram with injection into the right ventricle (RV) demonstrates how the right ventricle is rotated to the right. P, pulmonary artery. **D.** Slightly later phase demonstrates the position of both the right ventricle (RV) and the left ventricle (LV). The radiolucent septum lies between them. A, aorta.

drome (5), and intestinal malrotation (6) have been found in association with these syndromes.

In both asplenia and polysplenia syndromes, cardiac configurations often are bizarre, since serious and complex congenital anomalies exist. Many times, the pulmonary vascularity is severely diminished because of some form of right outflow tract obstruction. In addition, evidence of a midline liver or a small midline stomach also is present (Fig. 3.110). As for the lungs, even though bilateral right-side lungs (Fig. 3.111A) have been demonstrated in asplenia and bilateral left-side lungs have been demonstrated in polysplenia, these findings often are difficult to detect on plain films in infants. Exact delineation of the underlying cardiac abnormality and associated abnormalities is best accomplished with angiocardiography, MRI, or even CT (Figs. 3.111–3.113).

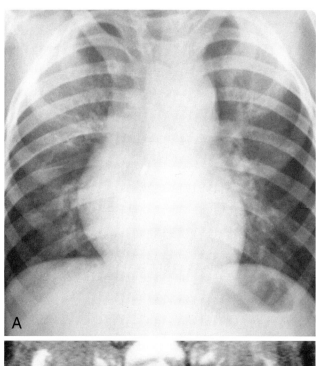

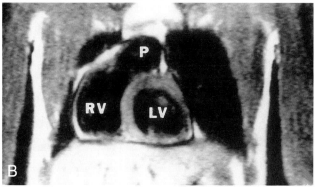

FIGURE 3.109. Mesocardia. A. The heart is incompletely rotated to the right. Right atrial enlargement may erroneously be suggested. **B.** Another patient whose coronal magnetic resonance image demonstrates the position of the right ventricle (RV) and the pulmonary artery (P). LV, left ventricle.

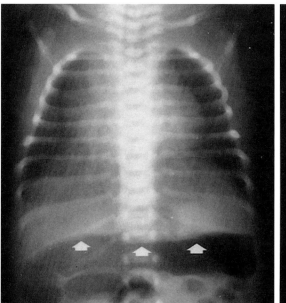

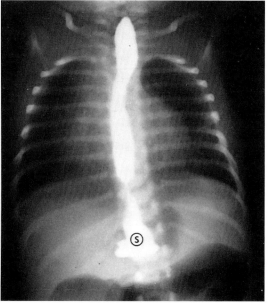

FIGURE 3.110. Polysplenia syndrome. A. First note the midline liver (arrows). Then note that the heart is a little enlarged and the vascularity is slightly congested. **B.** Barium swallow shows a small (microgastria) midline stomach (S).

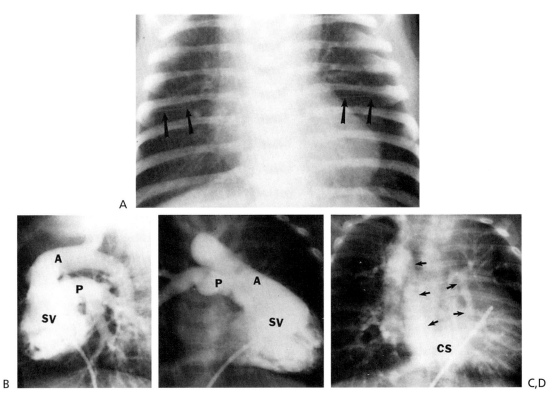

FIGURE 3.111. Asplenia syndrome. A. Note the bilateral minor fissures (arrows). The other cardiac findings are not particularly remarkable, but the vascularity is a little prominent. The liver was midline. **B. Cardioangiogram of another patient with suspected asplenia syndrome.** This lateral view demonstrates a single ventricle (SV) and a transposed aorta (A) and pulmonary artery (P). **C.** Frontal view with injection into the single ventricle (SV) demonstrates the congenitally corrected "L-transposition" configuration of the aorta (A). Note also the position of the pulmonary artery (P). The great vessels are inverted. **D.** Venous phase, after a pulmonary artery injection, demonstrates bilateral abnormal-draining pulmonary veins (arrows) into the coronary sinus (CS), which constitutes type II total anomalous pulmonary venous return.

Situs Inversus with Levocardia

Situs inversus with levocardia is a rare condition in which there is situs inversus but persistent levocardia. Systemic venous abnormalities such as absence or abnormal positioning of the inferior vena cava often are present. In addition, other congenital heart lesions, often with right outflow tract obstruction, are not uncommonly associated.

REFERENCES

Cardiac Malpositions
1. Rodin AE, Sloane JA, Nghiem QX. Polysplenia with severe con-genital heart disease and Howell-Jolly bodies. Am J Clin Pathol 1972;58:127–134.
2. Abramson SJ, Berdon WE, Altman RP, et al. Biliary atresia and non-cardiac polysplenic syndrome: US and surgical considerations. Radiology 1987;163:377–379.
3. Ditchfield MR, Hutson JM. Intestinal rotational abnormalities in polysplenia and asplenia syndromes. Pediatr Radiol 1998;28:303–306.
4. Krull F, Schulze-Neick I, Luhmer I. Polycystic kidneys in Ivemark's syndrome. Acta Paediatr 1992;81:562–563.
5. Schidlow DV, Moriber S, Turtz MG, et al. Polysplenia and Kartagener syndromes in sibship: association with abnormal respiratory cilia. J Pediatr 1982;100:401–403.
6. Horgan JG, Lock JH, Cloffi-Ragan D. Horseshoe adrenal in Ivemark (asplenia) syndrome. J Ultrasound Med 1995;14:785–786.

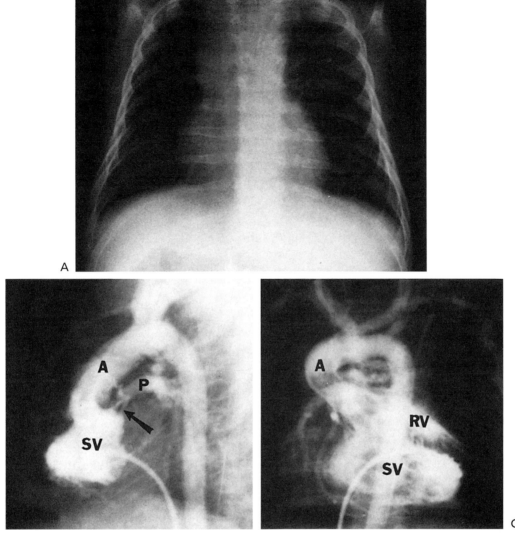

FIGURE 3.112. Polysplenia syndrome. A. Plain film demonstrates low normal pulmonary vascularity but a nonspecific cardiac configuration. Note the presence of a midline liver. **B.** Lateral view cardioangiogram demonstrates a single ventricle (SV), a transposed aorta (A), and a small, underdeveloped, and transposed pulmonary artery (P) with severe stenosis (arrow). **C.** Frontal view demonstrates the single ventricle (SV), the remaining rudimentary ventricle (RV), and the aorta (A). Although the ascending aorta is deviated to the right, it is not a right-sided aorta.

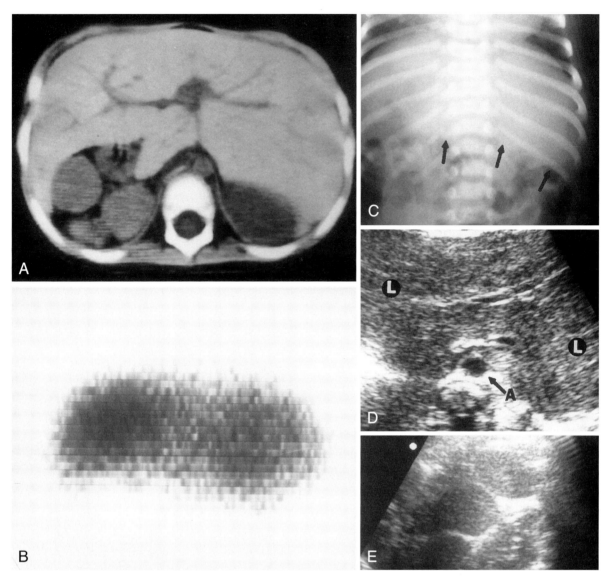

FIGURE 3.113. Polysplenia-asplenia syndromes: other imaging features. A. Computed tomography study of midline liver in polysplenia syndrome. Note the hepatic veins draining centrally. **B.** Another patient whose nuclear scintigraphy study demonstrates a midline liver. Same patient as in Fig. 3.110. **C.** This patient had asplenia and a midline liver that actually was more on the left than on the right (arrows). **D.** Subsequent transverse ultrasonogram demonstrates the liver (L) located in midline, and on the left, the aorta (A) is visualized, but there is no inferior vena cava. **E.** Ultrasonographic demonstration of multiple spleens.

VASCULAR RINGS AND OTHER ARTERIAL ABNORMALITIES

The term "vascular ring" is, at times, loosely used to include all anomalies of the aortic arch and great vessels, but, strictly speaking, it should be restricted to those entities in which actual encirclement of the trachea and esophagus occurs. For the most part, there are two true vascular rings: double aortic arch and right aortic arch with aberrant left subclavian artery and an encircling patent ductus arteriosus or ligamentum arteriosum. Other forms of vascular ring are extremely rare. In anomalies where a true ring is not present, symptoms may or may not occur and are dependent on the precise location of the anomalous vessel. In all cases where tracheal or bronchial compression occurs, wheezing, stridor, and overaeration can be seen. Concurrent esophageal compression leads to difficulty in feeding, regurgitation, choking, and aspiration pneumonia. Overall, however, respiratory symptoms predominate.

Initial demonstration and differentiation of the various vascular anomalies primarily is accomplished through the use of the chest film and the barium esophagram. In many cases, the underlying abnormality will become apparent from these studies alone. Indeed, it has been documented that if chest film findings are normal in patients who are symptomatic, a vascular ring is not likely to be present (1). After the plain film and barium esophagram, confirmation or acquisition of new data is usually relegated to MRI. A wide variety of vascular anomalies, both symptomatic and asymptomatic, are known to occur (Tables 3.6 and 3.7). However, before undertaking a discussion of these lesions, the right aortic arch itself needs to be addressed.

A right arch deviates the trachea and esophagus to the right (Fig. 3.114) and generally is readily detected on plain films. In this regard, there is absence of the normal left aortic knob silhouette and its replacement by a slightly higher bulge on the right. In addition, a slanted or oblique line running along the right paraspinal region is helpful in identifying a right aortic arch, when it then descends on the right (Fig. 3.114). Although all of these features are reason-

TABLE 3.6. VASCULAR ANOMALIES THAT PRODUCE NO SYMPTOMS

Anomalous (aberrant) right subclavian artery[a]
Right aortic arch, right descending aorta, mirror image branching[b]
Right aortic arch, right descending aorta, anomalous (aberrant) left subclavian artery[b]
Right aortic arch, left descending aorta[c]
Left aortic arch, right descending aorta[c]

[a]Most common.
[b]Next most common.
[c]Relatively rare.

TABLE 3.7. VASCULAR ANOMALIES THAT PRODUCE SYMPTOMS

Right or left double aortic arch[a]
Right aortic arch, right descending aorta, aberrant left subclavian artery, left ductus or ligamentum[a]
Left aortic arch, left descending aorta, aberrant right subclavian artery, right ductus or ligamentum[c]
Right aortic arch, left descending aorta, left ductus or ligamentum[c]
Left aortic arch, right descending aorta, right ductus or ligamentum[c]
Right aortic arch with isolated left subclavian artery (congenital subclavian steal)[c]
Anomalous innominate artery[b]
Anomalous left common carotid artery[c]
Vascular sling—aberrant left pulmonary artery[b]

[a]Most common.
[b]Next most common.
[c]Relatively rare.

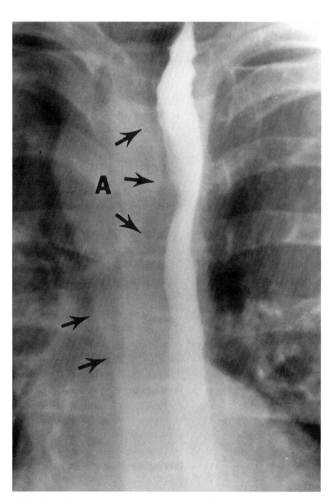

FIGURE 3.114. Right aortic arch. Note the right-side aorta (A) producing indentation and displacement (upper arrows) of the trachea and esophagus. Also note the slanted line below the aortic knob (lower arrows) representing the proximal portion of the descending aorta, which in this case is descending on the right.

ably easy to detect in the older child and adult, they often are more difficult to see in the neonate and young infant, especially when the trachea is not markedly displaced (2). This is especially prone to occur in young infants, and in these cases, it is worthwhile to obtain an inspiratory-expiratory view of the chest. With inspiration, the normal trachea moves to the right, and thus, if it remains fixed in the midline, an underlying right-side aortic arch should be suspected (Fig. 3.115, A and B). In addition, when the aorta is on the right and descends on the right, the latter finding can be seen to better advantage with slight rotation of the chest to the right (Fig. 3.115, C and D). High-voltage, selective filtration, and magnification techniques also are useful (3) but in most cases are not required.

When the aortic arch is right sided and descends on the right, the brachiocephalic vessels may originate in one of three ways: (a) mirror image branching, (b) aberrant left subclavian artery, and (c) isolated left subclavian artery. In

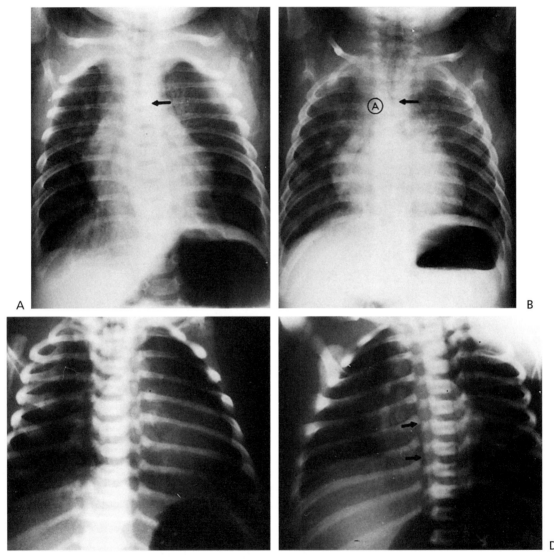

FIGURE 3.115. Right aortic arch: value of expiratory film. A. On this inspiratory view, note air trapping and a midline trachea (arrow). It would be difficult to determine whether a right-side aortic arch is present. **B.** Note, however, that with expiration, the trachea remains in the midline (arrow) and there is slight right-sided indentation resulting from a right aortic arch (A). Normally, the trachea should buckle to the right, but when a right aortic arch is present, it anchors the trachea in the midline. **C. Value of oblique film.** Frontal view with slight rotation to the left makes it difficult to determine whether a descending aorta is present on the right. **D.** Note, however, with obliquity to the right, how clearly the right-side descending aorta is seen (arrows). In normal individuals, of course, such a line is not seen, either on the frontal view or with obliquity to the right.

the latter case, the subclavian artery receives blood from the left vertebral artery via a "congenital subclavian steal," and finally when a right aortic arch descends in the midline, it can compress the left main bronchus and carina between itself and the left pulmonary artery, leading to obstruction of these structures (4). In addition, with any compressive vascular anomaly, underlying tracheomalacia or a frank stenotic area can be encountered.

ASYMPTOMATIC VASCULAR ANOMALIES

Anomalous or Aberrant Right Subclavian Artery

Anomalous or aberrant right subclavian artery is the most common vascular anomaly of all and most frequently is noted as an incidental finding during an upper gastrointestinal examination for some other reason. Anatomically, the aberrant right subclavian artery arises from a point just

distal to the left subclavian artery and, to reach the right upper extremity, must course across the mediastinum (Fig. 3.116, A and B). When it does so, it passes behind the esophagus to produce a characteristic oblique posterior esophageal indentation from lower left to upper right (Fig. 3.116, C and D). The configuration is characteristic, and further investigation is not necessary. Aberrant right subclavian artery rarely produces symptoms, although occasionally dysphagia (dysphagia lusoria) is said to occur. We have seen one such patient (Fig. 3.117).

Right Aortic Arch with Right Descending Aorta and Mirror Image Branching

Right aortic arch with right descending aorta and mirror image branching is one of the few aortic arch anomalies frequently associated with congenital heart disease. Tetralogy of Fallot is most common, and the plain film and esophagram findings are confined to those of a right-sided aortic

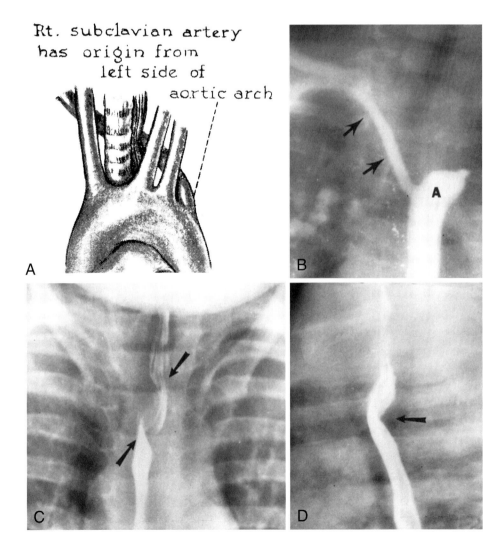

FIGURE 3.116. Aberrant right subclavian artery. A. The aberrant right subclavian artery arises as the most distal branch on the aortic arch and extends across the mediastinum behind the esophagus. **B.** Aortogram with injection into the descending aorta (A) demonstrates the characteristic course of the aberrant right subclavian artery (arrows). **C.** Note the characteristic oblique indentation of the esophagus (arrows) on frontal view. **D.** Lateral view demonstrates the typical finger-like, somewhat oblique indentation of the posterior aspect of the esophagus (arrow). (**A** reproduced with permission from Gross RE. The surgery of infancy and childhood. Philadelphia: Saunders, 1953).

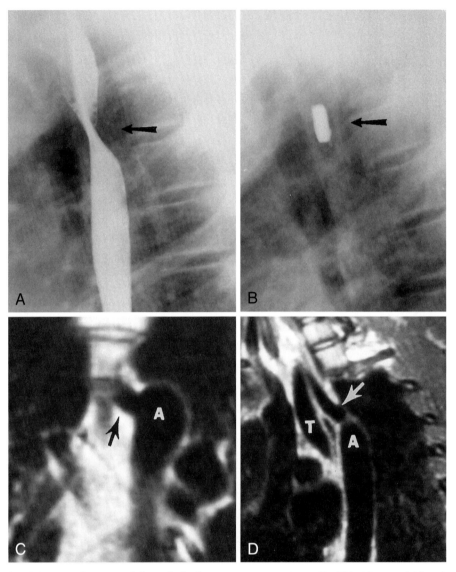

FIGURE 3.117. Aberrant right subclavian artery: symptomatic. This 15-year-old boy had symptoms of dysphagia all his life. In some instances with food lodging in the esophagus, respiratory compromise occurred. **A.** Typical oblique indentation on the posterior esophagus (arrow). **B.** Barium tablet (arrow) fails to pass the area of indentation. The tablet did not pass with multiple boluses of water. **C.** Coronal magnetic resonance imaging study demonstrates the descending aorta (A) and the aberrant right subclavian artery (arrow). **D.** Right anterooblique magnetic resonance imaging study. Note the descending aorta (A) and the aberrant right subclavian artery (arrow) passing posterior to the trachea (T) and esophagus. There is a small amount of air in the esophagus lying between the trachea and the aberrant left subclavian artery.

arch and right descending aorta. There is mirror image branching of the brachiocephalic vessels (Fig. 3.118), and posterior indentation of the esophagus is not seen. This arrangement of the brachiocephalic vessels generally is rather innocuous and only rarely associated with a vascular ring (5).

Right Aortic Arch and Right Descending Aorta with Aberrant Left Subclavian Artery

Right aortic arch and right descending aorta with aberrant left subclavian artery generally are not associated with con-

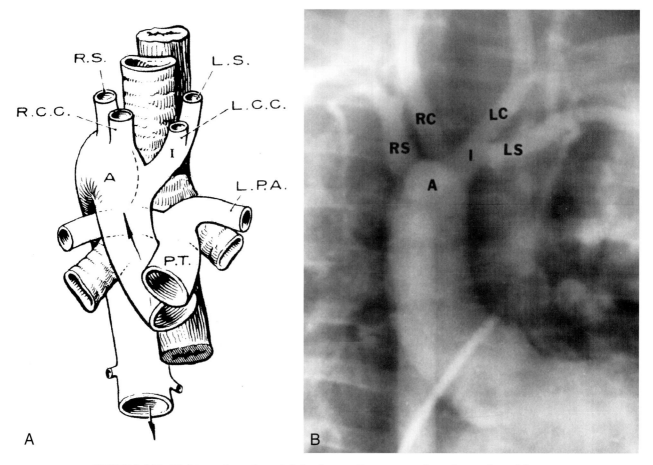

FIGURE 3.118. Right aortic arch and right descending aorta: mirror image branching. A. Diagrammatic representation. Note the aorta (A), innominate artery (I), right common carotid (R.C.C.), right subclavian (R.S.), left subclavian (L.S.), and left common carotid (L.C.C.) arteries. L.D., left ductus arteriosus; L.P.A., left pulmonary artery; P.T., pulmonary trunk. **B. Angiogram.** Note the right side aorta (A), mirror image branching of the left common carotid (LC), left subclavian (LS), and innominate (I) arteries. Also note the right common carotid (RC) and right subclavian (RS) arteries. (**A** reproduced with permission from Stewart JR et al. An atlas of vascular rings and related malformations of the aortic arch system. Springfield, IL: Thomas, 1964).

genital heart disease and can be considered the mirror image lesion of aberrant right subclavian artery with a normal left aortic arch (Fig. 3.119A). In these cases, the left subclavian artery originates as the most distal branch on the right aortic arch and to reach the left upper extremity must course across the mediastinum, posterior to the esophagus. There are no specific plain film findings, except for the right-sided arch and descending aorta, but the esophagram shows a characteristic oblique posterior indentation (Fig. 3.119B). The indentation is the mirror image of the indentation produced by an aberrant right subclavian artery.

Very often with an aberrant left subclavian artery, a diverticulum at the base of the artery is present (Fig. 3.119C). This is part of the anomaly and can be seen

whether the anomalous left subclavian artery exists alone or in association with a vascular ring. This diverticulum usually is referred to as the "diverticulum of Kommerell" (6) and can produce additional left-side esophageal indentation (7). Nonetheless, the diverticulum at the base of the aberrant left subclavian artery now is commonly referred to as a "Kommerell diverticulum."

Right or Left Aortic Arch with Contralateral Descending Aorta

In right or left aortic arch with contralateral descending aorta, there may be a right aortic arch with a left descending aorta or a left aortic arch with a right descending aorta.

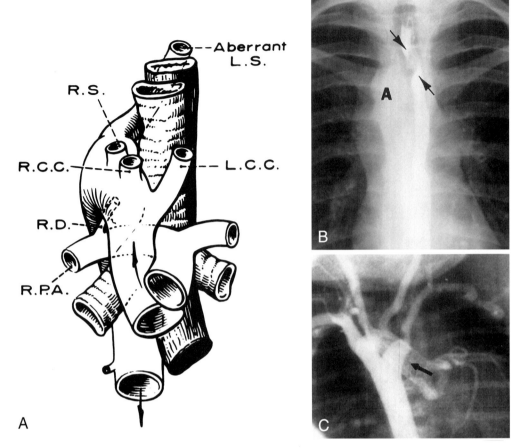

FIGURE 3.119. Right aortic arch, right descending aorta, and aberrant left subclavian artery. A. Diagrammatic representation. Note the aberrant left subclavian artery (L.S.) passing posterior to the esophagus. Also note the left common carotid (L.C.C.), right common carotid (R.C.C.), right pulmonary (R.P.A.), and right subclavian (R.S.) arteries. R.D., right ductus arteriosus. **B. Barium swallow.** Note the characteristic oblique indentation (arrows) on the posterior esophagus. A, aorta. **C.** Another patient with an aberrant left subclavian artery with a diverticulum of Kommerell (arrow) at its base. (**A** reproduced with permission from Stewart JR et al. An atlas of vascular rings and related malformations of the aortic arch system. Springfield, IL: Thomas, 1964).

In either case, a posterior indentation of the esophagus is produced, and little else is seen. The anomaly usually is asymptomatic and can readily be detected with angiography or MRI. Rarely, these patients may have persistence of the left or right ductus or ligamentum arteriosum and present with symptomatic vascular rings (2–4).

SYMPTOMATIC VASCULAR ANOMALIES

Double Aortic Arch

A double aortic arch always has a right-side aorta, an important plain film finding. Thereafter, as the arch splits, it encircles the trachea and esophagus and unites to form the descending aorta posterior to the esophagus (Fig. 3.120). In approximately 75% of these cases, the aorta eventually descends on the left, while in the remaining 25%, it remains on the right. In addition, most cases (80%) have a small anterior (left) arch and a large and higher posterior (right) arch. Focal tracheomalacia or actual stenosis of the trachea or bronchi also can co-exist.

On the posteroanterior roentgenogram, the right aortic arch usually is visible, but the smaller left arch may be a little more difficult to detect. In other cases, when it is visible, the two bulges representing the two aortic limbs can be seen. Thereafter, the barium esophagram provides the most useful information. Characteristically, a reverse S-shaped indentation of the esophagus is produced (Fig. 3.121, A

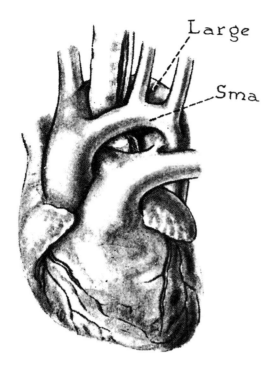

FIGURE 3.120. Double aorta and left descending aorta. Note the large (Large) posterior arch and the small (Sma) anterior arch. (Reproduced with permission from Gross RE. The surgery of infancy and childhood. Philadelphia: Saunders, 1953).

and B). The upper curve of the "S" is produced by the large posterior arch, while the lower curve is produced by the smaller anterior arch. This configuration is rather specific and usually is visible on all views. Aortography (Fig. 3.121C) and currently MRI (Fig. 3.122) clearly delineate the two arches.

Right Aortic Arch, Right Descending Aorta, Aberrant Left Subclavian Artery, and Left Ductus Arteriosus or Ligamentum

The presence of an encircling ductus arteriosus or ligamentum arteriosum will convert any asymptomatic vascular anomaly to a true vascular ring. Most commonly, this occurs with right aortic arch, a right descending aorta, and an aberrant left subclavian artery with a persistent left ductus arteriosus or ligamentum arteriosum (Fig. 3.123). The vascular ring in this condition is formed by the ascending right aortic arch, the left subclavian artery passing posterior to the esophagus, and the persistent ductus arteriosus or ligamentum arteriosus passing from the left subclavian artery to the left pulmonary artery. Since the pulmonary artery lies anterior to the trachea, a complete ring is formed. Occasionally, the ring can result in compression of the left bronchus to produce obstructive emphysema of the left lung (8).

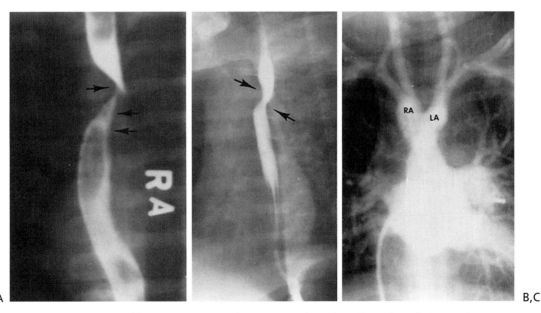

A   B,C

FIGURE 3.121. Double aorta. A. Note the reverse S-shaped configuration of the esophagus resulting from the larger posterior (right) arch (upper arrow) and the smaller anterior (left) arch (lower arrows). **B.** View of another patient demonstrates a similar esophageal configuration (arrows) on a left anterooblique view. **C.** Aortogram demonstrates the typical appearance of a double aortic arch. Note the slightly larger and higher right arch (RA) and the slightly lower and smaller left arch (LA).

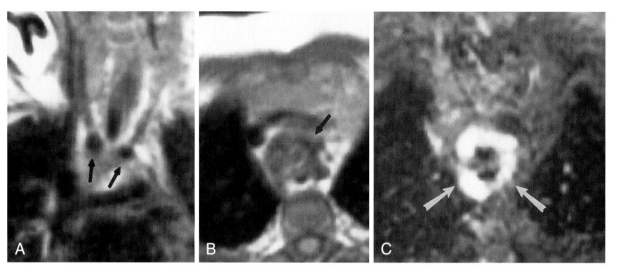

FIGURE 3.122. Double aortic arch: magnetic resonance imaging findings. A. Coronal view demonstrates the larger right and smaller left (arrows) branches of the double aortic arch. **B.** Axial view demonstrates the ring (arrow) surrounding the central trachea and esophagus behind it. **C.** Magnetic resonance angiography study more clearly demonstrates the encircling vascular ring (arrows).

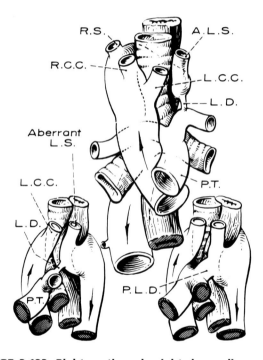

FIGURE 3.123. Right aortic arch, right descending aorta, aberrant left subclavian artery, and left ductus arteriosus. Note the right-sided aorta and aberrant left subclavian artery (A.L.S.) The left ductus arteriosus (L.D.) forms a ring by connecting the left pulmonary artery to the anomalous left subclavian artery. L.C.C., left common carotid artery; R.C.C., right common carotid artery; R.S., right subclavian artery; L.S., left subclavian artery; P.L.D., patent left ductus; P.T., pulmonary trunk. (Reproduced with permission from Stewart JR et al. An atlas of vascular rings and related malformations of the aortic arch system. Springfield, IL: Thomas, 1964).

The plain film and barium esophagram findings are similar, if not identical, to those seen with double aortic arch (Fig. 3.124). However, on aortography or MRI, the findings are different (Fig. 3.124). There will be a right-sided aortic arch, but then, the left subclavian artery, as it passes behind the esophagus, will be seen to be pulled and stretched to the left by the ductus arteriosus or ligamentum arteriosum (Fig. 3.124F). Most often, it is the ligamentum that is the problem, but this structure, as far as imaging is concerned, is invisible. Therefore, one must infer its presence by the stretched position of the aberrant left subclavian artery as it passes behind the esophagus (Fig. 3.124, C and D). In addition, as with double aortic arch, focal tracheomalacia or fixed tracheal stenosis (complete tracheal rings) can co-exist.

Isolated Left Subclavian Artery

An isolated left subclavian artery is relatively rare (Fig. 3.125) and usually asymptomatic in terms of producing stridor or dysphagia. However, since in this condition the left subclavian artery is atretic at its base, blood supply to the left upper extremity is somewhat tenuous and decreased pulses and ischemia of the extremity can occur. The isolated left subclavian artery receives blood from the aorta via retrograde flow through the ipsilateral vertebral artery (Fig. 3.126) and hence the term "congenital subclavian steal syndrome" (9, 10).

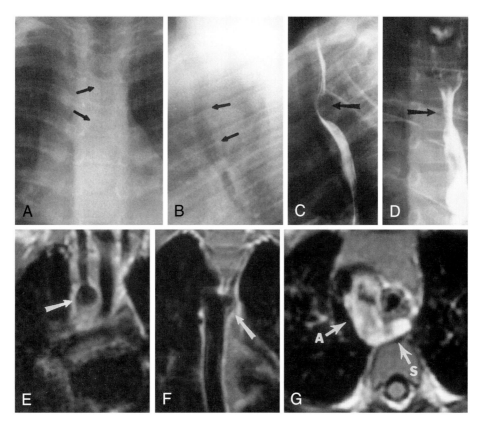

FIGURE 3.124. Right aortic arch, right descending aorta, aberrant left subclavian artery, and left ligamentum arteriosus. A. Note the right-side aortic arch producing displacement and indentation of the trachea (arrows). **B.** Lateral view demonstrates anterior displacement of the trachea (arrows). **C.** Lateral esophagram showing a pronounced posterior indentation (arrow). **D.** Frontal esophagram demonstrates bilateral opposing indentations (arrow). **E.** Coronal T1-weighted magnetic resonance study demonstrates the right aortic arch (arrow) indenting the trachea. It is giving rise to the right common carotid artery. **F.** Posterior coronal view demonstrates the takeoff (arrow) of the aberrant left subclavian artery. A small Kommerell diverticulum is present. **G.** Axial T1-weighted view with flow artifact enhancing visualization of the aorta (A) and aberrant left subclavian artery (S) passing behind and encircling the trachea and collapsed esophagus. The esophagus lies behind the trachea and is compressed.

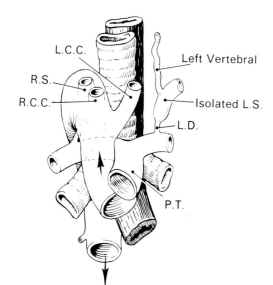

FIGURE 3.125. Right aortic arch with isolated left subclavian artery. Note that the aberrant, isolated left subclavian (L.S.) artery is completely isolated from the aorta. It receives its blood from the left vertebral artery. This results in the so-called "congenital subclavian steal syndrome" and ischemia of the left upper extremity. L.C.C., left common carotid artery; L.D., left ductus; P.T., pulmonary trunk; R.C.C., right common carotid artery; R.S., right subclavian artery

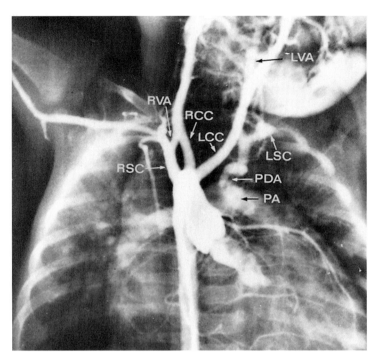

FIGURE 3.126. Right aortic arch, isolated left subclavian artery, and congenital left subclavian steal syndrome. Note the right-sided aortic arch, right subclavian (RSC), right vertebral (RVA), right common carotid (RCC), and left common carotid (LCC) arteries. The left vertebral artery (LVA) is filling retrogradely from the cranial circulation and is then delivering contrast material to the isolated left subclavian artery (LSC). This constitutes a congenital subclavian steal syndrome. There also is left-to-right shunting through the patent ductus arteriosus (PDA) to the pulmonary artery (PA). (Reproduced from Sunderland CO, Lees MH, Bonchek LI, et al. Congenital pulmonary artery—subclavian steal. J Pediatr 1972;81:927–931, with permission from C. V. Mosby, St. Louis, MO).

Isolated Right Subclavian Artery

Isolated right subclavian artery is a very rare anomaly but has been documented (11, 12). Findings in patients with this anomaly are similar to those in patients with isolated left subclavian artery, except that they exist in reverse.

Anomalous Innominate Artery and Anomalous Left Common Carotid Artery

Anomalous innominate artery and anomalous left common carotid artery are rather unique vascular abnormalities,

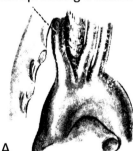

Innominate artery compressing trachea

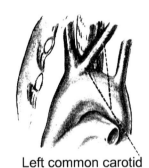

A

Left common carotid
B artery presses on trachea

FIGURE 3.127. A. Anomalous innominate artery. Note the anomalous innominate artery compressing the trachea. It originates too near the left common carotid artery. **B. Anomalous left common carotid artery.** The anomalous left common carotid artery compresses the trachea. It originates too near the innominate artery. (Reproduced with permission from Gross RE. The surgery of infancy and childhood. Philadelphia: Saunders, 1953).

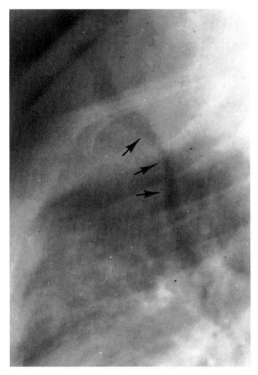

FIGURE 3.128. Anomalous left common carotid artery: lateral view. Note the marked posterior displacement and indentation of the trachea (arrows) at the level of the manubrium. This can result from either an anomalous left common carotid or innominate artery.

since they are the only ones that produce isolated anterior tracheal compression. In the former condition, the innominate artery arises from a point more distal than normal along the aortic arch, and in the latter condition, the left common carotid artery originates from a point more proximal than normal (Fig. 3.127). As these vessels cross the mediastinum to reach their respective destinations, they pass anterior to the trachea and, in so doing, compress the trachea. If the degree of tracheal compression is significant, symptoms in the form of respiratory distress, wheezing, stri-

dor, and occasionally difficulty in feeding become apparent. In a few cases, life-threatening apneic spells can occur.

The aortic arch in these cases is left sided, and tracheal indentation is always anterior. It is visualized on the lateral chest roentgenogram only and is best evaluated with the neck fully extended (Fig. 3.128). The degree of tracheal compression is dependent on the size, tautness, and exact position of the anomalous vessel. Aortography or MRI can identify either anomaly (Fig. 3.129), but currently, MRI is preferred. Indeed, with the use of MRI, it has been demon-

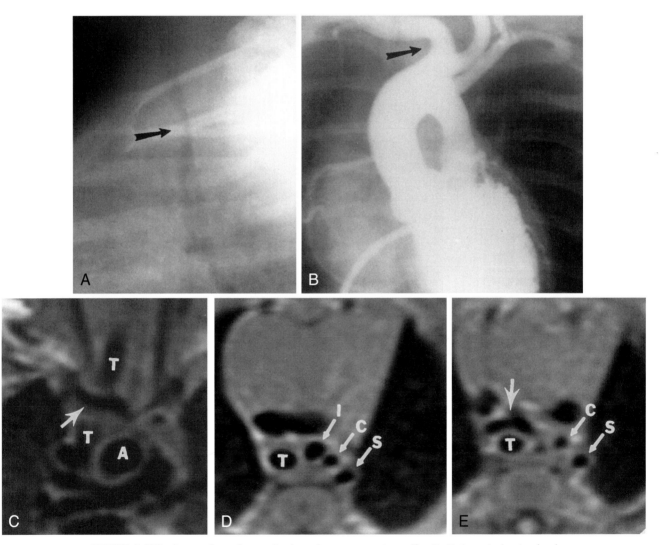

FIGURE 3.129. Anomalous innominate artery: asymptomatic. A. Note anterior tracheal indentation (arrow) in this asymptomatic infant. **B.** Arteriogram in another asymptomatic infant with a greater degree of anomalous origin of the innominate artery (arrow). **C.** Magnetic resonance study demonstrating an anomalous innominate artery (arrow) in another infant as it courses in front of the trachea (T). A, aorta. **D.** Axial view demonstrates the trachea (T), innominate artery (I), left common carotid artery (C), and left subclavian artery (S). The innominate vein is traveling in front of all of the mentioned structures. **E.** Slightly higher axial view demonstrates the anomalous innominate artery (arrow) traveling in front of the trachea (T). Note that the trachea is somewhat more oval (partially compressed) than in the previous figure. C, left common carotid artery; S, left subclavian artery.

strated that tracheomalacia or frank stenosis at the site of tracheal compression is present (13–15).

In terms of the symptoms in these patients, most are asymptomatic (16). In those with symptoms, it has been suggested that the small and crowded superior mediastinum of young infants results in compression of the trachea (17). In addition, the presence of normal thymus gland herniat-

ing into the thoracic inlet has been invoked in this crowding theory (18). In any case, close clinical correlation is necessary since it does appear that symptoms arise only when all of these factors become critical. Then, surgical intervention may be required. Otherwise, the finding of anterior tracheal indentation is of no particular consequence and with maturation tends to disappear (16, 17).

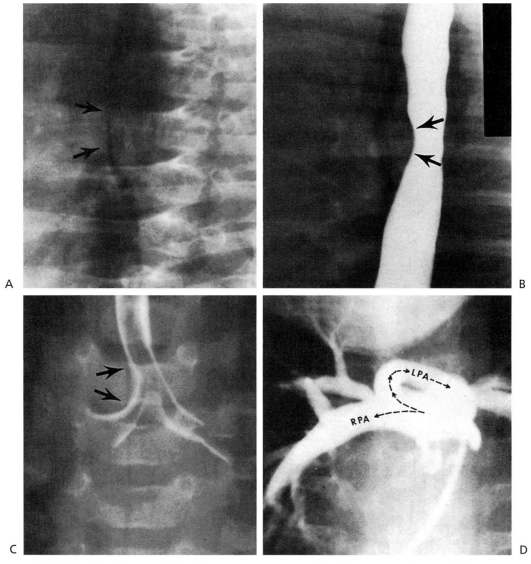

FIGURE 3.130. Aberrant left pulmonary artery: vascular sling. A. Note characteristic anterior displacement and indentation of the trachea produced by the aberrant left pulmonary artery (arrows). **B.** A corresponding indentation on the esophagus (arrows) is seen. **C.** Tracheogram demonstrates characteristic indentation of the trachea at the level of the carina (arrows). **D.** Pulmonary arteriogram, with angled view, demonstrates the course of the normal right pulmonary artery (RPA) and aberrant left pulmonary artery (LPA). The left pulmonary artery arises from the right pulmonary artery and circles around the trachea to produce the indentation seen in **C.** The artery must pass between the trachea and the esophagus to reach the left lung, resulting in the indentations seen in **A** and **B.** (Courtesy of Joe Jackson, M.D.).

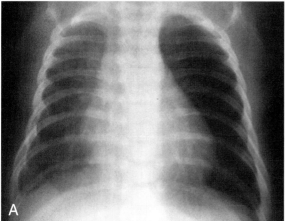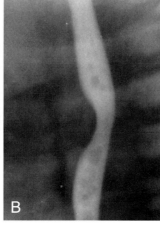

FIGURE 3.131. Aberrant left pulmonary artery and small right lung. A. Note that the right lung is clear but smaller than the left lung. **B.** Lateral view of the chest with barium in the esophagus demonstrates the characteristic tracheal and esophageal indentations of a pulmonary sling.

Vascular Sling or Aberrant Left Pulmonary Artery

Vascular sling, or aberrant left pulmonary artery, is a relatively rare vascular anomaly that is of special interest because of its unique effect on the trachea and esophagus. In this entity, the left pulmonary artery arises from the right pulmonary artery and, to reach the left lung, must cross the mediastinum. In doing so, it hooks around the carina just above the takeoff of the right bronchus (Fig. 3.130) and results in a variety of aeration disturbances of the right lung. The problem often takes the form of obstructive emphysema, but underaeration also can be seen. In addition, a small, probably hypoplastic right lung and pulmonary artery are seen in some patients (Fig. 3.131A). This finding may be more common than is generally appreciated.

After the aberrant left pulmonary artery hooks around the carina, it crosses the mediastinum between the esopha-

gus and the trachea. In so doing, it produces a characteristic indentation of the posterior aspect of the trachea just above the carina and a corresponding indentation of the anterior wall of the barium-filled esophagus (Figs. 3.130B and 3.131B). Aberrant left pulmonary artery is the only vascular anomaly to produce this configuration, but it is not necessarily clearly demonstrated in all patients. However, once seen, it is pathognomonic, and one should proceed with further imaging. In this regard, in the past, pulmonary arteriography (Fig. 3.130D) and CT were the imaging modalities used, but currently MRI (19, 20) is the modality of choice (Fig. 3.132).

A variation of the aberrant left pulmonary artery is the so-called "ring-sling" complex (21). In these cases, there is associated stenosis of the trachea (Fig. 3.133), resulting from complete cartilaginous rings. There may also be stenosis of the right bronchus, and again, hypoplasia of the right lung can occur. In addition, the anomaly known as "bridg-

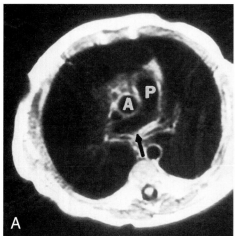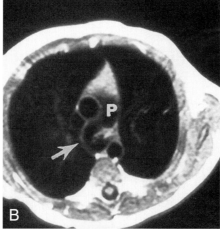

FIGURE 3.132. Aberrant left pulmonary artery: magnetic resonance imaging findings. A. Axial T1-weighted image demonstrates the main pulmonary artery (P) and right pulmonary artery branch (arrow). A, aorta. **B.** Note the aberrant left pulmonary artery first heading to the right and then encircling the trachea (arrow) as it passes posterior to the trachea and in front of the esophagus and descending aorta to supply the left lung. P, main pulmonary artery. (Courtesy of C. Keith Hayden, Jr., M.D.).

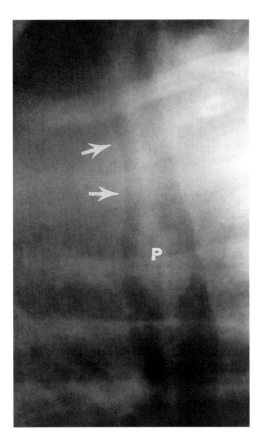

FIGURE 3.133. Ring-sling complex. Note tracheal stenosis (arrows), and then note the aberrant left pulmonary artery (P), between the trachea and esophagus. This anomaly has been termed the "ring-sling complex."

ing bronchus" also has been described with the ring-sling complex (22).

MISCELLANEOUS AORTIC ANOMALIES

Cervical Aortic Arch

Cervical aortic arch (circumflex aorta) is a relatively uncommon anomaly that results from an unusually high position of the aortic knob (Fig. 3.134A). Most often, it and the knuckle of the arch that protrudes into the base of the neck and causes a palpable, pulsatile mass (23). Aortography or MRI (Fig. 3.134, B and C) is necessary for identification of this lesion, but certain plain film findings can provide strong clues to its presence. For the most part, these consist of a high, right (usually) paratracheal mass or area of soft tissue prominence and deviation of the trachea to the left. On lateral view, anterior displacement of the trachea often is present, and with barium in the esophagus, a posterior indentation caused by the right aortic arch as it crosses the mediastinum to descend on the left is seen. The anomaly rarely is associated with a true vascular ring configuration (24).

REFERENCES

1. Pickhardt PJ, Siegel MJ, Gutierrez FR. Vascular rings in symptomatic children; frequency of chest radiographic findings. Radiology 1997;205:581–582.
2. Strife JL, Matsumoto J, Bisset GS III. The position of the trachea in infants and children with right aortic arch. Pediatr Radiol 1989;19:226–229.
3. Wolf EL, Berdon WE, Baker DH. Improved plain film diagnosis of right aortic arch anomalies: high kilovoltage selective filtration magnification technique. Pediatr Radiol 1978;7:141–146.
4. Donnelly LF, Bisset GS III, McDermott GS III, et al. Case report: anomalous midline location of the descending aorta: a cause of compression of the carina and left mainstem bronchus in infants. AJR 1995;164:705–707.
5. Schlesinger AE, Mendeloff E, Sharkey AM, et al. MR of right aortic arch with mirror image branching and a left ligamentum arteriosum: an unusual cause of a vascular ring. Pediatr Radiol 1995;25:455–457.
6. Kommerell B. Verlagerung des osophagus durch eine abnorm verlaufende arteria subclavia dextra (arteria lusoria). Fortschr Roentgenstr 1936;54:590–595.
7. Kleinman PK, Spevak MR, Nimkin K. Left-sided esophageal indentation in right aortic arch with aberrant left subclavian artery. Radiology 1994;191:565–567.
8. Pirtle T, Clarke E. Vascular ring: unusual cause of unilateral obstructive pulmonary hyperinflammation. AJR 1983;140:1111–1112.
9. Boroshok MJ, White RI Jr, Oh KS, et al. Congenital subclavian steal. AJR 1974;121:559–564.
10. Victorica BE, Van Mierop LHS, Elliott LP. Right aortic arch associated with congenital subclavian steal syndrome. AJR 1970;108:582–590.
11. Boroshok MJ, White RI Jr, Oh KS, et al. Congenital subclavian steal. AJR 1974;121:559–564.
12. Mathieson JR, Silver SF, Culham JAG. Case report. Isolation of the right subclavian artery. AJR 1988;151:781–782.
13. Fletcher BD, Cohn RC. Tracheal compression and the innominate artery: MR evaluation in infants. Radiology 1989;170:103–107.
14. Strife JL, Baumel AS. Tracheal compression by the innominate artery in infancy and childhood. Radiology 1981;139:73–75.
15. Vogl T, Wilimzig C, Hofmann U, et al. MRI in tracheal stenosis by innominate artery in children. Pediatr Radiol 1991;21:89–93.
16. Swischuk LE. Anterior tracheal indentation in infancy and early childhood: normal or abnormal? AJR 1971;112:12–17.
17. Berdon WD, Baker DH, Bordiuk J, et al. Innominate artery compression of trachea in infants with stridor and apnea. Radiology 1969;92:272–278.
18. Mandell GA, McNicholas KW, Padman R, et al. Innominate artery compression of the trachea: relationship to cervical herniation of the normal thymus. Radiology 1994;190:131–136.
19. Vogl TJ, Diebold T, Bergman C, et al. MRI in pre- and postoperative assessment of tracheal stenosis due to pulmonary artery sling. J Comput Assist Tomogr 1993;17:878–886.
20. Newman R, Meza MP, Towbin RB, et al. Left pulmonary artery sling: diagnosis and delineation of associated tracheobronchial anomalies with MR. Pediatr Radiol 1996;26:661–668.
21. Berdon WE, Baker DH, Wung J-T, et al. Complete cartilage ring tracheal stenosis associated with anomalous pulmonary artery: the ring-sling complex. Radiology 1984;152:57–64.
22. Wells TR, Stanley P, Pauda EM, et al. Serial section-reconstruc-

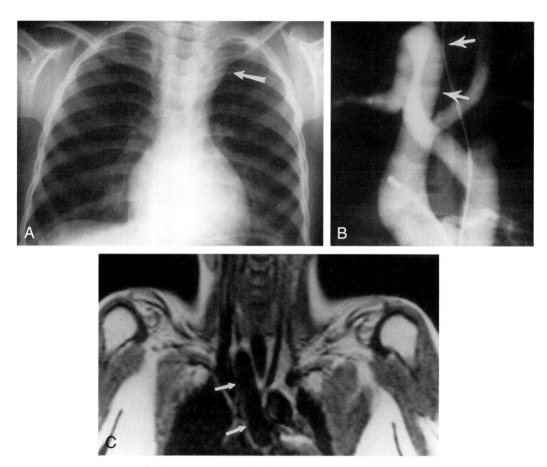

FIGURE 3.134. Cervical aorta. A. Note the high aortic knob on the left (arrow). **B.** Another patient with a high right cervical aorta (arrows) demonstrated with aortography. **C.** High right cervical aorta (arrows) demonstrated with magnetic resonance imaging.

tion of anomalous tracheobronchial branching patterns from CT scan images: bridging bronchus associated with sling left pulmonary artery. Pediatr Radiol 1990;20:444–446.

23. Shuford WH, Syvbers RG, Milledge RD, et al. The cervical aortic arch. AJR 1972;116:519–527.

24. McLeary MS, Fye LL, Young LW. Magnetic resonance imaging of a left circumflex aortic arch and aberrant right subclavian artery: the other vascular ring. Pediatr Radiol 1998;28: 263–265.

MISCELLANEOUS CONGENITAL CARDIAC PROBLEMS

Congenital Pericardial Defect

Congenital pericardial defect is a cardiac anomaly that rarely is appreciated because of its elusiveness on the plain film. In mild form, it probably is not recognized. Pericardial defects are much more common on the left than on the right, and of those occurring on the left, complete absence of the left pericardium is the most common (1). Fortunately, this particular anomaly is relatively benign and requires no specific treatment. Roentgenographically, the diagnosis of complete left pericardial defect might be suspected when there is a pronounced shift of the heart to the left. If the defect is partial, herniation of a portion of the heart, usually the left atrial appendage (2,3), occurs through the defect (Fig. 3.135).

REFERENCES

1. Tabakin BS, Hanso JS, Tapas JP, et al. Congenital absence of the left pericardium. AJR 1965;94:122–128.

2. Nogrady MB, Nemec J. Partial congenital pericardial defect in childhood: report of four cases. J Can Assoc Radiol 1970;21: 116–119.

3. Hoeffel JC, Henry M, Pernot C, et al. A new case of congenital partial pericardial defect with preoperative diagnosis. J Can Assoc Radiol 1973;24:261–264.

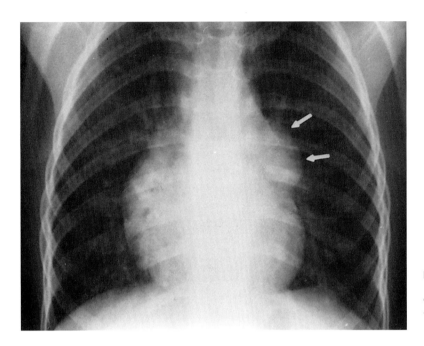

FIGURE 3.135. Partial left pericardial defect. Note the characteristic appearance of a partial pericardial defect through which the left atrial appendage has herniated (arrows). Surgically proven.

SUPERIOR AND INFERIOR VENA CAVA ABNORMALITIES

A number of vena caval abnormalities exist, and although most are mere curiosities, others can cause problems with differentiation from a mediastinal mass. One of the most common of these is idiopathic dilatation of the superior vena cava (1, 2), producing variable fullness of the right paratracheal region (Fig. 3.136). Persistence of the left superior vena cava (3) results in left-side widening of the superior mediastinum. Often, this widening mimics that caused by a normal thymus gland (Fig. 3.137). Persistence of the left superior vena cava can occur alone or in association with other congenital heart lesions.

Another interesting vena caval abnormality is that of intraabdominal interruption of the inferior vena cava and its

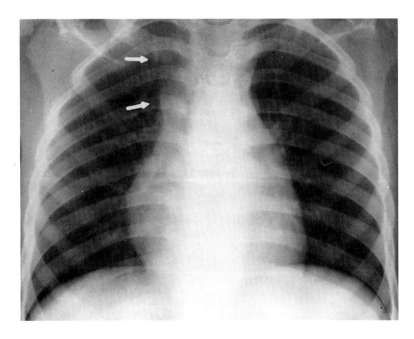

FIGURE 3.136. Prominent superior vena cava. Note prominence of the right paratracheal region (arrows) in this normal infant. The finding was the result of a dilated superior vena cava but could be confused with a mediastinal mass or prominent thymus gland.

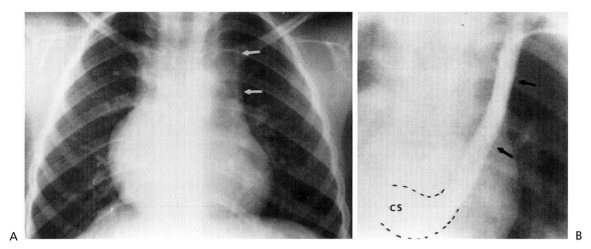

FIGURE 3.137. Persistent left superior vena cava. A. Note widening of the superior mediastinum and especially fullness along the left side (arrows). **B.** Venogram demonstrates the persistent left superior vena cava (arrows) draining into the coronary sinus (CS).

continuation into the azygos or, occasionally, hemiazygos vein in the chest (4). As with persistence of the left superior vena cava, this abnormality can be seen alone or in combination with other congenital heart lesions and is commonly associated with the polysplenia syndrome. On plain films, absence of the inferior vena cava (5) is manifest by loss of visualization of the inferior vena caval silhouette on lateral chest views and enlargement or prominence of the azygos vein on frontal pro-

jection (Fig. 3.138). If the interrupted inferior vena cava continues into the hemiazygos system, a similar superior mediastinal vascular prominence is seen on the left.

Angiography clearly can demonstrate these venous abnormalities (Fig. 3.139), and often they are found incidentally during cardiac catheterization. Ultrasonography, CT, and MRI also are useful in identifying these venous abnormalities.

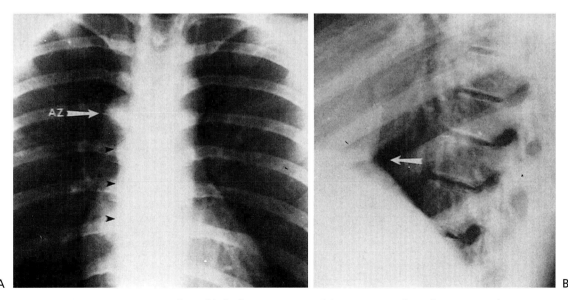

FIGURE 3.138. Interruption of inferior vena cava with azygos continuation. A. Note characteristic enlargement of the azygos vein (AZ) and the associated paraspinal stripe (arrowheads) resulting from continuation of the inferior vena cava into the azygos vein. **B.** Lateral view demonstrates the characteristic absence of the normal inferior vena caval silhouette just behind the lower heart border (arrow).

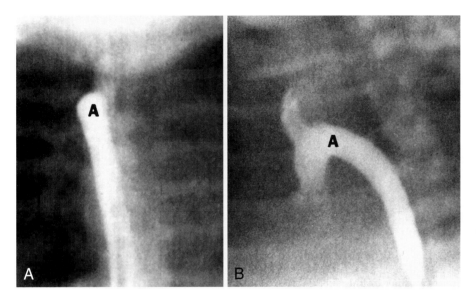

FIGURE 3.139. Azygos continuation of inferior vena cava. A. Interruption of the inferior vena cava results in its continuation into the azygos vein (A). **B.** Lateral view demonstrates typical appearance of this anomaly. A, azygos vein.

REFERENCES

1. Heil BJ, Felman AH, Talbert JL, et al. Idiopathic dilatation of the superior vena cava. J Pediatr Surg 1978;13:193.
2. Polansky S, Gooding CA, Potter B. Idiopathic dilatation of the superior vena cava. Pediatr Radiol 1974;21:67.
3. Cha EM, Khoury GH. Persistent left superior vena cava. Radiologic clinical significance. Radiology 1972;103:375–381.
4. Petersen RW. Infrahepatic interruption of inferior vena cava with azygos continuation (persistent right cardinal vein). Radiology 1965;84:304–307.
5. Berdon WE, Baker DH. Plain film findings in azygos continuation of the inferior vena cava. AJR 1968;104:452–457.

Levoposition of Right Atrial Appendage

The congenital levoposition of the right atrial appendage has been described with transposition of the great vessels (1). In this condition, instead of the right atrial appendage lying above and just slightly to the right of the right atrium proper, it lies to the left of midline and above the left atrial appendage. In so doing, it produces localized bulging just above the area of the normal left atrial appendage. In addition, there is decreased prominence of the right cardiac border. It is usually best demonstrated with angiocardiography.

REFERENCE

1. Tyrrell MJ, Moes CAF. Congenital levoposition of the right atrial appendage. Am J Dis Child 1971;121:508–510.

Cardiac Aneurysms and Diverticula

Congenital cardiac aneurysms or diverticula can occur in all cardiac chambers (1–4), but those of the ventricles are most common. Aneurysms also can be associated with midline thoracoabdominal defects (5). Cardiac diverticula or aneurysms may cause cardiac arrhythmias, and transventricular connections through the diverticula may produce intracardiac shunts. Cardiac diverticula can be delineated with ultrasonography or angiocardiography.

REFERENCES

1. Akkary S, Sahwi E, Kandil W. Congenital diverticulum of the left ventricle. J Pediatr Surg 1981;16:737–738.
2. Bandow GT, Rowe GG, Crummy AB. Congenital diverticulum of the right and left ventricles. Radiology 1975;117:19–20.
3. Hoeffel JC, Henry M, Pernot C. Heart diverticula in children: radiological aspects. Ann Radiol 1974;17:411–415.
4. Kadowaki MH, Berger S, Shermeta DW, et al. Congenital left atrial aneurysm in an infant. J Pediatr Surg 1989;24:306–308.
5. Gula G, Yacomb M. Syndrome of congenital ventricular diverticulum and midline thoraco-abdominal defects. Thorax 1977;3: 365–369.

Aneurysm of the Ductus Arteriosus

Spontaneous aneurysms of the ductus arteriosus occur primarily during the neonatal period (1), and fatal complications such as rupture and thromboembolic phenomena can occur. The etiology probably lies in aberrant closure of the ductus, and it is postulated that although normal closure at the pulmonary end occurs, the aortic end remains open or reopens. Consequently, blood from the aorta causes aneurysmal dilation of this remaining portion of the ductus arteriosus. Complications include pressure on the left recurrent laryngeal or phrenic nerve producing hoarseness and diaphragmatic leaflet paralysis (2), thromboemboli with peripheral arterial occlusive disease, and dissections with rupture. The abnormality might be suspected on plain films when an unusually large bulge is seen in the left upper mediastinum (3, 4). This is especially true if the bulge shows rapid and progressive enlargement (3). Angiocardiography, CT, or MRI can be used in demonstrating the aneurysmally dilated ductus arteriosus, and early operative intervention has been met with success (3).

REFERENCES

1. Kirks DR, McCook TA, Serwer GA, et al. Aneurysm of the ductus arteriosus in the neonate. AJR 1980;134:573–576.
2. Berger M, Ferguson C, Hendry J. Paralysis of the left diaphragm, left vocal cord, and aneurysm of the ductus arteriosus in the 7-week-old infant. J Pediatr 1960;56:800–802.
3. Heikkinen ES, Similauml S. Aneurysm of ductus arteriosus in infancy: report of two surgically treated cases. J Pediatr Surg 1972; 7:392–397.
4. Siragusa RJ, Cumming WA. Ductus arteriosus aneurysm: an unusual mediastinal mass. J Pediatr Surg 1989;24:309–310.

ACQUIRED CARDIOVASCULAR DISEASE

Myocardial Abnormalities: Myocarditis, Cardiomyopathy, and Endocarditis

Myocarditis can be bacterial or viral, but the latter is more common. Myocarditis also can be seen with cardiac involvement in rheumatic fever, but with better control of streptococcal infections, rheumatic fever is now not very common. With any form of myocarditis, the roentgenographic findings are nonspecific and consist of diffuse dilatation of the heart and passive congestion of the lungs (Fig. 3.140). Ultrasonography is useful in defining associated pericardial effusions and myocardial thickness and function (Fig. 3.140D). Residual valvular disease is not a problem with viral myocardial infections, but with rheumatic heart disease, mitral valve and aortic valve complications are common. In the child, the problem usually is insufficiency of these valves, leading to marked left atrial and left ventricular enlargement.

Endocarditis is less of a problem in children than is myocarditis. It can result from the use of long-term intravascular and intracardiac indwelling catheters. Most commonly, endocarditis in these cases results from bacterial infection, but it also can be seen with candida and other fungal infections. The roentgenographic findings are nonspecific and depend on the valves involved. Echocardiography is especially helpful in defining the valvular vegetations.

Idiopathic Cardiomyopathy

The left ventricle is most commonly affected in idiopathic cardiomyopathy. There are two forms of this condition: one in which the left ventricle is hypertrophic (thickened) and

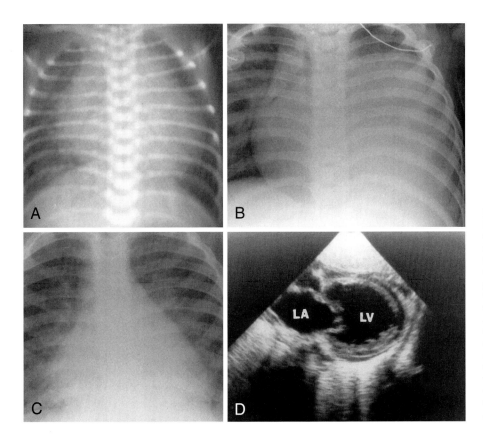

FIGURE 3.140. Myocarditis. A. Neonate with viral myocarditis leading to generalized cardiomegaly and passive congestion of the lungs. **B.** Acute viral myocarditis in an older child leading to diffuse cardiomegaly and marked passive congestion. **C.** Another patient with viral myocarditis and marked cardiomegaly. Some pulmonary edema also is present. Left ventricular dilatation predominates. **D.** Ultrasonogram demonstrating the enlarged left atrium (LA) and left ventricle (LV). Also note the thin rim of sonolucent pericardial fluid surrounding the left ventricle. The ventricle had virtually no muscular contractility during this study. (**D** courtesy of Wendy Wolf, M.D.).

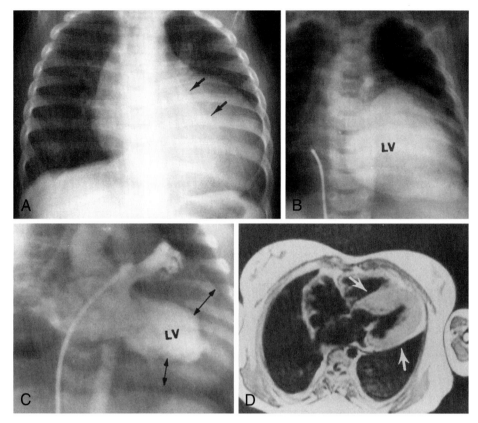

FIGURE 3.141. Cardiomyopathy. A. Hypertrophic cardiomyopathy presenting with an enlarged heart and a full left cardiac border. Compressive left lower lobe atelectasis also is present (arrows). **B.** Congestive cardiomyopathy demonstrating a large dilated left ventricle (LV). **C.** Another patient with constrictive cardiomyopathy demonstrating a small left ventricular cavity (LV) and a markedly thickened myocardium (arrows). **D.** Axial magnetic resonance image in a patient with Noonan's syndrome demonstrating marked hypertrophy of the left ventricular wall (arrows). The cavity of the left ventricle is markedly compromised.

the other where the left ventricle is dilated and thin walled (Fig. 3.141). For this reason, these two forms often respectively are referred to as restrictive and congestive cardiomyopathies. The term "restrictive" results from the fact that the thickened myocardium fosters poor systolic filling of the left ventricle, and the term "congestive" reflects the fact that the thinned left ventricular myocardium is ineffective in expulsion of blood from the left ventricle, and passive congestion results.

Congenital fibroelastosis, a disease now seldom seem, primarily was a congestive cardiomyopathy. Cardiomyopathy also can be seen with Friedreich's ataxia (1), Noonan's syndrome (Fig. 3.141D), and as a complication of steroid therapy (2). In addition, cardiomyopathy may be seen with glycogen storage disease (3).

REFERENCES

1. Sharatt GP, Jacob JC, Hobeika C. Friedreich's ataxia presenting as cardiac disease. Pediatr Cardiol 1985;6:41–42.

2. Alpert BS. Steroid-induced hypertrophic cardiomyopathy in an infant. Pediatr Cardiol 1984;5:117–118.

3. Ruttenberg HD, Steidl RM, Carey LS, et al. Glycogen-storage disease of the heart. Hemodynamic and angiocardiographic features in two cases. Am Heart J 1964;67:469–480.

Hypoxic (Ischemic) Cardiomyopathy of the Neonate

Neonatal hypoxia is extremely common, and it has been known for some time that, in association with acidosis, it can lead to pulmonary arteriolar vasoconstriction and pulmonary hypertension. Less well appreciated is that hypoxia also can lead to direct myocardial schemia, actual infarction, and, at the least, transient myocardial dysfunction (1–3). Very often, the problem is aggravated by papillary muscle necrosis (4, 5). Cardiac enlargement generally is nonspecific except when tricuspid insufficiency secondary to tricuspid valve papillary muscle necrosis is pronounced. In these cases, right atrial and right ventricular enlargement predominate.

REFERENCES

1. Brunson S, Nudel DB, Gootman N. Neonatal asphyxia and functional tricuspid atresia. Chest 1980;77:669–670.
2. Kilbride H, Way GL, Merenstein GB, et al. Myocardial infarction in the neonate with normal heart and coronary arteries. Am J Dis Child 1980;134:759–762.
3. Oh KS, Bender TM, Bowen A, et al. Transient myocardial schemia of the newborn infant. Pediatr Radiol 1985;15:29–33.
4. Donnelly WH, Bucciarelli RL, Nelson RM. Ischemic papillary muscle necrosis in stressed newborn infants. J Pediatr 1980;96:295–300.
5. Setzer E, Ermocilla R, Tonkin I, et al. Papillary muscle necrosis in a neonatal autopsy population; incidence and associated clinical manifestations. J Pediatr 1980;96:289–294.

Diabetic Cardiomyopathy of the Neonate

In diabetic cardiomyopathy of the neonate, occurring in infants of diabetic mothers, there is transient hypertrophy of the interventricular septum in the subaortic region of the left ventricle (1). The entity should not be confused with the genetic form of hypertrophic subaortic stenosis, for in infants of diabetic mothers, hypertrophy of the subaortic region is transient. Most likely, it occurs in conjunction with the generalized cardiomegaly and organomegaly seen in these patients. Similar hypertrophy occurs with hyperinsulinemia resulting from insulin-secreting neonatal pancreatic tumors (2). The heart, in some of these patients, can be quite large, and yet passive congestion minimal or not apparent at all. The septal, subaortic hypertrophy is readily demonstrable with ultrasound.

REFERENCES

1. Halliday HL. Hypertrophic cardiomyopathy in infants of poorly-controlled diabetic mothers. Arch Dis Child 1981;56:258–263.
2. Breitweser JA, Meyer RA, Sperling MA, et al. Cardiac septal hypertrophy in hyperinsulinemic infants. J Pediatr 1980;96:535–539.

MISCELLANEOUS CARDIAC DISEASES RESULTING IN CARDIAC FAILURE

Metabolic Disease Causing Cardiac Failure

Except for thyrotoxicosis, most metabolic conditions leading to cardiac failure are likely to do so in infancy. In this regard, neonatal hypoglycemia, de novo or as seen in infants of diabetic mothers, can lead to nonspecific cardiac enlargement and failure (1). Hypocalcemia also can cause cardiomegaly and cardiac failure in infants (2).

In terms of thyroid disease, both hyperthyroidism and hypothyroidism can lead to cardiomegaly. Cardiac failure is less common with hypothyroidism (3). With hyperthyroidism, both in the neonate and in the older child, thyro-toxic cardiomyopathy with cardiac enlargement and failure can occur (4, 5).

REFERENCES

1. Herrera M, Gil MD, Lucaya J. Cardiomegaly in association with neonatal hypoglycemia. Ann Radiol 1976;19:212.
2. Troughton O, Singh SP. Heart failure and neonatal hypocalcemia. Br Med J 1972;4:76–79.
3. Farooki ZQ, Hoffman WH, Perry BL, et al. Myocardial dysfunction in hypothyroid children. Am J Dis Child 1983;137:65–68.
4. Cavallo A, Casta A, Fawcett HD, et al. Is there a thyrotoxic cardiomyopathy in children? J Pediatr 1985;107:531–536.
5. Lightner ES, Allen HD, Loughlin G. Neonatal hyperthyroidism and heart failure. Am J Dis Child 1977;131:68–70.

Systemic Arteriovenous Fistula

Peripheral arteriovenous fistulas can lead to hyperkinetic heart failure. Many of these are congenital, but some are iatrogenic and can be seen after multiple vascular punctures or after dialysis procedures (1). In the neonate, one of the most common arteriovenous fistulas is the so-called "vein of Galen aneurysm." Arteriovenous fistulas also are a feature of angiomatous tumors of the liver in neonates and actually probably are the second most common arteriovenous fistula to produce heart failure in the neonate.

Arteriovenous fistulas also can be seen in bronchopulmonary vascular malformations associated with sequestration or bronchopulmonary foregut malformation, vascular tumors other than hemangiomas of the liver (2), vascular tumors or arteriovenous malformations of the placenta, and any number of peripheral arteriovenous fistulas (3). Peripheral arteriovenous fistulas can involve the umbilical vessels, either congenitally or iatrogenically after umbilical vein catheterization (1). Cardiomegaly in any of these patients is nonspecific, and increased pulmonary blood flow through the lungs causes increased pulmonary vascularity.

REFERENCES

1. Ontell SJ, Gauderer MWL. Iatrogenic arteriovenous fistula after multiple arterial punctures. Pediatrics 1985;76:97–98.
2. Sanyal SK, Saldivar V, Doburn TP, et al. Hyperdynamic heart failure due to A-V fistula associated with Wilms' tumor. Pediatrics 1976;57:564–568.
3. Woolley MM, Stanley P, Wesley JR. Peripherally located congenital arteriovenous fistulae in infancy and childhood. J Pediatr Surg 1977;12:165–176.

Intravascular Volume Overload and Myocardial Failure

Any time one is dealing with an expanded blood volume, cardiomegaly and vascular congestion can result. This can occur with primary polycythemia or, in newborns, polycythemia secondary to maternal-fetal hemorrhage, placental-to-fetal transfusion, and twin-to-twin transfusion. Of course, iatrogenic fluid overload is another cause of vascular congestion. In these patients, cardiomegaly often is not very pronounced.

In the past, in older children, one of the most common causes of fluid overloading was **acute glomerulonephritis** (1). Indeed, these patients frequently presented with cardiomegaly and passive vascular congestion, virtually indistinguishable from that seen with myocarditis.

REFERENCE

1. Macpherson RK, Banerjee AJ. Acute glomerulonephritis: a chest film diagnosis. J Can Assoc Radiol 1974;25:58–64.

Myocardial Infarction

Myocardial infarction in the pediatric age group is uncommon, especially in the neonate. However, in the neonate, it can be seen with coronary artery embolism resulting from paradoxical thrombi originating from the ductus venosus. Myocardial infarction secondary to atherosclerosis is seen in progeria, maternal cocaine abuse (1, 2), and the collagen vascular diseases such as systemic lupus erythematosus (3). The roentgenographic findings in myocardial infarction usually are nonspecific, and these patients often present with normal chest roentgenograms. In others, cardiomegaly with some degree of passive pulmonary vascular congestion is seen. In addition, calcification of the myocardium after infarction also can be encountered (4).

REFERENCES

1. Bulbul ZR, Rosenthal DN, Kleinman CS. Myocardial infarction in the perinatal period secondary to maternal cocaine abuse: a case report and literature review. Arch Pediatr Adolesc Med 1994;148:1092–1096.
2. Hoyme HE, Jones KL, Dixon SD, et al. Prenatal cocaine exposure and fetal vascular disruption. Pediatrics 1990;85:743–747.
3. Friedman DM, Lazarus HM, Fierman AH. Acute myocardial infarction in pediatric systemic lupus erythematosus. J Pediatr 1990;117:263–266.
4. Arndt RD, Smith LE, Po J, et al. Myocardial calcification of the infant heart following infarction; detected on the chest roentgenogram: a case report. AJR 1974;122:133–136.

Cardiac Tumors

Cardiac tumors may be asymptomatic, but they also can lead to a variety of symptoms associated with intracardiac blood flow obstruction. They are more common in the neonate and young infant, and of these tumors, the most common is a rhabdomyoma. This tumor often is associated with tuberous sclerosis and may be the presenting problem in the neonate (1–4). The tumor may present as a single mass or diffuse thickening of the myocardium (2, 3). In addition, diffuse thickening of the myocardium and interventricular septum may lead to subvalvular aortic stenosis (5). Other tumors, if located at this critical sight, also can lead to left ventricular obstruction (6, 7) and include myxoma (6, 8), fibroma (7), teratoma, rhabdomyosarcoma, hamartoma, hemangioma, and secondary metastases (9). Myxoma tends to occur in the atria and may involve the valves. In addition, it frequently disposes to the formation of thromboemboli. Finally, fibroma of the heart has been reported in the basal cell nevoid or Gorlin's syndrome (10, 11).

Occasionally, a cardiac tumor may produce a local bulge of the cardiac silhouette, but most often plain films are normal. Ultrasonography, MRI, CT, and angiocardiography all can demonstrates these tumors (Fig. 3.142), but currently ultrasonography is the diagnostic modality of choice for the initial study.

REFERENCES

1. Allison JW, Stephenson CA, Angtuaco TL, et al. Radiological case of the month—tuberous sclerosis with myocardial and central nervous system involvement at birth. Am J Dis Child 1991;145:470–471.
2. Coates TL, McGahan JP. Fetal cardiac rhabdomyomas presenting as diffuse myocardial thickening. J Ultrasound Med 1994;13: 813–816.
3. Kilman JW, Craenen J, Hosier DM. Replacement of entire right atrial wall in an infant with a cardiac rhabdomyoma. J Pediatr Surg 1973;8:317–321.
4. Kuehl KS, Perry LW, Chandra R, et al. Rhabdomyoma causing subaortic stenosis. Pediatrics 1970;46:464–468.
5. Shaher RM, Farina M, Alley R, et al. Congenital subaortic stenosis in infancy caused by rhabdomyoma of the left ventricle. J Thorac Cardiovasc Surg 1972;63:157–163.
6. Balsara RK, Pelias AJ. Myxoma of right ventricle presenting as pulmonic stenosis in a neonate. Chest 1983;83:145–146.
7. Oliva PB, Breckinridge JC, Johnson ML, et al. Left ventricular outflow obstruction produced by a pedunculated fibroma in a newborn. Chest 1978;74:590–593.
8. Dunnigan A, Oldham N, Serwer GA, et al. Left atrial myxoma. Am J Dis Child 1981;135:420–421.
9. Chan HSL, Sonley MJ, Moes CAF, et al. Primary and secondary tumors of childhood involving the heart, pericardium and great vessels. A report of 75 cases and review of the literature. Cancer 1985;56:825–836.
10. Cotton JL, Kavey R-EW, Palmier CE, et al. Cardiac tumors and the nevoid basal cell carcinoma syndrome. Pediatrics 1991;87: 725–728.
11. Herman TE, Siegel MJ, McAlister WH. Cardiac tumor in Gorlin's syndrome. Nevoid basal cell carcinoma syndrome. Pediatr Radiol 1991;21:234–235.

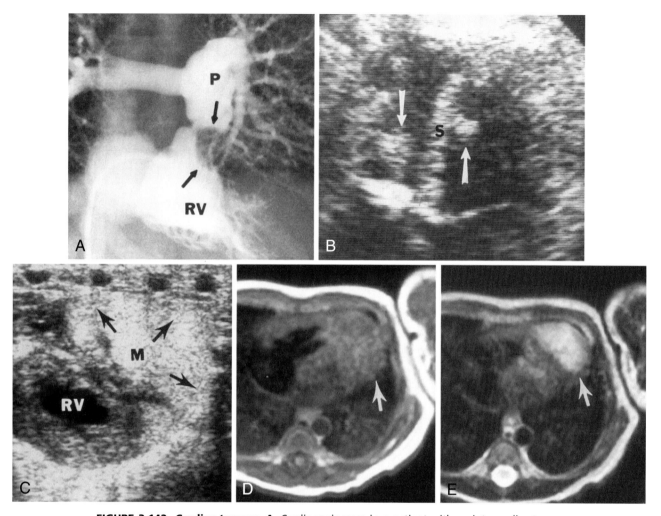

FIGURE 3.142. Cardiac tumors. A. Cardioangiogram in a patient with an intracardiac tumor arising in the ventricular septum and producing a filling defect (arrows) impinging on the right outflow tract. RV, right ventricle; P, pulmonary artery. **B.** Ultrasonogram in another infant demonstrates two echogenic intracardiac tumors (arrows). One was in the right ventricle and the other arose off the septum (S) and projected into the left ventricle. **C. Rhabdomyomas in tuberous sclerosis.** Note the large echogenic tumor mass (M) in the wall of the right ventricle (RV). **D.** T1-weighted axial magnetic resonance image demonstrates thickening of the myocardium at the tumor site (arrow). **E.** T2-weighted axial magnetic resonance study demonstrates increased signal in the same tumor (arrow) as demonstrated in **C.** (**B** courtesy of A. Casta, M.D.).

PERICARDIAL ABNORMALITIES

Pericarditis, Hemopericardium, and Pericardial Effusion

In terms of the etiology of pericarditis, viral pericarditis (1) is much more common than bacterial infection (2). However, pericarditis also can result from mycoplasma infections (3) and, of course, fungal and tuberculous infections. Constrictive pericarditis is uncommon in infancy, but it should be noted that when it is present, the heart is normal sized.

Hemopericardium often is secondary to chest trauma, either accidental or iatrogenic, or a generalized bleeding diathesis. Hemopericardium also can be seen with pericardial teratomas, rupture of cardiac aneurysms or diverticula, and perforation of the heart by indwelling catheters (4–6). Chylopericardium is extremely uncommon (7) but can be seen with cystic hygromas or other lymphangiomatous tumors of the mediastinum or pericardium. Serous pericardial effusions may be seen with the nephrotic syndrome, acute glomerulonephritis, erythroblastosis fetalis, and almost any other condition where excessive accumulation of body fluids is present. Pericardial effusions also have been associated with central diaphragmatic hernias into the pericardial sac in neonates (8, 9). Pericardial calcification after any type of insult to the pericardium is uncommon in children but can occur after infection, hemorrhage, or trauma.

Clinically, with gradual accumulations of fluid, symptoms are minimal, but if fluid accumulation is rapid, cardiac tamponade and severe respiratory distress may require immediate pericardial tap. Roentgenographically, no matter what type of fluid is present, changes are similar; there is globular enlargement of the cardiac silhouette with almost equal bulging to the left and right of the spine (Fig. 3.143A). The pulmonary artery and aortic silhouettes are obliterated as the pericardial sac distends over the base of the heart. The pulmonary vascularity in most cases is normal. Confirmation of the presence of a pericardial effusion is most readily accomplished with ultrasonography, and seldom is any other type of imaging required (Fig. 3.143B).

REFERENCES

1. Hutchison JS, Joubert GIE, Whitehouse SR, et al. Pericardial effusion and cardiac tamponade after respiratory syncytial viral infection. Pediatr Emerg Care 1994;10:219–221.
2. Stroobant J, Leanage R, Deanfield J, et al. Acute infective pericarditis in infancy. Arch Dis Child 1982;57:73–74.
3. Miller TC, Baman SI, Albers WH. Massive pericardial effusion due to *Mycoplasma hominis* in a newborn. Am J Dis Child 1982;136:271–272.
4. Agarwal KC, Khan A, Falla A, et al. Cardiac perforation from central venous catheters: survival after cardiac tamponade in an infant. Pediatrics 1984;73:333–338.
5. Kulkarni PB, Dorand RD, Simmons EM Jr. Pericardial tamponade: complication of total parenteral nutrition. J Pediatr Surg 1981;16:735–736.
6. Opitz JC, Toyama W. Cardiac tamponade from central venous

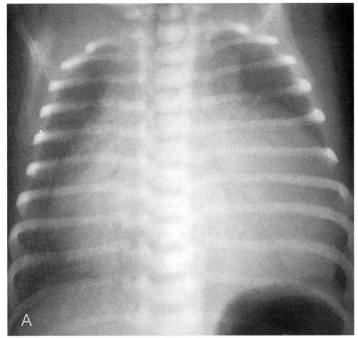

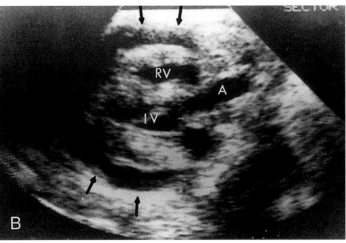

FIGURE 3.143. Pericardial fluid. A. Note marked broadening and enlargement of the cardiac silhouette secondary to pericardial fluid. Note especially the widened superior mediastinum as pericardial fluid extends around the great vessels. **B.** Long-axis peristernal ultrasonogram demonstrates a rim of fluid (arrows) around the heart of another patient with a pericardial effusion. RV, right ventricular cavity; LV, left ventricular cavity; A, aorta. (**B** courtesy of A. Casta, M.D.).

catheterization: two cases in premature infants with survival. Pediatrics 1982;70:139–140.

7. Museneche CA, Riveron FA, Backer CL, et al. Massive primary chylopericardium: a case report. J Pediatr Surg 1990;25:840–842.

8. Einzig S, Munson DP, Sharanjeet S, et al. Intrapericardial herniation of the liver: uncommon cause of massive pericardial effusion in neonates. AJR 1981;137:1075–1077.

9. Iliff PJ, Eyre JA, Westaby S, et al. Neonatal pericardial effusion associated with central eventration of the diaphragm. Arch Dis Child 1983;58:147–149.

Pneumopericardium

Pneumopericardium, except for that seen in the neonate, is rather uncommon in children. Of course, it can be seen with penetrating chest trauma and postoperatively, if the pericardium was entered. In the neonate, pneumopericardium usually is the result of positive pressure ventilation. It is not known just how air reaches the pericardial cavity in the foregoing cases, but it has been suggested that most often it tracts along the perivisceral fascia investing the trachea and esophagus (1). The fascia is continuous with the fibrous layer of the parietal pericardium and, as such, provides a ready route for the passage of air into the pericardial cavity.

The roentgenographic findings are characteristic in that there is a radiolucent halo (free air) of varying width around the heart (Fig. 3.144A), and very often, the pericardium itself is visible as a thin white stripe encircling the heart. When pericardial air is minimal, no therapy is required, but when the volume of air is substantial, cardiac tamponade results and immediate removal of the air is necessary.

REFERENCE

1. Varano LA, Maisels MJ. Pneumopericardium in the newborn; diagnosis and pathogenesis. Pediatrics 1974;53:941–945.

Pericardial Cysts and Tumors

The most common pericardial tumor noted in childhood, and especially in infancy, is pericardial teratoma (1–4). These tumors may be either cystic or solid, and some may

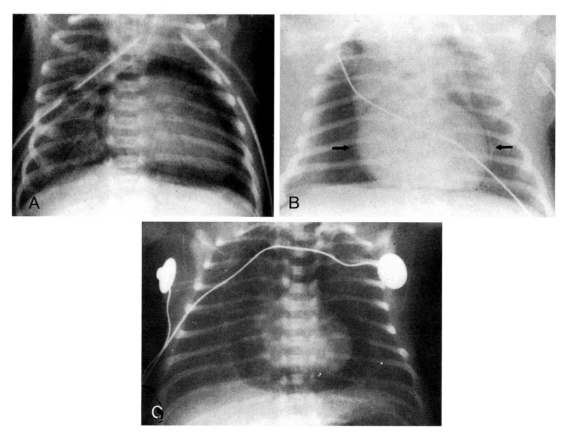

FIGURE 3.144. Pneumopericardium. A. Typical air surrounding the heart in a newborn infant with surfactant deficiency disease on respirator therapy. **B.** Less pronounced pneumopericardium encircling the heart. Note the pericardial sac, visible bilaterally (arrows). Air beneath the thymus gland is a result of a pneumomediastinum. A right medial pneumothorax also is present. **C.** Another patient with pneumopericardium encircling the heart and causing cardiac tamponade. Note how small the cardiac silhouette has become. There also is air in the soft tissues of the neck.

rupture into the pericardial sac. Hemopericardium and acute cardiac tamponade can result. Pericardial teratoma also can be associated with tamponading pericardial effusions (2) and has been noted to be a cause of fetal hydrops (1). Roentgenographically, enlargement of the cardiac silhouette may at first suggest congenital heart disease. Ultrasonography, CT scanning, and MRI all can identify these tumors, but MRI probably is the procedure of choice.

Pericardial cysts are rather uncommon but, when seen, present with localized bulging of the cardiac border. Most often, these cysts are right sided and lie in the cardiophrenic angle. However, a posterior mediastinal pericardial cyst also has been reported (5).

REFERENCES

1. Banfield F, Dick M II, Behrendt DM, et al. Intrapericardial teratoma: a new and treatable cause of hydrops fetalis. Am J Dis Child 1980;134:1174–1175.
2. Lubin BH, Friedman S, Miller WW. Intrapericardial teratoma associated with pericardial effusion. An acute surgical problem in infancy. J Pediatr Surg 1967;2:336–341.
3. Sumner TE, Crowe JE, Klein A, et al. Intrapericardial teratoma in infancy. Pediatr Radiol 1980;10:51–53.
4. Zerella JT, Halpe DCE. Intrapericardial teratoma—neonatal cardiorespiratory distress amenable to surgery. J Pediatr Surg 1980; 15:961–963.
5. Slasky BS, Hardesty RL. Midline pericardial cyst in the posterior mediastinum: sonographic and computed tomographic correlation. CT 1982;6:171–175.

VASCULAR ABNORMALITIES

Arterial Occlusions

Arterial occlusion secondary to thrombosis or embolism is not particularly common in childhood, except in infancy, where it is primarily a problem of the neonate. Any artery in the body can be involved, but in the neonate, frequently it is the aorta. Generally speaking, basic predisposing factors to thrombosis are dehydration and/or sepsis, but indwelling catheters also are a problem and are the main problem in neonates (1, 2). Infants of diabetic mothers also are prone to thromboses, and it is believed that the relatively water-depleted state predisposes them to this problem (3). Arterial embolization from thrombi related to a closing patent ductus arteriosus also can occur, and, of course, disseminated intravascular coagulation frequently leads to vascular and cardiac thromboses.

In any of these cases, the thrombus usually is best demonstrated with ultrasonography including color flow Doppler studies (4). Angiography also can be performed, but ultrasound usually suffices (Figs. 3.145 and 3.146). In the past, large arterial thrombi or emboli were removed surgically, but currently, fibrinolytic therapy often is first attempted (5). However, it should be remembered that smaller thrombi often resolve spontaneously.

Another feature of arterial thrombosis (renal) in the neonate is the development of systemic hypertension (6, 7) and congestive heart failure (Fig. 3.146A). Once again, the main contributing factor to the development of renal artery thrombosis in these patients is the presence of indwelling catheters. Interestingly, however, the hypertension problem in these infants usually resolves and has been shown to respond to aggressive antihypertensive therapy (8). In terms of long-term complications of aortic thrombi, in one study it was demonstrated that 3 of 10 patients developed hypertension, while 8 of 10 developed leg length discrepancies (9). In addition to the foregoing considerations, it should be remembered that thrombi can become infected and may, as such, lead to the development of mycotic aneurysms (10).

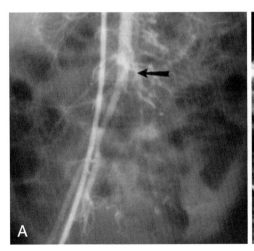
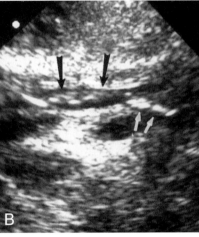

FIGURE 3.145. Arterial occlusions. A. Note complete occlusion of the left common iliac artery (arrow), an umbilical artery catheter complication. **B.** Another patient with a thrombus in the descending aorta (black arrows) just above the bifurcation. Thrombus also extends into the right common iliac artery (white arrows).

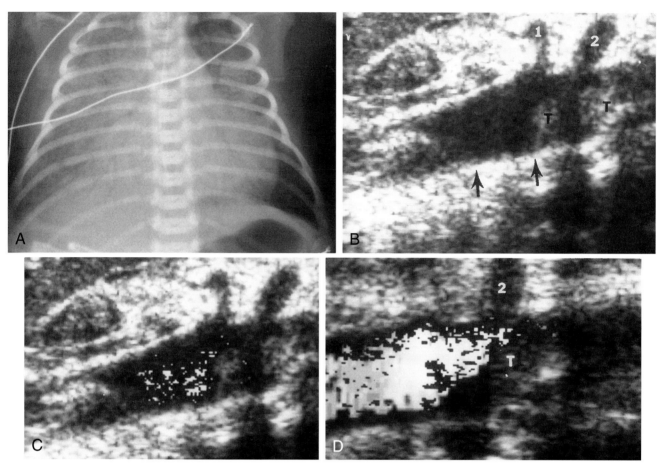

FIGURE 3.146. Aortic thrombus with systemic hypertension. A. Note the enlarged heart and marked pulmonary edema in this infant. **B.** Sagittal sonogram through the aorta (arrows) demonstrates multiple echogenic thrombi (T) within its lumen. Along the upper aspect, note the patent celiac (1) and superior mesenteric (2) arteries. **C.** Color flow Doppler demonstrates very little blood flow (white speckles) in the aorta. **D.** After anticoagulant therapy, color flow Doppler demonstrates markedly increased flow down to the level of the occluding thrombus (T), which lies just distal to the takeoff of the superior mesenteric artery (2).

REFERENCES

1. Goetzman BW, Stadalnik RC, Bogren HG, et al. Thrombotic complications of umbilical artery catheters; a clinical and radiographic study. Pediatrics 1975;56:374–379.
2. Henry CG, Gutierrez F, Lee JT, et al. Aortic thrombosis presenting as congestive heart failure: an umbilical artery catheter complication. J Pediatr 1981;98:820–822.
3. Ward TF. Multiple thromboses in an infant of a diabetic mother. J Pediatr 1977;90:982–984.
4. Deeg KH, Wolfel D, Tupprecht TH. Diagnosis of neonatal aortic thrombosis by colour coded Doppler sonography. Pediatr Radiol 1992;22:62–63.
5. Strife JL, Ball WS Jr, Towbin R, et al. Arterial occlusions in neonates: use of fibrinolytic therapy. Radiology 1988;166:395–400.
6. Baldwin CE, Holder TM, Ashcraft KW, et al. Neonatal renovascular hypertension—a complication of the aortic monitoring catheters. J Pediatr Surg 1981;16:820–821.
7. Skalina MEL, Kliegman RM, Fanaroff AA. Epidemiology and management of severe symptomatic neonatal hypertension. Am J Perinatol 1986;3:235–239.
8. Caplan MS, Cohn RA, Langman CB, et al. Favorable outcome of neonatal aortic thrombosis and renovascular hypertension. J Pediatr 1989;115:291–295.
9. Seibert JJ, Northington FJ, Miers JF, et al. Aortic thrombosis after umbilical artery catheterization in neonates: prevalence of complications on long-term follow-up. AJR 1991;156:567–569.
10. Lobe TE, Richardson CJ, Boulden TF, et al. Mycotic thromboaneurysmal disease of the abdominal aorta in preterm infants: its natural history and its management. J Pediatr Surg 1992;27:1054–1060.

Venous Thromboembolism

Spontaneous venous thromboembolism in infancy and childhood is not particularly common (1), but in the premature infant and other patients with long-term indwelling catheters, the incidence is much higher. Predisposing factors, much as with arterial thromboembolism, include sepsis, dehydration, and mechanical injury secondary to indwelling catheters. Thrombosis of the renal vein com-

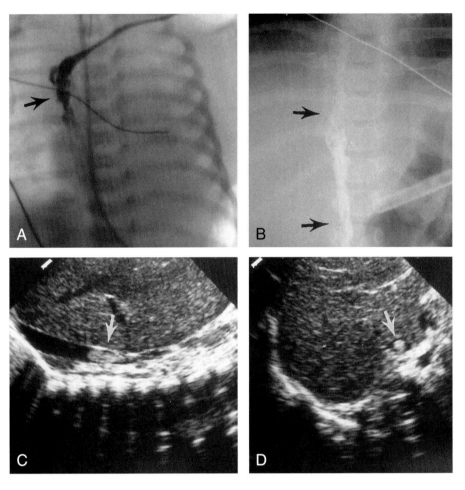

FIGURE 3.147. Venous thrombosis. A. Digital subtraction venogram demonstrates clot (arrow) in the superior vena cava. B. Another patient with extensive clot causing irregularity of the contrast column throughout the entire inferior vena cava (arrows). C. Same patient whose sagittal ultrasound through the superior vena cava demonstrates the superiormost extent of the echogenic clot (arrow). D. Cross-sectional view through the superior vena cava demonstrates the echogenic clot (arrow).

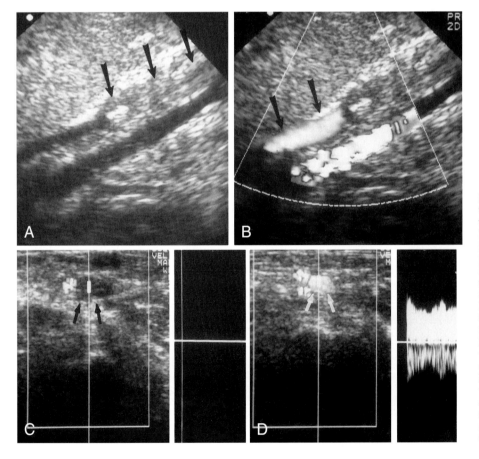

FIGURE 3.148. Venous thrombosis with color flow Doppler. A. Note the extensive echogenic clot in the lower inferior vena cava (arrows). The inferior vena cava above this level is patent. The patent aorta is seen below. B. With color flow Doppler, flow is seen in the superior vena cava (arrows) down to the level of the blood clot. Normal flow also is seen in the aorta. C. Femoral vein thrombosis, indirect findings: color flow Doppler. Note that there is no signal in the femoral vein (arrows) and no evidence of flow on the Doppler wave tracing. Normal flow is present in the adjacent femoral artery. This vein also was non-compressible. D. Normal side demonstrates flow in the normal femoral vein (arrows), and the Doppler wave tracing verifies the flow.

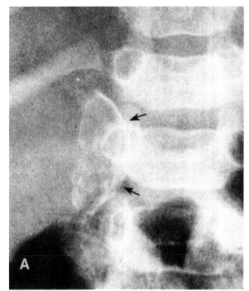
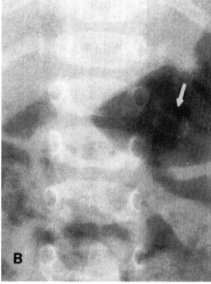
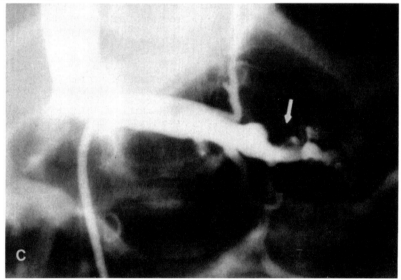

FIGURE 3.149. Venous thrombus calcification. A. Note the oval-shaped calcification (arrows) of a thrombus in the inferior vena cava. **B.** Note the small oval-shaped calcification on the left (arrow). This was an incidental finding. **C.** Subsequent renal venogram demonstrates filling defect (arrow) in the left renal vein. The defect corresponds to the calcified renal vein thrombus seen on plain films. (**A** reproduced with permission from Kassner EG, Baumstark A, Kinkhabwala MN, et al. Venous thrombus calcification in infancy. Pediatr Radiol 1976;4:167–171; **C** courtesy of R. Cavazos, M.D., and J. Arndt, M.D.).

monly is seen in the nephrotic syndrome, and thrombi in the cavae can extend into the heart. In the neonate, the problem often is a combination of thrombosis and fungal (candida) infection (2).

Venous thrombi, in the large veins, are best identified with ultrasonography (3, 4) and can be confirmed with venography (Figs. 3.147 and 3.148). Later, as the thrombi mature, they may calcify (5) and then produce characteristic oval or bullet-shaped calcifications in the various vessels involved (Fig. 3.149). In addition, it has been noted that with inferior venal obstruction, plain films show compensatory dilatation of the azygos vein (6). This occurs because collateral venous return must be accomplished through the azygos or hemiazygos venous systems when the inferior vena cava is obstructed.

REFERENCES

1. Nguyen LT, Laberge J-M, Guttman FM, et al. Spontaneous deep vein thrombosis in childhood and adolescence. J Pediatr Surg 1986;21:640–643.
2. Johnson DE, Bass JL, Thompson TR, et al. Candida septicemia and right atrial mass secondary to umbilical vein catheterization. Am J Dis Child 1981;135:275–277.
3. Stringer DA, Krysl J, Manson D, et al. The value of Doppler sonography in the detection of major vessel thrombosis in the neonatal abdomen. Pediatr Radiol 1990;21:30–33.
4. Rand T, Kohlhauser C, Popow C, et al. Sonographic detection of internal jugular vein thrombosis after central venous catheterization in the newborn period. Pediatr Radiol 1994;24:577–580.
5. Tarantino MD, Vasu MA, Von Drak TH, et al. Calcified thrombus in the right atrium: a rare complication of long-term parenteral nutrition in a child. J Pediatr Surg 1991;26:91–93.

6. Berdon WE, Baker DH. Azygos vein dilatation in acquired obstruction of the inferior vena cava. Pediatr Radiol 1974;2: 221–224.

Superior Vena Cava Syndrome

The superior vena cava syndrome is not particularly common in children (1). For the most part, it results from thrombosis of the superior vena cava, and predisposing causes are much the same as for venous thromboses in general (see preceding section). However, one can see peculiar complications with the superior vena caval syndrome including chylothorax (2), communicating hydrocephalus (3), and retropharyngeal soft tissue thickening (4). All of these findings probably are related to high retrograde venous back pressures. Currently, therapy can be accomplished with catheter-directed thrombolysis (5).

REFERENCES

1. Issa PY, Brihi ER, Jannin Y, et al. Superior vena cava syndrome in childhood: report of ten cases and review of the literature. Pediatrics 1983;71:337–441.
2. Kramer SS, Taylor GA, Garfinkel DJ, et al. Lethal chylothoraces due to superior vena caval thrombosis in infants. AJR 1981; 137:559–563.
3. Markowitz RI, Kleinman CS, Hellenbrand WE, et al. Communicating hydrocephalus secondary to superior vena caval obstruction. Am J Dis Child 1984;138:638–641.
4. Hayden CK Jr, Swischuk LE. Retropharyngeal edema, airway obstruction and caval thrombosis. AJR 1982;138:757–758.
5. Kee ST, Kinoshita L, Razavi MK, et al. Superior vena cava syndrome: treatment with catheter-directed thrombolysis and endovascular stent placement. Radiology 1998;206:187–193.

Pulmonary Embolism

Pulmonary embolism in infants and children is not common. If the pulmonary embolus is massive, the patient may die, but if multiple showers of small emboli occur, the patient may develop a picture of pulmonary hypertension. Roentgenographically, there will be cardiomegaly with right ventricular hypertrophy, prominence of the pulmonary artery, and diminution of the pulmonary vasculature. Pulmonary emboli also can calcify (1).

Pulmonary embolism is best identified with pulmonary angiography, but usually first is documented with nuclear scintigraphy using ventilation-perfusion scans. The findings are no different from those in adults where the perfusion scan is abnormal while the ventilation scan is normal. Plain films, when embolism is massive, tend to show decreased pulmonary vascularity and cardiomegaly with a right-side enlargement pattern. Most often, however, with pulmonary embolism, plain films are normal.

REFERENCE

1. Hourihane JB, O'Donnell JR, Costigan C, et al. Calcified pulmonary artery thrombus diagnosed on the plain radiograph. Br J Radiol 1980;53:1097–1099.

Intravascular Gas Embolism

Intravascular gas embolism was relatively common before surfactant therapy for surfactant deficiency disease was available. The complication resulted from positive pressure ventilation in patients who were very refractory to this form of treatment (1). Very often, other air block phenomena were present, and even then, the complication of intravascular gas embolism was uncommon. Nonetheless, the finding usually signaled a terminal event, and the appearance of gas in the vascular system is demonstrated in Fig. 3.150.

REFERENCE

1. Kogutt MS. Systemic air embolism secondary to respiratory therapy in the neonate; six cases including one survivor. AJR 1978; 131:425–429.

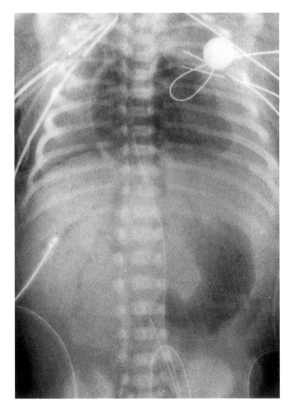

FIGURE 3.150. Massive air embolus. Note that the heart is full of air (pneumocardium) and that there is air in the various blood vessels around the shoulder and in the liver.

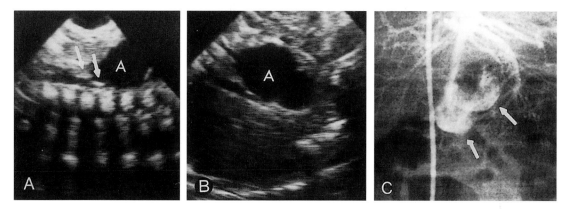

FIGURE 3.151. Mycotic aortic aneurysm in neonate. A. On this longitudinal sonogram of the aorta, note the large sonolucent aortic aneurysm (A). The two echogenic foci at the cranial end of the aneurysm represent the thrombus (arrows) and an intimal flap. **B.** Cross-sectional sonogram demonstrates the large aneurysm (A). **C.** Subsequent aortogram demonstrates the mycotic aneurysm (arrows).

Aortic and Arterial Aneurysms

Congenital and idiopathic aneurysms of the aorta or branch arteries are uncommon (1, 2), but aneurysms can be seen with periarteritis nodosa, fibromuscular dysplasia of the renal artery (3), neurofibromatosis (4), the mucocutaneous lymph node syndrome (5), Marfan's syndrome, homocystinuria, after trauma (6–8), and after renal dialysis or peripheral vascular catheterization. Mycotic aneurysms secondary to infection also occur in children, and most are encountered in neonates and young infants undergoing umbilical artery catheterization. Indeed, this is the most common cause of arterial aneurysm in the pediatric age group (9). However, aortic aneurysms also can be seen with Turner's syndrome (10), cystic medial necrosis (5), tuberous sclerosis (11, 12), Ehlers-Danlos syndrome, and other connective tissue disorders.

Aneurysms usually were demonstrated with arteriography but now also are demonstrable with ultrasonography (3) (Fig. 3.151). They also are vividly displayed with contrast-enhanced CT and especially well demonstrated with MRI.

REFERENCES

1. Saad SA, May A. Abdominal aortic aneurysm in a neonate. J Pediatr Surg 1991;26:1423–1424.
2. Stanley P, Gilsanz V. Aortic aneurysm in a 5-year-old girl. Pediatr Radiol 1985;15:418–419.
3. Bunchman TE, Walker HSJ III, Joyce F, et al. Sonographic evaluation of renal artery aneurysm in childhood. Pediatr Radiol 1991;21:312–313.
4. Pentecost M, Stanley P, Takahashi M, et al. Aneurysms of the aorta and subclavian and vertebral arteries in neurofibromatosis. Am J Dis Child 1981;135:475–477.
5. Millar AJW, Gilbert RD, Brown RA, et al. Abdominal aortic aneurysms in children. J Pediatr Surg 1996;31:1624–1628.
6. Lowe LH, Bulas DI, Eichelberger MD, et al. Traumatic aortic injuries in children: radiologic evaluation. AJR 1998;170:39–42.
7. Spouge AR, Burrows PE, Armstrong D, et al. Traumatic aortic rupture in the pediatric population. Role of plain film, CT and angiography in the diagnosis. Pediatr Radiol 1991;21:324–328.
8. Roche KJ, Genieser NB, Berger DK, et al. Traumatic abdominal pseudoaneurysm secondary to child abuse. Pediatr Radiol 1995;25:S247–S248.
9. Khoss AE, Ponhold W, Pollak A, et al. Abdominal aortic aneurysm in a premature neonate with disseminated candidiasis: ultrasound and angiography. Pediatr Radiol 1985;15:420–421.
10. Lin AE, Lippe BM, Geffner ME, et al. Aortic dilatation, dissection, and rupture in patients with Turner syndrome. J Pediatr 1986;109:820–826.
11. Baker PC, Furnival RA. Tuberous sclerosis presenting with bowel obstruction and an aortic aneurysm. Pediatr Emerg Care 2000;16:255–257.
12. Tsukui A, Noguchi R, Honda T, et al. Aortic aneurysm in a four-year-old child with tuberous sclerosis. Pediatr Anaesth 1995;5:67–70.

Venous Aneurysms

Venous aneurysms, except those seen with trauma, multiple catheterizations, or peritoneal dialysis, are not common. Idiopathic venous aneurysms can involve any vein but most commonly occur in the superior vena cava and jugular veins of children (1–3). The former produces right-side paratracheal mediastinal widening but no displacement of the trachea. With any venous aneurysm, the problem is believed to result from a congenital muscular defect of the venous wall.

REFERENCES

1. Danis RK. Isolated aneurysm of the internal jugular vein: a report of three. J Pediatr Surg 1982;17:130–131.

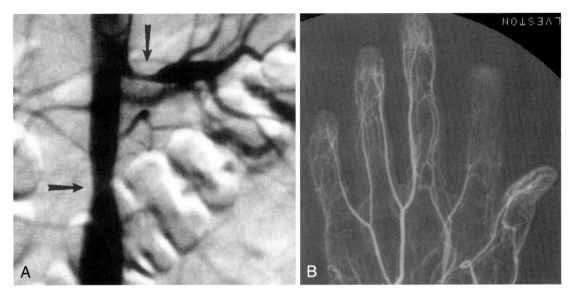

FIGURE 3.152. Takayasu's arteritis. A. Note narrowing of the proximal left renal artery (top arrow) and mild narrowing of the descending aorta (lower arrow). The other left renal artery is visualized, but both renal arteries on the right show poor flow. **B. Patient with nonspecific arteritis,** probably collagen vascular disease induced, demonstrating diffuse small vessel disease with poor circulation, obliteration of vessels, and irregularity of vessels involving primarily the second and fifth digits. Lesser changes are present in the fourth digit.

2. Nwako FA, Agugua NEM, Udeh CA, et al. Jugular phlebectasia. J Pediatr Surg 1989;24:303–305.
3. Yokomori K, Kubo K, Kanamori Y, et al. Internal jugular phlebectasia in two siblings: manometric and histopathologic studies of the pathogenesis. J Pediatr Surg 1990;25:762–765.

Vascular Stenoses and Arteritis

Stenoses of the systemic veins usually are asymptomatic and incidental, but arterial stenoses usually are symptomatic. Any vessel can be involved, including the aorta, where diffuse stenosis can be associated with renal artery stenosis and hypertension (1). Arterial stenoses also occur with neurofibromatosis and the infantile hypercalcemia syndrome. When such stenoses involve the renal artery, hypertension can be a problem. Fibromuscular hyperplasia also can be encountered in childhood (2) and usually involves the renal arteries. The nodular appearance of the involved vessels is no different from that seen in adults.

Takayasu's arteritis is uncommon in children but, when seen, produces a variety of stenotic lesions throughout the arterial tree (Fig. 3.152A). The disease is of unknown etiology and often is termed "pulseless disease." There is no specific cure, although corticosteroids have been used in some cases. Takayasu's arteritis also can involve the coronary arteries (3, 4), where delayed problems can occur (5).

Stenosis of the renal artery in renal transplantation is another cause of arterial narrowing, and these and other stenoses now usually are first treated with balloon angioplasty (6, 7). Arteritis also can occur with periarteritis

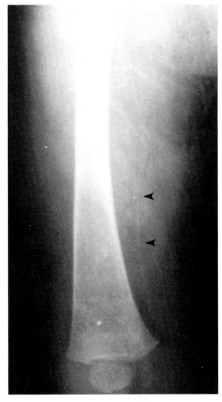

FIGURE 3.153. Arterial calcifications. Note calcifications of the arteries of the lower extremity (arrowheads). (Reproduced with permission from Weens HS, Marin CA. Infantile arteriosclerosis. Radiology 1956;67:168–174).

nodosa and nonspecifically with Raynaud's phenomenon (Fig. 3.152B).

REFERENCES

1. O'Neill JA Jr, Berkowitz H, Gellows KJ, et al. Midaortic syndrome and hypertension in childhood. J Pediatr Surg 1995;30:164–172.
2. Price RA, Vawter GF. Arterial fibromuscular dysplasia in infancy and childhood. Arch Pathol 1972;93:419–426.
3. Burke AP, Virmani R, Perry LW, et al. Fatal Kawasaki disease with coronary arteritis and no coronary aneurysms. Pediatrics 1998; 101:108–112.
4. McConnel ME, Hannon DW, Steed RD, et al. Fatal obliterative coronary vasculitis in Kawasaki disease. J Pediatr 1998;133: 259–261.
5. Burns JC, Shika H, Gordon JB, et al. Sequelae of Kawasaki disease in adolescents and young adults. J Am Coll Cardiol 1996;28: 253–257.
6. Spijkerboer AM, Mali WP, Donckerwolcke RAMG. Renal transplant artery stenosis in children: treatment with percutaneous transluminal angioplasty. Pediatr Radiol 1992;22:519–521.
7. Stanley P, Senac MO, Bakody P, et al. Percutaneous transluminal dilatation for renal artery stenosis in a 22-month-old hypertensive girl. AJR 1983;140:983–984.

Vascular Calcifications

Vascular calcifications in infancy are not common, but in an older child, one occasionally can see normal calcification of the ligamentum arteriosum. Otherwise, calcifications in the vessels are pathologic and can be seen with hyperparathyroidism, hypercalcemia, or with the so-called "infantile arteriosclerosis syndrome" (1–5). No metabolic etiology has been demonstrated in this latter condition, but it has been suggested that the abnormality may stem from a connective tissue disorder (3, 4). Spontaneous survival is rare (6), and more recently, the condition has been noted to respond to diphosphonate therapy (3–5). The calcifications occur primarily in the medial elastic tissue (4) and roentgenographically consist of linear or curvilinear calcifications in the vessel walls (Figs. 3.153 and 3.154).

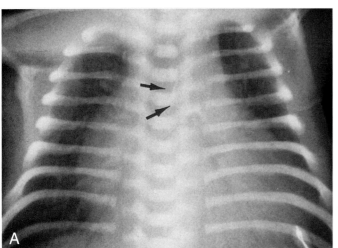

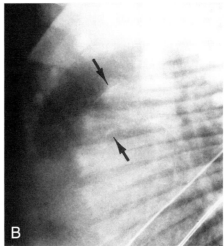

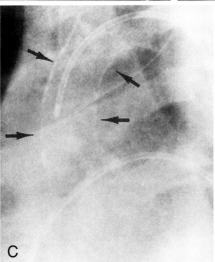

FIGURE 3.154. A and B. Idiopathic calcification of the arteries. Frontal and lateral views demonstrate delicate curvilinear calcifications within the great vessels (arrows) in this infant with cardiomegaly and congestive heart failure. The calcifications were of unknown etiology and, at postmortem examination, were present in both the aorta and pulmonary artery. Microscopic calcifications also were present in the peripheral pulmonary arterioles. None of the systemic blood vessels, except for the aorta, showed calcifications. **C. Singleton-Merten syndrome.** Note calcification of the aorta (arrows). (**A** and **B** courtesy of Sally Robinson, M.D., and Tom Allen, M.D.).

Calcification in congenital heart disease is rather uncommon in the general pediatric age group and virtually unheard of in the neonate. However, in the adolescent and young adult, one may see calcification of a stenotic aortic or pulmonary valve. In addition, postoperatively in tetralogy of Fallot, calcification of the patch used to correct the infundibular stenosis also can be seen. Similarly, calcification of aortic homografts can occur. Myocardial calcifications generally are rare in the pediatric age group but can be seen after infection or trauma. In addition, calcification of the heart has been noted with chronic renal failure (7), and calcification of the aorta has been seen in a storage disease known as the Singleton-Merten syndrome (8). We also have seen one such child (Fig. 3.154C). Aortic calcification also occurs with the candidiasis-endocrinopathy syndrome (9).

Venous calcifications are more common than arterial calcifications, and most are calcified venous thrombi. The most commonly involved veins are the inferior vena cava and renal vein (1). Most often, these calcifications are seen as incidental findings and typically are elliptical or bullet shaped. Their location and configuration identify them as such, and usually venography is not required for substantiation. They also can be visualized with ultrasound and, especially well, with CT scans.

REFERENCES

1. Bissett GS III. Gamut: cardiac and great vessel calcifications in childhood. Semin Roentgenol 1985;20:194–196.
2. Lussier-Lazaroff J, Fletcher BD. Idiopathic infantile arterial calcification: roentgen diagnosis of a rare cause of coronary artery occlusion. Pediatr Radiol 1973;1:224–228.
3. Meradji M, deVilleneuve VH, Huber J, et al. Idiopathic infantile arterial calcification in siblings; radiologic diagnosis and successful treatment. J Pediatr 1978;92:401–405.
4. Thiaville A, Smets A, Clercx A, et al. Idiopathic infantile arterial calcification: a surviving patient with renal artery stenosis. Pediatr Radiol 1995;24:506–508.
5. Vera J, Lucaya J, Garcia Conesa JA, et al. Idiopathic infantile arterial calcifications: unusual features. Pediatr Radiol 1990;20:585–587.
6. Sholler GF, Yu JS, Bale PM, et al. Generalized arterial calcification of infancy: three case reports, including spontaneous regression with long-term survival. J Pediatr 1984;105:257–260.
7. deMoraes CR. Calcification of the heart: a rare manifestation of chronic renal failure. Pediatr Radiol 1986;16:422–424.
8. Singleton EB, Merten DF. An unusual syndrome of widened medullary cavities of the metacarpals and phalanges, aortic calcification and abnormal dentition. Pediatr Radiol 1973;1:2–7.
9. Shikata A, Sugimoto T, Kosaka K, et al. Thoracic aortic calcification in 3 children with candidiasis-endocrinopathy syndrome. Pediatr Radiol 1993;23:100–103.

MISCELLANEOUS CARDIOVASCULAR DISEASES

Collagen Vascular Diseases

The vasculitis of the collagen vascular diseases can result in protean clinical manifestations. A complete discussion of these diseases is beyond the scope of this book, but it might be noted that periarteritis nodosa is more likely to be encountered in the neonate and young infant and lupus erythematosus in older children. Infants with periarteritis nodosa can present with transient skin rashes, conjunctivitis, prolonged fever, and abnormal renal function. Radiographically, the various findings result from a necrotizing angiitis, which leads to a bead-like arterial nodulation and aneurysm formation (1). Both systemic and coronary arteries can be involved, and myocardial infarction is a recognized complication. Recently, however, it has been noted that these coronary artery aneurysms can regress (2). Cardiomegaly and pericardial effusions also can be seen. In lupus erythematosus, pleural and pericardial effusions are common. Pulmonary manifestations are less pronounced, but if bleeding into the lungs occurs (secondary to the vasculitis), fluffy infiltrates or pseudoconsolidations can be seen (3).

With periarteritis nodosa, if the cranial vessels are involved, cerebral infarction can occur, and in the lungs, one may see cavitating nodules. Similar nodules, with or without cavitation, can be seen in lupus erythematosus. In rheumatoid arthritis, cardiovascular and pulmonary manifestations are much less common but can occur and are not unlike those seen with the other collagen vascular diseases.

REFERENCES

1. Eriksson BA, Foucard T, Lorelius LE, et al. Multiple aneurysm of visceral arteries in a child with polyarteritis nodosa. J Pediatr Surg 1980;15:347–348.
2. Glanz S, Bittner SJ, Berman MA, et al. Regression of coronary-artery aneurysms in infantile polyarteritis nodosa. N Engl J Med 1976;294:939–941.
3. Ramirez RE, Glasier C, Kirks D, et al. Pulmonary hemorrhage associated with systemic lupus erythematosus in children. Radiology 1984;152:409–412.

Mucocutaneous Lymph Node Syndrome

Originally a disease of the Japanese, mucocutaneous lymph node syndrome is now commonly reported on this continent. It is a disease of young children and infants, and the main features are fever lasting for 1 or 2 weeks, congestion of the conjunctiva, reddening of the lips and oral mucosa, and swelling of the cervical lymph nodes. Toward the end of a week, a macular, erythematous skin eruption develops, and there is marked hyperemia of the palms and soles. Thereafter, desquamation at the junction of the nails and skin occurs, but the heart and systemic artery complications are most devastating to these infants. Coronary artery and other vascular aneurysms are commonplace (1–3), and because of this, there has been some comparison to periarteritis nodosa (4).

Roentgenographically, the findings consist of cardiac silhouette enlargement in those cases with pericardial effusion, localized bulging of the cardiac silhouette in those cases with coronary artery aneurysms, and, on aortography, evidence of peripheral vasculitis with multiple aneurysm formation (Fig. 3.155). Deaths usually are related to the cardiovascular system, especially to the coronary arteries, but encephalopathy, gallbladder hydrops (5,6), and epiglottitis along with uvulitis (7) also have been reported. Indeed, almost every system of the body has been involved by this vasculitis.

In terms of the coronary artery aneurysms seen in these patients, 70% occur proximally and the larger ones tend to persist and may even calcify (8, 9). Smaller aneurysms tend to regress, and it has been noted that the larger aneurysms may, after they heal, contribute to adult coronary artery disease (10). Indeed, acute arteritis and its aftereffects are now being recognized as short- and long-term sequelae leading to myocardial schemia (11–13).

REFERENCES

1. Kato H, Koike S, Yamamoto M, et al. Coronary aneurysms in infants and young children with acute febrile mucocutaneous lymph node syndrome. J Pediatr 1975;86:892–898.
2. Kawasaki T, Kosaki F, Okawa S, et al. A new infantile acute febrile mucocutaneous lymph node syndrome (MLNS) prevailing in Japan. Pediatrics 1974;54:271–276.
3. Kuribayashi S, Ootaki M, Tsuji M, et al. Coronary angiographic abnormalities in mucocutaneous lymph node syndrome: acute findings and long-term follow-up. Radiology 1989;172:629–633.
4. Landing BH, Lason EJ. Are infantile periarteritis nodosa with coronary artery involvement and fatal mucocutaneous lymph node syndrome the same? Comparison of 20 patients from North America with patients from Hawaii and Japan. Pediatrics 1977;59:651–662.
5. Magilavy DB, Speert DP, Silver TM, et al. Mucocutaneous lymph node syndrome: report of two cases complicated by gallbladder hydrops and diagnosed by ultrasound. Pediatrics 1978; 61:699–702.

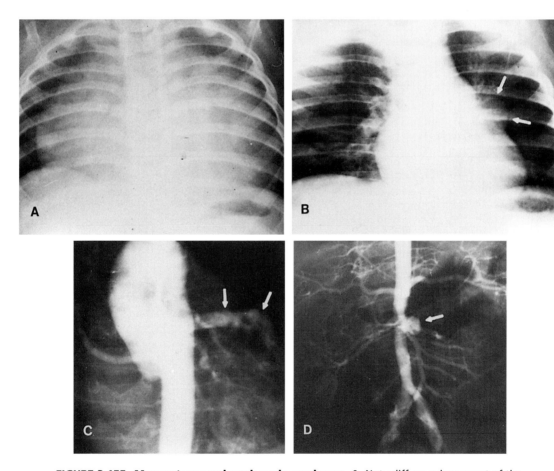

FIGURE 3.155. Mucocutaneous lymph node syndrome. A. Note diffuse enlargement of the cardiac silhouette resulting from pericardial effusion. **B.** The pericardial effusion has cleared, and the heart is now near normal in size. Note the localized bulge along the left cardiac border (arrows). This was a result of a coronary artery aneurysm. **C.** Aortogram demonstrating the aneurysmally dilated left coronary artery (arrows). **D.** Abdominal aortogram demonstrating another large aneurysm (arrow) and other smaller aneurysms and tortuosity of the aorta and systemic vessels. (Reproduced with permission from Cook A, L'Heureux P. Radiographic findings in the mucocutaneous lymph node syndrome. AJR 1979;132:107–109).

6. Slovis TL, Hight DW, Philippart AI, et al. Sonography in the diagnosis and management of hydrops of the gallbladder in children with mucocutaneous lymph node syndrome. Pediatrics 1980;65:789–794.
7. Kazi A, Gauthier M, Lebel MH, et al. Uvulitis and supraglottitis: early manifestations of Kawasaki disease. J Pediatr 1992;120:564–567.
8. Akagi T, Rose V, Benson LN, et al. Outcome of coronary artery aneurysms after Kawasaki disease. J Pediatr 1992;121:689–694.
9. Ino T, Shimazaki S, Akimoto K, et al. Coronary artery calcification in Kawasaki disease. Pediatr Radiol 1990;20:520–523.
10. Kato H, Inoue O, Kawasaki T, et al. Adult coronary artery disease probably due to childhood Kawasaki disease. Lancet 1992;230:1127–1129.
11. Burke AP, Virmani R, Perry LW, et al. Fatal Kawasaki disease with coronary arteritis and no coronary aneurysms. Pediatrics 1998;101:108–112.
12. McConnell ME, Hannon DW, Steed RD, et al. Fatal obliterative coronary vasculitis in Kawasaki disease. J Pediatr 1998;133:259–261.
13. Burns JC, Shika H, Gordon JB, et al. Sequelae of Kawasaki disease in adolescents and young adults. J am Coll Cardiol 1996;28:253–257.

Pulmonary Hypertension

Pulmonary hypertension is not as common in children (1) as in adults, but it does occur with longstanding left-to-right shunts and cardiac admixture lesions. It also can be seen with multiple thromboemboli, but, again, this is not as common in children as in adults. Pulmonary hypertension also occurs as a result of chronic pulmonary disease and is seen in the so-called "persistent fetal circulation syndrome" of infancy. Roentgenographically, the chest film findings in pulmonary hypertension vary, depending on the cause. In longstanding left-to-right shunts, the peripheral vascularity is diminished, while centrally the pulmonary artery and its proximal branches become large. When pulmonary hypertension results from pulmonary emboli, the lungs, in extreme cases, are undervascularized and the heart may show right-side enlargement.

REFERENCE

1. Perkin RM, Anas NG. Pulmonary hypertension in pediatric patients. J Pediatr 1984;105:511—522.

Pulmonary Artery Aneurysm

Pulmonary artery aneurysms on a congenital or acquired basis are uncommon. On an acquired basis, they can be seen after pulmonary infections (1) or percutaneous transluminal angioplasty (2).

REFERENCES

1. Moorthy C, Walser E, John SD, et al. Rupture of a solitary, erosive peripheral pulmonary artery aneurysm. Emerg Radiol 1996;3:253–257.
2. Simmons PL, Scavetta KL, McLeary MS, et al. Pulmonary artery pseudoaneurysm after percutaneous transluminal angioplasty in a pediatric patient. Pediatr Radiol 1997;27:760–762.

Microcardia

Microcardia, that is, an unusually small cardiac silhouette, is not uncommonly encountered in young infants (1). Most often, it is a temporary phenomenon resulting from excessive fluid loss. This usually occurs in infants with severe dehydration (vomiting, diarrhea) or massive blood loss. Characteristically, the cardiac silhouette is small, the pulmonary vascularity decreased, and the chest somewhat overaerated (Fig. 3.156). This latter finding is especially prevalent in those infants who are dehydrated and acidotic (1).

Apparent microcardia, the result of "stretching" of the mediastinum, can be seen with conditions leading to severe air trapping (e.g., bronchiolitis, asthma). Microcardia is also sometimes seen with adrenal insufficiency. In the neonate, this is usually part of the adrenogenital syndrome. Microcardia with actual loss of muscle bulk (atrophy) can be seen with chronic debilitating infection, severe malnutrition, or end-stage malignancy (1).

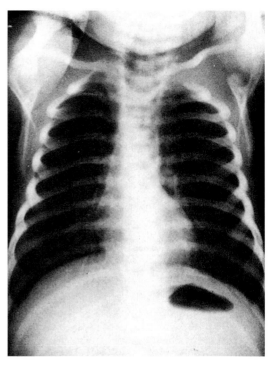

FIGURE 3.156. Microcardia. Note the small cardiac silhouette and thin pulmonary vessels in this infant with severe vomiting and diarrhea leading to marked dehydration.

REFERENCE

1. Swischuk LE. Microcardia: an uncommon diagnostic problem. AJR 1968;103:115–118.

Arteriovenous Fistulas

Arteriovenous fistulas can occur anywhere in the body. In the neonate, they are most commonly encountered with the vein of Galen malformation and as a manifestation of hemangiomatous tumors of the liver. However, they can also occur in the lung, anywhere in the abdomen, in the extremities, and in the neonate in the umbilical vessels. In this latter instance, the abnormality may be congenital in origin, resulting from persistent communication between the umbilical arteries and veins (1), or iatrogenically induced, after prolonged umbilical vessel canalization (2).

Arteriovenous fistulas may produce local symptoms, but in the infant, they not uncommonly lead to hyperkinetic congestive heart failure. They can also induce local overgrowth and hypertrophy of the surrounding tissues.

REFERENCES

1. Murray DE, Meyerowitz BR, Hutter JJ. Congenital arteriovenous fistula causing congestive heart failure in the newborn. JAMA 1969;209:770–771.
2. Reagan LC, James FW, Dutton RV. Umbilical artery-vein fistula. Am J Dis Child 1970;119:363–364.

Single Umbilical Artery

Over the years, considerable difference of opinion has existed as to whether the presence of a single umbilical artery predisposes the infant to an increased incidence of congenital anomalies, especially of the urinary tract. In the end, even if uncommon (1), some of the anomalies are significant, and now, since ultrasonography is so easy to obtain, it can be used to exclude these more rarely seen, but potentially serious, anomalies (2).

REFERENCES

1. Thummala MR, Raju TNK, Langenberg P. Isolated single umbilical artery anomaly and the risk for congenital malformations: a meta-analysis. J Pediatr Surg 1998;33:580–585.
2. Bourke WG, Clarke TA, Mathews TG, et al. Isolated single umbilical artery—the case for routine renal screening. Arch Dis Child 1993;68:600–601.

Systemic Hypertension

Systemic hypertension usually is diagnosed clinically, but radiographically, in some cases in older children, one may see evidence of left ventricular hypertrophy and a dilated aortic arch and descending aorta on chest films (Fig. 3.157). In this regard, while "physiologic" aortic dilatation may be common in adults, in the pediatric age group, undue aortic dilatation should be considered abnormal. In the workup of systemic hypertension, the radiologist usually is called upon to investigate the renal vascular system,

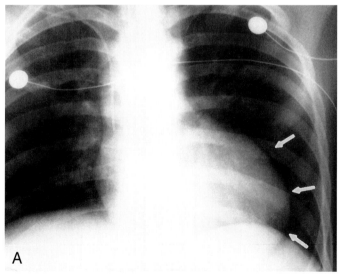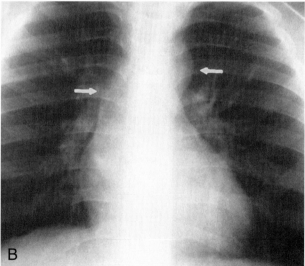

FIGURE 3.157. Systemic hypertension. A. Note left ventricular hypertrophy (arrows) and a prominent ascending aorta and aortic knob. **B.** Another patient demonstrating less hypertrophy but more prominence of the ascending aorta and aortic knob (arrows).

and this usually first entails ultrasonography, where morphology and size of the kidneys are documented as well as patency of the renal arteries. Nuclear scintigraphy also is useful, using the captopril-enhanced renal scan. Finally, however, arteriography usually is required, and abnormalities encountered include focal congenital renal artery stenosis, fibromuscular hyperplasia, and stenoses as seen with neurofibromatosis.

Vascular Catheter Complications

Complications arising from the use of indwelling catheters are numerous and result from thrombosis, embolization, or traumatic aneurysm formation. However, one may also perforate a blood vessel and produce bleeding (1). When the femoral artery is compromised, one can see complicating leg growth impairment or, on a more acute basis, skin and muscle necrosis (2, 3). Intravascular thrombi, catheter position (4), and vessel spasm of the larger vessels in neonates and young infants are readily evaluated with ultrasonography. Finally, it has been noted that medially deployed tubes for the treatment of pneumothoraces can compress the aorta and cause aortic obstruction in neonates (5).

REFERENCES

1. Johnson JF, Basilio FS, Pettett PG, et al. Radiographic exhibit: hemoperitoneum secondary to umbilical artery catheterization in the newborn. Radiology 1980;134:60.
2. Mortensson W. Effects of percutaneous femoral artery catheterization on leg growth in infants and children. Acta Radiol 1980;21:297–302.
3. Mann NP. Gluteal skin necrosis after umbilical artery catheterization. Arch Dis Child 1980;55:815–817.
4. Das Narla L, Hom M, Lofland GK, et al. Evaluation of umbilical catheter and tube placement in premature infants. Radiographics 1991;11:849–863.
5. Gooding CA, Kerlan RK Jr, Brasch RC, et al. Medially deployed thoracostomy tubes: cause of aortic obstruction in newborns. AJR 1981;136:511–514.

Cardiac Transplantation

Cardiac transplantation is not performed in all centers. In those centers where it is performed, those individuals dealing with the problem will be familiar with all the radiographic findings. The subject is too large to discuss here, but for those interested, references are provided (1–5).

REFERENCES

1. Armitabe JM, Fricker FJ, Kurland G, et al. Pediatric lung transplantation: expanding indications, 1985–1993. J Heart Lung Transplant 1993;12:S246–S254.
2. Backer CL, Zales VR, Idriss FS, et al. Heart transplantation in neonates and in children. J Heart Lung Transplant 1992;11:311–319.
3. Bailey LL, Gundry SR, Razzouk AJ, et al. Bless the babies: one hundred fifteen late survivors of heart transplantation during the first year of life. J Thorac Cardiovasc Surg 1993;105:805–815.
4. Chiavarelli M, Gundry SR, Razzouk AJ, et al. Cardiac transplantation for infants with hypoplastic left-heart syndrome. JAMA 1993;270:2944–2947.
5. Whitehead B, Helms P, Goodwin M, et al. Heart-lung transplantation for cystic fibrosis. 2. Outcome. Arch Dis Child 1991;66:1022–1026.

4

ALIMENTARY TRACT

A number of imaging modalities are available for evaluation of the abdomen and alimentary tract, but a preliminary plain film still is a usual starting point. Valuable data still can be obtained from this study, including the presence of free air, air in the bowel wall, level of intestinal obstruction, and location of masses. After this, one can proceed to upper gastrointestinal series, contrast enema, ultrasound, or computed tomography (CT). Magnetic resonance imaging (MRI) is useful on a selective basis.

In terms of the upper gastrointestinal (GI) series, contrast may be administered to the infant by a number of methods. Often, a simple baby bottle suffices, but in some cases, it may be more expedient and desirable to introduce contrast through a nasopharyngeal tube. Contrast should be introduced just over the base of the tongue so that the infant still will have to swallow. Contrast should not be delivered with the patient in the supine position. The infant should be in the lateral or right anterior-oblique position, because this guards against aspiration. Needless to say, the entire study should be fluoroscopically monitored and controlled.

With contrast enema examinations in newborn and young infants, the most important practical point is to have adequate occlusion of the anus. This can be facilitated by tightly squeezing the buttocks together and then taping them together with adhesive tape. A Foley catheter is preferred and should be inserted before taping of the buttocks. It is important to make a few points regarding the Foley balloon. When one is looking for low rectal pathology, such as Hirschsprung's disease, it is best not to blow up the balloon. However, once one demonstrates that the rectum is normal and one is looking for pathology higher in the colon, there is no doubt that, if one chooses not to inflate the balloon, **after a couple of patients evacuating prematurely, one will change one's ideas.** It is most important that snug occlusion be maintained, because without it, the study becomes prolonged, and radiation exposure is increased for the patient and physician. In most neonates and very young infants, it is best to inject the contrast material with a syringe, but in older patients, regular infusion is used. **With a syringe, one has a better idea of how much pressure is being applied to the colon.**

Preexamination preparation and intraexamination maneuvers are not usually as extensive as in older children and adults. In many cases, extensive preparation of the colon is not required and, in Hirschsprung's disease, is contraindicated. Similarly, with upper GI examinations in newborn and very young infants, all one should attempt is to omit the feeding before the examination. Overnight fasting is not required and is detrimental. In the neonate and young infant, fluid and electrolyte balance is delicate, and it is most important that these infants not be dehydrated for prolonged periods. Our preparation of infants and children for upper and lower examinations of the GI tract is presented in Table 4.1.

Contrast agents available for examination of the GI tract include barium, Gastrografin, and iso-osmolar (arionic) agents. Overall, barium still is the mainstay, but various aqueous, anionic contrast agents generally are used in infants and neonates. These contrast agents have virtually no deleterious effect on the GI, cardiovascular, or renal systems (1, 2). However, they are a little expensive but the preferred agents in neonates and premature infants and certainly in those with suspected GI perforations. One added benefit of these contrast agents is that they do remain as markers in the GI tract for prolonged periods. They are not absorbed as are the hypertonic aqueous contrast agents (3).

Hypertonic, hyperosmolar agents such as Gastrografin can lead to significant dehydration of the infant. These agents draw fluid into the colon and at the same time pass from the colon into the blood pool. Together, these factors lead to significant dehydration and electrolyte imbalance; any infant subject to a water-soluble, hyperosmolar contrast enema should be well hydrated before the examination, on intravenous fluids during the examination, and monitored carefully after the study is performed.

Another problem with hyperosmolar agents is that, if they are aspirated into the lungs, they cause marked irritation and pulmonary edema. Barium is not nearly as damaging to the lungs and, in fact, is innocuous. Because of this, the use of hypertonic, water-soluble contrast agents generally is discouraged when the upper GI tract is being examined, and now that iso-osmolar agents are available, hypertonic agents should not be used for examination of

TABLE 4.1. PREPARATION FOR CONTRAST STUDIES OF GASTROINTESTINAL TRACT

Upper GI series	
Infants ≤1 year	Omit AM feeding
Children >1 year	Nothing to eat or drink after PM meal
Contrast enema	
Infants ≤2 years	No preparation
Children 2–4 years	Whatever laxative used at home to be administered 1 day before examination; liquid diet all day
Children >4 years	Whatever laxative used at home to be administered 2 successive days before examination; on 2nd day, liquid diet
Air contrast barium enema	
Diet	For 2 days before the examination, low-residue diet; if possible, mostly clear liquids on last day
Cathartic	Magnesium citrate (4 ml/kg/dose) should be given at 2 PM on each of the 2 days before examination. (Magnesium citrate is not used in patients with renal insufficiency.)
Flush liquids	Total of three 8-oz glasses of clear liquids (e.g., tea, water, soft drinks) administered as follows: 1st glass 1 h before cathartic and then one glass each hour after the cathartic for 2 h. In infants (<4 years), reduce total volume of fluids to three 4-oz glasses.

the upper GI tract at all. In the lower intestinal tract, although barium enemas produce exceptionally sharp colonic outlines, hypertonic, water-soluble contrast enemas often are required. The reason for this is that hyperosmolar enemas are therapeutic in many of the conditions encountered in the first days of life (e.g., meconium plug syndrome, meconium ileus).

In terms of using a hypertonic, water-soluble agent for a therapeutic contrast enema, one usually is dealing with cases of suspected meconium ileus, the meconium plug syndrome, or the small left colon syndrome. The latter two syndromes probably are the same. In such cases, it probably is best to use Gastrografin (diatrizoate), which contains Tween 80 (polysorbate 80). This latter compound acts as a lubricant, emulsifier, and reducer of surface tension and as such plays a key role in the infant's ability to evacuate colon or small bowel contents in conditions in which the meconium is very sticky and tenacious. However, Gastrografin also can irritate the colonic mucosa. In our institution, for diagnostic enemas, Gastrografin is made isotonic with a 1:5 dilution with normal saline, and when used as a therapeutic enema, we dilute Gastrografin 1:3 with normal saline. Therapeutic Gastrografin enemas also can be used in chronic fecal impactions in older children, but it should not be employed if Hirschsprung's disease is suspected or diagnosed. Reactions to barium and latex are uncommon in children (4, 5).

REFERENCES

1. DiSessa TG, Zednikova M, Hiraishi S, et al. The cardiovascular effects of metrizamide in infants. Radiology 1983;148:687–691.
2. Harvey LA, Caldicott WJH, Kuruc A. The effect of contrast mediums on immature renal function: comparison of agents with high and low osmolality. Radiology 1983;148:429–432.
3. Cohen MD. Prolonged visualization of the gastrointestinal tract with metrizamide. Radiology 1982;144:327–328.
4. Llatser R, Zambrano C, Guillaumet B. Anaphylaxis to natural rubber latex in a girl with food allergy. Pediatrics 1994;94:736–737.
5. Stringer DA, Hassall E, Ferguson AC, et al. Hypersensitivity reaction to single contrast barium meal studies in children. Pediatr Radiol 1993;23:587–588.

ESOPHAGUS

Normal Features

The neonatal esophagus is a relatively simple structure easily studied with a barium swallow. Mucosal folds are not as prominent as in adults, but indentations by the aortic arch, left main stem bronchus, and normal left atrium are frequently noted, even in the neonate (Fig. 4.1). Normal peristaltic activity usually is evident at birth but may not be as pronounced as in later life. In the recumbent position, emptying of the esophagus may be somewhat prolonged.

In the neonate, the esophagus is flexible and can assume peculiar configurations during various phases of the respiratory cycle. The resulting bizarre, tortuous configuration of the esophagus at any level may at first appear startling, but repeat study usually demonstrates a normal esophagus (Fig. 4.2).

ESOPHAGEAL ABNORMALITIES

Air in the Esophagus (Pneumoesophagus)

Many infants demonstrate small amounts of air in the esophagus on regular chest films, and the finding is entirely normal. However, other infants demonstrate massive collections of air in the esophagus, or so-called **mega-aeroesophagus** (1). Such air collections are readily visible on plain chest films and can be startling (Fig. 4.3). In most of these cases, the underlying problem usually is gastroesophageal reflux (1), but excessive air in the esophagus also can be a sign of the presence of a tracheoesophageal fistula.

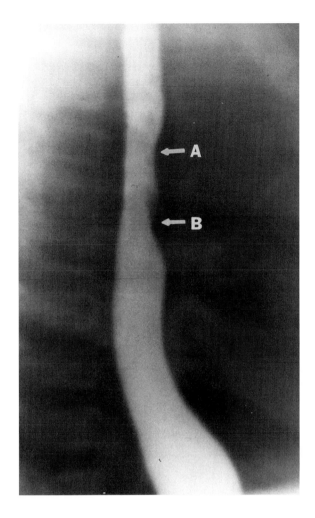

FIGURE 4.1. Normal esophagus. Lateral view showing normal indentations produced by aortic arch (A) and left main bronchus (B).

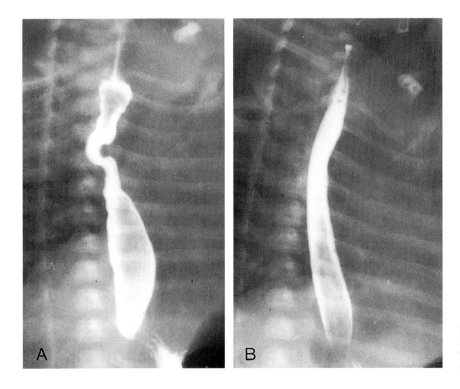

FIGURE 4.2. Tortuous esophagus. A. Bizarre, tortuous-appearing esophagus in young infant. **B.** Moments later, the esophagus appears normal.

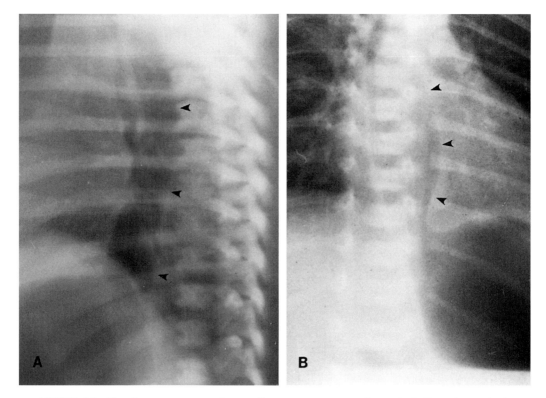

FIGURE 4.3. Massive pneumoesophagus (i.e., mega-aeroesophagus). A. Note the marked distention of the air-filled esophagus (arrows). This air is much more voluminous than that seen under normal circumstances. Most often, such massive distention of the esophagus is the result of gastroesophageal reflux. **B. Premature infant.** Supine position with air reflux from the stomach into the esophagus (arrows).

Patients with cerebral palsy and/or mental retardation also are likely to demonstrate massive volumes of air in the esophagus due to gastroesophageal reflux (1). Other causes of massive pneumoesophagus include obstruction of the distal esophagus, paralysis resulting from caustic burns, and vomiting such as may occur with acute gastroenteritis.

REFERENCE

1. Swischuk LE, Hayden CK Jr, Callie BD. Mega-aeroesophagus in children: a sign of gastroesophageal reflux. Radiology 1981;141: 73–76.

Transient Esophageal Hypotonia of the Neonate

In some newborn infants, the esophagus appears almost totally inactive, and even with prolonged examination, little peristaltic activity is noted (Fig. 4.4). These infants frequently have difficulty with swallowing, and regurgitation is common. This is why they are referred to the radiologist for examination. No obstructing lesions are found, and the phenomenon is transient. Within a week or less, normal

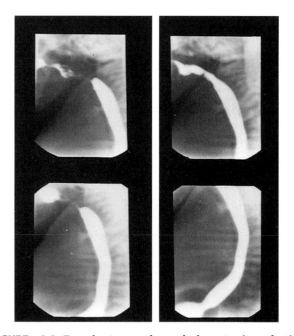

FIGURE 4.4. Transient esophageal hypotonia of the neonate. On these four spot films, taken in rapid sequence, note that there is no suggestion of peristaltic activity of the esophagus. Any one of the spot films could be interpreted as normal, but when it is noted that on none is there evidence of peristalsis of the esophagus, transient hypotonia should be suspected.

peristaltic activity prevails, feeding difficulties disappear, and the infant has no further problems. This lack of normal motility is simply a reflection of normal, but transient, neuromuscular immaturity.

Dysphagia Lusorum

Dysphagia lusorum is rare and often of questionable existence. However, it has been documented in children (1) and consists of mild to moderate dysphagia as a result of pressure on the esophagus by an aberrant right subclavian artery. The artery, because it anomalously arises as the last branch of the aortic arch, has to cross the mediastinum to get to the right. To do so, it must pass across the mediastinum, and it passes posterior to the esophagus and produces an indentation on the barium-filled esophagus. In the vast majority of cases, it is asymptomatic, but in some individuals, it can produce dysphagia (1), and we have seen one such child (see Fig. 3.117 in Chap. 3).

REFERENCE

1. Martin GR, Hillemeier C, Heyman MB. Dysphagia lusorum in children. Am J Dis Child 1986;140:815–816.

Gastroesophageal Reflux, Chalasia, and Hiatus Hernia

This has always been a controversial condition with discussion centering on (a) what degree of gastroesophageal reflux is significant, (b) the extent to which one should pursue its demonstration, (c) what exactly constitutes a hiatus hernia, and (d) how important is the demonstration of reflux in infants who already are known to be chronic vomiters.

Nuclear scintigraphy and pH monitoring (1) are most sensitive for the detection of reflux. However, since pH monitoring is invasive and time consuming, most settle for GE scintigraphy as the initial study. Ultrasonography also has been employed (3, 4) but has not come into common use across the board. **The upper GI series is not as sensitive as the other two studies but in our hands still produces good results and does detect most significant cases of gastroesophageal reflux.**

The pursuit of the demonstration of gastroesophageal reflux often is more exuberant than required. One reason for this is that one often forgets that serious complications such as stricture and significant esophagitis are rare and that most infants recover from reflux within a year, no matter what is done (5). Another reason for the overinvestigation of these patients is that often one fails to consider the fact that **if the patient is vomiting, regurgitating, or spitting up, then clearly the patient must be refluxing (6). Once this fact is accepted, there is little need in the vast majority of cases to verify that reflux is**

occurring with any imaging or clinical modality. There are, however, other times when the demonstration of reflux is of prime importance. For the most part, these cases consist of those patients where reflux is suspected in the absence of vomiting and regurgitation. **If one does not separate these patients from those who present because of vomiting, regurgitation, or excessive spitting up, one easily can see how overinvestigation of the latter patients can occur.** This is especially true with so many tests now being available for evaluating reflux.

Reflux can be primary and due to an immature and lax gastroesophageal sphincter. This is termed **chalasia.** Gastroesophageal reflux also occurs secondary to gastric outlet obstruction. Most commonly, the obstruction is due to pylorospasm but the next most common problem is pyloric stenosis. Thereafter, one can be dealing with gastric diaphragms or duodenal obstructing lesions. These lesions are readily detected with ultrasound, and only the latter need a confirmatory upper GI series.

In terms of determining severity of gastroesophageal reflux, a study attempting to grade it into five degrees or grades resulted in a final categorization of only two types: major and minor reflux (7). Minor reflux is reflux that occurs into the distal third of the esophagus only, whereas major reflux occurs above this level and frequently into the upper (cervical) esophagus. The latter is responsible for complications such as chronic aspiration and peptic stenosis. Minimal reflux is more difficult to assess, and in any given case, one often is unsure of just how significant it is. It probably is not significant.

The term **hiatus hernia** designates herniation of the stomach above the diaphragm into the thoracic cavity. Basically, there are two types of such herniation. The first is the sliding hiatus hernia, and the second is the paraesophageal hiatus hernia. The sliding hiatus hernia is more common and definitely the problematic lesion. Paraesophageal hiatus hernias, although often large, frequently also are asymptomatic. Both hernias are readily identified and differentiated one from the other roentgenographically (Fig. 4.5), and while the sliding hiatus hernia usually is associated with an incompetent lower esophageal sphincter, the paraesophageal hernia is not. The term "partial thoracic stomach" is an old term that, in essence, describes a fixed, sliding hiatus hernia. Often, it was used in conjunction with the term "congenitally short esophagus," but the latter probably does not exist. In most cases, the so-called congenitally short esophagus is an esophagus shortened by peptic esophagitis and stricture in utero. Overall, however, this lesion is rare, as is reflux-induced esophageal stenosis in infancy.

When dealing with infants who are vomiting, what is most important is that one evaluate the gastric outlet and determine whether it is normal or abnormal, for this determines whether treatment should be surgical or medical. For example, if the antral abnormality demonstrated is fixed (e.g., pyloric stenosis, gastric diaphragm, mass cyst), surgi-

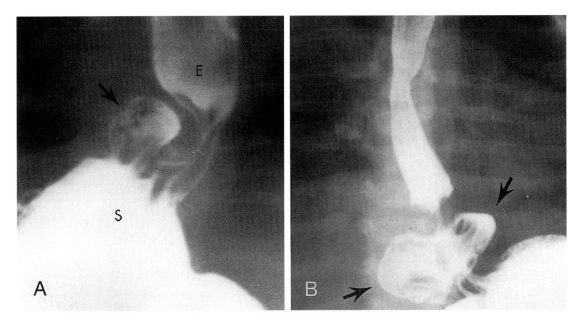

FIGURE 4.5. Hiatus hernia: paraesophageal versus sliding types. A. Small paraesophageal hiatus hernia (arrow). E, esophagus; S, stomach. **B.** Large, incarcerated, sliding hiatus hernia (arrows). The narrowing above the hernia is the esophageal sphincter, while that below is the result of puckering as the hernia passes through the diaphragmatic leaflet.

cal treatment is in order, but if a functional obstruction is demonstrated (e.g., pylorospasm, gastric ulcer disease), medical treatment is the choice (6). This is best evaluated with ultrasound because it can assess directly, the gastric lumen, mucosa, and muscle.

The upper GI series readily demonstrates gross reflux and demonstrates most cases of significant moderate reflux (Fig. 4.6). It also generically evaluates the status of the gastric outlet and can give one some idea of the state of gastric emptying. Gastroesophageal scintigraphy is sensitive for the demonstration of reflux (Fig. 4.7) but provides no data regarding antral anatomy. It can provide information regarding rates of gastric emptying, but no antroanatomic information is available. Ultrasound demonstrates both gross and lesser degrees of reflux (Fig. 4.8), but it is a little tedious to perform and probably will not replace the upper GI series, gastroesophageal scintigram, or pH monitoring.

As far as the technique for performing the upper GI series is concerned, the study should be initiated with the patient swallowing in the lateral position. This guards against any aspiration. Thereafter, the patient is turned into the right anterior-oblique position so that the gastric outlet and duodenum can be evaluated. At this point the patient can be placed supine on its back, and the gastroesophageal junction intermittently monitored for the presence of reflux. **At this stage, all must be alert to any noise or sound that the patient may make that suggests that reflux has occurred and that the patient may be aspirating.** The patient, under these circumstances, should be immediately flipped to the side or face down.

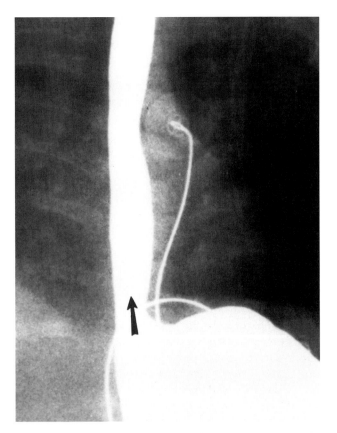

FIGURE 4.6. Gastroesophageal reflux. Note the straight, rigid-like appearance of the esophagus as barium refluxes (arrow) through the open distal esophageal sphincter. The straight appearance of the esophagus is due to lack of peristalsis during the sudden burst of reflux.

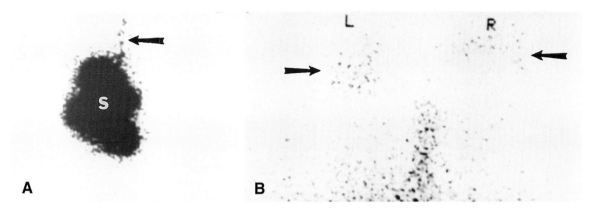

FIGURE 4.7. Gastroesophageal reflux: nuclear scintigraphy. A. Note reflux into the esophagus (arrows) from the stomach (S). **B.** Delayed image demonstrates aspiration into both lungs (arrows).

As far as gastroesophageal scintigraphy is concerned, after fasting for a minimum of 6 hours, formula or juice with technetium-99m sulfur colloid is administered to the patient. The patient is burped and placed in a supine position with a gamma camera under the table. Images of the upper abdomen and chest are obtained in the supine and left lateral decubitus positions. At 3–4 hours, a 5-minute image of the chest is obtained to determine whether aspiration has occurred into the lungs. All of these maneuvers are enhanced by the use of film format and computer-acquired, contrast-enhanced (single photon emission computed tomography [SPECT]) images.

With ultrasound, the patient is examined in the recumbent position but somewhat turned toward the examiner. In the longitudinal plane, the gastroesophageal junction easily can be visualized, and gross reflux in the form of free, sonolucent fluid is clearly visible (Fig. 4.8B). More often,

however, microbubble-induced streaks of echogenicity are seen as reflux into the esophagus (Fig. 4.8A).

In summary, when we deal with a patient who is vomiting or regurgitating, we go directly into the ultrasound study so that we can evaluate the gastric outlet. However, if there is any indication in the history that swallowing is a problem, we perform an upper GI series. In older children, no matter what the problem, we begin with the upper GI series because ultrasonography of the stomach is less productive. In infants, however, the ultrasound study is most informative, and thereafter, there is little need for an upper GI series, a gastroesophageal scintigram, or pH monitoring. If the patient is refractory to medical treatment (i.e., longer than 2–4 weeks), we reevaluate the patient with ultrasound.

In terms of esophagitis and esophageal stricture, although these are known complications of gastroesophageal reflux, they are not nearly as common as once

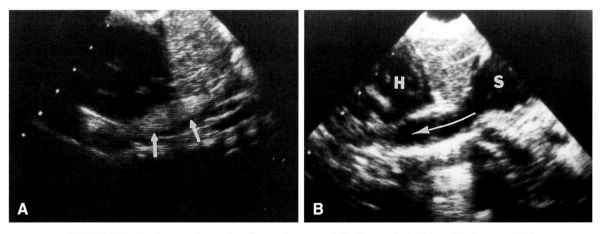

FIGURE 4.8. Gastroesophageal reflux, ultrasound findings. A. In this patient, on sagittal section through the gastroesophageal junction, note an echogenic bolus of fluid (arrows) being refluxed into the esophagus. **B.** Another patient with gross reflux (arrow). S, stomach; H, heart.

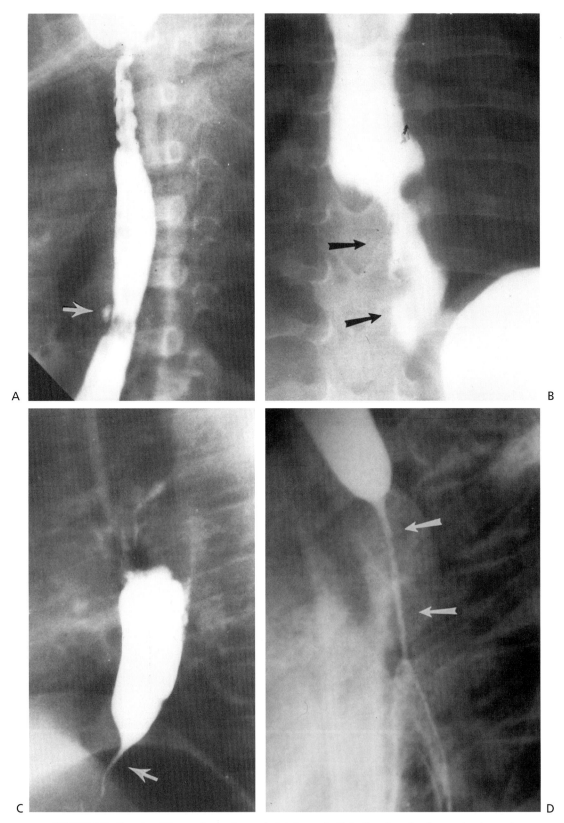

FIGURE 4.9. Esophagitis, and esophageal stricture. A. Note the discrete ulcer crater (arrow). **B.** Diffuse esophagitis leading to spasm and profound irregularity of the distal esophagus (arrows). **C.** Distal esophageal stenosis (arrow). **D.** Severe mid-esophageal stenosis (arrows).

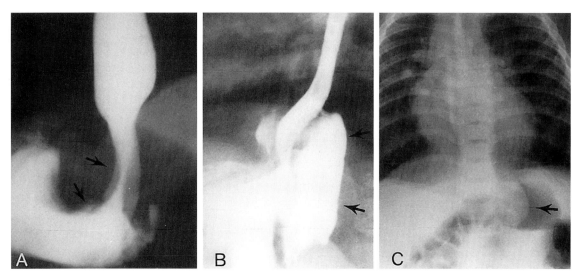

FIGURE 4.10. Fundoplication for hiatus hernia. A. Note the narrowed distal esophageal segment, located well below the diaphragm. It is narrowed because the fundus of the stomach has been wrapped around it. This causes a pseudotumor (arrows) of the stomach. **B.** Fundoplication procedure with recurrent herniation into the thoracic cavity (arrows). Reflux occurred in this patient, but it does not always recur with such reherniation. **C.** Characteristic fundal pseudotumor (arrows) in patient with fundoplication procedure.

suggested. Furthermore, most cases are mild and disappear with satisfactory medical treatment. In more severe cases with actual dysphagia, a barium swallow is in order, because severe esophagitis and complicating strictures are readily identified with this study (Fig. 4.9). Treatment of reflux primarily is medical and, in this regard, often involves nothing more than changing a milk formula to a nonallergenic formula, such as Nutramigen. If this fails and no surgical lesion is identified, the patient can be placed on frequent, thickened feedings and, if required, placed in an upright position in an antireflux sling. If this type of medical therapy fails, one can attempt drug therapy in the form of bethanechol (Bentyl).

If medical management is unsuccessful, surgical correction is required. Recently, it has been shown that pyloromyotomy is as effective as pyloroplasty in these patients (8). Associated fundoplication of the gastroesophageal junction also usually is performed. In this procedure, the esophagus is drawn below the diaphragm and a portion of the stomach wrapped around it. This reinforces the gastroesophageal vestibule and usually is curative. Roentgenographically, the mass-like appearance of the fundoplication should not be misinterpreted for a gastric tumor (Fig. 4.10A). In some cases, the hernia recurs and the fundoplicated portion of the stomach herniates into the thorax (9) (Fig. 4.10B). Very often, but certainly not always, the postoperative gastroesophageal junction again becomes incompetent. A rare complication of the procedure is reverse gastroesophageal intussusception (10). In addition, a very smooth esophageal mucosal pattern resembling a feline (smooth) esophagus has been demonstrated in patients with esophagitis (11).

REFERENCES

1. Andze GO, Brandt ML, St-Vil D, et al. Diagnosis and treatment of gastroesophageal reflux in 500 children with respiratory symptoms: the value of pH monitoring. J Pediatr Surg 1991;26:295–300.
2. Da Dalt L, Mazzoleni S, Montini G, et al. Diagnostic accuracy of pH monitoring in gastroesophageal reflux. Arch Dis Child 1989;64:1421–1426.
3. Gomes H, Lallemand A, Lallemand P. Ultrasound of the gastroesophageal junction. Pediatr Radiol 1993;23:94–99.
4. Gomes HL, Menanteau B. Gastroesophageal reflux: comparative study between sonography and pH monitoring. Pediatr Radiol 1991;21:168–174.
5. Nelson SP, Chen EH, Syniar GM, et al. Prevalence of symptoms of gastroesophageal reflux during infancy: a pediatric practice-based survey. Pediatric Practice Research Group. Arch Pediatr Adolesc Med 1997;151:569–572.
6. Swischuk LE, Fawcett HD, Hayden CK Jr. Gastroesophageal reflux: how much imaging is required? Radiographics 1988;8:1137–1145.
7. McCauley RGK, Darline DB, Leonidas JC, et al. Gastroesophageal reflux in infants and children: a useful classification and reliable physiologic technique for its demonstration. AJR 1978;130:47–50.
8. Okayama H, Urao M, Starr GA, et al. A comparison of the efficacy of pyloromyotomy and pyloroplasty in patients with gastroesophageal reflux and delayed gastric emptying. J Pediatr Surg 1997;32:316–320.
9. Festen C. Paraesophageal hernia: a major complication of Nissen's fundoplication. J Pediatr Surg 1981;16:496–499.
10. Post PJ, Robben SG, Meradji M. Gastro-oesophageal intussusception after Nissen-fundoplication. Pediatr Radiol 1990;20:282.
11. Rencken IO, Heyman MB, Perr HA, et al. Ringed esophagus (feline esophagus) in childhood. Pediatr Radiol 1997;27:773–775.

Gastroesophageal Reflux and Associated Conditions

Although gastroesophageal reflux generally is considered a condition attendant primarily with GI symptoms, it is becoming increasingly apparent that a wide variety of other symptom complexes can occur. One of the first such complexes recognized was **Sandifer's syndrome,** a condition in which peculiar torsion spasms of the head and neck mimic torticollis, opisthotonos, or "seizure" activity (1, 2). These symptoms definitely can cause one to focus on an underlying neurologic problem. However, the torsion spasms merely represent postural abnormalities used by the patient to avoid reflux of esophageal contents over the vocal cords. All of these abnormal motions dissipate once the gastroesophageal reflux is corrected.

Reflux of gastric acid contents over the vocal cords also can lead to cyanotic "seizures" or apneic spells or the sudden infant death syndrome (3–5). Reflux, by distending the esophagus, can cause vagal-induced bradycardia. Gastroesophageal reflux leading to chronic aspiration can result in refractory bronchitis or asthma. However, this is far less common than originally believed. The same could also be said for apneic spells induced by reflux. In terms of documenting aspiration into the lungs, the best imaging study probably is the gastroesophageal scintigram. It does, however, have variable results, and in our own hands, it has proved to be less sensitive than expected (6).

Rumination is another symptom of gastroesophageal reflux (7) and probably is more common than generally appreciated. It also should be noted that gastroesophageal reflux occurs more commonly in brain-damaged children and those with cerebral palsy (8, 9). Just why this should occur is not known, but decreased lower esophageal sphincter tone has been demonstrated in these individuals (8). In addition, the chronic supine position in which many of these patients live must be a causative factor. More recently, gastroesophageal reflux in retarded children has received special emphasis, because many of these patients undergo corrective surgery for scoliosis. Aspiration into the lungs with general anesthesia becomes a serious possible complication.

Finally, it might be recalled that reflux is a significant problem in many infants with esophageal atresia and seems to be a problem after surgical repair of congenital diaphragmatic hernia (10).

REFERENCES

1. Hadar A, Azizi E, Lernau O. Sandifer's syndrome: a rare complication of hiatal hernia. A case report. Z Kinderchir 1984;39: 202–203.
2. Murphy WJ Jr, Gellis SS. Torticollis with hiatus hernia in infancy. Am J Dis Child 1977;131:564–565.
3. Gomes H, Lallemand P. Infant apnea and gastroesophageal reflux. Pediatr Radiol 1992;22:8–11.
4. Jolley SG, Halpern LM, Tunell WP, et al. The risk of sudden infant death from gastroesophageal reflux. J Pediatr Surg 1991; 26:691–696.
5. Menon AP, Schefft GL, Thach BT. Apnea associated with regurgitation in infants. J Pediatr 1985;106:625–629.
6. Fawcett HD, Hayden CK, Adams JC, et al. How useful is gastroesophageal reflux scintigraphy in suspected childhood aspiration? Pediatr Radiol 1988;18:311–314.
7. Herbst J, Friedland GW, Zboralski F. Hiatal hernia and "rumination" in infants and children. J Pediatr Surg 1995;29: 1447–1451.
8. Halpern LM, Jolley SG, Johnson DG. Gastroesophageal reflux: a significant association with central nervous system disease in children. J Pediatr Surg 1991;26:171–173.
9. Swischuk LE, Hayden CK Jr, van Caillie BD. Mega-aeroesophagus in infancy and childhood—a sign of gastroesophageal reflux. Radiology 1981;141:73–76.
10. Nagaya M, Akatsuka H, Kato J. Gastroesophageal reflux occurring after repair of congenital diaphragmatic hernia. J Pediatr Surg 1995;29:1447–1451.

Esophageal Atresia and Tracheoesophageal Fistula

In this group of abnormalities, it is of some practical value to consider three types of abnormality: (a) simple esophageal atresia, (b) esophageal atresia with tracheoesophageal fistula, and (c) tracheoesophageal fistula with no esophageal atresia. A diagrammatic representation of the most common types is presented in Figure 4.11. Most often, esophageal atresia and tracheoesophageal fistula still are classified in this manner, but more complex classifications also are available. However, for diagnostic purposes **the durable and simple classification** presented in Figure 4.11 suffices.

The etiology of esophageal atresia and tracheoesophageal fistula generally is considered to be due to faulty separation of the primitive, embryonic trachea and esophagus. The failure of recanalization theory cannot be applied to the esophagus because no solid stage in the developing esophagus occurs. With faulty separation of the esophagus and trachea, segmental esophageal atresia occurs and may (most common) or may not be associated with a tracheoesophageal fistula. In regard to the latter, the fistulous connection usually occurs from the trachea to the distal esophageal pouch. On rare occasions, a fistula from the proximal pouch also may be present, and rarely, one may find multiple fistulas (1, 2). The next most common anomaly is esophageal atresia without fistula, followed by tracheoesophageal fistula without esophageal atresia (i.e., H-fistula). A rare form of esophageal atresia is that resulting from a membrane or web occurring alone or in association with an H-fistula (3, 4).

Esophageal atresia is not uncommonly associated with other anomalies of the GI tract, particularly imperforate (ectopic) anus and duodenal atresia or stenosis. In addition, cardiac anomalies, other tracheobronchial anomalies (5–7), renal anomalies, and anomalies of almost all other systems

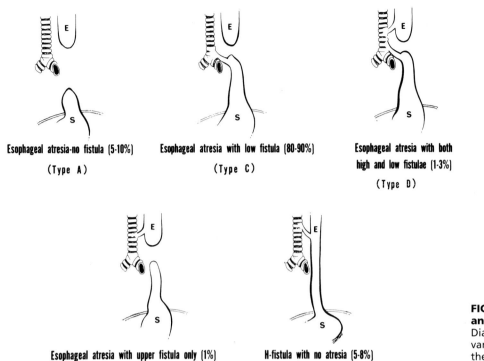

Esophageal atresia-no fistula (5-10%)
(Type A)

Esophageal atresia with low fistula (80-90%)
(Type C)

Esophageal atresia with both
high and low fistulae (1-3%)
(Type D)

Esophageal atresia with upper fistula only (1%)
(Type B)

H-fistula with no atresia (5-8%)
(Type E)

FIGURE 4.11. Esophageal atresia and tracheoesophageal fistula. Diagrammatic representation of the various anomalies encountered and their relative incidence. E, esophagus; S, stomach.

frequently are encountered (7, 8). One of the most curious associated anomalies, however, is that related to the vertebra and ribs. In approximately 25% of cases, 13 or more thoracic vertebral bodies and ribs or 6 or more lumbar vertebral bodies are present (9, 10). This associated abnormality also can signify the presence of a long gap between the proximal and distal esophageal pouches (10).

Clinically, infants with esophageal atresia, regardless of whether a fistula is present or not, present early. There is difficulty in handling normal secretions, choking, and drooling. Feeding is attendant with great difficulty, and regurgitation, aspiration, and respiratory distress all occur. In tracheoesophageal fistula with no atresia (H-fistula), initial symptoms may not appear as striking, and some patients may remain undiagnosed even into late childhood. On the other hand, if the fistula is large enough to allow contents from the esophagus to pass freely into the tracheobronchial tree, severe problems arise early. No distinct familial tendency has been documented in esophageal atresia, but a number of occurrences of more than one case in the same family have been noted (11, 12).

Roentgenographically, the findings vary from one type of abnormality to another. Aspiration pneumonia frequently is present and, in cases with esophageal atresia, often involves the right upper lobe. In many cases, one is able to identify the radiolucent, air-filled, blind-ending distended proximal esophageal pouch on chest films (Fig. 4.12). On frontal view, the radiolucency produced by this pouch should not be confused with a similar, but normal radiolucency resulting from

air in the suprasternal fossa (see Fig. 1.23 in Chap. 1). In cases of esophageal atresia with no fistula, no air enters the GI tract, and the abdomen is airless (Fig. 4.12). Since air usually is seen in the stomach within 15 minutes after birth, an airless abdomen in the neonate should suggest the strong possibility of esophageal atresia with no tracheoesophageal fistula. In cases in which a fistulous communication between the tracheobronchial tree and distal esophageal pouch exists, gas is present in the GI tract (Fig. 4.13).

Further delineation of the obstructed proximal pouch can be accomplished in a variety of ways, but it often is debatable as to whether any additional procedures are really necessary. It is a rare occasion when one can demonstrate a tracheal fistula from the proximal esophageal pouch, but if further delineation of the pouch is desired, it should be performed under fluoroscopic control. Only a small amount of barium or nonionic contrast material should be introduced (both are safe, but barium is cheaper) by way of a nasopharyngeal tube (Fig. 4.14A). This should be done with the infant in lateral position, and then, to facilitate demonstration of a possible associated fistula, the infant can be turned prone. The infant should not be put in the supine position, because aspiration may occur. When the examination is complete, instilled barium should be removed, and if the procedure is performed in this manner, there is little chance of barium aspiration. When fluoroscopy is not available or even before it is performed, simple passage of a soft opaque tube into the proximal pouch usually confirms the diagnosis (Fig. 4.14B).

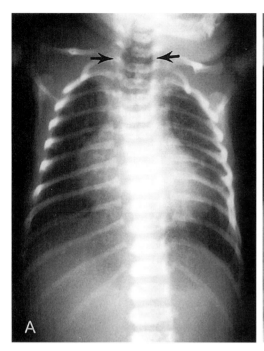

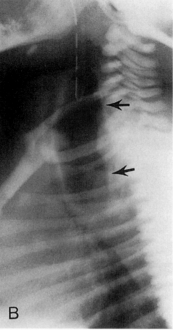

FIGURE 4.12. Esophageal atresia without a fistula: type A. A. Note the airless abdomen and dilated proximal esophageal pouch (arrows). This infant also had congenital heart disease. **B.** Lateral view in another infant demonstrates the classic air-filled proximal pouch (arrows). Note that the trachea is displaced forward and compressed. This leads to tracheomalacia, which can cause postoperative respiratory difficulty.

The distal pouch in cases of esophageal atresia without fistula can be delineated with barium or air. This is best accomplished by refluxing barium or air into the distal esophagus after a gastrostomy has been performed (Fig. 4.15). This is best accomplished in the left lateral position, and the subsequent combination of proximal and distal pouch delineation enables one to determine whether a direct end-to-end anastomosis is possible. This is of special value in cases for which elongation of the proximal pouch is contemplated.

In cases of H-fistula, the pattern of pneumonia usually is more widespread, and delineation of the fistula may be difficult. A dilated air-filled proximal esophageal pouch is not seen, but excessive air is seen in the esophagus as a result of air entering the esophagus through the fistula from the trachea. However, all of these findings are subtle, and the definitive diagnosis usually depends on contrast studies.

In examining infants with possible H-type fistula, contrast material should be introduced through a tube placed just over the base of the tongue. These infants, as those with esophageal atresia, should be examined in the lateral position, but not in the supine position. The tube must be placed high, for many of these fistulas are located in the lower cervical and upper thoracic areas. If the tube is placed too low, the fistula may be missed, but when seen, it characteristically assumes an upwardly oblique configuration (Fig. 4.16). It should be stressed that this is the characteristic slope of the fistula, rather than it being horizontal, as might be implied by the "H-fistula" connotation. In some infants, one also is able to demonstrate excessive air distention of the esophagus during inspiration (Fig. 4.17). Various degrees of hypoplasia of the esophagus in the area of the fistula also can be seen, and the fistula can be demonstrated endoscopically. This latter procedure is especially valuable with smaller, more elusive fistulas (13). With esophageal atresia, one occasionally can visualize the fistula from the trachea to the distal esophagus on plain films. In such cases, with inspiration, the fistula will dilate, and the distal esophagus will become distended with air (Fig. 4.18), and finally all these anomalies can be evaluated with three-dimensional CT (5, 14).

Congenital esophageal stenosis, with or without tracheobronchial remnants (15–17), can be a significant associated problem in esophageal atresia (Fig. 4.19). The distal esoph-

FIGURE 4.14. Esophageal atresia. A. A small amount of barium outlines the proximal pouch (arrows). **B.** The blind-ending proximal pouch (arrows) can also be identified with the introduction of an opaque catheter.

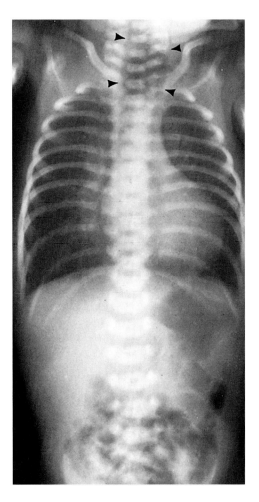

FIGURE 4.13. Esophageal atresia with a lower fistula: type C. Note the dilated air-filled esophageal pouch (arrows). However, also note that air is present in the GI tract. This indicates that a fistula to the distal esophagus is present.

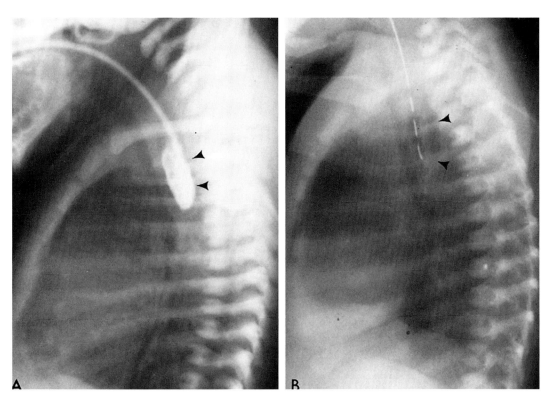

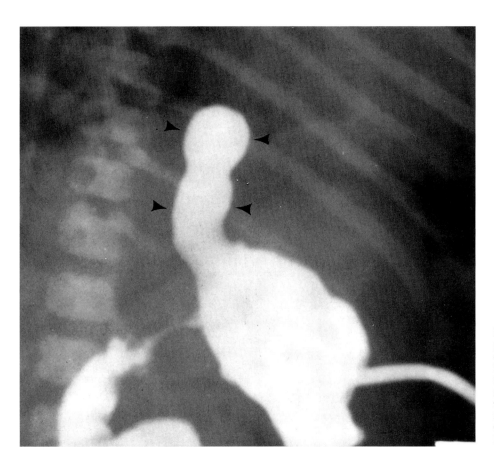

FIGURE 4.15. Distal esophageal pouch. Through a gastrostomy one can reflux barium from the stomach into the distal esophageal pouch (arrows). (Reproduced with permission from Swischuk LE. Demonstration of the distal esophageal pouch in esophageal atresia without fistula. Am J Roentgenol Radium Ther Nucl Med 1968;103:277–280.)

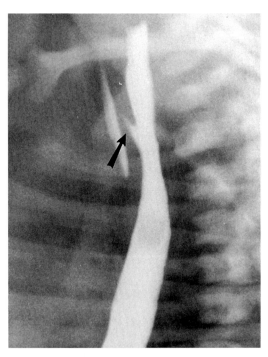

Figure 4.16. H-fistula. Note characteristic position and obliquity of the tracheoesophageal fistula (arrow). There is some aspiration of barium into the trachea.

agus often is hypoplastic in these patients, and motility in the distal segment usually is abnormal. Therefore, even though the fistula may be closed and the esophagus reanastomosed, problems with dysphagia often persist. It has been demonstrated by microdissection that the myenteric plexus of the esophagus and proximal stomach, along with that of the trachea, is abnormal in patients with esophageal atresia and tracheoesophageal fistula (18, 19).

Finally, in all cases, the surgeon requires information regarding the position of the aortic arch in these infants. It is important for the surgeon to know whether the aortic arch is right or left sided to facilitate surgical repair. This can be difficult to demonstrate in neonates, and magnification, high-kilovoltage techniques, and CT and MR examinations have been used to meet this end. Ultrasonography also can identify the aortic arch and determine whether it is left or right sided, but the study is not always easy to accomplish.

Postoperative Problems

The problems of dysphagia can occur postoperatively because of abnormal esophageal motility (20). Part of this problem lies in the inherent motility abnormality seen in these esophagi, but part may result from vagal nerve damage during mobilization of the esophagus. Fistulas, sinus tracts, and stenotic areas around the anastomotic site also are potential problems. The smaller fistulas and sinus tracts usually spontaneously regress and disappear (Fig. 4.19), but larger ones may require surgical intervention. Stenoses can be refractory and may require balloon dilation (21, 22) or surgical repair.

Shortening of the esophagus is a common problem in patients with esophageal atresia after surgical repair. Associated hiatus hernias and gastroesophageal reflux also are common. Another problem in these patients is that of focal tracheomalacia (Fig. 4.20). Tracheomalacia, or softening of the trachea, is believed to result from chronic intrauterine compression of the trachea by the distended upper esophageal pouch (23, 24). Such distention of the pouch is readily apparent on regular roentgenograms, and one easily can see how chronic pressure on the trachea could occur. However, although some of these patients initially are in serious respiratory difficulty, most seem to fare reasonably well, and eventually the trachea grows to a more normal

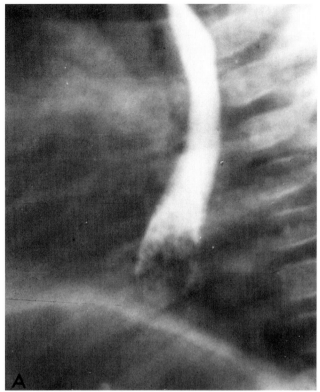

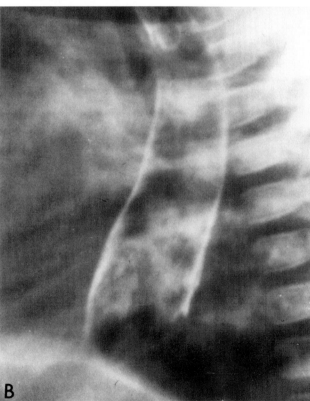

FIGURE 4.17. H-fistula. A. The esophagus is of normal diameter during expiration. B. During inspiration the esophagus is markedly dilated. Such distention occurs because air enters the esophagus through the tracheoesophageal fistula.

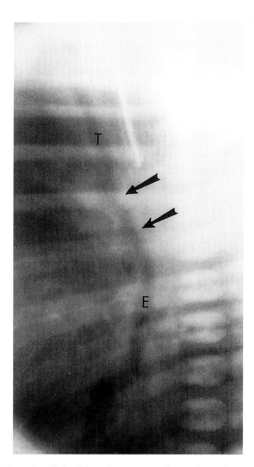

FIGURE 4.18. Plain film demonstration of tracheoesophageal fistula. Note the continuous column of air from the trachea (T), through the fistula (arrows), into the esophagus (E). An opaque tube is in the blind proximal pouch.

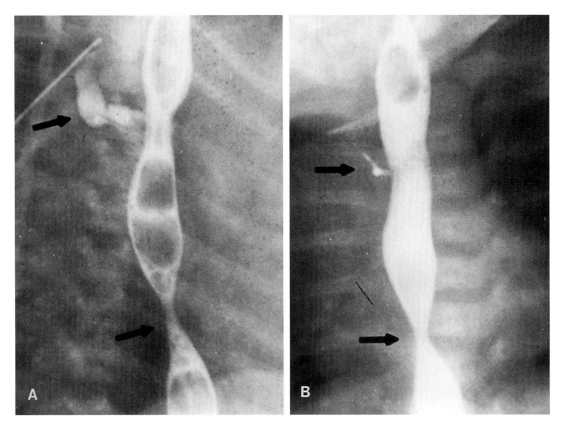

FIGURE 4.19. Postoperative sinus tract. A. Note the postoperative sinus tract at the anastomotic site (upper arrow). There is minimal narrowing of the esophagus at this point, but lower in the esophagus, an area of more pronounced stenosis (lower arrow) is present. **B.** A few weeks later, the sinus tract is barely detectable (upper arrow), but stenosis remains the same (lower arrow).

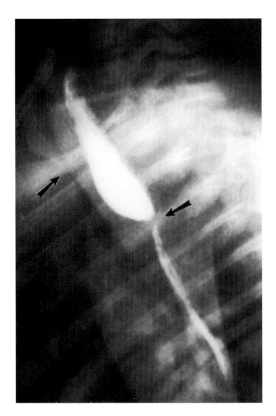

FIGURE 4.20. Tracheomalacia. Note the anteriorly displaced and narrowed trachea (arrows) being compressed by the air-filled and distended esophageal pouch.

diameter. A final interesting point regarding tracheomalacia is that it is not common when only esophageal atresia (without fistula) occurs (25).

REFERENCES

1. Yun KL, Hartman GE, Shochat SJ. Esophageal atresia with triple congenital tracheoesophageal fistulae. J Pediatr Surg 1992;27:1527–1528.
2. Johnson AM, Rodgers BM, Alford B, et al. Esophageal atresia with double fistula: the missed anomaly. Ann Thorac Surg 1984;38:195–200.
3. Gopal SC, Gangopadhyay AN, Pandit SK. Membranous atresia of the lower oesophagus. Pediatr Surg Int 1993;8:140–141.
4. Sharma AK, Sharma KK, Sharma CS, et al. Congenital esophageal obstruction by intraluminal mucosal diaphragm. J Pediatr Surg 1991;26:213–215.
5. Lam W-M, Tam PKH, Chan F-L, et al. Esophageal atresia and tracheal stenosis: use of three-dimensional CT and virtual bronchoscopy in neonates, infants, and children. AJR 2000;174:1009–1012.
6. Newman B, Bender TM. Esophageal atresia, tracheoesophageal fistula and associated congenital esophageal fistula and associated congenital esophageal stenosis. Pediatr Radiol 1997;27:530–534.
7. Ein SH, Shandling B, Wesson D, et al. Esophageal atresia with distal tracheo-esophageal fistula: associated anomalies and prognosis in the 1980s. J Pediatr Surg 1989;24:1055–1059.
8. Tovar JA, Frais EG, Martinez A, et al. Malformations of the spine and limbs in 120 cases of esophageal atresia and tracheo-oesophageal fistula. Ann Chir Infant 1974;15:29–37.
9. Hodson CJ, Shaw DG. Congenital atresia of the oesophagus and thirteen pairs of ribs. Pediatr Radiol 1973;1:248–249.
10. Kulkarni B, Rao RS, Oak S, et al. Pairs of ribs—a predictor of long gap atresia in tracheoesophageal fistula. J Pediatr Surg 1997;32:1453–1454.
11. Dennis NR, Nicholas JL, Kovar I. Oesophageal atresia: 3 cases in 2 generations. Arch Dis Child 1973;48:980–982.
12. Gibson BW, Moore R, Bianchine JW. Familial tracheoesophageal fistula in four members of a kindred. Am J Hum Genet 1974;26:34A.
13. Benjamin B, Pham T. Diagnosis of H-type tracheoesophageal fistula. J Pediatr Surg 1991;26:667–671.
14. Fitoz S, Atasoy C, Yagmurlu A, et al. Three-dimensional CT of congenital esophageal atresia and distal tracheoesophageal fistula in neonates: preliminary results. AJR 2000;175:1403–1407.
15. Neilson IR, Croitoru DP, Guttman FM, et al. Distal congenital esophageal stenosis associated with esophageal atresia. J Pediatr Surg 1991;26:478–482.
16. Olguner M, Ozdemir T, Akgur FM, et al. Congenital esophageal stenosis owing to tracheobronchial remnants: a case report. J Pediatr Surg 1997;32:1485–1487.
17. Yeung CK, Spitz L, Brereton RJ, et al. Congenital esophageal stenosis due to tracheobronchial remnants: a rare but important association with esophageal atresia. J Pediatr Surg 1992;27:852–855.
18. Yutaka N, Landing BH, Wells TR. Abnormal Auerbach plexus in the esophagus and stomach of patients with esophageal atresia and tracheoesophageal fistula. J Pediatr Surg 1986;21:831–837.
19. Yutaka N, Wells TR, Landing BH. Abnormal tracheal innervation in patients with esophageal atresia and tracheoesophageal fistula: study of the intrinsic tracheal nerve plexuses by a microdissection technique. J Pediatr Surg 1986;21:838–844.
20. Putnam TC, Lawrence RA, Wood BP, et al. Esophageal function after repair of esophageal atresia. Surg Gynecol Obstet 1984;158:344–348.
21. Kleinman PK, Waite RJ, Cohen IT, et al. Atretic esophagus: transgastric balloon-assisted hydrostatic dilation. Radiology 1989;171:831–833.
22. Sato Y, Frey EE, Smith WL, et al. Balloon dilation of esophageal stenosis in children. AJR 1988;150:639–642.
23. Griscom NT, Martin TR. The trachea and esophagus after repair of esophageal atresia and distal fistula: computed tomographic observations. Pediatr Radiol 1990;20:447–450.
24. Schwartz MZ, Filler RM. Tracheal compression as a cause of apnea following repair of tracheoesophageal fistula: treatment by aortopexy. J Pediatr Surg 1980;15:842–848.
25. Rideout DT, Hayashi AH, Gillis DA, et al. The absence of clinically significant tracheomalacia in patients having esophageal atresia without tracheoesophageal fistula. J Pediatr Surg 1991;26:1303–1305.

Peptic Esophagitis

Peptic esophagitis, in its early stages, is best assessed with endoscopy. By the time radiographic evidence of its presence is noted, disease is fairly advanced. Initially, there is lack of peristalsis of the esophagus, and then fine mucosal ulcerations are seen. Eventually, these ulcerations become more ragged, and the esophageal wall thickens (Fig. 4.9). Most of the changes occur in the distal one third or one half of the esophagus, and stricture formation eventually may be seen. Fortunately, however, the overall problem of advanced esophagitis and stricture formation is not very common. Most patients who have reflux cease to have reflux before advanced changes occur.

The complication of Barrett's esophagus is not common in childhood (1–4). In this condition, gastric mucosa lines the esophagus, and an area of stenosis is seen at its upper end (Fig. 4.21). This lesion has a malignant predisposition (5, 6), but for the most part, its occurrence in children is rare. With treatment, some patients can return to normal (7).

REFERENCES

1. Bar-Maor JA, He YR, Li D. Barrett's epithelium, with complete stricture of the esophagus: hypothesis of its etiology. J Pediatr Surg 1995;30:893–895.
2. Dahms BB, Rothstein FC. Barrett's esophagus in children: a consequence of chronic gastroesophageal reflux. Gastroenterology 1984;86:318–323.
3. Gorostiaga L, Tovar JA, Echeverry J, et al. Barrett's oesophagus in children and adolescents. Pediatr Surg Int 1993;8:389–394.
4. Othersen HB Jr, Ocampo RJ, Parker EF, et al. Barrett's esophagus in children: diagnosis and management. Ann Surg 1993;217:676–681.
5. Hassall E, Dimmick JE, Magee JF. Adenocarcinoma in childhood Barrett's esophagus: case documentation and the need for surveillance in children. Am J Gastroenterol 1993;88:282–288.
6. Hoeffel JC, Nihoul-Fekete C, Schmitt M. Esophageal adenocarci-

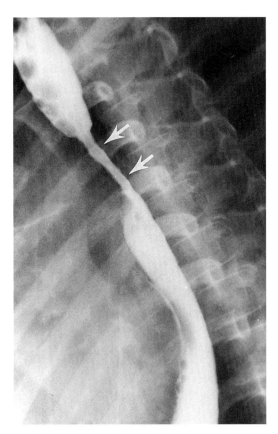

FIGURE 4.21. Barrett's esophagus. Note area of narrowing in the upper esophagus (arrows). In this case, narrowing is higher than usual. Most often, it occurs in the lower third of the esophagus, just above the diaphragm.

noma after gastroesophageal reflux in children. J Pediatr 1989; 115:259–261.
7. Beddow ECL, Wilcox DT, Drake DP, et al. Surveillance of Barrett's esophagus in children. J Pediatr Surg 1999;34:88–91.

Monilial Esophagitis (Thrush)

Although monilial infections in the neonate are common, esophageal involvement is rare. Similarly, monilial esophagitis in older children is uncommon, but it is a distinct problem in immunologically compromised children. Involvement can be diffuse or focal, although most often it is diffuse. The changes are best demonstrated with barium swallow and consist of extreme spasm leading to so-called pseudodiverticula (1), or mucosal edema and ulceration leading to cobblestoning (2, 3). In a few cases, superficial aphthous ulcers are seen (4), and complicating stricture occasionally develop. Most often, the findings are totally reversible with appropriate medical therapy. Examples of the various appearances of monilial esophagitis are presented in Figure 4.22.

REFERENCES

1. Markle BM, Hanson K. Esophageal pseudodiverticulosis: two new cases in children. Pediatr Radiol 1992;22:194–195.
2. Goldberg HI, Dodds WJ. Cobblestone esophagus due to monilial infection. AJR 1968;104:608–612.
3. Sam JW, Levine MS, Rubeshin SE, et al. The "foamy" esophagus: a radiographic sign of *Candida* esophagitis. Diagn Radiol 2001; 281–285.
4. Glick SN. Barium studies in patients with *Candida* esophagitis: pseudoulcerations simulating viral esophagitis. AJR 1994;163: 349–352.

Herpes Esophagitis

Herpes infection can involve the larynx and esophagus (1) and can be seen in the neonate. It also is seen in immunodeficient children, and the radiographic changes most often are focal and consist of esophageal spasm, lack of normal motility, and diffuse, small, aphthous ulcers (Fig. 4.23). While these findings can be seen with other viral infections of the esophagus, the most commonly appreciated is that resulting from herpes. Most often, the changes are self-limiting, but strictures occasionally develop.

REFERENCE

1. Lallemand D, Huault G, Laboureau JP, et al. Laryngeal and oesophageal lesions in patients with herpetic disease. Ann Radiol 1974;17:317–325.

Corrosive Esophagitis

Esophagitis secondary to ingestion of corrosive material such as sodium hydroxide, while a common problem in the past, is becoming less common with public awareness of the sequelae. In the usual case, however, extensive burns eventually result in stricture, and this is especially likely to occur when liquid caustic preparations are ingested (1). In the early stages, with more severe burns, necrosis and perforation of the esophagus can occur. With milder burns, no particular abnormalities of the esophagus are visible, except that the involved segment may be paralyzed and show aperistalsis. When stenosis occurs, it usually involves a long segment and is irregular, but short-segment stenosis and web strictures also can be seen (Fig. 4.24). In more severe cases, stricture of the distal end of the stomach can occur, but gastric strictures are more common with acid ingestion (2). Recently, it has been advocated that long-term stenting of these esophageal strictures can aid in their dissipation (3).

Focal, corrosive esophagitis also can occur from the ingestion of Clinitest tablets (4) and alkaline disc batteries (5–7). The hydroxide from these ingested articles can produce extensive burns to the esophagus and even result in tracheoesophageal fistulas (8). In older children, tetracy-

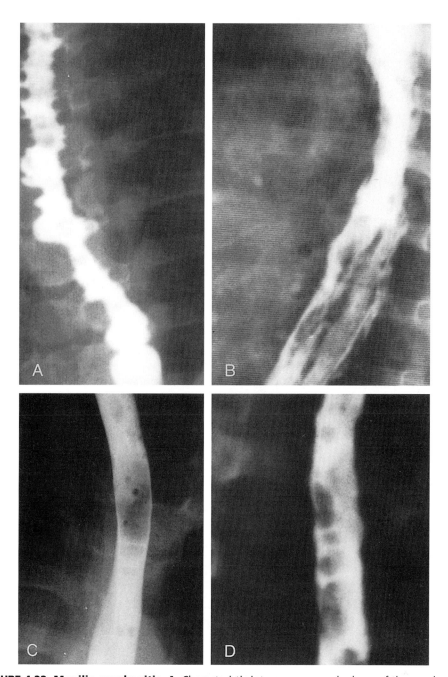

FIGURE 4.22. Monilia esophagitis. A. Characteristic intense spasm and edema of the esophagus producing widespread serrated, pseudodiverticular appearance in an 8-month-old infant. **B.** Another patient showing less spasm but more pronounced mucosal edema and cobblestoning. Ulceration also is suggested. **C.** Older patient with only a few small nodules in the esophagus. **D.** Another patient demonstrating large filling defects suggesting cobblestoning.

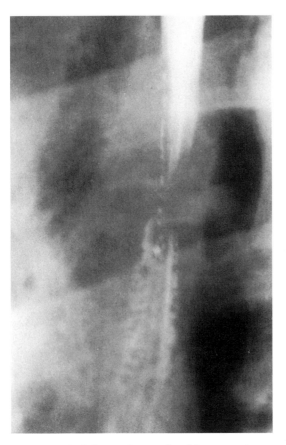

FIGURE 4.23. Viral herpetic esophagitis. Note the spasm, irregularity, and diffuse ulceration of the midportion of the esophagus.

cline can produce local esophagitis. The condition usually is self-limiting and produces changes similar to those seen with viral (herpes) esophagitis. This is especially worth remembering in older children who are treated for acne with tetracycline.

REFERENCES

1. Leape LL, Ashcraft KW, Scarpelli DG, et al. Hazard to health: liquid lye. N Engl J Med 1971;284;578–581.
2. Muhletaler CA, Gerlock AJ Jr, de Soto L, et al. Acid corrosive esophagitis: radiographic findings. AJR 1980;134:1137–1140.
3. Mutaf O. Treatment of corrosive esophageal strictures by long-term stenting. J Pediatr Surg 1996;31:681–685.
4. Burrington JD. Clinitest burns of the esophagus. Ann Thorac Surg 1975;20:400–404.
5. Litovitz TV. Button battery ingestions. A review of 56 cases. JAMA 1983;249:2495–2500.
6. Maves MD, Lloyd TV, Cariters JS. Radiographic identification of ingested disc batteries. Pediatr Radiol 1986;16:154–156.
7. Votteler TP, Nash JC, Rutledge JC. The hazard of ingested alkaline disk batteries in children. JAMA 1983;249:2504–2506.
8. Vaishnav A, Spitz L. Alkaline battery-induced tracheo-oesophageal fistula. Br J Surg 1989;76:1045.

Esophageal Stenosis

Congenital esophageal stenosis is uncommon but can be seen in association with tracheoesophageal fistula and on an isolated basis with the so-called cartilaginous ring (1) or tra-

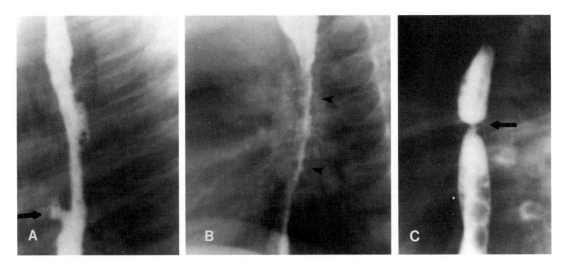

FIGURE 4.24. Corrosive esophagitis. A. Acute phase. Note intense spasm of the esophagus, numerous mucosal irregularities, and one large sinus tract extending into the mediastinum (arrow). **B.** Typical long segment, irregular stenosis (arrows). **C.** Focal stenosis produced by a resultant web (arrow).

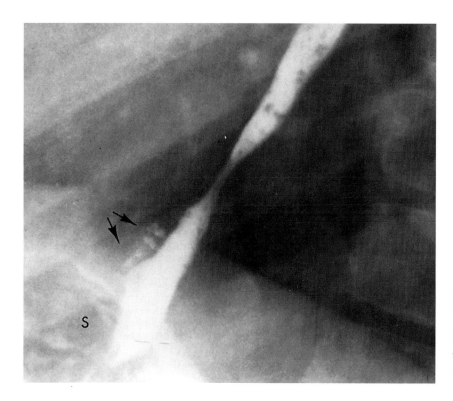

FIGURE 4.25. Tracheobronchial remnants. Older child with distal esophageal stenosis and barium-filled diverticular-like structures or clefts (arrows) representing the tracheobronchial remnants. These clefts are lined with respiratory epithelium and stenosis is the result of a cartilaginous ring. S, stomach. (Courtesy of W. H. McAlister, M.D.)

cheobronchial remnant syndromes (2, 3). Tracheobronchial remnants in the latter patients consist of aberrant cartilage or muscle and are associated with small diverticular-like structures. The lesion usually occurs in the lower esophagus (Fig. 4.25).

Overall, however, the most common cause of stenosis of the esophagus in childhood is acquired esophagitis. Most often, this is secondary to peptic esophagitis or corrosive material ingestion, but it also has been documented with chronic granulomatous disease (4). Esophageal stricture also can be seen with the Stevens-Johnson syndrome (2). Many of these strictures are dilated with intraluminal balloons (6–9), but the procedure is not free of complications such as perforation (10).

REFERENCES

1. Anderson LS, Shackelford GD, Mancilla-Jimenez R, et al. Cartilaginous esophageal ring: cause of esophageal stenosis in infants and children. Radiology 1973;108:665–666.
2. Nishina T, Tsuchida Y, Saito S. Congenital csophageal stenosis due to tracheobronchial remnants and its associated anomalies. J Pediatr Surg 1981;16:190–193.
3. Ohkawa H, Takahashi H, Hoshino Y, et al. Lower esophageal stenosis in association with tracheobronchial remnants. J Pediatr Surg 1975;10:453–457.
4. Renner WR, Johnson JF, Lictenstein JE, et al. Esophageal inflammation and stricture: complication of chronic granulomatous disease of childhood. Radiology 1991;178:189–191.
5. Edell DS, Davidson JJ, Muelenaer AA, et al. Unusual manifestation of Stevens-Johnson syndrome involving the respiratory and gastrointestinal tract. Pediatrics 1992;89:429–432.
6. Allmendinger N, Hallisey MJ, Markowitz SK, et al. Balloon dilation of esophageal strictures in children. J Pediatr Surg 1996;31:334–336.
7. Grabowski ST, Andrews DA. Upper esophageal stenosis: two case reports. J Pediatr Surg 1996;31:1438–1439.
8. Jayakrishnan VK, Wilkinson AG. Treatment of oesophageal strictures in children: a comparison of fluoroscopically guided balloon dilatation with surgical bouginage. Pediatr Radiol 2001;31:98–101.
9. Johnsen A, Jensen LI, Mauritzen K. Balloon-dilation of esophageal strictures in children. Pediatr Radiol 1986;16:388–391.
10. Kim IO, Yeon KM, Kim WS, et al. Perforation complicating balloon dilation of esophageal strictures in infants and children. Radiology 1993;189:741–744.

Esophageal Webs

Congenital esophageal webs are uncommon, and those that are seen usually are associated with tracheoesophageal fistu-

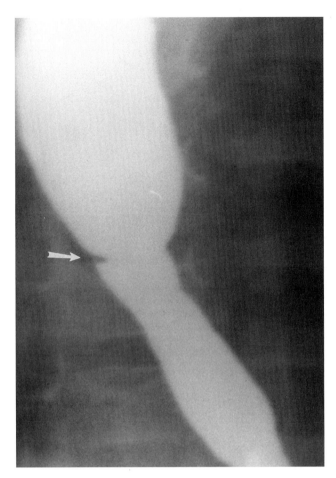

FIGURE 4.26. Esophageal web. Note a thin esophageal web (arrow) in the upper esophagus. The esophagus proximal to the web is distended. This patient had marked gastroesophageal reflux and esophagoscopic evidence of esophagitis.

las (1–3). Such webs or diaphragms are located across from the fistula and probably are a form of esophageal atresia. However, the esophagus appears normal externally. Esophageal webs also can be acquired secondary to lye burns, chronic esophageal reflux, or epidermolysis bullosa (4), but in any case, the web can be defined during barium swallow as a transverse or oblique, thin, radiolucent defect in the esophagus (Fig. 4.26).

REFERENCES

1. Grabowski ST, Andrews DA. Upper esophageal stenosis. Two case reports. J Pediatr Surg 1996;31:1438–1439.
2. Maclean AD, Houghton-Allen BW. Upper oesophageal web in childhood. Pediatr Radiol 1975;3:240–241.
3. Fox PF. Unusual esophageal atresia with tracheoesophageal fissure (membrane). J Pediatr Surg 1978;13:373.
4. Hillemeier C, Touloukian R, McCalluym R, et al. Esophageal web: a previously unrecognized complication of epidermolysis bullosa. Pediatrics 1981;67:678–682.

Esophageal Varices

Esophageal varices in the neonate and young infant are rare, and most cases are secondary to portal hypertension resulting from hepatic cirrhosis or portal vein obstruction. Portal vein obstruction is frequently the result of thrombosis secondary to sepsis and/or dehydration. In many such cases, subsequent cavernous transformation of the portal vein occurs, and a collateral circulation develops. Roentgenographically, esophageal varices on barium swallow appear as dilated, straight or serpentine tubular structures (Fig. 4.27A). Varices also can be detected with CT (Fig. 4.27C) and MRI, and they are especially well visualized with color-flow Doppler. Eventually, however, they are best demonstrated with dedicated positive contrast splenoportography (Fig. 4.27B).

Esophageal Diverticula and Duplications

Congenital esophageal diverticula are uncommon (1), but can produce dysphagia, regurgitation, and even airway obstruction. These diverticula probably represent incompletely separated duplication (neurenteric) cysts (2, 3), and the only connection to the spinal canal may be a fibrous band. Completely separated duplication cysts usually manifest as masses in the mediastinum and may or may not produce symptoms. In this regard, it should be noted that the esophagus is the second most common site of GI duplication, and on rare occasions, duplication of the esophagus can be associated with that of the stomach (4, 5). Multiple cysts can occur (6). Duplication cysts can be identified with any number of imaging modalities, and since many contain gastric mucosa, they are positive on technetium-99m isotope scans. Esophageal diverticula are best demonstrated with barium swallow (Fig. 4.28, A and B).

Traumatic diverticula in the neonate and young infant result from iatrogenic submucosal perforation of the esophagus and are a complication of intubation (7 –9). Most of these perforations arise just above the cricopharyngeus muscle and may more properly be considered pharyngeal diverticula. Symptoms consist of dysphagia, respiratory distress, and hematemesis, but some patients may be asymptomatic. In the symptomatic infant it is not unusual to first consider a congenital obstruction such as esophageal atresia (3). Treatment is conservative (8), for the diverticula or sinus tracts tend to obliterate with time (Fig. 4.28, C and D).

Complete duplication of the esophagus so as to produce a double esophagus is rare (2). Usually, one end is

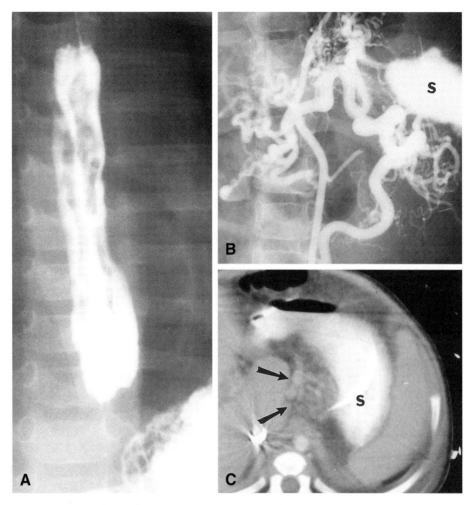

FIGURE 4.27. Esophageal varices. A. Note the broad, tortuous, radiolucent bands running throughout the length of the esophagus. These are characteristic of esophageal varices. **B.** Splenoportogram. Injection into the splenic pulp (S) demonstrates extensive varices upward into the gastroesophageal region, downward into the splenorenal area, and across midline around the distal stomach and duodenum. **C.** In another patient, CT demonstrates nodular and serpentine varices just below the gastroesophageal junction (arrows). S, stomach.

blind, but it may connect to the spinal canal with a fibrous band; the other opens into the stomach (Fig. 4.29).

REFERENCES

1. Ohbatake M, Muraji T, Yamazato M, et al. Congenital true diverticula of the esophagus: a case report. J Pediatr Surg 1997;32: 1592–1594.
2. Billmire DF, Allen JE. Duplication of the cervical esophagus in children. J Pediatr Surg 1995;30:1498–1499.
3. Superina RA, Ein SH, Humphreys RP. Cystic duplications of the esophagus and neurenteric cysts. J Pediatr Surg 1984;19:517–530.
4. Moir JD. Combined duplication of the esophagus and stomach. J Can Assoc Radiol 1970;21:257–262.
5. Mazziotti MV, Ternberg JL. Continuous communicating esophageal and gastric duplication. J Pediatr Surg 1997;32: 775–778.
6. Robison J, Paulina PM, Sherer LR, et al. Multiple esophageal duplication cysts. J Thorac Cardiovasc Surg 1987;94:144–147.
7. Armstron RG, Lindberg EF, Stanford W, et al. Traumatic pseudo-diverticulum of the esophagus in the newborn infant. Surgery 1970;67:844–846.
8. Astley R, Roberts KD. Intubation perforation of the esophagus in the newborn baby. Br J Radiol 1970;43:219–222.
9. Ducharme JC, Bertrand R, Debie J. Perforation of the pharynx in the newborn: a condition mimicking esophageal atresia. Can Med Assoc J 1971;104:785–787.

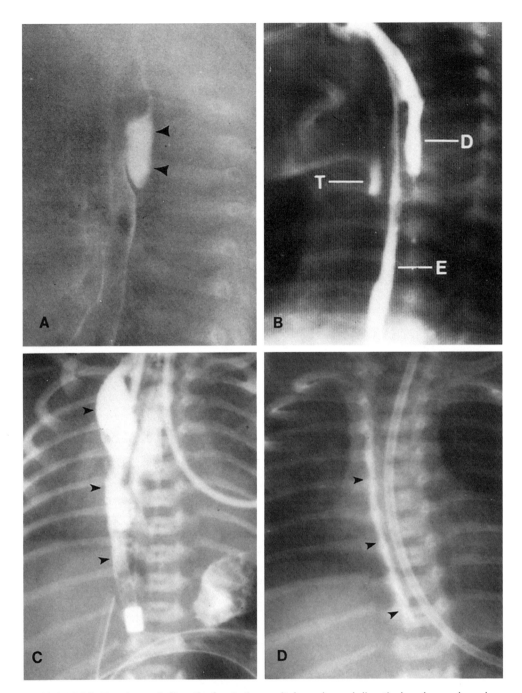

FIGURE 4.28. Esophageal diverticula. A. Congenital esophageal diverticulum (arrows), probably representing an incomplete esophageal duplication. A hemivertebra at the T4 level was present, and at surgery a fibrous band extending from the diverticulum to the cleft vertebra was present. **B.** Posttraumatic (perforation with tube) esophageal diverticulum (D), esophagus (E), trachea (T). **C.** Iatrogenic sinus tract or pseudodiverticulum of the esophagus. Note the large sinus tract (arrows). The nasogastric tube with a metallic (rectangular) bead at its distal end is present in the sinus tract. The true esophagus lies medial to the tract. This patient was relatively asymptomatic. **D.** Weeks later, only a thin strand of barium remains in the spontaneously obliterating sinus tract (arrows). (**A** reproduced with permission from Astley R, Roberts KD. Intubation perforation of the esophagus in the newborn baby. Br J Radiol 1970;43:219–222.)

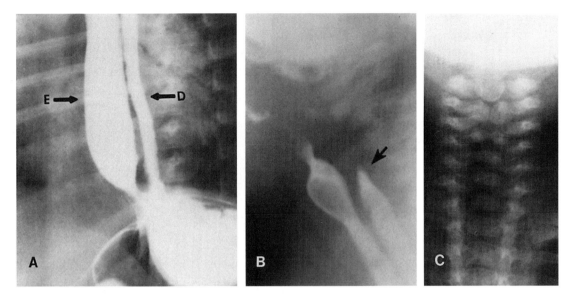

FIGURE 4.29. Esophageal duplication. A. Note the esophagus proper (E) and the duplicated esophagus posteriorly (D). **B.** Upper end demonstrating the blind-ending duplicated esophagus (arrow). At surgery, a thin fibrous strand extended from this blind-ending pouch to the body of C4. This was a vestigial remnant of the primitive neurenteric canal. **C.** Cervical spine in the same infant demonstrates anterior vertebral body defects, consistent with the hypothesis of abnormal neurenteric canal development.

MISCELLANEOUS ESOPHAGEAL LESIONS

Achalasia

Achalasia is rare in infancy and childhood (1). Familial cases have been documented and often are associated with selective adrenocorticotropic hormone (ACTH) insensitivity, alacrima, and neurologic abnormalities (2–4). Symptoms usually consist of chronic regurgitation of undigested food, aspiration pneumonia, and failure to thrive. The etiology of the condition is unknown, but in some cases, absence of ganglion cells in the distal esophagus has been noted (2).

Roentgenographically, plain film findings are scant in early infancy. The esophagus usually is not so dilated that it can be seen on plain chest roentgenograms. In older children, however, it often is dilated and filled with fluid and may show an air-fluid level in the upright position. Occasionally, one may see the entire esophagus filled with air, but generally, this is an uncommon presentation of achalasia in any age group. Most often, the dilated esophagus is full of fluid or food and may at first suggest a mediastinal mass, but it should be emphasized that this is a late stage finding and not commonly seen in infancy or early childhood. A barium swallow is required to demonstrate the dilated esophagus and characteristic distal beak deformity (Fig. 4.30). Lack of normal peristalsis or bizarre contractions of the esophagus above the beak also can be seen and

serve to distinguish achalasia from cardiospasm and peptic esophagitis.

Treatment usually consists of dilating the distal esophageal sphincter (5–7), but in infancy, this is often difficult to accomplish. Furthermore, one runs the risk of esophageal perforation or mucosal tears. For this reason, in the newborn infant at least, some prefer formal, surgical cardiomyotomy (3). Postoperatively, gastroesophageal reflux can be a significant problem.

REFERENCES

1. Berquist WE, Byrne WJ, Ament ME, et al. Achalasia: diagnosis, management and clinical course in 16 children. Pediatrics 1983; 71:798–805.
2. Ambrosino MM, Genieser NB, Bangaru BS, et al. The syndrome of achalasia of the esophagus, ACTH insensitivity and alacrima. Pediatr Radiol 1986;16:328–329.
3. Nihoul-Fekete C, Bawab F, Lortat-Jacob S, et al. Achalasia of the esophagus in childhood: surgical treatment in 35 cases with special reference to familial cases and glucocorticoid deficiency association. J Pediatr Surg 1989;24:1060–1063.
4. Tryhus MR, Davis M, Griffith JK, et al. Familial achalasia in two siblings: significance of possible hereditary role. J Pediatr Surg 1989;124:292–295.
5. Hammond PD, Moore DJ, Davidson GP, et al. Tandem balloon dilatation for childhood achalasia. Pediatr Radiol 1997;27: 609–613.

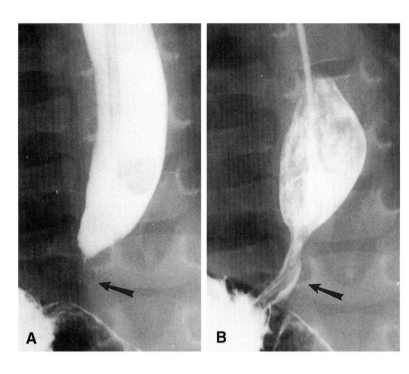

FIGURE 4.30. Achalasia. A. Note the distended esophagus and beak-like deformity (arrow) of its distal end. **B.** Barium passes into the stomach, but the distal end of the esophagus still remains abnormally narrow (arrow).

6. Perisic VN, Scepanovic D, Radlovic N. Nonoperative treatment of achalasia. J Pediatr Gastroenterol Nutr 1996;22:45–47.
7. Wilkinson AG, Raine PAM, Fyfe AHB. Pneumatic dilatation in childhood cardio-achalasia. Pediatr Radiol 1997;27:60–62.

Cardiospasm

Cardiospasm is a condition in which there is temporary, but intense, spasm of the distal esophagus. The etiology of cardiospasm is unknown, but successful treatment with antispasmodic therapy supports the concept of transient muscular spasm. In the newborn infant, cardiospasm may be a transient manifestation of immaturity of lower esophageal sphincter. However, the beak-like deformity is most difficult to differentiate from the one seen with achalasia (Fig. 4.31). Whereas bizarre peristaltic activity of the esophagus often is present in achalasia, such activity is not a feature of simple cardiospasm.

Chagas' Disease

Chagas' disease is extremely uncommon in our part of the world, but in the neonate, it can be acquired from the mother (1). The responsible organism is *Trypanosoma cruzi*, which in the neonate produces a generalized, systemic illness with hepatosplenomegaly, anemia, jaundice, edema, petechiae, neurologic symptoms, and GI problems. Later acquisition of the disease seems to ultimately focus on the GI tract, where histologically there is inflammation of the

mucosa and submucosa and destruction of the nerve cells of the myenteric plexus. Roentgenographically, the findings are difficult to differentiate from achalasia and, in the colon, from Hirschsprung's disease.

REFERENCE

1. Bittencourt AL. Congenital Chagas disease. Am J Dis Child 1976; 130:97–103.

Granulomatous Disease (Neutrophil Dysfunction)

In this condition, thickening and narrowing of the antrum is more common, but occasionally, a similar lesion can be seen in the esophagus (1, 2). Thickening is the result of a chronic, indolent inflammatory process common to these patients, whose basic problem lies in the presence of defective neutrophils, which results in difficulty mobilizing this line of defense against infection.

REFERENCES

1. Hiller N, Fisher D, Abrahamov A, et al. Esophageal involvement in chronic granulomatous disease. Case report and review. Pediatr Radiol 1995;25:308–309.
2. Renner WR, Johnson JF, Lictenstein JE, et al. Esophageal inflam-

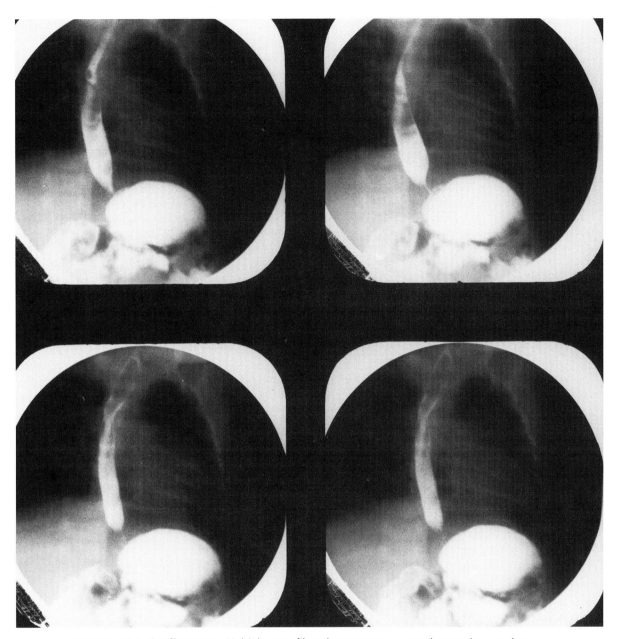

FIGURE 4.31. Cardiospasm. Multiple spot films demonstrate a normal-appearing esophagus but lack of relaxation of the lower esophageal sphincter. This was a temporary disturbance in this infant and resolved spontaneously.

mation and stricture: complication of chronic granulomatous disease of childhood. Radiology 1991;178:189–191.

Epidermolysis Bullosa

Epidermolysis bullosa is a rare, chronic, hereditary skin disease in which GI mucous membrane involvement is common. Bullae are commonly seen on the skin and on the mucosal surfaces of the mouth and oropharynx. The esoph-

agus can be involved in the dystrophic form, but dysphagia secondary to stenosis usually does not appear until later childhood. Characteristically, barium esophagram changes consist of various degrees of esophageal stenosis (Fig. 4.32), loss of normal esophageal motility, and occasionally, even mucosal ulcerations. Associated pyloric atresia of the same etiology also has been reported (1). The problem in the pylorus probably is the same as that in the esophagus (i.e., scarring after mucosal involvement).

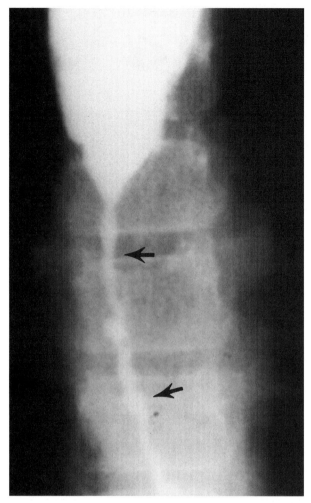

FIGURE 4.32. Esophageal stricture with epidermolysis bullosa. Note the extensive irregular structure of the esophagus (arrows) in this patient with epidermolysis bullosa.

REFERENCE

1. Cetinkursun S, Ozturk H, Celasun B, et al. Epidermolysis bullosa associated with pyloric, esophageal, and anal atresia: a case report. J Pediatr Surg 1995;30:1477–1478.

Esophageal Rupture and Perforation

Perforation of the esophagus in the pediatric age group is not particularly common. It can occur with ingestion of pointed objects and does occur on an iatrogenic basis with intraluminal tube insertions (1). Esophageal perforation secondary to peptic esophagitis is rare, but perforation secondary to extensive caustic burns of the esophagus may be a little more common. An uncommon cause of esophageal rupture is pneumatic rupture secondary to the voluminous ingestion of carbonated drinks (2). Esophageal perforation also can occur with inflicted trauma as part of child abuse (3).

Spontaneous esophageal rupture, also called Boerhaave's syndrome, is rare in children, and when it does occur, it tends to do so in the neonatal period (4). The etiology of such rupture is not always known, but the problem most likely centers on markedly increased intraluminal pressures encountered during delivery. Later, the same physiologic abnormality can occur with severe vomiting, which may or may not be associated with gastric outlet or duodenal obstruction.

Clinically, patients with esophageal rupture usually present with abrupt onset of symptoms of respiratory distress, choking spells, and difficulty in feeding. Hematemesis also can occur. Roentgenographically, mediastinal widening, pneumomediastinum and/or pneumothorax (often tension), pleural fluid, and pneumonia can be seen. In newborn infants, pneumothorax is believed to occur more frequently on the right side and to be more common than pneumomediastinum (5). The fact that it occurs more on the right than on the left probably is related to differences in the anatomic relationships of the pleural surfaces to the esophagus in the newborn (5). Contrast studies usually clearly demonstrate the site of the esophageal leak (Fig. 4.33).

REFERENCES

1. Gruenbaum M, Horodniceanu C, Wilunsky E, et al. Iatrogenic transmural perforation of the oesophagus in preterm infant. Clin Radiol 1980;31:257–261.
2. Meyerovitch J, Ami TB, Rozenman J, et al. Pneumatic rupture of the esophagus caused by carbonated drinks. Pediatr Radiol 1988; 18:468–470.
3. Morzaria S, Walton J, MacMillan A. Inflicted esophageal perforation. J Pediatr Surg 1998;33:871–873.
4. Dubos JP, Bouchez MC, Kacet N, et al. Spontaneous rupture of the esophagus in the newborn. Pediatr Radiol 1986;16:317–319.
5. Fleming PJ, Venugopal S, Lewins MJ, et al. Esophageal perforation into the right pleural cavity in a neonate. J Pediatr Surg 1980; 15:335–336.

Mallory-Weiss Syndrome

The Mallory-Weiss syndrome is extremely uncommon in the pediatric age group (1). The condition results from acute vomiting and increased intraluminal esophageal pressure. A mucosal tear occurs, but there is no mural perforation. Consequently, although hematemesis can be profound, there is no sign of an esophageal leak.

REFERENCE

1. Baptist EC, Arenberg ME, Baskin WM. Mallory-Weiss syndrome in a 16-week-old infant. Clin Pediatr 1981;20:59–60.

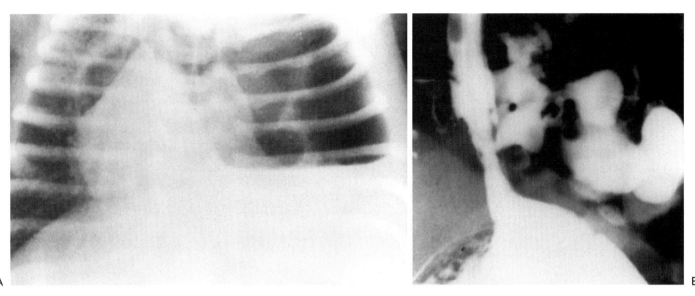

A   B

FIGURE 4.33. Esophageal rupture. A. Note the massive pneumohydrothorax on the left with pronounced shift of the mediastinal structures to the right. Most often, in the neonate, these findings are seen on the right. **B.** Esophagram demonstrating the site of the large extravasation of contrast material into the left pleural space. (Reproduced with permission from Harell GS, Friedland GW, Daily WJ, et al. Neonatal Boerhaave's syndrome. Radiology 1970;95:665–668.)

Esophageal Foreign Body

Almost everyone is familiar with the various types of foreign bodies ingested by infants. These can produce obstruction at the level of the cricopharyngeus muscle, aortic knob, or gastroesophageal junction (Fig. 4.34). If opaque, they may be demonstrated on plain films (Fig. 4.35, A and B); if not radiopaque, barium swallow is necessary (Fig. 4.35C). In some infants, foreign bodies may elude initial diagnosis, especially those that are not opaque and located high in the esophagus (Fig. 4.36) or in the hypopharynx. Such a foreign body can lead to chronic respiratory distress, recurrent pneumonia, or failure to thrive (1), and the true nature of the problem may not become apparent until roentgenograms of the neck and a barium swallow are obtained (1, 2). Smooth, small, and otherwise noninjurious foreign bodies such as coins can be removed retrogradely with the aid of Foley catheters (3–6). However, the procedure is not without hazard, including esophageal trauma, mucosal injury, reswallowing the foreign body, or having the foreign body flip and occlude the airway (7, 8). Nonetheless, it has become a popular procedure. Most often, the foreign body is extracted in retrograde fashion, but the foreign body also can be pushed into the lower esophagus with a Foley bulb (9). In addition, a forceps "penny pincher" technique under fluoroscopic control has been suggested (10).

Patient selection for Foley bulb removal of foreign bodies is important. Only those foreign bodies impacted less than 24–48 hours should be treated, and if there is any evidence of paraesophageal edema on the plain films, the pro-

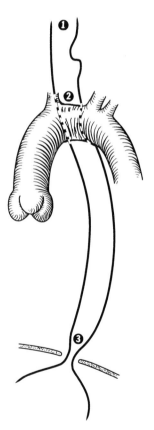

FIGURE 4.34. Sites of esophageal foreign body lodgment. 1. In the upper esophagus just above the cricopharyngeus muscle. **2.** In the upper chest just above the aortic knob. **3.** In the lower esophagus just above the esophageal junction. Most foreign bodies lodge just at the level of the aortic knob.

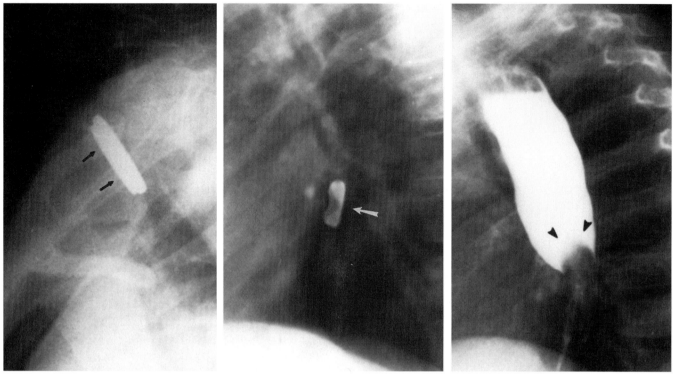

A

B,C

FIGURE 4.35. Esophageal foreign bodies. A. Note two coins (arrow) in the upper esophagus. **B.** Another patient with a metallic foreign body (arrow) in a somewhat unusual lower esophageal position. **C.** Foreign body (arrows) impacted in the distal esophagus at the site of an old stricture.

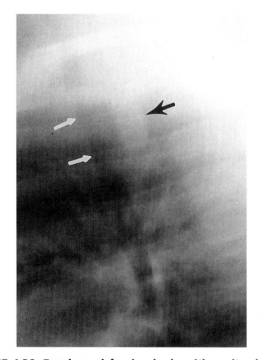

FIGURE 4.36. Esophageal foreign body with peritracheal edema. A barely visible foreign body (black arrow) is lodged in the upper esophagus. Note that the trachea (white arrows) at the site of lodgment is narrowed secondary to periesophageal edema.

cedure should not be performed. Chronically embedded foreign bodies in the esophagus can manifest with respiratory symptoms, and this problem is discussed in more detail in Chapter 2.

Button batteries are a special problem (11). These batteries are alkaline, and when they are chronically imbedded, the alkaline substance can leak out of the battery and cause erosion of the esophageal mucosa and the wall. This can lead to perforation, and in some instances of a chronically imbedded foreign body, an underlying vascular ring may be present (12).

REFERENCES

1. Smith PC, Swischuk LE, Fagan CJ. An elusive and often unsuspected cause of stridor or pneumonia (the esophageal foreign body). AJR 1974;122:80–89.
2. Macpherson RI, Hill JG, Othersen HB, et al. Esophageal foreign bodies in children: diagnosis, treatment, and complications. AJR 1966;166:919–924.
3. Kelley JE, Leech MH, Carr MG. A safe and cost effective protocol for the management of esophageal coins in children. J Pediatr Surg 1993;28:898–900.
4. Harned RK II, Strain JD, Hay TC, et al. Esophageal foreign bod-

ies: safety and efficacy of Foley catheter extraction of coins. AJR 1997;168:443–446.

5. Morrow SE, Bickler SW, Kennedy AP, et al. Balloon extraction of esophageal foreign bodies in children. J Pediatr Surg 1998;33: 266–270.
6. Schunk Je, Harrison AM, Corneli HM, et al. Fluoroscopic Foley catheter removal of esophageal foreign bodies in children: experience with 415 episodes. Pediatrics 1994;94:709–714.
7. Myer CM III. Potential hazards of esophageal foreign body extraction. Pediatr Radiol 1991;21:97–98.
8. Bonadio WA, Emslander H, Milner D, et al. Esophageal mucosal changes in children with an acutely ingested coin lodged in the esophagus. Pediatr Emerg Care 1995;10:333–334.
9. Alexander A, Swischuk LE, Hayden CK Jr. Letter to the Editor. AJR 1988;151:835.
10. Gauderer MWL, DeCou JM, Abrams RS, et al. The "penny-pincher": A new technique for fast and safe removal of esophageal coins. J Pediatr Surg 2000;35:276–278.
11. Samad L, Ali M, Rams H. Button battery ingestion: hazards of esophageal impaction. J Pediatr Surg 1999;34:1527–1531.
12. Currarino G, Nikaidoh H. Esophageal foreign bodies in children with vascular ring or aberrant right subclavian artery: coincidence or causation? Pediatr Radiol 1991;21:406–408.

Esophageal Neoplasms

Neoplasms in the esophagus are extremely uncommon in childhood and, for the most part, are unknown in the neonate. Occasionally, however, in infants and children, one may encounter tumors such as hamartomas (1), leiomyomas (2, 3), carcinomas (often associated with Barrett's esophagus) (4, 5), lipomas (6, 7), and ectopic gastric mucosa (8, 9). Any of these tumors, if large enough, can compromise the airway and manifest as respiratory distress (3, 6, 7).

REFERENCES

1. Beckerman RC, Taussig LM, Froede RC, et al. Fibromuscular hamartoma of the esophagus in an infant. Am J Dis Child 1980; 134:153–155.
2. Bourque MD, Spigland N, Bensoussan AL, et al. Esophageal leiomyoma in children: two case reports and review of the literature. J Pediatr Surg 1989;24:1103–1107.
3. Guest AR, Strouse PJ, Hiew CC, et al. Progressive esophageal leiomyomatosis with respiratory compromise. Pediatr Radiol 2000;30:247–250.
4. Aryya NC, Lahiri TK, Gangopadhyay AN, et al. Carcinoma of the esophagus in childhood. Pediatr Surg 1993;8:251–252.
5. Gangopadhyay AN, Mohanty PK, Gopal SC, et al. Adenocarcinoma of the esophagus in an 8-year-old boy. J Pediatr Surg 1997;32:1259–1263.
6. Hasan N, Mandhan P. Respiratory obstruction caused by lipoma of the esophagus. J Pediatr Surg 1994;29:1565–1566.
7. Samad L, Ali M, Ramzi H, et al. Respiratory distress in a child caused by lipoma of the esophagus. J Pediatr Surg 1999;34: 1537–1538.
8. Powell RW, Luck SR. Cervical esophageal obstruction by ectopic gastric mucosa. J Pediatr Surg 1988;23:632–634.
9. Karmak I, Senocak ME, Akcoren Z, et al. Ectopic gastric mucosa causing dysphagia due to strictures in a boy. Eur J Pediatr Surg 1999;9:413–415.

Acquired Tracheoesophageal Fistula

Tracheoesophageal fistula usually is congenital in origin, but it can be acquired on an iatrogenic basis after esophageal or tracheal perforation with tubes (1). It also can be acquired with tuberculosis (2) and caustic esophagitis (3).

REFERENCES

1. Szold A, Udassin R, Seror D, et al. Acquired tracheoesophageal fistula in infancy and childhood. J Pediatr Surg 1991;26:672–675.
2. Bhatia R, Mitra DK, Mukherjee S, et al. Bronchoesophageal fistula of tuberculous origin in a child. Pediatr Radiol 1992;22:154.
3. Vaishnav A, Spitz L. Alkaline battery-induced tracheo-oesophageal fistula. Br J Surg 1989;76:1045.

Miscellaneous Motility Problems

Esophageal motility can be disturbed and a cause of dysphagia. This can occur with congenital myotonic dystrophy (1) and with collagen vascular diseases such as scleroderma (2).

REFERENCES

1. Mabille JP, Giroud M, Athias P. Esophageal involvement in a case of congenital myotonic dystrophy. Pediatr Radiol 1982;12:89–91.
2. Flick JA, Boyle JT, Tuchman DN, et al. Esophageal motor abnormalities in children and adolescents with scleroderma and mixed connective tissue disease. Pediatrics 1988;82:107–111.

STOMACH

Normal Configurations

On plain films, the normal stomach in infants often is gas-filled, overdistended, and erroneously suggests obstruction (Fig. 4.37A). Similarly, when the stomach is fluid-filled, it may appear as a pseudotumor (Fig. 4.37B). In still other cases, milk curds may temporarily accumulate within the fundus and suggest a mass or abscess (Fig. 4.38). In older children, the barium-filled stomach appears much the same as in adults, but in young infants, mucosal folds are characteristically absent or sparse, and the stomach appears smooth. In addition, the antropyloric region and duodenum are somewhat more posterior in position than in older children and adults. This positioning is accentuated when the stomach is full and this makes it difficult to visualize these structures on anteroposterior views. With the barium upper GI series, right anterior-oblique or lateral views are helpful, whereas with ultrasound, one searches for the pylorus somewhere in the general vicinity of the right upper quadrant and mid-epigastric areas. It

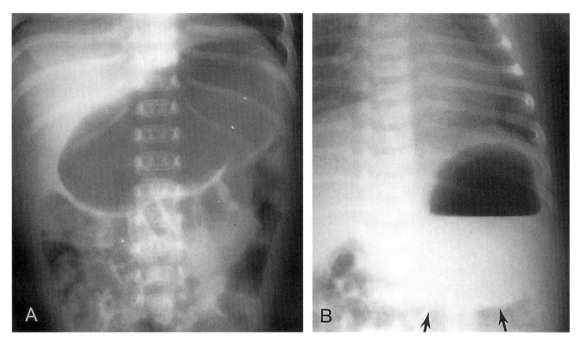

FIGURE 4.37. Normal distended stomach. A. Supine view showing pronounced distention of stomach. A similar configuration, perhaps with less gas in the remaining GI tract, can be seen with gastric outlet obstruction such as pyloric stenosis, but this infant was normal. **B.** Upright view in another infant showing a fluid- and air-filled stomach (arrows).

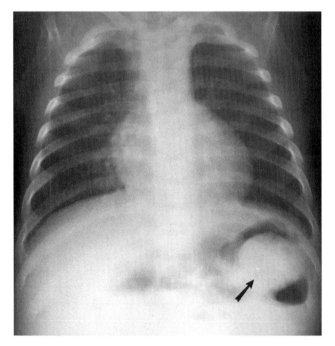

FIGURE 4.38. Gastric pseudotumor. Milk curds in the stomach produce a mass-like effect (arrow).

usually is helpful to have the patient rotated a little to his or her right. With barium studies, the antropyloric region and duodenal bulb are readily identified (Fig. 4.39A), but ultrasound is equally as good or even better for the investigation of the gastric antrum in infants. This is not so true in older children, and in any age group, it generally more difficult to examine the fundus of the stomach with ultrasound. However, this is not such a great problem since most diseases encountered in infants occur in the antrum. Using the left lobe of the liver as an acoustic window and with the infant swallowing glucose water, one readily can identify, using a 10–13 MHz transducer the lumen of the stomach, echogenic surface of the mucosa, sonolucent mucosa and muscularis mucosae layers, echogenic submucosa, and the sonolucent outer muscle layer (Fig. 4.39, B and C). In addition, one can observe peristaltic activity and gastric emptying, and in essence, one performs an ultrasonographic upper GI series.

The smooth, outer muscle layer is the layer of muscle involved in pyloric stenosis and in normal infants is 1 mm thick and many times is "too thin to measure" (1). By the same token, the combined gastric mucosa, muscularis mucosae, and submucosa usually are 2.5 to 3.5 mm thick (1, 2). The antrum also has been shown to increase in size and length from prematurity to full-term gestational age (3).

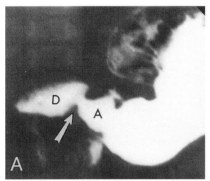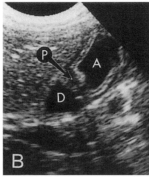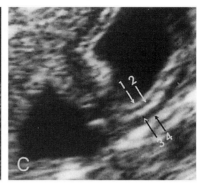

FIGURE 4.39. Normal stomach. A. Barium upper GI series demonstrates the normal antrum (A), pyloric canal (arrow), and duodenal bulb (D). **B.** Ultrasonogram demonstrating fluid in the antrum (A), the pyloric canal (P), and the duodenal bulb (D). Note the multiple layers of the gastric wall. **C.** Magnified view of the foregoing layers demonstrates the mucosa (1), muscularis mucosae (2), submucosa (3), and outer circular muscle (4). The mucosal layers are echogenic while the muscular layers are sonolucent.

REFERENCES

1. Hayden CK Jr, Swischuk LE, Lobe TE, et al. Ultrasound: the definitive imaging modality in pyloric stenosis. Radiographics 1984;4:517–530.
2. Stringer DA, Daneman A, Brunelle F, et al. Sonography of the normal and abnormal stomach (excluding hypertrophic pyloric stenosis) in children. J Ultrasound Med 1986;5:183–188.
3. Argyropoulou MI, Hadjigeorgi CG, Kiortsis DN. Antropyloric canal values from early prematurity to full-term gestational age: an ultrasound study. Pediatr Radiol 1998;28:9333–936.

ABNORMALITIES OF THE STOMACH

Hypertrophic Pyloric Stenosis

Hypertrophic pyloric stenosis generally is considered to be an acquired condition, rather than congenital. Most infants develop symptoms 2–8 weeks after birth, but some infants may present in the first week of life or even at birth (1, 2). Symptoms in the typical case of infantile hypertrophic pyloric stenosis consist of vomiting (usually projectile), regurgitation, difficulty in feeding, and if severe enough, weight loss. Bile is usually absent in the vomitus, and first-born males characteristically are more frequently afflicted. However, the condition also commonly occurs in females. Pyloric stenosis also is reported to be less common in black infants but has been noted with surprising frequency in triplets (3–5). A few instances of familial involvement have been noted (6, 7), and all of this probably is more than just coincidental. There most likely is a genetic predisposition to the development of pyloric stenosis in certain individuals. On the other hand, the disease does not seem to penetrate as a classic autosomal dominant condition. Nonetheless, it is difficult to overlook the recorded incidence of familial or multiple birth involvement and the numerous occasions when the parent relates to you that "the brother, sister, father, and others also had pyloric stenosis."

The precise etiology of infantile hypertrophic pyloric stenosis is unknown, but certain postulated mechanisms should be reviewed. One theory favors that the nerve cells of the myenteric plexus of the pylorus are abnormal in number or function (8–11). Another etiologic consideration may be that the problem is simply one of overactivity or prolonged spasm of the antropyloric muscle, leading to hypertrophy. If this is the case, many factors could lead to such prolonged muscle spasm, and in this regard, it is difficult to discuss muscle spasm without discussing the role of hyperacidity. Hyperacidity is common in the immediate postnatal period and, in any patient, leads to increased secretion of cholecystokinin and secretin, hormones that lead to both pyloric muscle spasm and hypertrophy.

In support of gastrin being one of the culprits in this disease is that gastrin administered to experimental animals has resulted in hyperacidity and pyloric muscle hypertrophy (12). It may be then that some infants are genetically more predisposed to either increased gastrin production or hypersensitivity to it. Stress also probably plays a part in this problem, for it has been noted that mothers stressed in the third trimester of pregnancy deliver more infants with pyloric stenosis than do mothers not stressed (13).

Considering all of these facts, prolonged pyloric muscle spasm leading to muscle hypertrophy may be the most important factor in the development of pyloric stenosis (14). Strong support for this hypothesis lies in the therapy of the condition, for whether therapy is medical or surgical, it is aimed at breaking the cycle leading to pyloric muscle spasm and hypertrophy. With medical, antispasmodic therapy used more in the past but recently revived with the use of atropine (15–17), the muscle was laid to rest. With surgical therapy, the muscle also is laid to rest, because its circumferential contractibility is destroyed when a pyloromyotomy is performed. In either case, the muscle no longer can go into spasm, and as it atrophies, it slowly returns to normal. The whole phenomenon could be considered an isometric exercise of the pyloric muscle, which can be interrupted by either medical or surgical therapy. This simply has to do with a basic principle of smooth muscle contractibility. As a result, it has become apparent that any condition or disease process that leads to persistent or repeated antropyloric muscle spasm can lead to frank pyloric stenosis. This is probably what happens in cases of pyloric stenosis developing secondary to irritating indwelling catheters (18), erythromycin-induced gastritis (19), gastric ulcer disease (20), eosinophilic gastroenteritis (21), prostaglandin-induced foveolar hyperplasia (22), and intraluminal obstructing lesions (23, 24).

The diagnosis of well-established and classic hypertrophic pyloric stenosis can be made on clinical grounds. The history is typical, complete with projectile vomiting, and on physical examination, the hypertrophied muscle mass, or olive, is readily palpable. In addition, exaggerated gastric peristalsis can be seen through the abdominal wall, and in most of these cases, imaging of the upper GI tract is not required. This occurs in a very small percentage of patients, but this approach is slowly fading (25) as the diagnosis of pyloric stenosis basically has been relegated to ultrasound. Ultrasound is so accurate that it has caused considerable erosion of the clinical detection of this disease by way of the physical examination. However, at the same time that this is regrettable, it is merely a sign of evolution of science and medicine. Ultrasound is so dependable at detecting pyloric stenosis that it almost obviates anything else

except the history. The old guard will stick to the concept that if an olive is palpable, then nothing else needs to be done. My experience, however, is that the definitely palpable olive was present in only a small percentage of cases, and thus, there always was equivocation. **With ultrasound, there is no equivocation.**

It has been questioned whether performing ultrasound is cost efficient (27–29). This concept has been titrated against physical examination and the barium upper GI series. Others have indicated that it is probably more effective and definitely more accurate to perform ultrasound in patients with suspected gastric outlet obstruction (25). We agree with this latter concept and believe that there is little place for the barium upper GI series in the evaluation of chronic vomiting in infancy. We probably have performed no more than six upper GI series in these patients over the last 2 years, and it was only when the ultrasonographic findings were confusing or normal in the face of significant vomiting. The reason we have adopted this posture is that ultrasound can accurately identify pyloric stenosis, pylorospasm, gastric diaphragms, duodenal obstructions, malrotation, and gastritis. **The upper GI series never was able to do this with confidence, but the ultrasound imaging study can.**

The classic appearance of pyloric stenosis on ultrasound (30–35) is that of (a) elongation of the pyloric canal; (b) persistent spasm of the pyloric canal with little, if any, fluid passing into the duodenum; (c) persistent thickening of the circular muscle in the elongated canal; and (d) a sonolucent donut (thickened muscle) on cross-section (Fig. 4.40). Mea-

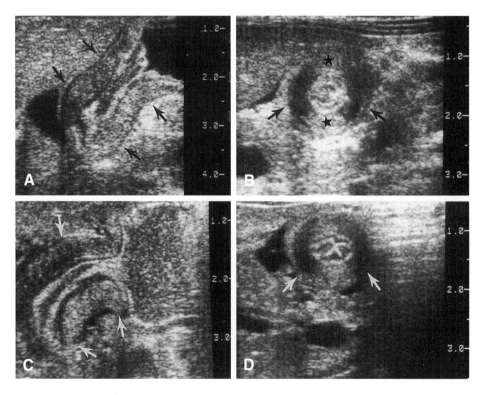

FIGURE 4.40. Pyloric stenosis: ultrasonographic features. A. On longitudinal section the pyloric canal is elongated and the muscle thickened. The muscle, however, is echogenic (arrows) because of the 6- and 12-o'clock echogenicity artifacts. Sonolucent fluid is seen in the center of the canal. **B.** Cross-sectional view demonstrates the sonolucent outer portions of the muscle (arrows). However, note that the muscle is echogenic at the 6- and 12-o'clock artifact positions (stars). **C.** Another patient with an elongated pyloric canal (arrows) with marked muscle thickening and two sonolucent streaks in the center. These represent fluid trapped in mucosal folds and constitute the double track sign. **D.** Cross-sectional image demonstrates the sonolucent muscle (arrows) and the central star-like configuration corresponding to the double track sign seen on longitudinal view.

surements have been devised to assist diagnosis, and in terms of muscle thickness, originally a measurement of 4 mm or greater was considered diagnostic. However, we (33) and others (34) have found that any measurement 3 mm or greater is diagnostic when all of the other findings are present. The accepted length for the elongated pyloric canal originally was 1.5 cm or longer but later was reduced to approximately 1.2 cm. Overall, however, neither measurement is that important, because if the muscle is pathologically thickened, the canal will be elongated and fixed in spasm, and its length makes no difference. Furthermore, only an abnormal pyloric canal can be measured for length, because a normal canal never stays fixed long enough to be measured. Therefore, if one can measure an elongated pyloric canal, it is abnormal, usually due to pylorospasm or pyloric stenosis.

Originally, one other measurement was included in the ultrasonographic diagnosis of pyloric stenosis: the diameter of the pylorus in cross-section. However, there was so much overlap between normal and abnormal that it is now generally not used. In addition, pyloric muscle length versus diameter or thickness ratios and volumes of the pyloric muscle mass have been advocated (34, 36, 37), but in practice, they probably will never be used. The diagnosis can be accomplished without such sophisticated approaches, even in the premature infant where the hypertrophied muscle is smaller than normal (38, 39).

Another finding that can be seen with ultrasonography is the so-called **double track sign** (40). This sign results from compressed mucosa showing numerous linear fluid accumulations within it. The fluid stripes appear sonolucent, and the mucosal stripes are echogenic on both longitudinal and cross-sectional views (Fig. 4.40, C and D). The finding is exactly the same as that seen on barium studies in the past where it also was known as the double track sign.

On ultrasonographic cross-section, the findings are typical and consist of a sonolucent donut. Often, there is echogenicity at the 6- and 12-o'clock positions (Fig. 4.40, A and B), and on longitudinal images made through this plane (midsagittal), the echogenic muscle may be relatively invisible. Echogenicity at the 6- and 12-o'clock positions has been determined to be the result of numerous acoustic interfaces being present as the circular muscle traverses the ultrasonographic beam (41). At the other sites (i.e., the 3- and 9-o'clock positions), the ultrasonographic beam passes through the longitudinal axis of the circular muscle fibers, and acoustic interfaces are scarce. As a result, the muscle appears hyperechoic.

In the past, pitfalls in the ultrasonographic diagnosis of pyloric stenosis were a problem. These basically consisted of imaging the antrum tangentially (resulting in erroneously thickened muscle and mucosal layers) and imaging the stomach that was so full of fluid that the antrum and pyloric canal were invisible. These problems have been circumvented, and the ultrasonographic diagnosis of pyloric stenosis remains intact and is virtually 100% accurate.

In the usual case of pyloric stenosis, pyloromyotomy is definitely the preferred form of therapy, and in the vast majority of cases, it is very successful. Failures are few and, when seen, usually are the result of incomplete transsection of the muscle on the gastric side. In the average case, normal emptying of the stomach occurs within 2 or 3 days after pyloromyotomy, but some muscle thickening may remain for longer periods, even up to 6 weeks (42). Ultrasound is excellent for this evaluation (43). Long-term results of pyloromyotomy are very good, and these patients usually pass into adulthood with no further difficulties (44). Recently, balloon dilatation has been advocated (45).

Jaundice is another interesting feature of some infants with pyloric stenosis (45), and while it probably results from liver immaturity and decreased glucuronyl transferase activity, the problem may be aggravated by the presence of pyloric stenosis. Glucuronyl transferase activity has been demonstrated to be inhibited by increased gastric acidity and starvation, and both are present in infants with pyloric stenosis.

REFERENCES

1. Ali KI, Haddad MJ. Early infantile hypertrophic pyloric stenosis: surgery at 26 hours of age. Eur J Pediatr Surg 1996:233–234.
2. Geer LL, Gaisie G, Mandell VS, et al. Evolution of pyloric stenosis in the first week of life. Pediatr Radiol 1985;15:205–206.
3. Gilespie JC, Peterson GH, Lehocky R, et al. Occurrence of pyloric stenosis in triplets. Am J Dis Child 1982;136:746–747.
4. Hicks LM, Morgan A, Anderson MR. Pyloric stenosis—a report of triplet females and notes on its inheritance. J Pediatr Surg 1981;16:739–740.
5. Janik JS, Nagaraj HS, Lehocky R. Pyloric stenosis in identical triplets. Pediatrics 1982;70:282–283.
6. Bilodeau RG. Inheritance of hypertrophic pyloric stenosis. AJR 1971;113:241–244.
7. Burmeister RE, Hamilton HB. Infantile hypertrophic stenosis in four siblings. Am J Dis Child 1964;108:617–624.
8. Kobayashi H, O'Briain DS, Puri P. Defective cholinergic innervation in pyloric muscle of patients with hypertrophic pyloric stenosis. Pediatr Surg Int 1994;9:338–341.
9. Kobayashi H, Wester T, Puri P. Age-related changes in innervation in hypertrophic pyloric stenosis. J Pediatr Surg 1997;32:1704–1707.
10. Langer JC, Berezin I, Daniel EE. Hypertrophic pyloric stenosis: ultrastructural abnormalities of enteric nerves and the interstitial cells of Cajal. J Pediatr Surg 1995;30;1535–1543.
11. Okazaki T, Yamataka A, Fujiwara T, et al. Abnormal distribution of nerve terminals in infantile hypertrophic pyloric stenosis. J Pediatr Surg 1994;29:655–658.
12. Karim AA, Morrison JE, Parks TG. The role of pentagastrin in the production of canine hypertrophic pyloric stenosis and pyloroduodenal ulceration. Br J Surg 1974;61:327.
13. Revill S, Dodge JA. Psychological determinants of infantile pyloric stenosis. Arch Dis Child 1978;53:66–68.
14. Wesley JR, DiPietro MA, Coran AG. Pyloric stenosis: evolution from pylorospasm? Pediatr Surg Int 1990;5:425–428.
15. Nagita A, Yamaguchi J, Amemoto K, et al. Management and ultrasonographic appearance of infantile hypertrophic pyloric stenosis with intravenous atropine sulfate. J Pediatr Gastroenterol Nutr 1996;23:172–177.

16. Yamamoto A, Kino M, Sasaki T, et al. Ultrasonographic follow-up of the healing process of medically treated hypertrophic pyloric stenosis. Pediatr Radiol 1998;28:177–178.

17. Yamataka A, Tsukada K, Yokoyama-Laws, et al. Pyloromyotomy versus atropine sulfate for infantile hypertrophic pyloric stenosis. J Pediatr 2000;35:338–342.

18. Latchaw LA, Jacir NN, Harris BH. The development of pyloric stenosis during transpyloric feedings. J Pediatr Surg 1989;24:823–824.

19. San Filippo JA. Infantile hypertrophic pyloric stenosis related to ingestion of erythromycin estolate: a report of five cases. J Pediatr Surg 1976;11:177–180.

20. Kelsey D, Stayman JW Jr, McLaughlin ED, et al. Massive bleeding in a newborn infant from a gastric ulcer associated with hypertrophic pyloric stenosis. Surgery 1968;64:979–982.

21. Hummer-Ehret BH, Rohrschneider WK, Oleszczuk-Raschke K, et al. Eosinophilic gastroenteritis mimicking idiopathic hypertrophic pyloric stenosis. Pediatr Radiol 1998;28:711–713.

22. Callahan MJ, McCauley RGK, Patel H, et al. The development of hypertrophic pyloric stenosis in a patient with prostaglandin-induced foveolar hyperplasia. Pediatr Radiol 1999;29:748–751.

23. Kim S, Chung CJ, Fordham LA, et al. Coexisting hyperplastic antral polyp and hypertrophic pyloric stenosis. Pediatr Radiol 1997;27:912–914.

24. Kao SCS, Muir LV, Kimura K. Combined hypertrophic pyloric stenosis and duodenal web in Down syndrome: sonographic and radiographic diagnosis. J Ultrasound Med 1996;15:475–477.

25. Chen EA, Luks FI, Gilchrist BF, et al. Pyloric stenosis in the age of ultrasonography: fading skills, better patients? J Pediatr Surg 1996;31:829–830.

26. Ozsvath RR, Poustchi-Amin M, Leonidas JC, et al. Pyloric volume: an important factor in the surgeon's ability to palpate the pyloric "olive" in hypertrophic pyloric stenosis. Pediatr Radiol 1997;27:175–177.

27. Hulka F, Campbell JR, Harrison MW, et al. Cost-effectiveness in diagnosing infantile hypertrophic pyloric stenosis. J Pediatr Surg 1997;32:1604–1608.

28. Olson AD, Hernandez R, Hirschl RB. The role of ultrasonography in the diagnosis of pyloric stenosis: a decision analysis. J Pediatr Surg 1998;33:676–681.

29. White MC, Langer JC, Don S, et al. Sensitivity and cost minimization analysis of radiology versus olive palpation for the diagnosis of hypertrophic pyloric stenosis. J Pediatr Surg 1998;33:913–917.

30. Davies RP, Linke RK, Robinson RG, et al. Ultrasound diagnosis of infantile hypertrophic pyloric stenosis. J Ultrasound Med 1992;11:603–605.

31. Haller JO, Cohen HL. Hypertrophic pyloric stenosis: diagnosis using US. Radiology 1986;161:335–339.

32. Hernanz-Schulman M, Sells LL, Ambrosino MM, et al. Hypertrophic pyloric stenosis in the infant without a palpable olive: accuracy of sonographic diagnosis. Radiology 1994;193:771–776.

33. Hayden CK Jr, Swischuk LE, Lobe TE, et al. Ultrasound: the definitive imaging modality in pyloric stenosis. Radiographics 1984;4:517–530.

34. Rohrschneider WK, Mittnacht H, Darge K, et al. Pyloric muscle in asymptomatic, infants: sonographic evaluation and discrimination from idiopathic hypertrophic pyloric stenosis. Pediatr Radiol 1998;28:429–434.

35. Stunden RJ, LeQuesne GW, Little KET. The improved ultrasound diagnosis of hypertrophic pyloric stenosis. Pediatr Radiol 1986;16:200–205.

36. Lowe LH, Banks WJ, Shyr Y. Pyloric ratio: efficacy in diagnosis of hypertrophic pyloric stenosis. J Ultrasound Med 1999;18:773–777.

37. Westra SJ, deGroot CJ, Smits NJ, et al. Hypertrophic pyloric stenosis: use of the pyloric volume measurement in early US diagnosis. Radiology 1989;172:615–619.

38. Bisset RAL, Gupta SC. Hypertrophic pyloric stenosis, ultrasonic appearances in a small baby. Pediatr Radiol 1988;18:405.

39. Cosman BC, Sudekum AE, Oakes DD, et al. Pyloric stenosis in a premature infant. J Pediatr Surg 1992;27:1534–1536.

40. Cohen HL, Schechter S, Mestel AL, et al. Ultrasonic "double track" sign in hypertrophic pyloric stenosis. J Ultrasound Med 1987;6:139–143.

41. Spevak MR, Ahmadjian JM, Kleinman PK, et al. Sonography of hypertrophic pyloric stenosis: frequency and cause of nonuniform echogenicity of thickened pyloric muscle. AJR 1992;158:129–132.

42. Sauerbrei EE, Paloschi GGB. The ultrasonic features of hypertrophic pyloric stenosis, with emphasis on the postoperative appearance. Radiology 1983;147:503–506.

43. Yamamoto A, Kino A, Sasaki T, et al. Ultrasonographic follow-up of the healing process of medically treated hypertrophic pyloric stenosis. Pediatr Radiol 1998;28:177–178.

44. Ludtke FE, Bertus M, Voth E, et al. Gastric emptying 16 to 26 years after treatment of infantile hypertrophic pyloric stenosis. J Pediatr Surg 1994;29:523–526.

45. Ogawa Y, Higashimoto Y, Nishijima E, et al. Successful endoscopic balloon dilatation for hypertrophic pyloric stenosis. J Pediatr Surg 1996;31:1712–1714.

Pylorospasm

Pylorospasm is the most common cause of gastric outlet obstruction in infancy and is multifactorial in its etiology. In many cases, it is secondary to milk allergy, but the etiology most often is similar to that of pyloric stenosis, and in fact, pylorospasm could be considered the precursor of pyloric stenosis. In most cases, the findings do not progress to true pyloric stenosis, but in some cases, they do. Overall, pylorospasm differs from pyloric stenosis in that there usually is no thickening of the pyloric muscle, but in some cases, minimal thickening (2–3 mm) may be seen (Fig. 4.41). With ultrasound and barium studies, the antropyloric canal is seen to be relatively fixed in spasm, but it eventually will open (Fig. 4.42). With milk allergy, associated thickening of the gastric mucosa can be seen (see Fig. 4.49).

Pylorospasm also can occur in the adrenogenital syndrome and has been documented with prostaglandin therapy where foveolar hyperplasia can lead to a picture mimicking pylorospasm or pyloric stenosis (1–5). Although foveolar hyperplasia has been documented with prostaglandin therapy it can also occur on an idiopathic basis (2).

REFERENCES

1. Babyn P, Peled N, Manson D, et al. Radiologic features of gastric outlet obstruction in infants after long-term prostaglandin administration. Pediatr Radiol 1995;25:41–43.

2. Holland AJA, Freeman JK, LeQuesne GW, et al. Idiopathic focal foveolar hyperplasia in infants. Pediatr Surg Int 1997;12:498–500.

3. Kriss VM, Desai NS. Relation of gastric distention to prostaglandin therapy in neonates. Radiology 1997;203:219–221.

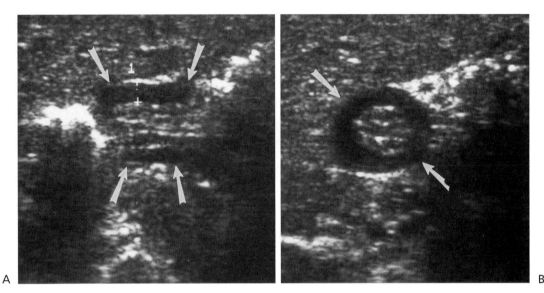

FIGURE 4.41. Pylorospasm with minimal thickening. A. Note the elongated pyloric canal (arrows) and minimal thickening (0.21 cm) of the muscle. **B.** The cross-sectional view demonstrates a thin sonolucent donut (arrows).

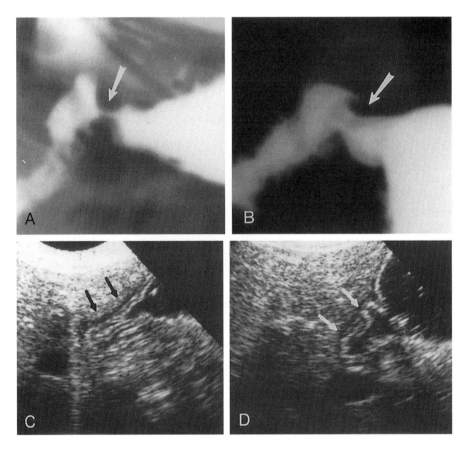

FIGURE 4.42. Pylorospasm. A. Note the persistent, short segment narrowing of the antropyloric canal (arrow). **B.** After antispasmodic therapy, the pyloric canal is of normal diameter (arrow). **C.** Ultrasonographic features consisting of a spastic pyloric canal (arrows) with normal muscle and mucosal layers. **D.** Five or 10 minutes later, the pyloric canal has opened (arrows), and peristaltic waves are propelling fluid through it.

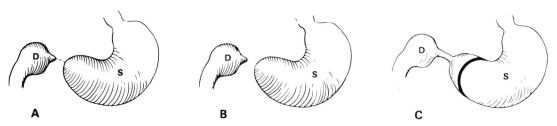

FIGURE 4.43. Pyloric atresia: various types. A. Atresia with fibrous connection. **B.** Complete atresia with no connection. **C.** Membranous atresia. D, duodenum; S, stomach. (Modified from Bronsther B, Nadeau M, Abrams M. Congenital pyloric atresia: a report of three cases and a review of the literature. Surgery 1971;69:130.)

4. Kobayashi N, Aida N, Nishimura G, et al. Acute gastric outlet obstruction following the administration of prostaglandin: an additional case. Pediatr Radiol 1997;27:57–59.
5. Mercado-Deane MG, Burton EM, Brawley AV, et al. Prostaglandin-induced foveolar hyperplasia simulating pyloric stenosis in an infant with cyanotic heart disease. Pediatr Radiol 1994;24:45–46.

Delayed Gastric Emptying

Gastric emptying can be assessed with nuclear scintigraphy, but a rough idea of emptying of the stomach can also be obtained during an ultrasound study. Generally, the normal stomach empties 60–75% of its load in 1 hour, but it has been suggested that imaging at the end of 1 hour is not adequate for this determination (1). However, others believe that 1 hour is satisfactory (2). Our own study (3) suggests that it is not so much the time factor as the position of the patient. Most patients are imaged in the semiupright supine position, and this does not enhance gastric emptying; in fact, it probably impedes emptying. We therefore suggested that the patients be carried around or laid on the right side to enhance gastric emptying (3). In this regard, with the barium upper GI series, it is standard to place the patient into the right anterior-oblique position to enhance emptying and outline the duodenum. We have found that, scintigraphic results are much more meaningful with such positioning, and false-positive studies basically do not occur. Delayed gastric emptying, on a prolonged, but reversible basis also has been seen after rotavirus infection of the GI tract (4).

REFERENCES

1. Gelfand MJ, Wagner GG. Gastric emptying in infants and children: limited utility of 1-hour measurement. Radiology 1991;178:379–381.
2. Tolia V, Kuhns L, Kauffman R. Correlation of gastric emptying at one and two hours following formula feeding. Pediatr Radiol 1993;23:26–28.
3. Villanueva-Meyer J, Swischuk LE, Cessani F, et al. Pediatric gastric emptying: value of right, lateral and upright positioning. J Nucl Med 1996;1356–1358.

4. Sigurdsson L, Flores A, Putman PE, et al. Postviral gastroparesis: presentation, treatment, and outcome. J Pediatr 1997;131:751–754.

Gastric Atresia and Antropyloric Membranes

Antropyloric membranes usually are considered congenital and a form of gastric atresia, because very few are acquired in infants and children. Gastric atresia is classified into three types: complete atresia with no connection between the stomach and duodenum, complete atresia with a fibrous band connecting the stomach and duodenum, and a gastric

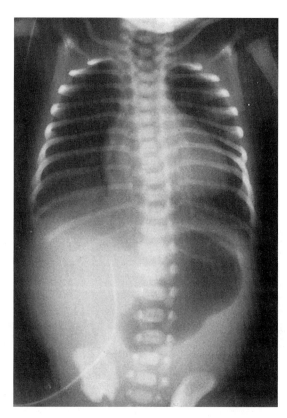

FIGURE 4.44. Gastric atresia. Note the air-filled, obstructed stomach, but no air distal to the stomach.

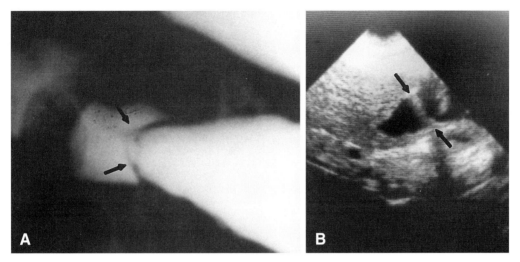

FIGURE 4.45. Antropyloric membrane. A. Note the crescent-shaped radiolucent defect, ballooning out, in the antrum (arrows). **B.** Ultrasound in another patient demonstrating an antropyloric membrane (arrows).

membrane or diaphragm (1, 2). The three types are diagrammatically depicted in Figure 4.43. With gastric atresia, since obstruction is complete, no air is seen distal to the stomach (Fig. 4.44). If the diaphragm has a hole in it, gas can be seen throughout the GI tract.

In the membranous type, obstruction usually is incomplete, because there is an opening in the center of the membrane or diaphragm. When this opening is large, no significant obstruction is present, but when it is small, the diaphragm is obstructive and will balloon or bulge out with gastric peristalsis (Fig. 4.45A). Nonobstructing diaphragms produce no such bulging. Gastric diaphragms also can be demonstrated ultrasonographically (6), but we confine the use of this imaging modality to infants. The echogenic diaphragms can be seen to cross the antrum (Fig. 4.45B), but care must be taken not to mistake the portion of the stomach distal to the membrane for the duodenal bulb. Incomplete diaphragms also can be readily imaged, and in this regard, it is important that any suspected diaphragm be imaged through the midsagittal plane of the stomach. The reason for this is that tangential imaging may erroneously suggest that a partial diaphragm is complete (Fig. 4.46). Incomplete diaphragms also are demonstrable with barium studies, and it should be noted that mucous strands can mimic diaphragms on barium upper GI series.

Most cases of gastric atresia are the result of an intrauterine vascular insult to the stomach. With healing, scarring is believed to occur, resulting either in atresia or a membrane (diaphragm). In support of this vascular theory is the fact that, in some cases, gastric atresia can be seen with atresia of other parts of the GI tract, where it also is believed to be ischemic in origin. A familial form of gastric atresia is

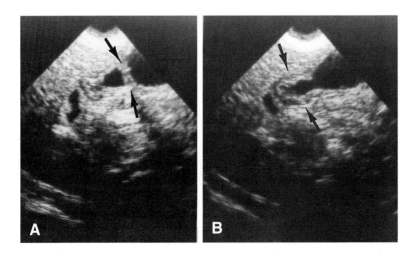

FIGURE 4.46. Pseudodiaphragm. A. Note this patient with an apparent diaphragm (arrow). However, this was a tangential cut. **B.** With a true midsagittal cut, the antrum (arrows) is normal.

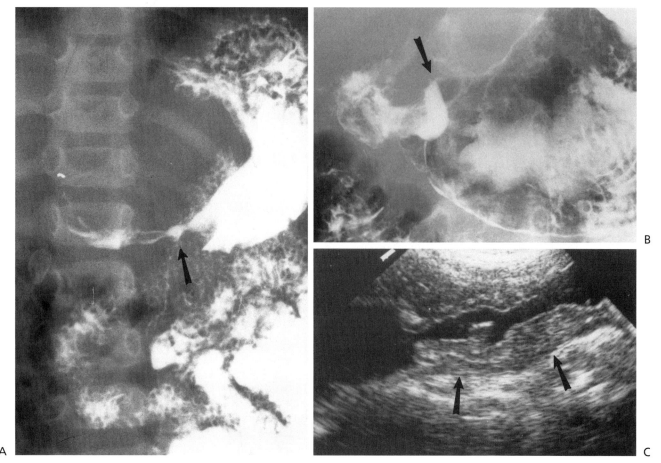

FIGURE 4.47. Gastric ulcer disease. A. Gastric ulcer (arrow) in a 7-month-old infant. Note the extensive edema and spasm of the stomach around the ulcer. **B.** Note a typical gastric ulcer (arrow) in the antrum. **C.** Ultrasonogram demonstrates the thickened gastric mucosa (arrows), in the center of which is a small ulcer crater. D, duodenal bulb. (**A** courtesy of R. Bombet, M.D.).

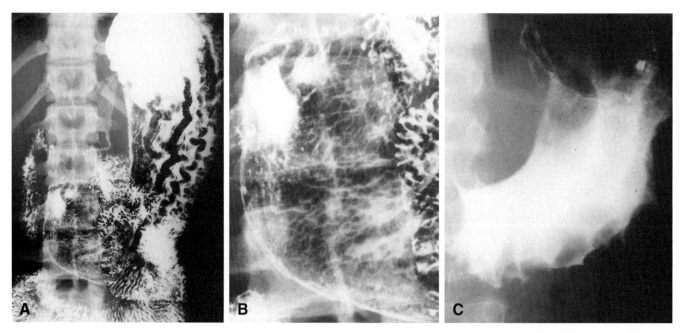

FIGURE 4.48. Gastritis. A. Note the markedly thickened gastric folds in the body and fundus of the stomach. **B.** In the antrum, multiple nodules and thickened folds are seen. **C.** Marked thumbprinting of the stomach secondary to eosinophilic gastroenteritis.

known to occur, but it probably results from failure of recanalization of the GI tract (2) rather than from an ischemic insult. Gastric atresia also can be seen as a complication (scarring) of epidermolysis bullosa (4–6).

REFERENCES

1. Grant HW, Hadley GP, Wiersma R. Membranous atresia of the body of the stomach. J Pediatr Surg 1994;29:1588.
2. Moore CCM. Congenital gastric outlet obstruction. J Pediatr Surg 1989;24:1241–1246.
3. Chew AL, Friedwald JP, Donovan C. Diagnosis of congenital antral web by ultrasound. Pediatr Radiol 1992;22:342–343.
4. Bull MJ, Norins AL, Weaver DD, et al. Epidermolysis bullosa—pyloric atresia. Am J Dis Child 1983;137:449–451.
5. Garcia Hernandez JB, Orense M, Celorio C, et al. Pyloric atresia associated with epidermolysis bullosa. Pediatr Radiol 1987;17:4335.
6. Rosenboom MS, Ratner M. Congenital pyloric atresia and epidermolysis bullosa letalis in premature siblings. J Pediatr Surg 1987;22:374–376.

Gastritis and Gastric Ulcer Disease

Gastric ulcer disease in infants and children is not particularly common, but affected patients can present with hematemesis, rectal bleeding, or vomiting only. If an upper GI series is obtained, unless an ulcer crater is visualized (Fig. 4.47) only secondary, nonspecific findings are present. These consist of spasm and deformity of the antrum and evidence of mucosal thickening. Chronic, fibrotic changes are not usually seen in infants and children. With gastritis, one can see diffuse, superficial ulceration and thick folds (Fig. 4.48).

Infants with gastritis and gastric ulcer disease also can be studied ultrasonographically (1, 2), which is probably the imaging modality of choice. The reason for this is that ultrasound allows one to assess the gastric mucosa directly, and hence, one can measure its thickness. In patients with gastritis, the mucosa is abnormally thickened (Fig. 4.47C), measuring 4 mm thick or more (1). Normal thickness is 2.5–3.5 mm (1). Some of these infants also may show muscle hypertrophy and minimal thickening (2–3 mm) but definitely not in the order of that seen with classic pyloric stenosis. Ulcer craters, if large enough, also can be detected (Fig. 4.47C) (2). The etiology of gastric ulcers in children probably is the same as that in adults (i.e., stress and hyperacidity), although in infants, milk allergy also can be a cause. Acute stress ulcers also can be seen in infants (3) and children, and gastric ulcers can occur in the neonate where gastric acidity is high for the first few days of life (4).

The most common cause of gastritis is viral infection of the intestinal tract, but few of these patients come to any form of imaging. It also can occur secondary to accidental acid ingestion and steroid therapy. Eosinophilic gastroenteritis is rare in children (5) and rare in infants. It manifests in one of two forms, and the most common is diffuse eosinophilic infiltration of the GI tract. Less commonly, the presentation is that of a solitary, polypoid granuloma impregnated with eosinophils. The former is associated with a peripheral eosinophilia. Roentgenographically, the findings consist of marked thickening and thumbprinting of the gastric mucosa (Fig. 4.48C). Milk allergy in young infants is another cause of gastritis, and ultrasonographically, the mucosa is seen to be thickened in these patients (Fig. 4.49).

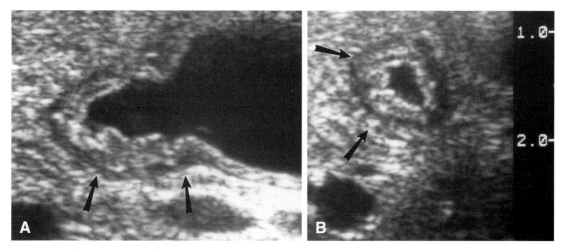

FIGURE 4.49. Milk allergy. A. Note eccentric thickening of the mucosa (arrows) in the antrum of the stomach. **B.** The cross-sectional view demonstrates the same eccentric thickening of the echogenic mucosa (arrows).

Menetrier's disease (6) also is uncommon in children and is virtually unheard of in infants. It can produce profound thickening of the mucosal folds of the stomach, and there has been considerable association between cytomegalovirus infection and Menetrier's disease (7, 8). Although not a true gastritis, chronic granulomatous disease of childhood can lead to thickening of the gastric antrum (Fig. 4.50, B and C) and obstruction (9–11). Similar thickening can occur in the esophagus (Fig. 4.50A) and less commonly elsewhere. Ultrasonography is excellent in identifying the hypoechoic, thickened mucosa (12, 13) (Fig. 4.50C).

Campylobacter pylori infections have been identified as a cause of recurrent abdominal pain and gastritis in children. Originally believed to be a cause of duodenal ulcer disease, there is growing evidence that the main problem is gastritis (14–16). The infection produces nonspecific thickening of the gastric mucosa, but the pattern often is delicate, with small nodules rather than massively thickened gastric folds. The carbon 13-labeled urea breath test is used for detection of *Helicobacter* infections (17), and the condition is treated with antibiotics. However, it has been noted that the infection in children is mostly asymptomatic (18).

REFERENCES

1. Hayden CK, Swischuk LE, Rytting JE. Gastric ulcer disease in infants: US findings. Radiology 1987;164:131–134.
2. Tomooka Y, Koga T, Shimoda Y, et al. The ultrasonic demonstration of acute multiple gastric ulcers in a child. Br J Radiol 1987;60:290–292.
3. Bell MJ, Keating JP, Ternberg JL, et al. Perforated stress ulcers in infants. J Pediatr Surg 1981;16:998–1002.
4. Kamagata S, Ishida H, Hayashi A, et al. Peptic ulcer disease in neonates. J Jpn Soc Pediatr Surg 1990;26:648–654.
5. Kravis LP, South MA, Rosenlund ML. Eosinophilic gastroenteritis in the pediatric patient. Clin Pediatr (Phila) 1982;21:713–717.
6. Bar-Ziv J, Barki Y, Weizman Z, et al. Transient protein losing gastropathy (Menetrier's disease) in childhood. Pediatr Radiol 1988;18:82–84.
7. Cieslak TJ, Mullett CT, Puntel RA, et al. Menetrier's disease associated with cytomegalovirus infection in children: report of two cases and review of the literature. Pediatr Infect Dis J 1993;12:3340–3343.
8. Sferra TJ, Pawel BR, Qualman SJ, et al. Menetrier disease of childhood: role of cytomegalovirus and transforming growth factor alpha. J Pediatr 1996;128:213–219.
9. Gassner I, Strasser K, Bart G, et al. Sonographic appearance of Menetrier's disease in a child. J Ultrasound Med 1990;9:537–539.
10. Dickerman JD, Colletti RB, Tampas JP. Gastric outlet obstruction in chronic granulomatous disease of childhood. Am J Dis Child 1986;140:567–570.
11. Hartenberg MA, Kodroff MB. Chronic granulomatous disease of childhood: probable diffuse gastric involvement. Pediatr Radiol 1984;14:57–58.
12. Smith FJ, Taves DH. Gastroduodenal involvement in chronic granulomatous disease of childhood. J Can Assoc Radiol 1992;43:215–217.
13. Kopen PA, McAlister WH. Upper gastrointestinal and ultrasound examinations of gastric antral involvement in chronic granulomatous disease. Pediatr Radiol 1987;14:192–195.
14. Gormally SM, Prakash N, Durnin MT, et al. Association of symptoms with *Helicobacter pylori* infection in children. J Pediatr 1995;126:753–756.
15. Levine MS, Rubesin SE. The *Helicobacter pylori* revolution: radiologic perspective. Radiology 1995;195:593–596.

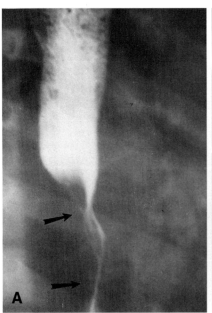

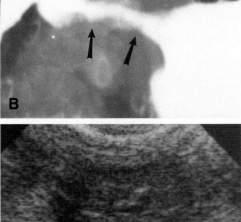

FIGURE 4.50. Granulomatous disease: gastrointestinal manifestation. A. Note narrowing of the esophagus (arrows). **B.** Same patient with circumferential narrowing of the antrum (arrows). **C.** Another patient with ultrasonographic evidence of thickening of the antrum in cross-section (arrows). (**C** reproduced with permission from Colpin PA, McAlister WH. Pediatr Radiol 1984;14:91–93.)

16. Morrison S, Dahms BB, Hoffenberg E, et al. Enlarged gastric folds in association with *Campylobacter pylori* gastritis. Radiology 1989;171:819–821.
17. Rowland M, Lambert I, Gormally S, et al. Carbon 13-labeled urea breath test for the diagnosis of *Helicobacter pylori* infection in children. J Pediatr 1997;131:815–820.
18. Bode G, Rothenbacher D, Brenner H, et al. *Helicobacter pylori* and abdominal symptoms: a population-based study among preschool children in Southern Germany. Pediatrics 1998;101: 634–637.

Gastric Perforation

Gastric perforation is uncommon in the pediatric age group but does occur with gastric ulcers, acute gastric distention, caustic burns to the stomach, and after blunt abdominal trauma. However, most commonly gastric perforation occurs in the neonate, and while such perforations at one time were considered to be the result of congenital deficiencies of the gastric wall, this etiology is no longer commonplace (1). Most probably, they are secondary to gastric ulcers or hypoxia-induced focal necrosis (2). However, overdistention of the stomach resulting from distal obstruction or proximal overinflation, as might be seen with mechanical ventilation, also is an etiologic factor (3, 4). Indomethacin therapy for ductal closure in premature infants also has been associated with gastric perforation, and the problem probably is secondary to focal vasospasm and schemia (5).

REFERENCES

1. Leone RJ Jr, Krasna IH. Spontaneous neonatal gastric perforation: is it really spontaneous? J Pediatr Surg 2000;35:1066–1069.
2. Rosser SB, Clark CH, Elechi EN. Spontaneous neonatal gastric perforation. J Pediatr Surg 1982;17:390–394.
3. Bruce J, Bianchi A, Doig CM, et al. Gastric perforation in the neonate. Pediatr Surg Int 1993;8:17–19.
4. Jones TB, Kirchner SG, Lee FA, et al. Stomach rupture associated with esophageal atresia, tracheoesophageal fistula, and ventilatory assistance. AJR 1980;134:675–677.
5. Nagaraj HS, Sandhu AS, Cook LN, et al. Gastrointestinal perforation following indomethacin therapy in very low birth weight infants. J Pediatr Surg 1981;16:1003–1007.

Gastric Duplication Cysts and Duplication

Gastric duplication cysts generally are uncommon and usually do not communicate with the stomach (1). Many are located in the antropyloric region (Fig. 4.51) and both clinically and on the upper GI series can mimic the findings of pyloric stenosis. However, now that ultrasound (2) is available, the latter should not occur because the cyst can be accurately identified as being a cyst. The walls of these cysts are composed of an inner echogenic mucosal lining and outer sonolucent muscle layer (Fig. 4.51C). Bleeding or even perforation can occur with these cysts, because they often contain aberrant pancreatic or gastric tissue leading to ulceration (3). Complete duplication (4, 5) or triplication (6) of the stomach is rare, as is duplication of the pylorus (7).

REFERENCES

1. Gupta AK, Berry M, Mitra DK. Gastric duplication cyst in children: report of two cases. Pediatr Radiol 1994;24:346–347.
2. Moccia WA, Astacio JE, Kaude JV. Ultrasonographic demonstration of gastric duplication in infancy. Pediatr Radiol 11:52–54, 1981.
3. Kleinhaus S, Boley SJ, Winslow P. Occult bleeding from a perforated gastric duplication in an infant. Arch Surg 1981;116:122.
4. Agha FP, Gabriele OF, Abdulla FH. Complete gastric duplication. AJR 1981;137:406–407.
5. Gray DH. Total reduplication of the stomach: a rare anomaly. Aust N Z J Surg 1971;41:130–133.
6. De la Torre, ML, Daza DC, Bustamante AP. Gastric triplication and peritoneal melanosis. J Pediatr Surg 1997;32:1773–1775.
7. Stannard MW, Currarino G, Splawski JB. Congenital double pylorus with accessory pyloric channel communicating with an intraluminal duplication cyst of the duodenum. Pediatr Radiol 1993;23:48–50.

Gastric Diverticula

Gastric diverticula are uncommon in any age group. They probably represent communicating duplications and, if seen, usually occur in the cardiofundal and antropyloric regions.

REFERENCE

1. Cifci AO, Tanyel FC, Hicsonmnez A. Gastric diverticulum: an uncommon cause of abdominal pain in a 12-year-old. J Pediatr Surg 1998;33:529–531.

Volvulus of the Stomach

Gastric volvulus can occur in early infancy and usually produces acute gastric obstruction. Most cases are of the mesenteroaxial type, in which the stomach twists and flips into an inverted position (1, 2). Roentgenographic findings usually consist of an inverted, distended stomach (3), and the condition can be seen as an isolated phenomenon or in association with paraesophageal diaphragmatic hernia. Gastric volvulus also has been described in association with asplenia (4), and a wandering spleen (5). In addition, the volved stomach can reside in the thorax (6), and gastric volvulus can occur with diaphragmatic hernias, both congenital and traumatic.

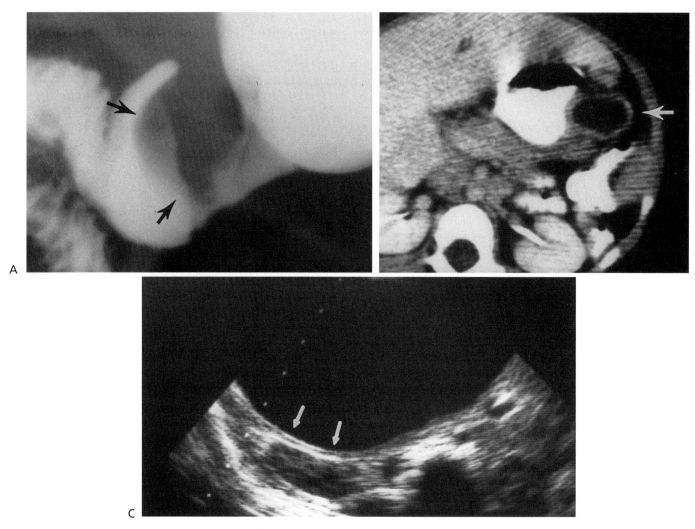

FIGURE 4.51. Gastric duplication cyst. A. Note the filling defect (arrows) caused by a duplication cyst in the antrum. **B.** Same patient, demonstrating a duplication cyst (arrow) on CT. **C.** Ultrasound study through a duplication cyst demonstrates the echogenic intramucosal lining (arrows) and the hypoechoic muscle layer next to it. (**A** and **B** courtesy of James Rytting, M.D.)

REFERENCES

1. Brzezinski W, Laskin MM, Wong KS. Acute mesenteroaxial gastric volvulus in an infant: a case report. Can J Surg 1993;36:233–235.
2. Honna T, Kamii Y, Tsuchida Y. Idiopathic gastric volvulus in infancy and childhood. J Pediatr Surg 1990;25:707–710.
3. Andiran F, Tanyel FC, Balkanci F, et al. Acute abdomen due to gastric volvulus: diagnostic value of a single plain radiograph. Pediatr Radiol 1995;25(Suppl 1):S240.
4. Aoyama K, Tateishi K. Gastric volvulus in three children with asplenic syndrome. J Pediatr Surg 1986;21:307–310.
5. Spector JM, Chappell J. Gastric volvulus associated with wandering spleen in a child. J Pediatr Surg 2000;35:641–642.
6. Mutabagani KH, Teich S, Long FR. Primary intrathoracic gastric volvulus in a newborn. J Pediatr Surg 1999;34:1869–1871.

Microgastria

Microgastria is a rare abnormality in which the stomach is midline in position and rudimentary in size (1, 2). Gastroesophageal reflux and aspiration are common, and it is as though the esophagus takes over the storage duties of the stomach. Microgastria also is commonly seen with the polysplenia-asplenia and Vater syndromes (Fig. 4.52). It also occurs as an isolated anomaly (3).

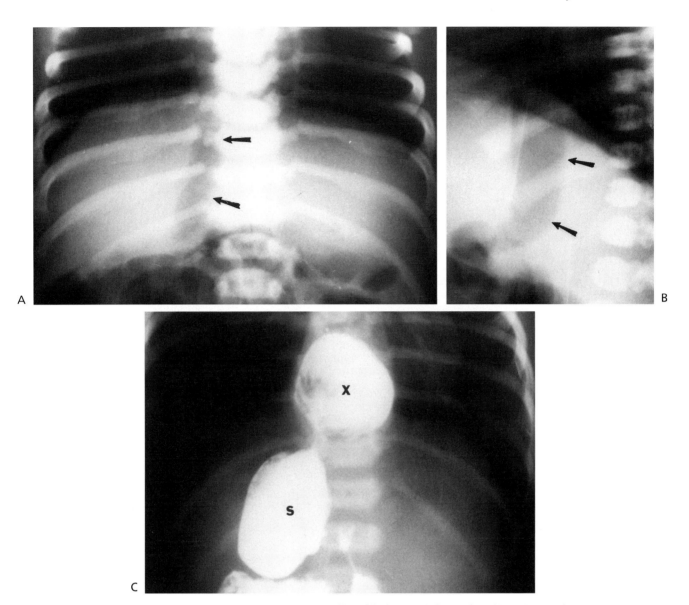

FIGURE 4.52. Microgastria. A. Note the small air-filled stomach (arrows) in this patient with a midline liver and asplenia. **B.** Lateral view shows the same air-filled small tubular stomach (arrows). **C.** Another patient with asplenia, showing a small stomach (S) with an intrathoracic component (X).

REFERENCES

1. Hoehner JC, Kimura K, Soper RT. Congenital microgastria. J Pediatr Surg 1994;29:1591–1593.
2. Moulton SL, Bouvet M, Lynch FP. Congenital microgastria in a premature infant. J Pediatr Surg 1994;29:1594–1595.
3. Ramos CT, Moss RL, Musemeche CA. Microgastria as an isolated anomaly. J Pediatr Surg 1996;31:1445–1447.

Bezoars

Bezoars, at one time, were primarily a problem of older children, and for the most part, they were trichobezoars (i.e., hair) (1) and phytobezoars (i.e., vegetable matter) (2, 3). However, recently lactobezoars have become more common, primarily in premature infants (4–7). In these cases, a dense milk coagulum forms when powdered milk is mixed with inadequate amounts of water. Polystyrene resin bezoars also have been reported in infants requiring exchange resin treatment (8). An antacid bezoar also has been documented (9).

Most frequently, bezoars cause gastric obstruction, but perforation and intussusception (10) also can occur. Gastrostomy frequently is necessary for removal, but in some

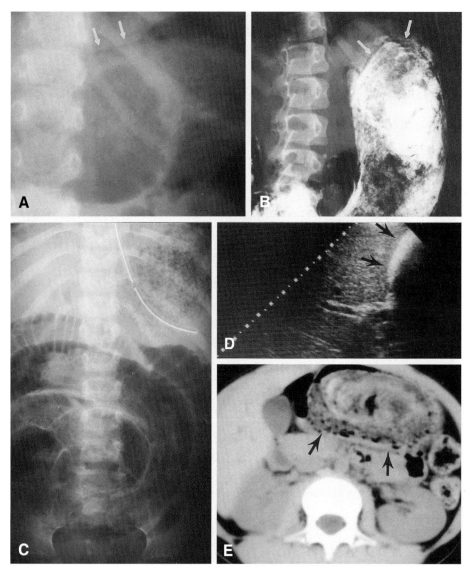

FIGURE 4.53. Gastric bezoar. A. The fundus is full of granular-appearing material, and there is a thin rim of air (arrows) interposed between the bezoar and the gastric wall. **B.** Another patient with a trichobezoar, demonstrating characteristic findings on upper GI series. Note the thin rim of air (arrows) in the fundus. **C.** Another patient with a bezoar in the stomach and a small bowel obstruction secondary to a portion of the bezoar breaking off and becoming impacted in the small bowel. **D.** Note the characteristic arc (arrows) produced by air trapped between the bezoar and gastric wall. Compare with the findings in **A** and **B. E.** CT demonstration of a bezoar (arrows) shows a characteristic bubbly appearance. (**D** and **E** reproduced with permission from Neumann B, Gerdani BR. Gastric trichobezoars—sonographic and computed tomographic appearance. Pediatr Radiol 1990;20:526–527.)

cases, the bezoar may break up, and portions may pass into the small bowel, producing small bowel obstruction. Radiographically, bezoars present as solid- or granular-appearing gastric masses that very often are outlined with air (Fig. 4.53A). Upper GI series clearly identify these lesions (Fig. 4.53B), but care should be taken not to misinterpret transient semisolid milk curds for a true bezoar (Fig. 4.54). This is not to say that all such milk curd collections are transient, because milk curd bezoars, or so-called lactobezoars, are common in infancy. Sonographically, bezoars also may have a reasonably characteristic appearance (1, 11), because air in and around the bezoar tends to produce a very strongly echogenic arc over the bezoar (Fig. 4.53D). Bezoars also are readily demonstrable with CT (1), where they will appear as a mass with air bubbles (Fig. 4.53E). In addition, gastric bezoars can break up and a portion may pass into the small bowel, causing small bowel obstruction (Fig. 4.53C). In

other cases, the bezoar can be very long and extend down to the terminal ileum , in which case the condition is referred to as the Rapunzel syndrome (12, 13).

REFERENCES

1. Newman B, Girdany BR. Gastric trichobezoars: sonographic and computed tomographic appearance. Pediatr Radiol 1991;20:526–527.
2. Choi S-O, Kang J-S. Gastrointestinal phytobezoars in childhood. J Pediatr Surg 1988;23:338–341.
3. Eshel G, Broide E, Azizi E. Phytobezoar following raisin ingestion in children. Pediatr Emerg Care 1988;4:192–193.
4. Bakken DA, Abramo TJ. Gastric lactobezoar: a rare cause of gastric outlet obstruction. Pediatr Emerg Care 1997;13:264–267.
5. Erenberg A, Shaw RD, Yousefzadeh D. Lactobezoar in the low-birth-weight infant. Pediatrics 1979;63:642–646.
6. Levkoff AH, Gadsden RH, Hennigar GR, et al. Lactobezoar and gastric perforation in a neonate. J Pediatr 1970;77:875–877.

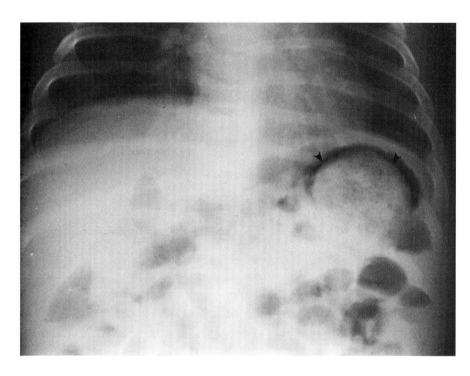

FIGURE 4.54. Transient milk curds in the stomach. Note the filling defect in the stomach of this infant (arrows). This was the result of a milk curd bolus.

7. Singer JI. Lactobezoar causing an abdominal triad of colicky pain, emesis and mass. Pediatr Emerg Care 1988;4:194–196.
8. Metlay LA, Klionsky BL. An unusual gastric bezoar in a newborn: polystyrene resin and *Candida albicans*. J Pediatr 1983; 102:121–123.
9. Portuguez-Malavasi A, Aranda JV. Antacid bezoar in the newborn. Pediatrics 1979;63:679–680.
10. Mehta MH, Patel RV. Intussusception and perforations caused by multiple trichobezoars. J Pediatr Surg 1992;27:1234–1235.
11. McCracken S, Jongeward R, Silver TM, et al. Gastric trichobezoar: sonographic findings. Radiology 1986;161:123–124.
12. Dalshaug GB, Wainer S, Hollaar GL. The Rapunzel syndrome (trichobezoar) causing atypical intussusception in a child. A case report. J Pediatr Surg 1999;34:479–480.
13. West WM, Duncan ND. CT appearance of the Rapunzel syndrome: an unusual form of bezoar and gastrointestinal obstruction. Pediatr Radiol 1998;28:315–316.

Interstitial Emphysema of the Stomach

Occasionally, one can encounter air within the wall of the stomach. In adults, the condition usually is the result of emphysematous gastritis, but in the infant, it frequently is a manifestation of schemia and necrotizing enterocolitis (Fig. 4.55). Intramural air also can be seen secondary to gastric or duodenal obstruction (1–4). In these cases, gas enters the intramural space through mucosal tears produced by overdistention of the stomach. This form of pneumatosis cystoides intestinalis (intramural air) often is termed benign, because it is not associated with bowel schemia and necrosis. Pneumatosis also can result from catheter perforation (5).

REFERENCES

1. Johnson JF, Woisard KK, Cooper GL. Diffuse neonatal gastric infarction. Pediatr Radiol 1988;18:161–163.
2. Franquet T, Gonzalez A. Gastric and duodenal pneumatosis in a child with annular pancreas. Pediatr Radiol 1987;17:262.
3. Gupta A. Interstitial gastric emphysema in a child with duodenal stenosis. Br J Radiol 1977;591:222–224.
4. Lester PD, Budge AF, Barnes JC, et al. Gastric emphysema in infants with hypertrophic pyloric stenosis. AJR 1978;131:421–423.
5. Mandell GA, Pinkelstein M. Gastric pneumatosis secondary to an intramural feeding catheter. Pediatr Radiol 1988;l18:418–420.

Gastric Infarction

Gastric infarction is a rare condition but has been reported in the neonate (1). In this one case, schemia secondary to yeast emboli was the cause of the problem, and the presenting problem was obstruction.

REFERENCE

1. Johnson JF, Woisard KK, Cooper GL. Diffuse neonatal gastric infarction. Pediatr Radiol 1988;18:161–163.

Foreign Bodies

Most foreign bodies that are swallowed and enter the stomach tend to pass spontaneously. However, if they are large, long, or pointed, they are much less likely to do so and, in fact, can lead to perforation. Furthermore, if a foreign body fails to leave the stomach, then one should consider an

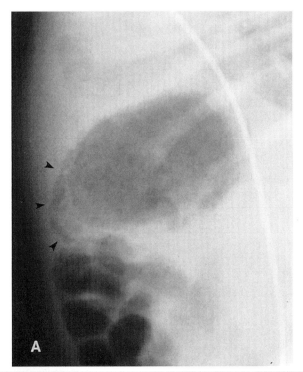

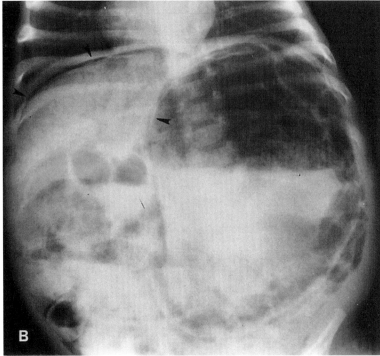

Figure 4.55. Gastric emphysema. A. Note the bubbly appearance of the fundus of the stomach and gas bubbles in the stomach wall (arrows). At laparotomy, similar findings were present throughout the small and large intestines. Most likely, the problem was necrotizing enterocolitis. **B.** Another infant with advanced necrotizing enterocolitis (ischemic gastroenteritis) demonstrating free intraperitoneal air (arrows), air in the portal veins of the stomach, air in the intestinal walls, and a rim of intramural air, outlining the entire gastric wall. (Courtesy of C. Stuart Houston, M.D.)

underlying obstruction and contrast studies are in order. The modern zinc-based penny may dissolve because of gastric acid activity and become invisible (1).

REFERENCE

1. O'Hara SM, Donnelly LF, Chuang E, et al. Gastric retention of zinc-based pennies: radiographic appearance and hazards. Radiology 1999;213:113–117.

Gastric Tumors

Gastric tumors in the pediatric age group are uncommon. Occasionally, one may encounter a young child with a gastric carcinoma (1), sarcoma (2), lymphoma, leiomyoma or leiomyoblastoma (3, 4), inflammatory pseudotumor (5, 6), hamartoma or hemangioma (7, 8), or polyps (8), but all are rare. Gastric leiomyoblastoma in association with paraganglioma and pulmonary chondroma constitute Carney's

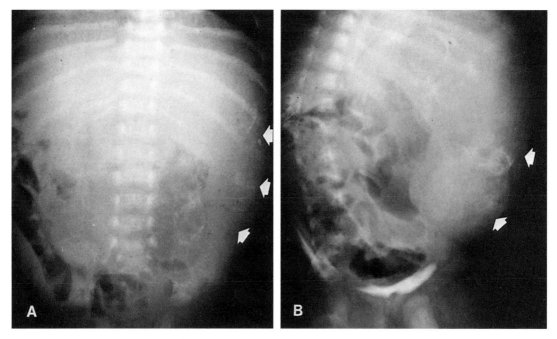

FIGURE 4.56. Gastric teratoma. A. Note the scattered irregular calcifications (arrows) in this large gastric teratoma presenting as a central abdominal mass. Some of the calcifications are curvilinear. **B.** Oblique view from intravenous pyelogram demonstrates the same calcification (arrows). (Reproduced with permission from Siegel MJ, Shackelford GD. Gastric teratomas in infants. Pediatr Radiol 1978;7:197–200.)

triad (9). In the neonate, gastric teratoma is the most common tumor seen (10–12) and often is very large on discovery. It usually contains calcification (Fig. 4.56). These teratomas usually occur in males but occurrence in females has been documented (12). Teratomas, as many other intraabdominal tumors, may extend into the chest (10, 13). Gastric tumors can be demonstrated with regular upper GI series but also are demonstrable with CT, ultrasound, and MRI. On ultrasound, sarcomas and lymphomas may appear sonolucent. Gastric polyps are uncommon in children but may be seen in association with intestinal polyposis syndromes such as the Peutz-Jeghers syndrome.

Ectopic pancreas often is an incidental lesion and, unless biopsied, not always proved. Characteristically it presents as a small nodular filling defect in the gastric antrum (14, 15) and bleeding can be a complication (14). Characteristically, a small collection of barium is seen in the center of the mass (Fig. 4.57), representing the dimple of the duct draining the

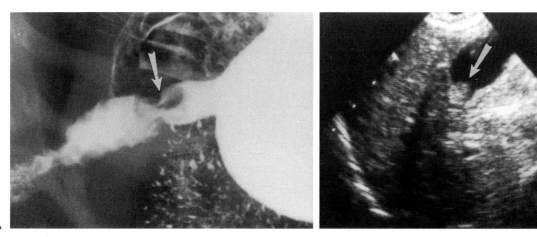

FIGURE 4.57. Ectopic pancreas. A. Note the small filling defect in the antrum (arrow). **B.** Sonographic demonstration of the same lesion (arrow).

ectopic pancreatic tissue. However, this "niche" is not always visualized, and frequently final diagnosis rests with endoscopy.

REFERENCES

1. McGill TW, Downey EC, Westbrook J, et al. Gastric carcinoma in children. J Pediatr Surg 1993;28:1620–1621.
2. Schneider K, Dickerhoff R, Bertele RM. Malignant gastric sarcoma—diagnosis by ultrasound and endoscopy. Pediatr Radiol 1986;16:69–70.
3. Gupta AK, Berry M, Mitra DK. Ossified gastric leiomyoma in a child: a case report. Pediatr Radiol 1995;25:48–49.
4. Tamate S, Lee N, Sou H, et al. Leiomyoblastoma causing acute gastric outlet obstruction in an infant. J Pediatr Surg 1994;29:1386–1387.
5. Maves CK, Johnson JF, Bove K, et al. Gastric inflammatory pseudotumor in children. Radiology 1989;173:381–383.
6. Taratuta E, Krinsky G, Genega E, et al. Case report. Pediatric inflammatory pseudotumor of the stomach: contrast-enhanced CT and MR imaging findings. AJR 1996;167:919–920.
7. Nagaya M, Kato J, Nimi N. Isolated cavernous hemangioma of the stomach in a neonate. J Pediatr Surg 1998;33:653–654.
8. Quinn FM Jr, Brown S, O'Hara D. Hemangiopericytoma of the stomach in a neonate. J Pediatr Surg 1991;26:101–102.
9. Argos MD, Ruiz A, Sanchez F, et al. Gastric leiomyoblastoma associated with extraadrenal paraganglioma and pulmonary chondroma: a new case of Carney's triad. J Pediatr Surg 1993;28:1545–1549.
10. Esposito G, Cigliano B, Paludetto R. Abdominothoracic gastric teratoma in a female newborn infant. J Pediatr Surg 1983;18:304–305.
11. Matias IC, Huang YC. Gastric teratoma in infancy: report of a case and review of world literature. Ann Surg 1973;178:631–636.
12. Senocak ME, Kale G, Buyukpamukco N, et al. Gastric teratoma in children including the third reported female case. J Pediatr Surg 1990;25:681–684.
13. Chiba T, Suzuki H, Habiguchi T, et al. Gastric teratoma extending into the mediastinum. J Pediatr Surg 1980;15:191–192.
14. Ishihara M, Yamazaki T, Aiwa R. Aberrant pancreatic tissue causing pyloric obstruction. Pediatr Surg Int 1990;5:140–141.
15. Hayes-Jordan A, Idowu O, Cohen R. Ectopic pancreas as the cause of gastric outlet obstruction in a newborn. Pediatr Radiol 1998;28:868–870.

Acute Gastric Dilatation

Acute gastric dilatation can occur with excessive air swallowing related to respiratory distress, improper endotracheal tube insertion, tracheoesophageal fistula, and with distal gastric or duodenal obstruction (1). In such cases, when the degree of gastric distention is profound, and acute, a vagal stimulus can be induced so as to cause the patient to have apnea.

REFERENCE

1. Veysi VT, Humphrey G, Stringer MD. Superior mesenteric artery syndrome presenting with acute massive gastric dilatation. Pediatr Surg 1997;32:1801–1803.

DUODENUM

Normal Configuration

The duodenum and duodenal bulb tend to be somewhat posteriorly directed and are best seen on right anterior-oblique or lateral views on the upper GI series (Fig. 4.58, A and B). The duodenum also can be assessed with ultrasound as fluid passes from the stomach into the duodenal bulb and duodenal sweep (Fig. 4.58, C and D). A variation of the "normal" duodenum is the duodenal loop that is incompletely fixed (1). In such cases, the duodenal sweep often lacks its normal curve and shows unusual indentations. Even though these indentations at first may appear sinister, it soon becomes apparent that no obstruction is present. Consequently, a simple duodenal indentation or peculiar configuration does not necessarily indicate symptomatic abnormality (Fig. 4.59).

Generally, the duodenum is considered in three sections: the duodenal bulb, the descending duodenum, and the third and fourth portions, crossing over the spine to the ligament of Treitz. It is important to appreciate these different portions of the duodenum, because certain abnormalities tend to occur at certain sites. Duodenal peristaltic activity usually is brisk, and once barium enters the bulb it is quickly propelled into the small bowel. This also is seen during ultrasound examination.

REFERENCE

1. Katz ME, Siegel MJ, Shackelford GD, et al. The position and mobility of the duodenum in children. AJR 1987;148:947–951.

DUODENAL ABNORMALITIES

Duodenal Atresia and Stenosis

In terms of the etiology of duodenal atresia and stenosis, the failure of recanalization theory is favored over intrauterine vascular schemia. Infants with duodenal atresia present with vomiting in the first few hours of life, but those with duodenal stenosis can present at more variable times, because the clinical findings depend on the degree of stenosis. Bile usually is absent in the vomitus of infants with duodenal atresia or stenosis for the area of obstruction usually is at, or proximal to the ampulla of Vater. In a very few cases, however, atresia occurs below the ampulla, and then, bile is present.

Clinically, abdominal distention is present, and roentgenographically, dilation of the stomach and duodenum produce the characteristic "double bubble" sign (Fig. 4.60).

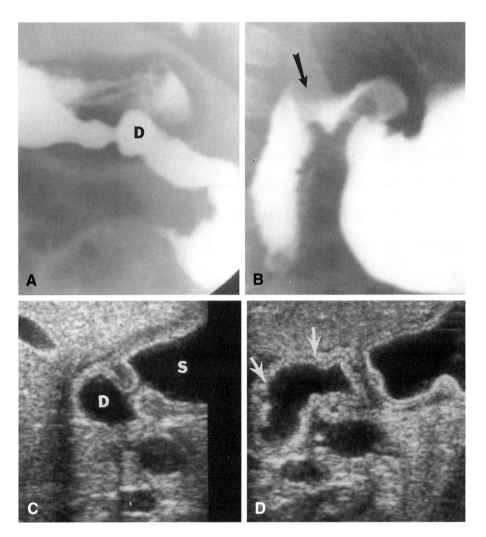

FIGURE 4.58. Normal duodenum. **A.** Note characteristic appearance of the duodenal bulb (D) and descending duodenum. **B.** Normal, incompletely filled duodenal bulb and finger-like indentation at the junction of the first and second portions of the duodenum (arrow). This probably is produced by the normal common bile duct. **C.** Ultrasonogram demonstrates a normal duodenal bulb (D) and the antrum of the stomach (S). In between is the pyloric canal. **D.** Another patient demonstrating the duodenal bulb and descending duodenum (arrows). Note the normal-appearing gastric antrum with its multilayered wall.

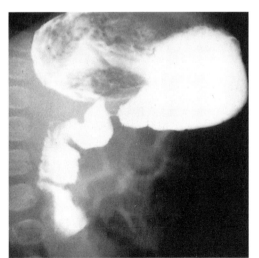

FIGURE 4.59. Duodenal indentations. Note that a number of duodenal indentations are present, but none produces obstruction. In other instances, the duodenal loop may appear more tortuous (greater degree of poor fixation). The indentations probably represent nonobstructing duodenal kinks. The important point with such indentations is to determine whether they are producing obstruction.

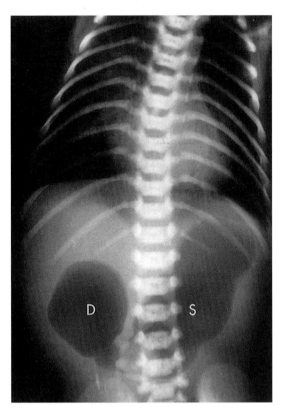

FIGURE 4.60. Duodenal atresia. Note that the stomach (S) and duodenal bulb (D) are distended, leading to the "double bubble" sign. No air is present distal to the duodenum.

This configuration most commonly is seen with duodenal atresia or annular pancreas, which usually is associated with duodenal atresia. Once this roentgenographic pattern is demonstrated, there is no need for further contrast studies. If not enough air is present to adequately demonstrate the obstruction, one can introduce more air through a nasogastric tube.

In a few cases of duodenal atresia gas, albeit scant, can be seen in the small bowel. The reason for this is that an associated anomaly of the hepaticopancreatic ducts occurs (1, 2). In the fetus, the hepaticopancreatic ducts pass through a normal phase where a double orifice is present. If this arrangement persists, one limb of the duct system opens into the duodenum above the point of atresia, and one below. Consequently, a Y-shaped connection is present, and gas can bypass the point of atresia. Because of this, one can have a classic double bubble with evidence of gas in the distal small bowel, and then the findings are indistinguishable from those seen with severe duodenal stenosis (Fig. 4.61, A and B) or other forms of incomplete duodenal obstruction. These findings are not specifically diagnostic, and contrast studies are required (Fig. 4.61C). However, even with contrast studies, it may be difficult to differentiate duodenal stenosis from a nearly completely occluding duodenal diaphragm, because in both cases, the duodenal bulb is

markedly enlarged (i.e., megabulbia). In other cases, the area of stenosis is located further down the duodenum.

Duodenal atresia and stenosis are more common in trisomy 21 (8), and both abnormalities can be associated with other GI and biliary tract anomalies (e.g., malrotation, esophageal atresia, ectopic anus, annular pancreas, gallbladder or biliary atresia [3], vertebral anomalies). Duodenal obstruction also can be seen in the VATER and VACTERL syndromes, and a few familial cases have been encountered (4–6).

When duodenal atresia is combined with esophageal atresia and no fistula, a peculiar set of roentgenographic findings result (7–9). No air is seen in the stomach, and since the stomach is obstructed at both ends, the infant presents with a large, opaque abdomen with evidence of a chest mass: the fluid-filled distal esophagus (Fig. 4.62). Ultrasound studies are even more useful and probably the studies of choice. These studies demonstrate a large echolucent fluid-filled stomach and duodenal bulb (Fig. 4.62B). In other cases, obstruction of the duodenum can lead to perforation of the stomach (10) or regurgitation of air through the sphincter of Oddi into the biliary tract (11).

REFERENCES

1. Kassner EG, Sutton AL, DeGroot TJ. Bile duct anomalies associated with duodenal atresia: paradoxical presence of small bowel gas. AJR 1972;116:577–583.
2. Knechtle SJ, Filston HC. Anomalous biliary ducts associated with duodenal atresia. J Pediatr Surg 1990;25:1266–1269.
3. Coughlin JP, Rector FE, Klein MD. Agenesis of the gallbladder in duodenal atresia: two case reports. J Pediatr Surg 1992;27:1304.
4. Gahukamble DB, Khamage AS, Shaheen. Duodenal atresia: its occurrence in siblings. J Pediatr Surg 1994;29:1599–1600.
5. Mitchell CE, Marshall DG, Reid WD. Preampullary congenital duodenal obstruction in a father and son. J Pediatr Surg 1993;28:1582–1583.
6. Milshalany HG, der Kaloustian VM, Ghandour M. Familial congenital duodenal atresia. Pediatrics 1970;46:629–632.
7. Crowe JE, Summer TE. Combined esophageal and duodenal atresia without tracheoesophageal fistula: characteristic radiographic changes. AJR 1978;130:167–168.
8. Hayden CK Jr, Schwartz MZ, Davis M, et al. Combined esophageal and duodenal atresia: sonographic findings. AJR 1983;140:225–226.
9. Spitz L, Ali M, Brereton RJ. Combined esophageal and duodenal atresia: experience of 188 patients. J Pediatr Surg 1981;16:4–7.
10. Takebayashi J, Asada K, Tokura K, et al. Congenital atresia of the duodenum with gastric perforation. Am J Dis Child 1975;129:1227–1228.
11. Kirks DR, Baden M. Incompetence of the sphincter of Oddi associated with duodenal stenosis. J Pediatr 1973;83:838–840.

Annular Pancreas

Annular pancreas (1) is not as common a cause of duodenal obstruction as is duodenal atresia, but it is the second most

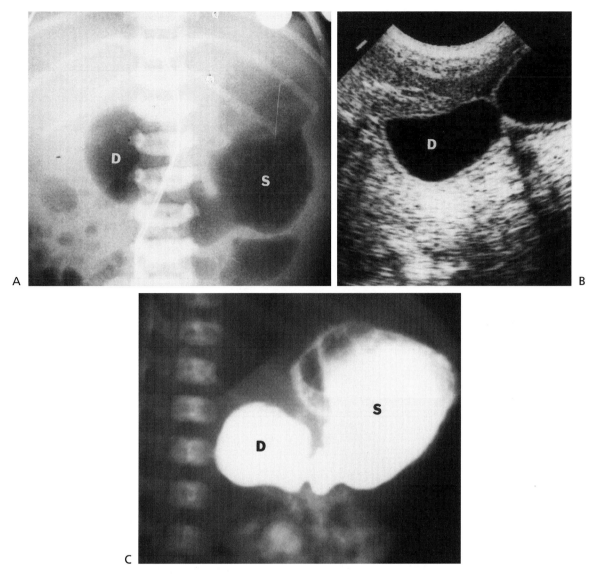

FIGURE. 4.61. Duodenal stenosis. A. Note the duodenal bulb configuration. Air is present in the small bowel. **B.** Ultrasound demonstrates the dilated duodenal bulb (D). **C.** Upper GI series demonstrates similar findings. D, duodenum; S, stomach.

common condition to produce the characteristic double bubble sign. The annular pancreas is believed to result from failure of embryonic pancreatic tissue to properly rotate around the duodenum. Consequently it grows in the form of an encircling ring. As in duodenal atresia, associated GI and other anomalies also can occur.

Some cases are asymptomatic until late adulthood, but in the neonatal period annular pancreas usually presents with findings similar to those of duodenal atresia or stenosis. Some degree of duodenal stenosis or atresia is present in all cases of annular pancreas, and it may be more proper to consider them the actual cause of obstruction (2). Roentgenographically, the findings are usually indistin-

guishable from those of duodenal atresia or stenosis (Fig. 4.63). Contrast studies are not required if obstruction is complete, and occasionally obstruction and the encircling soft tissue ring can be identified with ultrasound (3).

REFERENCES

1. Merrill JR, Raffensperger JG. Pediatric annular pancreas: twenty years' experience. J Pediatr Surg 1976;11:921–925.
2. Verga G. Is annular pancreas the true cause of duodenal obstruction in the newborn? Ann Chir Infant 1972;13:275–276.
3. Orr LA, Powell RW, Melhem RE. Sonographic demonstration of

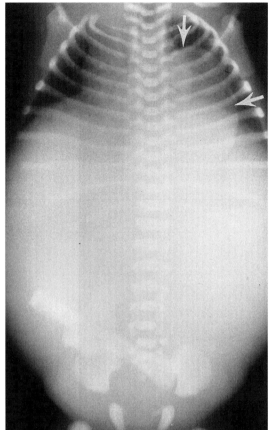

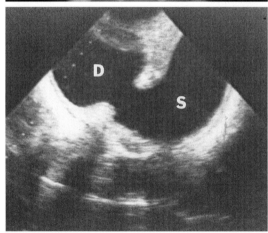

FIGURE. 4.62. Combined duodenal and esophageal atresia without fistula. A. Note the airless, distended abdomen. Also note the mass (arrows) projecting above the diaphragm. **B.** Ultrasonographic study demonstrates the dilated stomach (S) and duodenum (D). (**A** Reproduced with permission from Crow JE, Summer TE. Combined esophageal and duodenal atresia without tracheoesophageal fistula; characteristic radiographic changes. Am J Roentgenol Radium Ther Nucl Med 1987;131: 167–168.).

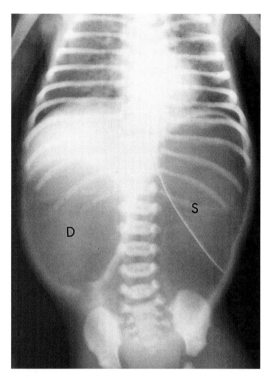

FIGURE 4.63. Annular pancreas. Note double bubble effect, indistinguishable from that seen with duodenal atresia. This infant had an annular pancreas and duodenal atresia. D, duodenum; S, stomach.

annular pancreas in the newborn. J Ultrasound Med 1992;11: 373–375.

Duodenal Bands and Abnormal Duodenal Fixation

Obstructing duodenal bands usually occur in the region of the third and fourth portions of the duodenum. However, they can also occur at higher levels. They often are referred to as Ladd's bands and are associated with various degrees of intestinal malrotation. The bands usually extend from the malplaced cecum to the distal duodenum, and although they most commonly produce obstruction to the third and fourth portions of the duodenum, they can also produce obstruction of the terminal ileum. Bands have also been described from the gallbladder to the cecum and in various other locations in the abdomen. However, most are located around the duodenum, and overall, it is impossible to discuss the problem of duodenal bands without discussing intestinal malrotation, absence of the ligament of Treitz, and complicating midgut volvulus. This whole problem is discussed in detail in the section dealing with malrotation and volvulus.

Incomplete rotation and fixation of the duodenum can produce a peculiar configuration of the duodenum, but it generally is not associated with any clinical symptoms (1). The descending duodenum appears more tortuous than usual and does not conform to its usual smooth C-shaped configuration.

REFERENCE

1. Firor HV, Harris VJ. Rotational abnormalities of the gut: re-emphasis of a neglected facet, isolated incomplete rotation of the duodenum. AJR 1974;120:315–321.

Duodenal Duplication Cysts and Diverticula

Duplication cysts of the duodenum are not as common as are those of the esophagus and small bowel. Occasionally, they are encountered and produce variable impressions on the duodenum, including a beak-like deformity that can erroneously suggest volvulus (1). The most definitive way to identify a duplication cyst, however, is with ultrasound (2). These sonolucent structures usually contain very little intraluminal debris and, as with all duplication cysts, one may be able to identify the echogenic mucosa and the sonolucent rim of muscle in the wall. In addition, peristalsis of the cyst wall can be seen, and some cysts can extend into the chest (3) (Fig. 4.64). Duodenal duplication cysts have produced duodeno-jejunal intussusception (4), and a case of intrapancreatic duodenal duplication cyst has been reported in association with reverse positioning of the superior mesenteric artery and vein (5).

Duodenal diverticula usually are congenital in origin, because in children pseudodiverticula resulting from ulcer disease and scarring are uncommon. Congenital diverticula can be large or small and are most dramatically demonstrated

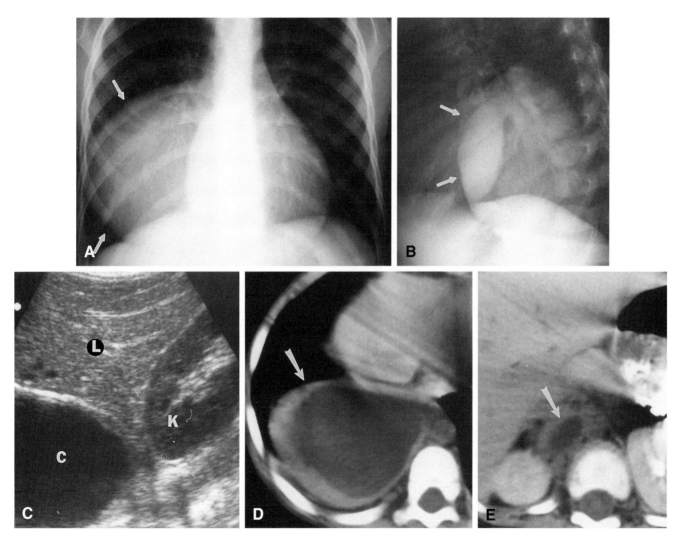

FIGURE 4.64. Duodenal duplication cyst extending into chest. A. Note the large mass on the right (arrows). **B.** Lateral view demonstrates the posterior position of the mass (arrows). **C.** Ultrasonogram demonstrates the large cyst (C) located in the chest above the diaphragm. L, liver; K, kidney. **D.** Axial CT demonstrates the large, intrathoracic component of the cyst (arrow). **E.** Abdominal CT demonstrates the lowermost extent of the duplication cyst (arrow).

with barium upper GI series. Most are located on the medial aspect of the descending duodenal sweep, near the ampulla.

REFERENCES

1. Blake NS. Beak sign in duodenal duplication cyst. Pediatr Radiol 1984;14:232–233.
2. Barr LL, Hayden CK Jr, Stansberry SD, et al. Enteric duplication cysts in children: are their ultrasonographic wall characteristics diagnostic? Pediatr Radiol 1990;20:326–328.
3. Kobayashi Y, Uetsuji S, Yamada T, et al. Transdiaphragmatic duodenal duplication in a premature infant. 1987;22:372–373.

Intraluminal Duodenal Diaphragm

Duodenal diaphragms usually occur in the descending portion of the duodenum, and the common bile duct frequently is incorporated into the diaphragm. The etiology of duodenal diaphragms probably is the same as for duodenal atresia: failure of recanalization. Clinically, various degrees of obstruction are encountered, bile is present in the vomitus, and plain abdominal roentgenograms often show obstruction of the descending duodenum, somewhat lower than with duodenal atresia (Fig. 4.65A). Air is seen in the small bowel if the diaphragm has a hole in it (1). If the hole

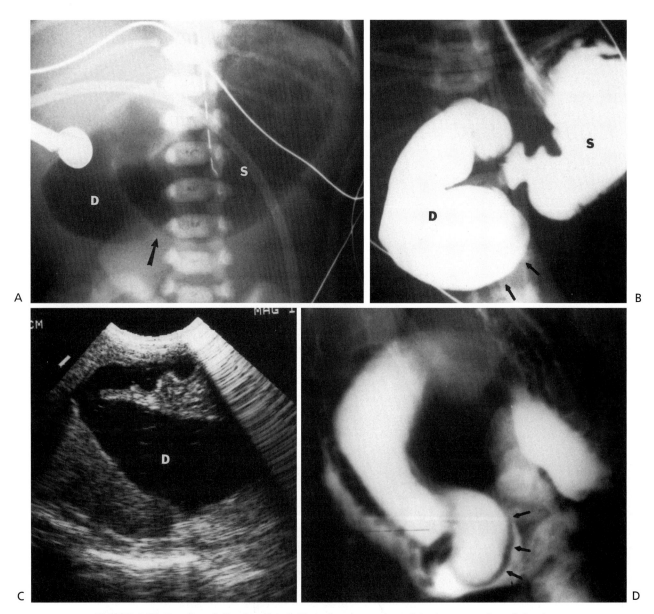

FIGURE 4.65. Duodenal diaphragm. A. Note the obstruction of the lower portion of the duodenum (arrow). D, duodenum; S, stomach. **B.** Same patient. Upper GI series shows the rounded, obstructing diaphragm (arrows). **C.** Ultrasound in the same infant demonstrates the dilated, obstructed duodenum and duodenal bulb (D). **D.** Wind sock duodenal diaphragm (arrows) in the duodenum.

is large, lesser degrees of obstruction and abnormal findings result. Barium studies clearly demonstrate the level of obstruction (Fig. 4.65B), but the findings also can be seen with ultrasound (Fig. 4.65C). The diaphragm itself often is difficult to demonstrate, but in some cases, it becomes so stretched that an "intraluminal" or "windsock" diverticulum is formed (Fig. 4.65D).

The most important practical feature of duodenal diaphragms is that they can occur in conjunction with such lesions as duodenal bands, midgut volvulus, and duodenal atresia and with obstructing diaphragms in other portions of the GI tract. Consequently, even though one demonstrates obstruction resulting from one of these lesions, it is mandatory that a search for a coexisting diaphragm be made during roentgenographic examination or surgical exploration. At the same time, when a diaphragm is encountered, these other lesions should be excluded, and this generally is accomplished during surgical exploration.

REFERENCE

1. Bickler SW, Harrison MW, Blank E, et al. Microperforation of a duodenal diaphragm as a cause of paradoxical gas in congenital duodenal obstruction. J Pediatr Surg 1992;27:747.

Preduodenal Portal Vein

The preduodenal portal vein is a rare anomaly that results from an abnormality of development of the portal vein, the right and left vitelline veins, and their anastomotic channels. As a result, the portal vein comes to lie anterior to the duodenum and, in so doing, can produce indentation and compression of the duodenum (1, 2). In a few cases, a preduodenal portal vein can occur as an isolated anomaly, but more frequently, it is part of a complex of anomalies involving the GI tract and other systems. Malrotation with duodenal bands is commonly associated, and the vein may be contained within such a band. Biliary atresia, intestinal atresia, esophageal atresia, annular pancreas, other portal vein anomalies, and dextrocardia often also coexist.

The most important feature of preduodenal portal vein obstruction is that the vein not be transected during surgery, especially if it is contained in a peritoneal band. Ultrasound can aid in identifying the vessel within such a band. Plain films often show nonspecific high duodenal obstruction. The condition usually is finally diagnosed at surgery.

REFERENCES

1. Fernandes ET, Burton EM, Hixson SD, et al. Preduodenal portal vein: surgery and radiographic appearance. J Pediatr Surg 1990; 25:1270–1272.
2. Patti G, Marrocco G, Mazzoni G, et al. Esophageal and duodenal atresia with preduodenal common bile duct and portal vein in a newborn. J Pediatr Surg 1985;20:167–168.

Duodenal Ulcers

Duodenal ulcer disease generally is believed to be rare in children, but it is much more common than is generally appreciated (1, 2). The etiology of duodenal ulcers in childhood is the same as that in adults. Factors such as stress and hyperacidity are important, and more recently, *Helicobacter* infection (3, 4) has been incriminated as a cause of peptic ulcer disease in adults and children. However, it would appear that with *Helicobacter* infection, the problem is more one of a gastritis than of duodenal ulcer disease.

Duodenal ulcer disease also is seen after steroid therapy (5) and with type I diabetes mellitus (6). Overall, there is nothing unique about childhood duodenal ulcers except that general teaching tends to dissuade one from considering them in children. One of the reasons for this is that children often do not present with typical complaints, and even if they did, the younger ones could not relate their symptoms accurately to a physician. Frank bleeding from the upper GI tract or blood in the stool may be the initial presenting problem in children.

Roentgenographically, the diagnosis of duodenal ulcer disease is subject to variable interpretation. If one is of the school that an ulcer crater needs be demonstrated before the disease entity is suggested, then one will miss many cases. Certainly the crater is almost foolproof evidence of the disease (Fig. 4.66A), but secondary findings are important and include mucosal edema (7), extreme spasm of the duodenal bulb and antrum, and deformity of the postbulbar region resulting from spasm and edema (i.e., thick folds—duodenitis) (Fig. 4.66B). It is worthwhile to pay attention to the secondary findings of duodenal ulcer disease, because even though one cannot demonstrate an ulcer, if the findings are taken in context with the clinical presentation, one often can arrive at a strong presumptive diagnosis and proceed with a trial of therapy, or endoscopy. Duodenal ulcer disease also can be demonstrated with ultrasonography (8, 9), but generally this imaging modality is not used for demonstrating this entity.

REFERENCES

1. Murphy MS, Eastham EJ, Jiminez M, et al. Duodenal ulceration: review of 110 cases. Arch Dis Child 1987;62:554–558.
2. Tsang T-M, Saing H, Yeung C-K. Peptic ulcer in children. J Pediatr Surg 1990;25:744–748.
3. Kilridge PM, Dahms BB, Czinn SJ. *Campylobacter pylori*-associated gastritis and peptic ulcer disease in children. Am J Dis Child 1988;142:1149–1152.
4. Yeung CK, Fu KH, Yuen KY, et al. *Helicobacter pylori* and associated duodenal ulcer. Arch Dis Child 1990;65:1212–1216.
5. Bickler SW, Harrison MW, Campbell JR. Perforated peptic ulcer

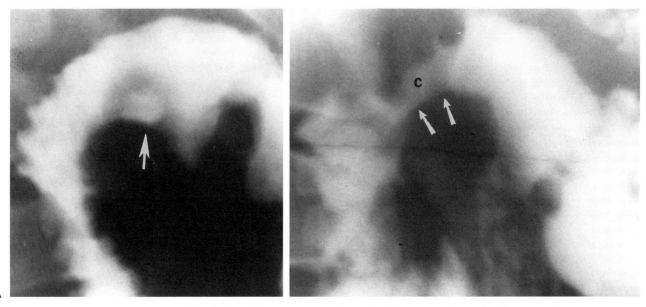

A   B

FIGURE 4.66. Duodenal ulcer disease. A. Note the typical ulcer crater (arrow) and surrounding edema. **B.** Older child with intense edema and spasm of the postapical portion of the duodenum (arrows) secondary to ulcer disease. The ulcer crater (C), however, is only faintly visible.

disease in children: association of corticosteroid therapy. J Pediatr Surg 1993;28:785–787.

6. Burghen GA, Murrell LR, Whitington GL, et al. Acid peptic disease in children with type I diabetes mellitus: a complicating relationship. Am J Dis Child 1992;146:718–722.
7. Long FR, Kramer SS, Markowitz RI, et al. Duodenitis in children: correlation of radiologic findings with endoscopic and pathologic findings. Radiology 1998;206:103–106.
8. Joharjy IA, Mustafa MA, Zaidi AJ. Fluid-aided sonography of the stomach and duodenum in the diagnosis of peptic ulcer disease in adult patients. J Ultrasound Med 1990;9:77–84.
9. Lim JH, Lee KH, Ko YT. Sonographic detection of duodenal ulcer. J Ultrasound Med 1992;11:91–94.

Duodenal Trauma and Hematoma

The most common cause of trauma to the duodenum is blunt abdominal trauma as sustained in seat belt accidents (1) or the battered child syndrome (2). In many of these cases there is associated injury to other organs, especially the pancreas. In any case, the hematoma may present as an abdominal mass, but, more often, it will present as vomiting. Ultrasonography is effective in demonstrating the hematoma (Fig. 4.67B), which in its early stages presents with a somewhat mixed echo pattern. Later, as it degener-

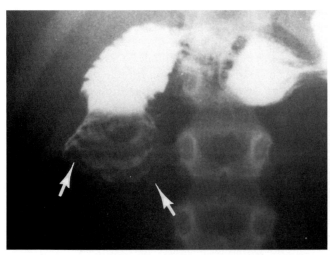

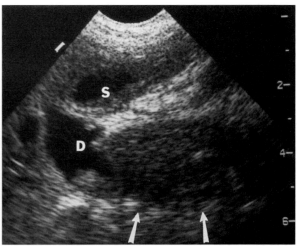

A   B

FIGURE 4.67. Duodenal hematoma. A. Characteristic appearance of an intramural duodenal hematoma (arrows). There is compression of the barium between the hematoma and wall of the duodenum. **B.** Ultrasonogram demonstrates a large echogenic duodenal hematoma (arrows). D, duodenum; S, stomach.

ates and liquefies, it becomes more hypoechoic. Upper GI series findings are more characteristic and consist of a various-sized mass that, because of its intramural location, produces typical, curved, compressive deformities of the duodenum. As a result, the duodenum appears spread out and the folds somewhat stretched and stacked (Fig. 4.67A). Most duodenal hematomas resolve and decompress into the lumen of the intestine. Hematomas also can occur with blood dyscrasia such as hemophilia (3).

REFERENCES

1. Sivit CJ, Taylor GA, Newman KD, et al. Safety-belt injuries in children with lap-belt ecchymosis: CT findings in 61 patients. AJR 1991;157:111–114.
2. Kleinman PK, Brill PW, Winchester P. Resolving duodenal-jejunal hematoma in abused children. Radiology 1986;160:747–750.
3. Nogues A, Elizaguirre I, Sunol M, et al. Giant spontaneous duodenal hematoma in hemophilia. Am J Pediatr Surg 1989;24:406–408.

Duodenal Foreign Bodies

If duodenal foreign bodies are small and smooth, they are of little consequence. It is only when they are long and pointed or of some otherwise problematic shape that they become a concern. In such cases, they may become embedded in the duodenum and lead to perforation. If a foreign body fails to pass out of the duodenum, no matter what its shape, an underlying intraluminal obstruction should be considered (1, 2). Most often, the problem is an intraluminal web, and in such cases, more than one foreign body may

be seen to remain at a fixed position for a prolonged period (Fig. 4.68).

REFERENCES

1. Kassner EG, Rose JS, Kottmeier PK, et al. Retention of a small foreign object in the stomach and duodenum. A sign of partial obstruction caused by duodenal anomalies. Radiology 1975;114:683–686.
2. Mandell GA, Rosenberg HK, Schnaufer L. Prolonged retention of foreign bodies in the stomach. Pediatrics 1977;60:460–462.
3. Swischuk LE. Fever, cough and irritability. Pediatric Emerg Care 1999;15:280–282.

Duodenal Tumors

Duodenal tumors are rare in the pediatric age group and, when seen, usually are of unusual pathology (1–5) and radiographically manifest with a variety of intraluminal filling defects. Tumors and cysts around the duodenum also can produce deformity of the duodenum and various degrees of obstruction. This circumstance probably is more common than obstruction resulting from an intraluminal tumor.

REFERENCES

1. Fleet M, Mellon AF, Lee JA, et al. Duodenal leiomyosarcoma presenting with iron deficiency anemia. J Pediatr Surg 1994;29:1601–1603.
2. Hammoudi SM, Corkery JJ. Congenital hemangiopericytoma of duodenum. J Pediatr Surg 1985;20:559–560.
3. Petit P, Panuel M, Scheiner C, et al. Calcifications in untreated

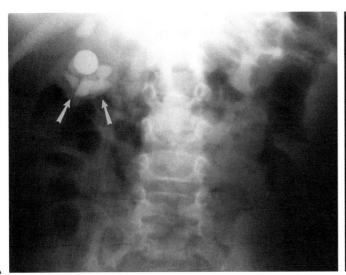
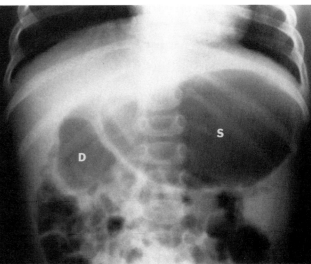

FIGURE 4.68. Foreign bodies trapped in duodenal diaphragm. A. Note the numerous foreign bodies in the abdomen (arrows). **B.** A prior abdominal film demonstrates a double bubble configuration. This patient had trisomy 21 and an occult diaphragm. D, duodenum; S, stomach.

primary duodenal lymphoma: an exceptional entity. Pediatr Radiol 1994;24:283–284.

4. Poplausky MR, Haller JO, Gerson LS. Congenital hemangiopericytoma of the duodenum. Pediatr Radiol 1992;22:344–345.
5. Riggle KP, Boeckman CR. Duodenal leiomyoma: a case report of a hematemesis in a teenager. J Pediatr Surg 1988;23:850–851.

Superior Mesenteric Artery Syndrome

The superior mesenteric artery syndrome consists of compression of the duodenum by the superior mesenteric artery as it crosses the spine. For the most part, it is seen in older children who are subject to a combination of prolonged recumbent positioning and poor nutrition with loss of retroperitoneal fat, which allows the mesenteric artery to compress the duodenum (Fig. 4.69). A rare complication is bezoar formation in the obstructed duodenum (1), and the condition occasionally can present with massive air distention of the stomach (2). The superior mesenteric artery syndrome generally is not seen in infants but has been documented on a familial basis (3).

REFERENCES

1. Doski JJ, Priebe CJ Jr, Smith T, et al. Duodenal trichobezoar caused by compression of the superior or mesenteric artery. J Pediatr Surg 1995;30:1598–1599.
2. Veysi VT, Humphrey G, Stringer MD. Superior mesenteric artery syndrome presenting with acute massive gastric dilatation. J Pediatr Surg 1997;32:1801–1803.
3. Ortiz C, Cleveland RH, Blickman JG, et al. Familial superior mesenteric artery syndrome. Pediatr Radiol 1990;20:588–589.

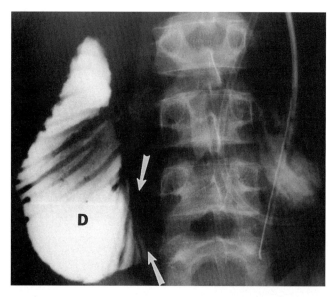

FIGURE 4.69. Superior mesenteric artery syndrome. Note the characteristic abrupt and finger-like indentation of the second-third portions of the duodenum (arrows) caused by the compressive effects of the superior mesenteric artery. D, duodenum.

SMALL INTESTINE

Normal Configurations

In older children, the small intestine appears the same as in adults, complete with a delicate and lacy normal mucosal pattern (Fig. 4.70A). In infants, however, the mucosal pattern may not be so clearly demonstrated. The small bowel intestinal mucosa also can be demonstrated and evaluated with ultrasound (Fig. 4.70B). On ultrasound, normal mucosa generally has a delicate pattern of tortuosity and usually is no more than 2 mm thick (1).

REFERENCE

1. Haber HP, Stern M. Intestinal ultrasonography in children and young adults: bowel wall thickness is age dependent. J Ultrasound Med 2000;19:315–321.

ABNORMALITIES OF THE SMALL BOWEL

Small Bowel Atresia and Stenosis

Small bowel atresia and stenosis combined, (i.e., jejunal, jejunoileal, or ileal) probably is more common than duodenal atresia. Clinically, if the infant has atresia or severe stenosis, abdominal distention and vomiting become apparent early. The vomitus characteristically contains bile.

Current concepts regarding the etiology of ordinary small bowel atresias and stenoses favor intrauterine intestinal schemia, not failure of recanalization. In support of schemia is the fact that small bowel atresias usually occur as isolated abnormalities and are associated with wedge-shaped mesenteric defects. Other anomalies of the GI tract or other systems seldom are encountered. Intestinal schemia can result from thromboemboli, vasospasm induced by fetal stress or hypoxia, and intrauterine volvulus (1). Other causes include internal hernia and fetal intussusception (2).

Small bowel atresia can be classified into four types (Fig. 4.71). Abdominal roentgenograms usually clearly demonstrate a pattern of small bowel obstruction, and if the obstruction is high in the jejunum, only one or two loops of small bowel are visualized (Fig. 4.72A). If atresia involves the mid-jejunum, more loops are seen (Fig. 4.72B), and when distal ileal atresia is present, many loops are present (Fig. 4.72C). Multiple air-fluid levels usually are present (Fig. 4.72D) and allow differentiation from obstruction secondary to meconium ileus where air-fluid levels are scarce because of the thick meconium present. This differentiation also can be accomplished with ultrasound (3). With meconium ileus thick meconium will be seen to encircle the intestinal lumen while with ileal atresia only fluid is seen in the lumen of the intestines. In some cases of distal ileal atresia, gas mixed with meconium can be seen in the distended small bowel loops, producing the so-called

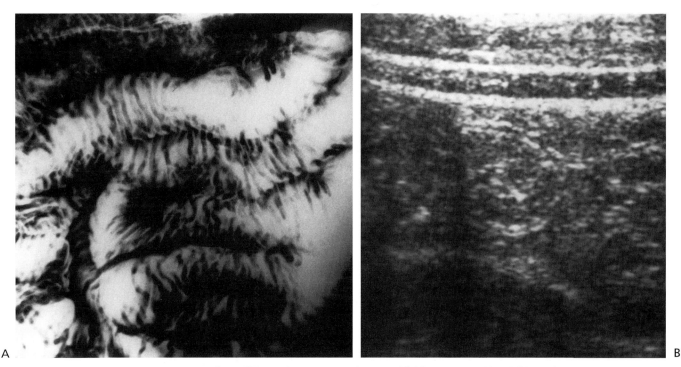

FIGURE 4.70. Normal small intestine. A. Normal mucosal fold pattern in older child. **B.** Ultrasound of normal bowel. Note the delicate granular appearance of the collapsed small bowel just under the abdominal wall.

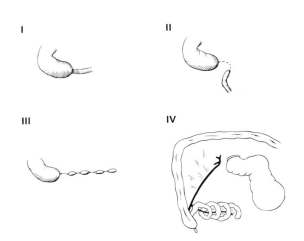

FIGURE 4.71. Small bowel atresia: classification. Type I. The atretic portion of the small bowel is in continuity with the dilated portion. **Type II.** There is discontinuity of the two parts of the intestine. The two parts may or may not be joined by a fibrous band. Many also will have a mesenteric defect and some degree of small bowel shortening often will be present. **Type III. Multiple atresias.** The bowel may or may not be in continuity. Multiple areas of atresia exist with interspersed areas of cyst-like small bowel segments. **Type IV. "Apple peel" small bowel.** The bowel ends are not in continuity. There is a large mesenteric defect and blood supply to the terminal (spiraled) small bowel is from the ileocolic artery. (Modified from Martin LW, Zerella JT. Jejunoileal atresia: a proposed classification. J Pediatr Surg 1976;11:399–403.)

soap bubble appearance (Fig. 4.73). However, this appearance is more common with meconium ileus.

If obstruction is judged to be in the high jejunum, no further roentgenographic studies are required, but if distal small bowel obstruction is suggested, a contrast enema usually is necessary. It is not possible to differentiate distal small bowel from colonic obstruction on the basis of plain abdominal roentgenograms, and consequently, contrast studies of the colon are necessary. Characteristically, in ileal atresia, the colon is small, spastic, and unused, the so-called microcolon (Fig. 4.74). Complete obstruction of the distal small bowel causes meconium to accumulate in the small intestine and not the colon, and consequently, the colon remains small and unused. If the obstruction is higher, some small bowel content does get into the colon, and intraluminal debris along with a more normal colon is seen.

In any of these cases, if intestinal perforation occurs meconium peritonitis can result and peritoneal calcifications can be seen on plain films. In intestinal atresia, intramural calcifications can occur. These calcifications can be clumpy and irregular (Fig. 4.74A), or linear (Fig. 4.75). Round or oval calcifications also can be seen with intestinal atresia, but these usually are seen in cases of multiple areas of atresia.

Multiple small bowel atresias are rare and, when they occur, seem to constitute a syndrome that is familial. It is

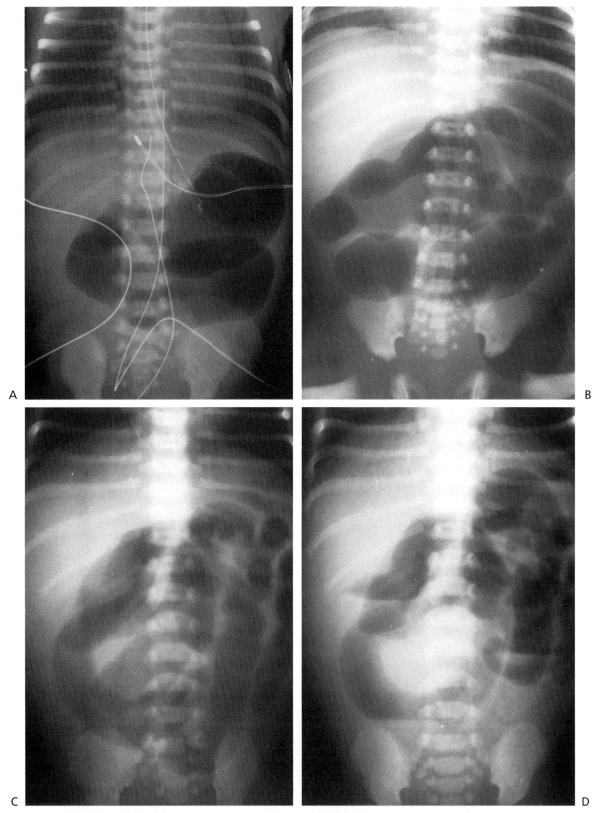

FIGURE 4.72. Small bowel atresia. A. High jejunal atresia with the stomach and one loop of large distended jejunum present. **B.** Mid-jejunal atresia with more loops of dilated jejunum visible. **C.** Low small bowel obstruction resulting from ileal atresia. **D.** Upright view demonstrates numerous air-fluid levels.

inherited on an autosomal recessive basis and along with multiple areas of atresia in a small bowel, atretic areas also can occur in the esophagus, stomach, duodenum, and colon (4–9). The etiology of this form of intestinal atresia probably lies in defective recanalization of the intestine (2). It probably does not result from multiple ischemic episodes or sites. Renal dysplasia also has been reported in association with multiple intestinal atresias (10), giving further credence to the problem being one of genetic predisposition and not the result of ischemic insult. However, multiple schemia-induced areas of small bowel atresia have been noted with cystic fibrosis (11). The problem is compressive schemia of the intestinal wall by intestinal distention or complicating volvulus.

Roentgenographically, in some of these cases, calcification of the intestinal contents in the small, viable, oval compartments between the areas of atresia (5, 9, 11) has led to the term "string of pearls sign" (12) (Fig. 4.76). Some of the areas of intestine between the stenotic areas can dilate and enlarge to form a cyst. Often, these are confused with true enteric, or duplication, cysts (13), and the same phenomenon can occur with regular intestinal atresia. In either case, the resultant cyst is not a true duplication cyst, but it often is referred to as such. Diverticula also have been reported in association with multiple intestinal atresias and the etiology is probably the same as for that offered to explain pseudocyst formation. In other words, while usually in between the areas of atresia a pseudocyst forms, in others, a diverticulum could result (14).

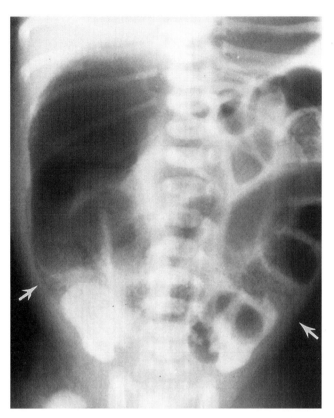

FIGURE 4.73. Ileal atresia: soap-bubble appearance. Note the numerous distended loops of intestine consistent with obstruction. In addition, some of these loops contain bubbly material (arrows), which represents air mixed with meconium.

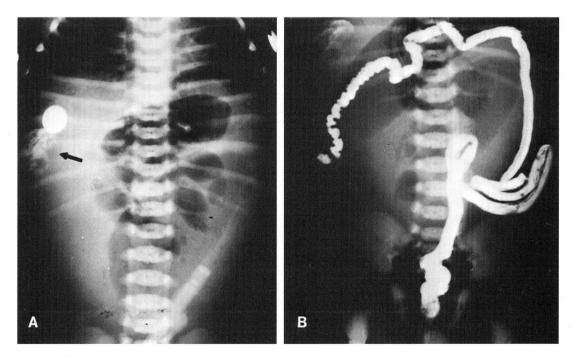

FIGURE 4.74. Ileal atresia, microcolon, and calcified small bowel. A. Note evidence of small bowel obstruction and a clumpy, irregular calcification in the right upper quadrant (arrow). **B.** Barium enema demonstrating typical microcolon. (Courtesy of Virgil Graves, M.D.)

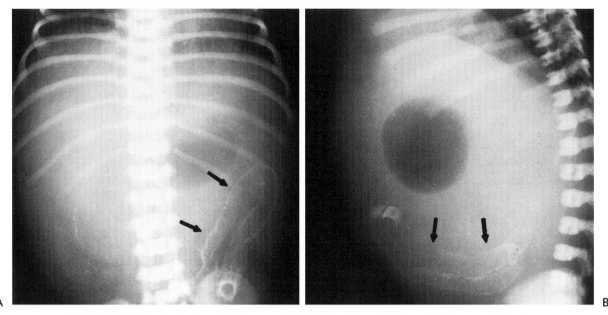

FIGURE 4.75. Ileal atresia with linear calcification. A and B. Note the linear calcification within the wall of the small intestine (arrows). (Reproduced with permission from Steinfeld JR, Harrison RB. Extensive intramural intestinal calcification in a newborn with intestinal atresia. Case report. Radiology 1973;107:405–406.)

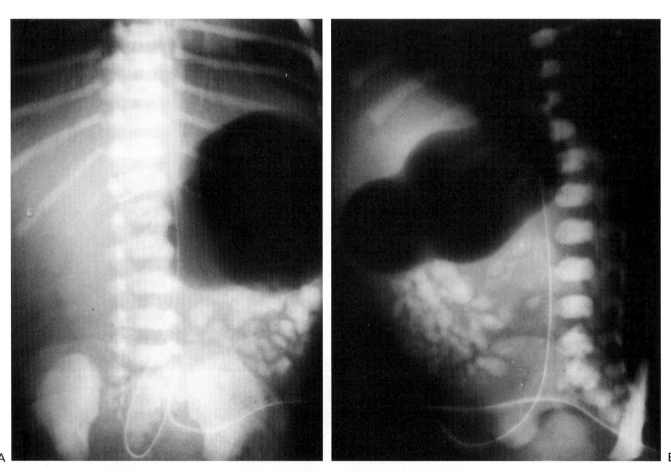

FIGURE 4.76. Familial multiple intestinal atresia with "string of pearls" sign. A and B. Note numerous oval calcifications (arrows) in the small intestine of this infant with multiple intestinal atresias. (Reproduced with permission from Martin C, Leonidas J, Amoury R. Multiple GI atresias, with intraluminal calcifications and cystic dilation of the bile ducts; a newly recognized entity resembling "'a string of pearls." Pediatrics 1976;57:268–272.)

A rare form of small bowel atresia is the so-called apple peel small bowel, or congenital short intestine (15–17). The etiology of this condition is probably in the realm of ischemic insult to the whole intestine. Associated with this condition is a large mesenteric defect and blood supply by the ileocolic, rather than by the superior mesenteric artery. Whatever the etiology, the small bowel is greatly contracted and very short. When the small bowel is allowed to dangle free, its spiral or helical appearance, secondary to the mesenteric defect, has led to the term "apple peel small bowel." The condition is basically incompatible with life and poses considerable difficulties for surgical management. Roentgenographically, these patients present with high small bowel obstruction, and the condition usually is not diagnosed until laparotomy.

REFERENCES

1. Black PR, Mueller D, Crow J, et al. Mesenteric defects as a cause of intestinal volvulus without malrotation and as the possible primary etiology of intestinal atresia. J Pediatr Surg 1994;29:1339–1343.
2. Adejuyigbe O, Odesanmi WO. Intrauterine intussusception causing intestinal atresia. J Pediatr Surg 1990;25:562–563.
3. Neal MR, Seibert JJ, Vanderzalm T, et al. Neonatal ultrasonography to distinguish between meconium ileus and ileal atresia. J Ultrasound Med 1997;16:263–266.
4. Guttmann FM, Braun P, Garance PH, et al. Multiple atresias and a new syndrome of hereditary multiple atresias involving the gastrointestinal tract from stomach to rectum. J Pediatr Surg 1973; 8:633–640.
5. Ponbo F, Arnal-Monreal F, Soler-Fernandez R, et al. Multiple gastrointestinal atresias with intraluminal calcification. Br J Radiol 1982;55:307–309.
6. Puri P, Guiney EJ, Carroll R. Multiple gastrointestinal atresia in three consecutive siblings: observations on pathogenesis. J Pediatr Surg 1985;20:22–24.
7. Puri P, Fujimoto T. New observations on the pathogenesis of multiple intestinal atresias. J Pediatr Surg 1988;23:221–225.
8. Gross E, Armon Y, Abu-Dalu K, et al. Familial combined duodenal and jejunal atresia. J Pediatr Surg 1996;31:1573–1578.
9. Lambrecht W, Kluth D. Hereditary multiple atresias of the gastrointestinal tract: report of a case and review of the literature. J Pediatr Surg 1998;33:794–797.
10. Herman TE, McAlister WH. Familial type 1: jejunal atresias and renal dysplasia. Pediatr Radiol 1995;25:272–274.
11. Oguzkurt P, Tanyel FC, Kotiloglu E, et al. Multiple atresias with extensive intraluminal calcifications in a newborn with cystic fibrosis. Pediatr Radiol 1998;28:174–176.
12. Martin C, Leonidas J, Amoury R. Multiple gastrointestinal atresias, with intraluminal calcifications and cystic dilation of bile ducts: a newly recognized entity resembling "a string of pearls." Pediatrics 1976;57:268–272.
13. Tabuse K, Hirota K, Tonoda S, et al. Congenital jejunal atresia associated with jejunal duplication. Jpn J Pediatr Surg 1977;9: 582–587.
14. Shenoy MU, Robson K, Broderick N, et al. Congenital small bowel diverticulosis and intestinal atresia: a rare association. J Pediatr Surg 2000;35:636–637.
15. Leonidas JC, Amoury RA, Ashcraft KW, et al. Duodenojejunal atresia with "apple peel" small bowel: a distinct form of intestinal atresia. Radiology 1976;118:661–665.
16. Schiavetti E, Massotti G, Torricelli M, et al. "Apple peel" syndrome. A radiological study. Pediatr Radiol 1984;14:380–383.
17. Seashore JH, Collins FS, Markowitz RI, et al. Familial apple peel jejunal atresia: surgical, genetic, and radiographic aspects. Pediatrics 1987;80:540–544.

Meconium Ileus

Meconium ileus usually is considered a manifestation of cystic fibrosis in the neonate. However, it occasionally can occur with pancreatic atresia or stenosis of the pancreatic duct. These rare cases not withstanding, meconium ileus usually is taken to be synonymous with cystic fibrosis and is the earliest manifestation of this disease. Even if the patient is of the black race (1), the condition still should be considered.

Obstruction in meconium ileus results from impaction of thick, tenacious meconium in the distal small bowel, and complications such as schemia-induced ileal atresia or stenosis, ileoperforation, and meconium peritonitis are common. Volvulus, with or without associated pseudocyst formation, can occur. Clinically, infants with meconium ileus present with vomiting (bile stained), abdominal distention, and failure to pass meconium. Pulmonary manifestations are not usually present at birth, but they may develop shortly thereafter (i.e., a bronchiolitis-like picture).

Plain abdominal roentgenograms frequently demonstrate a low small bowel obstruction with numerous air-filled loops of bowel (Fig. 4.77). Because of the tenacious meconium and the abnormality of mucous gland secretion, air-fluid levels usually are absent. However, some infants may demonstrate air-fluid levels, especially those with complications such as volvulus and stenosis or atresia. Consequently, while the absence of air-fluid levels strongly suggests meconium ileus, the presence of air-fluid levels does not exclude it. In some cases of meconium ileus, distention of the obstructed small bowel can be enormous, and one might misinterpret the findings for those of colon distention (Fig. 4.78). In other cases, the so-called soap bubble effect of gas mixed with meconium is seen (Fig. 4.78). Although the finding is not entirely pathognomonic of the condition, it most commonly is seen with meconium ileus. It can, however, also be seen with ileal atresia, colon atresia, Hirschsprung's disease, and the meconium plug syndrome. Similarly, while meconium peritonitis secondary to intestinal perforation can occur with any type of obstruction, it probably is most common with meconium ileus.

Once the diagnosis of meconium ileus is established, a contrast enema examination of the colon is required. Typically, this study demonstrates a microcolon (Fig. 4.79), but it is impossible to distinguish it from the one seen with ileal atresia or, for that matter, any other complete low small bowel intrauterine obstruction. However, when contrast is refluxed into the small bowel and meconium pellets are identified, the enema becomes diagnostic and at the same

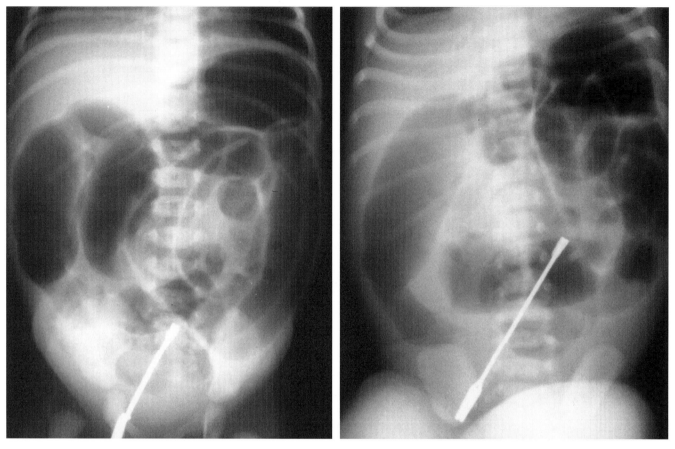

A

B

FIGURE 4.77. Meconium ileus. A. Supine view showing numerous distended loops of small bowel. Note that there is no gas in the rectum. **B.** Upright view shows only one or two ill-defined air-fluid levels. Compare with ileal atresia in Figure 4.72, C and D, in which more air-fluid levels are seen.

time therapeutic. For this reason, filling of the terminal ileum should be attempted in all cases, even though occasionally perforation can occur (2).

In terms of the type of contrast material used, it generally is agreed that it should be aqueous, and a variety of aqueous contrast agents including Gastrografin can be used (2), but Gastrografin diluted 3:1 with normal saline probably is best (3). This is what we use. The powerful osmotic effect of hyperosmolar agents such as Gastrografin cause added fluid to be drawn into the bowel, and this serves to lubricate the meconium mass and allow it to pass more easily, avoiding surgical intervention. Gastrografin also has further benefit, as it contains Tween 80, a surface tension reducing and emulsifying agent. We have always used Gastrografin and always attempt to relieve the obstruction (Fig. 4.80A) as long as it is uncomplicated (i.e., signs of perforation or peritonitis). However, hyperosmotic water-soluble contrast agents can, because of fluid shift, produce a temporary decrease in blood volume and associated changes in blood pressure and cardiac output. Therefore, while these

changes are temporary, they should and can be avoided, with adequate fluid and electrolyte balance being maintained before, during, and after the procedure is performed. This can be circumvented by diluting Gastrografin 3:1 with normal saline. Although we have not used it routinely, Mucomyst (N-acetylcysteine) also has been used in the nonsurgical treatment of meconium ileus, primarily because of its lytic effect on the meconium mass.

One other advantage of aqueous contrast materials over barium is that, if perforation occurs (Fig. 4.80B), it does not turn out to be such a dire consequence. This is important, because sooner or later, one will end up with a patient whose intestine will perforate. Most likely, the intestine is already compromised in these patients, and the added pressure of the enema leads to perforation. Even if this occasionally occurs, it should not dissuade one from always attempting treatment of meconium ileus as long as aqueous contrast agents, and not barium, are used.

In the older infant and child, chronic constipation can be a problem, and intestinal obstruction secondary to fecal

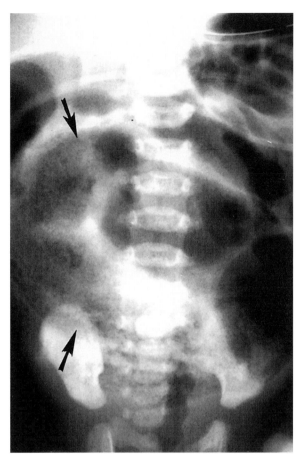

FIGURE 4.78. Meconium ileus: other plain film findings. Note the massively distended loops of small bowel. Often, such distention is misinterpreted as colonic distention. Also note the soap bubble effect (arrows).

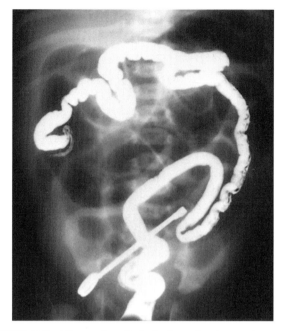

FIGURE 4.79. Microcolon. Typical microcolon in a patient with meconium ileus (same patient as in Figure 4.92). A similar configuration is seen with ileal atresia. A few mucous strands are seen in the descending colon. Note the somewhat high position of the cecum in this infant with no malrotation.

impaction, resulting in the so-called meconium ileus equivalent syndrome, can occur (4). These patients also may present with intussusceptions. Thickening, both linear and nodular, of the mucosa of the small and large bowel also occurs in cystic fibrosis but usually does so in the older patient. These changes probably are the result of the accumulation of mucus in the glands of the submucosa. Other manifestations include benign pneumatosis cystoides intestinalis (resulting from chronic obstruction), decreased bile secretion with a poorly functioning gallbladder, bile concretions in the biliary system, and cirrhosis of the liver with portal hypertension. In later childhood, a severe colitis resulting from the highly concentrated pancreatic enzyme meal given these patients as part of the treatment to prevent problems associated with meconium ileus equivalent syndrome can be seen (5).

REFERENCES

1. Flanigan RC, Stern RC, Izant RJ Jr, et al. Cystic fibrosis in the black infant: presentation with meconium ileus and volvulus. J Pediatr Surg 1978;13:435–436.
2. Ein SH, Shandling B, Reilly BJ, et al. Bowel perforation with non-operative treatment of meconium ileus. J Pediatr Surg 1987; 22:146–147.
3. Kao SCS, Franken EA Jr. Nonoperative treatment of simple meconium ileus: a survey of the Society for Pediatric Radiology. Pediatr Radiol 1995;25:97–100.
4. Matsehe JW, Go VLW, DiMagno EP. Meconium ileus equivalent complicating cystic fibrosis in postneonatal children and young adults: report of 12 cases. Gastroenterology 1977;72:732–736.
5. Schwarzenberg SJ, Wielinski CL, Shamieh I, et al. Cystic fibrosis—associated colitis and fibrosing colonopathy. J Pediatr 1995; 127:565–570.

Functional Obstruction of the Premature (Pseudomeconium Ileus)

Functional obstruction of the premature infant is becoming more common now that so many immature infants are being admitted to intensive care nurseries. This obstruction, as opposed to other neonatal obstructions, tends to occur some time after the immediate neonatal period (1–4). It is caused by immaturity of the small bowel, and intestine in general, leading to hypomotility and an inability to propel intestinal contents forward in a normal manner. As a result, there is impaction of meconium, or fecal material in the small bowel, and for this reason the condition has been compared to meconium ileus, but it is quite different. These patients do not suffer from cystic fibrosis.

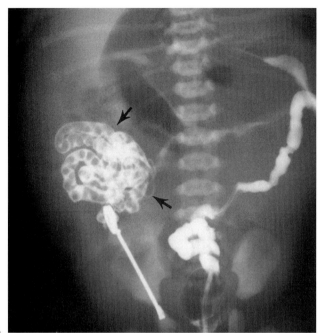

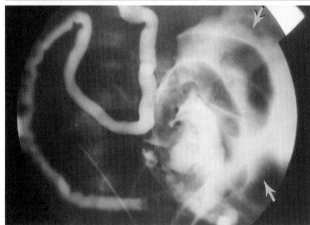

FIGURE 4.80. Meconium ileus: Gastrografin enema. A. Note the following: (1) microcolon, (2) massively distended small bowel loops, (3) soap bubble effect on the right side of the abdomen, and (4) Gastrografin refluxed into the terminal ileum (arrows). Inspissated meconium produces nodular and tubular filling defects. This infant spontaneously decompressed after the Gastrografin enema, and surgery was not required. **B.** Note the microcolon in another patient and extravasated Gastrografin (arrows) secondary to perforation.

Treatment usually is conservative and consists of irritating the colon with a variety of enema procedures. First, one could simply try saline enemas. If this does not work, Gastrografin (diluted) enemas can be employed (Fig. 4.81), and in other cases, Mucomyst enemas have been used. The end result is that the impaction is corrected and the patient is cured, but it may take many days for this to occur. Initially, the patients present with abdominal distention, variable distention of the intestines, and an overall picture that suggests low intestinal obstruction. Interestingly, most of these infants fail to show gas in the rectum, and this provides an important clue to the presence of the condition.

REFERENCES

1. Fakhoury K, Durie PR, Levison H, et al. Meconium ileus in the absence of cystic fibrosis. Arch Dis Child 1992;67:1204–1206.
2. Greenholz SK, Perez C, Wesley Jr, et al. Meconium obstruction in the markedly premature infant. J Pediatr Surg 1996;31:117–120.
3. Tomimoto Y. A histopathological study on the myenteric plexus in meconium ileus without mucoviscidosis. J Jpn Soc Pediatr Surg 1993;29:58–68.
4. Wilcox DT, Borowitz DS, Stovroff MC, et al. Chronic intestinal pseudo-obstruction with meconium ileus at onset. J Pediatr 1993;123:751–752.

Rotational Abnormalities and Midgut Volvulus

In the fetus, the GI tract is located outside the abdomen, but with time it is gradually withdrawn into the abdomen. At the same time, rotation occurs and the duodenum becomes fixed retroperitoneally on the right, the small bowel slung on a mesentery running from the left upper quadrant to the right lower quadrant, and the transverse colon comes to lie anterior to the stomach. The cecum is the last portion of the gastrointestinal tract to be fixed, and normally comes to lie in the right lower quadrant. When all, or part, of this fails to occur, a rotational abnormality results and for the most part consists of nonrotation, malrotation, or reversed rotation.

In nonrotation, usually an asymptomatic problem, the small bowel lies entirely on the right side and the colon on the left. This can be appreciated on plain abdominal roentgenograms but is best demonstrated with barium studies (Fig. 4.82). The bowel, although misplaced, is not particularly mobile and volvulus is not a common complication. The whole problem frequently is discovered incidentally. Malrotation, on the other hand, is a different matter and generally requires thorough investigation.

In malrotation, final positioning of the GI tract is somewhere between normal and complete nonrotation. Generally, the cecum and terminal ileum are displaced upward and medial, but in very mild cases, the cecum may merely be hypermobile. Normal small bowel mesenteric attachment is lost and the poorly fixed small bowel is floppy and lies predominantly on the right. Duodenal bands, commonly known as Ladd's bands, running from the duodenum to the cecum, are a part of the anomaly, as is absence of the ligament of Treitz. The bands usually are obstructing in themselves, but since the bowel also is poorly attached and floppy, it is prone to volve and add to the problem. When this occurs, the entire gut twists or corkscrews around the superior mesenteric artery and vascular compromise ensues. Volvulus may be intermittent or perma-

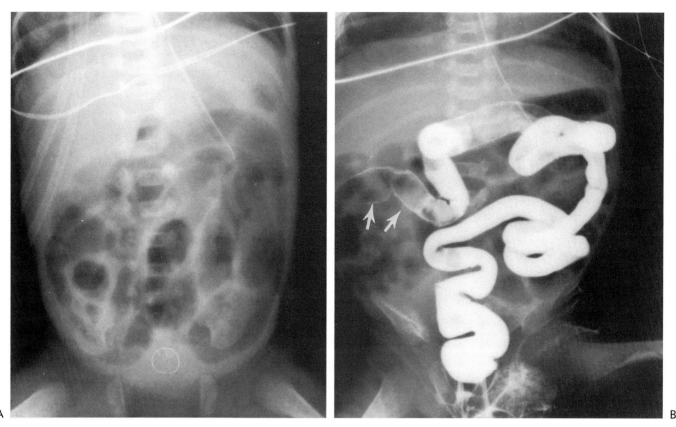

A   B

FIGURE 4.81. Functional obstruction of the premature. A. Note numerous loops of distended, obstructed intestine. **B.** Gastrografin enema outlining a solid intracolonic fecal plug (arrows).

nent, and complications all are dire and include necrosis, perforation, and gangrene. Intestinal malrotation usually occurs as an isolated problem but also can be seen, with or without complicating volvulus, in such conditions as diaphragmatic hernia (1), omphalocele, and gastroschisis. After repair of congenital diaphragmatic hernia it is believed that the subsequent, inherent, abdominal adhesions prevent the development of volvulus. This probably also occurs in the post-operative patient with an omphalocele or with gastroschisis.

Reversed intestinal rotation is rare (2) and renders the hepatic flexure and left transverse colon posterior in position. These portions of the colon lie behind the descending duodenum and the superior mesenteric artery. The cecum is usually malrotated and medially placed, and the small bowel is more right-sided than normal. Obstructing bands and midgut volvulus also can occur.

Clinically, infants with malrotation and obstructing duodenal bands (with or without volvulus) present with bilious vomiting. Although other causes such as sepsis and other distal duodenal obstructions may result in such vomiting, one first must exclude the presence of malrotation and associated midgut volvulus. If midgut volvulus is not recognized early, serious complications ensue. Most cases present early, usually during the first few days of life, and the presence of bilious vomiting in these infants constitutes an emergency that requires immediate investigation.

Roentgenographically, in infants with intestinal malrotation and obstructing duodenal bands, with or without complicating volvulus, a high GI obstruction usually is seen. The actual configuration is one of the stomach, but especially the descending duodenum being distended with air. The air column of the distended duodenum ends to the right of the vertebral column and this finding is very important (Fig. 4.83A). The reason for this is that it signifies that the obstruction is due to associated duodenal bands and that the normal ligament of Treitz is absent. All of this is part of the constellation of findings seen with malrotation.

Once one notes the foregoing plain film findings, one should either proceed to surgery or further verification with other imaging studies. The reason for this is that when obstruction is determined to be present at the level of the third-fourth portions of the duodenum, malrotation with associated duodenal bands and potential midgut volvulus are the primary, and number one diagnosis. There is no time for hesitation or discussion in these cases. Surgery

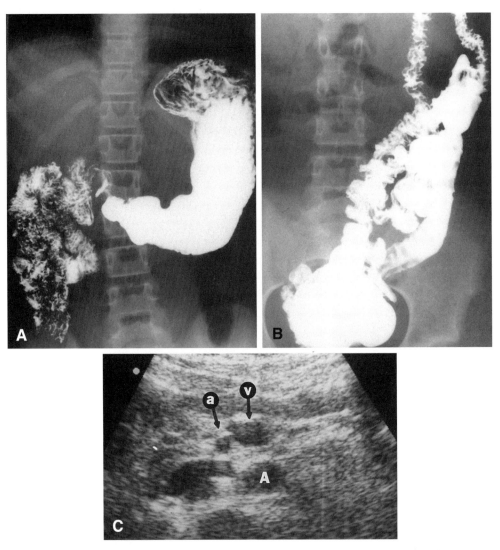

FIGURE 4.82. Intestinal nonrotation. A. The small bowel is entirely on the right side. **B.** Barium enema demonstrates the colon to be totally on the left side. **C.** Transverse sonogram demonstrates inverse positioning of the superior mesenteric artery (a) and the superior mesenteric vein (v). A, aorta.

should be performed promptly. Nonetheless, in some instances there will be temporization and some other imaging study will be requested. In this regard, a barium upper GI series can confirm the level of obstruction and if midgut volvulus is present, demonstrate a beaked or tapering deformity, virtually diagnostic for the presence of volvulus (Fig. 4.83B). Similar findings can be demonstrated with ultrasound (3) (Fig. 4.84).

Usually, in cases of malrotation, it is difficult to determine whether or not associated midgut volvulus is present on plain films alone. The findings are variable and can range from a normal-appearing abdomen to one suggesting a gastric outlet obstruction (Fig. 4.85A), or small bowel obstruction (Fig. 4.85, B and C). When a gastric outlet

obstruction is suggested, one may have to position the patient with the left side down, in the lateral decubitus position to allow air to enter the duodenum.

In the more distant past, the barium enema often was the first study performed in infants with suspected midgut volvulus whereupon one is looking for a medially and upwardly displaced cecum. However, mere medial positioning of the cecum is not indicative of midgut volvulus (Fig. 4.86); it simply indicates that the cecum is poorly fixed. To diagnose midgut volvulus the cecum must be tucked high under the transverse colon (Fig. 4.87). Ultimately, the degree of displacement of the cecum depends on the number of twists present in the volvulus—the larger the number of twists, the higher and more displaced is the cecum.

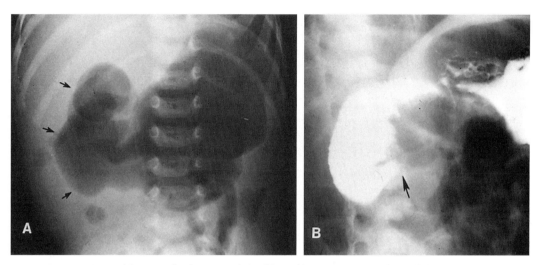

FIGURE 4.83. Midgut volvulus. A. Plain films demonstrating a distended stomach and descending duodenum (arrows). This indicates the presence of distal duodenal obstruction. **B.** Upper GI series demonstrates the distended descending duodenum and the typical tapered narrowing of the obstructed duodenum (arrow). Surgically confirmed midgut volvulus.

Because of these problems, the barium enema, for the most part, has been replaced with the barium upper GI study. This study provides much more definitive information and almost always delivers the correct diagnosis.

The upper GI series accurately demonstrates the level and nature of the duodenal obstruction (i.e., third-fourth portions of the duodenum). In addition, if volvulus is present, a beaked deformity of the obstructed duodenum is seen, and in many cases, there is associated spiraling of the small bowel around the superior mesenteric artery (Fig.

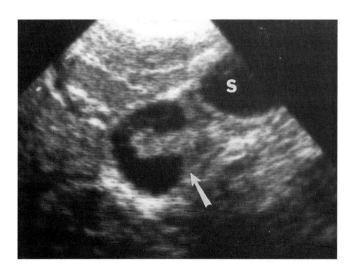

FIGURE 4.84. Midgut volvulus: ultrasonographic findings. Note the obstructed, distended duodenal C-loop with an almost beak-like, tapered end (arrow). S, stomach.

4.88). In other cases, intestinal edema is seen (Fig. 4.89). Another finding seen with duodenal bands and midgut volvulus is absence of the ligament of Treitz. Normally, the ligament of Treitz is located to the left of the spine, but when duodenal bands are present, the ligament of Treitz is absent and obstruction of the duodenum, by a band, occurs to the right of the spine (Fig. 4.90).

Recently, considerable attention has been devoted to the position of the superior mesenteric artery and veins in malrotation problems. These vessels are especially well demonstrated with color-flow Doppler ultrasonography (4–7), and with malrotation they are reversed from their normal orientation (Fig. 4.91). However, it should be noted that a normal arrangement of these vessels does not exclude malrotation (8) and also that abnormal positioning of the vessels simply indicates the presence of malrotation and not necessarily the presence of volvulus. However, volvulus can be inferred when only one pulsating vessel, the artery, is seen (9). In such cases, it is believed that the superior mesenteric vein is not visualized because it is squeezed by the volved intestine. Still another ultrasonographic finding recently described is that of the so-called whirlpool sign (10, 11). With this sign, twisting of the intestine around the vascular pedicle with a swirling effect of the mesentery and vessels is seen (Fig. 4.92). Inversion of the superior mesenteric vessels also can be demonstrated with CT and MR (12).

Most of the preceding comments apply to the usual case of malrotation with midgut volvulus that presents early in infancy, if not during the first few days of life (13). However, once beyond this age period, and in the older infant

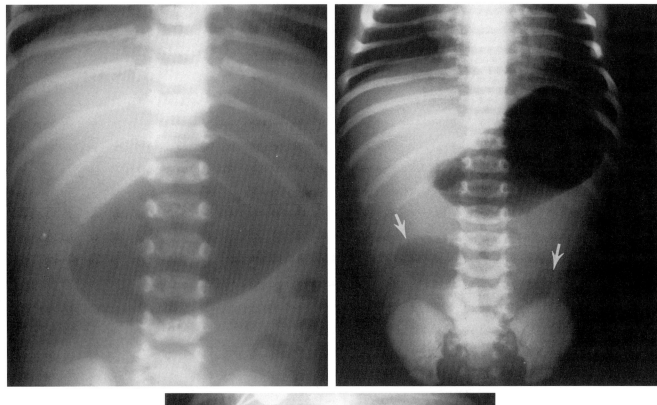

A

B

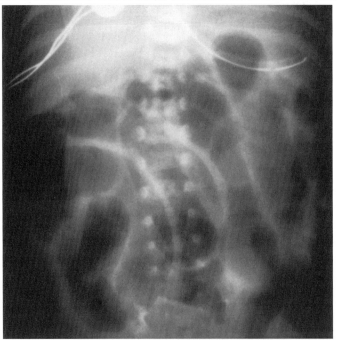

C

FIGURE 4.85. Midgut volvulus: various plain film findings. A. Note the distended stomach and absence of duodenal distention. This might erroneously suggest gastric outlet obstruction. However, this infant had an obstructing duodenal band and midgut volvulus. **B.** Note gastric distention and a virtually airless abdomen in this patient with midgut volvulus. However, two loops of small bowel are seen in the mid-abdomen (arrows). These loops were fixed from film to film and represented necrotic bowel. **C.** Another patient with numerous distended loops of small bowel, with thickened walls, suggesting a low small bowel obstruction with intestinal compromise. Surgically confirmed midgut volvulus.

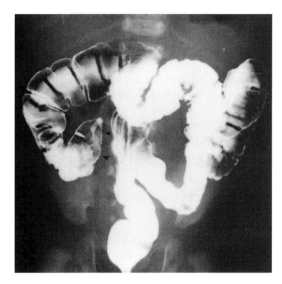

FIGURE 4.86. Normal medial cecum. Note the high, medial position of the cecum (arrows) in this patient with no malrotation of the small intestine and no symptoms or obstruction.

and child, the diagnosis of midgut volvulus can be difficult (14–18). Symptoms often are not characteristic and may include one or more of the following: recurrent vague abdominal pain, vomiting, diarrhea, bleeding per rectum, and malabsorption (9). In such cases, if one cannot come

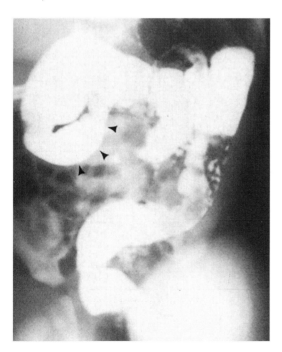

FIGURE 4.87. Midgut volvulus: barium enema. Note the high position of the cecum (arrows). The cecum is tucked under the transverse colon.

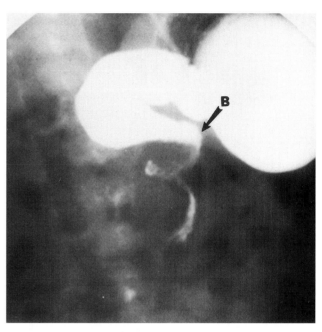

FIGURE 4.88. Midgut volvulus: beak and spiral signs. Note the typical beak (arrow) secondary to twisting of the intestine, and early small bowel spiraling.

up with another etiology for the symptoms, imaging of these patients should be pursued, and it is in such cases that ultrasonographic examination of the position of the superior mesenteric vein and artery are of most use. In terms of contrast studies in these patients, one seldom sees characteristic findings and, therefore, one must be suspicious of any deviation, whatsoever, from the normal position of the duodenum, small bowel, or cecum (Fig. 4.93). Once one notices any of these findings, the patient requires surgical intervention for correction of the problem (19). This is very important because patients with delayed volvulus often suffer catastrophic consequences.

Malrotation is not uncommonly seen in the asplenia-polysplenia syndromes (20), and the duodenal-jejunal junction can be displaced to the right in cases of left lobe liver transplantation (21).

REFERENCES

1. Levin TL, Liebling MS, Ruzal-Shapiro C, et al. Midgut malfixation in patients with congenital diaphragmatic hernia: what is the risk of midgut volvulus? Pediatr Radiol 1995;25:259–261.
2. Valioulis I, Anagnostopoulos D, Sfougaris D. Reversed midgut rotation in neonate: case report with a brief review of the literature. J Pediatr Surg 1997;32:643–645.
3. Hayden CK Jr, Boulden TF, Swischuk LE, et al. Sonographic demonstration of duodenal obstruction with midgut volvulus. AJR 1984;142:9–10.

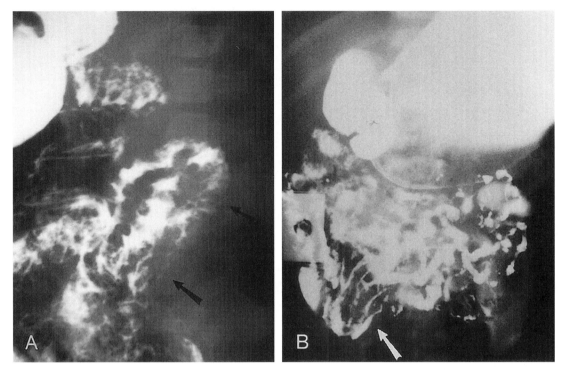

FIGURE 4.89. Midgut volvulus: edema of intestine. A. Note thickened, nodular mucosal folds (arrows). This indicates the presence of small bowel edema secondary to venous obstruction. **B.** In this infant, w Another patient with very thin streaks of barium, resulting from markedly edematous loops of bowel (arrow).

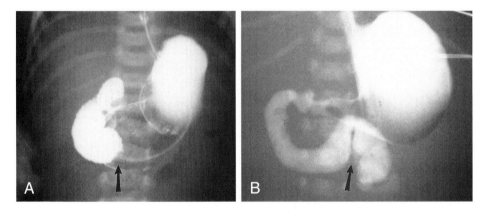

FIGURE 4.90. Malrotation and abnormal ligament of Treitz. A. In this patient with malrotation and midgut volvulus, the obstructed duodenum ends at a point medial to the left vertebral body pedicles (arrow). **B. Normal ligament of Treitz.** In this infant, who was septic and had an atonic bowel, the normal position of the ligament of Treitz, to the left of the spine, is vividly demonstrated (arrow).

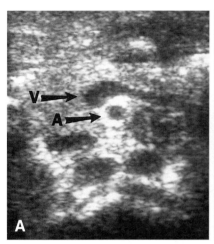
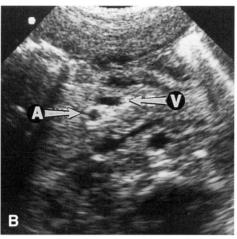

FIGURE 4.91. Normal and abnormal positions of the superior mesenteric artery and vein. A. Normal relationship of the superior mesenteric artery (A) and vein (V). The splenic vein runs anterior to the superior mesenteric artery as it joins the superior mesenteric vein. **B.** Malrotation causes reverse positioning of the superior mesenteric artery (A) and vein (V).

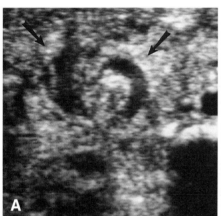
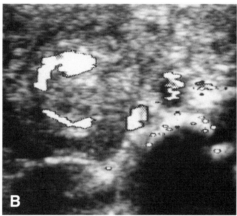

FIGURE 4.92. Malrotation with sonographic "whirlpool" sign. A. Note the whirlpool-like configuration of the superior mesenteric artery and vein (arrows) as they are twisted by the volvulus. **B.** Color-flow Doppler identifies the spiraled vessels. (Courtesy of Kenneth Martin, M.D.)

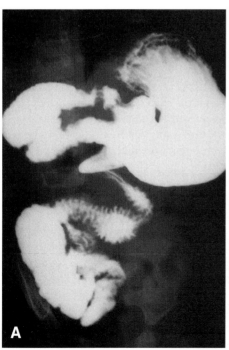
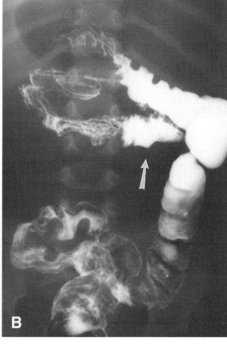

FIGURE 4.93. Malrotation in older patients. A. Note the peculiar configuration of the duodenum and the abnormal position of the small bowel. **B.** In this patient, the cecum (arrow) is abnormally placed under the transverse colon and the hepatic flexure seems to have made a bizarre loop.

4. Chao H, Kong M, Chen J, et al. Sonographic features related to volvulus in neonatal intestinal malrotation. J Ultrasound Med 2000;19:371–376.

5. Loyer E, Eggli KD. Sonographic evaluation of superior mesenteric vascular relationship in malrotation. Pediatr Radiol 1989;19:173–175.

6. Weinberger E, Winters WD, Liddell RM, et al. Sonographic diagnosis of intestinal malrotation in infants: importance of the relative positions of the superior mesenteric vein and artery. AJR 1992;159:825–828.

7. Zerin JM, DiPietro MA. Superior mesenteric vascular anatomy at US in patients with surgically proved malrotation of the midgut. Radiology 1992;183:693–694.

8. Dufour D, Delaet MH, Dassonville M, et al. Midgut malrotation, the reliability of sonographic diagnosis. Pediatr Radiol 1992;22:21–23.

9. Smet MH, Marchal G, Ceulemans R, et al. The solitary hyperdynamic pulsating superior mesenteric artery: an additional dynamic sonographic feature of midgut volvulus. Pediatr Radiol 1991;21:156–157.

10. Pracos JP, Sann L, Genin G, et al. Ultrasound diagnosis of midgut volvulus: the "whirlpool" sign. Pediatr Radiol 1992;22:18–20.

11. Shimanuki Y, Aiharat, T, Takano H, et al. Clockwise whirlpool sign at color Doppler US: an objective and definite sign of midgut volvulus. Radiology 1996;199:261–264.

12. Shatzkes D, Gordon DH, Haller JO, et al. Malrotation of the bowel: malalignment of the superior mesenteric artery-vein complex shown by CT and MR. J Comput Assist Tomogr 1990;14:93–95.

13. Long FR, Kramer SS, Markowitz RI, et al. Radiographic patterns of intestinal malrotation in children. Radiographics 1996;16:547–556.

14. Ablow RC, Hoffer FA, Seashore JH, et al. Z-shaped duodenojejunal loop: sign of mesenteric fixation anomaly and congenital bands. AJR 1983;141:461–464.

15. Berdon WE. The diagnosis of malrotation and volvulus in the older child and adult: a trap for the radiologist. Pediatr Radiol 1995;25:101–103.

16. Brandt ML, Pokorny WJ, McGill CW, et al. Late presentations of midgut malrotations in children. Am J Surg 1985;150:767–771.

17. Jackson A, Bisset R, Dickson AP. Case report. Malrotation and midgut volvulus presenting as malabsorption. Clin Radiol 1989;40:536–537.

18. Spigland N, Brandt ML, Yazbeck S. Malrotation presenting beyond the neonatal period. J Pediatr Surg 1990;25:1139–1142.

19. Prasil P, Flageole H, Shaw KS, et al. Should malrotation in children be treated differently according to age? J Pediatr Surg 2000;365:756–758.

20. Ditchfield MR, Hutson JM. Intestinal rotational abnormalities in polysplenia and asplenia syndromes. Pediatr Radiol 1998;28:303–306.

21. Benya EC, Ben-Ami TE, Whitington PF, et al. Duodenum and duodenal-jejunal junction in children: position and appearance after liver transplantation. Radiology 1998;207:233–236.

Small Bowel Volvulus without Malrotation

Midgut volvulus is the most common form of small bowel volvulus and has been discussed in the preceding section. In other types of small bowel volvulus, a short segment of intestine is volved, the level of obstruction depends on the exact site of volvulus, and it can occur before birth (1). In this regard, antenatal small bowel volvulus is a common complication of meconium ileus and subsequent stenosis or atresia is believed an aftermath of intestinal schemia at the points of twisting.

Plain films usually demonstrate nothing more than a small bowel obstruction. Complications include intestinal infarction, gangrene, and perforation, and late sequelae include stenosis, atresia, and pseudocyst formation. In those cases with pseudocyst formation, it is postulated that the intestine trapped between the two points of twisting accumulates secretions and eventually enlarges to produce a cystic mass or pseudocyst. Most cases of small bowel volvulus proceed to surgery after plain films showing obstruction are obtained. However, if contrast studies are obtained from above or below, they may demonstrate the typical beaked deformity of a volvulus (2). In addition, omphalomesenteric duct remnants may predispose to cecal and terminal ileal volvulus (3).

REFERENCES

1. Usmani SS, Keningsberg K. Intrauterine volvulus without malrotation. J Pediatr Surg 1991;26:1409–1410.

2. Siegel MJ, Shackelford GD, McAlister WH. Small bowel volvulus in children: its appearance on the barium enema examination. Pediatr Radiol 1980;10:91–93.

3. Fenton LZ, Buonomo C, Share JC, et al. Small intestinal obstruction by remnants of the omphalomesenteric duct: findings on contrast enema. Pediatr Radiol 2000;30:165–167.

Duplication Cysts

In the abdomen duplication cysts most commonly occur in the small bowel (1). Many contain ectopic gastric or pancreatic tissue, and because of this, bleeding, ulceration, and perforation often occur. Because gastric mucosa commonly is present in these cysts, technetium-99m pertechnetate scanning is of diagnostic value (1, 2). However, most often these patients present with an abdominal mass.

The etiology of duplication cysts is believed to be congenital (1) and lies in faulty recanalization of the solid state of the fetal intestine and its separation from the neurenteric canal. In the latter instances, persistent fibrous connections to the spinal canal can exist or the cyst itself can extend into the spinal canal. In such cases, relatively rare in the abdomen, anterior vertebral body segmentation anomalies are seen. Another theory often invoked in explaining the duplication cysts is one of schemia to the intestine. In these cases it is believed that the infarcted portion of bowel contains a small viable area in its center and that, as the infarcted area becomes sequestered, the viable area grows and forms a cyst. This probably does occur but the end result most likely does not represent a true, congenital duplication cyst.

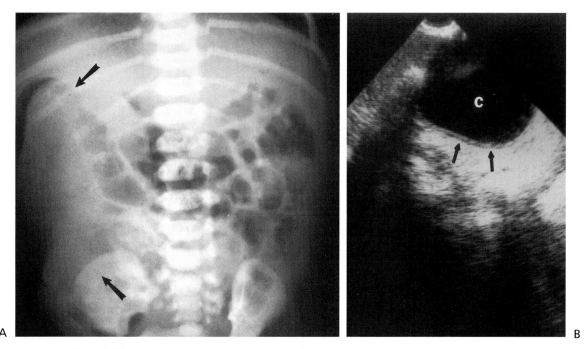

FIGURE 4.94. Duplication cyst. A. Note the large mass occupying the right side of the abdomen (arrows). **B.** Another patient where ultrasonography demonstrates a sonolucent cyst (C) with its wall composed of an inner thin lining of echogenic mucosa and an adjacent, outer, thin, sonolucent layer representing muscle (arrows).

Most duplication cysts of the small bowel are solitary, but multiple cysts can occur, either in the small bowel (2), or throughout the GI tract. In addition some cysts are so long and tubular that they can present as a fluctuant abdominal mass mimicking ascites. Transdiaphragmatic extension also can occur, and in such cases the portion of the cyst in the chest may be the predominant part of the mass. Larger duplication cysts may be seen on plan films (Fig. 4.94A) but are best evaluated with ultrasound (3, 4), where characteristically the cyst is hypoechoic but may contain debris. The most important feature, however, is the so-called "rim" sign (3) where both muscle and mucosal layers can be identified in the wall of the cyst (Fig. 4.94B). Another interesting ultrasonographic finding of duplication cysts is peristalsis of the cyst wall (5). Duplication cysts also can be demonstrated with CT, but the findings are less specific than with ultrasound.

Malignant degeneration can occur with duplication cysts (6, 7) and in addition retrograde intussusception has been documented (8). In addition, it might be recalled that duplication cysts can become lead points for antegrade intussusception.

REFERENCES

1. Macpherson RI. Gastrointestinal tract duplications: clinical pathologic, etiologic and radiologic considerations. Radiographics 1993;
13:1063–1080.
2. Gilchrist AM, Sloan JM, Logan CJH, et al. Gastrointestinal bleeding due to multiple ileal duplications diagnosed by scintigraphy and barium studies. Clin Radiol 1990;41:134–136.
3. Barr LL, Hayden CK Jr, Stansberry SD, et al. Enteric duplication cysts in children: are their ultrasonographic wall characteristics diagnostic? Pediatr Radiol 1990;20:26–28.
4. Segal SR, Sherman NH, Rosenberg HK, et al. Ultrasonographic features of gastrointestinal duplications. J Ultrasound Med 1994; 13:863–870.
5. Spottswood SE. Peristalsis in duplication cyst: a new diagnostic sonographic finding. Pediatr Radiol 1994;24:344–345.
6. Orr MM, Edwards AJ. Neoplastic change in duplications of the alimentary tract. Br J Surg 1975;62:269–274.
7. Rice CA, Anderson TM, Sepahdari S. Computed tomography and ultrasonography of carcinoma in duplication cysts. J Comput Assist Tomogr 1986;10:233–235.
8. Norton KI, Luhmann KC, Dolgin SE. Retrograde jejunal-duodenal intussusception associated with a jejunal duplication cyst in a newborn. Pediatr Radiol 1993;23:360–361.

Small Bowel Diverticula including Meckel's Diverticulum

Small bowel diverticula in general are rare and usually are incidental findings, but if large, they can lead to problems such as the blind loop syndrome, bleeding, or even obstruction. These diverticula are congenital in origin and develop much the same as duplication cysts.

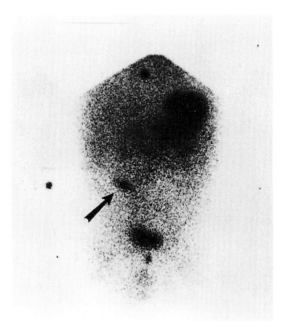

FIGURE 4.95. Meckel's diverticulum: positive technetium-99m pertechnetate scan. Note the localized collection of isotope in the Meckel's diverticulum (arrow). Scintigraphic activity also is present in the stomach and urinary bladder.

Meckel's diverticulum, although seen more frequently than other small bowel diverticula, still is relatively rare (1). It is unusual to demonstrate these diverticula on plain films, or for that matter with barium studies. With ultrasound, the diverticulum usually is not easy to identify for it is collapsed and may appear no different from any other loop of intestine. However, when inflamed the findings, including fluid within the lumen generally resemble those of acute appendicitis (2, 3). On the other hand, if the diverticulum is large, then the findings will differ from those of appendicitis, primarily on the basis of the size of the fluid-filled loop. Torsion of Meckel's diverticulum also can occur (3).

Meckel's diverticula frequently contain ectopic gastric mucosa, and as a result, ulceration and associated bleeding are common complications. Evidence of the presence of gastric mucosa usually is confirmed with nuclear scintigraphy using technetium-99m pertechnetate (4), which accumulates in the gastric mucosa (Fig. 4.95). However, the study is not always positive, because if scant gastric mucosa is present or if no gastric mucosa is present, there is little or no uptake of the isotope. In such cases, one may resort to arteriography (5), and if bleeding is excessive, arterial embolization can be attempted (6). Most of these diverticula are located in the right lower quadrant, but they rarely can extend to the left (7). False-positive scans can occur and result from the accumulation of isotope in lesions such as

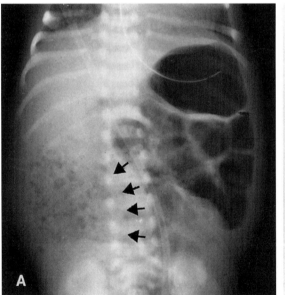
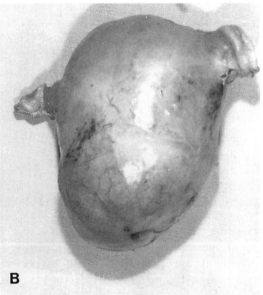

FIGURE 4.96. Giant Meckel's diverticulum. A. Note the large area of air mixed with bowel contents, producing a granular or soap bubble-like appearance (arrows). This represents air mixed with intestinal contents in a large Meckel's diverticulum. The findings can be mimicked in certain cases of colon atresia or meconium ileus, and a large abscess could produce similar findings. **B.** Pathologic specimen demonstrating the size of this large diverticulum. (Reproduced with permission from Cross VF, Wendth AJ, Phelan JJ, et al. Giant Meckel's diverticulum in a premature infant. Am J Roentgenol Radium Ther Nucl Med 1970;108:591–597.)

intussusception and inflammatory or ischemic disease of the intestine.

One can enhance visualization of the Meckel's diverticulum on a technetium-99m scan by premedicating the patient with gastrin or pentagastrin. This has not received universal acceptance but can enhance visualization. Similarly, it also has been suggested that, by administering cimetidine to the patient before the scan, one can inhibit secretion of technetium into the gastric lumen (8). In these cases, although pertechnetate accumulates in the parietal cells, it is not excreted into the lumen and therefore enhances visualization of the ectopic gastric mucosa.

Perforation is another recognized complication of Meckel's diverticulum, and in such cases, the findings may mimic those of perforated appendicitis or necrotizing enterocolitis (9). They also can be diagnosed with ultrasound and CT. Large diverticula can produce intestinal obstruction (10, 11). In such cases, usually neonates, the diverticulum may be visible on plain films as a large area of air mixed with granular bowel content (Fig. 4.96). The findings mimic those of meconium ileus and colon atresia and, occasionally, the granular collection of air and bowel contents may be misinterpreted for a large abscess. Rarely, the diverticulum may be air-filled and seen on plain abdominal films. In some cases, stones can be seen in these diverticula. A rare complication of Meckel's diverticulum is so-called inversion or invagination of the diverticulum (12, 13), resulting in a polypoid mass, which can be visualized with contrast enema, ultrasound and occasionally CT.

REFERENCES

1. St-Vil D, Brandt ML, Panic S, et al. Meckel's diverticulum in children: a 20-year review. J Pediatr Surg 1991;26:1289–1292.
2. Goyal MK, Bellah RD. Neonatal small bowel obstruction due to Meckel diverticulitis: diagnosis by ultrasonography. J Ultrasound Med 1993;12:119–122.
3. Gallego-Herrero C, del Pozo-Garcia G, Marin-Rodriguez C, et al. Torsion of a Meckel's diverticulum: sonographic findings Pediatr Radiol 1998;28:599–601.
4. Swaniker F, Soldes O, Hirschl RB. The utility of technetium 99m pertechnetate scintigraphy in the evaluation of patients with Meckel's diverticulum. J Pediatr Surg 1999;34:760–765.
5. Routh WD, Lawdahl RB, Lund E, et al. Meckel's diverticula: angiographic diagnosis in patients with non-acute hemorrhage and negative scintigraphy. Pediatr Radiol 1990;20:152–156.
6. Okazaki M, Higashihara H, Yamasaki S, et al. Case report: arterial embolization to control life-threatening hemorrhage from a Meckel's diverticulum. AJR 1990;154:1257–1258.
7. Fink AM, Alexopoulou E, Carty H. Bleeding Meckel's diverticulum in infancy: unusual scintigraphic and ultrasound appearances. Pediatr Radiol 1995;25:155–156.
8. Baum S. Pertechnetate imaging following cimetidine administration in Meckel's diverticulum of the ileum. Am J Gastroenterol 1981;76:464–465.
9. Gandy J, Byrne P, Lees G. Neonatal Meckel's diverticular inflammation with perforation. J Pediatr Surg 1997;32:750–751.
10. Galifer RB, Noblet D, Ferran JL. "Giant Meckel's diverticulum":
report of an unusual case in a child with preoperative x-ray diagnosis. Pediatr Radiol 1981;11:217–218.
11. Miller DL, Becker MH, Eng K. Giant Meckel's diverticulum: a cause of intestinal obstruction. Radiology 1981;14:93–94.
12. Gaisie G, Kent C, Klein RL, et al. Radiographic characteristics of isolated invaginated Meckel's diverticulum. Pediatr Radiol 1993;23:355–356.
13. Johnson JF III, Lorenzetti RJ, Ballard ET. Plain film identification of inverted Meckel diverticulum. Pediatr Radiol 1993;23:551–552.

Intussusception

Intussusception presents with crampy abdominal pain, vomiting, bloody (currant jelly) stools, and often a palpable mass. In some cases, palpable emptiness in the right flank or lower right quadrant is present, but not all of the findings are present in all patients. In addition, some patients can appear normal and others may present with atypical findings such as apathy, altered consciousness, and virtually no pain (1–3). Just why the apathy and altered consciousness should occur is not known but it is not rare and it has been suggested that endotoxins from the ischemic intestine alter the blood-brain barrier and depress brain activity (2), leading to lethargy.

Intussusception is most common between the ages of 6 months and 4 years, but can be seen in the older child. Neonatal intussusception is rare (4, 5) and often associated with a lead point. Similarly, intussusception in older children usually is associated with a lead point (6–10). Consequently intussusceptions in the neonate and older child are more difficult to reduce, and in older children a good case could be made for immediate surgical intervention. Lead points include Meckel's diverticula (6, 7), polyps, lymphoma, and the appendix (10). Focal pneumatosis intestinalis in the colon has also been described as a lead point in colocolic intussusception (11).

A Meckel's diverticulum can be suspected when the intussusception is associated with a tubular or bulbous mass, often a double mass (6, 7) (Fig. 4.97). The appendix itself can act as a lead point and can be identified with ultrasound or contrast enema (Fig. 4.98). Most intussusceptions are ileocolic, but ileo-ileo and ileo-ileocolic intussusceptions also occur. These latter cases probably account for no more than 10% of intussusceptions, but at the same time are more difficult to diagnose and reduce. Intrauterine intussusceptions also can occur and frequently lead to bowel death and subsequent intestinal atresia (5).

Plain film radiographic findings of intussusception are variable and depend to some extent on the duration of symptoms and presence or absence of complications. In some cases, the abdominal gas pattern may be entirely normal, and in this regard, plain films have been found to be of no help in up to 50% of cases (12, 13). Eventually, if the problem is unresolved, evidence of small bowel obstruction becomes apparent and is associated with a paucity of gas on

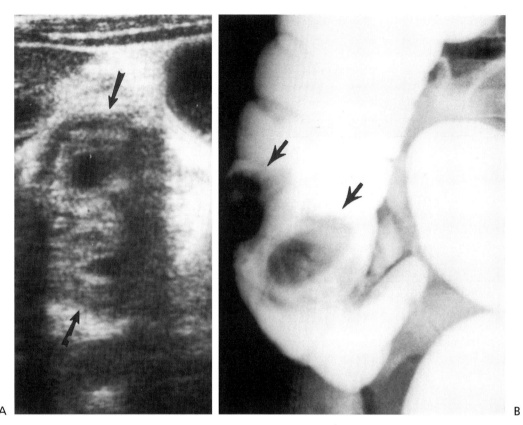

FIGURE 4.97. Intussusception: Meckel's diverticulum. A. Ultrasound. Note the two separate lead points (arrows). They are indistinct but still present. **B.** Barium enema demonstrates two lead points (arrows).

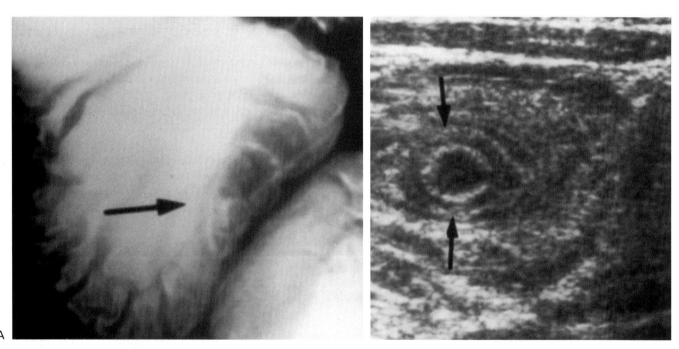

FIGURE 4.98. Intussusception; appendix. A. Note the intussuscepted appendix (arrow). **B.** Ultrasound demonstrates the fluid-filled appendix (arrows) on cross-section. (Reproduced with permission from Koumanidou C, Vakaki M, Theofanopoulou M, et al. Appendiceal and appendiceal-ileocolic intussusception: sonographic and radiographic evaluation. Pediatr Radiol 2001;31:180–183.)

the right (Fig. 4.99A). In other cases, one can see the actual head of the intussusception as a soft tissue mass within the colon (Fig. 4.9, B and C). It is interesting that the mass within the colon often is seen as a relatively isolated finding (13). The mass causes an abrupt cut-off of the air column in the transverse colon and hence the "interrupted air column sign" has been proposed (14). In our experience, the visible head of the intussusception usually is seen in the absence of high-grade obstruction (13). Another finding on plain films consists of the "target" or "crescent" sign (15, 16). Both are the result of mesenteric fat being layered between the intussuscepted intestine, but the finding usually is subtle (Fig. 4.100). On ultrasound, this finding has been termed the crescent in donut sign (17).

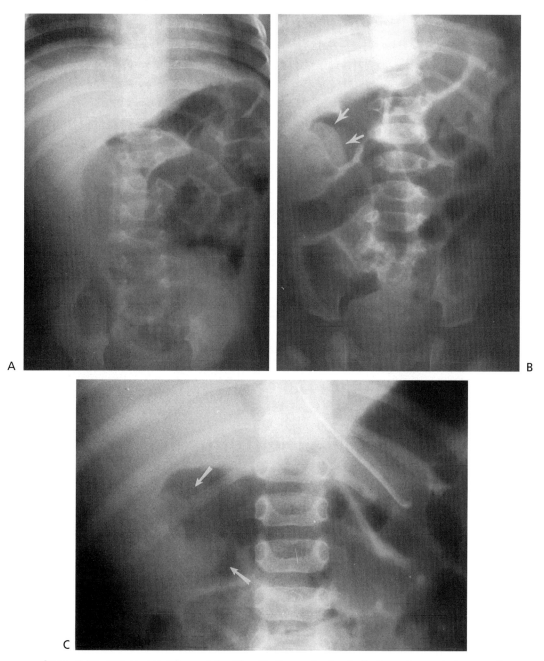

Figure 4.99. Intussusception, plain film findings. A. Classic findings demonstrate a small bowel obstruction and paucity of gas on the right side of the abdomen. This corresponds to the so-called empty right lower quadrant on physical examination. **B.** Another patient with a non-specific intestinal gas pattern but visualization of the head of the intussusception (arrows) in the transverse colon. **C.** In this patient, the intracolonic mass (arrows) is lobular.

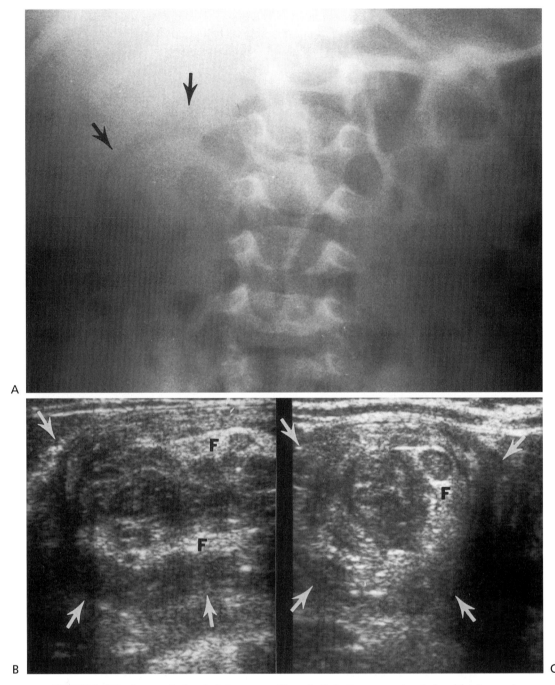

FIGURE 4.100. Crescent sign in intussusception. A. Note the crescent or halo of fat (arrows) around the head of the intussusception. **B.** Longitudinal sonogram demonstrates the circle of fat (F), embedded lymph node, and the oval, multilayered intussusception (arrows). **C.** Cross-sectional view demonstrates the same layer of fat (F), the associated lymph nodes, and the characteristic concentric ring configuration of an intussusception (arrows).

Because of the variability of plain film findings and the fact that the plain film findings often are normal (13), one needs to proceed to some type of imaging study for further identification of an intussusception suspected clinically. In the past, this was relegated, almost exclusively, to the barium enema where the findings typically consisted of a smooth, convex, or lobulated filling defect (Fig. 4.101), which at times assumed the so-called coiled spring configuration (Fig. 4.101C). A mass also is seen with air reduction (Fig. 4.101B). However, over the last two decades, ultrasound has proven to be useful and very accurate in the detection and demonstration of intussusception (18–20). It

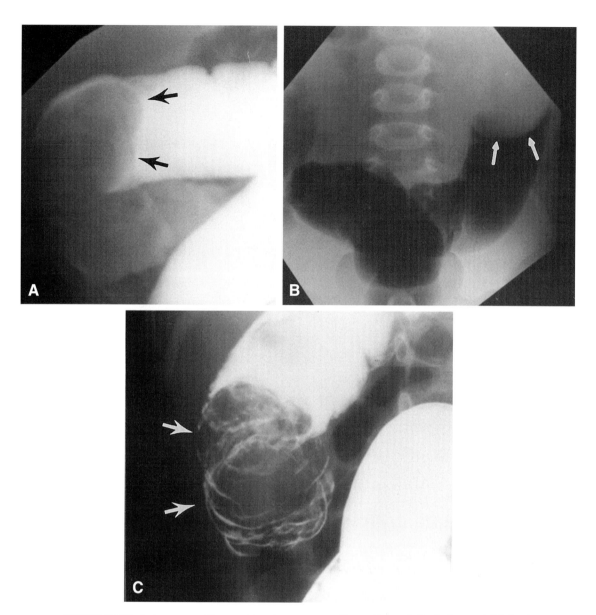

FIGURE 4.101. Intussusception: contrast enema configurations. A. Typical smooth bilobed filling defect (arrows) produced by intussusception on positive contrast enema. **B.** Similar finding (arrows) with air contrast enema. **C.** Coiled spring appearance (arrows) of intussusception in another patient.

has been shown to have sensitivity of 100% and specificity of 88% (21). In our institution we use it exclusively, as the first imaging procedure after plain films. A question remains, however, as to whether the ultrasound study should be performed in all cases, or only those where clinical (history and physical findings) and radiographic findings are inconclusive (22, 23). The argument is that if one is sure clinically and radiographically that intussusception is present, one should proceed directly to a contrast study of the colon. In our institution, however, we proceed to ultrasound in all cases, either to initially diagnose intussusception or to confirm our clinical and radiographic findings.

In the earlier days of the ultrasonographic detection of intussusception, because high-frequency linear transducers were not universally available, intussusceptions appeared as a sonolucent donut or a sonolucent pseudokidney (24). Although these basic configurations still exist, high-frequency linear transducers allow for the demonstration of the various layers of the intussusception, and as a result, rather than a sonolucent donut or a sonolucent pseudokidney appearance, one sees a round or oval mass (depending on the plane of imaging) with layering. In addition, fluid in the inner lumen and associated edematous mesenteric fat along with adenopathy can be encountered (Fig. 4.102).

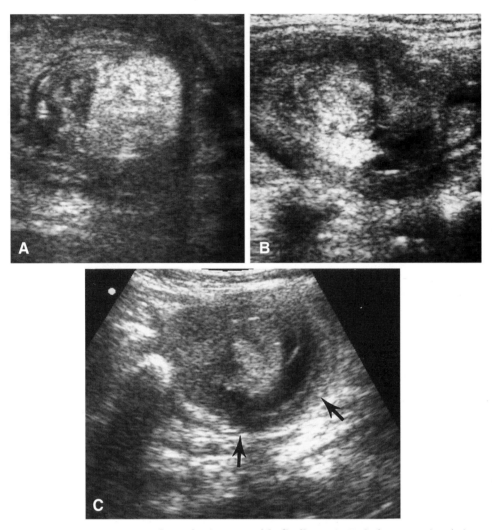

FIGURE 4.102. Intussusception: ultrasonographic findings. A. Typical cross-sectional view demonstrates concentric rings and echogenic mesenteric fat in the intussusception. **B.** Another patient with a more oval-appearing mass. **C.** In this patient, some hypoechoic fluid (arrows) is present in the intussusception.

Adenopathy is a common feature of intussusception (Fig. 4.100) and it has been demonstrated that its presence may inhibit nonsurgical reduction (25). Overall, the findings are characteristic and basically, if intussusception is not found with ultrasound, it is not present. We have not missed an intussusception in nearly twenty years. Intussusception also can be demonstrated with CT (26) (Fig. 4.103, A and B), but most often this occurs fortuitously rather than on purpose.

Color-flow Doppler also has been employed in the evaluation of intussusception and has been used, with some success, to determine whether reduction is likely (27, 28). The concept here is that, if no blood flow is seen to the intussusception, it would be less likely to be reduced nonsurgically. There is considerable validity in this line of rea-

soning, but it is not foolproof. If the intussusception wall is more than 10 mm thick, there is less of a chance for reduction (22). By the same token, if fluid (peritoneal) is trapped within the intussusception (Fig. 4.102C), it also has been suggested that there is less likelihood of successful, nonsurgical reduction (29).

Another benefit of ultrasound in the investigation of intussusception is its ability to document spontaneous reduction (30–32). This is helpful, because in the past, one could only suspect that intussusception initially was present in such patients. With ultrasound, however, one can clearly document that intussusception was present even though, when one finally attempts to reduce it, no intussusception is found (Fig. 4.104). Ultrasound also is useful in detecting transient intussusception which commonly is seen with gas-

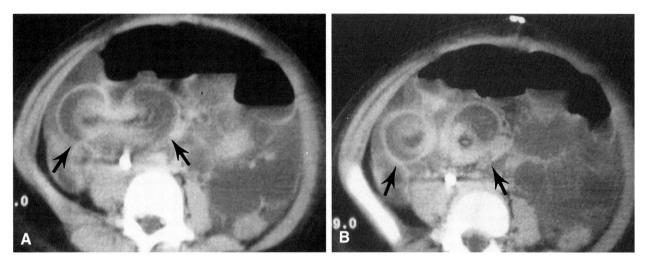

FIGURE 4.103. Intussusception: CT findings. A. In this patient with a postoperative intussusception, note its typical appearance (arrows) on cross-sectional imaging. **B.** Another slice demonstrates the two loops of the intussusception (arrows) along with fluid in one loop and a concentric appearance in another.

troenteritis (Fig. 4.105A). Transient intussusceptions also can be seen with CT (Fig. 4.105B) and also have been documented with celiac disease (33). All of these usually are small and do not resemble the larger, edematous true intussusception. Inversion of the superior mesenteric vessels has been seen with distal ileocolic intussusception (34).

Ultrasound also has been valuable in documenting that a small amount of peritoneal fluid is a normal finding with intussusception (35). It is important to appreciate this and the fact that the fluid is of small volume with no debris (Fig. 4.106). When debris (fibrin) is seen (Fig. 4.106, C and D), one should suspect bowel compromise and the finding should constitute a contraindication to the nonsurgical reduction of the intussusception. When only a small amount of non-debris-containing fluid is present, and there are no clinical or radiographic findings of bowel death or perforation, one can proceed with nonsurgical reduction.

In terms of reduction, as mentioned earlier, in the past this routinely was relegated to the hydrostatic barium enema. Currently, however, there is a preference for air reduction but hydrostatic reduction with ultrasound guidance also has been used (36–39). Even air reduction under ultrasound guidance has been suggested (40). Being that perforation can occur, it is probably best not to use barium. Air, water, or aqueous contrast agents are much more satisfactory in this regard. By and large, one can attain reduction rates of 80–90% with air contrast and ultrasound-guided reduction. Barium reduction rates were lower and often were in the 45–50% bracket (36–39, 41). These low reduction rates probably reflected a reluctance to be aggressive and bold when barium was used because of the possibility of perforation and barium peritonitis. Proponents of air or

ultrasound guided reduction emphasize that when barium or aqueous contrast agents are used, radiation to the patient becomes a factor. However, such radiation is not that significant (41).

One of the reasons that air became so popular is that there was a tendency to be somewhat cautious when barium was used. The reason for this was that with perforation one could induce barium peritonitis. Since this is not a problem with air, one could afford to be bolder, and the mechanics of air reduction themselves led to much higher reduction rates. In this regard and to attain higher reduction rates we began to use aqueous contrast agents, Gastrografin diluted 5:1 with saline before air became popular. We did this because we realized that it was safer to use an aqueous contrast agent when a perforation occurred. Our reduction rates were comparable to those seen with gas reduction and so we have continued to use this form of reduction. It takes a little longer than when one is using air but still quite satisfactory. In the end, there are different ways to reduce an intussusception and all but barium reduction seem to be satisfactory.

Whatever contrast material one uses, the head of the intussusception during reduction must be followed to the ileocecal valve and then seen to pass into the dilated (obstructed) small bowel (Fig. 4.107). Very often, however, one encounters difficulty at the ileocecal valve, or earlier at the hepatic flexure and in all such cases one must be persistent. In this regard, as long as there is progression of reduction, be it ever so little, one should continue. However, if no change occurs within 4 to 5 minutes at any one location, we usually stop or lower the reservoir of Gastrografin, drain the bowel, and try again. This, in effect, mimics the plunger

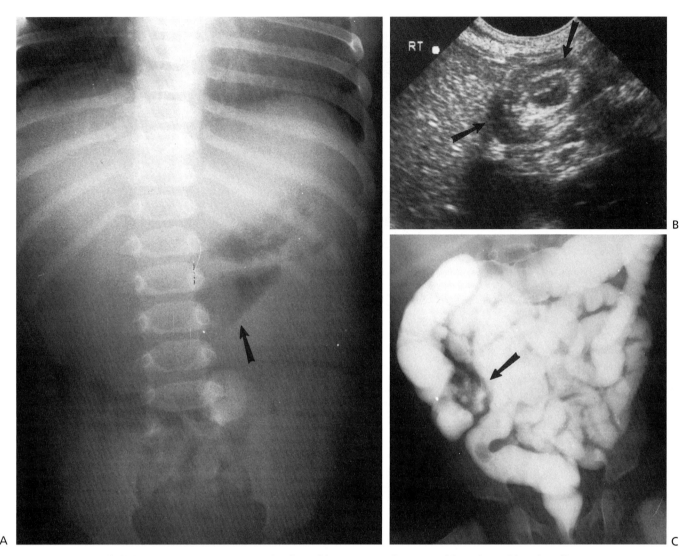

FIGURE 4.104. Spontaneous reduction of intussusception. A. In this patient with a virtually airless abdomen, note the head of the intussusception (arrow) in the transverse colon. **B.** Cross-sectional ultrasonographic image through the intussusception (arrows) confirms its presence. **C.** The intussusception, however, could not be demonstrated with subsequent contrast enema, because it had spontaneously reduced in the interval. Nonetheless, characteristic deformity of the terminal ileum (arrow), resulting from persistent edema after reduction of the intussusception is seen. Thereafter, the intussusception was not detected with ultrasound, attesting to the fact that it reduced spontaneously.

FIGURE 4.106. Free peritoneal fluid with intussusception. A. Patient with an intussusception (arrows). **B.** Free fluid (F) is seen between the liver (L) and kidney (K). This patient had an uncomplicated intussusception. **C.** Another patient with an intussusception demonstrating blood flow with color-flow Doppler (arrows) in the wall of the intussusception. **D.** However, just over the spleen, considerable fluid (arrows) with fibrin strands was noted. This patient had an ischemically compromised intussusception.

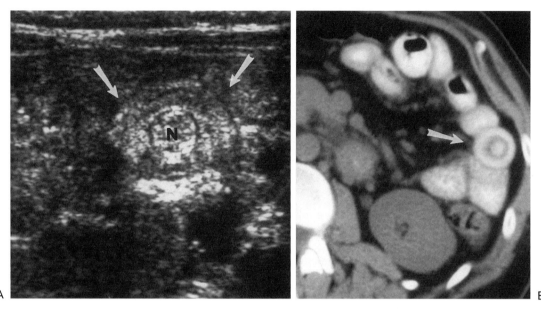

FIGURE 4.105. Transient intussusception: ultrasound and CT findings. A. On this ultrasound study note the intussusceptum (arrows) and a small, central intussuscepted head (H) of an intussusception. **B.** Note a transient, incidental intussusception (arrow) demonstrated with CT.

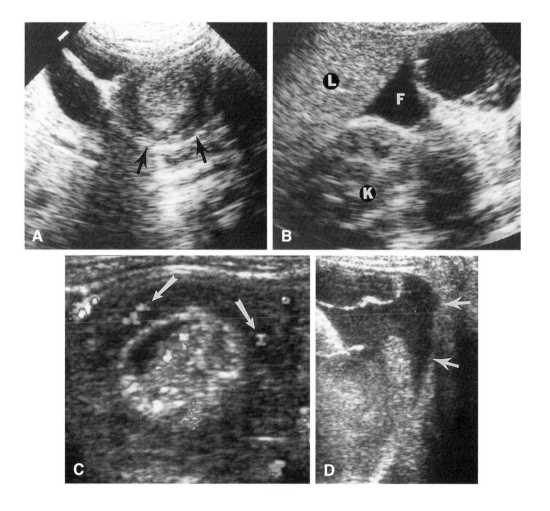

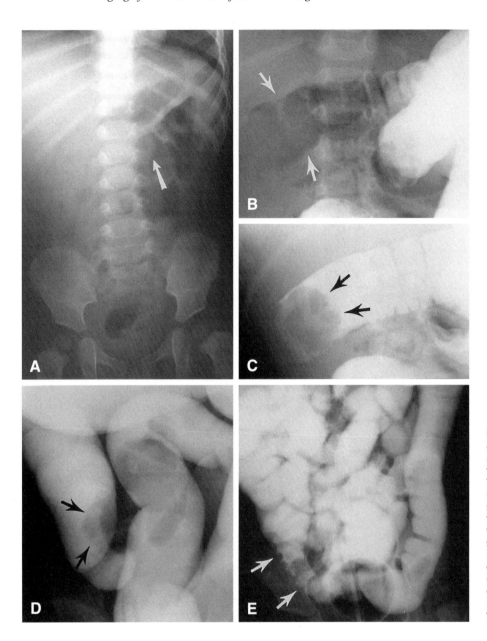

FIGURE 4.107. Intussusception: successful reduction. A. Plain film demonstrates the head of the intussusception (arrow) in the transverse colon. There is little air in the abdomen. **B.** Contrast enema reduction demonstrates the head of the intussusception (arrows) outlined by air. This would be the appearance of the intussusception with air reduction. **C.** A little later, the head of the intussusception (arrows) is outlined by Gastrografin. **D.** The head of the intussusception (arrows) now is lodged in the ileocecal valve. **E.** With reduction, Gastrografin fills the small bowel.

effect present with air reduction. Usually, three or four tries allow one to reduce the intussusception, but we have gone up to seven or eight decompressions and recompressions.

When reduction has occurred, there will be flooding of the dilated small bowel with the contrast agent used (Figs. 4.107 and 4.108). Once this occurs, one can assume that reduction has been accomplished. However, with air it has been noted that premature flooding of the small bowel can be seen before successful reduction has been accomplished (42). When positive contrast agents are used, postreduction deformity of the cecum and edema of the terminal ileum frequently are seen and are to be expected (Fig. 4.109). Although in simple intussusception the head of the intussusception is somewhat smooth and round, it has been

noted that with ileo-ileo colic intussusceptions a multilobulated configuration is seen (43).

The arrival of air as a suitable contrast agent for reducing intussusception caused all concerned to reexamine the factors involved in the nonsurgical reduction of intussusception. First it became apparent that, with air, greater pressures were instantaneously generated in the colon, and it was subsequently documented that, to reach the 120-mm Hg peak air pressures used for air reduction, one needed to elevate the reservoir of barium to 3.5 feet and with diluted aqueous contrast agents to 5 feet (44). In terms of pressures used with air reduction, pressures of at least 60 mm Hg are required for reduction, and pressure beyond 120 mm Hg should be avoided (45). In addition it has been demon-

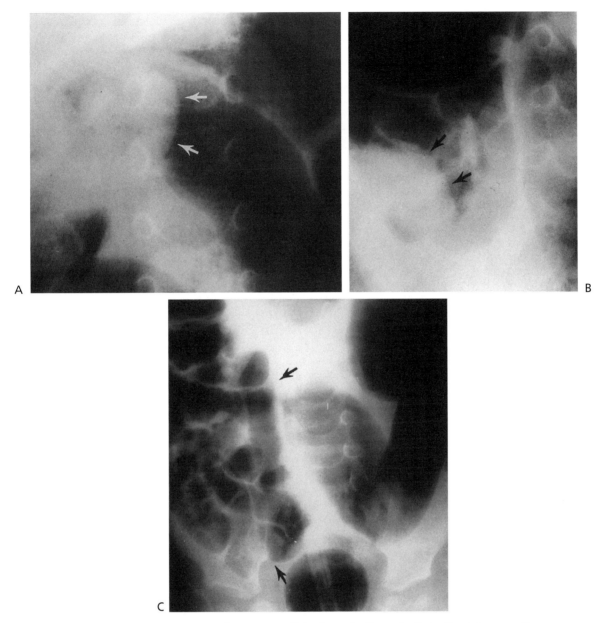

FIGURE 4.108. Intussusception: successful air reduction. A. Note the intussusception (arrows) outlined by air. **B.** The intussusception (arrows) has moved into the ascending colon. **C.** Later, with reduction, air fills numerous loops of small bowel (arrows).

strated that if one cannot make any progress after 4 minutes, reduction is less likely to occur (46).

Perforation rates now hover somewhere between 1 and 3%, and perforation is less of a problem when air or aqueous contrast agents, rather than barium, are used. The reason for this is that, when barium is not used, one does not need to worry about perforation and barium peritonitis. As a result, one can become more aggressive. In terms of the perforation, it probably is not the procedure itself that causes the perforation but rather the fact that the bowel is compromised and when reduction occurs and exposes this

bowel to the increased luminal pressures, perforation occurs.

When perforation occurs, contrast material is seen to flood the peritoneal cavity and, in this regard, positive contrast agents are easier to see than negative contrast agents. However, no matter what contrast agent is used, once perforation occurs, one must stop the procedure and decompress the colon. Thereafter, the patient must be treated surgically and, in this regard, **before attempting nonsurgical reduction, one always should have the surgical service present. With this close collaboration, perforations**

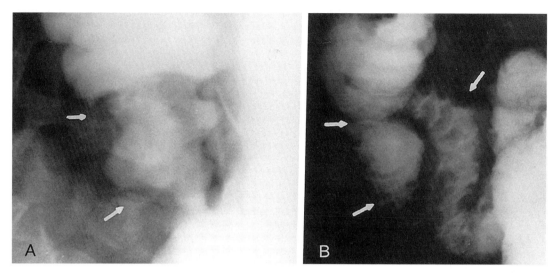

FIGURE 4.109. Postreduction: cecal and terminal ileal edema. A. Note deformed edematous cecum after reduction (arrows). **B.** Another patient with edema of the cecum and terminal ileum resulting in coarse nodularity (arrows).

occurring during reduction generally are not a serious problem, at least as long as one does not use barium.

In terms of measures used to enhance nonsurgical reduction of intussusception, it has been demonstrated that temporary peaks of high pressure are generated in patients with air reduction (47). This probably also occurs with other forms of reduction and most likely is related to the Valsalva maneuver as the patient grunts against the enema. This speaks against the use of sedation for relaxing the patient. Sedation was at one time in vogue but has lost considerable support. Glucagon was also once used, but now is generally not used.

All of the foregoing is important, but I have found that the most important factor leading to the success of nonsurgical reduction of intussusception is that the anus be totally occluded so that proper pressures can be built up in the colon. In this regard, we have always used a Foley bulb (inflated after contrast has been introduced into the colon and the intussusception identified) and **taped the buttocks with many strips of good adhesive tape.** Taping of the buttocks must be thorough, because one must ensure adequate occlusion of the anus. Thereafter, the Foley bulb can be inflated and pulled back against the solidly sealed anus. As a result, even with the patient's subsequent straining, tight occlusion is achieved and each time this occurs the Foley bulb is pushed against the strapped buttocks and intracolonic pressures increase. Occluding the anus completely is the most important part of the reduction procedure no matter what contrast agent is used, and in this regard, it has been demonstrated that a larger tube is better

than a smaller tube (48) and we have certainly found this to be true. We use as large a tube as we can comfortably insert into the patient's rectum.

As a final adjunctive measure in the reduction of intussusceptions, it recently has been suggested that manual palpation of the intussusception should be attempted in refractory cases (49). We have performed this in a few patients and believe that it can help. This is contrary to teaching of the past where palpation of the intussusception generally was discouraged. However, now that air, water, and aqueous contrast material are used for intussusception reduction, one can be more aggressive and this can include manual palpation in refractory cases.

Postreduction films still are important. If positive contrast aqueous material is used, and if the reduction is complete, almost all of the contrast material will evacuate. However, if reduction is incomplete, the intussusception will be seen to persist, and the colon distal to the obstruction will show intense spasm, reflecting the irritability and spastic nature of intestine distal to any obstruction. These findings are more difficult to see with air, but a postreduction film still should be obtained to determine whether the gas pattern in the abdomen has returned to normal.

Recurrence rates always have been between 4 and 10% and generally occur within a few days (50). If recurrence occurs, nonsurgical reduction should be attempted again, at least once (49). A third attempt may also be useful, but surgical exploration would probably be required at this stage. Over the years, numerous contraindications to nonsurgical reduction of intussusception have been proposed. Currently, however, these consist primarily of evidence of bowel necrosis, free air, or peritonitis. The presence of obstruction or the fact that obstruction has been present for 24 hours or more are not contraindications for nonsurgical reduction (51).

Finally, intussusceptions are more common in patients with cystic fibrosis (52), giving rise to the so-called meconium ileus equivalent syndrome. Postoperative intussusceptions also can occur (53) in patients having undergone abdominal surgery. Often, these intussusceptions are elusive and discovered only when CT studies are obtained to determine what is going on in the abdomen (54) (see Fig. 4.103). They also can be detected with ultrasound (55, 56). Intussusceptions also have been identified around gastrojejunostomy tubes (57, 58).

REFERENCES

1. Avinoam R, Rosenbach Y, Amir J, et al. Apathy as an early manifestation of intussusception. Am J Dis Child 1983;137:701.
2. Conway EE Jr. Central nervous system findings and intussusception: how are they related? Pediatr Emerg Care 1993;9: 15–18.
3. Barr LL, Stansberry SD, Swischuk LE. Significance of age, duration, obstruction, and the dissection sign. Pediatr Radiol 1990;20:454–456.
4. Patriquin HB, Afshani E, Effman E, et al. Neonatal intussusception: report of 12 cases. Radiology 1977;125:463–466.
5. Mooney DP, Steinthorsson G, Shorter NA. Perinatal intussusception in premature infants. J Pediatr Surg 1996;31:695–697.
6. Daneman A, Myers M, Shuckett B, et al. Sonographic appearance of inverted Meckel diverticulum with intussusception. Pediatr Radiol 1997;27:295–298.
7. Kim G, Daneman A, Alton DJ, et al. The appearance of inverted Meckel diverticulum with intussusception on air enema. Pediatr Radiol 1997;27:647–650.
8. Ong N-T, Beasley DW. The leadpoint in intussusception. J Pediatr Surg 1990;25:640–643.
9. Reijnen JAM, Joosten HJM, Festen C. Intussusception in children 5 to 15 years of age. Br J Surg 1987;74:692–693.
10. Koumanidou C, Vakaki M, Theofanopoulou M, et al. Appendiceal and appendiceal-ileocolic intussusception: sonographic and radiographic evaluation. Pediatr Radiol 2001;31:180–183.
11. Navarro O, Daneman A, Alton DJ, et al. Colo-colic intussusception associated with pneumatosis cystoids intestinalis. Pediatr Radiol 1998;28:515–517.
12. Sargent MA, Babyn P, Alton DJ. Plain abdominal radiography in suspected intussusception: a reassessment. Pediatr Radiol 1994; 24:17–20.
13. Hernandez JA, Swischuk LE, Hendrick EP, et al. Plain films in intussusception: an analysis of findings. (In preparation).
14. Lazar L, Rathaus V, Erez I, et al. Interrupted air column in the large bowel on plain abdominal film: a new radiological sign of intussusception. J Pediatr Surg 1995;30:1551–1553.
15. Lee JM, Kim H, Byun JY, et al. Intussusception: characteristic radiolucencies on the abdominal radiograph. Pediatr Radiol 1994;24:293–295.
16. Ratcliffe JF, Fong S, Cheong L, et al. The plain abdominal film in intussusception: the accuracy and incidence of radiographic signs. Pediatr Radiol 1992;22:110–111.
17. del-Poza G, Albillos JC, Trejedor D. Intussusception: US findings with pathologic correlation—the crescent-in-doughnut sign. Radiology 1996;199:688–692.
18. Bhisitkul DM, Listernick R, Shkolnik A, et al. Clinical applications of ultrasonography in the diagnosis of intussusception. J Pediatr 1992;121:182–186.
19. Shanbhogue RLK, Hussain SM, Meradji M, et al. Ultrasonography is accurate enough for the diagnosis of intussusception. J Pediatr Surg 1994;29:324–328.
20. Harrington L, Connolly B, Wesson DE, et al. Ultrasonographic and clinical predictors of intussusception. J Pediatr 1998;132: 836–839.
21. Kaste SC, Wilimas J, Rao BN. Post-operative small bowel intussusception in children with cancer. Pediatr Radiol 1995;25: 21–23.
22. John SD. The value of ultrasound in children with suspected intussusception. Emerg Radiol 1998;5:297–305.
23. Verschelden P, Filiatrault D, Garel L, et al. Intussusception in children: reliability of US in diagnosis—a prospective study. Radiology 1992;184:741–744.
24. Swischuk LE, Hayden CK, Boulden T. Intussusception: indications for ultrasonography and an explanation of the donut and pseudokidney signs. Pediatr Radiol 1985;15:388–391.
25. Koumanidou C Vakaki M, Pitsoulakis G, et al. Sonographic detection of lymph nodes in the intussusception of infants and young children: clinical evaluation and hydrostatic reduction. AJR 2002;178:445–450.
26. Cox TD, Winters WD, Weinberger E. CT of intussusception in the pediatric patient: diagnosis and pitfalls. Pediatr Radiol 1996; 26:26–32.
27. Lim HK, Bae SH, Lee KH, et al. Assessment of reducibility of ileocolic intussusception in children: usefulness of color Doppler sonography. Radiology 1994;191:781–785.
28. Kong-M-S, Wong H-F, Lin S-L, et al. Factors related to detection of blood flow by color Doppler ultrasonography in intussusception. J Ultrasound Med 1997;16:141–144.
29. del-Pozo G, Gonzalez-Spinola J, Gomez-Anson B, et al. Intussusception: trapped peritoneal fluid detected with US—relationship to reducibility and schemia. Radiology 1996;201:379–383.
30. Swischuk LE, John SD, Swischuk PN. Spontaneous reduction of intussusception: verification with US. Radiology 1994;192: 269–271.
31. Kornecki A, Daneman A, Navarro O, et al. Spontaneous reduction of intussusception: clinical spectrum, management and outcome. Pediatr Radiol 2000;30:458–63.
32. Morrison SC, Stork E. Documentation of spontaneous reduction of childhood intussusception by ultrasound. Pediatr Radiol 1990;20:358–359.
33. Mushtaq N, Marven S, Walker J, et al. Small bowel intussusception in celiac disease. J Pediatr Surg 1999;34:1833–1835.
34. Papadopoulou F, Efremidis SC, Raptopoulou A, et al. Distal ileocolic intussusception: another cause of inversion of superior mesenteric vessels in infants. AJR 1996;167:1243–1246.
35. Swischuk LE, Stansberry SD. Ultrasonographic detection of free peritoneal fluid in uncomplicated intussusception. Pediatr Radiol 1991;21:350–351.
36. Chan KL, Saing H, Peh WCG, et al. Childhood intussusception: ultrasound-guided Hartmann's solution hydrostatic reduction or barium reduction? J Pediatr Surg 1997;323:3–6.
37. del-Pozo G, Albillos JC, Tejedor D, et al. Intussusception in children: current concepts in diagnosis and enema reduction. Radiographics 1999;19:299–319.
38. Ein SH, Alton D, Palder SB, et al. Intussusception in the 1990s: has 25 years made a difference? Pediatr Surg Int 1997;12: 374–376.
39. Hadidi AT, El Shal N. Childhood intussusception: a comparative

study of nonsurgical management. J Pediatr Surg 1999;34: 304–307.

40. Yoon CH, Kim YJ, Goo HW. Intussusception in children: US-guided pneumatic reduction—initial experience. Radiology 2001;218:85–88.

41. Persliden J, Schuwert P, Mortensson W. Comparison of absorbed radiation doses in barium and air enema reduction of intussusception: a phantom study. Pediatr Radiol 1996;26:329–3332.

42. Hedlung GL, Johnson JF, Strife JL. Ileocolic intussusception: extensive reflux of air preceding pneumatic reduction. Radiology 1990;174:187–189.

43. Hogan M, Johnson JF III. Multipolypoid intussusceptum: a distinctive appearance of ileo-ileocolic intussusception at the ileocecal valve. Pediatr Radiol 1996;26:405–408.

44. Shiels WE II, Maves CK, Hedlund GL, et al. Air enema for diagnosis and reduction of intussusception: clinical experience and pressure correlates. Radiology 1991;181:169–171.

45. Shiels WE II, Kirks DR, Keller GL, et al. Colonic perforation by air and liquid enemas: comparison study in young pigs. AJR 1993;160:931–935.

46. Iui K-W, Wong H-F, Cheung Y-C, et al. Air enema for diagnosis and reduction of intussusception in children. Clinical experience and fluoroscopy time correlation. J Pediatr Surg 2001;36: 479–481.

47. Zambuto D, Bramson RT, Blickman JG. Intracolonic pressure measurements during hydrostatic and air contrast barium enema studies in children. Radiology 1995;196:55–58.

48. Schmitz-Rode T, Muller-Leisse C, Alzen G. Comparative examination of various rectal tubes and contrast media for the reduction of intussusceptions. Pediatr Radiol 1991;21:341–345.

49. Grasso SN, Katz ME, Presberg HJ, et al. Transabdominal manually assisted reduction of pediatric intussusception: reappraisal of this historical technique. Radiology 1994;191:777–779.

50. Daneman A, Alton DJ, Lobo A, et al. Patterns of recurrence of intussusception in children: a 17-year review. Pediatr Radiol 1998;28:913–919.

51. Fecteau A, Flageole H, Nguyen LT, et al. Recurrent intussusception: safe use of hydrostatic enema. J Pediatr Surg 1996;31: 858–861.

52. Okuyama H, Nakai H, Okada A. Is barium enema reduction safe

and effective in patients with a long duration of intussusception? Pediatr Surg Int 1990;15:105–107.

53. Holsclaw DS, Rocmans C, Schwachman H. Intussusception in patients with cystic fibrosis. Pediatrics 1971;48:51–58.

54. Allbery SM, Swischuk LE, John SD, et al. Post-operative intussusception: often an elusive diagnosis. Pediatr Radiol 1998;28: 271.

55. Beek FJ, Rovekamp MH, Bax NM, et al. Ultrasound findings in post-operative jejunojejunal intussusception. Pediatr Radiol 1990;20:601.

56. Connolly BL, Chait PG, Silva-Nandan R, et al. Recognition of intussusception around gastrojejunostomy tubes in children. AJR 1998;170:467–470.

57. Hughes UM, Connolly BL, Chait PG, et al. Further report of small-bowel intussusceptions related to gastro-jejunostomy tubes. Pediatr Radiol 2000;30:614–617.

58. Carnevale E, Graziani M, Fasanelli S. Postoperative ileo-ileal intussusception: sonographic approach. Pediatr Radiol 1994;24: 161–163.

Inspissated Milk or Milk Curd Syndrome

Intestinal obstruction by milk curds (1, 2) almost always occurs in premature infants and results from feeding them a high-calorie or concentrated powdered milk formula. It differs from other causes of neonatal intestinal obstruction in that it is somewhat delayed in onset. There is a period of normal meconium passage before obstructive symptoms develop. Plain abdominal roentgenograms in these infants show obstructive patterns, and the inspissated milk curds can frequently be seen as masses in the dilated air-filled bowel (Fig. 4.110). The fact that the inspissated bowel contents are not adherent to the mucosa (i.e., air can be seen between the intestinal wall and the milk curd inspissations) is strongly suggestive of the condition. However, such air can mimic the findings of pneumatosis cystoides intestinalis

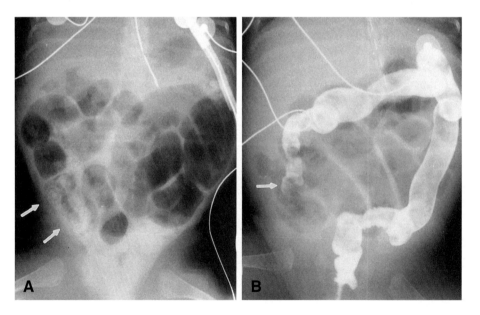

FIGURE 4.110. Inspissated milk curd syndrome. A. In this premature infant an intestinal obstruction is suggested and inspissated milk curds (arrows) are seen in the right lower quadrant. **B.** Contrast enema demonstrates the filling defect (arrow) produced by the milk curds. Dilated loops of small bowel attest to the presence of obstruction.

as seen in necrotizing enterocolitis (3). Therapeutic Gastrografin enema (diluted 3:1), much as in meconium ileus, can be used in these infants.

REFERENCES

1. Cremin BJ, Smythe PM, Cywes S. The radiological appearance of the "inspissated milk syndrome." A cause of intestinal obstruction in infants. Br J Radiol 1970;43:856–858.
2. Friedland GW, Rush WA Jr, Hill AJ. Smythe's "inspissated milk" syndrome. Radiology 1972;103:159–161.
3. Berkowitz GP, Buntain WL, Cassady G. Milk curd obstruction mimicking necrotizing enterocolitis. Am J Dis Child 1980;134: 989–990.

Inguinal Hernia

Inguinal hernia is a very common problem in young infants. However, it is usually readily detectable clinically and little roentgenographic investigation is necessary. On the other hand, if incarceration occurs, bowel obstruction may be the presenting problem as seen on initial plain abdominal films (Fig. 4.111). In such cases, it is important to look for gas bubbles in the incarcerated loop of bowel (Fig. 4.111, A and B). In cases in which a hernia is present but the loops of intestine do not contain air, prominence of the inguinal fold (1) may provide a clue to the diagnosis (Fig. 4.111C).

In the past, herniography was variably employed to demonstrate inguinal hernias in some cases, but now if a hernia extends into the scrotum or inguinal canal, and there is question as to whether it is a hernia, ultrasound is used. It will demonstrate the presence of intestine in the inguinal canal or scrotum, as the intestinal wall will demonstrate its characteristic echogenic mucosal layer and hypoechoic muscular layer (Fig. 4.112). In addition, the presence of omentum or mesentery can be detected. Color-flow Doppler can be used to demonstrate the presence or absence of blood flow to an incarcerated inguinal hernia. Postoperatively, after inguinal hernia repair, the scrotal and intrascrotal soft tissues may become edematous, and nonspecific fluid collections or hematomas also may be seen. These generally are considered normal postoperative findings.

REFERENCE

1. Currarino G. Incarcerated inguinal hernia in infants: plain films and barium enema. Pediatr Radiol 1974;2:247–250.

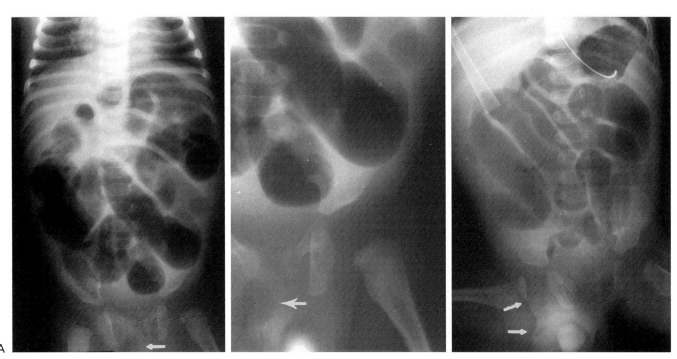

A   B,C

FIGURE 4.111. Intestinal obstruction secondary to incarcerated hernia. A. Note numerous distended loops of small bowel consistent with an intestinal obstruction. Also note an air bubble (arrow) in the right scrotum. **B.** Magnified view of the air bubble (arrow). **C.** Another patient with a similar pattern of obstruction. No air is seen in the scrotum but a prominent right inguinal fold (arrows) is seen.

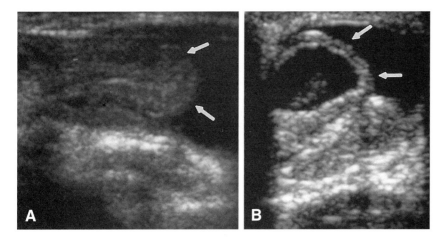

FIGURE 4.112. Inguinal hernia, ultrasound findings. A. Note the loop of compressed intestine (arrows) extending down into the inguinal canal and scrotal regions. It is surrounded by echogenic fluid of a hydrocele. **B.** Another view demonstrates a fluid-filled loop of intestine

Other Hernias

Umbilical hernia is discussed later with abdominal wall problems, but other hernias that might be encountered include Richter's hernia (1), femoral hernia and Spigelian hernias. Umbilical hernias are easy to detect clinically but the other hernias may be more difficult to detect and demonstrate. Ultrasound or CT, however, can be helpful.

REFERENCE

1. Shanbhogue LKR, Miller SS. Richter's hernia in the neonate. J Pediatr Surg 1986;21:881–882.

Miscellaneous Small Bowel Obstructions in the Neonate

Other causes of small intestinal obstruction include total colon and terminal small bowel Hirschsprung's disease (discussed later with Hirschsprung's disease), compression of the intestine by abdominal masses or cysts and by peritoneal bands and omphalomesenteric or vitelline duct remnants (1). In most cases, the abdominal findings are nonspecific but do show evidence of small bowel obstruction.

Another uncommon cause of intestinal obstruction in the newborn is **absence of the intestinal musculature** (2, 3). The condition often is segmental, and once again the abdominal findings are relatively nonspecific, but in congenital **segmental dilation of the jejunum or ileum** (4–6), a single, massively dilated loop of small bowel may provide a clue to proper diagnosis (Fig. 4.113). No definite etiology has been determined for this condition, but it probably is similar to that considered with segmental dilation of the colon. Small bowel obstruction also can occur secondary to plexiform neurofibromatosis (7).

Another uncommon and somewhat poorly defined entity is the idiopathic pseudoobstruction syndrome (8, 9).

The key to diagnosis of these problems is to be aware of the fact that they exist and begin to think of them when other, more common problems do not appear to be the cause of the patient's problems. The etiology may have to do with abnormality of the myenteric plexus of the intestine (10–12). Chronic intestinal dilation in these patients can lead to marked intestinal obstruction and even benign pneumatosis cystoides intestinalis and pneumoperitoneum (13).

REFERENCES

1. Gaisie G, Curf JH, Croom RD, et al. Neonatal intestinal obstruction from omphalomesenteric duct remnants. AJR 1985;144:109–112.
2. Alawadhi A, Chou S, Carpenter B. Segmental agenesis of intestinal muscularis: a case report. J Pediatr Surg 1989;24:1089–1090.
3. McCarthy DW, Qualman S, Besner GE. Absent intestinal musculature: anatomic evidence of an embryonic origin of the lesion. J Pediatr Surg 1995;29:1476–1478.
4. Balik E, Taneli C, Yazici M, et al. Segmental dilation of intestine: a case report and review of the literature. Eur J Pediatr Surg 1993; 3:118–120.
5. Kuint J, Avigad I, Husar M, et al. Segmental dilation of the ileum: an uncommon cause of neonatal intestinal obstruction. J Pediatr Surg 1993;28:1637–1639.
6. Ratcliffe J, Tait J, Lisle D, et al. Segmental dilation of the small bowel: report of three cases and literature review. Radiology 1989;171:827–830.
7. Takahaski M, Katsumata K, Yokoyama J, et al. Plexiform neurofibromatosis of the ileum in an infant. J Pediatr Surg 1977; 12:571–574.
8. Glassman M, Spivak W, Mininberg D, et al. Chronic idiopathic intestinal pseudoobstruction: a commonly misdiagnosed disease in infants and children. Pediatrics 1989;83:607–608.
9. Goulet O, Jobert-Giraud A, Michel J-L, et al. Chronic intestinal pseudo-obstruction syndrome in pediatric patients. Eur J Pediatr Surg 2000;9:83–90.
10. Krishnamurthy S, Heng Y, Schuffler MD. Chronic intestinal pseudo-obstruction in infants and children caused by diverse

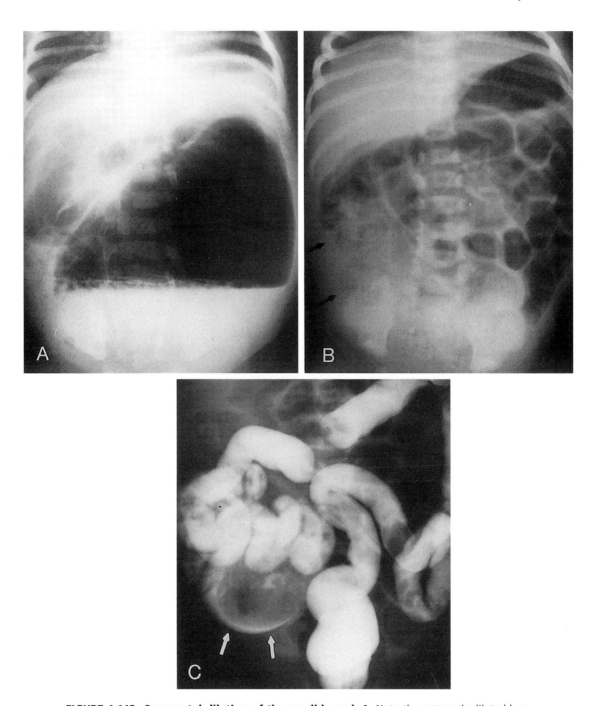

FIGURE 4.113. Segmental dilation of the small bowel. A. Note the extremely dilated loop of small bowel, which on this upright view has a long air-fluid level. **B.** Another infant with a collection of granular material on the right (arrows). **C.** Subsequent barium enema, with reflux into the small bowel, outlines the segment of dilated intestine (arrows). It was this loop that contained the granular air and meconium seen in **B.** (**A** reproduced with permission from Irving IM, Lister J. Segmental dilation of the ileum. J Pediatr Surg 1977;12:103–112.).

abnormalities of the myenteric plexus. Gastroenterology 1993; 104:1398–1408.

11. Yamagiwa I, Ohta M, Obata K, et al. Intestinal pseudoobstruction in a neonate caused by idiopathic muscular hypertrophy of the entire small intestine. J Pediatr Surg 1988;23:866–869.

12. Yamataka A, Ohshiro K, Kobayashi H, et al. Abnormal distribution of intestinal pacemaker (C-KIT-positive cells in an infant with chronic idiopathic intestinal pseudoobstruction. J Pediatr Surg 1998;33:859–862.

13. Luks FI, Chung MA, Brandt ML, et al. Pneumatosis and pneumoperitoneum in chronic idiopathic intestinal pseudoobstruction. J Pediatr Surg 1991;26:1384–1386.

MISCELLANEOUS SMALL BOWEL DISEASE

Celiac Disease (Gluten Enteropathy)

The roentgenographic changes in celiac disease are somewhat variable, depending on the age of the patient. In older children, typically there is dilation of the small bowel and stretching of the mucosal folds. This pattern is typical but merely reflects the effects of dilation (Fig. 4.114A). In some cases, the mucosal folds are thicker, presumably because of coating with secretions. In infants, this discrete pattern of fold abnormality often is less apparent and replaced by nonspecific clumping and dilution of the barium (Fig. 4.114C). The disease results from a sensitivity to gluten in the diet and usually finally is diagnosed by small bowel biopsy, which shows atrophy of the villi. Findings return to normal with removal of gluten from the diet (Fig. 4.114, B and D), and finally an association between celiac disease and trisomy 21 has recently come to the forefront (1–3).

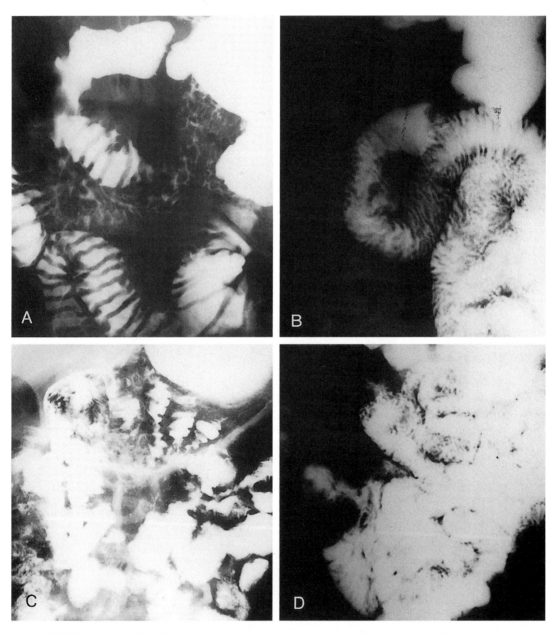

FIGURE 4.114. Celiac disease. A. Typical straight, slightly thickened folds of dilated bowel. Both the duodenum and jejunum are involved. **B.** Normal pattern after treatment. **C.** Infant with thickened straight loops in the upper portion of the small bowel and formless loops in the lower intestine. **D.** Normal intestine after successful therapy.

REFERENCES

1. Gale L, Wimalaratna H, Brotodiharjo A, et al. Down's syndrome is strongly associated with celiac disease. Gut 1997;40:492–496.
2. Jansson U, Johansson C. Down syndrome and celiac disease. J Pediatr Gastroenterol Nutr 1995;21:443–445.
3. Zubillaga P, Vitoria JC, Arrieta A, et al. Down's syndrome and celiac disease. J Pediatr Gastroenterol Nutr 1993;16:168–171.

Food Allergy

Cow's milk intolerance (allergy) is not an uncommon problem in infants, and often may involve the colon more than the small bowel. It is a common cause of intestinal bleeding in neonates and young infants (1). These infants also can present with vomiting and diarrhea, and if a small bowel series is obtained, the mucosal folds can be seen to be thickened. In the stomach, antral spasm (pylorospasm) with thickening of the mucosa and minimal thickening of the pyloric muscle also can be encountered. All of these changes disappear once the milk formula is changed and the diagnosis often comes to the forefront after milk feeding challenge (1). In terms of the mucosa in food allergy, thickening, on ultrasound, usually measures greater than the normal 2 mm intestinal mucosa. Ultrasound can readily detect mucosal thickening and can be used to monitor these patients as they are treated (2).

REFERENCES

1. Willetts IE, Dalzell M, Puntis JWL, et al. Cow's milk enteropathy: surgical pitfalls. J Pediatr Surg 1999;34:1486–1488.
2. Kino M, Kojima T, Yamamoto A, et al. bowel wall thickening in infants with food allergy. Pediatr Radiol 2002;32:31–33.

Inflammatory Bowel Disease

There are a number of conditions that can lead to both acute and chronic inflammatory disease of the small intestine. Those producing chronic findings include tuberculosis (1), atypical tuberculosis (2), and regional enteritis, or Crohn's disease. The latter is most common in North America and the findings are the same as they are in adults. For the most part, they consist of variable thickening of the terminal ileum and deformity of the cecum (Fig. 4.115). Spasm and edema may lead to the "string sign" during the acute phase (Fig. 4.116) and sinus tracks, fistulas, and abscesses are common complications (Fig. 4.117). Regional enteritis most commonly involves the terminal ileum but other "skip" areas in the small bowel can be encountered. The disease also can involve the stomach, duodenum, and even the esophagus. Ultrasonography, in the classic case, shows transmural thickening of the intestinal wall of the terminal ileum (Fig. 4.117B). Color-flow Doppler demon-

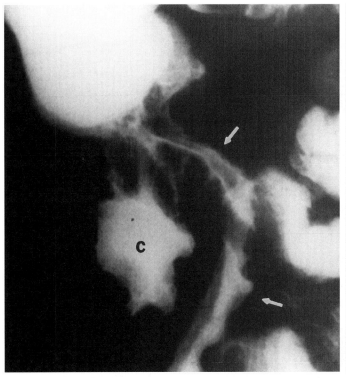

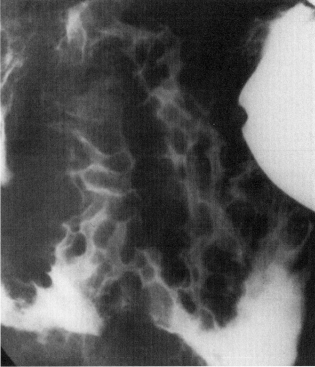

A B

FIGURE 4.115. Regional enteritis. A. Note the cone-shaped, deformed cecum (C) and the thickened and nodular rigid-appearing edematous terminal ileum (arrows). **B.** Another patient with nodular thickening of the terminal ileum.

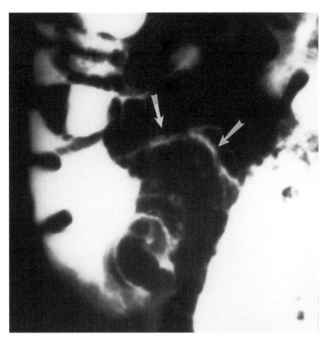

FIGURE 4.116. Regional enteritis; string sign. Note the deformed cecum and the spastic terminal ileum (arrows) constituting the string sign.

strates increased blood flow to the area (Fig. 4.117C) and can be used as an indicator of disease activity (3, 4). Adenopathy is not commonly seen, and this can be used to differentiate the findings from tuberculosis for which one often sees associated adenopathy and mesenteric thickening.

In addition to the foregoing inflammatory problems, there are a number of other acute or chronic entities that can involve the terminal ileum and cecum, including *Yersinia* (5, 6,), pathogenic *Escherichia coli*, and viral (acute) infections. In these latter cases the problem often is associated with mesenteric adenitis. This is especially prone to occur with viral infections. In addition, while the terminal ileum often is primarily involved, other segments of the jejunum and ileum also can be involved and this whole problem is discussed later with mesenteric adenitis.

As far as imaging of the foregoing entities is concerned, ultrasonography is becoming more and more dominant in its use for their detection and post therapy monitoring (7–10). In addition, color-flow Doppler is valuable in demonstrating increased blood flow to the inflamed intestine, mesentery, and lymph nodes (3, 4). CT also can demonstrate some of these findings (11, 12) and nuclear scintigraphy also has been used to identify inflammatory bowel disease (13).

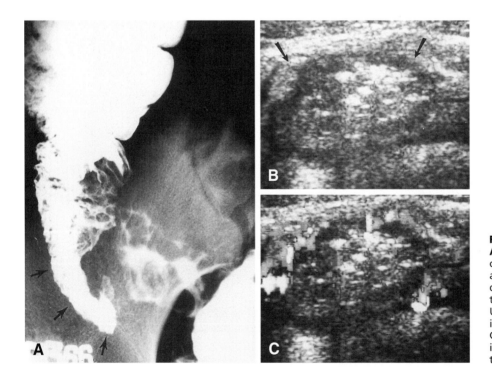

FIGURE 4.117. Regional enteritis. A. In this patient, the cecum is totally deformed and cone-shaped (arrows), and the terminal ileum is markedly deformed with numerous sinusoidal tracts and typical linear ulcerations. **B.** Ultrasonogram demonstrates the inflamed terminal ileum (arrows). **C.** Color-flow Doppler demonstrates the increased blood flow (white blotches) to this inflammatory lesion.

REFERENCES

1. Ablin DS, Jain KS, Azouz EM. Abdominal tuberculosis in children. Pediatr Radiol 1995;24:473–477.
2. Lee DH, Ko YT, Yoon Y, et al. Sonographic findings of intestinal tuberculosis. J Ultrasound Med 1993;12:537–540.
3. Giovagnorio F, Diacinti D, Vernia P. Doppler sonography of the superior mesenteric artery in Crohn's disease. AJR 1998;170:123–126.
4. Spalinger J, Patriquin H, Miron M-C, et al. Doppler US in patients with Crohn disease: vessel density in the diseased bowel reflects disease activity. Radiology 2000;217:787–791.
5. Grant H, Rode H, Cywes S. *Yersinia* pseudotuberculosis affecting the appendix. J Pediatr Surg 1994;29:1621.
6. Sue K, Nishimi T, Yamada T, et al. A right lower abdominal mass due to *Yersinia* mesenteric lymphadenitis. Pediatr Radiol 1994;24:70–71.
7. Faure C, Belarbi N, Mougenot JF, et al. Ultrasonographic assessment of inflammatory bowel disease in children: comparison with ileocolonoscopy. J Pediatr 1997;130:147–151.
8. Frisoli JK, Desser TS, Jeffrey RB. Thickened submucosal layer: a sonographic sign of acute gastrointestinal abnormality representing submucosal edema or hemorrhage. AJR 2000;175:1595–1599.
9. Siegel MJ, Friedland JA, Hildebolt CF. Bowel wall thickening in children: differentiation with US. Radiology 1997;203:631–635.
10. Ruess L, Black ARN, Bulas DI, et al. Inflammatory bowel disease in children and young adults: correlation of sonographic and clinical parameters during treatment. AJR 2000;175:79–84.
11. Jabra AA, Fishman EK, Taylor GA. Pictorial essay. CT findings in inflammatory bowel disease in children. AJR 1994;162:975–979.
12. Hyer W, Beattie RM, Walker-Smith JA. Computed tomography in chronic inflammatory bowel disease. Arch Dis Child 1997;76:428–431.
13. Charron M, Orenstien SR, Bhargava S. Detection of inflammatory bowel disease in pediatric patients with technetium-99m-HMPAO labeled leukocytes. J Nucl Med 1994;35:451–455.

Zollinger-Ellison Syndrome

This condition is uncommon in children and virtually undocumented in infants, and the basic problem is severe peptic ulcer disease of the intestinal tract, primarily the stomach and duodenum. There is pronounced diarrhea and often one sees ulceration and marked edema of the duodenal and proximal small bowel mucosal folds. The condition results from a gastrin-producing tumor of the pancreas, which leads to severe hyperacidity. It also can be one manifestation of the multiple endocrine adenoma syndrome. Radiologic findings consist mostly of the demonstration of ulcers in the stomach and duodenum and thickening of the duodenal and jejunal mucosal folds.

Scleroderma

Scleroderma and some of the other collagen vascular diseases may involve the intestine in childhood. In such cases, one sees extreme dilation of the involved loops of intestine and marked stretching and thinning of the mucosal folds.

Diffusely Thickened Intestinal Mucosal Folds

Diffuse thickening of small intestinal mucosal folds can result from any number of inflammatory or infiltrative disorders, and on barium studies such thickening may be either nodular or straight. Thickening tends to be nodular with conditions such as intestinal lymphangiectasia, cystic fibrosis, giardiasis, strongyloidiasis, and the odd case of Whipple's disease (Fig. 4.118). The latter is seldom seen in

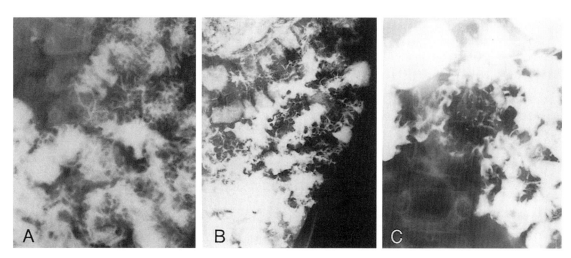

FIGURE 4.118. Thickened mucosal folds: nodular pattern. A. Typical nodular thickening in lymphangiectasia. **B.** Nodular thickening in giardiasis. **C.** Nodular thickening of the proximal small bowel, just distal to the duodenum, in cystic fibrosis.

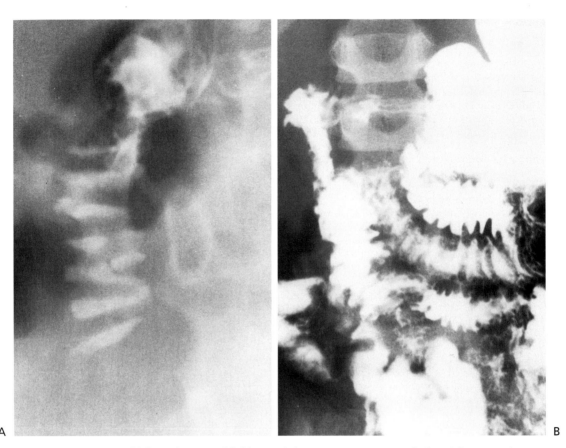

A   B

FIGURE 4.119. Thickened mucosal folds: straight pattern. A. Note typical straight mucosal fold thickening in a patient with eosinophilic gastroenteritis **B.** Straight fold thickening in gastroenteritis.

childhood. Straight, thick mucosal folds usually result from mucosal edema and can be seen in conditions such as protein-losing enteropathy, nephrotic syndrome, cirrhosis, abetalipoproteinemia (1), gastroenteritis, eosinophilic enteritis, hyperacidity (Zollinger-Ellison syndrome), celiac disease (Fig. 4.114), and allergic eosinophilic enteritis. The findings are much the same from condition to condition (Fig. 4.119).

mia (4) and, while the problem might not at first glance suggest necrotizing enterocolitis, the condition almost could be considered focal necrotizing enterocolitis. One of the key features clinically is the **bluish discoloration of the abdomen reflecting extravasation of meconium from the compromised bowel within** (1, 2). Cytomegalic inclusion virus and *Candida* infections have been implicated in this condition (5–7).

REFERENCE

1. Weinstein MA, Pearson KD, Agus SG. Abetalipoproteinemia. Radiology 1973;108:269–273.

Spontaneous Small Bowel Ulceration and Perforation in Premature Infants

This is an increasingly common entity whose etiology is unknown, but it is suspected that the problem is focal ischemia to the intestine of the premature infant (1–3). Indomethacin therapy has been associated with such sche-

REFERENCES

1. Harms K, Ludtke F-E, Lepsien G. Idiopathic intestinal perforations in premature infants without evidence of necrotizing enterocolitis. Eur J Pediatr Surg 1995;5:30–33.
2. Mintz AC, Applebaum H. Focal gastrointestinal perforations not associated with necrotizing enterocolitis in very low birth weight neonates. J Pediatr Surg 1993;28:857–860.
3. Huang S-F, Vacanti J, Kozakewich H. Semental defect of the intestinal musculature of a newborn. Evidence of acquired pathogenesis. J Pediatr Surg 1996;31:721–725.
4. Tatakawa Y, Muraji T, Imai Y, et al. the mechanism of focal intestinal perforation in neonates with low birth weight. Pediatr Surg Int 1999;15:549–552.

5. Adderson EE, Pappin A, Pavia AT. Spontaneous intestinal perforation in premature infants: a distinct clinical entity associated with a systemic candidiasis. J Pediatr Surg 1998;33:1463–1467.
6. Huang Y-C, Lin T-Y, Huang C-S, et al. Ileal perforation caused by congenital or perinatal cytomegalovirus infection. J Pediatr 1996;129:931–934.
7. Reyes C, Pereira S, Warden MJ, et al. Cytomegalovirus enteritis in a premature infant. J Pediatr Surg 1997;32:1545–1547.

Parasitic Infestation

Infestation by parasites can occur with *Giardia* (1, 2), *Strongyloides*, *Ascaris*, and *Anisakis* (3). *Anisakiasis* represents an uncommon entity that results from the eating of raw fish. It manifests in thickening of intestinal mucosa. Giardiasis frequently produces a fine nodular pattern in the small bowel (Fig. 4.120A) and frequently is associated with immunodeficiency diseases. With ascariasis, the worm may be seen on plain films or an upper GI series (Fig. 4.120, B and C) or even with ultrasound (4) *Ascaris* may pass into the biliary tract, bore through the intestine and produce peritonitis (5), or form a conglomerate of worms in the intestines, leading to obstruction (6, 7).

REFERENCES

1. Burke JA. Giardiasis in childhood. Am J Dis Child 1975;129: 1304–1310.
2. Gunasekaran TS, Hassal E. Giardiasis mimicking inflammatory bowel disease. J Pediatr 1992;120:424–426.

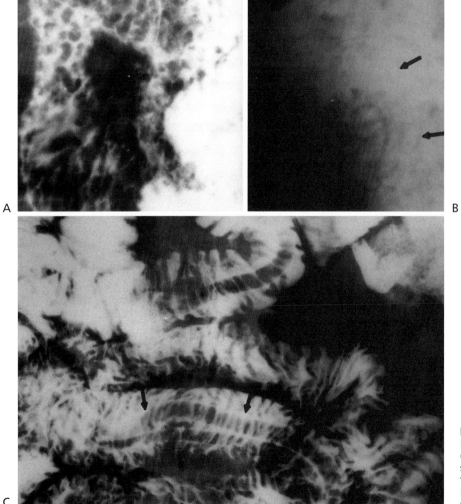

FIGURE 4.120. Parasitic disease. A. Nodular and tortuous mucosal fold thickening in giardiasis. **B.** Plain films demonstrating numerous roundworms (arrows) in the intestine. **C.** Same patient demonstrating linear-tubular small bowel filling defects (arrows) typical of ascariasis.

3. Shirahama M, Koga T, Ishibashi H, et al. Intestinal anisakiasis: US in diagnosis. Radiology 1992;185:789–793.
4. Ozmen MN, Oguzkurt L, Ahmet B, et al. Ultrasonographic diagnosis of intestinal ascariasis. Pediatr Radiol 1995;25:S171–S172.
5. Mello CMG, Briggs M, do Carno F, et al. Granulomatous peritonitis by *Ascaris*. J Pediatr Surg 1992;27:1229–1230.
6. Mohta A, Bagga D, Malhotra CJ, et al. Intestinal obstruction due to roundworms. Pediatr Surg Int 1993;8:226–228.
7. Rode H, Cullis S, Millar A, et al. Abdominal complications of *Ascaris lumbricoides* in children. Pediatr Surg Int 1990;5:397–401.

Henoch-Schönlein Purpura

In this acute bleeding problem resulting from an acute vasculitis, intramural intestinal hematomas are common (2). Findings on the upper GI series include thumbprinting, a stacked coin appearance (Fig. 4.121A), and nonspecific mural thickening suggesting submucosal edema. The condition is self-limiting and, while the radiographic findings are nonspecific, in the proper clinical setting they are highly suggestive of the diagnosis. In a few cases, intestinal necrosis can lead to entero-entero fistulas (1).

Ultrasound is very useful in detecting the intestinal findings in this condition (2–4). This is important because ultrasound is increasingly being used for the evaluation of acute abdominal problems in childhood. **Many times, Henoch-Schönlein purpura presents with abdominal pain rather than the typical purpuric rash.** In such cases, if one identifies segments of intestine with thickened mucosa (Fig. 4.121, B and C), one should be suspicious of diagnosis. Thickening usually is circumferential but can be eccentric. In addition, fluid in the abdomen can be seen, and in some cases, an intramural hematoma may mimic an

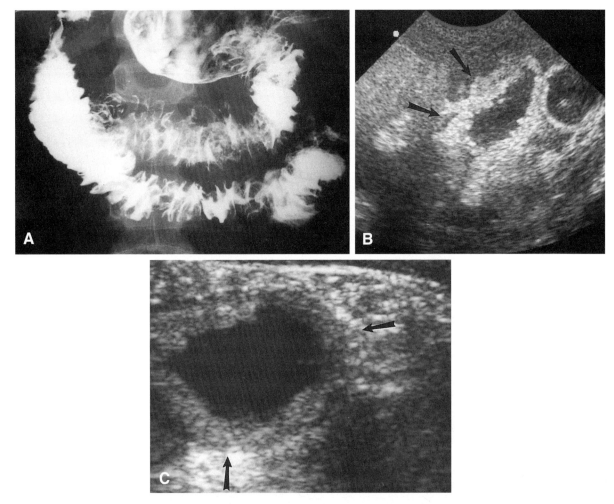

FIGURE 4.121. Henoch-Schönlein purpura. A. Typical thickening of the small intestine mucosa. **B.** Early mucosal thickening (arrows) as seen with ultrasound. **C.** Another patient demonstrating circumferential thickening of the mucosa (arrows) of an involved loop of intestine.

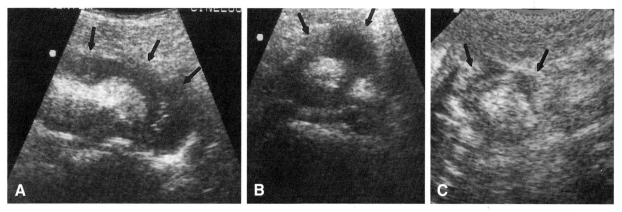

FIGURE 4.122. Henoch-Schönlein purpura: intramural hematoma mimicking intussusception. A. Longitudinal view demonstrates the intramural hematoma (arrows) centrally compressing the echogenic mucosa. The findings resemble those of intussusception. **B.** Similar findings (arrows) on cross-sectional view. **C.** Approximately 10 days later, the hematoma has almost completely resolved (arrows).

intussusception (3) (Fig. 4.122). This is important, because intussusception is a relatively common complication of Henoch-Schönlein purpura, but confusion was more common in the past when sector ultrasound scanners were used. With high-frequency linear scanners, one usually can differentiate a hematoma from the multilayered appearance of an intussusception. With Henoch-Schönlein purpura, other organ systems can be involved, including the kidney. In these cases a nonspecific hemorrhagic nephritis is seen, and on ultrasound the kidneys demonstrate increased echogenicity. Stenosing ureteritis also has been documented with Henoch-Sch^nlein purpura (5).

REFERENCES

1. Gow KW, Murphy JJ III, Blain GK, et al. Multiple entero-entero fistulae: an unusual complication of Henoch-Schönlein purpura. J Pediatr Surg 1996;31:809–811.
2. Coputure A, Veyrac C, Baud C, et al. Evaluation of abdominal pain in Henoch-Schonlein syndrome by high frequency ultrasound. Pediatr Radiol 1992;22:12–17.
3. John SD, Swischuk LE, Hayden CK. Gastrointestinal sonographic findings in Henoch-Schonlein purpura. Emerg Radiol 1996;3:4–8.
4. Kagimoto S. Duodenal findings on ultrasound in children with Schonlein-Henoch purpura and gastrointestinal symptoms. J Pediatr Gastroenterol Nutr 1993;16:178–182.
5. Smet M-H, Marchal G, Oyen R, et al. Stenosing hemorrhagic ureteritis in a child with Henoch-Schonlein purpura: CT appearance. J Comput Assist Tomogr 1991;15:326–328.

Hemolytic Uremic Syndrome

The GI tract can be involved in the hemolytic uremic syndrome, in which nonspecific thickening of the mucosa of the intestines is seen (1).

REFERENCE

1. Siegler RL. Spectrum of extrarenal involvement in postdiarrheal hemolytic-uremic syndrome. J Pediatr 1994;125:511–518.

Lymphoid Hyperplasia

Lymphoid hyperplasia usually is seen in the colon, but it also can be seen in the small bowel where it produces small submucosal nodules (Fig. 4.123). The finding, however, is nonspecific and also can be seen with immunologic deficiency, allergy, and as a normal finding.

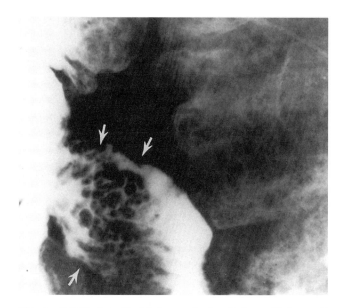

Figure 4.123. Lymphoid hyperplasia. Note multiple small nodules (arrows) in the terminal ileum and less well-seen nodules in the poorly filled more proximal small bowel.

Tumors and Tumorous Conditions of the Small Bowel

Intestinal lymphangiectasia and lymphoma probably are the most common tumors of the small bowel in young infants, but occasionally one can encounter sarcomas (1, 2), adenocarcinoma (3), leiomyomas (1), solitary or multiple hemangiomas (4), AV malformations (5, 6), hamartomas, fibromas (7, 8), and solitary or multicentric lymphoma. Polyps are relatively uncommon, except in the Peutz-Jeghers syndrome. This condition is usually seen in older children (10) but has been documented in an infant as young as 11 months (9) and in a neonate (10). The polyps often are large and nodular and relatively easily detected both with ultrasound and GI series (Fig. 4.124). Bleeding and intussusception with obstruction are common presentations.

Localized tumors can present with obstruction, perforation, or bleeding, whereas intestinal lymphangiectasia often presents as a problem of hypoproteinemia secondary to protein-losing enteropathy (11). Roentgenographically, the small bowel in intestinal lymphangiectasia usually shows thickened, tortuous, or nodular mucosal folds (see Fig. 4.118A). If protein-losing enteropathy supervenes, edema of the folds can cause them to become straighter.

Lymphoma of the small bowel in the older child and adult often is segmental, but in young infants, it tends to be more diffuse, and some cases are familial. Small bowel contrast studies show areas of segmental narrowing, bowel rigidity, and nodular filling defects (Fig. 4.125). Some of these cases may represent lymphoma of the mesentery with secondary involvement of the intestine. Ultrasonographically lymphoma tends to be somewhat hypoechoic and the masses produced can be rather extensive.

REFERENCES

1. Gupta AK, Berry M, Mitra DK. Gastrointestinal smooth muscle tumors in children: report of three cases. Pediatr Radiol 1995; 24:498–499.
2. Kennedy AP Jr, Cameron B, Dorion RP, et al. Pediatric intestinal leiomyosarcomas. Case report and review of the literature. J Pediatric Surg 1997;32:1234–1236.
3. Tankel JW, Galasko CSB. Adenocarcinoma of small bowel in a 12-year-old girl. J R Soc Med 1984;77:693–694.

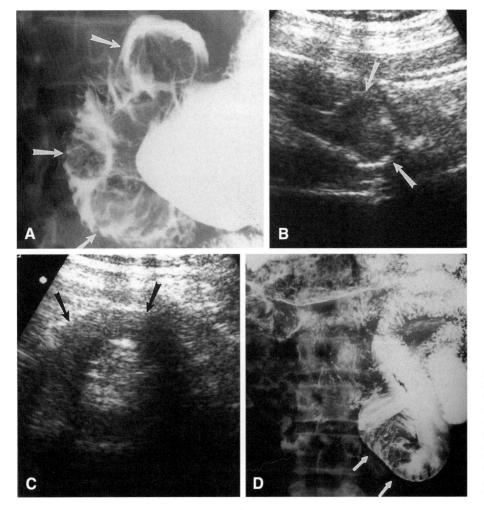

FIGURE 4.124. Peutz-Jeghers syndrome. A. Typical polyps (arrows) in the duodenum. **B.** Ultrasonographic demonstration of one of these polyps (arrows). **C.** Ultrasound also demonstrates the presence of an intussusception (arrows). **D.** Upper GI series demonstrates the intussusception in the distal small bowel (arrows). In addition the stomach was carpeted with small polyps.

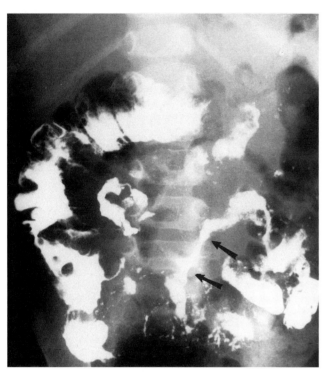

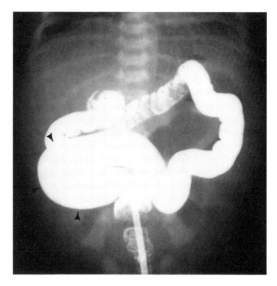

FIGURE 4.126. Normal colon. Rectal tube with distended Foley bulb is in the rectum. Note the redundancy and normal right-sided positioning of the sigmoid colon (arrows). The remainder of the colon is of normal caliber, and a few haustral markings are seen in the transverse colon.

FIGURE 4.125. Lymphosarcoma of small bowel. Note the stenotic, deformed segment of small bowel in the distal jejunum (arrows).

4. Scafidi DE, McLeary MS, Young LW. Diffuse neonatal gastrointestinal hemangiomatosis: CT findings. Pediatr Radiol 1998;28: 512–514.

5. Park JM, Yeon KM, Han MC, et al. Diffuse intestinal arteriovenous malformation in a child. Pediatr Radiol 1991;21:314–315.

6. Fremond B, Yazbeck S, Dubois J, et al. Intestinal vascular anomalies in children. J Pediatr Surg 1997;32:873–877.

7. Basak D, Roy SKS. Congenital fibromatosis of the ileum. Pediatr Surg Int 1992;7:300–302.

8. Chang WWL, Griffith KM. Solitary intestinal fibromatosis: a rare cause of intestinal obstruction in neonate and infant. J Pediatr Surg 1991;26:1406–1408.

9. Morens DM, Garvey SP. An unusual case of Peutz-Jeghers syndrome in an infant. Am J Dis Child 1975;129:973–976.

10. Fernandez Seara MJ, Martrinez Soto MI, Fernandez Lorenzo Jr, et al. Peutz-Jeghers syndrome in a neonate. J Pediatr 1995;126: 965–967.

11. Kingham JGC, Moriarty KJ, Furness M, et al. Lymphangiectasis of the colon and small intestine. Br J Radiol 1982;55:774–777.

COLON

Normal Configuration

The colon in infants and young children appears a little different from that seen in adults, and one of the most important of these differences is generalized redundancy (Fig. 4.126). The colon also shows less prominent haustral folds, and the cecum often is high and more medially located than one would expect (see Fig. 4.86). More importantly, perhaps, is that one appreciate redundancy of the sigmoid flexure (1) which often presents itself as a "fixed loop" mimicking the fixed loop of sigmoid volvulus in necrotizing enterocolitis (Fig. 4.127).

REFERENCE

1. Fiorella DJ, Donnelly LF. Frequency of right lower quadrant position of the sigmoid colon in infants and young children. Radiology 2001;219:91–94.

ABNORMALITIES OF THE COLON

Hirschsprung's Disease (Aganglionosis of the Colon)

Aganglionic megacolon (i.e., Hirschsprung's disease) most frequently presents in the neonate where the infants usually are full term and, except for cases of total aganglionosis usually male. In total aganglionosis, females predominate. Initial symptoms in Hirschsprung's disease may be atypical in the neonatal period. Obstruction may not be striking, and in some cases, the main problem may be diarrhea. In others, however, obstruction with vomiting is the major presenting feature, and failure to pass meconium within the first 24 hours of life should be treated with considerable concern.

Aganglionosis of the colon most commonly involves the distal colon, specifically the rectal and rectosigmoid regions.

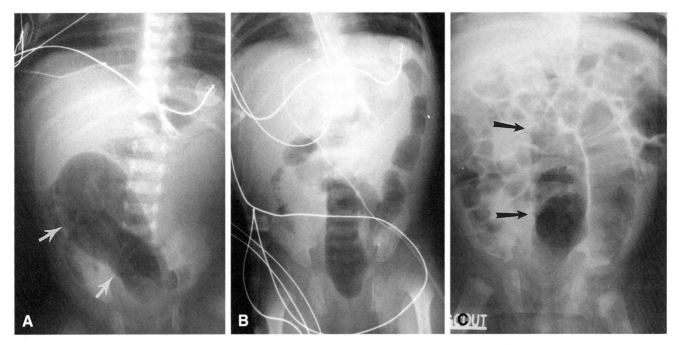

FIGURE 4.127. Normal redundant sigmoid colon. A. In this infant, the air-filled sigmoid colon (arrows) may erroneously suggest the fixed loop of necrotizing enterocolitis or even sigmoid volvulus. **B.** With prone positioning, air is redistributed in the colon and now is in the rectum and descending colon, confirming that the air-filled sigmoid colon in **A** is normal. **C.** Older infant with a prominent redundant, but normal, sigmoid colon (arrows).

Total colon aganglionosis is rare and usually associated with aganglionosis, or rarely, atresia (1) of a variable length of distal small bowel. In addition, cases have been documented with aganglionosis up to the level of the duodenum (2–4), and there is some suggestion that such cases (total intestinal aganglionosis) are inherited as an autosomal recessive condition (3). Hirschsprung's disease also may be familial (5–8).

Skip areas in Hirschsprung's disease, if they occur, must be extremely uncommon and, if current concepts of neuroblast migration down the GI tract are accepted (9), would seem unlikely to exist. It is more likely that such areas represent areas of intrauterine ischemic insult where, among other things, ganglion cells are destroyed. Support for this concept lies in the fact that some cases of Hirschsprung's disease have been described in association with colon or small bowel atresia (10–12). Complications of undiagnosed Hirschsprung's disease are serious and include enterocolitis (13, 14), perforation of the appendix in the neonate (15–17), exudative enteropathy, and failure to thrive. Enterocolitis problems also can arise after pull-through procedures (18), and in all cases the etiology of enterocolitis probably lies in the realm of impaired mucosal defense mechanisms resulting from schemia secondary to chronic overdistention of the intestine (19).

The precise etiology of Hirschsprung's disease is not known, but it has been accepted for some time that the problem stems from the absence of ganglion cells in the myenteric plexus of the involved segment. This results from failure of normal caudal migration of neuroblasts in the developing embryo and fetus (9). Normally, neuroblasts descend down the GI tract until they reach the anus. However, their descent can be arrested at any level but it is not known why this should occur. Nonetheless, it does get arrested, and most often this occurs in the rectosigmoid region. In addition it has been noted that in the normal maturation of neuroblast ganglion cells the last neuroblasts to fully mature are those of the distal colon (20), a concept not out of keeping with the failure of neuronal descent theory.

After Hirschsprung's disease is suspected clinically, contrast enema examination is mandatory, but it must be stressed that this examination alone does not produce a definitive diagnosis in every case. In this regard, the younger the infant, the more difficult the diagnosis and in the neonate the diagnosis may be very subtle. Studies have documented normal results in 20–30% of cases (21–22). Nonetheless, whatever the circumstances, once Hirschsprung's disease is suspected clinically, even though suspicions may be low, rectal biopsy usually becomes necessary. Suction mucosal biopsy without general anesthesia is a valuable procedure, because if it demonstrates abundant normal ganglion cells, the diagnosis of Hirschsprung's disease can, for the most part, be dismissed. However, if no ganglion cells are present, there is no way to determine whether they are absent or the biopsy was too shallow. For this reason full-thickness biopsy under general anesthesia then is required. A suggested approach to the investigation of patients with suspected Hirschsprung's disease is presented in Table 4.2. Manometric measurements of intrarectal pressures also can be used in the diagnosis of Hirschsprung's disease in equivocal cases, and biochemically, acetylcholinesterase activity in biopsies of Hirschsprung's disease has been noted to be abnormally high (23).

In the neonate, plain abdominal roentgenograms in the typical case of Hirschsprung's disease usually show some degree of low small bowel or colonic obstruction. Colonic obstruction can be massive (Fig. 4.128A), and rectal gas may be absent. In other cases, less pronounced findings are seen (Fig. 4.128B). In any case, once Hirschsprung's disease is suspected one should proceed to contrast enema examination.

In terms of subsequent contrast enema examination, one does not necessarily need to fill the colon past the tran-

sition zone, which is the point at which the colon becomes dilated. If one elects to use water-soluble contrast agents (21), then it is best to use anionic rather than hyperosmolar ones such as Gastrografin. The reason for this is that, if one overfills the intestine with Gastrografin, one can encounter a fluid shift into the colon and accompanying dehydration and electrolyte disturbances. In our institution we start with barium, and when we encounter findings that suggest Hirschsprung's disease as the most likely possibility, we stop the study. If we believe that the meconium plug syndrome is the most likely possibility, we change to Gastrografin diluted 3:1 and proceed with a therapeutic enema.

If one can demonstrate a transition zone with clarity (Fig. 4.129), the diagnosis of Hirschsprung's disease can be made with reasonable certainty. Many times, the involved segment demonstrates peculiar contractions (Fig. 4.129). However, it cannot be overstressed that the characteristic transition zone

TABLE 4.2. HIRSCHSPRUNG'S DISEASE—SUGGESTED MANAGEMENT

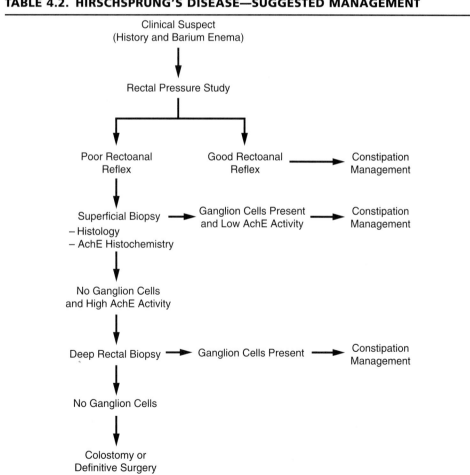

AchE, acetylcholinesterase.
Adapted from Morikawa Y, Donahoe PK, Hendren WH. Manometry and histochemistry in the diagnosis of Hirschsprung's disease. *Pediatrics* 1979;63:865–871, with permission.

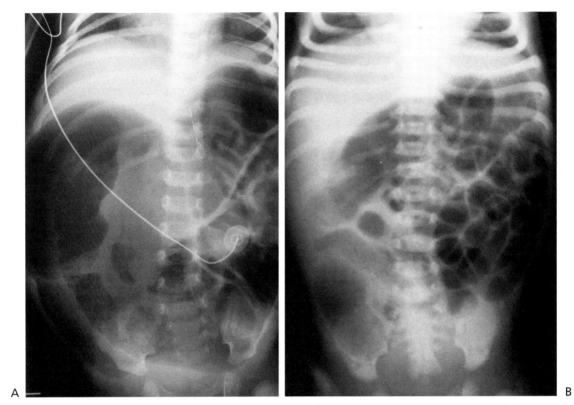

FIGURE 4.128. Hirschsprung's disease: plain film findings. A. Note considerable dilatation of the air-filled colon. **B.** Less pronounced changes in another patient with most of the distended colon being in the right lower quadrant.

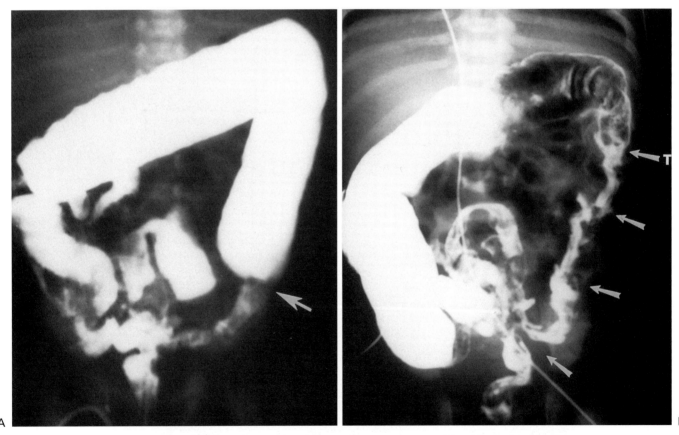

FIGURE 4.129. Hirschsprung's disease: transition zone. A. In this patient, the transition zone (arrow) is clearly defined in the lower descending colon. **B.** In this patient, there is a long segment of aganglionic descending colon (arrows) with a high transition zone (T). Note the peculiar contractions of the involved segment, which extend to the rectum.

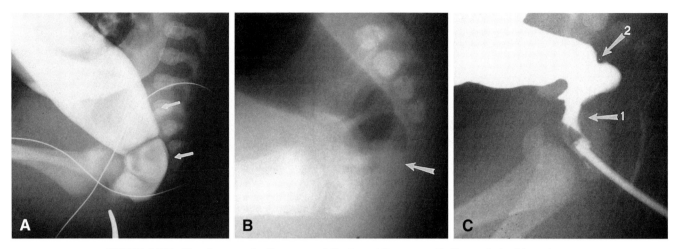

FIGURE 4.130. Hirschsprung's disease: subtle transition zone findings. A. In this patient, the abnormal rectosigmoid region simply demonstrates mild tapering (arrows). **B.** In another patient there is absence of gas in the very distal rectum (arrow) but distention of the more proximal rectum and colon. **C.** A subsequent contrast enema demonstrates a partially contracted distal rectal segment. A prominent puborectalis sling indentation (1) is seen but has nothing to do with the diagnosis of Hirschsprung's disease. A transition zone may be suggested at level 2 (2), but overall, the findings are less than pathognomonic.

between the abnormal aganglionic and normal ganglionic colon is not always precisely demarcated (Fig. 4.130). In still other cases, especially in the neonate, the aganglionic segment may show abnormal contractions manifesting in spastic corrugation or serration (24) of the involved colonic segment (Fig. 4.131). In still other cases, again in neonates and very young infants, the rectosigmoid region may appear surprisingly normal (Fig. 4.132). In many of these cases, very straight transverse bands are seen in the involved segment of colon (Fig. 4.133). These bands probably represent areas of persistent spasm, and can serve as additional positive clues to the presence of Hirschsprung's disease in difficult cases.

The rectosigmoid index (25) also can be used in the diagnosis of Hirschsprung's disease. In these cases, the

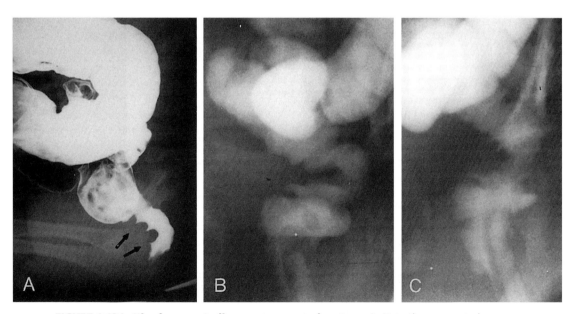

FIGURE 4.131. Hirschsprung's disease: corrugated rectum. A. Note the corrugated appearance of the rectum (arrows). A transition zone is present. **B.** Another patient with no clear-cut transition zone but a peculiar convoluted or corrugated-appearing rectum. **C.** Lateral view of the same patient.

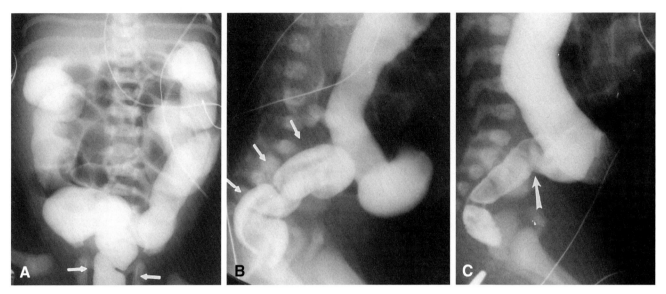

FIGURE 4.132. Hirschsprung's disease: false-normal findings. A. On this contrast enema, note that the rectum (arrows) has a near-normal appearance. **B.** Lateral view again suggests that the rectum (arrows) is normal. **C.** On another film, the rectosigmoid region is narrowed, and a transition zone (arrow) is suggested.

transverse measurement of the rectum is compared with that of the sigmoid colon. Normally, these measurements demonstrate either a 1:1 relationship or the rectal diameter is greater. If, however, the rectal diameter is less than the sigmoid diameter (i.e., less than a 1:1 ratio), even if not very striking, Hirschsprung's disease should be suspected (Fig. 4.133D). Short segment, distal rectal aganglionosis always is a problem (26). In the older infant, it may be impossible to distinguish the findings from those of functional megacolon but this is not such a problem because both are treated the same (27). Treatment primarily consists of dilatation of the anal sphincter.

Twenty-four hour delay films still are a good method with which to judge degree of colon emptying but they are helpful only when most of the contrast agent is retained. Although we obtain 24-hour delay films, we assess them with some caution. Nonetheless, these delayed films are still useful, especially in puzzling cases (Fig. 4.134).

Total colon aganglionosis also can present considerable difficulty in diagnosis. In these cases, plain films demonstrate a low small bowel, rather than colonic obstruction, and although in some cases the contrast-filled colon appears normal, in others, it may be shorter and smoother than normal. It has a more adult-like configuration, because the various flexures become less redundant, the haustral markings become sparser, and overall, the colon shows generalized peculiar contractions and convolutions throughout (Fig. 4.134). In addition to these configurations, in one study, a microcolon (spastic empty colon) was demonstrated in 38% of cases, and a normal colon in 22% of cases (28). The terminal ileum may or may not be involved (29, 30). Reflux

of barium in large volumes into the terminal ileum and small bowel frequently occurs in these infants and is a useful diagnostic feature (Fig. 4.134).

Enterocolitis, as previously noted, is a definite problem in Hirschsprung's disease and, although not overly common, can be devastating when it occurs. These patients present with profound diarrhea, often bloody, and the contrast enema findings can be striking. Generally, they show intense spasm and mucosal edema, irregularity, cobblestoning, and ulceration (Fig. 4.135). In some cases, pneumatosis cystoides intestinalis can develop.

Hirschsprung's disease in older children usually presents with a constipation (Fig. 4.136A). In some cases, acute gaseous dilatation can occur but most often the problem is chronic constipation. In some of these cases a clearcut transition zone is identified but in most cases the findings are those of low segment Hirschsprung's disease (Fig. 4.136C) and difficult to differentiate from those of functional megacolon. However, the point may be moot as the treatment is usually the same.

Associated anomalies in Hirschsprung's disease are generally considered to be fortuitous, and associated urinary tract abnormality, although not entirely uncommon, is generally not believed to be the result of associated aganglionosis of the urinary tract. The changes are believed to more likely be secondary to displacement of the bladder and ureters by the distended rectum with resulting abnormal trigone function. Hirschsprung's disease also has been documented, probably as an incidental finding with imperforate anus (31) and as a part of the complex of neuroblastoma, Ondine's curse, and neurocristopathy (32–35).

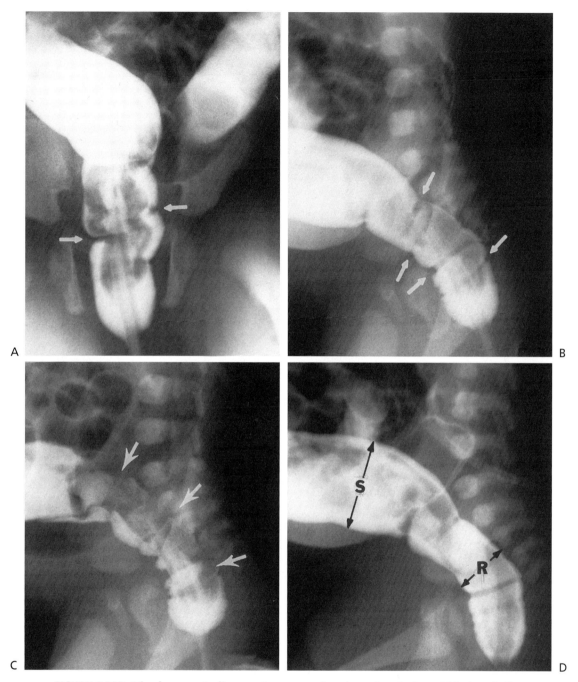

FIGURE 4.133. Hirschsprung's disease: transverse bands and rectosigmoid index. A. On this anteroposterior view, note the transverse folds (arrows) in the partially distended rectum. **B.** Lateral view demonstrates the same folds (arrows). **C.** Later, irregular contractions are seen in the involved segment (arrows). **D.** Another patient with similar transverse folds. **The rectosigmoid index** in this patient is abnormal. The diameter of the rectum (R) is much less than the diameter of the sigmoid colon (S).

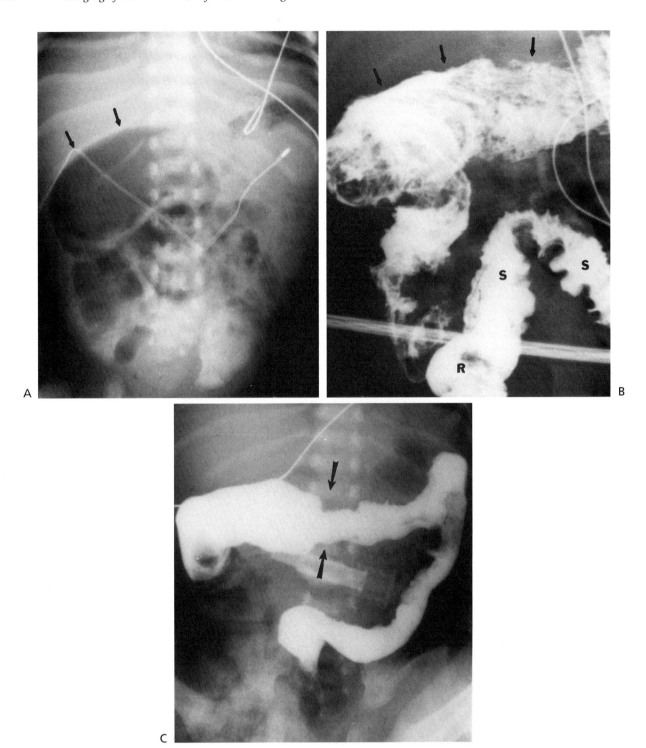

FIGURE 4.134. Hirschsprung's disease: value of 24-hour delay film. A. Newborn infant demonstrating dilatation of the proximal transverse colon (arrows). The ascending colon also is dilated. **B.** Contrast enema demonstrates a dilated transverse colon (arrows) without an obvious transition zone. The ascending colon is irregular and contracted. Similarly, the rectum and sigmoid colon are contracted and narrow. **C.** Twenty-four hours later, most of the contrast remains in the colon, but now a clear-cut transition zone (arrows) is demarcated.

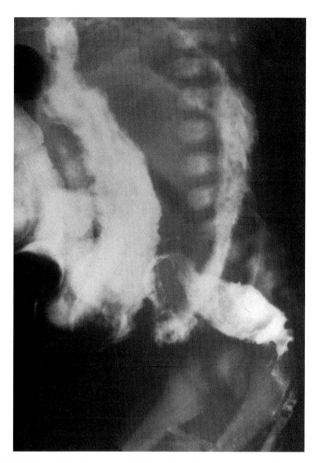

FIGURE 4.135. Enterocolitis with Hirschsprung's disease.
Note the spastic colon with widespread mucosal ulceration and edema.

REFERENCES

1. Janik JP, Wayne ER, Janik JS, et al. Ileal atresia with total colonic aganglionosis. J Pediatr Surg 1997;32:1502–1503.
2. Ahmed S, Cohen SJ, Jacobs SI. Total intestinal aganglionosis presenting as duodenal obstruction. Arch Dis Child 1971;46:868–869.
3. Caniano DA, Ormsbee HS III, Polito W, et al. Total intestinal aganglionosis. J Pediatr Surg 1985;20:456–460.
4. Stringer MD, Brereton RJ, Drake DP, et al. Meconium ileus due to extensive intestinal aganglionosis. J Pediatr Surg 1994;29:501–503.
5. Engum SA, Petrites M, Rescorla FJ, et al. Familial Hirschsprung's disease: 20 cases in 12 kindreds. J Pediatr Surg 1993;28:1286–1290.
6. Reyna CTM. Familial Hirschsprung's disease: study of a Texas cohort. Pediatrics 1994;94:347–349.
7. Schiller M, Levy P, Shawa RA, et al. Familial Hirschsprung's disease: a report of 22 affected siblings in four families. J Pediatr Surg 1990;25:322–325.
8. Stannard VA, Fowler C, Robinson L, et al. Familial Hirschsprung's disease: report of autosomal dominant and probable recessive X-linked kindreds. J Pediatr Surg 1991;26:591–594.
9. Okamoto E, Ueda T. Embryogenesis of the intramural ganglia of the gut and its relation to Hirschsprung's disease. J Pediatr Surg 1967;2:437–443.
10. Kim PCW, Superina RA, Ein S. Colonic atresia combined with Hirschsprung's disease: a diagnostic and therapeutic challenge. J Pediatr Surg 1995;30:1216–1217.
11. Moore SW, Rode H, Millar AJW, et al. Intestinal atresia and Hirschsprung's disease. Pediatr Surg Int 1990;5:182–184.
12. Weinberg RJ, Klish WJ, Smalley JR, et al. Acquired distal aganglionosis of the colon. J Pediatr 1982;101:406–409.
13. Elhalaby EA, Coran AG, Blane CE, et al. Enterocolitis associated with Hirschsprung's disease: a clinical-radiological characterization based on 168 patients. J. Pediatric Surg 1995;30:76–83.
14. Teich S, Schisgall RM, Anderson KD. Ischemic enterocolitis as a complication of Hirschsprung's disease. J Pediatr Surg 1986;21:143–145.
15. Arliss J, Holgersen LO. Neonatal appendiceal perforation and Hirschsprung's disease. J Pediatr Surg 1990;25:694–695.
16. Martin LW, Perrin EV. Neonatal perforation of the appendix in association with Hirschsprung's disease. Ann Surg 1967;166:799–802.
17. Stringer MD, Drake DP. Hirschsprung's disease presenting as neonatal gastrointestinal perforation. Br J Surg 1991;78:188–189.
18. Blane CE, Elhalaby E, Coran AG. Enterocolitis following endorectal pull-through procedure in children with Hirschsprung's disease. Pediatr Radiol 1994;24:164–166.
19. Wilson-Storey D, Scobie WG. Impaired gastrointestinal mucosal defense in Hirschsprung's disease: a clue to the pathogenesis of enterocolitis? J Pediatr Surg 1989;24:462–464.
20. Smith B. Pre- and postnatal development of the ganglion cells of the rectum and its surgical implications. J Pediatr Surg 1968;3:386–391.
21. O'Donovan AN, Habra G, Somers S, et al. Diagnosis of Hirschsprung's disease. AJR 1996;167:517–520.
22. Smith GHH, Cass D. Infantile Hirschsprung's disease—is a barium enema useful? Pediatr Surg Int 1991;6:318–321.
23. Meier-Ruge W, Lutterbeck PM, Herzog B, et al. Acetylcholinesterase activity in suction biopsies of the rectum in the diagnosis of Hirschsprung's disease. J Pediatr Surg 1972;7:11–17.
24. Swischuk LE, Barr LL, Stansberry SD. The corrugated rectum in infantile Hirschsprung's disease. Appl Radiol 1989;18:52–53.
25. Pockaczevsky R, Leonidas JC. The "rectosigmoid index": a measurement for the early diagnosis of Hirschsprung's disease. AJR 1975;123:770–777.
26. Neilson IR, Yazbeck S. Ultrashort Hirschsprung's disease: myth or reality. J Pediatr Surg 1990;25:1135–1138.
27. Nissan S, Bar-Maor JA. Further experience in the diagnosis and surgical treatment of the short-segment Hirschsprung's disease and idiopathic megacolon. J Pediatr Surg 1971;6:738–741.
28. DeCampo JF, Mayne V, Boldt DW, et al. Radiological findings in total aganglionosis coli. Pediatr Radiol 1984;14:205–209.
29. Takada Y, Aoyama K, Goto T, et al. The association of imperforate anus and Hirschsprung's disease in siblings. J Pediatr Surg 1985;20:271–273.
30. Fekete CN, Ricour C, Martelli H, et al. Total colonic aganglionosis (with or without ileal involvement): a review of 27 cases. J Pediatr Surg 1986;21:251–254.
31. Ikeda K, Goto S. Total colonic aganglionosis with or without small bowel involvement: an analysis of 137 patients. J Pediatr Surg 1986;21:319–322.
32. Essman E-H, Coran AG. Hirschsprung's disease associated with

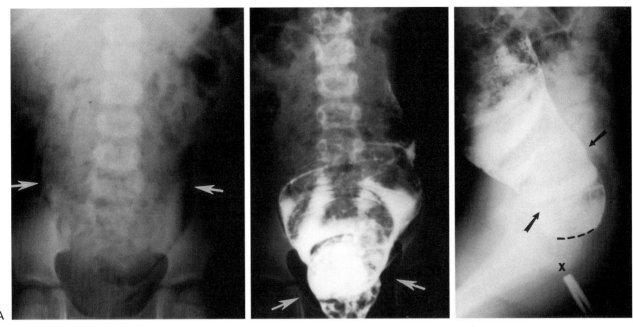

FIGURE 4.136. Hirschsprung's disease: older patient. A. Note the markedly distended rectum (arrows) full of fecal material. **B.** Anteroposterior view of barium enema demonstrates similar findings but note that the rectum (arrows) is not as dilated in its distal portion as it is proximally. This constitutes a reversed rectosigmoid index. **C.** Lateral view demonstrates similar findings in the rectum (arrows). The doted line represents the end of the opacified rectum. The tip of the forceps identifies the location of the anus (X). The space between the doted line and the anus is not filled because of puborectalis spasm. This patient had low-segment Hirschsprung's disease, often impossible to differentiate from functional megacolon.

Ondine's curse: report of three cases and review. J Pediatr Surg 1994;29:530–534.

33. Nakahara S, Yokomori K, Tamura K, et al. Hirschsprung's disease associated with Ondine's curse: a special subgroup? J Pediatr Surg 1995;30:1481–1484.
34. Roshkow JE, Haller J, Berdon WE, et al. Hirschsprung's disease, Ondine's curse and neurocristopathy. Pediatr Radiol 1988;19:45–49.
35. Stovroff M, Dykes F, Teague WG. The complete spectrum of neurocristopathy in an infant with congenital hypoventilation, Hirschsprung's disease, and neuroblastoma. J Pediatr Surg 1995;30:1218–1221.

Conditions Mimicking Hirschsprung's Disease

A number of conditions can mimic Hirschsprung's disease clinically and radiologically; of these, the best known is the neonatal meconium plug or small left colon syndrome. The roentgenographic findings can be indistinguishable, but as opposed to Hirschsprung's disease, the latter entity simply represents a problem of transient functional immaturity of the colon. This problem is discussed in more detail in the next section.

Another group of infants mimicking those with Hirschsprung's disease are those patients with a neuronal colonic dysplasia, a rare condition in which there is hyper-plasia of the ganglion cells in the myenteric plexus (1–5). Plexiform neurofibromatosis (6, 7) also can produce roentgenographic findings that are indistinguishable from those of Hirschsprung's disease (Fig. 4.137).

REFERENCES

1. Gillick J, Tazawa H, Puri P. Intestinal neuronal dysplasia: results of treatment in 33 patients. J Pediatr Surg 2001;36:777–779.
2. Gittes GK, Kim J, Yu G, et al. Severe constipation with diffuse intestinal myenteric hyperganglionosis. J Pediatr Surg 1993;28:1630–1632.
3. Kobayashi H, Hirakawa H, Puri P. Is intestinal neuronal dysplasia a disorder of the neuromuscular junction? J Pediatr Surg 1996;31:575–579.
4. Mya GH, Ng WF, Cheng W, et al. Colonic hyperganglionosis presenting as neonatal enterocolitis and multiple strictures. J Pediatr Surg 1994;29:1628–1630.
5. Simpser E, Kahn E, Kenigsberg K, et al. Neuronal intestinal dysplasia: quantitative diagnostic criteria and clinical management. J Pediatr Gastroenterol Nutr 1991;12:61–64.
6. Staple TW, McAlister WH, Anderson MS. Plexiform neurofibromatosis of the colon simulating Hirschsprung's disease. AJR 1964;91:840–845.
7. Stone MM, Weinberg B, Beck AR, et al. Colonic obstruction in a child with von Recklinghausen's neurofibromatosis. J Pediatr Surg 1986;21:741–743.

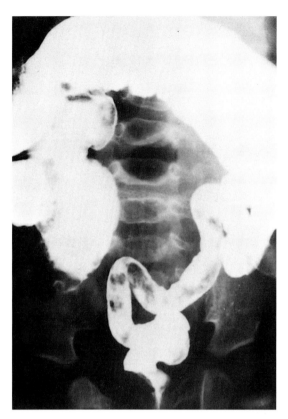

Figure 4.137. Plexiform neurofibromatosis mimicking Hirschsprung's disease. Note the distended transverse colon and small left colon. A transition zone is suggested. The findings would be most difficult to differentiate from Hirschsprung's disease. (Courtesy of Al Felman, M.D.)

Functional Megacolon

Functional megacolon is not a problem of the neonate, but it is commonly encountered thereafter, where often it is the result of intense anorectal spasm secondary to anal fissures. Roentgenographically, in these patients the hypertrophied puborectalis muscle or sling (1) produces a pronounced posterior indentation on the lower rectum (Fig. 4.138). However, it often is difficult to differentiate these patients from those with extremely low, short segment Hirschsprung's disease (see Fig. 4.136), but the distinction may be moot, because treatment of the two conditions generally is the same and conservative. It usually consists of the administration of laxatives and dilation of the distal rectum and anus (2).

REFERENCES

1. Hosie GP, Spitz L. Idiopathic constipation in childhood is associated with thickening of the internal anal sphincter. J Pediatr Surg 1997;32:1041–1044.
2. Kottmeir PK, Clatworthy HW Jr. Aganglionic and functional megacolon in children: diagnostic dilemma. Pediatrics 1965;36: 572–582.

Meconium Plug Syndrome, Small Left Colon Syndrome, and Colon Immaturity

The three conditions, meconium plug syndrome, small left colon syndrome, and colon immaturity refer to the same problem: functional immaturity of the ganglion cells of the colon. The problem probably is more common than generally realized, but in most cases symptoms are so mild and transient that they pass unnoticed. If, however, significant obstruction develops, symptoms become more profound and complications such as perforation may result. Most infants with this form of colonic obstruction present within the first 24–36 hours of life with abdominal distention, vomiting (with bile), and failure to initiate the normal passage of meconium. In some cases, the distal meconium plug is dislodged from the rectum, and a few pieces of meconium may be passed, but normal and continuous meconium evacuation is not established. In this regard, the term **meconium plug syndrome** is a misnomer because the plug which is passed, is not the problem. The plug is there during intrauterine life to ensure that the colon will not evacuate. When it is passed, however, the remainder of the meconium in the colon is not evacuated and while a variable length of the descending colon remains empty and contracted, the colon proximal to this area is distended and full of meconium. This leads to a pseudotransition zone, but the problem is transient, and simply speaking, the colon is not quite ready for "prime time."

The meconium plug syndrome is especially common in infants delivered of diabetic mothers (1), and also can be seen in any infant who is depressed or hypotonic (2). In this regard, hypermagnesemia has been incriminated as a cause of such hypotonia (3). In addition, sepsis can lead to bowel immotility and, as such, can masquerade as the meconium plug syndrome. All of these pieces of information seem to underscore the fact that the overall problem in these infants is one of transient colon inertia or immaturity (4).

Diagnosis of the meconium plug and small left colon syndromes is radiologic and depends on contrast enema examination. Plain films are nonspecific and usually show findings of a low small bowel obstruction (Fig. 4.139A). On upright view, there is a paucity of air-fluid levels and, in most cases, there is no gas in the rectum. Contrast enema examination results in a characteristic appearance of the colon, which to the uninitiated may at first suggest an air contrast barium enema of a normal colon (Fig. 4.139B). This configuration results from barium being trapped between the solid column of inspissated meconium and the colon wall. If a portion of the meconium is passed before or during the examination, that part of the colon from which it was evacuated appears narrowed, and

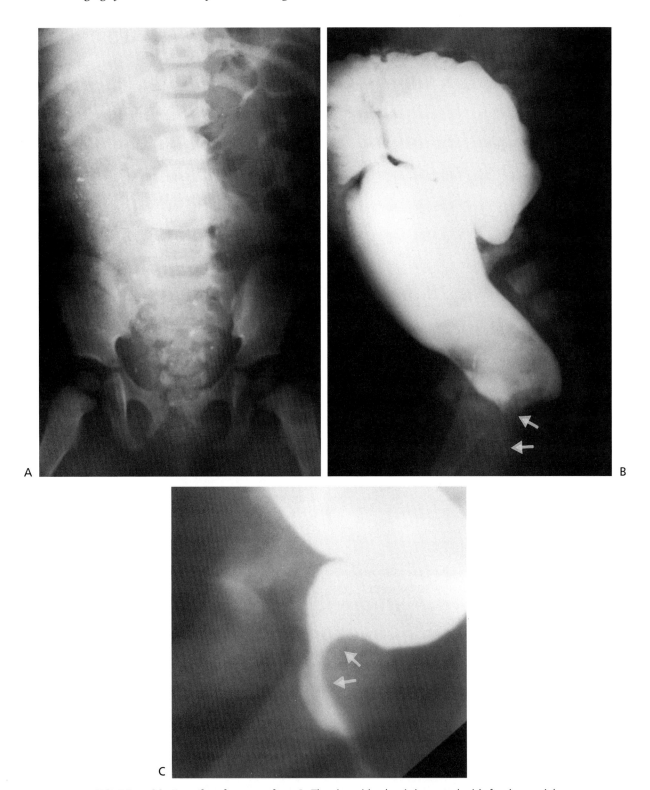

FIGURE 4.138. Functional megacolon. A. The sigmoid colon is impacted with fecal material. It also contains scattered opaque material (pica). The findings were at first misinterpreted for neuroblastoma. **B.** Lateral view demonstrates the distended fecal-filled rectum and the typical configuration of the puborectalis sling (arrows). **C.** Another patient with a prominent puborectalis sling indentation (arrows).

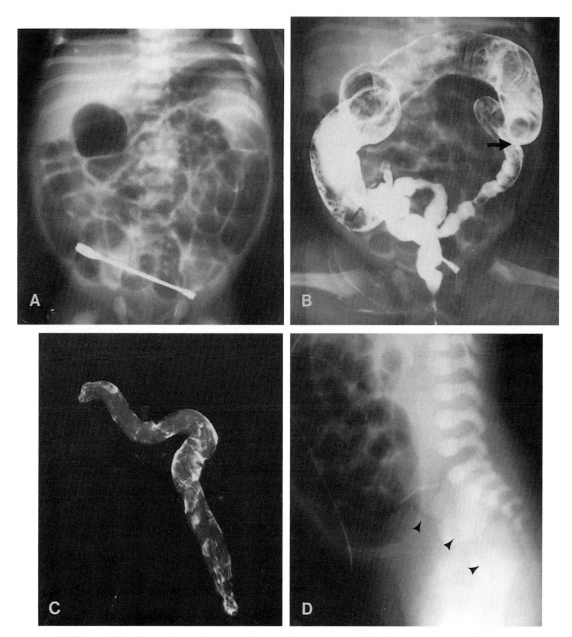

FIGURE 4.139. Meconium plug syndrome. A. Abdominal film shows numerous distended loops of small bowel. On the upright view, no air-fluid levels were seen. **B.** Barium enema shows a contracted, narrowed distal colonic segment. A transition zone is suggested (arrow), and above it, inspissated meconium is seen in a dilated colon. **C.** Meconium cast that was passed during the time of barium enema from the contracted segment of the colon seen in B. **D.** Meconium plug (arrows) outlined by air in the rectum. (Reproduced with permission from Swischuk LE. Meconium plug syndrome, a cause of neonatal intestinal obstruction. Am J Roentgenol Radium Ther Nucl Med 1968;103:339–346.)

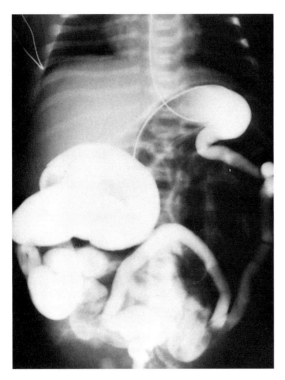

FIGURE 4.140. Small left colon syndrome. Note the small, contracted left colon. It is this configuration that led to the term "small left colon syndrome."

a transition zone of Hirschsprung's disease is mimicked (Fig. 4.139B). Other infants may pass meconium early and show these features from the onset (Fig. 4.140). The presence of the small, contracted portion of the descending colon in these infants has led to the term "neonatal small left colon syndrome" (1). In any of these cases, meconium proximal to the apparent transition zone may take the form of one solid, cylindrical mass extending to the cecum, lumps of solid meconium scattered throughout the colon, or granular (mixed with air)-appearing meconium. The contrast enema examination differentiates meconium plug syndrome from the usual case of meconium ileus or ileal atresia for in the latter conditions, one usually sees a microcolon, and only occasionally is an infant with meconium ileus reported to have meconium plug-like findings (5).

If small bowel gas is forced, by peristalsis, into the colon and mixes with the meconium, a granular or bubbly appearance mimicking the findings of pneumatosis cystoides intestinalis and necrotizing enterocolitis results (Fig. 4.141). However, if one remembers that necrotizing enterocolitis presents beyond the immediate neonatal period, one can be more certain that delayed meconium passage, rather than necrotizing enterocolitis, is the problem. In this regard, I have used the following rule: if a bubbly pattern is

seen within the first 12 hours of life, the meconium plug syndrome should be the problem, but if it arises 12–18 hours or later, necrotizing enterocolitis is most likely. Between is a gray zone where individual assessment of the patient is most important.

Treatment of the meconium plug or small left colon syndromes is conservative and consists of irritation of the rectum or colon in some manner. In many cases, simple finger examination of the rectum or insertion of a rectal thermometer produces enough irritation to induce peristalsis and promote evacuation of the meconium. In other cases, a saline enema may suffice, but if these fail, a contrast enema, preferably with a hypersomic water-soluble contrast agent such as Gastrografin can be used. It should be remembered, however, that such contrast agents require precautions regarding fluid and electrolyte balance. In addition the contrast agents may be irritable to the colonic mucosa. To circumvent these problems, we dilute Gastrografin 3:1 with normal saline. With the conservative treatment just outlined, complete decompression usually occurs within hours but, in some infants, may take up to 2 or 3 days to be complete (the minority). The meconium is rather sticky and tenacious and passes slowly, but, with persistence, complete decompression is usually eventually accomplished. However, it must be emphasized that it is most important to follow these patients closely, because if they do have Hirschsprung's disease, they will return with intestinal problems, usually constipation or diarrhea.

It should be remembered that the meconium plug syndrome is different from meconium ileus. Meconium ileus is a problem of distal small bowel obstruction as seen in infants with cystic fibrosis. Nonetheless, there have been a few cases of meconium plug syndrome secondary to cystic fibrosis documented (6, 7).

REFERENCES

1. Davis WS, Allen RP, Favara BE, et al. Neonatal small left colon syndrome. AJR 1974;120:322–329.
2. Falterman CG, Richardson CJ. Small left colon syndrome associated with maternal ingestion of psychotrophic drugs. J Pediatr 1980;97:308–310.
3. Cooney DR, Rosevear W, Grosfeld JL. Maternal and postnatal hypermagnesemia and the meconium plug syndrome. J Pediatr Surg 1976;11:167–172.
4. LeQuesne GW, Reilly BJ. Functional immaturity of the large bowel in the newborn infant. Radiol Clin North Am 1975;13: 331–342.
5. Siegel MJ, Shackelford GD, McAlister WH. Neonatal meconium blockage in the ileum and proximal colon. Radiology 1979;132: 79–82.
6. Ellerbroek C, Smith WL. Neonatal small left colon in an infant with cystic fibrosis. Pediatr Radiol 1986;16:162–163.
7. Hen J Jr, Dolan TF Jr, Touloukian RJ. Meconium plug syndrome associated with cystic fibrosis and Hirschsprung's disease. Pediatrics 1980;66:466–469.

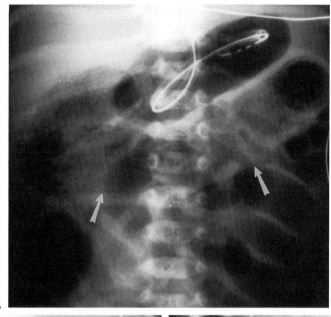

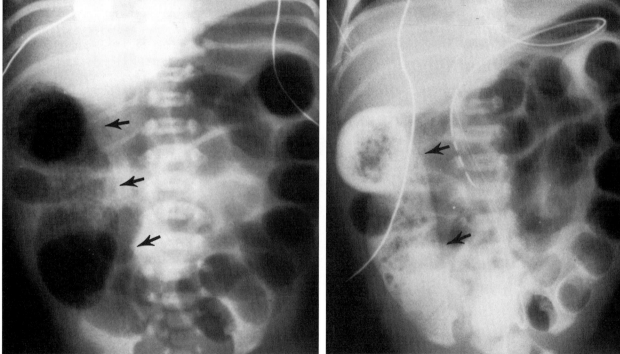

FIGURE 4.141. Meconium plug syndrome: pseudonecrotizing enterocolitis. A. Note the numerous distended loops of small bowel and a bubbly appearance of meconium mixed with air in the transverse colon (arrows). Necrotizing enterocolitis may erroneously be suggested. **B.** Another infant with similar findings, suggesting obstruction and a granular-appearing collection of meconium and air in the ascending colon and hepatic flexure (arrows). Pneumatosis cystoides intestinalis is erroneously suggested. **C.** Contrast enema in the same infant demonstrates that the findings are the result of meconium mixed with air (arrows) in a slightly dilated colon.

TABLE 4.3. ANORECTAL ANOMALIES

1. Ectopic anus	The hindgut opens ectopically at an abnormally high location (i.e., perineum, vestibule, urethra, bladder, vagina, or cloaca). There is failure of normal descent of the hindgut.
2. Imperforate anus	The terminal bowel ends blindly, and there is no opening or fistula. Two basic types are included: a. Membranous imperforate anus b. Anorectal or anal atresia
3. Rectal atresia	The anus is present and open, but a variable segment of rectum is atretic. No fistula is present.
4. Anal and rectal stenosis	Incomplete atresia of either structure

Adapted from Gans SL. Classification of anorectal anomalies: a critical analysis. *J Pediatr Surg* 1970;5:511–513, with permission.

Anorectal Anomalies (Imperforate Anus, Ectopic Anus)

A wide variety of abnormalities is encompassed by the term "anorectal anomalies," including imperforate anus, anorec-

tal atresia or stenosis, and ectopic anus. Various classifications and reviews of these conditions are available, but that of Gans (Table 4.3) is both simple and helpful. In this classification, rectal atresia is considered separate from imperforate or ectopic anus, because in rectal atresia the anus is present and open, but a variable segment of rectum above it is atretic. No fistula is present, and the anomaly probably results from an ischemic insult to the anorectal region. Anal or anorectal stenosis represents incomplete degrees of rectal atresia, and in membranous imperforate anus, the problem is believed to lie with failure of involution of the embryonic membrane between the hindgut and anus.

Ectopic anus, often also referred to as imperforate anus, is the most common anorectal anomaly encountered in neonatal infants and probably results from failure of normal descent of the hindgut through the puborectalis sling. As a result, the hindgut fails to reach the anal dimple and in females opens ectopically through a fistula, onto the perineum, vestibule, vagina, urethra, bladder, or cloaca (1) (Fig. 4.142). In males it opens into the bladder, urethra, or perineum (2) (Fig. 4.143). This abnormal termination of the hindgut in all these cases has led to the term "ectopic anus," a term now generally preferred, but not always used for this particular anomaly.

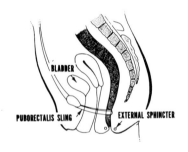

NORMAL FEMALE

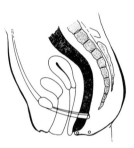

ANOPERINEAL FISTULA

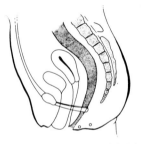

RECTOVESTIBULAR FISTULA

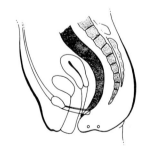

LOW RECTOVAGINAL FISTULA

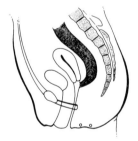

HIGH RECTOVAGINAL FISTULA

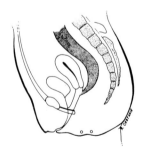

RECTOCLOACAL FISTULA

FIGURE 4.142. Types of ectopic anus: female. Diagrammatic representation of various types of ectopic anus in females. Note the position of puborectalis sling in each case. (Modified from Santulli TV, Schullinger JN, Amoury RA, et al. Malformations of the anus and rectum. Surg Clin North Am 1965;45:1253–1271.)

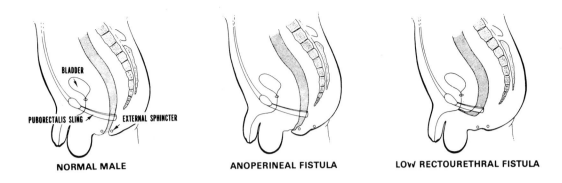

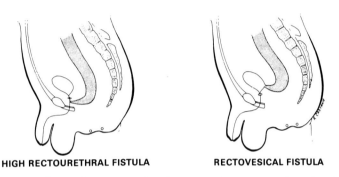

FIGURE 4.143. Types of ectopic anus: male. Diagrammatic representation of various types of ectopic anus in males. Note position of puborectalis sling in each case. (Modified from Santulli TV, Schullinger JN, Amoury RA, et al. Malformations of the anus and rectum. Surg Clin North Am 1965;45:1253–1271).

Generally, one fistula is present, but double fistulas occasionally are encountered (3, 4). The latter are seen almost exclusively in females. Covered anus in males can be considered a form of ectopic anus where the fistula runs as far as the base of the penis and is covered by skin. Another variation of fistula formation is the so-called H-type fistula (5), a condition where likely, there is persistence of the primitive communication between the urinary and rectal portions of the cloaca (i.e., persistent defect in the urorectal septum). Familial cases occasionally occur (6), and males appear to predominate in the general incidence of anorectal anomalies. In addition, cardiovascular malformations are not uncommonly associated, and in terms of GI abnormalities the most commonly associated ones are duodenal and esophageal atresia. There also is an increased incidence in Down's syndrome (7).

A wide range of associated genital and urinary anomalies also occur, as do spine and spinal cord abnormalities. Often, these associated abnormalities, including those involving the spinal cord (8) are silent. Therefore, MRI has come into standard use for the evaluation of the spine and spinal cord in these patients (9–14). However, in the newborn infant, ultrasound is very useful in delineating interspinal problems such as tethered cord or lipoma. Spine anomalies, usually involving the sacrum, are visible on plain films where evidence of colonic obstruction also will be present (Fig. 4.144).

Colonic aganglionosis also is sporadically reported with anorectal atresia and ectopic anus (15), and colonic atresia. In some of these latter cases, a short portion of the distal colon remains in tact and the term "colon pouch syndrome" is applied (16, 17). Another interesting association with anorectal malformations is the coexistence of sacral anomalies and presacral masses. The sacrum in these patients is deformed and the sacral mass may be a meningocele, enteric cyst, or teratoma (18, 19). The association is called the Currarino triad (20, 21), and it has been suggested that the problem in these cases lies in faulty separation of the hindgut from the primitive neural canal (19).

In terms of the investigation of this group of anomalies, if the ectopic hindgut ends on the perineum or the vestibule, or even in the low vagina, the opening can be seen clinically and little in the way of contrast studies is required. However, if the opening is not readily visible, then one must assume that the hindgut has been arrested at a higher level and has not traversed the puborectalis sling. In such cases, the opening will be into the vagina or cloaca in females, and the urethra or bladder in males.

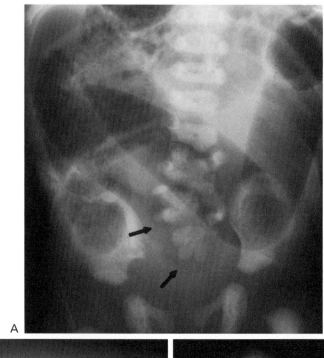

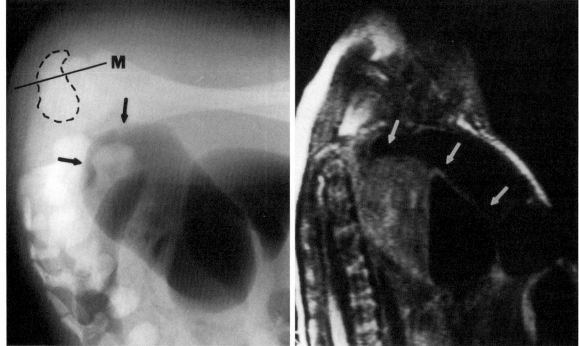

FIGURE 4.144. Imperforate anus: sacral findings, upside down film, and MRI. A. Note the distended, obstructed colon. There is no air in the rectum. Also note extensive sacral anomalies (arrows). **B.** Upside-down film demonstrates the distal air-filled pouch (arrows). It ends well above the M line (M), which signifies a high lesion. **C.** T1-weighted MR study in the midsagittal plane. In the supine position, the fluid-filled distal pouch (arrows) is demonstrated. Note that the sacrum is short and underdeveloped.

Arrest of the hindgut may be high, low, or intermediate, and in cases of high arrest, the colon ends at or above the puborectalis sling, and the sling is hypoplastic or even absent. Consequently, it usually is functionally inadequate and surgical correction is more difficult to accomplish. If colon arrest is low, the colon will have passed through the puborectalis sling, and the sling then usually is well developed and functional. As such, surgical repair is more often favorably accomplished. This is a most important consideration, because it is the integrity of the puborectalis sling of the levator ani muscle that eventually determines both the

specific surgical approach to the correction of this anomaly and the subsequent chances of attaining anorectal continence. The anal sphincters are usually underdeveloped and functionally inadequate in ectopic anus, and subsequently, continence falls to the puborectalis sling.

In terms of surgical repair, the higher the arrest of the hindgut, the more likely is it that a combined abdominal perineal approach, with subsequent hindgut pull-through, will be necessary. In the lower fistulas, especially those ending on the perineum, since the puborectalis muscle is more developed, simple dilation of the ectopic perineal opening

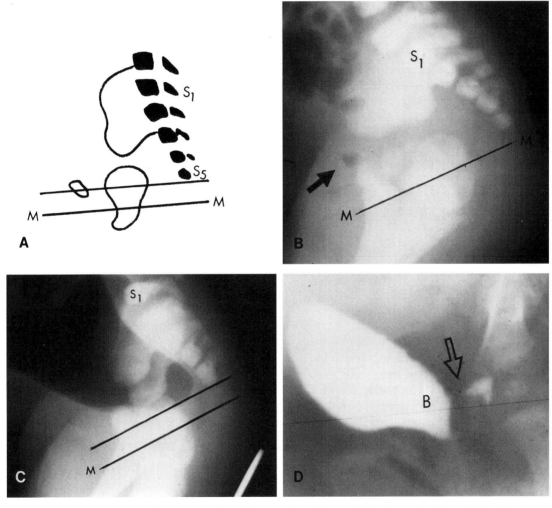

FIGURE 4.145. Ectopic anus: various lines and problems in their application. A. The M line of Cremin is drawn through the junction of the upper two thirds and lower one third of the ischia. This line corresponds to the level of the puborectalis sling. The line above it is in the old pubococcygeal line. **B.** Male with ectopic anus. Inverted film fails to clearly outline the distal pouch with air. The M line is drawn as a reference point, but because air is present in the bladder (arrow), one is clearly dealing with a high rectovesicular fistula. If the fistula emptied into the urethra, air would most likely not be present in the bladder. **C.** Another male with a grossly distended distal hindgut pouch ending just at the level of the old pubococcygeal line (top line). Using this line, an intermediate hindgut arrest is suggested. The M line, however, indicates a high fistula. **D.** A subsequent cystogram clearly shows a high rectovesical fistula (arrow). Bladder (B). The M line, because it corresponds to the level of the puborectalis sling, is of more practical value than the old pubococcygeal line.

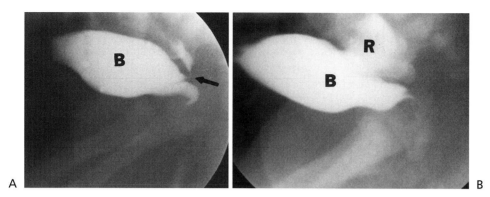

FIGURE 4.146. Ectopic anus: demonstration of rectovesical fistula. A. Contrast was introduced into the bladder (B). Note the fistula (arrow) between the base of the bladder and the rectum. Note the early filling of the rectum. **B.** Later, there is more contrast material in the rectum (R).

and/or a "cutback" procedure or anoplasty usually suffices. These procedures may require subsequent repeated dilatations. In simple imperforate membrane, all that is usually required is incision of the membrane, whereas in anorectal atresia, since no fistula or opening is present, colostomy with later pull-through is required.

Plain films in imperforate or ectopic anus reveal a colonic obstruction (Fig. 4.144A). In males, air bubbles can occasionally be seen in the bladder (Fig. 4.144B). Less commonly, air may be seen in the vagina of female infants. In either case, the presence of such air provides evidence of an internal fistula. Sacral anomalies also can be seen (Fig. 4.144A). Upside-down films still are helpful in the diagnosis of ectopic anus, even though they have some problems. This study originally was designed to enable one to outline the distal rectum with air and thereby estimate the level of termination of the hindgut. However, because the distal colon is not always filled with air (films may be taken too early, before gas reaches the distal colon or the colon is impacted with meconium), erroneous interpretations as to the exact termination of the hindgut can arise. For this reason the study has over the years had variable acceptance but is not totally useless. Information similar to that seen on upside-down views can be obtained with cross-table prone "butt-up" views (22) (Fig. 4.144B).

After either of these views is obtained, the pubococcygeal line (drawn approximately from the sacrococcygeal junction to the midpubic bone) originally was constructed and, depending on whether the air-filled hindgut ended above or below this line, the lesion was classified as being high or low (Fig. 4.145, A and B). This line eventually was believed to have been drawn at too high a level, and a substitute line, the "M" line of Cremin (Fig. 4.145, C and D), running horizontally through the junction of the lower and upper two thirds of the ischia, is now used. This latter line seems to correspond more closely to the level of the puborectalis muscle and, consequently, is of more practical value.

With high fistulas, further delineation of the fistula can be achieved by the injection of contrast material into the bladder, male urethra, or female genital tract. These studies can be accomplished by direct catheter injection or, in the female, by flush retrograde vaginography (Figs. 4.146 and 4.147). Fistulas also can be demonstrated after colostomy by pressure injection into the distal portion of the colon. In addition, CT and ordinary or rectal coil MR imaging can be used to locate the pouch and, even more importantly, to assess the integrity of the all important puborectalis muscle both preoperatively and postoperatively (23–27) (Fig. 4.148). With either study, one can determine the bulk of the puborectalis muscle, its location, and after surgery, whether the hindgut has been placed through it.

Preoperatively, transanal and perineal sagittal and coronal ultrasonography (28–29) can be used to identify the location and extent of the blind-ending pouch (Fig. 4.149). Identifying an underlying fistula is more difficult with ultrasound. As far as technique is concerned, with transverse scans, with the transducer in the anal dimple, the distance from the end of the pouch to the skin surface can be measured, and in this regard, low lesions tend to have a pouch-perineum distance of less than 1.5 cm. However, it is doubtful that these ultrasonographic measurements will be any more helpful than any of the radiographic lines proposed in the past. Sacral anomalies, spinal cord abnormalities, and urinary and genital tract abnormalities, generally more common with high fistulas, can be evaluated with ultrasound. In addition, neurogenic bladder and neurogenic colon are common complicating factors in ectopic anus and can result from inherent neurologic abnormality or from nerve root injury during corrective surgery.

At the far end of the hindgut abnormality spectrum is the so-called mermaid deformity or caudal regression syndrome (Fig. 4.150). The etiology of this condition probably lies in a fetal vascular insult (30, 31). Expanding on this hypothesis, it has been alternately suggested that the prob-

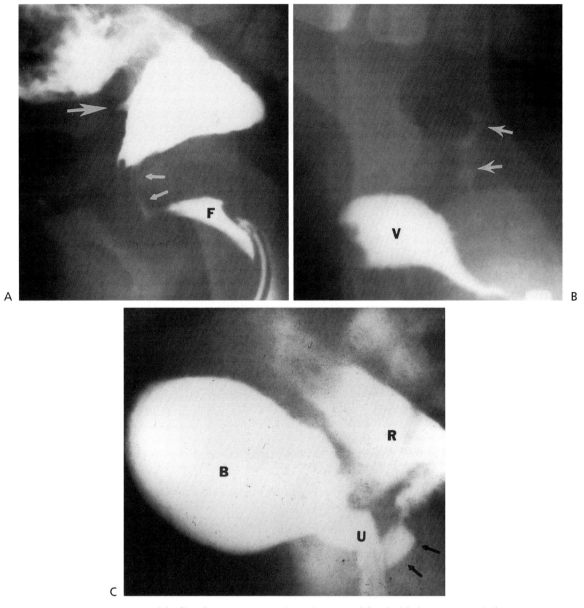

FIGURE 4.147. Double fistula. A. Injection through perineal fistula (F) demonstrates indentation produced by the puborectalis sling (small arrows) and early filling of rectovaginal fistula (large arrow). **B.** Retrograde vaginogram (same patient) demonstrates the vagina (V) and filling of the rectovaginal fistula (arrows). Note the cervix indenting the superior aspect of the vagina. **C.** Rectourethral fistula. Retrograde cystogram showing the bladder (B), posterior urethra (U), high rectourethral fistula (arrows), and rectum (R) in a male infant.

lem actually is one of an abnormal vessel draining blood away from the distal part of the body (32). This vessel, a primitive vitelline artery, arises high in the aorta and then passes through the umbilicus as the umbilical artery. When present, it is large, and siphons blood away from the body distal to its origin from the aorta. As a result, this portion of the body is undervascularized and prone to underdevelopment as seen in the mermaid or sirenomelia syndrome.

Finally, it might be noted that calcified enteroliths can be encountered with ectopic anus. These usually are seen in females (33, 34) and require fistulous connection to the urinary tract so that urine can pass to the GI tract. In some way this appears to induce the calcifications.

REFERENCES

1. Jaramillo D, Lebowitz RL, Hendren WH. The cloacal malformation: radiologic findings and imaging recommendations. Radiology 1990;177:441–448.

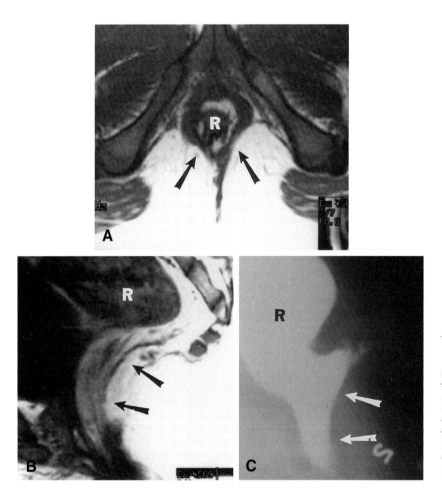

FIGURE 4.148. Ectopic anus: postoperative MR findings. A. Axial view. Note the underdeveloped and hypoplastic puborectalis muscle (arrows). This patient, however, still was continent. **B.** Lateral view demonstrates the pronounced posterior indentation (arrows) by the puborectalis muscle. **C.** Defecography demonstrates the same puborectalis sling indentation (arrows). R, rectum.

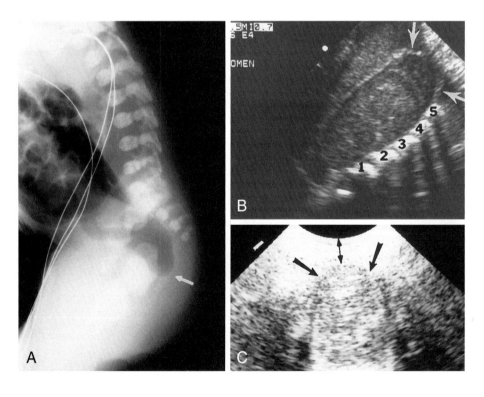

FIGURE 4.149. Imperforate anus: ultrasonographic findings. A. Lateral view of the sacrum demonstrates the low-lying distal rectal pouch (arrow). **B.** Ultrasound demonstrates a low-lying distal rectal pouch (arrows). The sacral vertebral bodies are numbered 1 through 5. **C.** Ultrasonogram through perineum demonstrates the same pouch (arrows). The distance from the skin to the pouch can be measured (small arrows).

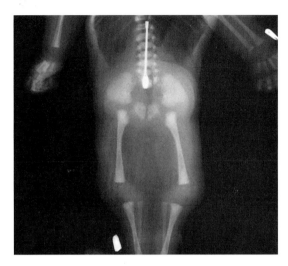

FIGURE 4.150. Ectopic anus: caudal regression. Postmortem film showing sacral agenesis, fusion of the lower extremities (mermaid deformity), and generalized underdevelopment of the lower half of the body. Infant had ectopic anus and numerous genitourinary anomalies.

2. Currarino G. the various types of anorectal fistula in male imperforate anus. Pediatr Radiol 1996;26:512–522.

3. Chatterjee SK, Talukder BC. Double termination of the alimentary tract in female infants. J Pediatr Surg 1969;4:237–243.

4. Tsuchida Y, Saito S, Honna T, et al. Double termination of the alimentary tract in females: a report of 12 cases and a literature review. J Pediatr Surg 1984;19:292–296.

5. Rintala RJ Mildh L, Lindahl H. H-type anorectal malformations: incidence and clinical characteristics. J Pediatr Surg 1996;31: 559–562.

6. Naveh Y, Friedman A. Familial imperforate anus. Am J Dis Child 1976;130:441–442.

7. Torres r, Levitt MA, Tovilla JM, et al. Anorectal malformations and Down's syndrome. J Pediatr Surg 1998;33:194–197.

8. Tsakayannis DE, Shamberger RC. Association of imperforate anus with occult spinal dysraphism. J Pediatr Surg 1995;30: 1010–1012.

9. Beek Fja, Boemers TML, Witkamp TD, et al. Spine evaluation in children with anorectal malformations. Pediatr Radiol 1995; 25:S28–S32.

10. Gudinchet F, Maeder P, Laurent T, et al. Magnetic resonance detection of myelodysplasia in children with Currarino triad. Pediatr Radiol 1997;27:903–907.

11. Levitt MA, Patel M, Rodriguez G, et al. The tethered spinal cord in patients with anorectal malformations. J Pediatr Surg 1997;32: 462—468.

12. Long FR, Hunter JV, Mahboubi S, et al. Tethered cord and associated vertebral anomalies in children and infants with imperforate anus: evaluation with MR imaging and plain radiography. Radiology 1996;200:377–382.

13. McHugh K, Dudley Ne, Tam P. Pre-operative MRI of anorectal anomalies in the newborn period. Pediatr Radiol 1995;25: S33–S36.

14. Rivosecchi M, Lucchetti MC, Zaccara A, et al. Spinal dysraphism detected by magnetic resonance imaging in patients with anorectal anomalies: incidence and clinical significance. J Pediatr Surg 1995;30:488–490.

15. Watanatittan S, Suwatanaviroj A, Limprutihum T. Association of Hirschsprung's disease and anorectal malformation. J Pediatr Surg 1991;26:192–195.

16. Wardhan H, Gangopadhyay AN, Singhal GD, et al. Imperforate anus with congenital short colon (pouch colon syndrome). Review of eighteen cases. Pediatr Surg Int 1990;5:124–126.

17. Yuejie W, Rong D, Guie Z, et al. Association of imperforate anus with short colon: a report of eight cases. J Pediatr Surg 1990;25: 282–284.

18. Currarino G, Coln D, Votteler T. Triad of anorectal, sacral, and presacral anomalies. AJR 1981;137:395–398.

19. Kirks DR, Merten DF, Filston HC, et al. The Currarino triad: complex of anorectal malformation, sacral body abnormality, and presacral mass. Pediatr Radiol 1984;14:220–225.

20. Lee S-C, Chun Y-S, Jung SE, et al. Currarino triad: anorectal malformation, sacral bony abnormality, and presacral mass—a review of 11 cases. J Pediatric Surg 1997;32:58–61.

21. Pfluger T, Czekalla R, Koletzko S, et al. MRI and radiographic findings in Currarino's triad. Pediatr Radiol 1996;26:524–527.

22. Narasimharao KL, Prasad GR, Katariya S, et al. Prone cross-table lateral view: an alternative to the invertogram in imperforate anus. AJR 1983;140:227–229.

23. Husberg B, Rosenborg M, Frenckner B. Magnetic resonance imaging of anal sphincters after reconstruction of high or intermediate anorectal anomalies with posterior sagittal anorectoplasty and fistula-preserving technique. J Pediatr Surg 1997; 32:1436–1442.

24. Taccone A, Martucaciello G, Dodero P, et al. New concepts in preoperative imaging of anorectal malformation. Pediatr Radiol 1992;22:196–199.

25. Fukuya T, Honda H, Kubota M, et al. Postoperative MRI evaluation of anorectal malformations with clinical correlation. Pediatr Radiol 1993;23:583–586.

26. deSouza NM, Gilderdale DJ, MacIver DK, et al. High resolution MR imaging of the anal sphincter in children: a pilot study using endoanal receiver coils. AJR 1997;169:201–206.

27. deSouza NM, Ward HC, Williams AD, et al. Transanal MR imaging after repair of anorectal anomalies in children: appearances in pull-through versus posterior sagittal reconstruction. AJR 1999;173:723–728.

28. Kim I-O, Tae H II, Woo Sun K, et al. Transperineal ultrasonography in imperforate anus: identification of the internal fistula. J Ultrasound Med 2000;19:211–216.

29. Han T, Kim I-O, Kim WS, et al. US identification of the anal sphincter complex and levator ani muscle in neonates: infracoccygeal approach. Radiology 2000;217:392–394.

30. Guidera KJ, Raney E, Ogden JA, et al. Caudal regression: a review of seven cases, including the mermaid syndrome. J Pediatr Orthop 1991;11:743–747.

31. Passarge E, Lenz W. Syndrome of caudal regression in infants of diabetic mothers: observations of further cases. Pediatrics 1966; 37:672–675.

32. Stevenson RE, Jones KL, Phelan MC, et al. Vascular steal: the pathogenic mechanism producing sirenomelia and associated defects of the viscera and soft tissues. Pediatrics 1986;78: 451–457.

33. Mandell J, Lillehi CW, Greene M, et al. The prenatal diagnosis of imperforate anus with rectourinary fistula: dilated fetal colon with enterolithiasis. J Pediatr Surg 1992;27:82–84.

34. Taccone A, Marzoli A, Martucaciello G, et al. Intraabdominal calcifications in the newborn: an unusual case with anorectal malformation and other anomalies. Pediatr Radiol 1992;22: 309–310.

Necrotizing Enterocolitis

This serious condition most commonly affects premature infants and, for the most part, is a sporadic disease. However, it also can be seen in full-term infants (1), where one more often than not is dealing with the epidemic form of the disease (2). In addition, necrotizing enterocolitis also can be seen in older infants and children where the main predisposing factor is hypoperfusion of the bowel secondary to severe dehydration. This is important, for, as will be seen later, hypoperfusion of the bowel is the basic and most important factor in the development of necrotizing enterocolitis.

In terms of the etiology of necrotizing enterocolitis, it is now generally accepted that the three most important etiologic factors are (a) intestinal schemia or hypoperfusion leading to altered mucosal integrity, (b) bacterial overgrowth with gas formation in the bowel wall, and (c) continued irritation of the bowel by oral feedings. Oral feedings per se are not the cause of necrotizing enterocolitis (3), but rather, if continued, they add significant burden to the injured bowel. Bacteria involved include *E. coli*, *Klebsiella*, and *Clostridium*. In the end, almost any condition or situation which leads to hypoperfusion of the intestine can lead to necrotizing enterocolitis. These include hyperviscosity, sepsis with hypotension, the hypoplastic left heart syndrome, cardiopulmonary bypass surgery and shock. In addition, the usually present distention of the intestines can complicate the problem by further compromising vascular flow (4).

Once schemia or hypoperfusion occurs in any of these infants, a definite cycle of events develops (Fig. 4.151). First, there is paralysis of the intestine and, as intraluminal gas accumulates, intestinal and abdominal distention occur. Intestinal distention in a paralytic ileus pattern is the most common early finding in terms of the radiograph, and clinically the problem often first manifests as deterioration of pulmonary function (5). This probably is secondary to shock. In addition to these problems the patient may manifest with poor feeding, vomiting, and at times vomiting with bile. After this initial period of decreased bowel activity, the bowel becomes more active, and bleeding into the lumen occurs and diarrhea with occult or overt blood in the stools is seen. Frequently, the diarrhea is intractable and feedings should be stopped so as to rest the bowel. Once the disease reaches this stage, there is loss of normal mucosal integrity, both mechanical (i.e., mucosal necrosis) and immunologic (i.e., loss of topical enteric immunity), and together these factors allow for an overgrowth of intestinal bacterial flora. The gases produced from this overgrowth lead to further distention of the intestines and entrance of bacterial by way of mucosal tears into the bowel wall. This then leads to intramural bacterial proliferation and the formation of gas in the intestinal wall, or so-called pneumatosis cystoids intestinalis. Eventually, the gas also enters the portal veins, a point to be addressed later.

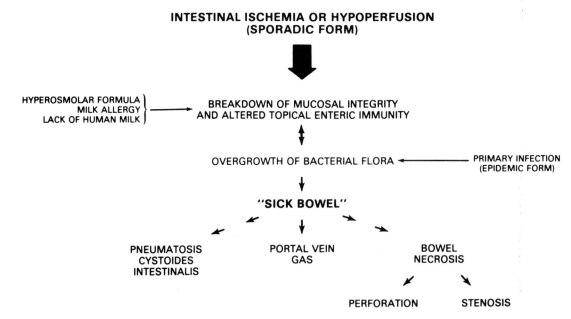

FIGURE 4.151. Necrotizing enterocolitis: pathogenesis. The pathogenesis of necrotizing enterocolitis is summarized in this scheme. The primary insult is intestinal schemia or hypoperfusion. This leads to breakdown of mucosal integrity. Thereafter, infection sets in, and there is an overgrowth of intestinal bacterial flora. This leads to gas formation in the bowel wall and so-called pneumatosis cystoides intestinalis and portal vein gas. Other complications include bowel necrosis, perforation, and stenosis. Aggravating factors include oral feeding and lack of normal topical enteric immunity. Food allergy or intolerance and hyperosmolar formulas also are significant factors, but their precise role is not clearly elucidated.

The sporadic and usual form of necrotizing enterocolitis usually develops toward the end of the first week of life or later, and males seem to predominate. There is a definite spectrum of severity to the disease, from very mild to severe and fulminant. In this regard, it cannot be overstated that the radiologist should not wait until intramural gas (pneumatosis cystoides intestinalis) is present to suggest the diagnosis of necrotizing enterocolitis; mere dilation of the intestines should make one suspicious. In such cases, the intestinal gas pattern also become organized (Fig. 4.152). A similar configuration can be seen with early sepsis, but the overlap of the two diseases is not so problematic because both are treated much in the same way. However, if guaiac-positive stools or bleeding from the GI tract are present, necrotizing enterocolitis is the diagnosis.

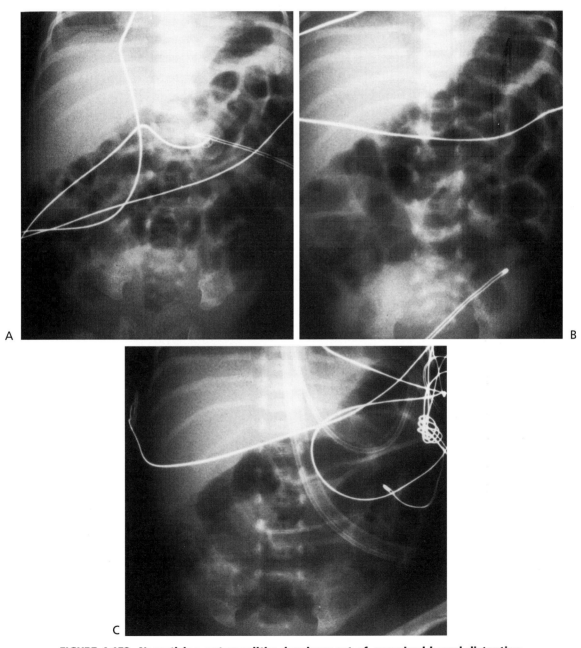

FIGURE 4.152. Necrotizing enterocolitis: development of organized bowel distention.
A. The intestinal gas pattern is completely normal. **B.** Early changes consist of slight dilation of the loops of intestine and early organization. **C.** Late changes demonstrate a number of dilated loops of intestine that now have become organized and stacked.

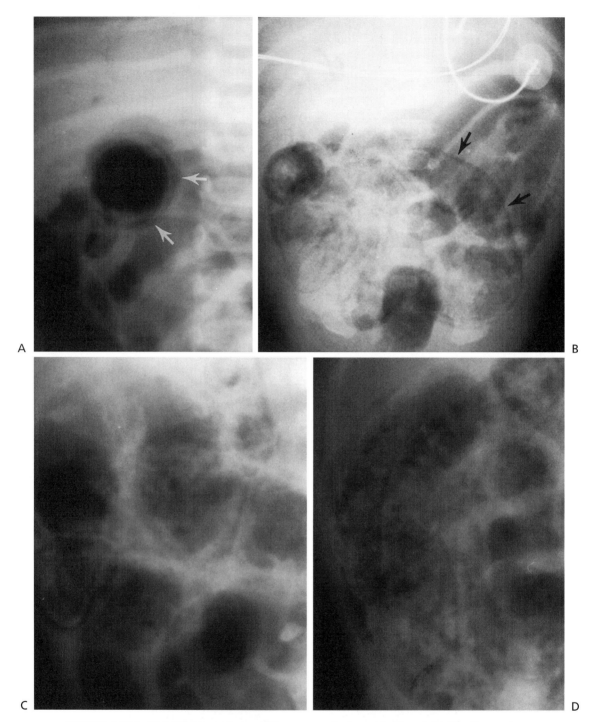

FIGURE 4.153. Necrotizing enterocolitis pneumatosis cystoides intestinalis: various configurations. A. Note curvilinear gas collections (arrows) in the hepatic flexure. This patient also has portal vein gas. **B.** Curvilinear air collections are present in the ascending colon and hepatic flexure while a long linear collection (arrows) is present in the transverse colon. **C.** Numerous curvilinear and bubbly collections of gas are seen. **D.** Predominately bubbly collections of gas are noted.

Medical therapy usually consists of stopping all gastric feedings, gastric decompression, antibiotics, and supportive intravenous fluid and nutrition. Blood replacement also may be necessary, and many times with these simple measures, the condition is abruptly aborted. However, one must be careful not to cease therapy too soon and begin feeding the infant too early, because recurrence of symptoms can be precipitated. Surgical therapy usually is relegated to those cases demonstrating complications such as free intraperitoneal air, peritonitis with the accumulation of peritoneal fluid, generalized or localized abdominal wall induration (diffuse peritonitis or locally adhesive necrotic bowel), and the presence of persistent focally dilated loops of intestine (i.e., dead bowel) (6). It is important not to confuse a normal sigmoid colon (see Fig. 4.127) for a persistently fixed inflamed loop of intestine. Once necrotizing enterocolitis is suspected clinically, abdominal films should be obtained immediately and regularly thereafter. In the more severe cases, these films should be obtained every 6 hours or even more frequently, and some type of gravity-dependent view should be included to detect free air. Most often, this is a cross-table, lateral, or decubitus view.

The first roentgenographic finding in necrotizing enterocolitis is generalized intestinal distention resulting from paralytic ileus, but at any point along the course of the disease, one can see the most pathognomonic finding of all: pneumatosis cystoides intestinalis. Pneumatosis cystoides intestinalis can assume a variety of configurations, including linear, curvilinear, bubbly, or foamy collections of gas (Fig. 4.153). One must be familiar with all of these patterns if one is to diagnose the condition early, and linear accumulations must be differentiated from the normal properitoneal fat line. Linear and curvilinear gas collections usually are easier to assess than the bubbly or foamy ones. These latter gas collections must be differentiated from fecal material or meconium mixed with air, but this point notwithstanding, **any infant suspected of having necrotizing enterocolitis who demonstrates the slightest hint of linear, curvilinear, foamy, or bubbly abdominal gas configurations should be assumed to have pneumatosis cystoides intestinalis until proven otherwise.** Pneumatosis cystoides intestinalis often is best visualized in the colon, but can occur anywhere from the stomach to the rectum. This serves to underscore that, although the disease often arises first in the terminal small bowel and ascending colon, it does have the potential of involving the entire GI tract.

The presence of portal vein gas once was considered an extremely ominous finding, and it still tends to be a finding seen with advanced disease. However, with current therapy so improved, no longer does its presence indicate that the entire disease process is irreversible. Usually, it is relatively easy to detect on plain films (Fig. 4.154A), but can come and go from one examination to another. In addition, it can be demonstrated with ultrasound as echogenic intravascular foci in the liver (7, 8). Under real-time examination the bubbles of air can be seen to actually move in the portal veins (Fig. 4.154B), and the bubbles can be seen in the absence of visible air in the portal system on plain films. Ultrasound also can detect gas in the bowel wall as an echogenic arc or circle (9). Thickened, edematous bowel also is readily detected with ultrasound (10).

When pneumoperitoneum occurs, there is clear indication for surgical intervention, but it must be stressed that many times free intraperitoneal air is not massive and one must inspect the decubitus views diligently for small collections. In addition, in many infants whose bowel perforates,

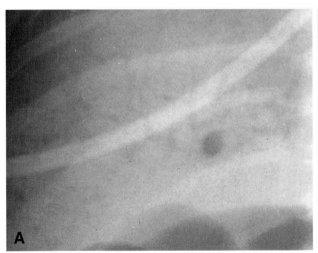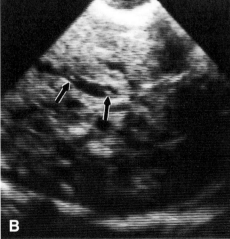

Figure 4.154. Necrotizing enterocolitis: portal vein gas. A. Note the branching appearance of portal vein gas. **B.** Another patient with bubbles of gas in the portal vein (arrows) demonstrated with ultrasound.

no free air at all is detected; rather, there is diminution of gas within the intestines but a concomitant increase in density of the abdomen resulting from the development of peritonitis and accumulation of peritoneal fluid. It is most important that this sequence of events be appreciated, because one can misinterpret the disappearance of bowel air as a sign of improvement. To guard against this pitfall, it is a wise policy to measure abdominal girth regularly and to correlate the findings with those seen on the abdominal film obtained at the same time. **When the infant improves, both abdominal girth and gaseous intestinal distention subside together.** Another sign of deterioration is the development of thickened loops of bowel (Fig. 4.155).

Once peritonitis develops, the abdomen becomes opaque, and in some cases, the abdominal wall becomes thickened and erythematous, suggesting that surgical intervention will be required. Another finding mitigating in favor of surgical intervention is the presence of a focally dilated loop of intestine persisting from examination to examination (6). This is an especially ominous finding if the remainder of the intestinal gas is disappearing, because it indicates the presence of necrotic bowel (Fig. 4.156). In many of these cases, there also is associated localized edema, redness, and thickening of the overlying abdominal wall (Fig. 4.157). Generally, it is not until one or other of these complications becomes apparent that surgical intervention occurs.

Problems encountered during convalescence from necrotizing enterocolitis include transient malabsorption, reactivation of the disease resulting from the premature reinstitution of oral feedings, and persistent, low-grade focal inflammation and bleeding. The transient malabsorption problems probably are related to mucosal damage, while the reinstitution of oral feedings too early probably overtaxes a sick intestine. In fact, in some infants it is difficult to institute normal feedings for weeks. Continued low-grade bleeding suggests subacute, smoldering disease, and on barium enema examination, these infants frequently demonstrate areas of inflammatory narrowing or stenosis (Fig. 4.158). These areas of narrowing, early on are not true fibrotic strictures, and many resolve spontaneously (Fig. 4.159) with appropriate medical therapy. On the other hand, when these strictures become fibrotic, they are fixed and require surgical intervention. Alternatively, the strictures can be treated with balloon dilation (11, 12), and overall, it probably is worthwhile to obtain a barium enema in all patients who first suffer from necrotizing enterocolitis in an effort to detect any occult strictures (13).

Another complication noted in some patients is the formation of enterocolic fistulas and enterocysts (14, 15), and occasionally even inflammatory polyps (16). Fistula formation is easy to conceive, but the development of enterocysts might require some explanation, and in this regard, it is believed that the portion of intestine between two ischemically compromised segments becomes cystic while the damaged areas become stenotic or atretic.

Finally, a word regarding benign pneumatosis cystoides intestinalis is in order. This topic is discussed later, but it should be noted here that, although pneumatosis cystoides intestinalis is the hallmark of necrotizing enterocolitis in neonates, air in the bowel wall also can be seen under other,

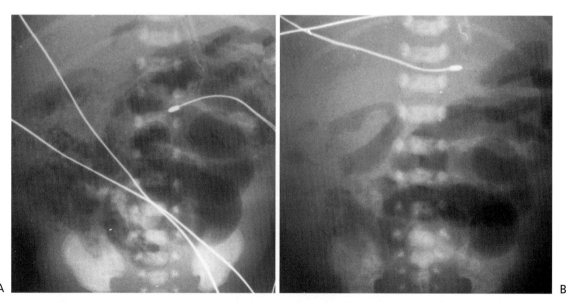

FIGURE 4.155. Necrotizing enterocolitis: development of thickened loops of intestine.
A. A few distended loops of intestine and scattered granular to curvilinear gas collections representing pneumatosis cystoides intestinalis are seen on the right. **B.** Later, pneumatosis clears but residual loops of intestine with thickened walls are seen.

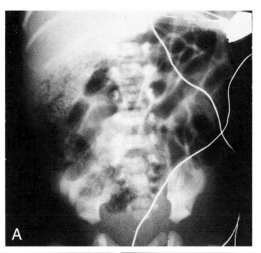

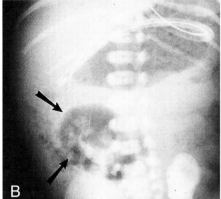

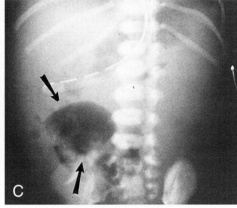

FIGURE 4.156. Necrotizing enterocolitis: fixed, necrotic loop of bowel. A. Note typical findings of early necrotizing enterocolitis. Granular or foamy pneumatosis cystoides intestinalis is present on the right. **B.** The next day, with treatment, intestinal gas has disappeared, but a large, locally distended loop of intestine remains in the right lower quadrant (arrows). **C.** The next day, the gas pattern is essentially unchanged but the loop of intestine in the right lower quadrant persists (arrows). Surgically confirmed necrotic loop of small bowel.

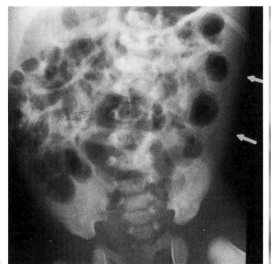
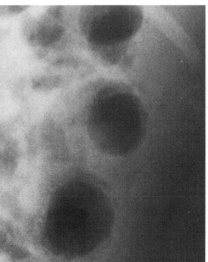
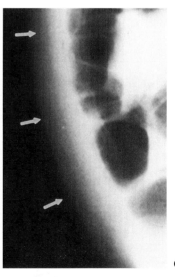

A,B   C

FIGURE 4.157. Necrotizing enterocolitis: fixed loops of necrotic intestine and abdominal wall edema. A. Note fixed loops with thickened walls and pneumatosis cystoides intestinalis on the left. The abdominal wall, over the loops, is thickened (arrows). **B.** Magnified view demonstrates the curvilinear intramural gas collections more clearly. Note that the loops of bowel are separated because of edema. **C.** Another patient with fixed loops and clearly visible abdominal wall thickening (arrows).

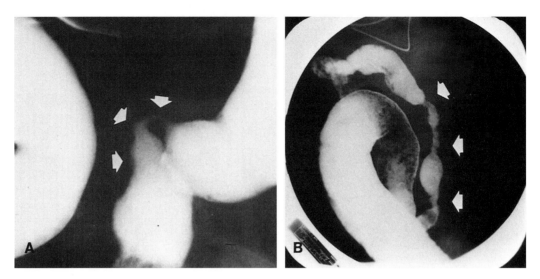

FIGURE 4.158. Necrotizing enterocolitis: colon strictures. A. Note the stricture in the sigmoid area (arrows). This patient had persistent guaiac-positive stools. **B.** Another infant demonstrating long segment, irregular stenosis of the descending colon (arrows). These strictures can spontaneously regress or go on to complete fibrotic obstruction.

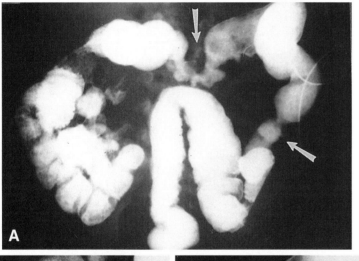

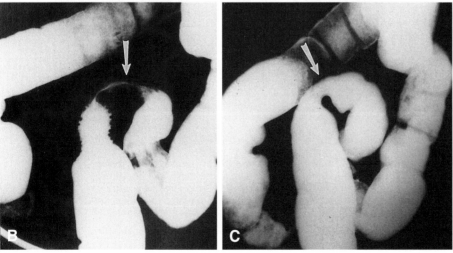

FIGURE 4.159. Necrotizing enterocolitis: inflammatory (incomplete) strictures. A. In this patient with continued guaiac-positive stools, two areas of persistent spasm (arrows) are identified in the colon. These are areas of inflammatory and not fibrotic stricturing. **B.** Another patient with an area of narrowing, which appears as a stricture (arrow). **C.** However, a little later, the same area opens up (arrow) but not to normal diameter. This is an irritable, spastic segment of colon. Segmental inflammation, not fixed stricture, is the problem.

innocuous circumstances. This usually occurs with chronic overdistention of the intestine. In these cases there are tears of the mucosa, and colonic gas enters the intramural space. The problem is not one of loss of mucosal integrity and bacterial overgrowth, and the condition therefore is benign.

REFERENCES

1. Wiswell TE, Robertson CF, Jones TA, et al. Necrotizing enterocolitis in full-term infants. Am J Dis Child 1988;142:532–535.
2. Guinan M, Schaberg D, Bruhn FW, et al. Epidemic occurrence of neonatal necrotizing enterocolitis. Am J Dis Child 1979;133:594–597.
3. Ostertag SG, LaGamma EF. Early enteral feeding does not affect the incidence of necrotizing enterocolitis. Pediatrics 1986;77:275–280.
4. Kazez A, Kucukaydin N, Kucikaydin M, et al. A model of hypoxia-induced necrotizing enterocolitis: the role of distension. J Pediatr Surg 1997;32:1466–1469.
5. Dolgin SE, Shlasko E, Levitt MA, et al. Alterations in respiratory status: early signs of severe necrotizing enterocolitis. J Pediatr Surg 1998;33:856–858.
6. Wexler HA. The persistent loop sign in neonatal necrotizing enterocolitis: a new indication for surgical intervention? Radiology 1978;126:201–204.
7. Avni EF, Rypens F, Cohen E, et al. Pericholecystic hyperechogenicities in necrotizing enterocolitis: a specific sonographic sign? Pediatr Radiol 1991;21:179–181.
8. Patel U, Leonidas JC, Furie D. Sonographic detection of necrotizing enterocolitis in infancy. J Ultrasound Med 1990;9:673–675.
9. Goske MJ, Goldblum Jr, Applegate KE, et al. The "circle sign": a new sonographic sign of pneumatosis intestinalis-clinical, pathologic and experimental findings. Pediatr Radiol 1999;29:530–535.
10. Kodroff MB, Hartenberg MA, Goldschmidt RA. Ultrasonographic diagnosis of gangrenous bowel in neonatal necrotizing enterocolitis. Pediatr Radiol 1984;14:168–170.
11. Ball WS Jr, Seigel RS, Goldthorn JF, et al. Colonic strictures in infants following intestinal ischemia: treatment by balloon catheter dilation. Radiology 1983;149:469–472.
12. Renfrew DL, Smith WL, Pringle KC. Perianal balloon dilation of a post-necrotizing enterocolitis stricture of the sigmoid colon. Pediatr Radiol 1986;16:320–321.
13. Brand IR, Arthur RJ. Contrast enemas after necrotising enterocolitis: a case for prophylaxis? Pediatr Radiol 1992;22:571–572.
14. Levin TL, Brill PW, Winchester P. Enteric fistula formation secondary to necrotizing enterocolitis. Pediatr Radiol 1991;21:309–311.
15. Stringer MD, Cave E, Puntis JWL, et al. Enteric fistulas and necrotizing enterocolitis. J Pediatr Surg 1996;31:1268–1271.
16. Iofel E, Kahn E, Lee TK, et al. Inflammatory polyps after necrotizing enterocolitis. J Pediatr Surg 2000;35:1246–1247.

MISCELLANEOUS COLON ABNORMALITIES

Colon Agenesis, Atresia, and Stenosis

Segmental congenital atresias or stenoses of the colon are relatively rare (1, 2) and colon atresia can assume one of four forms: (a) membranous atresia—type I, (b) atresia connected by a thin fibrous band—type II, (c) complete atresia

with no connecting band—type III, and (d) multiple atresias—type IV (Fig. 4.160). In the latter three types, an associated mesenteric defect also is present.

Roentgenographically (2), the colon proximal to the point of atresia often is massively dilated and contains a mixture of air and meconium (Fig. 4.161A). Barium enema examination usually reveals the colon distal to the area of atresia to be of the microcolon variety (Fig. 4.161B). In addition, it has been noted that in many of these cases, the blind, ending portion of the distal colon turns around on itself or assumes a so-called hook configuration (3). The case demonstrated in Figure 4.161C demonstrates a large, poorly formed hook. In the membranous form of colonic atresia, the membrane can bulge outward and result in the "windsock sign" (Fig. 4.161C). If the obstructed end of the colon (i.e., the portion just proximal to the diaphragm) is markedly dilated, the windsock sign is more vividly demonstrated. In cases of colon stenosis, the stenotic portion can be demonstrated with contrast material (Fig. 4.162), and in any of these cases, perforation of the colon during barium enema examination can occur. In this regard, it is probably better to use water-soluble, anionic contrast agents.

The etiology of colon atresia and stenosis currently is considered to lie with intrauterine vascular insult. As with the small bowel, this etiology now is favored over the failure of recanalization theory, and atresia can be single, multiple, or long segment. In addition, the colon proximal to the obstruction can become overdistended and ischemic secondary to compression by the massive intraluminal contents.

Colon atresia also has been documented in association with Hirschsprung's disease (4, 5). However, this must be

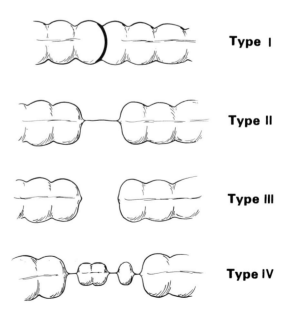

FIGURE 4.160. Colon atresia: classification. In type I colon atresia, a membrane is present. Type II colon atresia is associated with a fibrous band connecting the two ends of the large bowel. Type III atresia shows no fibrous connection. Type IV is multiple.

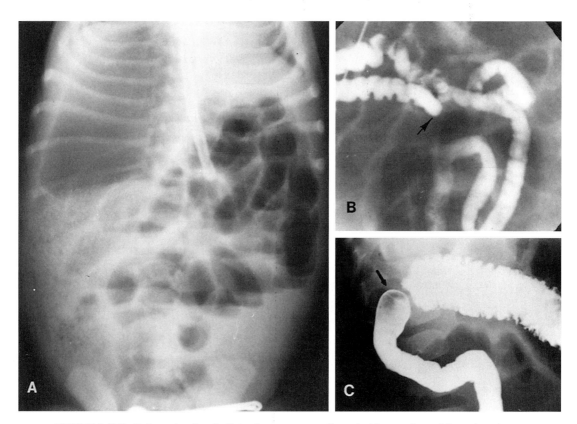

FIGURE 4.161. Colon atresia. A. Note the numerous distended loops of small bowel and one large distended loop, with bubbly meconium, on the right side of the abdomen. **B.** Barium enema shows a microcolon ending abruptly at a point designated by the arrow. Surgical exploration showed this to be the point of segmental colonic atresia, and the massively distended loop of intestine to be the ascending colon. **C. Membranous colon atresia.** Note the bulbous, bulging end of the obstructed distal portion of the colon (arrow). This type of bulbous distention signifies the presence of membranous atresia.

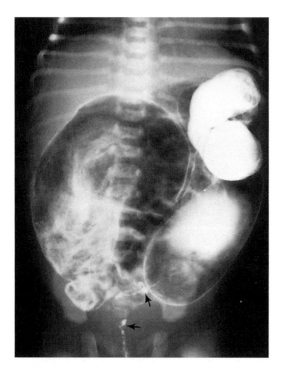

FIGURE 4.162. Colon stenosis. Note the massively dilated colon proximal to the stenotic segment (arrows).

an unusual circumstance, because the two conditions generally are held separate. It may be that the vascular insult rendering the colon atretic also renders the involved segment aganglionic. In one of the reported cases, the microcolon distal to the site of atresia was aganglionic (5), probably attesting to the fact that initial vascular insult was less focal, and more widespread than one would initially consider.

REFERENCES

1. Powelly RW, Raffensperger JG. Congenital colonic atresia. J Pediatr Surg 1982;17:171–174.
2. Winters WD, Weinberger E, Hatch E. Pictorial essay. Atresia of the colon in neonates: radiographic findings. AJR 1992;159:1273–1276.
3. Selke AC Jr, Jona JZ. The hook sign in type 3 congenital colonic atresia. AJR 1978;131:350–351.
4. Akgur FM, Tanyel FC, Buyukpamukcu N, et al. Colonic atresia and Hirschsprung's association shows further evidence of migration of enteric neurons. J Pediatr Surg 1993;28:635–636.
5. Williams MD, Burrington JD. Hirschsprung's disease complicating colon atresia. J Pediatr Surg 1993;28:637–639.

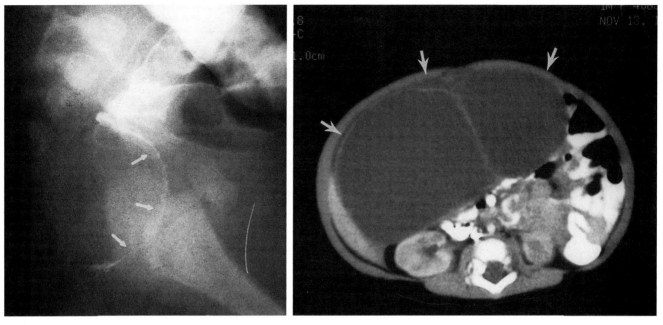

A

B

FIGURE 4.163. Duplication cyst. A. Note the marked indentation of distal rectum produced by duplication cyst (arrows). **B.** Another patient with CT demonstration of a large duplication cyst (arrows) of the colon. (**A** courtesy of R. Hagen, M.D., and C. Critchfield, M.D.)

Duplication Cysts

Duplication cysts of the colon are uncommon, but if large enough, they can produce pressure deformities (Fig. 4.163), and obstruction (1, 2). Ectopic gastric or pancreatic tissue may be present in these cysts and may lead to ulceration, bleeding, or perforation (3). Some of these duplications may be long and tubular (4) and diverticula, probably incomplete duplications, also can be encountered (5).

REFERENCES

1. Amjadi K, Poenaru D, Soboleski D, et al. Anterior rectal duplication: a diagnostic challenge. J Pediatr Surg 2000;35:613–614.
2. Shin K-S, Lee N-H, Kim S-Y. An unusual case of colonic duplication causing constipation in a child. J Pediatr Surg 1999;34:1410–1412.
3. Dutheil-Duco A, Le Pointe HD, Larroquet M, et al. a case of perforated cystic duplication of the transverse colon. Pediatr Radiol 1998;28:20–22.
4. Yousefzadeh DK, Bickers GH, Jackson JH Jr. Tubular colonic duplication—review of 1976–1981 literature. Pediatr Radiol 1983;13:65–71.
5. Sener RN, Melikoglu M, Kaya A. Rectal diverticulum in an infant. Pediatr Radiol 1991;21:433.

Colon Duplication

Duplication of the colon is rare and is often associated with duplication and numerous other anomalies of the genitourinary system and spinal canal (1, 2). Total duplication of the colon can present a most startling roentgenographic picture (Fig. 4.164), and in these cases, obstructing lesions such as imperforate (ectopic) anus or colon stenosis can also be present. In some cases, duplication involves the anorectum only (3).

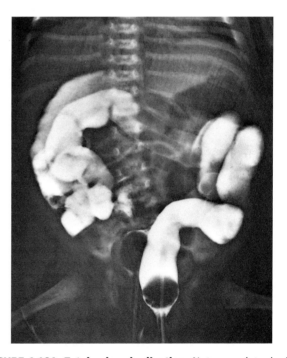

FIGURE 4.164. Total colon duplication. Note complete duplication of colon. This infant also had duplication of the genitourinary tract. (Reproduced with permission from Beach PD, Brascho DJ, Hein WR, et al. Duplication of the primitive hindgut of the human being. Surgery 1961;49:779–793.)

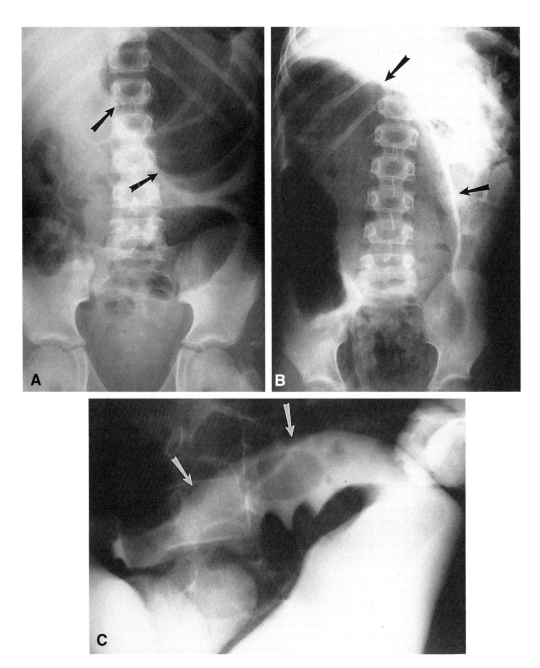

FIGURE 4.165. Colonic volvulus. A. Typical left upper quadrant placement of the cecum (arrows) in cecal volvulus. **B.** Typical location of the sigmoid colon (arrows) in sigmoid volvulus. **C.** Another patient, demonstrating thumbprinting (arrows) of a segment of sigmoid colon after spontaneous devolving.

REFERENCES

1. Dominguez R, Rott J, Castillo M, et al. Caudal duplication syndrome. Am J Dis Child 1993;147:1048–1052.
2. Shearer LT, Holt HA Jr, Young LW. Radiological case of the month: duplication of the bladder and colon. Am J Dis Child 1981;135:661–662.
3. La Quaglia MP, Feins N, Eraklis A, et al. Rectal duplications. J Pediatr Surg 1990;25:980–984.

Volvulus

Volvulus of the colon in children usually involves the sigmoid colon (1), but cecal volvulus also can be encountered (2, 3). Volvulus of the transverse colon is very rare (4). In terms of sigmoid volvulus, a predisposition exists in that the sigmoid colon often is redundant in infants and children and prone to twist.

Plain film findings in children generally are the same as those in adults, and with cecal volvulus the closed loop of the volved cecum usually comes to lie in the left upper quadrant (Fig. 4.165A). Sigmoid volvulus is more common and the twisted loop of sigmoid colon tends to point to the right upper quadrant (Fig. 4.165B). Sigmoid volvulus has a propensity to occur in chronically recumbent and retarded patients. The edematous loop of volved sigmoid colon also can be demonstrated with ultrasound, but usually is demonstrated with a barium enema where thumbprinting and spasm of the colonic segment is seen (Fig. 4.165C). This is after the volvulus has been reduced, which often occurs with the barium enema. Before reduction, the barium enema demonstrates a typical beak deformity (5) of the twisted colon. Finally, it is important to reiterate that the normally redundant sigmoid colon in infants often appears as if it had undergone volvulus (see Fig. 4.127).

REFERENCES

1. Salas S M, Angel CA, Salas N, et al. Sigmoid volvulus in children and adolescents. J Am Coll Surg 2000;190:717–723.
2. Kirks DR, Swischuk LE, Merten DF, et al. Cecal volvulus in children. AJR 1981;136:419–422.
3. Khope S, Rao PLNG. Cecal volvulus in a 2-month-old baby. J Pediatr Surg 1988;23:1038.
4. Houshian S, Sorensen JS, Jensen KE. Volvulus of the transverse colon in children. J Pediatr Surg 1998. 33:1399–1401.
5. Mellor MFA, Drake DG. Colonic volvulus in children: value of barium enema for diagnosis and treatment in 14 children. AJR 1994;162:1157–1159.

Megacystis-Microcolon-Intestinal Hypoperistalsis Syndrome

This relatively uncommon condition appears to predominate in female infants (1, 2) but also occasionally is seen in males (3). It is characterized by a massively distended bladder and a small colon (i.e., microcolon). The intestinal tract shows hypoperistalsis and this feature usually is refractory to any form of therapy. No focal GI-obstructing lesions have been demonstrated, but shortening of the bowel with malrotation is a common feature. Histologically, a visceral myopathy has been suggested to be the problem (3, 4).

No mechanical bladder neck or urethral obstruction is present and ureteral reflux usually does not occur. However, the kidneys can be hydronephrotic. The condition generally is refractory to therapy and, in severe form, usually results in demise of the infant. Roentgenographically, the large distended bladder usually is readily apparent on plain films, and barium enema clearly demonstrates the microcolon (Fig. 4.166).

REFERENCES

1. Kirtane J, Talwalker V, Dastur DK. Megacystis, microcolon, intestinal hypoperistalsis syndrome: possible pathogenesis. J Pediatr Surg 1984;19:206–208.
2. Puri P, Tsuji M. Megacystis-microcolon-intestinal hypoperistalsis syndrome (neonatal hollow visceral myopathy). Pediatr Surg Int 1992;7:18–22.
3. Krook OM. Megacystis-microcolon-intestinal hypoperistalsis syndrome in a male infant. Radiology 1980;136:649–650.
4. Ciftci AO, Cook RCM, van Velzen D. Megacystis microcolon intestinal hypoperistalsis syndrome: evidence of a primary myocellular defect of contractile fiber synthesis. J Pediatr Surg 1996; 31:1706–1711.

Segmental Dilation of the Colon

This condition probably is the same as segmental dilation of the small bowel (1, 2). These patients present with findings similar to those of Hirschsprung's disease but on barium enema, demonstrate a variably long segment of overly dilated colon. The dilated portion of the colon also can be seen on plain films (Fig. 4.167). Generally, this portion of the colon is hypertrophied and shows decreased motility and subsequent obstruction. Removal of the involved portion is curative.

REFERENCES

1. Ngai RLC, Chan AKH, Lee JPK, et al. Segmental colonic dilation in a neonate. J Pediatr Surg 1992;27:506–508.
2. Nguyen L, Shandling B. Segmental dilation of the colon: a rare cause of chronic constipation. J Pediatr Surg 1984;19:539–540.

Colon Inflammatory Disease (Colitis)

Inflammatory disease of the colon (i.e., colitis) can be seen with a number of entities, but most are infectious or ischemic in nature. In addition, apart from granulomatous

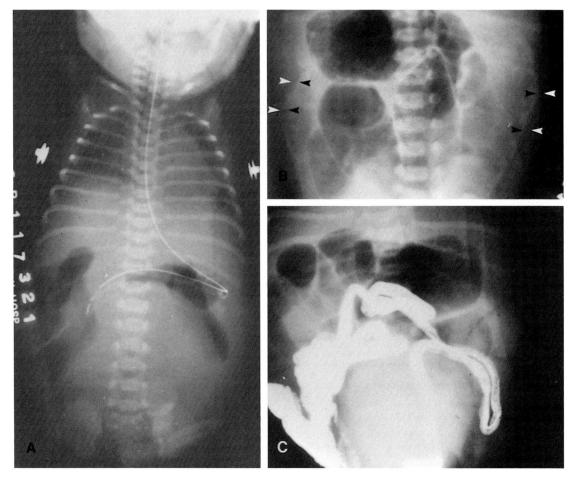

FIGURE 4.166. Microcolon-megacystis syndrome. A. Note the soft tissue mass rising out of the pelvis. This is the distended bladder. **B.** Intravenous pyelogram demonstrates rim signs in the bilaterally hydronephrotic kidneys (arrows). **C.** Barium enema demonstrates a typical microcolon being displaced by the distended bladder. (Reproduced with permission from Amoury RA, Fellows RA, Goodwin CD, et al. Megacystis-microcolon-intestinal hypoperistalsis syndrome; a cause of intestinal obstruction in the newborn period. J Pediatr Surg 1977;12:1063–1065.)

colitis (i.e., regional enteritis), which can involve the colon transmurally, most of the other conditions involve the colon mucosa. Differentiation of mucosal from transmural disease is relatively easily accomplished with ultrasound. With mucosal disease, increased echogenicity and thickening of the mucosa is seen, while with transmural disease, thickening of the entire intestinal wall occurs and it also tends to be somewhat hypoechoic (Fig. 4.168). These findings also can be seen with CT (Fig. 4.169).

In the neonate, inflammatory problems of the colon usually center on necrotizing enterocolitis, the enterocolitis of Hirschsprung's disease, and the colitis seen with milk allergy (1–3). These latter patients present with blood in the stool and short-segment areas of extreme spasm, usually in the rectosigmoid colon (Fig. 4.170). On endoscopy, spasm often is so pronounced that the sigmoidoscope cannot be passed through the area and overall the condition can be confused with Hirschsprung's disease (3). In older infants and children, colitis may be the result of infection such as *Shigella*, rotavirus, amebiasis, and *Clostridium difficile* infection. Pseudomembranous colitis also occurs (Fig. 4.169), and interestingly, a form of ulcerative colitis can be seen with *epidermolysis bullosa* (4). Inflammatory colitides such as those resulting from *Shigella* and rotavirus infections seldom are investigated beyond the plain film. However, many times on the plain film, dilated fluid-filled loops of intestine, primarily colon, will be seen and may mimic a surgical abdomen.

The barium enema also frequently is used to investigate inflammatory diseases of the colon, and in terms of amebiasis the findings usually consist of diffuse mucosal ulcerations that, early in the course of the disease, mimic those of granulomatous colitis. Later, ameboma formation around the cecum can lead to the so-called cone-shaped cecum, but

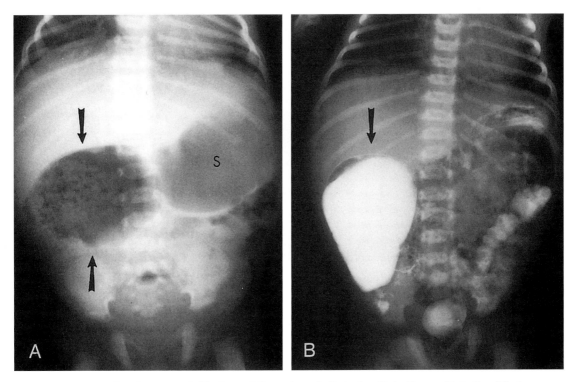

FIGURE 4.167. Segmental dilation of the colon. A. Note the dilated loop of intestine filled with granular material (arrows). S, stomach. **B.** Subsequent contrast enema demonstrates the dilated segment (arrow) of the ascending colon.

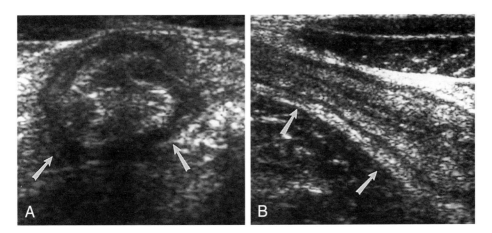

FIGURE 4.168. Colitis: ultrasonographic findings. A. Cross-sectional view through the rectum demonstrates thickening of the rectal wall and mucosa (arrows). **B.** Longitudinal view of the sigmoid colon (arrows) demonstrates markedly thickened echogenic mucosa.

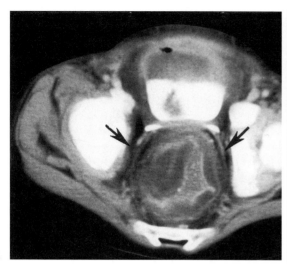
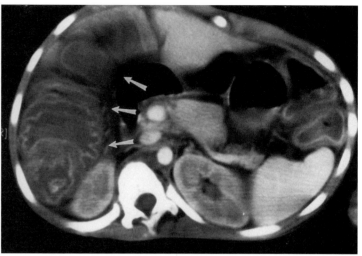

A

B

FIGURE 4.169. Colitis: CT findings. A. Note marked edema and thumbprinting of the rectum (arrows). **B.** Edema also extends into the ascending colon (arrows) in this case of pseudomembranous colitis.

it should be noted that the most common cause of a cone-shaped cecum in North America is granulomatous colitis.

Ulcerative colitis usually is a disease of older children. In the early stages, delicate superficial ulcers of the colon are seen (Fig. 4.171A), but with chronicity the so-called shortened, lead-pipe colon develops (Fig. 4.171B). In between these stages one can see variable edema, nodular mucosal thickening, and mucosal ulceration (Fig. 4.171C). Backwash colitis is common, and the overall findings are no different from those seen in adults. Toxic megacolon is a complication of ulcerative colitis more so than with granulomatous colitis. However, it can occur with almost any form of colitis. On plain films, it is the transverse colon that shows maximal distention and distention can be associated with thumbprinting (Fig. 4.172). Pseudopolyp formation also is seen in ulcerative colitis. Complicating malignancy is more common with ulcerative colitis.

Granulomatous colitis, or regional ileitis, also is uncommon in infants but is not an uncommon problem in older children. In fact, it is more common than ulcerative colitis. Findings in these patients are the same as findings in adults and consist of narrowing of the terminal ileum (string sign due to spasm and mucosal edema, a cone-shaped cecum, nodular thickening of the colon (Fig. 4.173B), deep linear undermining ulcers (Fig. 4.173A) and filiform polyposis (Fig. 4.173C). Stricture and sinus tract or fistula formation also occur and are common in this condition. Another common presentation is that of a perianal cutaneous fistula. Fistulas also can develop to other portions of the intestine, the urinary tract, or the genital tract. The thickened, edematous terminal ileum can be demonstrated with ultra-

sound, but the findings are not entirely specific (see Fig. 4.117). Similar findings can be seen with tuberculosis and lymphoma, but in the correct setting they are relatively specific for granulomatous colitis.

The colitis seen in the hemolytic uremic syndrome occurs mostly in older children (5). The findings on ultrasound and contrast enema examination are those of edema and thickening of the mucosa. Colitis also has been demonstrated in the Kawasaki-mucocutaneous lymph node syndrome (6) and with cystic fibrosis as a result of high dose enzyme therapy (7, 8). Strictures are not uncommon in this condition. In addition, in cystic fibrosis, patients with clostridium difficile colitis may lack the usual watery diarrhea component seen in otherwise normal children (8). One can also encounter pseudomembranous colitis in children and the mucosal changes can be quite profound (Fig. 4.169).

REFERENCES

1. Hill SM, Milla PJ. Colitis caused by food allergy in infants. Arch Dis Child 1990;65:132–133.
2. Swischuk LE, Hayden CK Jr. Barium enema findings (? segmental colitis) in four neonates with bloody diarrhea—possible cow's milk allergy. Pediatr Radiol 1985;15:34–37.
3. Bloom DA, Buonomo C, Fishman SJ, et al. Allergic colitis: a mimic of Hirschsprung disease. Pediatr Radiol 1999;29:37–41.
4. Smith PK, Davidson GP, Moore L, et al. Epidermolysis bullosa and severe ulcerative colitis in an infant. J Pediatr 1993;122:600–603.
5. Kawanami T, Bowen A, Girdany GR. Enterocolitis: prodrome of the hemolytic-uremic syndrome. Radiology 1984;151:91–92.

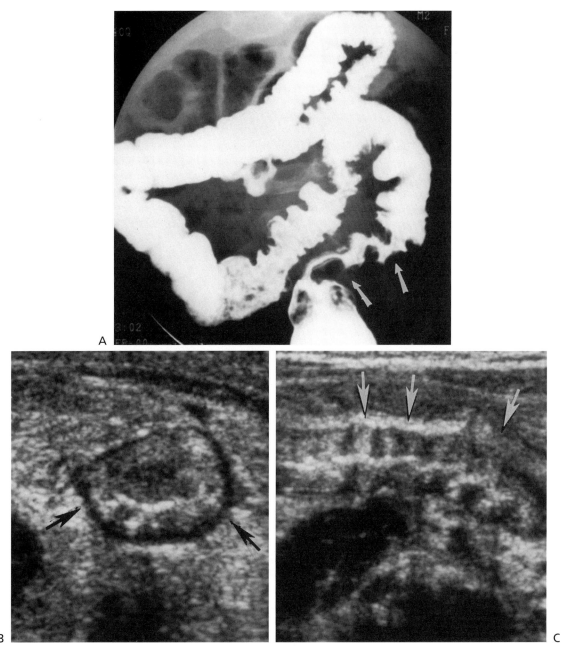

FIGURE 4.170. Segmental colitis: cow's milk allergy. A. Note the area of spasm and irregularity of the rectosigmoid colon (arrows). **B.** Another patient with an ultrasound study demonstrating mucosal thickening (arrows) on cross-section. **C.** Longitudinal view of the same portion of the colon demonstrates the extensive mucosal thickening (arrows).

6. Chung CJ, Rayder S, Meyers W, et al. Kawasaki disease presenting as focal colitis. Pediatr Radiol 1996;26:455–457.
7. Reichard KW, Vinocur CD, Franco M, et al. Fibrosing colonopathy in children with cystic fibrosis. J Pediatr Surg 1997;32:237–242.
8. Binkovitz LA, Allen E, Bloom D, et al. Atypical presentation of *Clostridium difficile* colitis in patients with cystic fibrosis. AJR 1999;172:517–521.

Behçet's Syndrome

Behçet's syndrome is not particularly common in children (1, 2), but the overall GI findings are similar to those seen with regional enteritis. It is a vasculitis that also presents with genital and oral mucosal ulcerations.

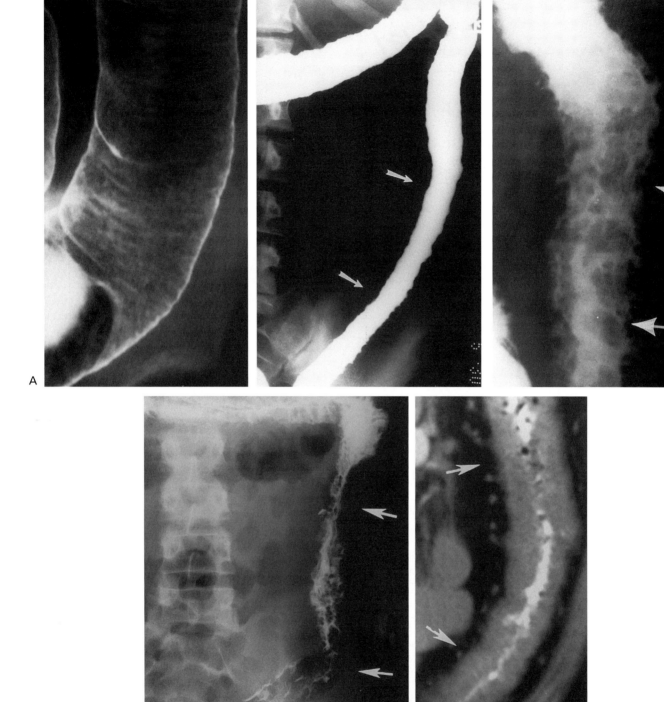

FIGURE 4.171. Ulcerative colitis. A. Early findings demonstrate diffuse amorphous ulceration of colonic mucosa. **B.** Late stages demonstrating a thin pipestem colon (arrows) with no haustral markings. **C.** This patient demonstrates diffuse nodularity and ulceration of the descending colon (arrows). **D.** In this patient, there is diffuse ulceration, nodular mucosal thickening, and spasm of the colon (arrows). **E.** CT study demonstrating similar findings (arrows).

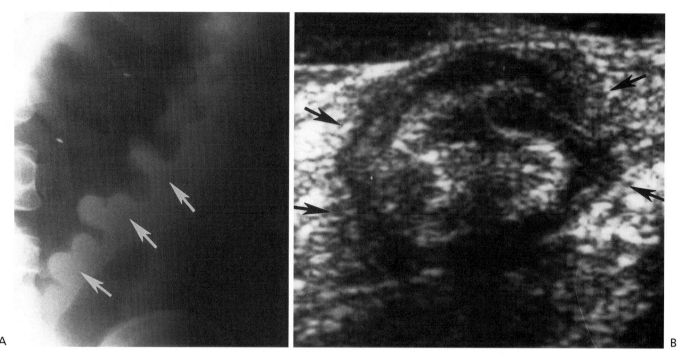

A   B

FIGURE 4.172. Ulcerative colitis: other findings. A. Toxic megacolon with thumbprinting. The colon is dilated, and there is pronounced thumbprinting (arrows) present. **B.** Ultrasound study demonstrates the markedly thickened mucosa (arrows).

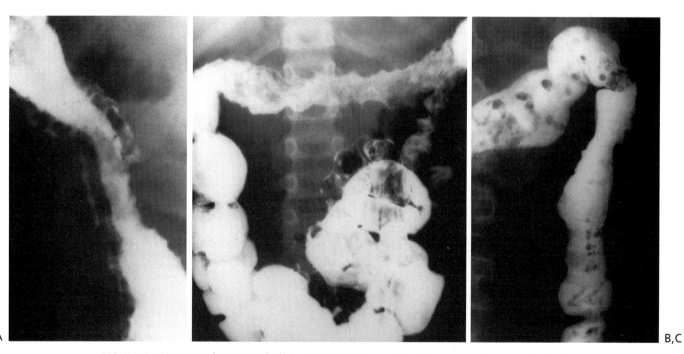

A   B,C

FIGURE 4.173. Granulomatous colitis. A. Typical deep undermining ulcers of regional enteritis (i.e., granulomatous colitis). **B.** Advanced mucosal changes with mucosal irregularity, thumbprinting, and shortening of the transverse and descending portions of the colon. **C.** Multiple filling defects resulting from filiform polyposis and longstanding granulomatous colitis.

REFERENCES

1. Ammann AJ, Johnson A, Fyfe GA, et al. Behçet syndrome. J Pediatr 1985;107:41–43.
2. Stringer DA, Cleghorn GJ, Durie PR, et al. Behçet's syndrome involving the gastrointestinal tract—a diagnostic dilemma in childhood. Pediatr Radiol 1986;16:131–134.

Typhlitis (Neutropenic Colitis)

This condition, also termed the ileocecal syndrome, is an affliction of patients with leukemia (1, 2). It is characterized by a profound necrotizing inflammation of the terminal ileum, appendix, and cecum. Very often it is a terminal event but it is unknown as to just why it occurs. The clinical findings mimic those of acute appendicitis. Thickening of the mucosa, along with increased echogenicity (1), although nonspecific findings, are characteristic in the appropriate clinical situation. Although most commonly neutropenic colitis involves the cecum (Fig. 4.174, A and B), it can involve other portions of the colon (Fig. 4.174, C and D) and even the small bowel (Fig. 4.174, E and F). All of these findings also are demonstrable with CT (Fig.

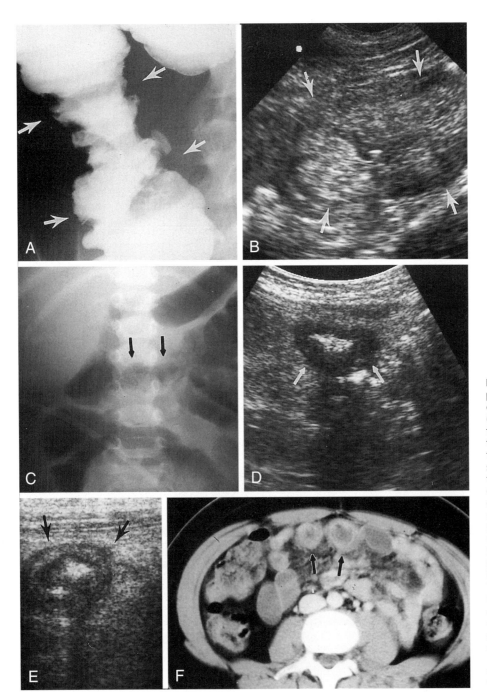

FIGURE 4.174. Typhlitis (neutropenic colitis). A. Note the deformity of the cecum and ascending colon (arrows). This area was spastic, and there are superficial mucosal ulcerations present. **B.** Ultrasonogram of the same area demonstrates the oval-shaped mass (arrows) representing the cecum. It is filled with thickened echogenic mucosa. **C.** Plain film demonstrates narrowing of a segment of transverse colon in this patient with neutropenic colitis. **D.** Cross-sectional ultrasonographic image through the area demonstrates marked hypoechoic thickening of the intestinal wall (arrows). The echogenic mucosa is compressed in the center. **E.** Another patient with a thickened loop of small bowel (arrows) demonstrated with ultrasound. **F.** CT study in the same patient demonstrates thickened small bowel loops (arrows). Compare with adjacent normal fluid-filled, but thin-walled, loops of intestine.

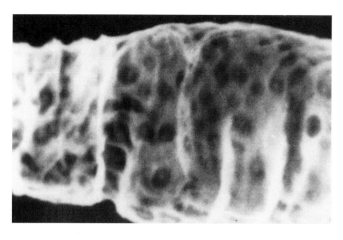

FIGURE 4.175. Lymphoid hypoplasia. Note the typical small filling defects with umbilicated centers.

4.174F). In addition, occasionally, one can encounter toxic megacolon and pneumatosis (3).

REFERENCES

1. Alexander JE, Williamson SL, Seibert JJ, et al. The ultrasonographic diagnosis of typhlitis (neutropenic colitis). Pediatr Radiol 1988;18:200–204.
2. Katz JA, Wagner ML, Gresik MV, et al. Typhlitis: an 18-year experience and post-mortem review. Cancer 1990;65:1041–1047.
3. Kamal M, Wilkinson AG, Gibson B. Radiological features of fungal typhlitis complicating acute lymphoblastic leukaemia. Pediatr Radiol 1997;27:18–19.

Lymphoid Hyperplasia

Lymphoid hyperplasia of the colon in children is common (1, 2), and now that double contrast air studies are being performed more frequently, these small nodules with their characteristically umbilicated centers are seen very often (Fig. 4.175). It is important, however, to note that these nodules do not always clearly demonstrate their umbilicated centers, but, whatever the case, they are benign. They are most commonly seen in older children but also are seen in infants and can be seen in exaggerated form with immunologic disturbances, infections, and milk allergy. Although every so often there is some attempt in adults to consider these lesions as precursors of malignancy, this does not seem to be the case in childhood.

REFERENCES

1. Atwell JD, Burge D, Wright D. Nodular lymphoid hyperplasia of the intestinal tract in infancy and childhood. J Pediatr Surg 1985; 20:25–29.
2. Riddlesberger MM Jr, Lebenthal E. Nodular colonic mucosa of childhood: normal or pathologic? Gastroenterology 1980;79: 265–270.

Tumors and Polyps of the Colon

Neoplasia of the colon is rare in childhood in general and extremely rare in the infant. Occasional cases of carcinoma of the colon occur in older children (1, 2), but in young infants, a colonic tumor is more likely to be an angiofibroma, leiomyoma, leiomyosarcoma, lymphosarcoma, some other sarcoma, or even a teratoma (3). Polyps are common in children, but rare in the neonate. Even in familial adenomatous polyposis the lesions do not become roentgenographically apparent until 6–12 months of age. At this stage, polypoid formation is so small that it may be difficult to differentiate the findings from those of lymphoid hyperplasia. Often, these polyps are very uniform in size, but eventually, some become larger. In the early stages, however, it is the number and virtual carpeting of the colonic mucosa with the polyps that is characteristic of familial adenomatous polyposis (Fig. 4.176A). As time goes by, malignant degeneration becomes an increasingly common risk in these patients.

Benign, nonadenomatous or juvenile polyps can present in children with bleeding, intussusception, or an abdominal mass. Bleeding is the most common presentation. These polyps usually are located in the lower colon and can be sessile or pedunculated (Fig. 4.176B). Many times, their stalks are clearly visible and they can be solitary or multiple. The vast majority of these cases are sporadic but familial cases also can occur. The condition generally is believed to be benign, but some cases of multiple juvenile non-adenomatosis polyposis with malignant potential have been documented (4). These polyps are inflammatory in etiology and inflammatory polyps also can be seen in the Canada-Cronkhite syndrome.

Adenomatous polyps also occur in Gardner's and Turcot syndromes but the polyps seen in the Peutz-Jeghers syndrome are hamartomatous polyps. In the Peutz-Jeghers syndrome, as in the other syndromes, the polyps usually are seen in the small bowel, rather than in the colon but also can be seen in the duodenum and stomach. Being that these

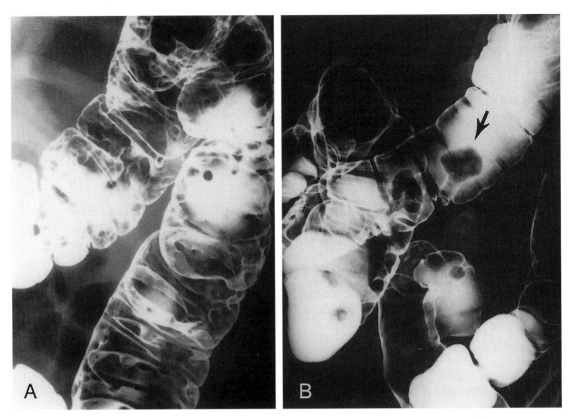

FIGURE 4.176. Colon polyposis. A. Familial polyposis. Small, uniform polyps virtually carpet the colon. This patient had familial adenomatous polyposis. **B.** Juvenile polyps. Note the numerous polyps of various sizes that are scattered in the colon and one with a stalk (arrow) in the transverse colon.

polyps occur in the small bowel, intussusception is a common complicating problem. In addition, osteo-arthropathy has been noticed with hamartomatous polyps (5).

REFERENCES

1. Borger JA, Barbosa J. Adenocarcinoma of the rectum in a 15-year-old. J Pediatr Surg 1993;28:1594–1596.
2. Karnak I, Ciftci AO, Senocak ME, et al. Colorectal carcinoma in children. J Pediatr Surg 1999;34:1499–1504.
3. Shah RS, Kaddu SJ, Kirtane JM. Benign mature teratoma of the large bowel: a case report. J Pediatr Surg 1996;31:701–702.
4. Heiss KF, Schaffner D, Ricketts RR, et al. Malignant risk in juvenile polyposis coli: increasing documentation in the pediatric age group. J Pediatr Surg 1993;28:1188–1193.
5. Erkul PE, Ariyurek OM, Altinok D, et al. Colonic hamartomatous polyposis associated with hypertrophic osteoarthropathy. Pediatr Radiol 1994;24:145–146.

GALLBLADDER AND BILE DUCTS

Normal Configuration, Variations, and Anomalies

The normal gallbladder and bile ducts appear the same in newborn and infants as in older children and adults, except

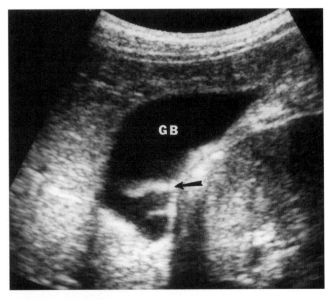

FIGURE 4.177. Normal gallbladder. Normal ultrasonographic appearance of the gallbladder (GB). The echogenic linear structure in the neck (arrow) is the valve of Heister.

that they are proportionately smaller. Currently, the best method with which to study the gallbladder is ultrasonography. The gallbladder appears hypoechoic and somewhat elongated, and occasionally the circular valves of Heister are visualized as echogenic areas in the neck of the gallbladder (Fig. 4.177), and in patients not being fed orally the gallbladder often becomes abnormally distended and can even present as an abdominal mass (1, 2). Ultrasound can readily establish that the mass is a normal gallbladder (Fig. 4.178). As far as anomalies of the gallbladder are concerned, in any age group one can encounter anomalies such as diaphragms, multiseptate gallbladders (3), duplication, or even triplication of the gallbladder (4).

The normal common bile duct also is readily visualized and in children (Fig. 4.179) is a little smaller than in adults. Maximum measurements in childhood have been estimated to be approximately 3 mm, while under 3 months the bile duct measures approximately 1 mm (5).

REFERENCES

1. Liechty EA, Cohen MD, Lemonas JA, et al. Normal gallbladder appearing as abdominal mass in neonates. Am J Dis Child 1982;136:468–469.
2. El-Shafie M, Mah CL. Transient gallbladder distension in sick pre-

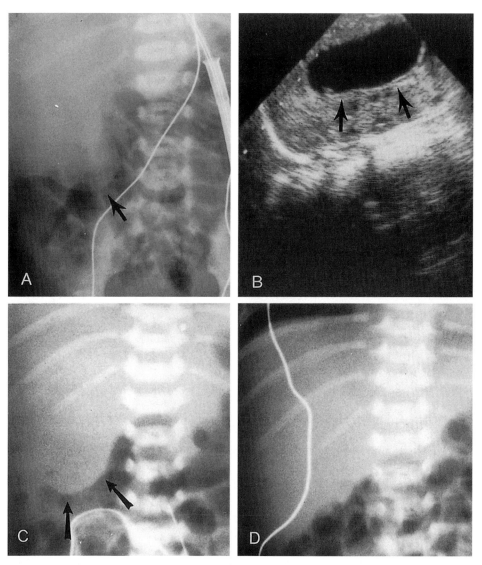

FIGURE 4.178. Transient gallbladder distention in the neonate. A. Note the readily visible and clinically palpable distended gallbladder (arrow). **B.** Ultrasonogram demonstrates the distended gallbladder (arrows), and a small sludge ball in it. **C.** Another patient with a distended gallbladder (arrows). **D.** Next day, gallbladder distention has disappeared.

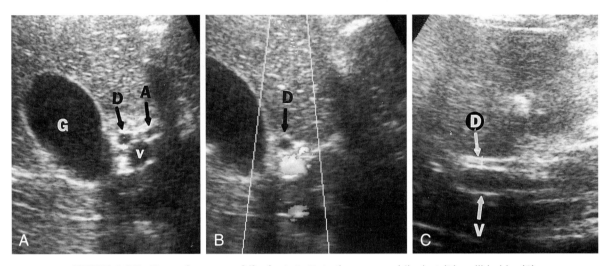

FIGURE 4.179. Normal common bile duct. A. Note the common bile duct (D), gallbladder (G), portal vein (V) and hepatic artery (A). **B.** Color-flow Doppler demonstrates flow in the portal vein and hepatic artery but no flow in the common bile duct (D). **C.** Longitudinal view demonstrating the portal vein (V) and the common bile duct (D).

mature infants: the value of ultrasonography and radionuclide scintigraphy. Pediatr Radiol 1986;16:468–471.

3. Strauss S, Starinsky R, Alon Z. Partial multiseptate gallbladder: sonographic appearance. J Ultrasound Med 1993;12:201–203.

4. Ross RJ, Sachs MD. Triplication of the gallbladder. AJR 1968;104:656–661.

5. Hernanz-Schulman M, Ambrosino MM, Freeman PC, et al. Common bile duct in children: sonographic dimensions. Radiology 1995;195:193–195.

ABNORMALITIES OF THE GALLBLADDER AND BILE DUCTS

Biliary Atresia

For the most part, biliary atresia can be considered as intrahepatic or extrahepatic. Intrahepatic atresia is less common (1), and generally the clinical course in these individuals is more protracted and liver enlargement slower to evolve. In an effort to explain this phenomenon, Ahrens et al. (2) suggested that, because there is absence of intrahepatic ducts, there is no backflow of bile, no intrahepatic ductal distention, and hence, no periductal inflammation. This form of biliary atresia can be inherited on an autosomal recessive basis (3), and there is now considerable feeling that this is the type of biliary atresia seen in the arteriohepatic dysplasia, or Alagille, syndrome (see next section). Biliary atresia also can coexist with polysplenia, and in these cases, cardiac disease need not necessarily be present (4, 5).

Infants with extrahepatic biliary atresia present with jaundice early, and while initially there may be some confusion with physiologic jaundice of the newborn, this is temporary. Bile is absent in the stools, and jaundice may wax and wane. Intrahepatic bile duct dilation and subsequent biliary cirrhosis usually develop quickly, and the disease is progressive. Early in the course, however, the real problem is to differentiate biliary atresia from neonatal hepatitis. Often, this is difficult, because the two conditions have certain similarities (6), and there is now considerable feeling that most cases of biliary atresia are the result of neonatal hepatobiliary infection and an ensuing chronic cholangiohepatitis (7, 8). However, there are reported cases of noninflammatory extrahepatic biliary atresia (9), and it appears that, although most cases represent the result of infection and inflammation, some cases are the result of congenital stenosis of the bile ducts. All of this notwithstanding, the end result on the liver is the same.

In terms of infection, it is theorized that in any given infant a viral infection first induces a cholangiohepatitis and, in response, an immune response is invoked (10). This entails the production of α-fetoprotein (11), an immune response regulator that attempts to control the disease process. Characteristically, it is elevated in infants with neonatal hepatitis (11), but not in infants with biliary atresia. This is of considerable importance, because it also has been demonstrated that those patients with elevated α-fetoprotein generally do not go on to develop biliary atresia, while those with low levels do (11). This would suggest that some infants are able to control the initial viral infection better than others, and that those who can do not develop biliary atresia.

Taking this concept one step further, one can see that, depending on just when the patient is examined, different degrees of biliary duct obliteration will be seen. In other words, one can see infants with reasonably well-preserved ducts, infants with ducts that appear hypoplastic and are visible only on microscopic examination, infants with no remaining bile ducts at all, and finally a few with cystic transformation of the intrahepatic bile ducts. The milder of these cases often are referred to as cases of biliary hypoplasia.

In terms of the imaging investigation of biliary atresia, final diagnosis often still usually is accomplished with an intraoperative cholangiogram, but considerable preliminary data can be obtained both with ultrasonography and nuclear scintigraphy. Ultrasonography yields data regarding the presence of a gallbladder, its size, and whether there is associated intrahepatic ductal dilation (Fig. 4.180A). In most cases of biliary atresia, hepatic parenchymal signals are nonspecific, and most times the liver is of normal echogenicity. With the

rarer intrahepatic biliary atresia, however, considerable echogenicity, resulting from fibrosis and scarring, can be seen in the periportal area (Fig. 4.181). This represents the recently demonstrated triangular cord sign on ultrasonography (12–16). This finding also can be seen on T2-weighted MR images as an increased area of triangular density in the porta hepatis (15). In most cases of extrahepatic biliary atresia, the gallbladder is small and neither the extrahepatic nor intrahepatic bile ducts are dilated (Fig. 4.180), but there are a few rare instances where intrahepatic cystic ductal dilation (17) can be seen (Fig. 4.180E). MR can be used to detect the presence of normal bile ducts and aid in excluding biliary atresia (18).

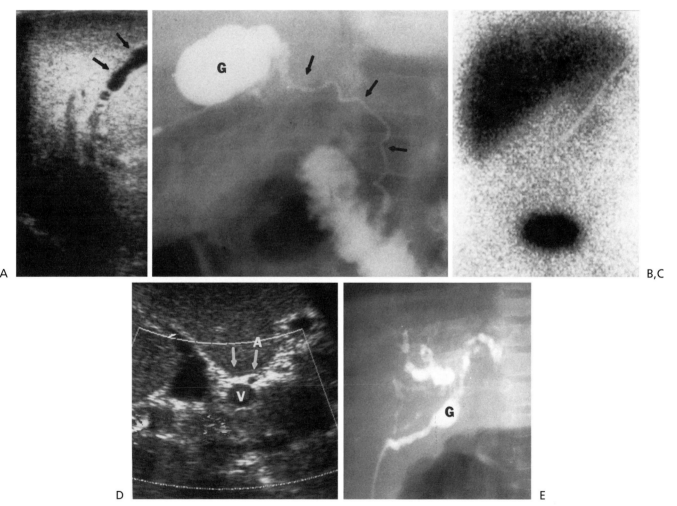

FIGURE 4.180. Extrahepatic biliary atresia: various configurations. A. The gallbladder (arrows) is very small in this patient. **B.** Operative cholangiogram demonstrates the small gallbladder (G) and the thin common bile duct (arrows). No intrahepatic radicals are demonstrated. **C.** Delayed hepatobiliary scintigram demonstrates activity in the liver but no activity in the intestine, consistent with biliary tract obstruction. **D.** Another patient, demonstrating a normal portal vein (V), a hepatic artery (A) but absence of the common bile duct (arrow). Compare with normal configuration of these structures in Fig. 4.179. **E.** Rare case of extrahepatic biliary atresia, demonstrating a small gallbladder (G) and numerous dilated, tortuous interhepatic biliary radicals.

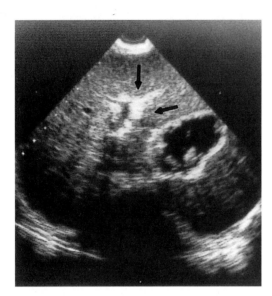

FIGURE 4.181. Interhepatic biliary atresia: Alagille syndrome. Note the echogenic, fibrotic area in the periportal region (arrows).

In terms of scintigraphy, the development of technetium-99m IDA analogs has led to considerable improvement in the differentiation of hepatitis from biliary atresia. In biliary atresia, hepatocyte function usually is intact early in the course of the disease, and the isotope is picked up by the liver cells. However, because of bile duct atresia, there is no excretion of the isotope into the intestine (Fig. 4.180C). With neonatal hepatitis, uptake by the liver cells is sluggish, although excretion of isotope into the bile and subsequently the GI tract eventually occurs. The oral administration of phenobarbital for 5 days before the study is said to enhance biliary excretion of the isotope and therefore increase the discriminatory value of the scintigram.

Eventually, however, final diagnosis of biliary atresia usually is made with intraoperative cholangiography and liver biopsy. In this regard, it should be emphasized that one not be tardy in progressing to diagnostic laparotomy, because it is important that cases of biliary atresia be treated early, before the ducts are totally obliterated. Currently, the preferred surgical procedure is the Kasai portoenterostomy, and if performed early enough, it results are reasonably encouraging. In untreated cases, biliary fibrosis (cirrhosis) and portal hypertension become significant chronic problems, and afflicted infants are plagued by recurrent ascites, esophageal varices, GI bleeding, and later, biliary rickets.

In terms of the cholangiogram, one makes the distinction between neonatal hepatitis and biliary atresia on the basis of the size of the gallbladder, size of the bile ducts, and the demonstration of filling of the hepatitic radicles. In neonatal hepatitis, the gallbladder is normal or near normal in size and usually contains bile. The cystic duct, common bile duct, and hepatic radicles are normal, but they may

appear somewhat thin, reflecting diminution in caliber secondary to decreased hepatic excretion and subsequent bile flow. In many cases, there also is very poor filling of the hepatic radicles, and biliary atresia may erroneously be suggested. However, with occlusion of the distal common bile duct or with endoscopic retrograde cholangiopancreatography (ERCP), reflux into the hepatic radicles often occurs (Fig. 4.182). If this does not occur, the diagnosis should be biliary atresia. Overall, then, if the gallbladder is normal or near normal in size, and hepatic bile duct filling occurs, even if it is minimal, the preferred diagnosis is neonatal hepatitis. Another interesting manifestation seen in the biliary tract in patients with biliary atresia is cystic dilation of the bile ducts in the liver after the Kasai procedure (19, 20). It is believed that an ascending cholangitis is the underlying problem (19).

REFERENCES

1. Engelskirchen R, Holschneider AM, et al. Biliary atresia—a 25-year survey. Eur J Pediatr Surg 1991;1:154–160.
2. Ahrens EH Jr, Harris RC, MacMahon HE. Atresia of the intrahepatic bile ducts. Pediatrics 1951;8:628–647.
3. Smith BM, Laberge J-M, Schreiber R, et al. Familial biliary atresia in three siblings including twins. J Pediatr Surg 1991;26:1331–1333.
4. Davenport M, Savage M, Mowat AP, et al. Biliary atresia splenic malformation syndrome: an etiologic and prognostic subgroup. Surgery 1993;113:662–668.
5. Karrer FM, Hall RJ, Lilly JR. Biliary atresia and the polysplenia syndrome. J Pediatr Surg 1991;26:524–527.
6. Lai M, Chang M, Hsu S, et al. Differential diagnosis of extrahepatic biliary atresia from neonatal hepatitis: a prospective study. J Pediatr Gastroenterol Nutr 1994;18:121–127.
7. Hart MH, Kaufman SS, Vanderhoof JA, et al. Neonatal hepatitis and extrahepatic biliary atresia associated with cytomegalovirus infection in twins. Am J Dis Child 1991;145:302–305.
8. Park W-H, Kim S-P, Park K-K, et al. Electron microscopic study of the liver with biliary atresia and neonatal hepatitis. J Pediatr Surg 1996;31:367–374.
9. Schwartz MZ, Hall RJ, Reubner B, et al. Agenesis of the extrahepatic bile ducts: report of five cases. J Pediatr Surg 1990;25:805–807.
10. Landing BH. Consideration of the pathogenesis of neonatal hepatitis, biliary atresia and choledochal cyst: the concept of infantile obstructive cholangiopathy. Prog Pediatr Surg 1974;6:113–139.
11. Zeltzer PM. Alpha-fetoprotein in the differentiation of neonatal hepatitis and biliary atresia: current status and implications for the pathogenesis of these disorders. J Pediatr Surg 1978;12:381–387.
12. Kendrick TAP, Phua KB, Subramaniam R, et al. Making the diagnosis of biliary atresia using the triangular cord sign and gallbladder length. Pediatr Radiol 2000;30:69–73.
13. Choi SO, Park WH, Lee HJ, et al. Triangular cord: a sonographic finding applicable in the diagnosis of biliary atresia. J Pediatr Surg 1996;31:363–366.
14. Park W-H, Choi S-O, Lee H-J, et al. A new diagnostic approach to biliary atresia with emphasis on the ultrasonographic triangular cord sign: comparison of ultrasonography, hepatobiliary scintigraphy, and liver needle biopsy in the evaluation of infantile cholestasis. J Pediatr Surg 1997;32:1555–1559.

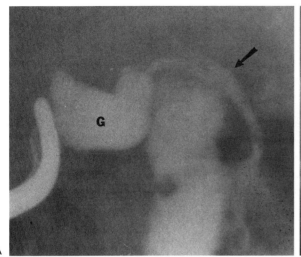
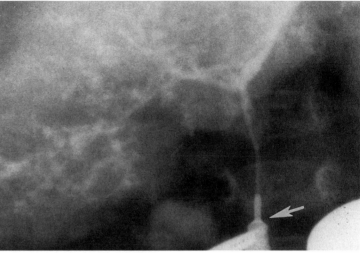
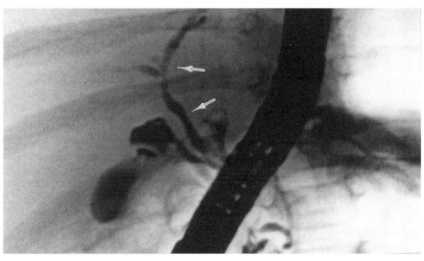

FIGURE 4.182. Hepatitis with false suggestion of absence of interhepatic bile ducts. A. Note the gallbladder (G). It is not particularly small. The common bile duct is identified (arrows), but no interhepatic bile duct biliary radicals are seen. The common bile duct is not as thin as seen with biliary atresia. **B.** With occlusion of the common bile duct (arrow), there is retrograde filling of intrahepatic biliary radicals. **C.** With endoscopic retrograde cholangiopancreatography, the intrahepatic bile ducts (arrows) are more clearly visualized.

15. Kim M-J, Park YN, Han SJ, et al. Biliary atresia in neonates and infants: triangular area of high signal intensity in the porta hepatis at T2-weighted MR cholangiography with US and histopathologic correlation. Radiology 2000;215:395–401.

16. Koth MA, Kotb A, Sheba MF, et al. Evaluation of the triangular cord sign in the diagnosis of biliary atresia. Pediatrics 2001;108: 416–420.

17. Takahashi A, Tsuchida Y, Hatakkeyama S, et al. a peculiar form of multiple cystic dilatation of the intrahepatic biliary system found in a patient with biliary atresia. J Pediatr Surg 1997;32: 1776–1779.

18. Twei-Shiun J, Yu-Ting K, Gin-Chung L, et al. MR cholangiography in the evaluation of neonatal cholestasis. Radiology 1999; 212:249–256.

19. Betz BW, Bisset GS III, Johnson ND, et al. MR imaging of biliary cysts in children with biliary atresia: clinical associations and pathological correlation. AJR 1994;162:167–171.

20. Tsuchida Y, Honna T, Kawarasaki H. Cystic dilation of the intrahepatic biliary system in biliary atresia after hepatic portoenterostomy. J Pediatr Surg 1994;29:630–634.

Arteriohepatic Dysplasia (Alagille's Syndrome)

This relatively rare condition consists of intrahepatic ductal dysplasia or atresia, peripheral pulmonary artery stenosis, chronic cholestasis, renal abnormalities, growth retardation, mental retardation, hypogonadism, and vertebral anomalies (1–3). Not all of these features need be present in every individual, and the condition is believed to be inherited on an autosomal recessive basis. The extrahepatic bile ducts are normal but the intrahepatic ducts are dysplastic or frankly atretic. Ultrasonographically one may see increased echogenicity (the triangular cord sign) in the periportal region resulting from fibrosis (Fig. 4.181).

REFERENCES

1. Levin SE, Zarvos P, Milner S, et al. Arteriohepatic dysplasia: association of liver disease with pulmonary arterial stenosis as well as facial and skeletal abnormalities. Pediatrics 1980;66:876–883.
2. Pombo F, Isla C, Gayol A, et al. Aortic calcification and renal cysts demonstrated by CT in a teenager with Alagille syndrome. Pediatr Radiol 1995;25:314–315.
3. Singcharoen T, Partridge J, Jeans WD, et al. Arteriohepatic dysplasia. Br J Radiol 1986;59:509–511.

Choledochal Cysts

Choledochal cysts can present in infants with fluctuating jaundice, pain, and at times, fever. A right upper quadrant mass often is palpable, rounding out the classic diagnostic triad of jaundice, pain, and a right upper quadrant mass. However, this classic triad is not always present and may be less common than generally considered (1). It also should be noted that choledochal cysts can present later in life, even in adulthood, and there is a definite spectrum of severity. Overall, a female predominance seems to exist, and more severe cases seem to be seen in infants.

In the past, the cause of choledochal cyst usually was considered to lie in the realm of congenital weakness or deficiency of the bile duct wall or, less likely, from congenital ductal obstruction. However some time ago Babbitt et al. (2) suggested a theory invoking anomalous development of the common bile and pancreatic ducts. In their cases, the common bile duct entered anomalously into the duct of Wirsung, and the ampulla of Vater was distal to the junction of the two ducts. Because of this, regurgitation of pancreatic secretions into the bile duct occurred. This, then, led to an ascending cholangitis and, subsequently, to inflammatory changes and cyst formation. This theory, more and more, has been supported by others (3–5) and also may well explain those cases of choledochal cyst associated with pancreatitis.

The classification of choledochal cyst often is more complicated than is necessary because there always is an attempt to include all bile duct dilations under the umbrella of choledochal cyst (Fig. 4.183). For example, the so-called choledochocele often is included in the discussion of choledochal cyst, yet there are those who feel that it is a separate entity (6, 7). It probably is a separate entity and consists of dilation of the bile duct, in its terminal portion, in the wall of the duodenum (Fig. 4.184). It is a very uncommon problem both in children and the population in general, and frequently it is asymptomatic.

The most common form of choledochal cyst, accounting for 80–90% of cases (8), is the form in which there is fusiform dilation of a portion of the biliary tree. Very rarely there may be multiple areas of dilation, and in some cases, there may be associated dilation of the intrahepatic bile ducts. In some cases, dilation may be enormous, and then many feel that one is dealing with Caroli's disease. Whether this is true or not remains debatable, but there is no question that some cases of choledochal cyst are associated with intrahepatic biliary duct dilation. It has been suggested that

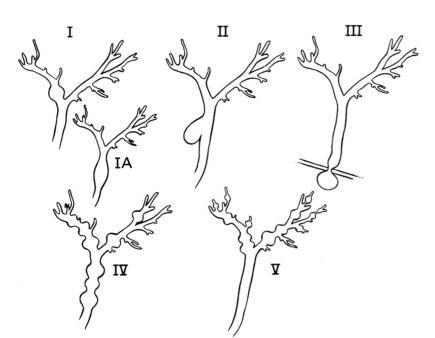

FIGURE 4.183. Choledochal cyst: diagrammatic representation. Note the configurations of the various types. The type I abnormality is the most common form of choledochal cyst. The type III abnormality, the choledochocele, often is not considered a true choledochal cyst. Type V represents Caroli's disease.

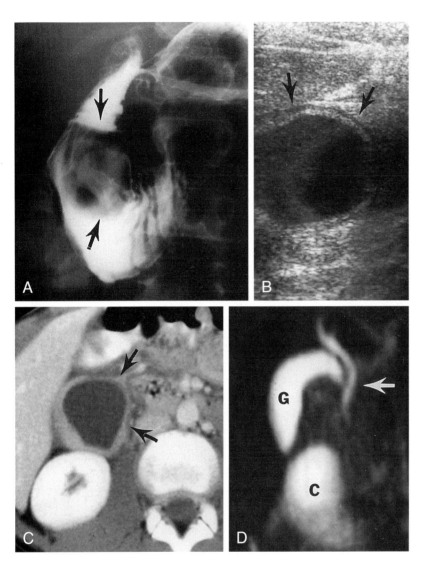

FIGURE 4.184. Choledochocele. A. Note the filling defect (arrows) in the duodenum. **B.** Ultrasonogram demonstrates the choledochocele (arrows) with an echogenic mucosal lining. **C.** Choledochocele demonstrated with CT (arrows). **D.** MR cholangiography demonstrates the choledochocele (C), gallbladder (G), and common bile duct (arrow).

two thirds of choledochal cysts are associated with such dilation (8). A rare form of choledochal cyst consists of a diverticulum off the biliary tract. In infancy and childhood, the type 1 anomaly, a fusiform dilation of a portion of the common bile duct, is seen most often.

Roentgenographically, strong presumptive, if not definitive, diagnosis can be made using a combination of ultrasound and nuclear scintigraphy. In terms of ultrasonography, once a sonolucent, extrahepatic cystic structure is identified in the right upper quadrant, it is most important that the gallbladder be sought for. If a normal gallbladder is not visualized, then most likely one is dealing with hydrops of the gallbladder, but if one is found, the diagnosis should be choledochal cyst. In addition, one should look for dilated biliary ducts and, in rare cases, one even may be able to demonstrate the ducts joining the cyst. MR cholangiography also can be employed and is becoming increasingly useful (9–12).

Choledochal cysts may be large or small and once anatomic details are delineated with ultrasound, a strong presumptive diagnosis of choledochal cyst is established. However, it usually is confirmed with technetium-99m IDA nuclear scintigraphy studies. With this scintigraphic agent, excretion by the liver of the isotope into the choledochal cyst or choledochocele occurs (Fig. 4.185). Such accumulation of isotope in a cystic structure does not occur with hydrops of the gallbladder nor with duplication cysts, which also can be confused with choledochal cysts.

In a few cases, a choledochal cyst may rupture (13, 14) and present with bile ascites, and occasionally choledochal cysts can be associated with cirrhosis of the liver (15). Bleeding resulting from pseudoaneurysm formation also has been documented (16), and carcinomatous change in choledochal cysts also has been noted (17). Furthermore, choledochal cysts can be associated with biliary atresia (18).

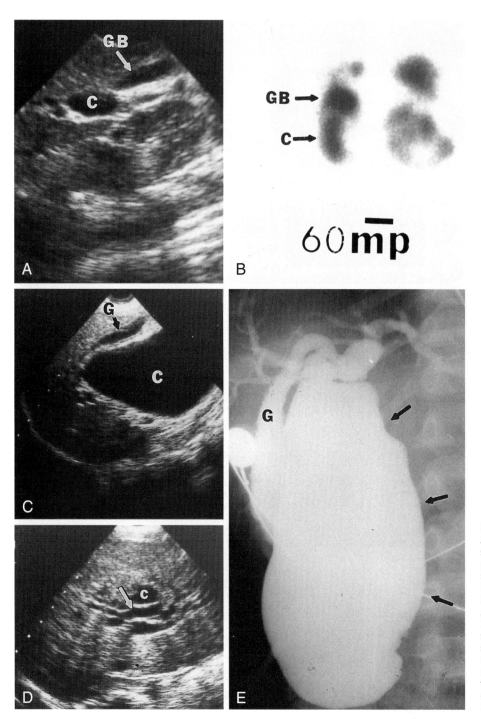

FIGURE 4.185. Choledochal cyst.
A. Ultrasonogram demonstrating a small choledochal cyst (arrow) and a gallbladder (GB) above it. **B.** Nuclear scintigraphy demonstrating accumulation of isotope in the gallbladder (GB), and the choledochal cyst (C). Also note isotope in the GI tract. **C.** Large choledochal cyst (C) is demonstrated with ultrasound. Note the small gallbladder (G). **D.** Ultrasonography demonstrates a dilated common bile duct (arrow) and a small portion of the cyst (C). **E.** Intraoperative cholangiogram demonstrates the large choledochal cyst (arrows).

REFERENCES

1. Samuel M, Spitz L. Choledochal cyst: varied clinical presentations and long-term results of surgery. Eur J Pediatr Surg 1996; 6:78–81.
2. Babbitt DP, Starshak RJ, Clemett AR. Choledochal cyst: concept of etiology. AJR 1973;119:57–62.
3. Han SJ, Hwang EH, Chung KS, et al. Acquired choledochal cyst from anomalous pancreatobiliary duct union. J Pediatr Surg 1997;32:1735–1738.
4. Suarez F, Bernard O, Gauthier F, et al. Bilio-pancreatic common channel in children. Pediatr Radiol 1987;17:206–211.
5. Wong KC, Lister J. Human fetal development of the hepato-pancreatic duct junction—a possible explanation of congenital dilation of the biliary tract. J Pediatr Surg 1981;16:139–145.
6. Schimpl G, Sauer H, Goriupp U, et al. Choledochocele: importance of histological evaluation. J Pediatr Surg 1993;28: 1562–1565.
7. Wearn FG, Wiot JF. Choledochocele: not a form of choledochal cyst. J Can Assoc Radiol 1982;33:110–112.

8. Crittenden SL, McKinley MJ. Choledochal cyst—clinical features and classification. Am J Gastroenterol 1985;80:643–647.

9. Arshanskiy Y, Vyas PK. Type IV choledochal cyst presenting with obstructive jaundice: role of MR cholangiopancreatography in preoperative evaluation. AJR 1998;171:457–459.

10. Lam WWM, Lam TPW, Saing H, et al. MR cholangiography and CT cholangiography of pediatric patients with choledochal cysts. AJR 1999;173:401–405.

11. van Heurn-Nijsten EWA, Snoep G, Kootstra G, et al. Preoperative imaging of a choledochal cyst in children: non-breath-holding magnetic resonance cholangiopancreatography. Pediatr Surg Int 1999;15:546–548.

12. Yamataka A, Kuwatsuru R, Shima H, et al. Initial experience with non-breath-hold magnetic resonance cholangiopancreatography: a new noninvasive technique for diagnosis of choledochal cyst in children. J Pediatr Surg 1997;32:1560–1562.

13. Ando H, Ito T, Watanabe Y, et al. Spontaneous perforation of choledochal cyst. J Am Coll Surg 1995;181:125–128.

14. Karnak I, Tanyel FC, Buyukpamukcu N, et al. Spontaneous rupture of choledochal cyst: an unusual cause of acute abdomen in children. J Pediatr Surg 1997;32:736–738.

15. Evans-Jones G, Cudmore R. Choledochal cyst and congenital hepatic fibrosis. J Pediatr Surg 1990;25:1259–1260.

16. Eliscu EH, Weiss GM. Case report. Hematobilia due to a pseudoaneurysm complicating a choledochal cyst. AJR 1988; 151:783–784.

17. Iwai N, Deguchi E, Yanagihara J, et al. Cancer arising in a choledochal cyst in a 12-year-old girl. J Pediatr Surg 1990;25: 1261–1263.

18. Torrisi JM, Haller JO, Velcek FT. Choledochal cyst and biliary atresia in the neonate: imaging findings in five cases. AJR 1990; 155:1273–1276.

Caroli's Disease

Caroli's disease is a condition characterized by saccular dilation of the major intrahepatic bile ducts without evidence of distal obstruction. However, there are some who classify Caroli's disease with choledochal cyst (see previous section). Stasis in the ducts leads to infection and stone formation and eventually biliary cirrhosis. Presentation of the disease in infancy is very uncommon although the condition has been reported in childhood (1). Caroli's disease usually is diagnosed preoperatively with ultrasound, hepatic scintigraphy (1, 2), or MR (3). Ultrasound demonstrates the cystic dilations within the liver (Fig. 4.186), while technetium-99m IDA isotope studies first demonstrate defects in the liver, which later fill in with isotope. What one is seeing in the early stage is the dilated ducts, and in the later stage, the same ducts being filled with excreted isotope (4). Caroli's disease also can be seen in association with infantile (autosomal recessive) cystic disease of the kidneys (3, 5), and choledochal cyst (5).

REFERENCES

1. Marchal GJ, Desmet VJ, Proesmans WC, et al. Caroli disease: high frequency US and pathologic findings. Radiology 1986;158: 507–511.

2. Miller WJ, Sechtin AG, Campbell WL, et al. Pictorial essay. Imaging findings in Caroli's disease. AJR 1995;165:333–337.

3. Jung g, Benz-Bohm G, Kugel H, et al. MR cholangiography in children with autosomal recessive polycystic kidney disease. Pediatr Radiol 1999;29:463–466.

4. Sty JR, Hubbard AM, Starshak RJ. Radionuclide hepatobiliary imaging in congenital biliary tract ectasis (Caroli disease). Pediatr Radiol 1982;12:111–114.

5. Pinto RB, Lima JP, da Silveira TR, Scholl JG, et al. "Caroli's disease." Report of 10 cases in children and adolescents in southern Brazil. J Pediatr Surg 1998;33:1531–1535.

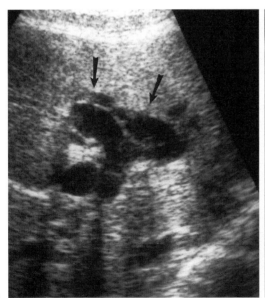 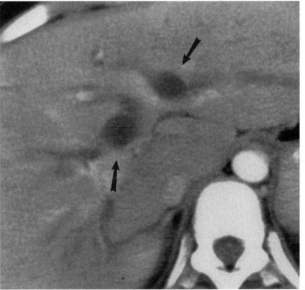

FIGURE 4.186. Caroli's disease. A. On this ultrasound study, note the dilated intrahepatic bile ducts (arrows). **B.** CT more clearly demonstrates the large, dilated intrahepatic bile ducts (arrows).

Bile Plug Syndrome

Inspissated bile plugs, either in the intrahepatic or extrahepatic biliary system, can produce a clinical picture resembling that of bile duct atresia. The biliary system proximal to the obstructing plugs usually is variably dilated and, along with the echogenic intraductal plugs, can be demonstrated with ultrasound (1) (Fig. 4.187). Overall, the condition is not particularly common and usually resolves spontaneously (2, 3). In other cases, however, infusion of the mucolytic agent acetylcysteine into the bile ducts has proved successful (4, 5). In its mildest form, the bile plug syndrome is manifested in so-called cholestatic jaundice.

REFERENCES

1. Mahr MA, Hugosson C, Nazer HM, et al. Bile-plug syndrome. Pediatr Radiol 1988;19:61–64.
2. Holgersen LO, Stolar C, Berdon WE, et al. Therapeutic and diagnostic implications of acquired choledochal obstruction in infancy: spontaneous resolution in three infants. J Pediatr Surg 1990;25:1027–1029.
3. Lang EV, Pinckney LE. Case report. Spontaneous resolution of bile-plug syndrome. AJR 1991;156:1225–1226.
4. Brown DM. Bile plug syndrome: successful management with a mucolytic agent. J Pediatr Surg 1990;25:351–352.
5. Evans JS, George DE, Zmollit D. Biliary infusion therapy in the inspissated bile syndrome of cystic fibrosis. J Pediatr Gastroenterol Nutr 1991;12:131–135.

Bile Duct Perforation

Bile duct perforation occasionally can occur secondary to obstructive lesions of the bile duct such as congenital stenoses or obstructing membranes. However, most cases are not associated with obstruction and are spontaneous (1). It is interesting that most often the perforation occurs anteriorly, just at the junction of the common and cystic bile ducts. There is no known etiology for these ruptures, but their rather constant location brings up the possibility of focal congenital deficiency of the ductal wall.

Bile duct perforation usually first is detected sonographically and then substantiated with nuclear scintigraphy. Sonographically, free fluid will be seen around the liver (Fig. 4.188). Most often, dilated bile ducts are not seen, but the usual clinical presentation of a chronic or subacute illness, with abdominal distention and jaundice, should suggest the diagnosis. Thereafter, technetium-99m IDA scintigraphy will show accumulation of isotope in the fluid around the liver (Fig. 4.188C).

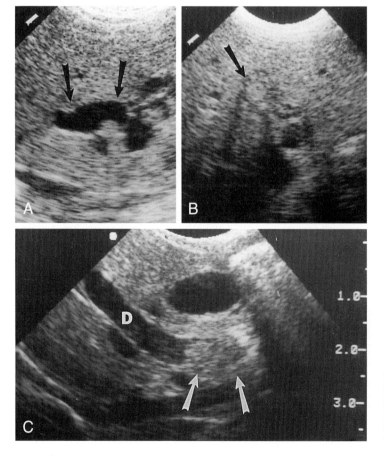

FIGURE 4.187. Bile plug syndrome. A. The common bile duct is markedly dilated (arrows) in this patient. **B.** More distally, a bile plug (arrow) obstructs the common bile duct. **C.** Another patient with a markedly dilated common bile duct (D) with inspissated bile (arrows) at its distal end.

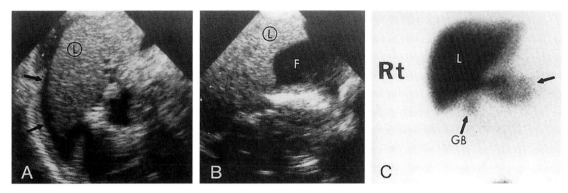

FIGURE 4.188. Idiopathic bile duct leak. A. Ultrasonogram demonstrates fluid (arrows) around the liver (L). **B.** Another cut demonstrates fluid (F) under the liver (L). **C.** Ten-minute scintigram demonstrates isotope in the liver (L) and gallbladder (GB) and extravasation into the peritoneal cavity (arrow).

REFERENCE

1. Banani SA, Bahador A, Nezakatgoo N. Idiopathic perforation of the extrahepatic bile duct in infancy: pathogenesis, diagnosis and management. J Pediatr Surg 1993;28:950–952.

Cholelithiasis and Cholecystitis

Cholelithiasis and cholecystitis are not as common in children as in adults; however, with the advent of ultrasound, gallstones have been discovered more frequently than previously anticipated. Whereas it was once considered that in childhood gallstones occurred primarily in patients with hematologic disorders such as sickle cell disease and other hemolytic anemias, it has become apparent that gallstones also are common in children without these conditions. Many of these latter cases were idiopathic (1), just as it is in adults. Overall, with the advent

of ultrasound, gallstones are no longer considered rare in children without underlying hematologic disease. Most of these stones are located in the gallbladder or in the extrahepatic biliary system, but occasionally they can be seen in the intrahepatic biliary system (2). Most cases of cholecystitis are associated with cholelithiasis and/or biliary obstruction, but so-called noncalculous (acalculous) cholecystitis also occurs (3). It is more common in infancy and probably is secondary to infection including human immunodeficiency virus (HIV) infection (4). Spontaneously resolving gallstones have been documented in the fetus (5).

Ultrasonography and technetium-99m IDA scintigraphy are the most useful imaging studies in investigating cholecystitis and cholelithiasis. Ultrasonography demonstrates stones that are echogenic and produce variable acoustic shadowing (Fig. 4.189), and if one is fortunate, imaging may even demonstrate a stone impacted in the bile

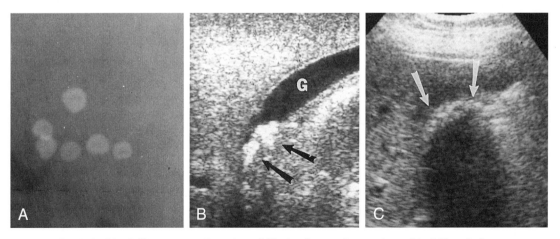

FIGURE 4.189. Gallstones. A. Note the calcified gallstones in a patient with sickle cell disease. **B.** A conglomeration of gallstones (arrows) located in the neck of the gallbladder (G). **C.** Sonogram of the gallbladder demonstrates an echogenic arc (arrows) characteristic of a gallbladder completely filled with gallstones.

duct. In such cases, one most often notes only that the bile duct is dilated (Fig. 4.190). In infants and young children the normal bile duct measures 2–4 mm, but when it becomes obstructed, it becomes dilated and usually measures 5–6 mm or more in diameter.

Other findings in acute cholelithiasis include distention of the gallbladder and thickening of its wall (Fig. 4.191). However, mural thickening is not present in all cases and indeed also can be seen with hypoalbuminemic states and systemic venous hypertension (6). The finding is entirely nonspecific, and in addition to the aforementioned associated conditions it can be seen with hepatitis, HIV infection (4), sepsis, and other conditions. Ordinarily, the normal gallbladder wall is 3 mm thick or less. With nuclear scintigraphy using IDA analogue studies, the gallbladder in acute cholecystitis, because the cystic duct is obstructed, shows nonfilling (Fig. 4.191B).

Gallbladder sludge can be seen in some cases of cholecystitis, but it should be appreciated that gallbladder sludge, probably a precursor to stone formation, is not exclusively

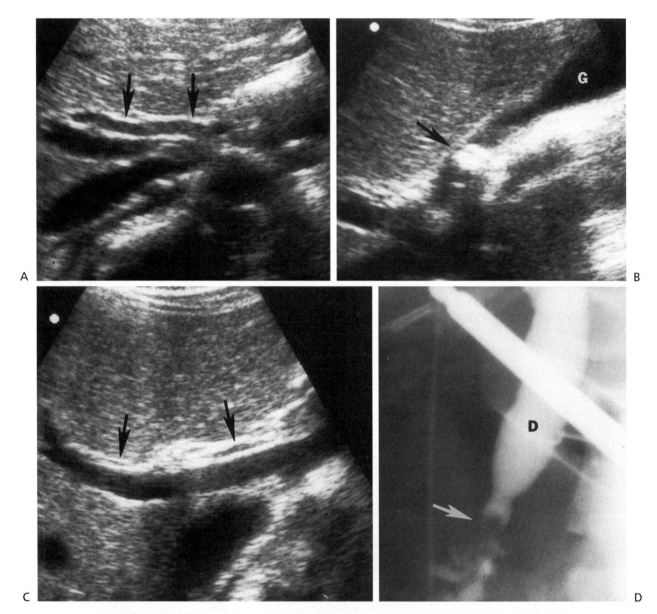

FIGURE 4.190. Obstructed common bile duct. A. Note the dilated common bile duct (arrows). No stone is seen, but its presence or recent presence is inferred. **B.** A gallstone (arrow) is seen in the gallbladder (G). **C.** Later, with resolution of symptoms the common bile duct (arrows) now is normal. This patient had spontaneous passage of a common bile duct stone. **D.** Another patient with an impacted stone (arrow) and a dilated common bile duct (D).

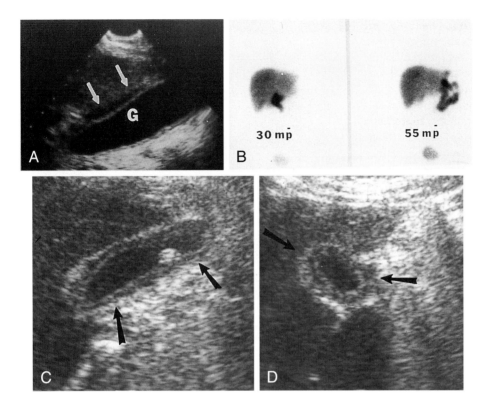

FIGURE 4.191. Acute cholecystitis: ultrasonographic and scintigraphic features. A. Note the distended gallbladder (G) with edematous thickening of the wall (arrows). **B.** Nuclear scintigraphy demonstrates no accumulation of isotope in the gallbladder. Isotope is visible in the liver and GI tract. **C.** Edema of the gallbladder wall (arrows) in another patient. Also note the presence of a single echogenic gallstone. **D.** Cross-sectional view demonstrates similar findings (arrows).

associated with gallbladder infection. Stasis due to any cause can lead to sludge and eventually gallstone formation. Gallbladder sludge is seen in sickle cell disease (7–9), cystic fibrosis, with third-generation cephalosporins (10), and in infants or children on total parenteral nutrition. In these cases it is believed that hyperalimentation puts the GI tract to rest, and hence there is no impulse for the gallbladder to contract and empty. As a result, there is stasis of bile and increased sludge and stone formation. In addition to the aforementioned factors, there also is some association with

furosemide (diuretic) treatment in these patients. Gallstones also can be seen with any form of ileal dysfunction leading to inadequate bile salt absorption, depletion of the hepatic bile salt pool, and subsequent supersaturation of bile with cholesterol and stone formation (11). The findings on ultrasonography are characteristic, with a sludge-bile fluid level being typical (Fig. 4.192).

Increasing experience with gallstones and gallbladder sludge in infants has demonstrated that very often both can disappear spontaneously (12, 13). It is not known exactly

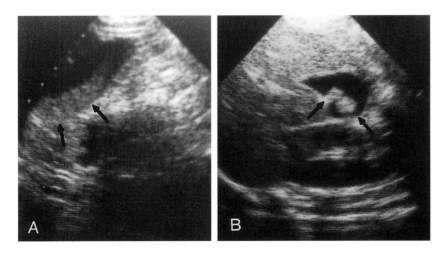

FIGURE 4.192. Gallbladder sludge and sludge balls. A. Note the layering of sludge in the gallbladder (arrows). **B.** Infant with sludge balls (arrows).

why this should occur, but with gallbladder sludge, once the gallbladder begins to function normally, the sludge is evacuated. As far as stone formation is concerned, it may be that the stones in these patients are not dense and hard and may, in fact, be more in the order of firm sludge balls. As a result, as gallbladder function improves, it is likely that the sludge balls break up and pass. In addition, a cautious approach to sludge in sickle cell disease has been suggested (7). It has been suggested that symptomatic gallstones are a definite indication for surgery, but that sludge formation and asymptomatic gallstones should be monitored with ultrasound and surgery performed only if symptoms develop (7, 8).

Porcelain gallbladder (a calcified bladder wall after inflammation) is rare in infants and children (12). Cholangitis, with or without associated cholecystitis also occurs in infants and children but is relatively rare (15) except with HIV infection (16). Emphysematous cholecystitis and porcelain gallbladder are rare in children.

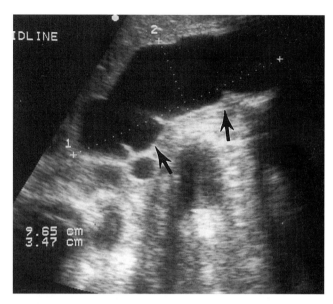

FIGURE 4.193. Hydrops in Kawasaki disease. Note the markedly distended gallbladder (arrows).

REFERENCES

1. Reif S, Sloven DG, Lebenthal E. Gallstones in children: characterization by age, etiology and outcome. Am J Dis Child 1991; 145:105–108.
2. Enriquez G, Lucaya J, Allende E, et al. Intrahepatic biliary stones in children. Pediatr Radiol 1992;22:283–286.
3. Imamoglu M, Sarihan H, Sari A, et al. acute acalculous cholecystitis in children: diagnosis and treatment. J Pediatr Surg 2002; 37:36–39.
4. Chung CJ, Sivit CJ, Rakusan TA, et al. Hepatobiliary abnormalities on sonography in children with HIV infection. J Ultrasound Med 1994;13:205–210.
5. Stringer MD, Lim P, Cave M, et al. Fetal gallstones. J Pediatr Surg 1996;31:1589–1591.
6. Patriquin HB, DiPietro M, Barber FE, et al. Sonography of thickened gallbladder wall: causes in children. AJR 1983;141: 57–60.
7. Al-Salem, AH, Qaisruddin S. The significance of biliary sludge in children with sickle cell disease. Pediatr Surg Int 1998;13: 14–16.
8. Walker TM, Serjeant GR. Biliary sludge in sickle cell disease. J Pediatr 1996/129:443–445.
9. Winter SS, Kinney TR, Ware RE. Gallbladder sludge in children with sickle cell disease. J Pediatr 1994;8:747–749.
10. Blais C, Duperval R. Biliary pseudolithiasis in a child associated with 2 days of ceftriaxone therapy. Pediatr Radiol 1994;24: 218–219.
11. Kirks DR. Lithiasis due to interruption of the enterohepatic circulation of bile salts. AJR 1979;133:383–388.
12. Jacir NN, Erson KD, Eichelberger M, et al. Cholelithiasis in infancy: resolution of gallstones in three of four infants. J Pediatr Surg 1986;21:567–569.
13. Keller MS, Markle BM, Laffey PA, et al. Spontaneous resolution of cholelithiasis in infants. Radiology 1985;157:345–348.
14. Casteel HB, Williamson SL, Golladay ES, et al. Porcelain gallbladder in a child: a case report and review. J Pediatr Surg 1990; 25:1302–1303.
15. Debray D, Pariente D, Urvoas E, et al. Sclerosing cholangitis in children. J Pediatr 1994;124:49–56.

16. Rusin JA, Sivit CJ, Rakusan TA, et al. Case report. AIDS-related cholangitis in children: sonographic findings. AJR 1992;159: 626–627.

Hydrops of the Gallbladder

Hydrops of the gallbladder is not particularly common in children but frequently is seen in the mucocutaneous lymph node syndrome (1, 2) (Fig. 4.193). In such cases, obstruction of the cystic duct probably occurs because of enlarged lymph nodes. However, obstruction resulting from other causes (e.g., temporary accumulation of sludge in the bile ducts; mechanical problems such as kinking of the ducts, webs, areas of stenosis) account for most cases of hydrops in the pediatric age group (3). There is very little inflammation associated with this abnormality, but the gallbladder can become quite large. Often, it is clinically palpable as a mass and is best detected with ultrasonography. If technetium-99m IDA studies are performed, there will be absence of uptake of isotope in the dilated gallbladder, but excretion of isotope into the GI tract will occur (Fig. 4.194).

REFERENCES

1. Grisoni E, Fisher R, Izant R. Kawasaki syndrome: report of four cases with acute gallbladder hydrops. J Pediatr Surg 1984;19:9–11.
2. Slovis TL, Hight DW, Philippart AI, et al. Sonography in the diagnosis and management of hydrops of the gallbladder in children with mucocutaneous lymph node syndrome. Pediatrics 1980;65: 789–794.
3. Rumley TO, Rodgers BM. Hydrops of the gallbladder in children. J Pediatr Surg 1983;18:138–140.

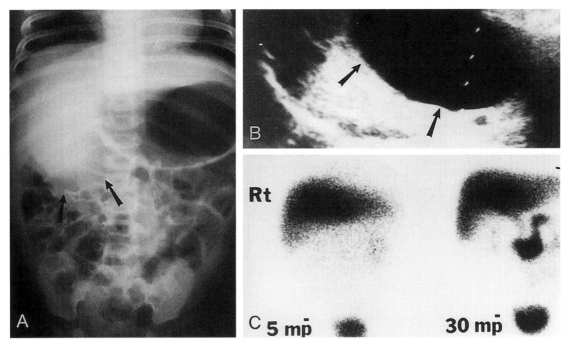

FIGURE 4.194. Hydrops of the gallbladder. A. Note the soft tissue mass in the right upper quadrant (arrows). **B.** Sonography demonstrates a cystic structure, the gallbladder (arrows). **C.** Nuclear scintigraphy demonstrates no accumulation of isotope in the gallbladder. Isotope is seen in the liver and GI tract.

Incompetence of the Sphincter of Oddi

Incompetence of the sphincter of Oddi in the newborn is relatively rare (1). On plain films, gas is seen in the biliary tract and, with barium studies, barium is seen to reflux into the bile duct system. Most often, these cases are associated with duodenal obstruction distal to the ampulla of Vater.

REFERENCE

1. Atkinson GO, Gay BB Jr, Patrick JW, et al. Incompetence of the sphincter of Oddi in the newborn: report of two cases. AJR 1977; 128:861–862.

Miscellaneous Diseases of the Gallbladder and Bile Ducts

Congenital bronchobiliary fistula is an uncommon problem that most often presents with respiratory distress and recurrent pneumonia. In some cases, the diagnosis can be made if bile is coughed up with mucus, but definitive diagnosis is usually made with bronchoscopy or bronchography. Gastric heterotopia in the biliary tract also can occur (1, 2) and can be a cause of abdominal pain. Tumors of the bile ducts are extremely rare in the pediatric age group in general and virtually unheard of in the neonate. However, rhabdomyosarcoma (3, 4), along with papilloma (5), polyps (6), adenoma

(7), adenocarcinoma (8), and granular cell tumor (9) all have been documented in childhood. Ascariasis of the biliary tract is best demonstrated with ultrasound (10–13), with the worms being demonstrated as a concentric configuration on cross-section and echogenic linear structures on longitudinal view (Fig. 4.195).

Infarction of the gallbladder has been documented in the neonate (14), and I have encountered one peculiar case of giant cystic malformation of the gallbladder (15). In this case, there was progressive enlargement of a large, rather flaccid cystic structure anterior to the liver.

Posttraumatic torsion of the gallbladder also can occur (16).

REFERENCES

1. Lamont N, Winthrop AL, Cole FM, et al. Heterotopic gastric mucosa in the gallbladder: a cause of chronic abdominal pain in a child. J Pediatr Surg 1991;26:1293–1295.
2. Martinez-Urrutia MJ, Vazquez Estevez J, Larrauri J, et al. Gastric heterotopy of the biliary tract. J Pediatr Surg 1990;25:356–357.
3. Roebuck DJ, Yang WT, Lam WWM, et al. Hepatobiliary rhabdomyosarcoma in children: diagnostic radiology. Pediatr Radiol 1998;28:101–108.
4. Verstandig A, Bar-Ziv J, Abu-Dalu KI, et al. Sarcoma botryoides of the common bile duct: preoperative diagnosis by coronal CT and PTC. Pediatr Radiol 1991;21:152–153.
5. Sirinelli D, Vanthournout I, Robert M, et al. Ultrasound diag-

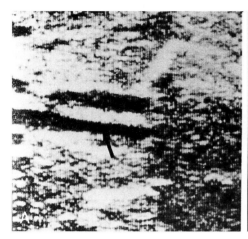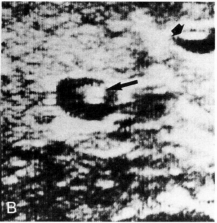

FIGURE 4.195. Biliary Ascaris: ultrasonographic findings. A. Longitudinal section demonstrating a dilated common bile duct with a worm in the center (arrow). **B.** Cross-section demonstrating the bull's-eye sign with the echogenic worms in the center (arrows) of the dilated bile duct. (Reproduced with permission from Cerri GG, Leite GJ, Simoes JB, et al. Ultrasonographic evaluation of *Ascaris* in the biliary tract. Radiology 1983;146:753–754).

nosis of gallbladder papilloma in childhood. Pediatr Radiol 1989; 19:203.

6. Barzilai M, Lerner A. Gallbladder polyps in children: a rare condition. Pediatr Radiol 1997;27:54–56.

7. Mogilner JG, Dharan M, Siplovich L. Adenoma of the gallbladder in childhood. J Pediatr Surg 1991;26:223–224.

8. Andiran F, Tanyel FC, Kale G, et al. Obstructive jaundice resulting from adenocarcinoma of the ampulla of Vater in an 11-year-old boy. J Pediatr Surg 1997;32:636–637.

9. Reynolds EM, Tsivis PA, Long JA. Granular cell tumor of the biliary tree in a pediatric patient. J Pediatr Surg 2000;35:652–654.

10. Cerri GG, Leite GJ, Simoes JB, et al. Ultrasonographic evaluation of *Ascaris* in the biliary tract. Radiology 1983;146:753–754.

11. Hoffmann H, Kawooya M, Esterre P, et al. In vivo and in vitro studies on the sonographical detection of *Ascaris lumbricoides*. Pediatr Radiol 1997;27:226–229.

12. Mahmood T, Mansoor N, Quraishy S, et al. Ultrasonographic appearance of *Ascaris lumbricoides* in the small bowel. J Ultrasound Med 2001;20:269–274.

13. Ozmen MN, Oguzkurt L, Ahmet B, et al. Ultrasonographic diagnosis of intestinal ascariasis. Pediatr Radiol 1995;25: S171–S172.

14. Yazdani M, Quinby GE, Gottschalk SK. Infarction of the gallbladder—an unusual cause of acute abdomen in the neonate. J Pediatr Surg 1983;18:630–631.

15. Lobe TE, Hayden CK Jr, Merkel M. Giant congenital cystic malformation of the gallbladder. J Pediatr Surg 1986;21:447–448.

16. Salman AB, Yildirgan MI, Gelebi F. Posttraumatic gallbladder torsion in a child. J Pediatr Surg 1996;31:1586.

LIVER

Normal Configuration and Variations

The liver usually is seen as a large triangular shadow in the right upper quadrant. Its inferior edge is visualized when adjacent air-filled loops of bowel are present. Unless the liver is markedly enlarged, it is roentgenographically difficult to appreciate hepatomegaly. In this regard, ultrasound, CT, and MR imaging are more useful (1, 2). In more pronounced cases, however, on plain films there is elevation of the ipsilateral diaphragmatic leaflet, downward displace-

ment of the adjacent loops of bowel, and medial displacement of the stomach.

With ultrasound, the normal liver has a uniform, finely speckled echo pattern, and structures such as the portal vein, hepatic veins, inferior vena cava, gallbladder, and even the hepatic artery branches are identified with ease. The liver also is readily identified with CT and MR imaging. Although one can measure the liver to determine its size, one usually makes this judgment more on a subjective than objective basis, and it is perhaps easier to make this determination on CT (2) and MR than with ultrasound (1).

As far as the portal vein is concerned, it has been demonstrated that at birth it measures approximately 3–5 mm, 4–8 mm at 1 year of age, 6–8 mm at 5 years of age, and 6–9 mm at 10 years of age (3).

REFERENCES

1. Konus OL, Ozdemir A, Akkaya A, et al. Normal liver, spleen, and kidney dimensions in neonates, infants, and children: evaluation with sonography. AJR 1998;171:1693–1698.

2. Noda T, Todani T, Watanabe Y, Yamamoto S. Liver volume in children measured by computed tomography. Pediatr Radiol 1997; 27:250–252.

3. Patriquin HB, Perreault G, Grignon A, et al. Normal portal venous diameter in children. Pediatr Radiol 1990;20:451–453.

ABNORMALITIES OF THE LIVER

Liver Trauma

In the neonate, trauma to the liver is encountered occasionally and most often these infants are delivered from abnormal fetal presentations. There also is a preponderance of premature and large infants. Perinatal hypoxia also has been implicated as an etiologic factor in some cases, because it is believed that hypoxia renders organs such as the liver and spleen more congested and therefore more susceptible

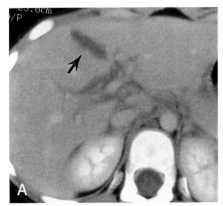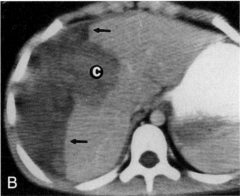

FIGURE 4.196. Liver trauma. A. Note the contusion (arrow) in the right lobe of the liver. Periportal tracking also is present. **B.** Another patient with a large parenchymal contusion (C) and an even larger subcapsular hematoma (arrows).

to rupture. In older infants and children, liver rupture usually results from blunt abdominal trauma, either accidental or as part of the battered child syndrome. However, no matter what the age group or the cause, the imaging findings are the same.

On plain films, the liver silhouette may appear enlarged and, as such, seen to displace adjacent bowel. Once suspected, however, the documentation of liver hemorrhage should be pursued with some other imaging modality. Although almost all the modalities have been used to demonstrate the abnormality, most success is achieved with CT, contrast-enhanced scanning. This approach most clearly delineates lacerations, hematomas, subcapsular bleeds, and perihepatic accumulations of blood. The findings in liver trauma in children are no different from those seen in adults (Fig. 4.196). However, it might be noted that "periportal tracking," (Fig. 4.196A), once thought to result from bleeding around the portal space in liver trauma, now is believed to be the result of the extravasation of fluid secondary to bolus injection of contrast material and/or massive intravenous resuscitation of these patients (1–3). Posttraumatic liver cysts are rare (4).

Ultrasonography, although able to demonstrate some of these abnormalities, is not nearly as useful as CT and probably should not be used as an initial investigative imaging modality. Nuclear scintigraphy is seldom required except in cases of suspected bile duct trauma and leakage. Ultrasonographically, lacerations and fresh hematomas produce echogenic areas in the liver, but later, as the hematoma matures and liquefies, a cystic appearance is seen.

REFERENCES

1. Patrick LE, Ball TI, Atkinson GO, et al. Pediatric blunt abdominal trauma: periportal tracking at CT. Radiology 1992;183: 689–691.
2. Siegel MJ, Herman TE. Periportal low attenuation at CT in childhood. Radiology 1992;183:685–688.
3. Sivit CJ, Taylor GA, Eichelberger MR, et al. Significance of peri-
portal low-attenuation zones following blunt trauma in children. Pediatr Radiol 1993;23:388–390.
4. Chuang J-H, Huang S-S. Post-traumatic hepatic cyst—an unusual sequela of liver injury in the era of imaging. J Pediatr Surg 1996; 31:272–274.

Hepatitis

Hepatitis in infants and children generally is of viral origin and usually results from type B hepatitis virus. In addition, in the neonate there is considerable feeling that neonatal hepatitis is closely related to biliary atresia. The overlapping aspects of these conditions have been discussed with biliary atresia and will not be repeated here. Hepatitis also can be seen with congenital lues (1), herpes (2), and in the α_1-antitrypsin deficiency syndrome, as well as lupus erythematosus (3). Calcifications after nonbacterial infectious hepatitis are occasionally encountered (1, 2), and with ultrasonography in the early stages enlarged lymph nodes can be seen in the region of the porta hepatis (4) (Fig. 4.197A). In addition one can encounter periportal edema and edema of the gallbladder wall (Fig. 4.197, B and C). In severe cases of hepatitis, usually viral in origin, the liver assumes a markedly hypoechoic appearance on ultrasound and the periportal areas show increased echogenicity, similar to that seen with hepatic necrosis (see Fig. 4.199A).

Differentiation of neonatal hepatitis from biliary atresia often is difficult, but for the most part, hepatitis can be suspected when certain ultrasonographic and scintigraphic findings are present. Ultrasonographically, the liver usually is of normal echogenicity and the bile ducts are not dilated. The gallbladder usually is visible and may be small (Fig. 4.198A), normal, or a little enlarged. With scintigraphy, using IDA analogs, accumulation of isotope in the liver parenchyma is slow, but eventual excretion into the biliary tract occurs (Fig. 4.198B). With biliary atresia, no radionuclide is excreted into the biliary tract, and hence, technetium-99m IDA scintigraphy remains the best imaging modality with which to attempt to differentiate neonatal hepatitis from biliary atresia. However, even with this study

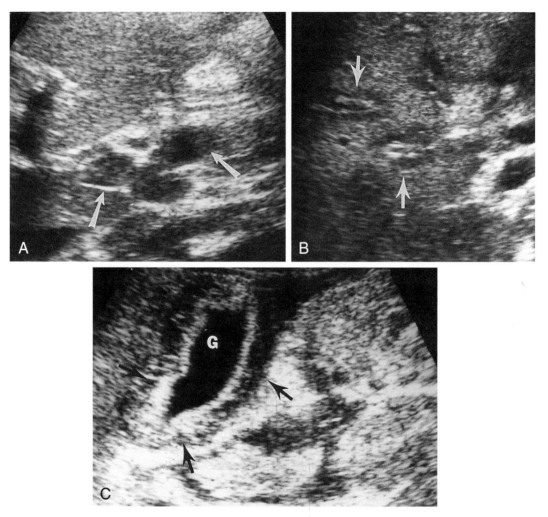

FIGURE 4.197. Hepatitis. A. Periportal adenopathy (arrows) is present in this patient. **B.** In another patient, ultrasonography demonstrates periportal edema (arrows). **C.** Same patient, demonstrating marked thickening of the wall (arrows) of the gallbladder (G).

many cases remain unresolved. During intraoperative cholangiography, the bile ducts often are very thin (Fig. 4.198C).

REFERENCES

1. Herman TE. Extensive hepatic calcification secondary to fulminant neonatal syphilitic hepatitis. Pediatr Radiol 1995;25:120–122.
2. Mannhardt W, Schumacher R. Progressive calcifications of lung and liver in neonatal herpes simplex virus infection. Pediatr Radiol 1991;21:236–237.
3. Laxer RM, Roberts EA, Gross KR, et al. Liver disease in neonatal lupus erythematosus. J Pediatr 1990;116:238–242.
4. Toppet V, Souayah H, Delplace O, et al. Lymph node enlargement as a sign of acute hepatitis A in children. Pediatr Radiol 1990;20:249–252.

Hepatic Necrosis and Infarction

Hepatic necrosis usually is the result of a fulminant viral infection, and ultrasonographically the findings consist of

FIGURE 4.199. A. Liver necrosis. Note the hypoechoic liver and marked periportal echogenicity surrounding all of the portal triads. **B. Liver infarct.** Contrast-enhanced CT study demonstrates a large geographic area of low signal (arrows).

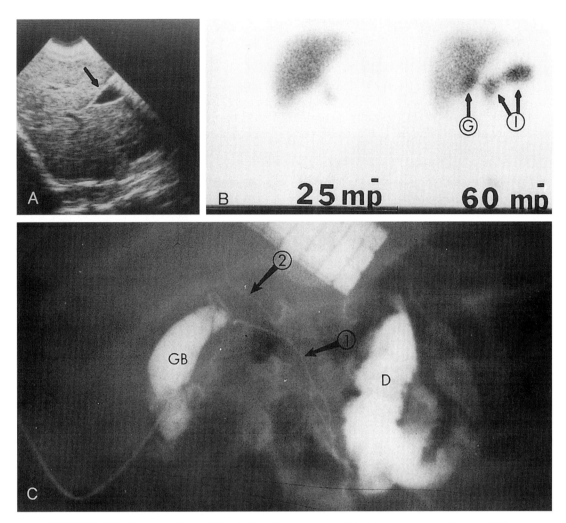

FIGURE 4.198. Neonatal hepatitis. A. Note the normal gallbladder (arrow) on ultrasound. The liver shows normal echogenicity and no dilated bile ducts. **B.** Technetium-99m iminodiacetate (IDA) isotope study demonstrates, at 25 minutes after injection, early excretion of isotope by the liver. At 60 minutes, isotope is present in the gallbladder (G) and in the intestine (I). **C.** Another patient with an intraoperative cholangiogram demonstrating a normal gallbladder (GB), and a thin (low-flow pattern) common bile duct (1). There is some early retrograde filling of the hepatic radicals (2). D, duodenum.

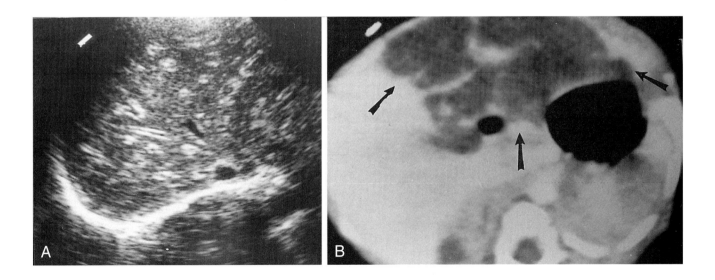

marked hyperlucency of the liver along with increased periportal echogenicity (Fig. 4.199A). The findings, as noted in the previous section, are difficult to differentiate from severe hepatitis. Hepatic infarction in the pediatric age group in general is rare. In the older patient it occurs with liver transplants, but it also can be seen with other hepatic surgery where hepatic arterial blood supply is compromised. In addition, we have seen a case of liver necrosis secondary to thrombus formation from indwelling venous catheters. This patient also had transposition of the great vessels, and the intracardiac communications allowed embolization of the venous thrombi to the hepatic artery (Fig. 4.199B).

In any patient with liver infarction the liver will enlarge on plain films, and on all imaging modalities the infarcted portion of the liver produces a "pseudomass." The pseudomass occurs because, while the lesion may be extensive, there is no displacement of normal adjacent liver tissue and no expansion or bulging of the capsule. The lesion is geographic rather than one with an epicenter and bulging edges (Fig. 4.199B). The lesion is hypodense on CT and does not enhance with contrast material. It is echogenic on ultrasonography (1), and with MR imaging it demonstrates low signal on T1-weighted images and increased signal on T2-weighted images. Long-term follow-up usually demonstrates resolution of the infarct, but atrophy may result.

REFERENCE

1. Lev-Toaff AS, Friedman AC, Cohen LM, et al. Hepatic infarcts: new observations by CT and sonography. AJR 1987;149:87–90.

Cirrhosis and Fibrosis

In the neonate and young infant, cirrhosis of the liver is usually secondary to long-standing biliary tract obstruction (e.g., biliary atresia, choledochal cyst) or neonatal hepatitis, but, in any case, the effects of cirrhosis are seldom seen in the immediate neonatal period. They usually appear gradually, over weeks, months, or even years; roentgenographically, problems center on complications such as portal hypertension and esophageal varices. Byler's disease also can present in early infancy and later result in cirrhosis. This disease is characterized by a deficiency in bile acid metabolism and resultant intrahepatic cholestasis, portal fibrosis, inflammatory changes, and eventually cirrhosis (1).

Hepatic fibrosis also is seen with autosomal recessive polycystic disease of the kidneys (2). In this regard, however, although many of these infants present with profound kidney disease in the neonatal period (infantile polycystic kidney), others have a minimal renal lesion and present in adolescence with progressive hepatic fibrosis, portal hypertension, and GI bleeding secondary to varices. This is referred to as the juvenile form of the disease.

Cirrhosis of the liver also has been documented in association with α_1-antitrypsin deficiency and focal biliary cirrhosis occurs with cystic fibrosis. In addition, in any case of cirrhosis, pulmonary AV shunts can be induced (3). These lead to desaturation and hypoxia, and on plain films, a very delicate reticular appearance to the lung parenchyma. Ultrasonography of a cirrhotic or fibrotic liver demonstrates increased echogenicity and a coarser pattern than the fine granular one seen in a normal liver. In addition, the liver usually is small, and ascitic fluid is seen. Associated varices also can be demonstrated with ultrasound, but usually are more readily visible with CT scanning and upper GI series. Eventually, however, the portal system is assessed with direct visualization through splenoportography.

REFERENCES

1. Linarelli LG, Williams CN, Phillips MJ. Byler's disease: fatal intrahepatic cholestasis. J Pediatr 1972;81:484–492.
2. Davies CH, Stringer DA, Whyte H, et al. Congenital hepatic fibrosis with saccular dilation of intrahepatic bile ducts and infantile polycystic kidneys. Pediatr Radiol 1986;16:302–305.
3. Barbe T, Losay J, Grimon G, et al. Pulmonary arteriovenous shunting in children with liver disease. J Pediatr 1995;126: 571–579.

Portal Vein Thrombosis and Portal Hypertension

Portal hypertension can result from hepatic abnormalities such as cirrhosis or fibrosis of the liver, but in infancy it more commonly is the result of portal vein thrombosis. In the vast majority of cases, thrombosis results from sepsis or omphalitis, but in older children, it may result from other intraabdominal infections such as perforated appendicitis or intestinal inflammatory disease (1, 2).

Characteristically, portal hypertension leads to the formation of esophageal and gastric varices, splenic enlargement, and hypersplenism. Spontaneous splenorenal shunts also may develop and, in infancy, in cases of portal vein thrombosis, a complex network of collateral veins can develop and the term "cavernous transformation of the portal vein" often is employed.

Portal hypertension now usually first is investigated with color-flow Doppler imaging (3, 4). It is relatively easy to demonstrate centrifugal versus centripetal flow in the portal vein, and in addition, with ordinary ultrasonography one can see increased echogenicity around the area of the portal vein and absence or poor visualization of the normal portal vein. In some cases, small venous channels are seen within this echogenic area and these represent the new channels of the cavernous transformation (Fig. 4.200, A–C). These also are clearly demonstrable with splenoportography (Fig. 4.200D). Echogenicity itself probably represents fibrosis and perhaps edema in response to the inflammatory

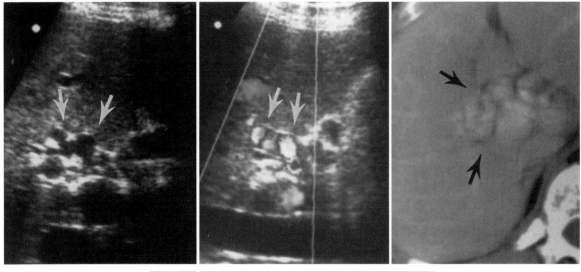

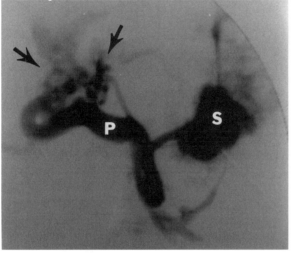

FIGURE 4.200. Cavernous transformation: portal vein thrombosis. A. Characteristic hypoechoic areas (arrows) resulting from collateral vessels as part of cavernous transformation. The vessels are surrounded by echogenic fibrosis (arrows). **B.** Color-flow Doppler demonstrates the collateral channels (arrows). **C.** Another patient whose contrast-enhanced CT study demonstrates the tortuous vessels of cavernous transformation (arrows). **D.** Splenoportography in still another patient demonstrates the spleen (S), portal vein (P), and the vessels (arrows) of the cavernous transformation.

process. One also can detect varices with ultrasound, CT, or barium swallow, and splenorenal shunts can be detected with ultrasound, CT or MR. The transjugular intrahepatic portosystemic shunt (TIPS) procedure commonly performed in adults with portal hypertension, also can be performed in children (5), but is difficult to perform in infants.

REFERENCES

1. Casals S, Enriquez G, Gomez JM, et al. Sonographic diagnosis of pylephlebitis in children. Pediatr Radiol 1993;23:567–568.
2. Slovis TL, Haller JO, Cohen HL, et al. Complicated appendiceal inflammatory disease in children: pylephlebitis and liver abscess. Radiology 1989;171:823–825.
3. Deeg K-H, Glockel U, Richter R, et al. Diagnosis of veno-occlusive disease of the liver by color-coded Doppler sonography. Pediatr Radiol 1993;23:134–136.
4. Tessler FN, Gehring BJ, Gomes AS, et al. Diagnosis of portal vein thrombosis: value of color Doppler imaging. AJR 1991;157:293–296.
5. Kerns SR, Hawkins IF Jr. Case report. Transjugular intrahepatic portosystemic shunt in a child with cystic fibrosis. AJR 1992;159:1277–1278.

Cysts of the Liver

Congenital cysts of the liver generally are uncommon, but when discovered, they often are massive (1–3) and, in the neonate, can produce respiratory distress (2). Cysts are best demonstrated with ultrasonography but also can be seen with CT or MR scanning. With ultrasonography, they are sonolucent. Plain abdominal roentgenographic findings are nonspecific and merely suggest the presence of a right upper quadrant mass.

Parasitic cysts, namely echinococcal cysts, also are uncommon in infants, except in endemic areas. On ultrasound they assume a variety of cystic, sonolucent configurations (4). Because of this, a classification has been proposed (5), consisting of types I, IR, II, and III cysts. Type I cysts are simple and fluid filled, while IR lesions also contain undulating membranes. Type II lesions contain daughter cysts and scattered echogenic matrix, while type III are dead, densely calcified lesions that are highly echogenic. Ultrasound guided drainage of the cysts has been demonstrated to be safe (6).

REFERENCES

1. Athey PA, Lauderman JA, King DE. Massive congenital solitary nonparasitic cyst of the liver in infancy. J Ultrasound Med 1986; 5:586–587.
2. Merine D, Nussbaum AR, Sanders RC. Solitary nonparasitic hepatic cyst causing abdominal distension and respiratory distress in a newborn. J Pediatr Surg 1990;25:349–350.
3. Quillin SP, McAlister WH. Congenital solitary nonparasitic cyst of the liver in a newborn. Pediatr Radiol 1992;22:543–544.
4. Haliloglu M, Saatci I, Akhan O, et al. Pictorial essay. Spectrum of imaging findings in pediatric hydatid disease. AJR 1997;169: 1627–1631.
5. Lewall DB, McCorkell SJ. Hepatic echinococcal cysts: sonographic appearance and classification. Radiology 1985;155: 773–776.
6. Dilsiz A, Acikogozoglu S, Gunel E, et al. Ultrasound-guided percutaneous drainage in the treatment of children with hepatic hydatid disease. Pediatr Radiol 1997;27:230–233.

Liver Tumors

Tumors of the liver in neonates and young infants can be benign or malignant, but benign tumors are more common. Malignant tumors are more common in older infants and children. Of the benign tumors, the most common is the hemangioma or hemangioendothelioma and then the mesenchymal hamartoma (1). With malignant lesions in young infants, the most common tumor is the hepatoblastoma, while in older infants and children hepatocellular carcinoma is the tumor to be considered. Ultrasonography, including color-flow Doppler imaging, has come to play the dominant role in the initial investigation of liver tumors. CT also is of value, especially with the arrival of helical scanning and has placed it in a competitive mode with MRI. Before that, MRI generally was considered superior to CT. In terms of any of these imaging modalities, what is important is that they identify whether: (a) the tumor is hemangiomatous or solid and probably malignant, (b) the location of the tumor in the liver, and (c) its relationship to blood vessels.

With hemangioma or hemangioendothelioma, the lesion may be single or multiple, and in the neonate, these tumors often are very large and predisposed to extensive arteriovenous shunting and hyperkinetic heart failure. Indeed, these infants frequently first come to the attention of a physician because of this problem (Fig. 4.201). On the other hand, some of these tumors either are so small or have so little blood flow that they go undetected. In addition, with infantile hemangioma spontaneous involution can occur (2). With the larger tumors, other clinical findings include a bruit over the enlarged liver and bleeding problems because of associated coagulation defects. Malignant degeneration is rare (3) and calcifications may be seen in some cases. When present, the calcifications are irregular and indistinguishable from those seen with other tumors such as hepatoblastoma and metastatic neuroblastoma. In addition, some of these patients may have associated hemangiomas elsewhere, including the skin, but most do not.

In terms of imaging hemangiomatous tumors, as has been noted earlier, ultrasonography usually is the first modality used. However, the findings are variable and depend on the nature of the hemangioma. In some cases, it is echogenic (Fig. 4.202, A and B) and this probably results

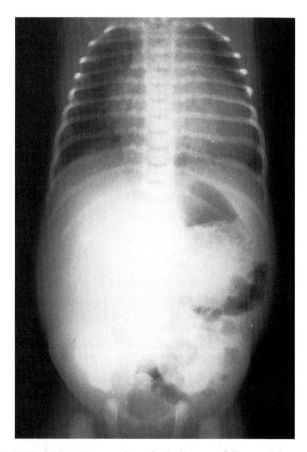

FIGURE 4.201. Hemangioendothelioma of liver with cardiac failure. Note the large mass in the right upper quadrant and flank displacing the stomach and intestines to the left. Also note that the heart is enlarged and the vascularity is engorged.

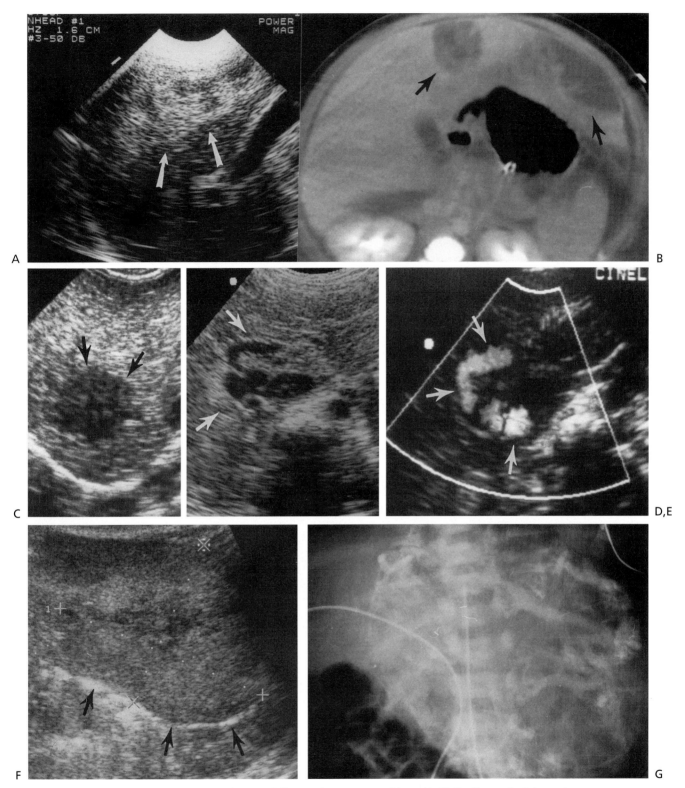

FIGURE 4.202. Hemangioma of liver: ultrasonographic and CT findings. A. Echogenic hemangioma (arrows). **B.** CT study with contrast enhancement demonstrates the low-density lesions (arrows). **C.** Another patient with a hypoechoic hemangioma (arrows). **D.** Echogenic hemangioma (arrows) with sinusoids and vessels. **E.** Color-flow Doppler demonstrates exuberant blood flow (arrows) corresponding to the hypoechoic sinusoids and vessels seen in **D. F.** Large, echogenic hemangioma (arrows) with multiple, small, hypoechoic sinusoids. **G.** Drainage phase of the arteriogram demonstrates the very vascular hemangioma located in the left lobe of the liver. Same patient as in **F.**

from the presence of numerous small vessels and thrombi, while in others the tumor is relatively hypoechoic (Fig. 4.202C). If large sinusoids are present, multiple sonolucencies are seen (Fig. 4.202, D and F), and color-flow Doppler can demonstrate flow within these vessels (Fig. 4.202E).

In cases in which significant arteriovenous shunting occurs, one also can see enlarged and early filling hepatic veins, an enlarged hepatic artery, and diminution in caliber of the aorta distal to the feeding hepatic artery. All of these latter findings previously were demonstrable with arteriography but also can be seen with ultrasonography (Fig. 4.203). In terms of the vascularity of these tumors, it should be noted that the presence of increased blood flow is not pathognomonic, because increased blood flow also can be seen with hamartomas and malignant liver tumors. However, when blood flow is exuberant, and there is diminution in caliber of the aorta distal to the hepatic artery, an hemangiomatous tumor should be the first consideration. Confusion on the basis of hypervascularity is more likely to occur with hamartoma than with malignant liver tumors.

On CT, the tumor usually is hypodense but enhances (from the periphery of the lesion) after contrast administration (Fig. 4.204). In some cases, one may be able to see the sinusoids and feeding vessels, but these are not usually as clearly visualized as with ultrasound. However, with helical scanning, definition of the vascularity of these tumors is more readily accomplished. MRI also vividly demonstrates these tumors where, on heavily T1-weighted (inversion recovery) images, hemangiomas are of low signal, while on T2-weighted images, they are of high signal. Furthermore, as do hemangiomas in general, hepatic hemangiomas retain high signal on heavily weighted (second echo) T2 images (Fig. 4.205). With Gadolinium the hemangiomas have been noted to fill in from the periphery (4).

Treatment of hemangioma or hemangioendothelioma is variable, depending on the extent of the disease. If the tumor is isolated to one lobe, lobectomy can be performed (5) and may need to be performed on an emergent basis. Corticosteroid therapy also is useful in promoting involution of these lesions, and if these measures are unsuccessful,

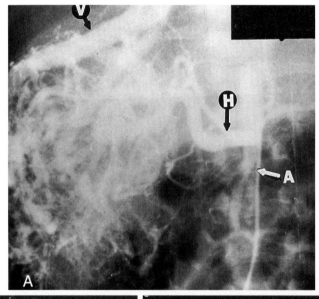

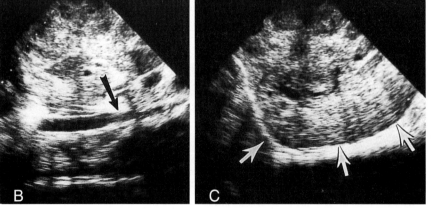

FIGURE 4.203. Hemangioma of liver: decrease in size of aorta. A. Note the large vascular hemangioma in the liver. There is a large hepatic artery (H), and the draining hepatic veins (V) are large. Note that the aorta (A) diminishes in caliber just after the take-up of the hepatic artery. **B.** Ultrasonogram in another patient demonstrates similar diminution in the caliber of the aorta (arrow). **C.** The liver in this patient demonstrates a mixed pattern of echogenicity (arrows). Some hypoechoic areas representing venous sinusoids are seen. Same patient as in Fig. 4.204, C and D.

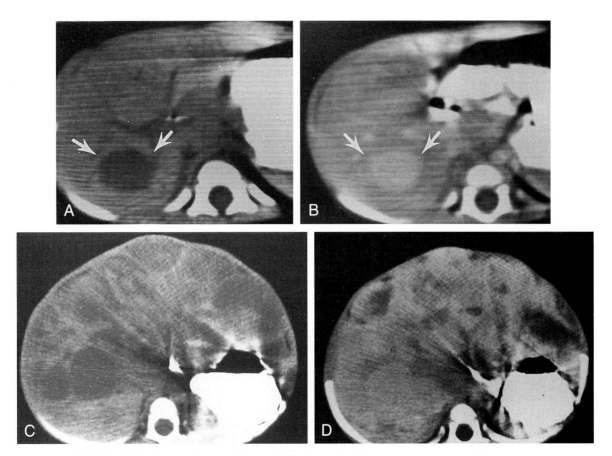

FIGURE 4.204. Hemangioma of liver: CT findings. A. Solitary hemangioma produces a hypo-dense mass (arrows) on this noncontrast study. **B.** With contrast enhancement the hemangioma (arrows) becomes as dense as the liver. **C.** Multiple hemangiomas in the liver produce multiple hypodense spherical masses (same case as Fig. 4.203, B and C). **D.** With contrast enhancement the multiple nodules show increase in density.

radiation therapy can be used. However, before radiation therapy is attempted, one also should consider embolization (5–7) or hepatic artery ligation (5). Unless the clinical situation represents an emergency though, conservative measures usually are employed, because the course of these tumors is to slowly involute and disappear. Hemangiomas also can be treated with interferon alpha-2a (8).

The next most common benign tumor of the liver in infancy is the mesenchymal hamartoma (9–14). This tumor almost always has a strong cystic component and often is very large when first discovered. The cystic component is the most useful finding (Fig. 4.206A), for it generally is not seen in other liver tumors, either benign or malignant. An exception would be the rare primary hepatic lymphangioma. On the other hand, an occasional hamartoma can be solid (Fig. 4.206, B and C). Calcification also may be noted, and all of this is different from any other liver mass and, therefore, highly suggestive of the lesion. CT and MR scanning (10, 11) also demonstrate the cystic and generally heterogeneous nature of this tumor. If arteriography is per-

formed, since many of these tumors are vascular, differentiation from hemangioma may be difficult unless cystic change is present. However, there is usually little in the way of sinusoid formation and sinusoidal pooling in hamartomas. Furthermore, there is little evidence of early filling of hepatic veins, and finally, although the lesion is quite vascular, cardiac failure is uncommon (13). Nuclear scintigraphy using IDA scans also has been helpful in the identification of these tumors. It is useful because the reticuloendothelial cells are preserved and accumulate isotope. With malignant tumors these cells usually are destroyed or so altered that they do not accumulate the isotope. Hamartomas have been noted to spontaneously regress (15), and although usually benign, malignant degeneration can occur (16).

Focal nodular hyperplasia, although not a true tumor of the liver, occurs after some type of insult to the liver and can pose a diagnostic problem (17–19). The lesion can be single or multiple and can be confused with adenoma of the liver. Sonographically, focal nodular hyperplasia can be

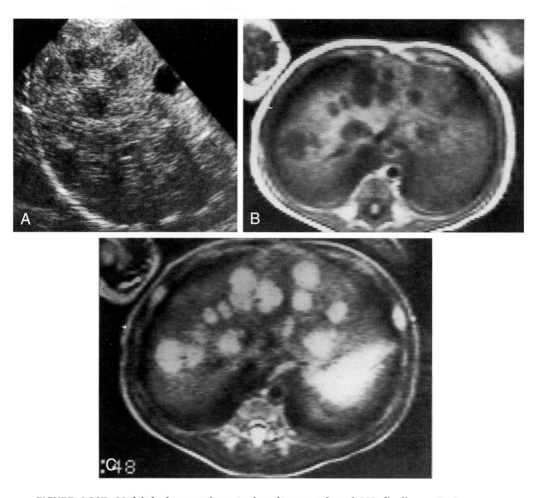

FIGURE 4.205. Multiple hemangiomatosis: ultrasound and MR findings. A. Sonogram demonstrating multiple intrahepatic sonolucencies. This patient was asymptomatic. **B.** Heavily T1-weighted, inversion recovery image shows multiple nodules of low signal. **C.** Heavily T2-weighted image (second echo) shows that the nodules are of high signal.

hypoechogenic or hyperechogenic (probably resulting from central scarring but usually has a well-defined margin (Fig. 4.207). Occasionally, however, echogenicity can be similar to that of normal liver and the lesion "invisible." Fortunately, however, scintigraphy of these lesions is diagnostic, because the lesion usually does not remain cold but accumulates isotope. This occurs because these lesions contain Kupffer cells. With CT the lesion is hypodense but enhances with contrast. On MR the scar is hyperintense on T2-weighted images. This is probably a result of increased blood flow to the scar, which also can be seen with color-flow Doppler imaging (20). If angiography is performed, the vascular pattern often takes the form of a spoked wheel. Because of this, the angiogram and hepatoiminodiacetic acid (HIDA) scintigram have become the most definitive studies in this relatively rare lesion of childhood.

A few comments regarding the hepatic adenoma are in order. This lesion is extremely uncommon and almost invariably is seen in association with glycogen storage disease (21, 22). Adenomas, on ultrasonography, are hyperechoic, but when seen with glycogen storage disease, the sonographic findings are less typical, as the liver itself may show increased echogenicity (Fig. 4.208). Scintigraphy usually demonstrates an area of photon deficiency, and arteriographic and CT findings are variable. On MR with gadolinium, washout occurs on delayed studies (22). Fortunately, the lesion is uncommon in the general pediatric population, and when a mass of any type is encountered in the liver of a patient with glycogen storage disease, hepatic adenoma should be the first diagnostic choice. Carcinoma of the liver in these patients is rare (21).

Malignant tumors of the liver in infants are less common than are benign tumors, and this is especially true in neonates. In younger infants the most common tumor is hepatoblastoma, while in older infants and children the tumor usually is a hepatocellular carcinoma. Most often,

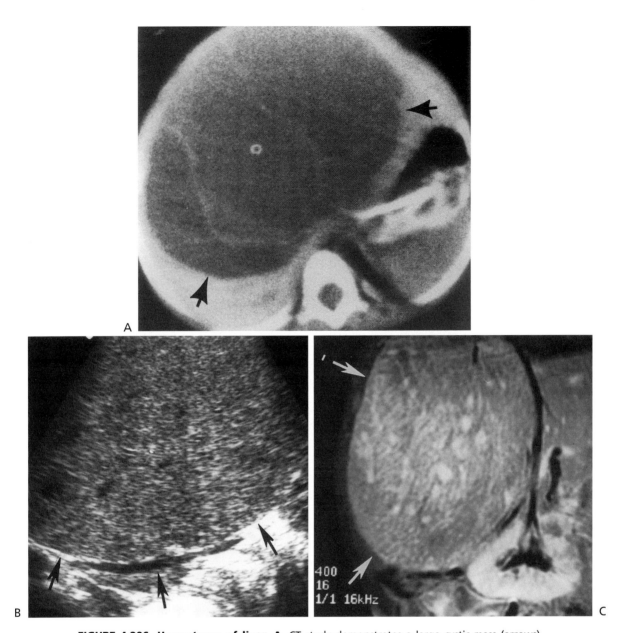

FIGURE 4.206. Hamartoma of liver. A. CT study demonstrates a large cystic mass (arrows). (Reproduced with permission from Ross PR, Goodman ZD, Ishak KG, et al. Mesenchymal hamartoma of the liver; radiologic and pathologic correlation. Radiology 1986;158:619–624.) **B.** Another patient with a solid hamartoma visualized on ultrasound (arrows). **C.** T1-weighted MR image demonstrates the solid hamartoma (arrows) causing marked displacement of the kidney.

infants with these tumors present with an enlarging abdomen, a right upper quadrant mass, anorexia, fever, and failure to thrive. Increased α-fetoprotein also is commonly present but, because arteriovenous shunting is rare, cardiac failure is not a presenting feature. In terms of the α-fetoprotein level it should be noted that it can be low in some of these patients (23), and in addition, that in the neonate and young infant elevated levels often are normal. Irregular calcifications can be seen in some patients and only rarely do these tumors have a cystic component (24). More often what appear to be cysts actually are areas of necrosis. Most

of these tumors are solitary, but occasionally they may be multiple, and rarely, the liver will be diffusely and homogeneously involved (Fig. 4.209). In these latter cases there is no definite tumor mass but rather the entire liver is enlarged and involved with tumor and finally, hepatocellular carcinoma can be seen as a sequel of biliary atresia with associated cirrhosis (25).

In the usual case of malignant liver tumor, a solid, solitary hepatic mass is identified (Fig. 4.210), but hypoechoic areas resulting from necrosis also can be seen. On CT, the tumor is hypodense and shows irregular opacifi-

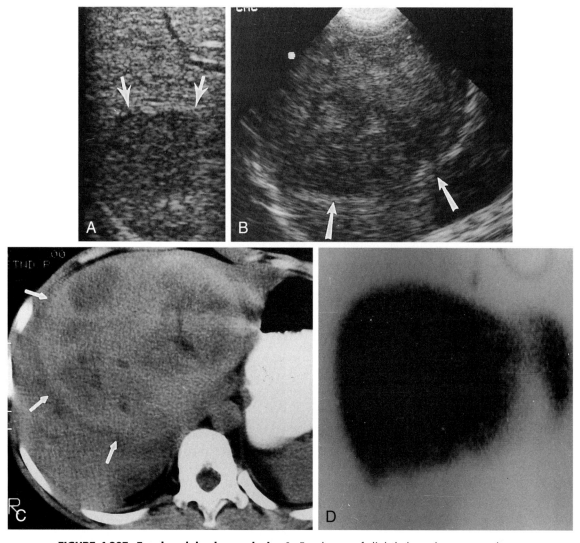

FIGURE 4.207. Focal nodular hyperplasia. A. Focal area of slightly hypodense parenchyma (arrows) representing focal nodular hyperplasia. **B.** Another patient with a large, heterogenous mass (arrows). **C.** CT scan demonstrates a large mass with some hypodense areas (arrows). **D.** Sulfur colloid liver scan demonstrates uniform uptake in the liver, indicating that the mass contains functioning liver tissue.

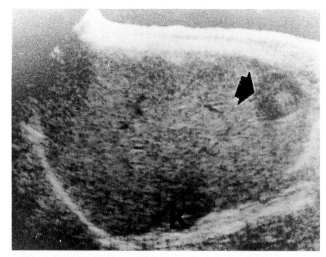

FIGURE 4.208. Hepatic adenoma in association with glycogen storage disease. Note the primarily hypoechoic mass with an echogenic center (arrow). K, kidney.

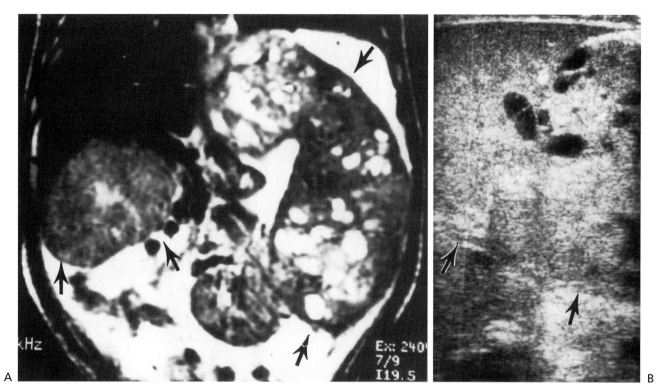

FIGURE 4.209. Diffuse hepatoblastoma. A. Note the extensive tumor involving both lobes of the liver (arrows) on this T2-weighted MR image. Multiple, high-signal-intensity cystic areas are seen in the tumor. **B.** Ultrasound study demonstrates the large tumor (arrows) occupying nearly the entire abdomen. Cystic areas are seen in its upper portion. This patient had Beckwith-Wiedemann syndrome.

cation after the administration of contrast material (Fig. 4.211). With MRI, the tumor is of low signal on T1-weighted images but may show spotty high signal resulting from bleeding or necrosis. On T2-weighted images, the tumor increases in signal (Fig. 4.212). CT and MRI are used more to demonstrate the geographic features of this tumor rather than for diagnosis. It is important that one demonstrate the boundaries of the tumor and blood vessel involvement before surgery is undertaken and while in the past, MR was considered slightly better than

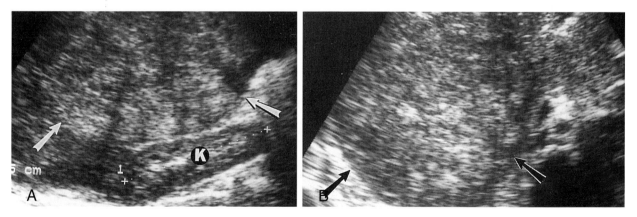

FIGURE 4.210. Hepatoblastoma: ultrasound findings. A. Note the large echogenic mass (arrows) compressing the right kidney (K). **B.** Cross-sectional view of the mass (arrows) demonstrates extensive heterogenicity of the echo pattern.

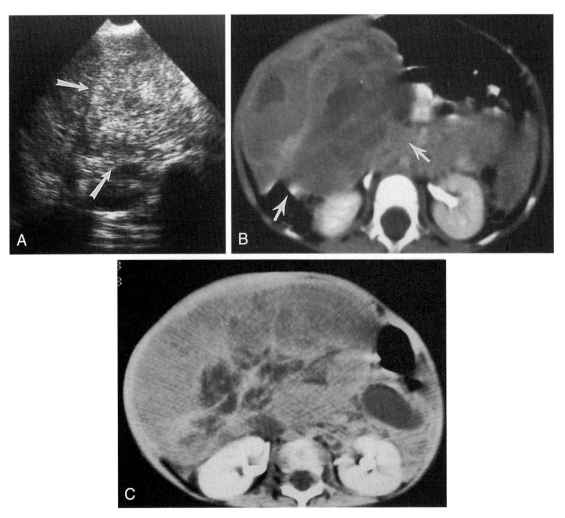

FIGURE 4.211. Hepatoblastoma: CT findings. A. Preliminary ultrasound demonstrates typical heterogeneous echogenicity of the mass (arrows). **B.** CT scan with contrast enhancement demonstrates the large mass (arrows) with many hypodense areas. The pattern is very heterogeneous. **C.** Another patient with a heterogenous mass after contrast enhancement. Numerous hypodense areas are present.

CT for this job, helical CT now is quite competitive. Arteriography now plays a minor or no role in the evaluation of these tumors.

Finally, it should be noted that metastatic deposits within the liver of infants almost always are the result of neuroblastoma. However, they can result from other primary malignancies and generally produce multiple areas of decreased echogenicity, but in some cases, the lesions may be hyperechoic. With CT scanning, liver metastases usually manifest as hypodense areas, while on MR imaging they appear as areas of low signal on T1-weighted images but are bright on T2-weighted images. Lymphoma, when it involves the liver, produces a solid hyperechoic mass on ultrasonography and a mass of increased signal on MRI studies, more so on T2-weighted images. The findings are nonspecific with CT imaging.

A rare tumor appearing in childhood is the so-called undifferentiated embryonal sarcoma (26). On ultrasonography the pattern is mixed with solid tissue and "cystic" areas of necrosis. CT and MR reveal a similar heterogeneous pattern and basically these tumors are avascular (Fig. 4.213). Finally it should be noted that patients with HIV infection are prone to develop spindle-cell tumors, primarily leiomyoma and leiomyosarcoma (27, 28).

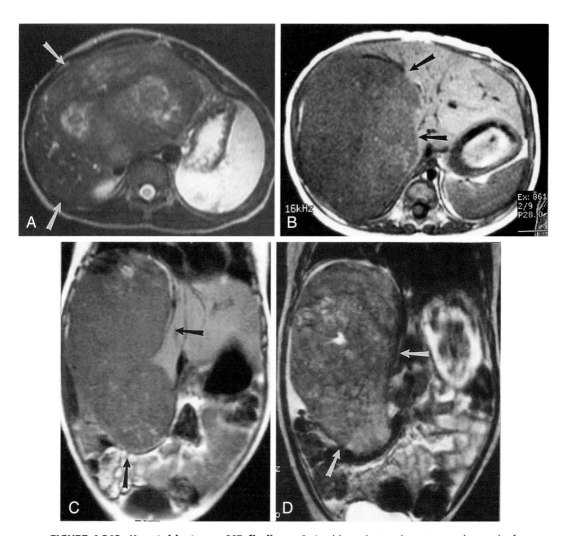

FIGURE 4.212. Hepatoblastoma: MR findings. A. In this patient, a large tumor (arrows) of low signal is present on this T2-weighted image. Scattered areas of increased signal (bleeding, necrosis) are seen throughout the mass. **B.** Another patient with an axial view through a large tumor (arrows) of low signal intensity. Compare with the normal signal of the liver, which is being displaced to the left, over the stomach. **C.** Coronal view demonstrates similar findings (arrows). **D.** T2-weighted image demonstrates spotty increased signal intensity throughout the mass (arrows).

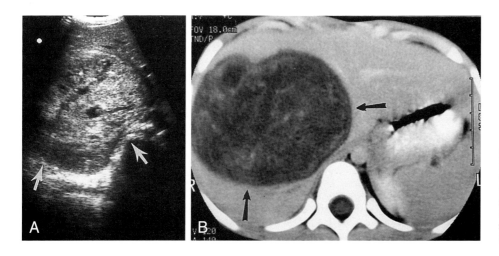

FIGURE 4.213. Undifferentiated liver sarcoma. A. Ultrasonogram demonstrates an echogenic mass (arrows) with sonolucent areas and some areas that appear as vessels. **B.** Contrast-enhanced CT study demonstrates a basically hypodense but very heterogeneous mass (arrows).

REFERENCES

1. Luks FI, Yazbeck S, Brandt ML, et al. Benign liver tumors in children: a 25-year experience. J Pediatr Surg 1991;26: 1326–1330.
2. Pardes JG, Bryan PJ, Gauderer MWL. Spontaneous regression of infantile hemangioendotheliomatosis of the liver: demonstration by ultrasound. J Ultrasound Med 1982;1:349–353.
3. Kirchner SG, Heller RM, Kasselberg AG, et al. Infantile hepatic hemangioendothelioma with subsequent malignant degeneration. Pediatr Radiol 1981;11:42–45.
4. Mortele KJ, Mergo PJ, Urrutia M, et al. MR findings in infantile hepatic hemangioendothelioma. J Comput Assist Tomogr 1998; 22:714–717.
5. Davenport M, Hansen L, Heaton ND, et al. Hemangioendothelioma of the liver in infants. J Pediatr Surg 1995;30:44–48.
6. Burrows PE, Rosenberg HC, Chuang HS. Diffuse, hepatic hemangiomas: percutaneous transcatheter embolization with detachable silicone balloons. Radiology 1985;156:85–88.
7. Johnson DH, Vinson AM, Wirth FH, et al. Management of hepatic hemangioendotheliomas of infancy by transarterial embolization: a report of two cases. Pediatrics 1984;73:546–549.
8. Chung T, Hoffer FA, Burrows PE, et al. MR imaging of hepatic hemangiomas of infancy and changes seen with interferon alpha-2a treatment. Pediatr Radiol 1996;26:341–348.
9. DeMaioribus CA, Lally KP, Sim K, et al. Mesenchymal hamartoma of the liver: a 35-year review. Arch Surg 1990;125: 598–600.
10. Frederici S, Gali G, Sciutti R, et al. Cystic mesenchymal hamartoma of the liver. Pediatr Radiol 1992;22:307–308.
11. Wholey MH, Wojno KJ. Pediatric hepatic mesenchymal hamartoma demonstrated on plain film, ultrasound and MRI, and correlated with pathology. Pediatr Radiol 1994;24:143–144.
12. Alwaidh MH, Woodhall CR, Carty HT. Mesenchymal hamartoma of the liver a case report. Pediatr Radiol 1997;27:247–249.
13. Kaufman RA. Is cystic mesenchymal hamartoma of the liver similar to infantile hemangioendothelioma and cavernous hemangioma on dynamic computed tomography? Pediatr Radiol 1992;22:582–583.
14. Balmer B, LeCoultre C, Feldges A, et al. Mesenchymal liver hamartoma in a newborn: case report. Eur J Pediatr Surg 1996;6:303–305.
15. Barnhart DC, Hirschl RB, Garver KA, et al. Conservative management of mesenchymal hamartoma of the liver. J Pediatr Surg 1997;32:1495–1498.
16. Ramanujam TM, Ramesh JC, Goh DW, et al. Malignant transformation of mesenchymal hamartoma of the liver: case report and review of the literature. J Pediatr Surg 2000;34:1684–1686.
17. Cheon J-E, Kim WS, Kim I-O, et al. Radiological features of focal nodular hyperplasia of the liver in children. Pediatr Radiol 1998;28:878–883.
18. Mortele KJ, Praet M, Villerberghe H, et al. Pictorial essay. CT and MR imaging findings in focal nodular hyperplasia of the liver: radiologic-pathologic correlation. AJR 2000;175:687–692.
19. Trenschel GM, Schubert A, Dries V, et al. Nodular regenerative hyperplasia of the liver: case report of a 13-year-old girl and review of the literature. Pediatr Radiol 2000;30:64–68.
20. Learch TJ, Ralls PW, Johnson MB, et al. Hepatic focal nodular hyperplasia: findings with color Doppler sonography. J Ultrasound Med 1993;12:541–544.
21. Grossman H, Ram PC, Coleman RA, et al. Hepatic ultrasonography in type I glycogen storage disease (Von Gierke disease): detection of hepatic adenoma and carcinoma. Radiology 1981; 141:753–756.
22. Brummett D, Burton EM, Sabio H. Hepatic adenomatosis: rapid sequence MR imaging following gadolinium enhancement: a case report. Pediatr Radiol 1999;29:231–234.
23. Tsuchida Y, Ikeda H, Suzuki N, Takahashi A, et al. A case of well-differentiated fetal-type hepatoblastoma with very low serum alpha-fetoprotein. J Pediatr Surg 1999;34:1762–1764.
24. Men S, Hekimol B, Tuzun M, et al. Unusual US and CT findings in hepatoblastoma: a case report. Pediatr Radiol 1995;25: 507–508.
25. Kohno M, Kitatani H, Wada H, et al. Hepatocellular carcinoma complicating biliary cirrhosis caused by biliary atresia: report of a case. J Pediatr Surg 1995;30:1713–1716.
26. Moon WK, Kim IO, Yeon KM, et al. Undifferentiated embryonal sarcoma of the liver: US and CT findings. Pediatr Radiol 1995;24:500–503.
27. Ha C, Haller JO, Rollins NK. Smooth muscle tumors in immunocompromised (HIV negative) children. Pediatr Radiol 1993;23:413–414.
28. Levin TL, Adam HM, van Hoeven K, et al. Hepatic spindle cell tumors in HIV positive children. Pediatr Radiol 1994;24:78–79.

Liver Abscess

Abscesses in and around the liver are uncommon in the neonate (1), but they are frequently seen in older infants and children. In the neonate, these abscesses usually are the consequence of either neonatal sepsis or umbilical vein catheterization. In older infants and children, liver abscess may be pyogenic or amebic. Most are pyogenic, unless one is in an endemic area for amoebiasis. Pyogenic abscesses also can result from perforated appendicitis or granulomatous disease of childhood (2), but some are primary.

Liver abscess usually presents with a large, tender liver, which may be visible on plain films. In addition to enlargement of the liver, there is elevation of the right diaphragmatic leaflet, and in some cases, an associated pleural effusion may be present. Thereafter, one should press on to ultrasound, which has become the primary imaging modality in liver abscess. Sonographically the appearance of hepatic abscess is variable (Fig. 4.214). In many cases, it presents as a purely hypoechoic lesion, but in other cases debris may be present within the abscess and, on upright positioning, a debris fluid level may be seen. In still other cases the abscess may be multilocular or solid in appearance. Amebic abscess is said to be typically sonolucent, although we (3), have found some to be echogenic (Fig. 4.214A), and in fact, others have shown that differences in amebic and bacterial abscesses are minimal (4). Overall, however, amebic abscesses have a tendency to contain less debris and are prone to rupture through the diaphragm into the chest, or through the pericardium into the pericardial cavity. In the past, drainage of amebic abscess was not considered proper, but now there are those who suggest percutaneous drainage, especially for cases where the abscess is next to

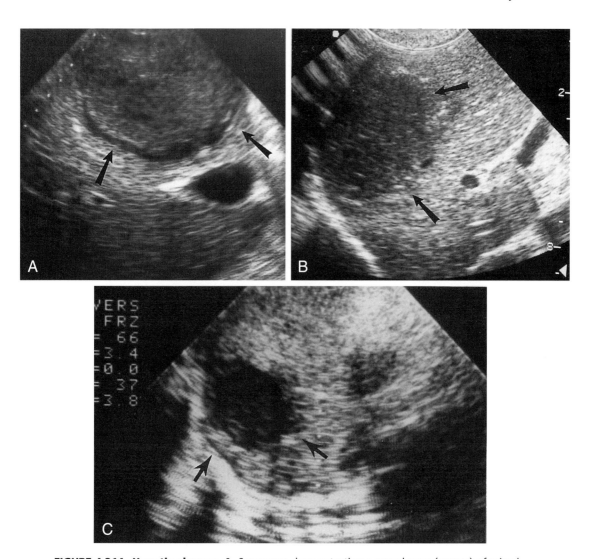

FIGURE 4.214. Hepatic abscess. A. Sonogram demonstrating a round mass (arrows) of mixed echogenicity and with a sonolucent rim. This was an amebic abscess. **B.** Another patient with an echogenic abscess, but in this case the abscess is a little more hypoechoic (arrows). **C.** Another patient with a basically hypoechoic abscess (arrows).

the pericardium or pleural cavity. With pyogenic abscess, treatment may be conservative, but increasingly, percutaneous drainage is advocated. Hepatic abscess also can be demonstrated with CT, which demonstrates a hypodense lesion in the liver (Fig. 4.215). On MRI, abscesses show increased signal on both T1- and T2-weighted images. Most hepatic abscesses, whether pyogenic or amebic, are single, but in some cases, multiple abscesses are seen (Fig. 4.215C). On ultrasonography, the latter present with multiple sonolucent lesions in the liver. We also have seen one such case with amebic involvement (Fig. 4.216).

REFERENCES

1. Kumar A, Srinivasan S, Sharma AK. Pyogenic liver abscess in children—South Indian experiences. J Pediatr Surg 1998;33: 417–421.
2. Garel LA, Pariente DM, Nezelof C, et al. Liver involvement in chronic granulomatous disease: the role of ultrasound in diagnosis and treatment. Radiology 1984;153:117–122.
3. Hayden CK Jr, Toups M, Swischuk LE, et al. Sonographic features of hepatic amebiasis in childhood. J Can Radiol 1984;35: 279–282.
4. Ralls PW, Barnes PF, Radin DR, et al. Sonographic features of

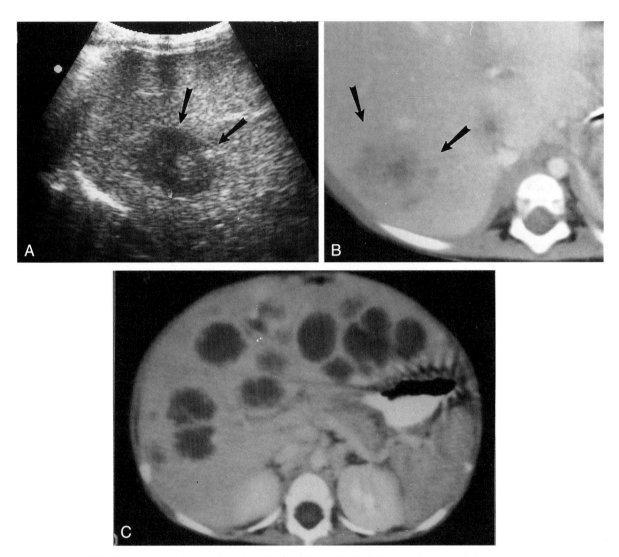

FIGURE 4.215. Hepatic abscess: CT findings. A. Preliminary ultrasound demonstrates a hypoechoic abscess (arrows). **B.** CT with contrast enhancement demonstrates the abscess to be of low density (arrows). It did not fill in on later sequences. **C.** Multiple, low-density abscesses (amebic) scattered throughout the liver. (Courtesy of Deborah Ablin, M.D.)

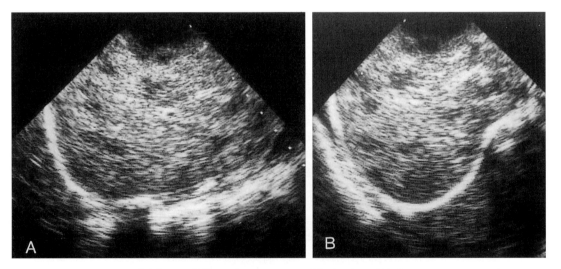

FIGURE 4.216. Multiple small liver abscesses: amebiasis. A and B. Note numerous sonolucent areas in the liver caused by amebiasis. Similar findings can be seen with visceral larva migrans and cat-scratch disease (see Fig. 4.217).

amebic and pyogenic liver abscesses: a blinded comparison. AJR 1987;149:499–501.

Cat-Scratch Disease and Other Granulomas

Over the last few years, it has become apparent that cat-scratch disease not only involves the lymph nodes of the extremities and the neck but also can involve the liver and spleen (1–5). The findings in both the liver and spleen consist of multiple granulomas that on ultrasonography appear as hypoechoic lesions and, on CT studies, as hypodense lesions (Fig. 4.217). Granulomas in the liver, single or multiple, also can be seen with visceral larva migrans, tuberculosis (6) fungal disease (Fig. 4.218), candidiasis, and toxocariasis (7). Calcifications of these granulomas can occur as they heal (8).

REFERENCES

1. Danon O, Duval-Arnould M, Osman Z, et al. Hepatic and splenic involvement in cat-scratch disease: imaging features. Abdom Imaging 2000;25:182–183.
2. Hopkins KL, Simoneaux SF, Patrick LE, et al. Pictorial essay. Imaging manifestations of cat-scratch disease. AJR 1996;166: 435–438.
3. Larsen CE, Patrick LE. Abdominal (liver, spleen) and bone manifestations of cat-scratch disease. Pediatr Radiol 1992;22:353–355.
4. Port J, Leonidas JC. Granulomatous hepatitis in cat-scratch disease. Pediatr Radiol 1991;21:598–599.
5. Port J, Leonidas JC. Granulomatous hepatitis in cat-scratch disease. Pediatr Radiol 1991;21:598–599.
6. Crover SB, Taneja DJ, Bhatis A, et al. Sonographic diagnosis of congenital tuberculosis: an experience with four cases. Abdom Imaging 2000;25:622–626.
7. Baldisserotto M, Conchin CF, Soares Mda G, et al. Ultrasound findings in children with toxocariasis: report on 18 cases. Pediatr Radiol 1999;29:316–319.
6. Talenti E, Cesaro S, Scapinello A, et al. Disseminated hepatic and splenic calcifications following cat-scratch disease. Pediatr Radiol 1994;24:342–343.

Fatty (Radiolucent) Liver

When the liver is massively replaced by fat, it becomes radiolucent and visible on plain films of the abdomen (1–3). For the most part, such deposition of fat in the liver must be chronic and the most common causes are kwashiorkor and cystic fibrosis. In both cases, chronic protein malnutrition leads to replacement of the cytoplasm of the hepatocytes with large, intracellular fat droplets (Fig. 4.219). In acute hepatic necrosis, although fatty degeneration occurs,

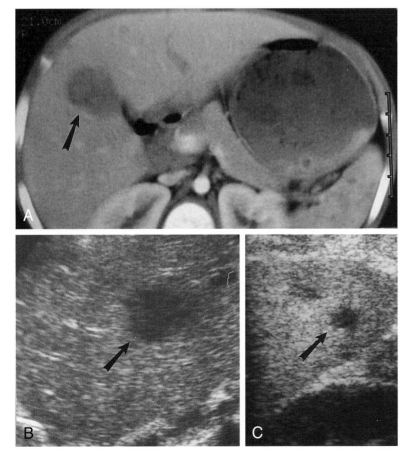

FIGURE 4.217. Cat-scratch disease. A. Note the low-density granuloma (arrow) in the liver on this contrast-enhanced scan. **B.** Ultrasonogram demonstrates the relatively hypodense granuloma (arrow). **C.** A small, similar granuloma (arrow) is seen in the spleen.

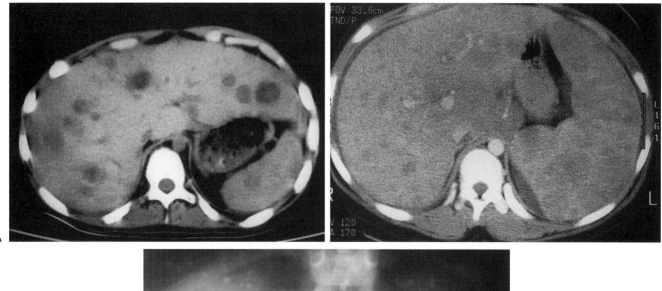

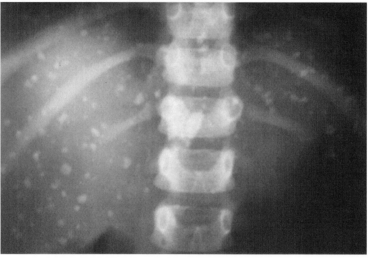

FIGURE 4.218. Liver granulomas. A. Note the numerous, hypodense granulomas in the liver and spleen secondary to coccidiomycosis. B. Multiple granulomas in the liver and spleen in this patient are due to histoplasmosis. C. Calcifications from old histoplasma granulomas.

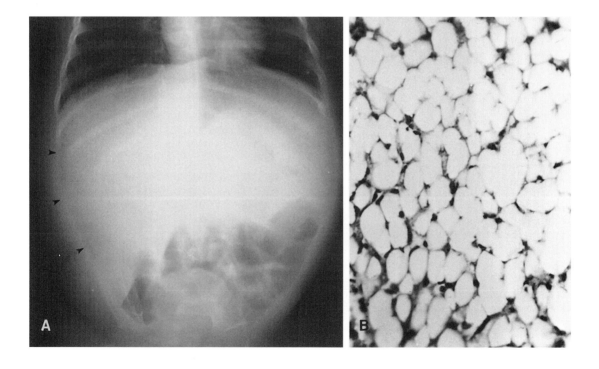

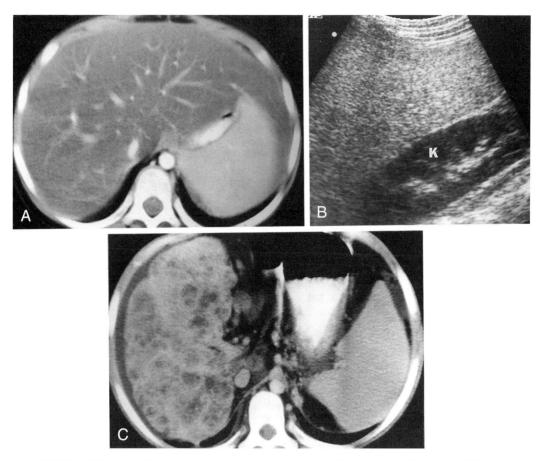

FIGURE 4.220. Fatty liver. A. Note marked hypodensity (radiolucency) of the enlarged liver in this patient with L-asparaginase toxicity. **B.** Same patient, demonstrating diffuse, fine, peppery, increased echogenicity of the right lobe of the liver. K. right kidney. **C.** Cystic fibrosis with nodular fatty degeneration of the liver. The spleen is enlarged. (**C** courtesy of Jiles Perreault, M.D.)

the fat droplets are microdroplets, which neither greatly distort the cells nor totally replace their cytoplasm. Because of this, enough liver tissue remains to obscure the presence of fat, and the same problem occurs with conditions such as Reye's syndrome, diabetes mellitus, galactosemia, tyrosinosis, fructosemia, and abetalipoproteinemia. Focal fatty infiltration in healthy children is rare (4).

Roentgenographically, the appearance of advanced fatty infiltration of the liver is characteristic, for the normal whiteness of the liver becomes more gray or radiolucent. The liver blends with the normally gray or radiolucent properitoneal fat stripe, and together these structures extend, as a diffuse grayness (radiolucency), to the inner edge of the normally more dense (white) abdominal muscles (Fig. 4.219A).

Fatty liver also is vividly demonstrable with CT and MR scanning. With CT scanning the liver is markedly hypodense (Fig. 4.220A), while with MR imaging it is high in signal. With ultrasound, a fatty liver shows increased echogenicity with a very fine grainy pattern resulting in the so-called bright liver (Fig. 4.220B). CT, however, is much more sensitive with early fatty infiltration. With cystic fibrosis, fatty liver may be less homogeneous in advanced cases and quite nodular (Fig. 4.220C).

FIGURE 4.219. Fatty (radiolucent) liver. A. Note typical radiolucency of the fat-infiltrated liver (arrows). **B.** Histologic material demonstrates the large fat-containing liver cells. (Reproduced with permission from Swischuk LE, McConnell RF Jr. The radiographic demonstration of fatty liver in children (a clue to protein malnutrition). J Pediatr 1978;88:452–454.)

REFERENCES

1. Swischuk LE. A new and unusual roentgenographic finding of fatty liver in infants. AJR 1974;122:159–164.
2. Swischuk LE, McConnell RF Jr. The radiographic demonstration of fatty liver in children (a clue to protein malnutrition). J Pediatr 1978;88:452–454.
3. Yousefzadeh DK, Lupetin AR, Jackson JH Jr. The radiographic signs of fatty liver. Radiology 1979;131:351–355.
4. Labuski MR, Eggli KD, Boal DKB, et al. Focal fatty infiltration of the liver in a healthy child. Pediatr Radiol 1992;22:281–282.

Intrahepatic Calcifications

Intrahepatic calcifications usually are irregular and can be seen with malignant tumors such as hepatoblastoma, hepatocellular carcinoma, and metastatic neuroblastoma. They also can be seen with benign hemangiomas of the liver, and in the portal vein or its radicals as calcified thromboemboli from umbilical vein catheterization (1). In addition, one can see postinflammatory calcifications from any number of viral infections, and calcifications in the ductus venosus also have been noted (3). In some cases, an etiology is not determined, but if the finding is isolated, and no mass is associated, no further investigation is necessary. Calcifications in the liver also have been documented with cystic fibrosis (4).

REFERENCES

1. Richter E, Globl H, Holthusen W, et al. Intrahepatic calcifications in infants and children following umbilical vein catheterization. Ann Radiol 1984;27:117–124.
2. Rigsby CK, Donnelly LF. Fetal varicella syndrome: association with multiple hepatic calcifications and intestinal atresia. Pediatr Radiol 1997;27:779.
3. Rizzo AJ, Haller JO, Mulvihill DM, et al. Calcification of the ductus venosus: a cause of right upper quadrant calcification in the newborn. Radiology 1989;173:89–90.
4. Magruder MJ, Munden MM. Intrahepatic microlithiasis: another gastrointestinal complication of cystic fibrosis. J Ultrasound Med 1997;16:763–765.

Budd-Chiari Syndrome

This is an uncommon problem in children and results from obstruction of the hepatic veins or inferior vena cava. Obstruction can be the result of membranes or webs, stenoses, thrombi, or compressive tumors and cysts (1). Often, however, no cause is identified. Symptoms usually consist of refractory ascites with normal liver function tests. Ultrasound can demonstrate the dilated veins proximal to the area of obstruction. Dilation of stenotic veins can be performed percutaneously (2).

REFERENCES

1. Gentil-Kocher S, Bernard O, Brunelle F, et al. Budd-Chiari syndrome in children: report of 22 cases. J Pediatr 1988;113:30–38.

2.. Lois JF, Hartzman S, McGlade CT, et al. Budd-Chiari syndrome: treatment with percutaneous transhepatic recanalization and dilation. Radiology 1989;170:791–793.

Glycogen Storage Disease

The liver can enlarge with a number of hematologic conditions and also enlarges in Gaucher's disease and glycogen storage disease, especially type I (von Gierke's disease) and type III (Cori's disease). In these cases the liver may show increased echogenicity on ultrasound. Liver enlargement is not usually seen in type II glycogen storage disease (i.e., Pompe's disease). Cardiomegaly and muscle changes predominate in this type. Finally, it should be recalled that adenomas of the liver are a common problem in glycogen storage disease.

Peliosis Hepatis

This is a rare condition where a peculiar vascular abnormality of the liver causes it to enlarge. The liver is riddled with large and small vascular sinusoids (1–3). Its etiology is unknown, but it has been reported after the use of anabolic steroids (3). It may represent some form of reparative process in the liver. The findings can be demonstrated with ultrasound, CT, and MR but are perhaps more vividly demonstrated with ultrasound including color-flow Doppler imaging. Calcifications also can occur (4).

REFERENCES

1. Bracero LA, Gambon TB, Evans R, et al. Ultrasonographic findings in a case of congenital peliosis hepatitis. J Ultrasound Med 1995;14:483–486.
2. Maves CK, Caron KH, Bisset GS III, et al. Case report. Splenic and hepatic peliosis: MR findings. AJR 1992;158:75–76.
3. Saatci I, Coskun M, Boyvat F, et al. MR findings in peliosis hepatis. Pediatr Radiol 1995;25:31–33.
4. Muradali D, Wilson SR, Wanless IR, et al. Peliosis hepatis with intrahepatic calcifications. J Ultrasound Med 1996;15:257–260.

Hemochromatosis

Primary and secondary forms of hemochromatosis exist. The primary form is rare and is characterized by deposition of hemosiderin in the liver parenchyma (1). It results from an underlying metabolic defect while the secondary form results from the breakdown of blood products after transfusion, muscle damage, or hemolytic anemias (1, 2). In the secondary form, deposition of hemosiderin occurs in the reticuloendothelial system. On plain films, in advanced cases, the liver will become more opaque, but this is unusual and most often the findings are detected with CT or MRI. With ultrasonography, increased echoes in the liver are seen, but with CT a characteristically high-density liver is present, and on MR images, because of the iron in the liver, marked loss of signal occurs, especially on T2-weighted images (Fig. 4.221).

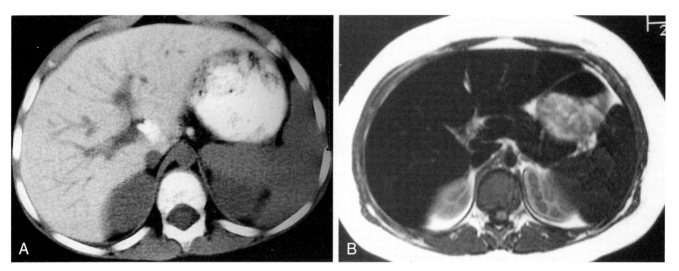

FIGURE 4.221. Hemachromatosis of liver. A. CT study demonstrates markedly increased density of the liver. **B.** T1-weighted MR study in another patient demonstrates low signal intensity, or so-called black liver.

REFERENCES

1. Siegelman ES, Mitchell DG, Rubin R, et al. Parenchymal versus reticuloendothelial iron overload in the liver: distinction with MR imaging. Radiology 1991;179:361–366.
2. Villari N, Caramella D, Lippi A, et al. Assessment of liver iron overload in thalassemic patients by MR imaging. Acta Radiol 1992;33:347–350.

Portal Vein Gas

Portal vein gas is characteristic of necrotizing enterocolitis and secondary to pneumatosis cystoides intestinalis. It also can occur on a benign basis with benign pneumatosis. Although a hallmark of necrotizing enterocolitis of the premature infant, it can be seen in any patient with bowel necrosis and gas formation in the bowel wall. Usually, it is clearly visible on plain films, but in subclinical cases the detection of air (gas) in the portal venous system can be accomplished with ultrasonography (1, 2). Echogenic bubbles of air will be seen to float through the portal vein.

REFERENCES

1. Avni EF, Rypens F, Cohen E, et al. Pericholecystic hyperechogenicities in necrotizing enterocolitis: a specific sonographic sign? Pediatr Radiol 1991;21:179–181.
2. King S, Shuckett B. Sonographic diagnosis of portal venous gas in two pediatric liver transplant patients with benign pneumatosis intestinalis. Case reports and literature review. Pediatr Radiol 1992;22:577–578.

Torsion of Accessory Lobe and Wandering Liver

These are uncommon conditions resulting from poor fixation of the liver or a portion thereof. Presentation can be that of an acute abdomen (1–3). The findings may be puzzling but the torsed accessory liver segment can be demonstrated with any imaging modality, including ultrasound.

REFERENCES

1. al-Ali F, Macpherson RI, Othersen HB, et al. A "wandering liver" in an infant. Pediatr Radiol 1997;27:287.
2. Elmasalme F, Aljudaibi A, Matbouly S, et al. Torsion of an accessory lobe of the liver in an infant. J Pediatr Surg 1995;30:1348–1350.
3. Sanguesa C, Esteban MJ, Gomez J, et al. Liver accessory lobe torsion in the infant. Pediatr Radiol 1995;25:153–154.

Congenital Arterial-Portal Venous Malformation

This is a rare abnormality (1, 2) often discovered incidentally. On the other hand, when high flow occurs through the fistula, portal hypertension can result. The abnormality is readily detected with ultrasonography, and embolization can be used for treatment of symptomatic cases.

REFERENCES

1. Martin LW, Benzing G, Kaplan S. Congenital intrahepatic arteriovenous fistula: report of a successfully treated case. Ann Surg 1965;161:209–212.
2. Routh WD, Keller FS, Cain WS, et al. Transcatheter embolization of a high-flow congenital intrahepatic arterial-portal venous malformation in an infant. J Pediatr Surg 1992;27:511–514.

Liver Transplant

This subject is beyond the scope of this book, but a number of references (1–7) are provided for the interested reader. In summary, however, preoperatively it is most important that normal vascular and biliary anatomy of the liver be documented. After transplantation, one monitors the patient, primarily with ultrasound, for the development of complications such as hepatic artery thrombosis, liver infarction, portal vein thrombosis, cystic duct mucocele formation, fluid collections around the operative site, and biliary tract obstructions. The findings associated with these complications are no different than when they occur de novo or as complications of other hepatobiliary surgical disease.

REFERENCES

1. Ametani F, Itoh K, Shibata T, et al. Spectrum of CT findings in pediatric patients after partial liver transplantation. Radiographics 2001;21:53–63.
2. Bilik R, Yellen M, Superina RA. Surgical complications in children after liver transplantation. J Pediatr Surg 1992;27:1371–1375.
3. Griffith JF, John PR. Imaging of biliary complications following pediatric liver transplantation. Pediatr Radiol 1996;26:388–394.
4. Lallier M, St-Vil D, Luks FI, et al. Biliary tract complications in pediatric orthotopic liver transplantation. J Pediatr Surg 1993;28:1102–1105.
5. Peclet MH, Ryckman FC, Pedersen SH, et al. The spectrum of bile duct complications in pediatric liver transplantation. J Pediatr Surg 1994;29:214–220.
6. Rollins NK, Sheffield EG, Andrews WS. Portal vein stenosis complicating liver transplantation in children: percutaneous transhepatic angioplasty. Radiology 1992;182:731–737.
7. Westra SJ, Zaninovic AC, Hall TR, et al. Imaging in pediatric liver transplantation. Radiographics 1993;13:1081–1099.

SPLEEN

Normal Configuration

The splenic silhouette is reasonably well visualized on both abdominal and chest roentgenograms, but as with the liver, it is difficult to be absolute about splenic size. Many times, splenic enlargement occurs primarily in a posterior direction and enlargement is not appreciated on the usual abdominal roentgenogram. The normal spleen may be mostly posterior in location and can appear as a retrogastric pseudotumor on lateral roentgenograms. The spleen is more readily assessed with CT or MR scanning, but ultrasonography also can be used to identify the spleen. Normal measurements both with ultrasound (1) and CT (2, 3) are available, but usually one's first assessment of splenic enlargement is subjective.

REFERENCES

1. Rosenberg HK, Markowitz RI, Kolberg H, et al. Normal splenic size in infants and children: sonographic measurements. AJR 1991;157:119–121.
2. Schlesinger AE, Edgar KA, Boxer LA. Volume of the spleen in children as measured on CT scans: normal standards as a function of body weight. AJR 1993;160:1107–1109.
3. Schlesinger AE, Hildebolt CF, Siegel MJ, et al. Splenic volume in children: simplified estimation at CT. Radiology 1994;193:578–580.

ABNORMALITIES OF THE SPLEEN

Splenic Enlargement

Splenic enlargement, no matter what the cause, usually produces some elevation of the ipsilateral diaphragmatic leaflet, medial or anterior displacement of the stomach, and downward displacement of the splenic flexure and loops of small intestine. Splenic enlargement can be seen with such conditions as portal hypertension, splenic trauma, the reticuloendothelioses, hematologic disease, infection, and occasionally with tumors and cysts. The spleen also enlarges in ECMO therapy and this is secondary to the extensive breakdown of red blood cells and other blood products (1). With ultrasound, enlarged spleens tend to extend over the anterior surface of the left kidney rather than stop at the upper pole.

REFERENCE

1. Klippenstein DL, Zerin JM, Hirschl RB, et al. Splenic enlargement in neonates during ECMO. Radiology 1994;190:411–412.

Splenic Inflammation and Infection

Most commonly, the spleen becomes inflamed or infected with systemic viral diseases, the most common of which is infectious mononucleosis. It also can become involved in patients with HIV infection, but bacterial infections (abscesses) of the spleen are rare. However, it is becoming increasingly apparent that the spleen can, as can the liver, become involved in cat scratch disease (1). The findings are the same as in the liver and consist of numerous hypoechoic granulomas on ultrasound and hypodense lesions on CT (See Fig. 4.218). Similar findings, as in the liver, can be seen with fungal disease, tuberculosis, visceral larva migrans, and toxocariasis.

REFERENCE

1. Danon, O, Duval-Arnould M, Osman Z, et al. Hepatic and splenic involvement in cat-scratch disease. Imaging features. Abdom Imaging 2000;25:182–183.

Splenic Trauma

In older infants and children the most common causes of splenic trauma are injury to the abdomen after motor vehicle accidents and blunt trauma to the upper abdomen from accidents such as handlebar injuries. Splenic trauma also can be seen in the battered child syndrome. In the neonatal period, it is the large babies who are prone to splenic rup-

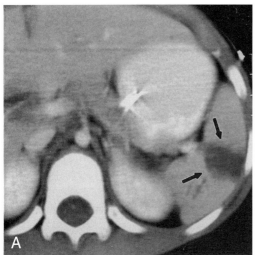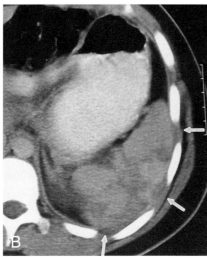

FIGURE 4.222. Splenic trauma. A. Note the splenic laceration (arrows). **B.** Another patient with a fractured or crushed spleen (arrows).

ture or hematoma formation. In addition, infants subject to hypoxia, which renders the liver and spleen more congested, also are prone to splenic injury. Similarly spleens enlarged from infection also are prone to rupture (1). Management of splenic injuries is conservative, no matter what the cause, and resolution is the rule. Currently, splenectomy is reserved for those cases where hemorrhage cannot be controlled or complications requiring removal of the spleen arise. This conservative attitude is necessary so as to avoid problems with immunity and infection later in life.

Splenic injury is best detected with CT, contrast-enhanced scans. On these studies the area of injury usually is hypodense (Fig. 4.222) and does not fill in after contrast administration. Fluid (blood) may accumulate in the subcapsular region, and actual fracturing of the spleen with fluid around the spleen can be seen. In addition, fluid (blood) can be present in the abdomen at large. Ultrasonography also can be employed but is less specific than CT scanning. It can demonstrate disorganized echoes, and fluid collections also can be documented. However, lesions can be missed by ultrasound scans, and the best imaging modality for splenic trauma is CT. Splenic injury can be evaluated and monitored with ultrasound during healing and resolution (2).

On plain films with splenic injury, as with any splenic mass, the splenic silhouette may appear enlarged, and there may be elevation of the left diaphragmatic leaflet, medial displacement of the gastric air bubble, and downward displacement of the splenic flexure. Fluid also may be present in the ipsilateral hemithorax.

REFERENCES

1. Ali J. Spontaneous rupture of the spleen in patients with infectious mononucleosis. Can J Surg 1993;36:49–52.
2. Emery KH, Babcock DS, Borgman AS, et al. Splenic injury diagnosed with CT: US follow-up and healing rate in children and adolescents. Radiology 1999;212:515–518.

Wandering Spleen and Torsion

When the normal ligaments that affix the spleen in the left upper quadrant are absent or deficient, poor fixation of the spleen results. The spleen then becomes ectopic and, as such, on any imaging modality, is missing from its usual left upper quadrant position. These ectopic spleens are quite mobile, and hence the term "wandering spleen" is used to describe them (1). However, because they are so hypermobile they are subject to torsion (2, 3). These patients present with an acute abdomen, and the imaging findings, especially with ultrasonography, can be confusing (3). However, no matter which imaging modality is used, the first clue to the problem is that the spleen cannot be located in its normal position. In addition, a "whorled" configuration of the twisted splenic pedicle has been described and can be of help (3) (Fig. 4.223). Although usually an isolated problem, torsion of a wandering spleen has been reported in association with gastric volvulus (4).

REFERENCES

1. Allen KB, Gay BB, Skandalakis JE. Wandering spleen: anatomic and radiologic considerations. South Med J 1992;85:976–984.
2. Herman ZW, Friedwald JP, Donovan C, et al. Torsion of a wandering spleen in a one month old, with a confusing ultrasound examination. Pediatr Radiol 1991;21:442–443.
3. Swischuk LE, Williams JB, John SD. Torsion of wandering spleen: the whorled appearance of the splenic pedicle on CT. Pediatr Radiol 1993;23:476–477.
4. Garcia JA, Garcia-Fernandez M, Romance A, et al. Wandering spleen and gastric volvulus. Pediatr Radiol 1995;24:535–536.

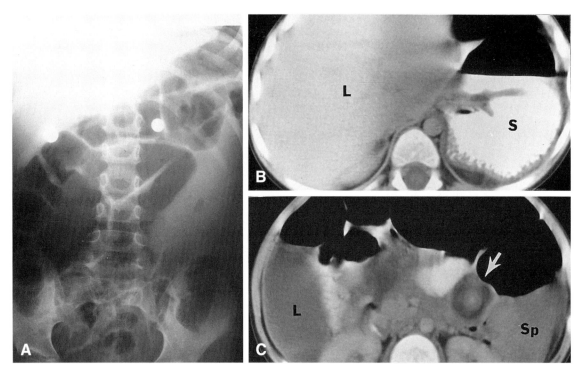

FIGURE 4.223. Wandering spleen. A. Note the soft tissue mass of the ectopic spleen in the left lower flank area. **B.** Through this high axial cut, note the liver (L) and stomach (S) but no evidence of the spleen. **C.** Slightly lower cut demonstrates the whorled appearance of the twisted pedicle (arrow) of the spleen (SP). L, liver. (Reproduced with permission from Williams JB et al. Torsion of the wandering spleen: the whorled appearance of the splenic pedicle on CT. Pediatr Radiol 1993;23:476–477.)

Splenic Tumors and Cysts

Splenic tumors and cysts are extremely uncommon in the pediatric group. Most cysts are epithelial or epidermoid in origin, and multiple cysts can be familial (1). Tumors include entities such as lymphangioma (2), hemangioma (3), and hamartoma (4–6). Ultrasonography usually is one's best initial imaging tool for investigating any of these masses. With this modality cysts are primarily sonolucent (unless hemorrhage or infection supervene), lymphangiomas are multicystic, and hemangiomas are solid but variably hypoechoic or hyperechoic. Perhaps they more often are hypoechoic (Fig. 4.224A) and with color-flow Doppler imaging will demonstrate increased blood flow (Fig. 4.224B). Hamartomas, as they are elsewhere in the body, demonstrate a very heterogeneous tissue pattern and numerous cysts.

REFERENCES

1. Iwanaka T, Nakanishi H, Tsuchida Y, et al. Familial multiple mesothelial cysts of the spleen. J Pediatr Surg 1995;30: 1743–1745.
2. Wadsworth DT, Newman B, Abramson SJ, et al. Splenic lymphangiomatosis in children. Radiology 1997;202:173–176.
3. Panuel M, Ternier F, Michel G, et al. Splenic hemangioma— report of three pediatric cases with pathologic correlation. Pediatr Radiol 1992;22:213–216.
4. Kassarjian A, Patenaude YG, Bernard C, et al. Symptomatic splenic hamartoma with renal, cutaneous, and hematological abnormalities. Pediatr Radiol 2001;31:111–114.
5. Iozzo RV, Haas JE, Chard RL. Symptomatic splenic hamartoma: a report of two cases and literature. Pediatrics 1980;66:261–265.
6. Thompson SE, Walsh EA, Cramer BC, et al. Radiological features of a symptomatic splenic hamartoma. Pediatr Radiol 1996;26: 657–660.

Splenic Hypoplasia, Agenesis, and Multiple Spleens

Splenic hypoplasia and splenic agenesis are uncommon and are difficult to diagnose from abdominal roentgenograms. Absence of the spleen is seen in the asplenia syndrome and, although multiple and accessory spleens can be seen in normal infants, they are more often associated with the polysplenia syndrome. Most times these accessory or multiple spleens are most expediently demonstrated with nuclear scintigraphy, but they also can be detected with ultrasound and CT (Fig. 4.224, C and D). An interesting case of ectopic spleen mimicking an abdominal lymphoma has

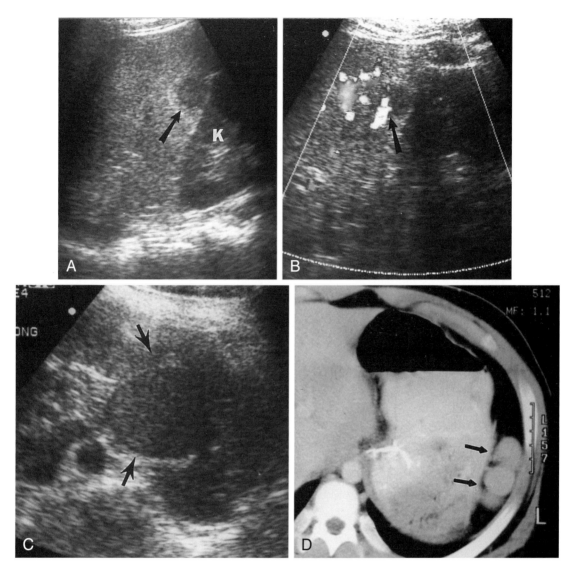

FIGURE 4.224. Hemangioma of spleen. A. Note the slightly hypoechoic nodule (arrow) in the spleen. K, kidney. **B.** Color-flow Doppler demonstrates increased flow (arrow) to the nodule. **C. Accessory spleen.** Note the round appearance of accessory splenic tissue (arrows). **D.** Another patient who on CT scan demonstrates a number of accessory splenic nodules (arrows).

been documented (1), but while this could occur with CT examination, it should not occur with ultrasound imaging, because lymphomas usually are hypoechoic, while ectopic splenic tissue has the normal echogenicity of spleen. Finally, it should be noted that accessory splenic tissue can undergo torsion and present as an acute abdomen (2).

REFERENCES

1. Mathurin J, Lalemand D. Splenosis simulating an abdominal lymphoma. Pediatr Radiol 1990;21:69–70.
2. Seo T, Ito T, Watanabe Y, et al. Torsion of an accessory spleen presenting as an acute abdomen with an inflammatory mass. US, CT, and MRI findings. Pediatr Radiol 1995;24:532–534.

Splenogonadal Fusion

Splenogonadal fusion is a rare anomaly that usually is discovered at surgery (1–4). It arises from embryonic fusion of the spleen with the gonads. As a result, there is tissue extending down to the gonads and accessory splenic tissue may be found in the area. This can be demonstrated with ultrasound (3). It is important to appreciate this anomaly for knowledge of its occurrence can avoid unnecessary orchiectomy (2).

REFERENCES

1. Jequier S, Hanquinet S, Lironi A. Splenogonadal fusion. Pediatr Radiol 1998;28:526.

2. Karaman MI, Gonzales ET Jr. Splenogonadal fusion: report of two cases and review of the literature. J Urol 1996;155:309–311.
3. Nimkin K, Kleinman PK, Chappell JS. Abdominal ultrasonography of splenogonadal fusion. J Ultrasound Med 2000;19: 345–347.
4. Patel RV. Splenogonadal fusion. J Pediatr Surg 1995;30:873–874.

PANCREAS

Normal Configuration

The pancreas, in the past, has been one of the most difficult organs in the body to image. However, with the advent of ultrasound, CT, and MR imaging, it has become a little more accessible. In children, the primary imaging modality for pancreatic lesions is ultrasound. CT and MR are used when ultrasonographic changes are equivocal or confusing. We have found that the pancreas is slightly larger in children than in adults and that on ultrasound it is moderately echogenic (Fig. 4.225A). It also is clearly seen with CT and MR as it lies anterior to the splenic vein (Fig. 4.225B). In normal premature and newborn infants, slight increase in echogenicity has been noted (1). With ultrasound (2), the normal diameter of the pancreatic duct in children has been determined to be approximately 1.65 mm. With chronic pancreatitis, the duct enlarges proportionately to age. Diameters greater than 1.5 mm in children 1–6 years and 1.9 mm in children 7–12 years were highly correlative with pancreatitis (2). The same was true of children 13–18 years where the pancreatic duct measured 2.2 mm or greater (2).

REFERENCES

1. Walsh E, Cramer B, Pushpanathan C. Pancreatic echogenicity in premature and newborn infants. Pediatr Radiol 1990;20: 323–325.
2. Chao H-C, Lin S-J, Kong M-S, et al. Sonographic evaluation of the pancreatic duct in normal children and children with pancreatitis. J Ultrasound Med 2000;19:757–763.

ABNORMALITIES OF THE PANCREAS

Congenital Abnormalities

Congenital abnormalities of the pancreas include annular pancreas, pancreas divisum, absence of the pancreas, and ectopic pancreas. Ectopic pancreatic tissue usually consists of a small nodule located in the gastric antrum (1) or duodenum. It can be demonstrated with barium studies of the upper GI tract but also can be seen with ultrasound (Fig. 4.226). It should be remembered that ectopic pancreatic tissue can be located almost anywhere along the GI tract and also has been documented in association with congenital jejunal atresia (2). In cases of absence of the pancreas, diabetes mellitus and findings mimicking those of cystic fibrosis (i.e., meconium ileus) can be seen.

With annular pancreas, obstruction of the proximal duodenum, usually resulting from associated duodenal atresia leads to the double bubble sign (Fig. 4.60). Pancreas divisum occurs when the pancreatic head forms in two parts and both contain a pancreatic duct that joins with the duodenum in anomalous fashion.

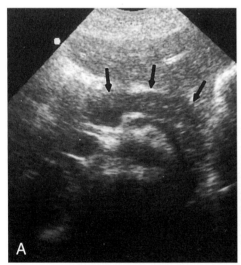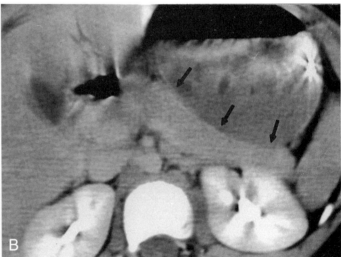

FIGURE 4.225. Normal pancreas. A. Ultrasound, cross-sectional view. Note the typical texture of the normal pancreas (arrows). The tubular structure just below it is the splenic vein. **B.** Contrast-enhanced CT study demonstrates similar findings, with the body and tail of the pancreas being clearly identified (arrows).

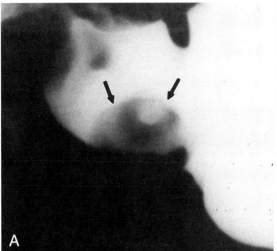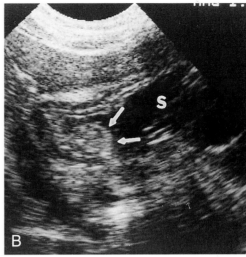

FIGURE 4.226. Ectopic pancreas. A. Typical configuration of ectopic pancreatic tissue producing an antral filling defect (arrows) with a central, barium-filled nidus. **B.** Ultrasonogram shows a nodular filling defect (arrows) in the antrum of the stomach (S), which proved to be ectopic pancreatic tissue.

REFERENCES

1. Ozcan C, Celik A, Guclu C, et al. A rare cause of gastric outlet obstruction in the newborn: pyloric ectopic pancreas. J Pediatr Surg 2002;3;7:119–120.
2. Suzuki H, Ohi R, Kasai M. Congenital jejunal atresia due to a septum containing ectopic pancreatic tissue. J Pediatr Surg 1973; 8:981.

Pancreatitis

Pancreatitis is very rare both in the newborn and in infancy and may present as unexplained ascites. In older children, pancreatitis is a little more common and, while many cases are idiopathic (1), most are seen with viral infections such as mumps (2) or as part of some multisystemic disease. Traumatic pancreatitis also is common, especially as it occurs in the battered child syndrome and pancreas divisum (3–5), choledochal cysts (6), enteric duplication cysts (7–9), and other bile duct anomalies all can be associated with pancreatitis. Pancreatitis now also is frequently seen with HIV infection (10). In addition, a hereditary form has been described (11), and pancreatitis also can be seen secondary to administration of drugs such as steroids, valproic acid (12), L-asparaginase (13), and tetracycline (14). It also has been documented with insecticide intoxication (15), organic acidemias (16), and on a chronic basis with cystic fibrosis (see next section). Chronic relapsing pancreatitis is uncommon in childhood (17).

Ultrasonographically, acute pancreatitis has been said to produce an enlarged, hypoechoic pancreas (Fig. 4.227A), and in one series this finding was seen in up to 50% of cases

(2). Our own experience, however, suggests that the pancreas very often is normal in size and its echogenicity so minimally abnormal that definitive diagnosis is not possible. Pancreatic duct dilation, when seen, is a useful additional finding (Fig. 4.227D), but unfortunately it is not that common. In the past, delineation of the pancreatic and biliary ducts eventually was relegated to retrograde endoscopic cholangiopancreatography (18), but currently magnet resonance cholangiopancreatography (MRCP) is deemed best (19–23). This study is relatively easy to perform and probably will replace retrograde cholangiopancreatography. In the end, however, in many, if not most cases, serum amylase and lipase determinations initially, often are more important.

Another ultrasonographic finding seen in some cases of pancreatitis is increased echogenicity of the pararenal space (24). This is seen on the right more than on the left, but in any case, since in most normal infants and young children little fat is present around the kidneys, the pararenal space is not very echogenic. With pancreatitis, however, the liberation of pancreatic enzymes leads to lipolysis and edema of the retroperitoneal and perinephric soft tissues, and as this space expands, it becomes visible as a highly echogenic halo around the kidney (Fig. 4.227B). Pleural effusions also can be seen with pancreatitis (25) and are readily demonstrable on plain films or with CT. In chronic pancreatitis, fatty replacement and calcifications also can be seen. The pancreas, in these cases, also becomes smaller than normal.

Parapancreatic fluid collections are not uncommonly encountered with acute pancreatitis and, while some of these proceed to actual pseudocyst formation, others disap-

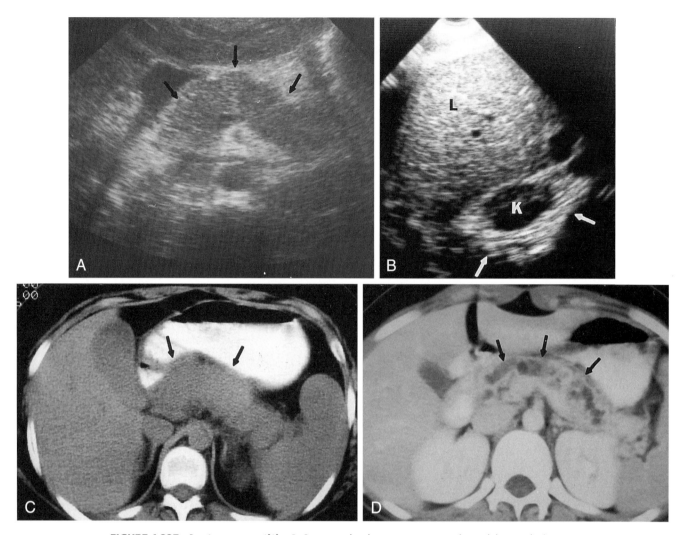

FIGURE 4.227. Acute pancreatitis. A. Sonography demonstrates an enlarged, hypoechoic pancreas (arrows). **B.** Another patient with increased perirenal echogenicity (arrows) resulting from pancreatic enzyme activity on normal fat, causing an increase in the volume of fat (lipolysis). K, kidney; L, liver. **C.** CT in this patient demonstrates an enlarged, edematous pancreas (arrows) with ragged edges. **D.** Another patient with chronic pancreatitis and dilation of the pancreatic duct (arrows). (**D** courtesy of C. Keith Hayden, Jr., M.D.)

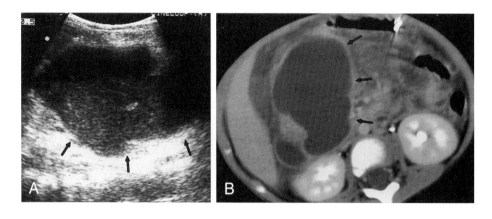

FIGURE 4.228. Pancreatic pseudocyst. A. Sonogram demonstrates a large, lobulated cystic mass (arrows) containing some debris. **B.** CT demonstrates the pseudocyst (arrows) more clearly. It has a well-defined margin, whereas acute fluid collections are ill-defined.

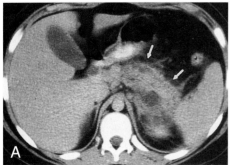 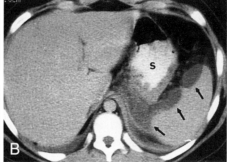

FIGURE 4.229. Pancreatitis with phlegmon. A. Note the enlarged pancreatic bed (arrows) with a poorly defined pancreas, small fluid collections, and inflammatory stranding into the neighboring soft tissues. **B.** Slightly higher slice demonstrates extension of the phlegmon into the subcapsular portion of the spleen (arrows) and the gastric wall. S, stomach.

pear as the patient improves. These fluid collections, when they mature into pseudocysts with a rind (Fig. 4.228), can be drained percutaneously (26, 27). All of these fluid collections and developing phlegmons are readily demonstrable with ultrasound and CT (Fig. 4.229). It also should be remembered that pancreatic pseudocysts can extend anywhere in the abdomen and even into the chest (28). Furthermore, as these cysts mature, their walls become thicker, and some may contain debris. Interestingly, pancreatic pseudocysts have been described prenatally (29–31), but the etiology of these cysts is not known.

REFERENCES

1. Mader TJ, McHugh TP. Acute pancreatitis in children. Pediatr Emerg Care 1992;8:157–161.
2. Haddock G, Coupar G, Youngson GG, et al. Acute pancreatitis in children: a 15-year review. J Pediatr Surg 1994;29:719–722.
3. Manfredi R, Costamagna G, Brizi MG, et al. Pancreas divisum and "Santorinicele": diagnosis with dynamic MR cholangiopancreatography with secretin stimulation. Radiology 2000;217:403–408.
4. Mori K, Nagakawa T, Ohta T, et al. Pancreatitis and anomalous union of the pancreaticobiliary ductal system in childhood. J Pediatr Surg 1993;28:67–71.
5. Tuggle DW, Smith EI. Pancreas divisum, pancreatic pseudocyst, and choledochal cyst in an 8-year-old child. J Pediatr Surg 1989;24:52–53.
6. Lee CC, Levine DA, Tunik MG, et al. A case report. Type I choledochal cyst induced pancreatitis in a 15-month-old child. Pediatr Emerg Care 2000;16:265–267.
7. Halilouglu M, Oto A, Karnak I, et al. Intrapancreatic duodenal duplication cyst with inversion of the superior mesenteric vessels: CT findings. Pediatr Radiol 2001;31:187–188.
8. Magnano GM, Occhi M, Mattioli G, et al. Pancreatitis caused by duodenal duplication. Pediatr Radiol 1998;28:524–526.
9. Materne R, Clapuyt P, Saint-Martin C, et al. Gastric cystic duplication communicating with a bifed pancreas: a rare cause of recurrent pancreatitis. J Pediatr Gastroenterol Nutr 1998;27:102–105.
10. Miller TL, Winter HS, Luginbuhl LM, et al. Pancreatitis in pediatric human immunodeficiency virus infection. J Pediatr 1992;120:223–227.
11. Spencer JA, Lindsell DRM, Isaacs D. Hereditary pancreatitis: early ultrasound appearances. Pediatr Radiol 1990;20:293–295.
12. Levin TL, Berdon WE, Seigle RR, Nash MA. Valproic-acid associated pancreatitis and hepatic toxicity in children with endstage renal disease. Pediatr Radiol 1997;27:192–193.
13. Sadoff J, Hwang S, Rosenfeld D, et al. surgical pancreatic complications induced by L-asparaginase. J Pediatr Surg 1997;32:860–863.
14. Nicolau DP, Mengedoht DE, Kline JJ. Tetracycline-induced pancreatitis. Am J Gastroenterol 1991;86:1669–1671.
15. Weizman Z, Sofer S. Acute pancreatitis in children with anticholinesterase insecticide intoxication. Pediatrics 1992;90:204–206.
16. Kahler SG, Sherwood WG, Woolf D, et al. Pancreatitis in patients with organic acidemias. J Pediatr 1994;124:239–243.
17. Ghishan FK, Greene HL, Avant G, et al. Chronic relapsing pancreatitis in childhood. J Pediatr 1983;120:154–158.
18. Iinuma Y, Narisawa R, Iwafuchi M, et al. The role of endoscopic retrograde cholangiopancreatography in infants with cholestasis. J Pediatr Surg 2000;35:545–549.
19. Arcement CM, Meza MP, Arumanla S, et al. MRCP in the evaluation of pancreaticobiliary disease in children. Pediatr Radiol 2001;31:92–97.
20. Chan Y-L, Yeung C-K, Lam WWM, et al. Magnetic resonance cholangiography—feasibility and application in the paediatric population. Pediatr Radiol 1998;28:307–311.
21. Hirohashi S, Hirohashi R, Uchida H, et al. Pancreatitis: evaluation with MR cholangiopancreatography in children. Radiology 1997;203:411–415.
22. Norton KI, Glass RBJ, Kogan D, et al. MR cholangiography in children and young adults with biliary disease. AJR 1999;172:1239–1244.
23. Shinji H, Hirohashi R, Uchida H, et al. Pancreatitis: evaluation with MR cholangiopancreatography in children. Radiology 1997;203:411–416.
24. Swischuk LE, Hayden CK Jr. Pararenal space hyperechogenicity in childhood pancreatitis. AJR 1985;145:1985–1986.
25. Simmons MZ, Miller JA, Zurlo JV, et al. Pleural effusions associated with acute pancreatitis. Incidence and appearance based on computed tomography. Emerg Radiol 1997;4:287–289.
26. Hendrickson M, Matlak ME, Jaffe RB, et al. Treatment of traumatic pancreatic pseudocysts in children: the role of percutaneous catheter drainage. Pediatr Surg Int 1990;5:347–349.
27. Jaffe RB, Arata JA Jr, Matlak ME. Percutaneous drainage of traumatic pancreatic pseudocyst in children. AJR 1989;152:591–595.
28. Crombleholme TM, deLorimic AA, Adzick NS, et al. Mediastinal pancreatic pseudocysts in children. J Pediatr Surg 1990;25:843–845.
29. Kebapci M, Aslan O, Kaya T, et al. Prenatal diagnosing of giant congenital pancreatic cyst of a neonate. AJR 2000;175:1408–1410.
30. Kurrer MO, Ternberg JL, Langer JC. Congenital pancreatic

pseudocyst: report of two cases. J Pediatr Surg 1996;31: 1581–1583.
31. Crowley JJ, McAlister WH. Congenital pancreatic pseudocyst: a rare cause of abdominal mass in a neonate. Report of two cases. Pediatr Radiol 1996;26:210–211.

Cystic Fibrosis

Cystic fibrosis is relatively common in children and, while initially most attention is focused on the respiratory tract, the pancreas slowly undergoes degenerative changes, and pancreatic insufficiency, both exocrine and endocrine, becomes a problem. For the most part, in advanced disease, the pancreas becomes smaller, scarred, nodular, and infiltrated with fat (1). Calcifications also can develop and, at the same time, ductal ectasia, even to the point of multiple, ductal pseudocyst formation, is seen. These cysts probably result from secretions becoming impacted in the ducts and causing backpressure ductal dilation. Ultrasonographically the pancreas becomes hyperechoic, and on MR imaging it shows increased signal on T1-weighted images secondary to fatty infiltration (2). Calcifications are best seen with CT but also can be seen with ultrasound. Ductal dilation can be demonstrated with ultrasound, CT, MR, or ERCP.

REFERENCES

1. Soyer P, Spelle L, Pelage J-P, et al. Cystic fibrosis in adolescents and adults. Fatty replacement of the pancreas-CT evaluation and functional correlation. Radiology 1999;210:611–615.
2. Murayama S, Robinson AE, Mulvihill DM, et al. MR imaging of pancreas in cystic fibrosis. Pediatr Radiol 1990;20:536–539.

Pancreatic Trauma

In the pediatric age group, pancreatic trauma can occur with motor vehicle accidents, blunt abdominal trauma, and in the battered child syndrome. With motor vehicle accidents, seat belt injuries often are the cause, but whatever the cause, pancreatic trauma is best evaluated with CT (1, 2). This modality can demonstrate enlargement of the pancreas, parapancreatic fluid collections, and lacerations or fractures of the pancreas (Fig. 4.230). Later, pseudocyst formation with traumatic pancreatitis is not an uncommon complication. Transection of the pancreatic ducts also can occur,[3] leading to peripancreatic fluid collections that can be drained percutaneously.

REFERENCES

1. Hiliter CL, Holgersen LO. Massive chylous ascites and transected pancreas secondary to child abuse: successful nonsurgical management. Pediatr Radiol 1995;25:117–119.
2. Sivit CJ, Eichelberger MR, Taylor GA, et al. Blunt pancreatic trauma in children: CT diagnosis. AJR 1992;158:1097–1100.
3. Ohno Y, Ohgami H, Nagasaki A, et al. Complete disruption of the main pancreatic duct. A case successfully managed by percutaneous drainage. J Pediatr Surg 1995;30:1741—1742.

Pancreatic Hydatid Disease

Hydatid disease of the pancreas is rare but the findings are the same as when other organs are involved (1).

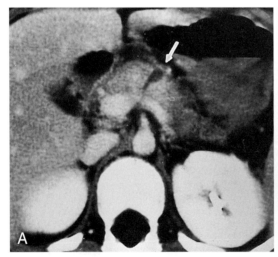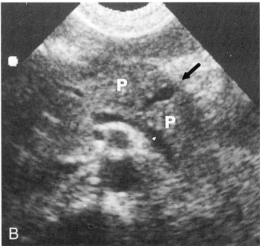

FIGURE 4.230. Pancreatic laceration: traumatic pancreatitis. A. On the CT study, note the oval-like collection of fluid (arrow) in the enlarged pancreas. **B.** Ultrasound study demonstrates the same fluid collection (arrow) in the enlarged pancreas (P).

REFERENCE

1. Barrera MC, Villanua J, Barrena JF, et al. Pancreatic hydatid disease. Pediatr Radiol 1995;25:S169–S170.

Pancreatic Tumors and Cysts

Congenital pancreatic cysts are extremely rare but do occur (1, 2), and they also have been seen in the von Hippel-Lindau syndrome (3). They appear as do cysts anywhere in the body and can be demonstrated with any imaging modality. Pancreatic pseudocysts are much more common and have been discussed previously with pancreatitis.

Primary malignant tumors are very uncommon in the pediatric age group, but still one can encounter lesions such as carcinoma (4, 5) and pancreatoblastoma (4–11). The

imaging features of these tumors are nonspecific because they merely reflect a solid lesion. Benign tumors also are not particularly common, but those that can be encountered include papillary cystadenoma (Fig. 4.231), insulinoma, hamartoma, lipoma, lymphangioma, and hemangioma. However, of these, the most significant in the pediatric age group, and certainly in the neonate, is the insulinoma or islet cell tumor. This functioning tumor can be a cause of severe neonatal hypoglycemia, but it is most difficult to identify, even at laparotomy. The lesion can be focal or diffuse (4, 5), and the latter form is referred to as nesidioblastosis. Nesidioblastosis probably represents a precursor lesion of an actual adenoma and can occur alone or in association with the Beckwith-Wiedemann syndrome. It usually produces enlargement of the pancreas and on ultrasound diffuse increase in echogenicity (Fig. 4.232).

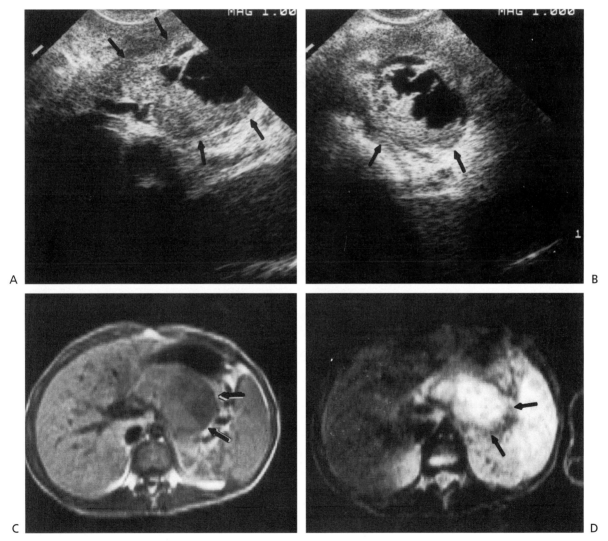

FIGURE 4.231. Pancreatic cystadenoma. A. Note the solid mass (arrows) containing large cysts. **B.** Another view of the same cystic mass (arrows). **C.** T1-weighted MRI demonstrates low signal intensity in the fluid portion of the mass (arrows). **D.** T2-weighted image demonstrates characteristic high signal intensity of the fluid within the cysts of this tumor (arrows).

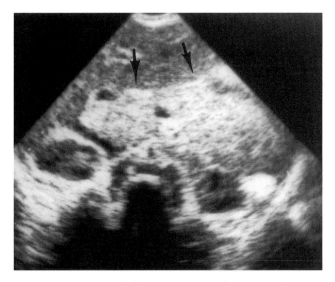

FIGURE 4.232. Nesidioblastosis. Note the enlarged, echogenic pancreas (arrows).

Pancreatoblastoma also has been noted to occur in the Beckwith-Wiedemann syndrome but also can occur alone (4–11). Generally, the tumor is solid but has a heterogeneous pattern on ultrasound examination. The margins usually are indistinct and at times it is difficult to determine whether the tumor is arising from the pancreas or the liver (4–11).

The so-called papillary cystic carcinoma or tumor deserves some extra attention in the pediatric age group. This low-grade malignancy (12) characteristically occurs in young females and usually arises in the tail of the pancreas. It usually is a silent lesion and can be very large when discovered. It is the cystic component (Fig. 4.233) that should suggest the diagnosis in this rare, yet definitive, tumor with a relatively good prognosis. Pancreatic pseudotumor is rare (13).

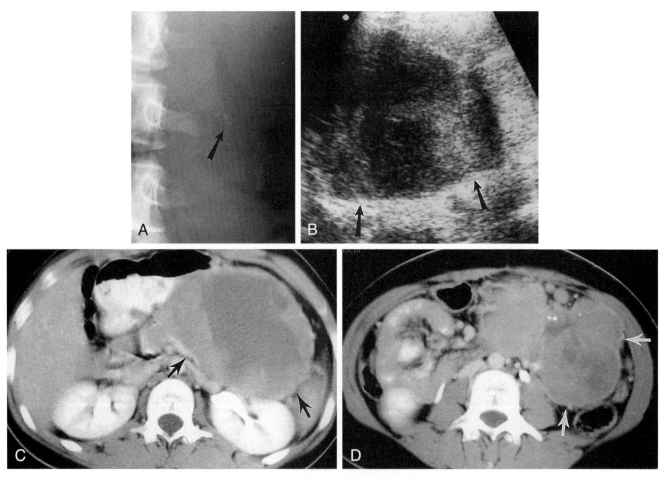

FIGURE 4.233. Papillary cystic tumor of the pancreas. A. Plain film demonstrating calcifications (arrow). **B.** Sonogram demonstrates a large mass (arrows), which is primarily sonolucent but also has mixed echoes. **C.** CT study, contrast-enhanced, demonstrates the large, heterogeneous mass (arrows) with multiloculated fluid collections. **D.** Slightly lower view demonstrates the large multiloculated tumor (arrows) with stippled calcifications. The tumor extends across midline and lies anterior to the aorta.

In terms of imaging, most solid or cystic tumors of the pancreas can be identified with ultrasound, CT, or MR, but the findings are nonspecific. The islet cell tumor, or insulinoma, on the other hand, is a different problem. Even with angiography it is difficult to identify, and it has been suggested that, even though a tumor is not palpated at surgery, partial pancreatectomy should be performed in the hope that the excised portion of the pancreas contains the tumor. Partial pancreatectomy also can be performed for nesidioblastosis.

REFERENCES

1. Auringer ST, Ulmer JL, Sumner TE, et al. Congenital cyst of the pancreas. J Pediatr Surg 1993;28:1572–1574.
2. Baker LL, Hartman GE, Northway WH. Sonographic detection of congenital pancreatic cysts in the newborn: report of a case and review of the literature. Pediatr Radiol 1990;20:488–490.
3. Neumann HPH, Dinkel E, Brambs H, et al. Pancreatic lesions in the von Hippel-Lindau syndrome. Gastroenterology 1991;101:465–471.
4. Grochowski J, Malek T, Miezynski W, et al. Pancreatic tumours in children. Pediatr Surg Int 1996;11:174–176.
5. Jaksic T, Yaman M, Thorner P, et al. A 20-year review of pediatric pancreatic tumors. J Pediatr Surg 1992;27:1315.
6. Gupta AK, Mitra DK, Berry M, et al. Original report. Sonography and CT of pancreatoblastoma in children. AJR 2000;174:1639–1641.
7. Inomata Y, Nishizawa T, Takasan H. Pancreatoblastoma resected by delayed primary operation after effective chemotherapy. J Pediatr Surg 1992;27:1570–1572.
8. Lumkin B, Anderson MW, Ablin DS, et al. CT, MRI and color Doppler ultrasound correlation of pancreato-blastoma: a case report. Pediatr Radiol 1993;23:61–62.
9. Montemarano H, Lonergan GJ, Bulas DI, et al. Pancreatoblastoma: imaging findings in 10 patients and review of literature. Radiology 2000;214:476–482.
10. Wang KS, Albanese C, Dada F, et al. Papillary cystic neoplasm of the pancreas: a report of three pediatric cases and literature review. J Pediatr Surg 1998;33:842–845.
11. Willnow U, Willberg B, Schwammborn D, et al. Pancreatoblastoma in children: case report and review of the literature. Eur J Pediatr Surg 1997;32:1132.
12. Poustchi-Amin M, Leonidas JC, Valderrama E, et al. Papillary-cystic neoplasm of the pancreas. Pediatr Radiol 1995;25:509–511.
13. McClain MB, Burton EM, Day DS. Pancreatic pseudotumor in 11-year-old child: imaging findings. Pediatr Radiol 2000;30:610–613.

Pancreatic Hemochromatosis (Hemosiderosis)

Hemochromatosis or hemosiderosis of the pancreas is much less common than is hemochromatosis of the liver or spleen. However, it results from the same problems, and in this regard, hemochromatosis of the pancreas has been documented after repeated transfusions (1). In such cases, the pancreas becomes hyperechoic on ultrasonography, hyperdense on CT, and "black" on MR images.

REFERENCE

1. Flyer MA, Haller JO, Sundaram R. Transfusional hemosiderosis in sickle cell anemia: another cause of an echogenic pancreas. Pediatr Radiol 1993;23:140–142.

ABDOMEN

Normal Configuration

A typical normal abdominal roentgenogram in an older infant, and for that matter, a child, is illustrated in Figure 4.234. Specifically notice the nonspecific distribution of gas in the intestinal tract. In the neonate, gas is usually noted within the stomach by 10 or 15 minutes of life (Fig. 4.235A). Almost as soon as the infant begins breathing, swallowing begins, and unless there is esophageal obstruction, air enters the stomach. If no air is present within the

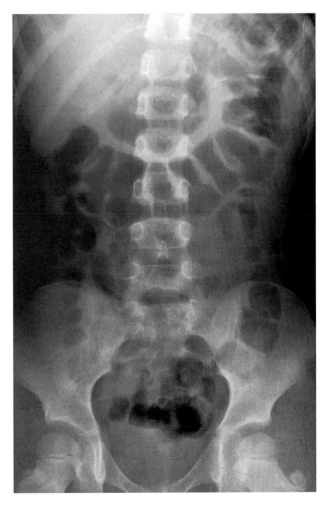

FIGURE 4.234. Normal abdomen. Note the normal gas distribution in the stomach, transverse colon and scattered throughout the small bowel.

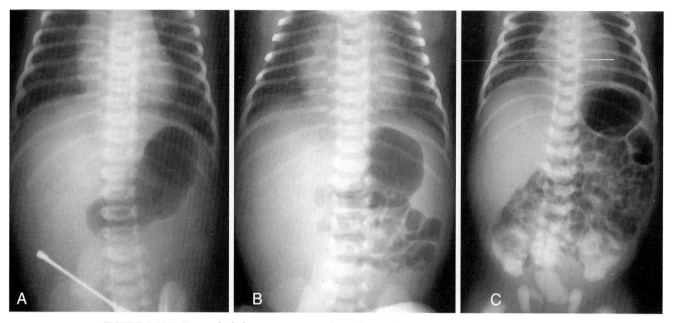

FIGURE 4.235. Normal abdomen, progression of gas through intestinal tract. A. Gas is present in the stomach at 15 minutes of age. **B.** By 30 to 60 minutes, gas is seen in the proximal small bowel. **C.** By 4 to 6 hours of age, gas is seen throughout the entire small intestine. Note the liver edge in the right upper quadrant.

abdomen of an infant who is 30 minutes to 1 hour old, one must strongly suspect esophageal obstruction in the form of esophageal atresia with no fistula. After initial filling of the stomach, gas progresses rapidly through the infant's GI tract; by 30–60 minutes, the stomach, duodenum, and proximal small bowel are well visualized (Fig. 4.235B). By 6 hours of age, gas is usually present in most of the small intestine (Fig. 4.235C), and by 12–24 hours of age gas begins to outline the colon. Transit of air and meconium through the colon is variable, but in most cases, meconium is passed by 12–24 hours of age.

The plain film is still valuable for evaluating abnormal gas patterns (1), but for other data one must turn to other imaging modalities. In this regard, the GI tract itself still is best studied with barium or aqueous contrast agents and in neonates with anionic aqueous contrast agents. On the other hand, ultrasound has come to play a dominant role in the investigation of acute abdominal problems in infants and children. CT also is useful, but ultrasound is easier to perform. MRI, along with CT and ultrasound, all are used for abdominal mass evaluation.

REFERENCE

1. Rothrick SG, Green SM, Harding M, et al. Plain abdominal radiography in the detection of acute medical and surgical disease in children: a retrospective analysis. Pediatr Emerg Care 1991;7: 281–285.

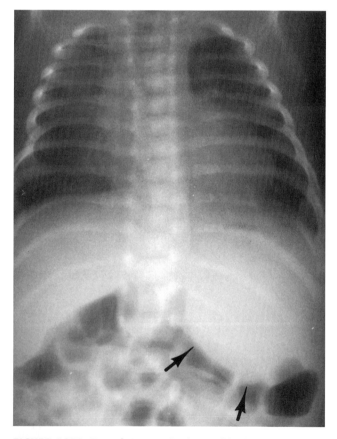

FIGURE 4.236. Pseudotumor. Supine positioning results in the fluid-filled fundus of the stomach presenting as a rounded mass in the left upper quadrant (arrows).

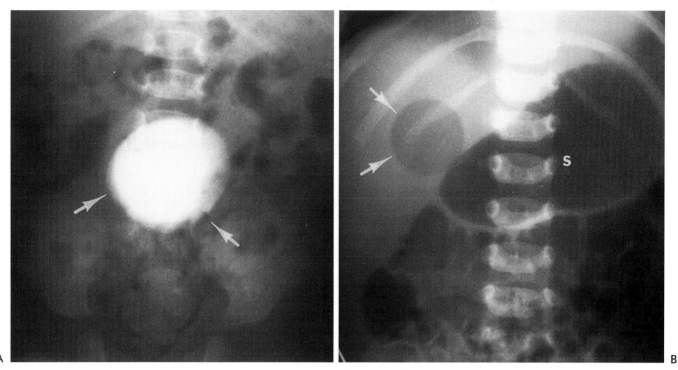

A   B

FIGURE 4.237. Pseudotumor, umbilical hernia. A. Round, opaque, mass-like configuration of umbilical hernia. These are characteristically located in the mid-abdomen and often contain loops of bowel. **B. Pseudocyst artifact.** Plastic hole in incubator so overlies the abdomen that an air-filled duodenal bulb is mimicked (arrows). S, stomach.

Plain Film Pseudotumors and Pseudocysts

Frequently, one can encounter fluid-filled portions of the GI tract that, on supine positioning, falsely present as tumors in the abdomen. Most often, this occurs in the fundus of the stomach (Fig. 4.236) and, if food is mixed with air, the findings might suggest an abscess or bezoar. In most cases, a pseudotumor is an unexpected finding, and once appreciated as a variation of normal, poses little practical difficulty. Similar pseudotumors can be produced by fluid-filled loops of bowel.

Umbilical hernias and umbilical stumps can project as round or oval soft tissue masses, which often also erroneously suggest intraabdominal masses (Fig. 4.237). Lumbosacral meningomyeloceles can produce a similar configuration, but most of these infants have obvious spinal column abnormality.

Gasless (Airless) Abdomen

An airless abdomen usually results either from excessive vomiting or prolonged nasogastric suction. The former is common in acute appendicitis and some cases of gastroenteritis. However, it should be noted that many cases of gastroenteritis show normal or excessive gas in the intestines. Decreased intestinal gas also can be seen when there is

decreased swallowing secondary to endotracheal intubation, CNS depression, or the use of paralytic drugs (1, 2).

REFERENCES

1. Coradello H, Ponhold W, Lubec G, et al. Disappearance of bowel gas in newborn infants on mechanical ventilation. Pediatr Radiol 1982;12:11–14.
2. Dillard RG, Crowe JE, Sumner TE. Pancuronium and abnormal abdominal roentgenograms. Am J Dis Child 1980;134:821–823.

ABNORMAL GAS PATTERNS

Mechanical Obstruction versus Paralytic Ileus

Although the term "ileus" means obstruction, it most commonly is used in association with paralyzed intestines and hence the term "paralytic ileus." When the word "obstruction" is used, it usually is done so in combination with the word "mechanical" and hence the term "mechanical obstruction." Therefore, although not completely correct, this section deals with the differences between mechanical obstruction and paralytic ileus and in most cases one usually can determine whether intestinal distention is due to mechanical obstruction or paralytic ileus. If one still remains puzzled, however, one can obtain prone (1), rather than supine films, whereupon redistribution of fluid and gas in the intestinal tract often leads one away from one's initial consideration that the abdominal gas pattern is abnormal.

In paralytic ileus, even though distention is often marked, small to large bowel proportions remain the same. In other words, the large bowel, because it is normally greater in diameter, is more distended than the small bowel (Fig. 4.238A).

Upright views usually show multiple, sluggish-appearing air-fluid levels and isolated loops are difficult to identify (Fig. 4.238B). The picture is much less organized than the one seen with mechanical obstruction and the "sluggish" air-fluid levels appear to be present everywhere.

In mechanical obstruction differential distention of intestine is seen (Fig. 4.238C). In other words, the bowel proximal to the obstruction is markedly distended, while that distal to the obstruction contains little or no air. This

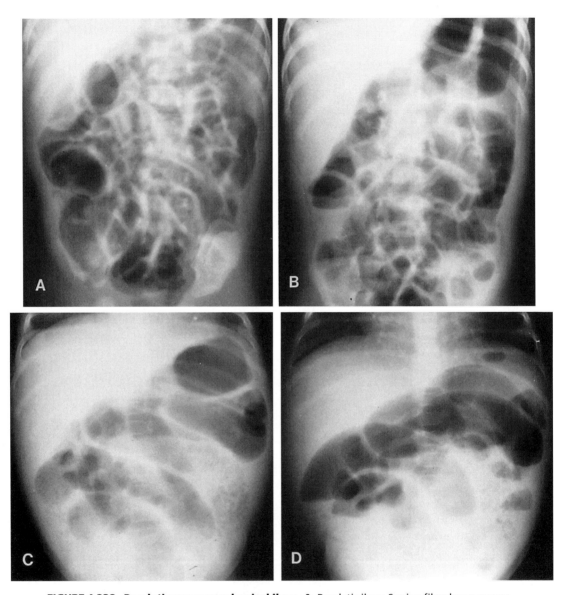

FIGURE 4.238. Paralytic versus mechanical ileus. A. Paralytic ileus. Supine film shows numerous distended loops of both small and large bowel. There is no differential distention; neither the small bowel nor colon is distended out of proportion to each other. **B.** Upright view shows "sluggish" air-fluid levels in both the small bowel and colon. Note bilateral properitoneal fat lines. Infant had gastroenteritis. **C.** Mechanical ileus. Note markedly distended small intestine arranged in an orderly fashion (stepladder effect). Some loops contain fluid intestinal contents mixed with air. There is no gas in the colon. **D.** Upright view shows a number of inverted "hairpin" loops of distended small bowel. Numerous discrete, air-fluid levels are seen, and characteristically, the two fluid levels in any given loop are at different levels. Obstruction is secondary to an incarcerated hernia.

is the key to the plain film diagnosis of mechanical obstruction but, in addition, infants with mechanical obstruction usually show a more orderly pattern of bowel distention such as stacking, or the stepladder effect (Fig. 4.238C). Individual loops are more easily recognized, and on upright films isolated "acute" inverted U-shaped loops with short air-fluid levels can be seen (Fig 4.238D). Another useful finding is that, in any given loop, air-fluid levels in each limb of the loop are at different heights. This stems from the pronounced peristaltic churning activity present in intestinal obstruction. Distended loops of intestine, either obstructed or paralyzed, also are readily visible with ultrasound and CT. They are fluid-filled and, when obstruction is the problem, demonstrate hyperperistalsis (Fig. 4.239A). When paralytic ileus is the problem, hypoperistalsis is present (Fig. 4.239A).

In neonates, excessive but normal gas may at first suggest obstruction or ileus. There are many causes for excessive gas in neonates, including excessive air swallowing with respiratory distress or resuscitative measures and sepsis. However, in any of these cases, if one sees a pattern of bowel distention that resembles honeycombing (Fig. 4.240A), the findings still are considered normal. Once this changes to a more organized pattern one should be suspicious of an underlying obstruction (Fig. 4.240, B and C).

Once it has been determined that mechanical obstruction is present, the radiologist's next job is to determine the level of obstruction. As a rule, the more loops visualized, the lower the obstruction. In neonates, low small bowel obstruction is difficult to differentiate from large bowel obstruction, but if one clearly sees a large distended colon in its characteristic location, then one can presume that

obstruction is low in the colon. After the level of obstruction is determined, one must decide whether to proceed to contrast studies. In high, complete obstruction, such as occurs with duodenal atresia, annular pancreas, or pyloric atresia, contrast studies generally are not required. In high, incomplete obstruction, such as seen with pyloric stenosis, duodenal bands, midgut volvulus, duodenal stenosis, duodenal diaphragm, and preduodenal portal vein, an upper GI series or ultrasound study usually is required.

Obstruction of the midportion of the small bowel (i.e., jejunal atresia) usually does not require either an upper GI series or barium enema, but if a low small bowel or colonic obstruction is suggested, a contrast study of the colon is mandatory. This is most important, because one usually cannot tell from the plain film findings whether the problem is a low small bowel or colonic obstruction. Under such circumstances the contrast enema can, and usually does differentiate conditions such as ileus atresia, meconium ileus, meconium plug syndrome, Hirschsprung's disease, and colon stenosis.

Generally, in the past, barium was the contrast agent of choice when a contrast enema was necessary. Gastrografin also has been used and has proved to be therapeutic in certain conditions (i.e., meconium plug syndrome, meconium ileus). However, when employed, proper precautions should be taken against this hypertonic contrast agent and its potential to cause fluid and electrolyte shift into the intestinal lumen. Currently, however, with the arrival of nonionic contrast agents there is a general tendency to use these agents in neonates and very young infants. In the older infant and child, however, barium still is the mainstay of the various contrast agents available.

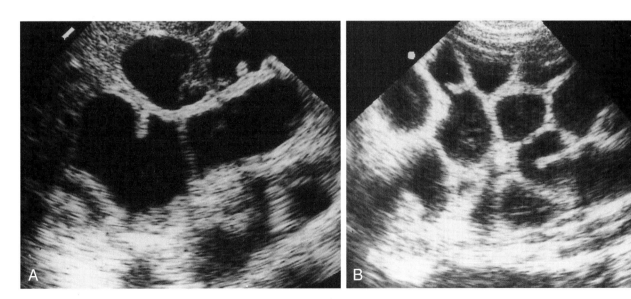

FIGURE 4.239. Paralytic versus mechanical ileus: ultrasound findings. A. Mechanical obstruction presents with more dynamic-appearing loops of intestine that are markedly distended and on real time show constant peristaltic activity. **B.** Paralytic ileus. Note the numerous dilated loops of bowel, which on real time showed very little peristaltic activity.

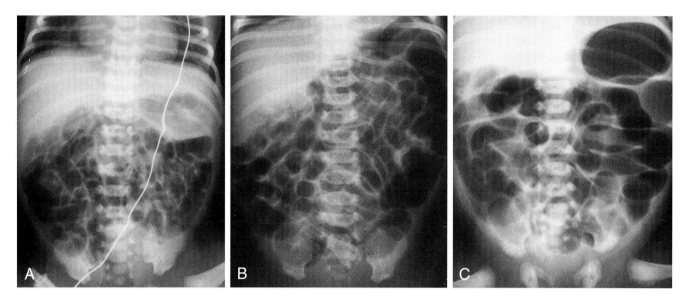

FIGURE 4.240. Upper limits of normal intestinal distention versus early obstruction. A. Upper limits of normal intestinal distention. Note the honeycomb appearance of the loops of intestine. This pattern often is seen in infants with delayed meconium passage, respiratory distress with excessive air swallowing, or with a combination of the two factors. This is upper normal. **B.** Early obstruction. First note that there is no gas in the rectum. Then note that the honeycomb pattern is yielding to a pattern of more organized U-shaped loops and long intestinal loops. This patient had mild meconium plug syndrome. **C.** Definite obstruction. There is no air in the rectum, but the loops of intestine now are clearly distended and much more organized. This pattern is clearly pathologic and indicates definite obstruction.

REFERENCE

1. Lorenzo RL, Harolds JA. The use of prone films in suspected bowel obstruction in infants and children. AJR 1977;129: 617–622.

ABDOMINAL MASSES: IMAGING APPROACH

Abdominal masses in neonates and young infants are common and, as in older children, imaging plays an important part in the diagnosis and evaluation of these lesions. Overall, renal masses are most common, and of these, the vast majority are benign and consist primarily of renal cystic lesions and hydronephrosis. Generally, malignant intraabdominal tumors, whether intrarenal or extrarenal, are much less common in newborn infants than in older infants and children.

Ultrasound, CT, and MR all are available for the evaluation of abdominal masses in infants and children, but ultrasound is the main and dominant initial imaging modality. It usually provides instant information about whether the lesion is cystic or solid, and it requires no patient preparation and is noninvasive.

A plain abdominal radiograph still probably should be obtained before any special imaging investigation is undertaken. Plain films can help in localizing masses and also

may show extension into the chest or the presence of calcifications. After ultrasound evaluation one can proceed to CT or MR, depending on what further information is required. MR has the advantage of providing images in multiple planes and being very good in terms of soft tissue imaging. However, it has a significant disadvantage in that deep sedation may be required. This can be obviated with fast, helical CT with reconstructed images and this has rendered this modality competitive with MR. Another drawback to MR is that there is, as yet, no satisfactory GI contrast agent, while with CT, diluted Gastrografin has proved useful for many years.

Arteriography seldom is required in this day and age, as information it yielded now is readily available with contrast-enhanced helical CT or MR imaging. Technetium-99m IDA analogs are useful in the evaluation of right upper quadrant masses related to the biliary tract (i.e., choledochal cysts, hydrops), but otherwise nuclear scintigraphy is seldom used in the evaluation of abdominal masses.

SPECIFIC ABDOMINAL MASSES

Renal, Pararenal, and Adrenal Masses

See Chapter 5 for an account of renal, pararenal, and adrenal masses.

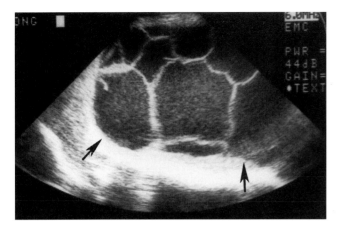

FIGURE 4.241. Abdominal lymphangioma. Note the multilocated lymphangioma (arrows), with some of the locules containing debris, probably blood. (Courtesy Scott Lile, M.D.)

Gastrointestinal Masses

Many of these masses have been individually discussed at various points in this chapter, depending on their organ of origin. This section therefore deals with the remaining abdominal masses encountered.

Mesenteric and Omental Cysts and Abdominal Lymphangiomatosis

In the past, mesenteric (1) and omental cysts were believed to be chylous cysts resulting from some form of congenital obstruction of the lymphatic ducts, and abdominal lymphangiomatosis was thought to result from a benign tumor of the lymphatic system. However, it is now believed by most that both conditions are manifestations of the same problem that is a benign, congenitally induced, obstructive malformation of the lymphatic system. Therefore the lesion can range from a solitary mesenteric or omental cyst, a multiloculated cyst, or diffuse abdominal lymphangiomatosis. Some of these cysts may contain debris such as blood (Figs. 4.241 and 4.242), and CT also can demonstrate these lesions (Fig. 4.242). MR imaging also usually clearly identifies the lesion, which, because of its high protein count, usually produces high signal on both T1- and T2-weighted images.

Calcifications are rare (2), but in some cases, the cyst is so thin-walled that it virtually fills the entire abdomen and mimics ascites (3, 4). The discrete mass is not palpable, and roentgenographically, only ascites or a picture of a shifting mass is suggested. In other instances, diffuse lymphangioma may extend through the patent processus vaginalis and present as an inguinal hernia (5). Rarely, trauma to the abdomen can result in rupture of a previously undetected mesenteric cyst (6).

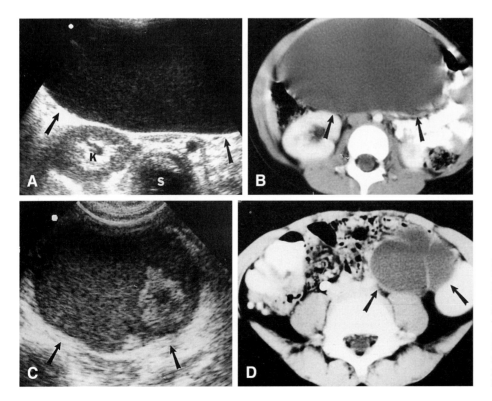

FIGURE 4.242. Mesenteric cyst. A. Ultrasonogram demonstrates a large hypoechoic mesenteric cyst (arrows) lying above the right kidney (K) and spine (S). **B.** CT study demonstrates the same cyst (arrows). **C.** Another patient whose sonogram demonstrates a mesenteric cyst containing debris (arrows). **D.** Multiloculated mesenteric cyst (arrows) demonstrated by CT.

REFERENCES

1. Chung MA, Brandt ML, St-Vil D, et al. Mesenteric cysts in children. J Pediatr Surg 1991;26:1306–1308.
2. Hatten MT, Hamrick-Turner JE, Smith DB. Mesenteric cystic lymphangioma: radiologic appearance mimicking cystic teratoma. Pediatr Radiol 1996;26:458—460.
3. Gyves-Ray K, Hernandez RJ, Hillemeier AC. Pseudoascites: unusual presentation of omental cyst. Pediatr Radiol 1990;20:560–561.
4. Lugo-Olivieri CH, Taylor GA. CT differentiation of large abdominal lymphangioma from ascites. Pediatr Radiol 1993;23:129–130.
5. Kafka V, Novak K. Multicystic retroperitoneal lymphangioma in an infant appearing as in inguinal hernia. J Pediatr Surg 1970;5:573.
6. Klein MD. Traumatic rupture of an unsuspected mesenteric cyst: an uncommon case of an acute surgical abdomen following a minor fall. Pediatr Emerg Care 1996;12:40.

Teratomas and Dermoid Cyst

Abdominal teratomas most frequently arise retroperitoneally, in the presacral region, or from the ovary, but they can arise anywhere in the abdomen (1). Dermoid cysts are

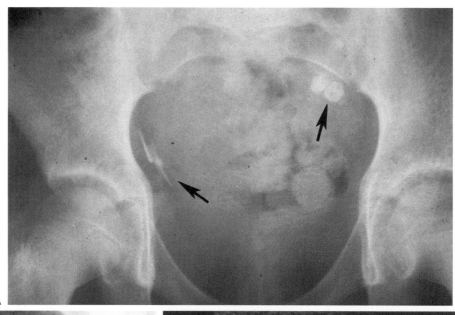

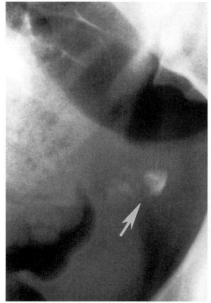

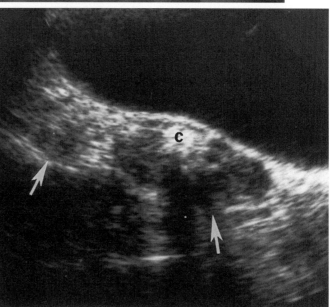

FIGURE 4.243. Dermoid. A. Note the formed, tooth-like, and curvilinear calcifications (arrows). **B.** Another patient with a tooth-like calcification (arrow). **C.** Same patient, demonstrating a heterogeneous mass (arrows) and the calcification (C) producing acoustical shadowing.

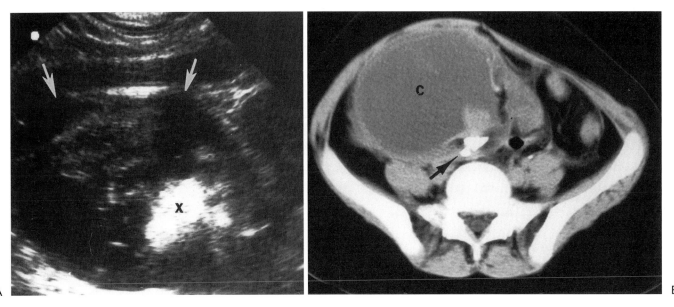

A   B

FIGURE 4.244. Dermoid. A. Large cystic dermoid (arrows) with a large area of echogenicity in the center (X) representing calcification and/or fat. **B.** CT study in another patient demonstrates a large cystic dermoid (C). Calcification (arrow) also is present.

most likely to arise from the ovaries in girls and, while some consider dermoid cysts to be separate from teratoma because they contain only two germinal layers (teratomas contain all three), others consider them the same.

Calcifications often are present in these lesions and, in dermoid cysts, teeth and other formed elements commonly are

seen (Figs. 4.243 and 4.244). Formed bony elements also are seen in more benign teratomas (Fig. 4.245), and in addition these tumors usually contain fat. On plain films, when flake, or shard-like calcifications are seen (2), malignancy usually is present. In such cases, the tumor usually arises from the ovary and is a **large**, malignant teratoma (Fig. 4.246).

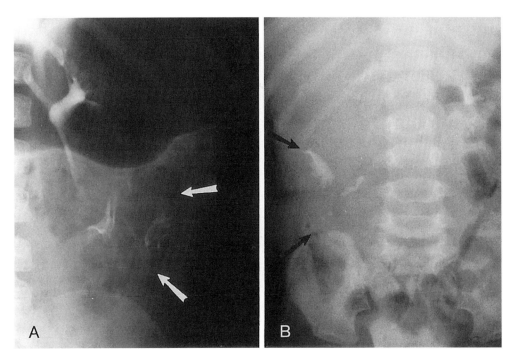

A   B

FIGURE 4.245. Teratoma. A. Formed calcifications in an abdominal teratoma (arrows). **B.** Another patient with formed calcifications in a teratoma.

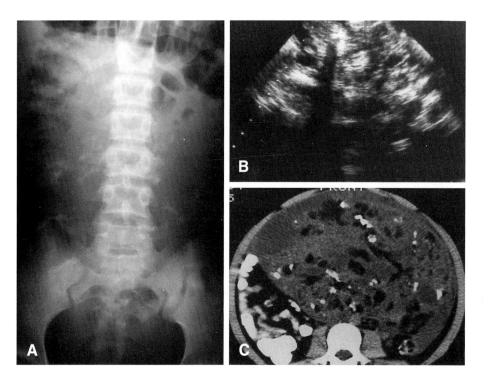

FIGURE 4.246. Large malignant teratoma. A. Note the large mass with flake-like, irregular calcifications. **B.** Ultrasonogram demonstrates a very mixed pattern with numerous cystic components. **C.** CT demonstrates the heterogeneous nature of this tumor with scattered hypodense areas of fat and hyperechogenic areas of calcium.

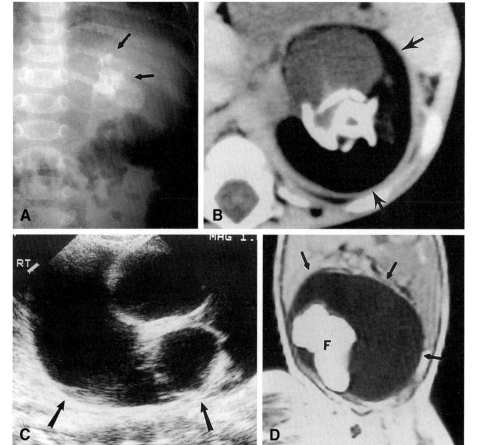

FIGURE 4.247. Teratoma: CT, ultrasound, and MR findings. A. Note the formed calcification in the left upper quadrant (arrows). **B.** CT study demonstrates the large mass (arrows) to contain fat (black area), bones (white structures) and nonspecific soft tissue (gray area). **C.** Another patient with a mass (arrows) demonstrating numerous fluid-filled cysts. **D.** T1-weighted MR image demonstrates a large, fluid-filled mass (arrows) with high-signal-intensity fat (F) within it. The fluid surrounding it typically is of low signal intensity (i.e., black) on T1-weighted images.

All of these tumors and cysts are readily demonstrable with ultrasound in which the cystic areas are hypoechoic while the calcium and fat collections are echogenic (Figs. 4.243C and 4.244A). Fat and bone are even more vividly demonstrated with CT (Figs. 4.244B). MR also is excellent in delineating fat and the heterogeneous nature of these tumors (Fig. 4.247). With MRI, fat produces high signal on T1-weighted images while fluid in the cysts shows medium signal on T1-weighted images and high signal on T2-weighted images.

REFERENCES

1. Chiba T, Iwami D, Kikuchi Y. Mesenteric teratoma in an 8-month-old girl. J Pediatr Surg 1995;30:120.
2. Schey WL, Vesely JJ, Radkowski MA. Shard-like calcifications in retroperitoneal teratomas. Pediatr Radiol 1986;16:82–84.

Fetus-in-Fetu

In this abnormality, there is a reasonably well-formed but aborted fetus in the infant's abdomen (1–3). Identifiable bones and fat may be seen on plain films (Fig. 4.248), but these findings are more vividly demonstrated with CT or MR studies (Fig. 4.248). The fact that identifiable body parts are present has led to the trend to separate fetus-in-fetu from teratoma, but the conditions probably represent a spectrum of abnormalities (4, 5). It also has been suggested that if spinal elements are absent, the lesion is a teratoma, while if they are present the tumor is a fetus-in-fetu (5). Unusual manifestations of this tumor include twin feti-in-fetu (6), postnatal growth of the tumor (7), or delayed malignant degeneration (8).

REFERENCES

1. Bernal-Sprekelsen JC, Bernal-Cascales M. Fetus-in-fetu: case report of an extremely uncommon cause of an abdominal mass in the neonate. Z Kinderchir 1990;45:317–318.
2. Eng H-L, Chuang J-H, Leem T-Y, et al. Fetus in fetu: a case report and review of the literature. J Pediatr Surg 1989;24:296–299.
3. Thakral CL, Maji DC, Sajwani MJ. Fetus-in-fetu: a case report and review of the literature. J Pediatr Surg 1998;33:1432–1434.

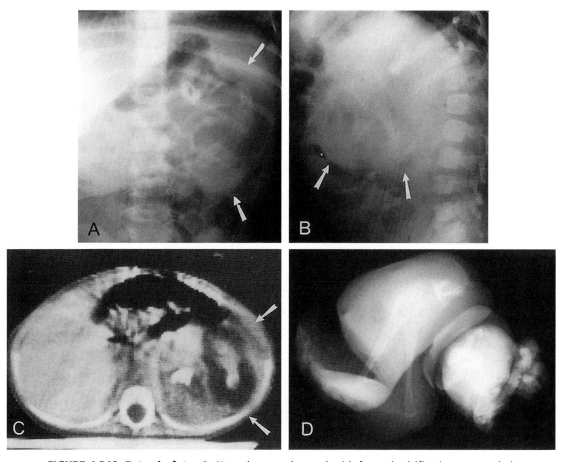

FIGURE 4.248. Fetus-in-fetu. A. Note the mass (arrows) with formed calcification surrounded by fatty density. **B.** Lateral view demonstrates the same fatty density of the mass (arrows). Also note the formed calcification. **C.** CT study demonstrates the radiolucent fat in the mass (arrows). Also note the bones. **D.** Specimen of removed tumor.

4. de Lagausie P, de Napoli CS, Stempfle N, et al. Highly differentiated teratoma and fetus-in-fetu: a single pathology? J Pediatr Surg 1997;32:115–116.

5. Kumar AN, Chandak GR, Rajasekhar A, et al. Fetus-in-fetu: a case report with molecular analysis. J Pediatr Surg 1999;34:641–644.

6. Luzzatto C, Talenti E, Tregnaghi A, et al. Double fetus in fetu: diagnostic imaging. Pediatr Radiol 1994;24:602–603.

7. Kim OH, Shinn KS. Postnatal growth of fetus-in-fetu. Pediatr Radiol 1993;23:411–412.

8. Hopkins KL, Dickson PK, Ball TI, et al. Fetus-in-fetu with malignant recurrence. J Pediatr Surg 1997;32:1476–1479.

Conjoined Twins and Twin Parasites

The study of conjoined twins is complicated, and the condition is included here primarily for the sake of completeness. The most common type of fusion is anterior union, either through the thorax or abdomen. The presurgical roentgenographic assessment of these infants centers on the delineation of the anatomy of each twin and the shared structures. All imaging modalities usually are employed

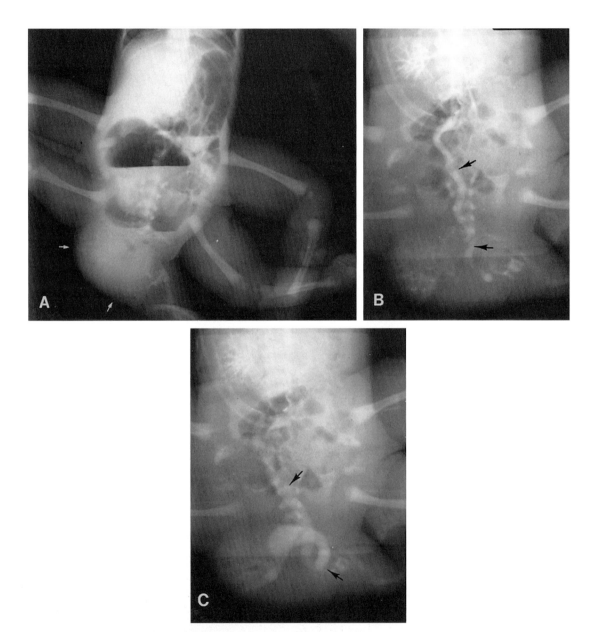

FIGURE 4.249. Conjoined twin (i.e., twin parasite). A. Note the malformed twin parasite (arrows). The lower two legs belong to the parasite, and the upper two legs belong to the otherwise normal upper infant. These infants were joined by the buttocks, and one can see two separate sets of pelvic structures and spines. The genitourinary tract was also duplicated. **B.** Arteriogram shows large feeding vessel (arrows) to the twin parasite. **C.** Drainage phase shows a large draining vessel (arrows).

including arteriography, because one must provide complete anatomic information before surgical correction is contemplated. Not all of these patients survive, and many die shortly after birth. When one of the twins is only partially formed the term "twin parasite" is employed (Fig. 4.249).

Lymphoma and Leukemia

Neonatal lymphoma is very rare and in the young infant lymphoma usually is a lymphosarcoma or reticulum cell sarcoma. Calcifications (1) do not usually occur in lymphomas, and from the radiographic standpoint, it is not possible to differentiate Hodgkin's from non-Hodgkin's lymphoma except with ultrasound, where sclerosing Hodgkin's lymphoma may be more echogenic. Typically, most lymphomas are hypoechoic, but in the end, definitive diagnosis rests with biopsy. In most cases abdominal lymphomas present as retroperitoneal masses (Fig. 4.250), but lymphoma can occur almost anywhere in the abdomen and involve any organ. In addition, mesenteric involvement can occur and be massive (Fig. 4.251). Another interesting feature of lymphoma is its association with Epstein-Barr virus, both in HIV-infected children and children without this infection (2, 3). Finally, nuclear scintigraphy, in the form of gallium, and Tl-201 scans (4) can be used to detect initial and residual disease but overall, either CT or MR is best for detecting lymphomas. Residual, small masses with no evidence of tumor activity elsewhere can be watched (5). In addition, PET scanning is useful in determining whether these masses represent residual fibrosis or active tumor tissue. With leukemia, adenopathy may be seen in the retroperitoneum or pelvis. However, once again, any organ in the abdomen can be involved, and the imaging findings usually are much the same as those of lymphoma. Similar findings can be seen with Castleman disease (6).

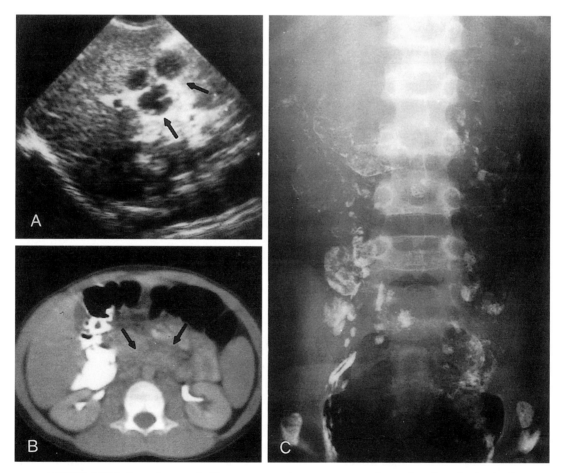

FIGURE 4.250. Lymphoma. A. Ultrasonogram demonstrates sonolucent lymph nodes (arrows) in the portahepatis. **B.** Same patient, whose CT study demonstrates increased nodular soft tissue resulting from a lymphoma in the retroperitoneum (arrows). **C.** Another patient, whose lymphangiogram demonstrates large lymph nodes being replaced by lymphoma. The soap bubble appearance and expanded periphery is characteristic.

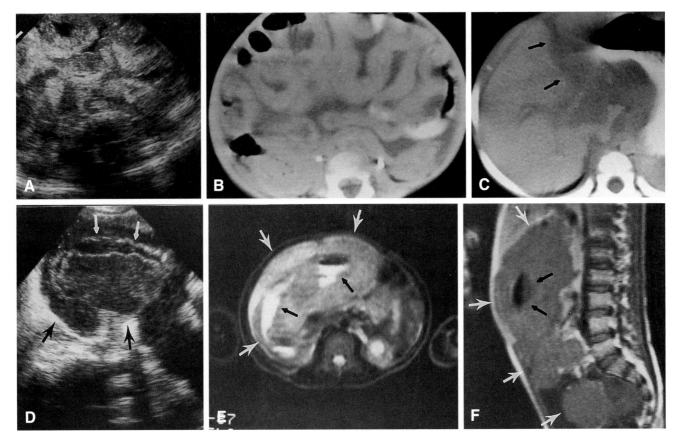

FIGURE 4.251. Lymphoma of the mesentery. A. Note the numerous, thickened loops of intestine with some fluid in between the loops. **B.** CT study demonstrates numerous loops of intestine embedded in low-density lymphomatous tissue (gray areas between loops of intestine). **C.** Lymphoma has extended into the falciform ligament (arrows) and is present between the stomach and liver. It is hypodense. **D.** Another patient with a large lobular lymphoma (black arrows) encasing the transverse colon (white arrows). **E.** Proton density axial MR study demonstrates the large lymphoma (white arrows) in which lies embedded intestine (black arrows) containing fluid and air. **F.** Sagittal T1-weighted MR study demonstrates the extensive lymphoma tumor mass (white arrows) in which is embedded the fluid and air-filled transverse colon (black arrows).

REFERENCES

1. Laufer L, Barki Y, Schulman H, et al. Calcification in an untreated case of Burkitt's lymphoma: radiographic, ultrasound and CT diagnosis. Pediatr Radiol 1994;24:180–181.
2. Katz BZ, Berkman AB, Shapiro ED. Serologic evidence of active Epstein-Barr virus infection in Epstein-Barr virus-associated lymphoproliferative disorders of children with acquired immunodeficiency syndrome. J Pediatr 1992;120:228–232.
3. Weinreb M, Day PJ, Murray PG, et al. Epstein-Barr virus (EBV) and Hodgkin's disease in children: incidence of EBV latent membrane protein in malignant cells. J Pathol 1992;168:365–369.
4. Fletcher BD, Kauffman WM, Kaste SC, et al. Use of Tl-201 to detect untreated pediatric Hodgkin's disease. Radiology 1995;196:851–855.
5. Karmazyn B, Ash S, Goshen Y, et al. Significance of residual abdominal masses in children with abdominal Burkitt's lymphoma. Pediatr Radiol 2001;31:801–805.
6. Moon WK, Kim WS, Kim I-O, et al. Castleman disease in the child: CT and ultrasound findings. Pediatr Radiol 1994;24:182–184.

Miscellaneous Abdominal Tumors and Cysts

Amongst the other, usually uncommon abdominal tumors one may encounter in children are the intraperitoneal or extraperitoneal lipomatous group of lesions (i.e., liposarcoma, lipoma, and lipoblastoma) (1–3), leiomyoma (4), mesothelioma (5–7), rhabdomyosarcoma, embryonal sarcoma, mesenchymal hamartoma (8), fibrous histiocytoma (9), mesenteric neurofibromatosis (10, 11), and pseudotumor (12). Hamartomas, although usually cystic, can be solid, and they often are quite vascular (Fig. 4.252).

Another relatively common mass encountered in the abdomen is the so-called pseudocyst after ventriculoperitoneal shunting. These pseudocysts are a common cause of shunt malfunction and usually are readily identifiable with ultrasound (Fig. 4.253). They can be aspirated percutaneously or surgically removed, and ultrasound usually is the

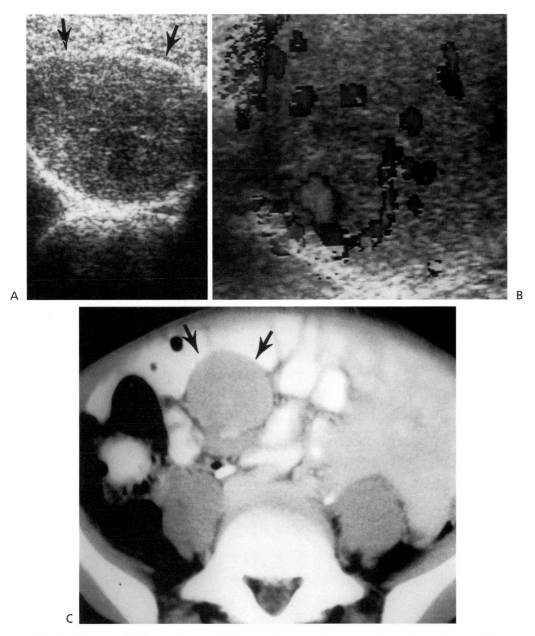

FIGURE 4.252. Solid hamartoma. A. Ultrasound demonstrates an echogenic mass (arrows). **B.** Doppler ultrasound demonstrates increased vascularity to the mass. **C.** CT study demonstrates the homogenous mass (arrows).

only imaging modality needed to demonstrate their presence. One also can encounter enteric cysts and these can be identified by the presence of a mucosal lining (13) (Fig. 4.254). These enteric or duplication cysts also can extend into the chest (Fig. 4.255).

REFERENCES

1. Beebe MM, Smith MD. Omental lipoblastoma. J Pediatr Surg 1993;28:1626–1627.
2. Ilhan H, Tokar B, Isiksoy S, et al. Giant mesenteric lipoma. J Pediatr Surg 1999;34:639–640.
3. Yalcin B, Ozurk H, Kismer E, et al. Giant retroperitoneal lipoma in a child. Pediatr Radiol 2001;31:304.
4. O'Brien JG, Allen JE, Queen TA. Leiomyoma of the omentum in a child. J Pediatr Surg 1986;21:981–982.
5. Kovalivker M, Motovic A. Malignant peritoneal mesothelioma in children: description of two cases and review of the literature. J Pediatr Surg 1985;20:274–275.
6. Haliloglu M, Hoffer FA, Fletcher BD. Malignant peritoneal mesothelioma in two pediatric patients: MR imaging findings. Pediatr Radiol 2000;30:251–255.

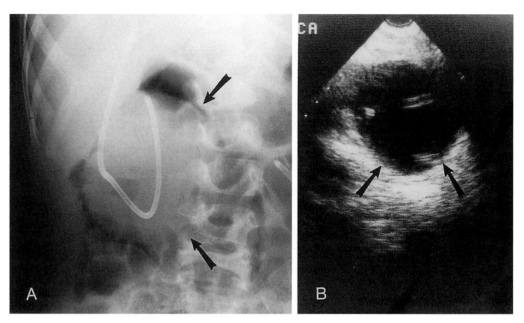

FIGURE 4.253. Postshunt pseudocyst. A. Note the shunt tubing in the abdomen, and associated mass (arrows). **B.** Ultrasound demonstrates a multiloculated pseudocyst (arrows).

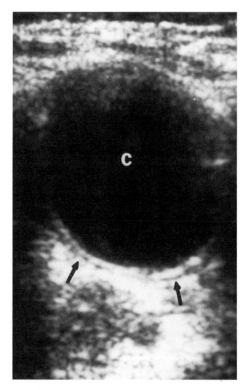

FIGURE 4.254. Duplication cyst. Note the hypoechoic cyst (C) with an echogenic inner mucosal lining (arrows) signifying that the cyst is a duplication cyst.

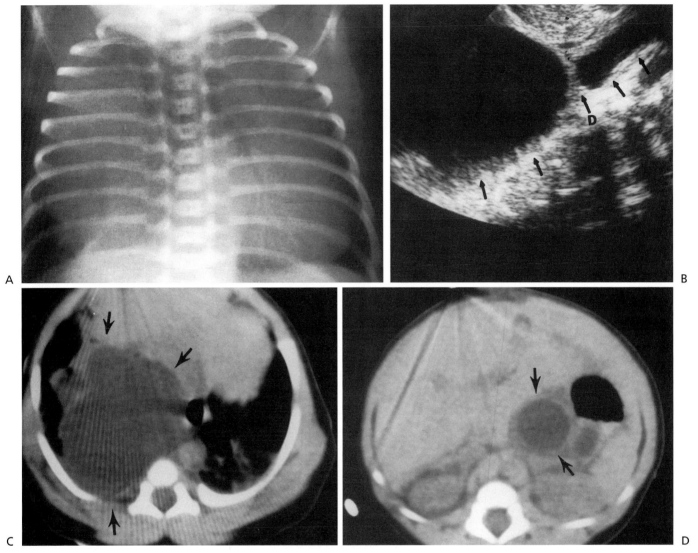

FIGURE 4.255. Duplication cyst: extension into chest. A. Note distortion and widening of the mediastinum and the cardiac silhouette. A large mass is suggested, and the heart is displaced to the left. **B.** Ultrasound demonstrates a large, hypoechoic structure (upper arrows) above and a small, elongated, hypoechoic structure (lower arrows) below the diaphragm (D). **C.** CT study shows a large, homogenous mass (arrows) in the right hemithorax. **D.** Lower axial slice demonstrates a small portion of the mass (arrows) below the diaphragm in the abdomen.

7. Silberstein MJ, Lewis JE, Blair JD, et al. Congenital peritoneal mesothelioma. J Pediatr Surg 1983;18:243–246.

8. George JC, Cohen MD, Tarver RD, et al. Ruptured cystic mesenchymal hamartoma: an unusual cause of neonatal ascites. Pediatr Radiol 1994;24:304–305.

9. Kim OH, Lee KY. Malignant fibrous histiocytoma of primary omental origin in an infant. Pediatr Radiol 1994;24:285–287.

10. Frawley KJ, Cohen R, O'Loughlin EV, et al. Neurofibromatosis os the small intestine mesentery in a child with neurofibromatosis type 1. J Pediatr Surg 1997;32:1783–1785.

11. Matsuki K, Kakitsubata Y, Watanabe K, et al. Mesenteric plexiform neurofibroma associated with Recklinghausen's disease. Pediatr Radiol 1997;27:255–256.

12. Sanders BM, West KW, Gingalewski C, et al. Inflammatory pseudotumor of the alimentary tract: clinical and surgical experience. J Pediatr Surg 2001;36:169–173.

13. Barr LL, Hayden CK Jr, Stansberry SD, et al. Enteric duplication cysts in children: are their ultrasonographic wall characteristics diagnostic? Pediatr Radiol 1990;20:26–28.

EXTRAINTESTINAL AIR COLLECTIONS

Pneumoperitoneum

Before the advent of mechanically assisted ventilation in premature infants with respiratory problems, most cases of pneumoperitoneum in the newborn and young infant were the result of perforation of the GI tract. After the advent of such therapy, pneumoperitoneum more often was a complication of positive pressure ventilation. Currently, however, because of downward modifications in positive pressure therapy, this cause of pneumoperitoneum is much less common, and GI perforation again has risen to be the most common cause.

In the newborn, pneumoperitoneum often is massive and when due to GI perforation most often involves the stomach or colon. Gastric perforations usually occur within the first few hours, or day or two of life, and in the past, deficiency or absence of the gastric musculature was invoked as the underlying problem. More likely, however, gastric perforations probably are secondary to acute gastric ulceration or focal necrosis secondary to perinatal hypoxia. In the latter instance, it is believed that hypoxia leads to shunting of blood away from the GI tract (diving reflex) and subsequently to GI schemia, focal necrosis, and perforation. There also is some suggestion that indomethacin therapy, because it leads to GI hypoperfusion (1), also can result in perforation. Gastric perforations also can result from simple gastric overdistention. Colon perforations occasionally are spontaneous, but most result from iatrogenic perforation with a thermometer or some similar object. Pneumoperitoneum also can be seen as a complication of pneumatosis cystoides intestinalis and GI obstruction.

Massive pneumoperitoneum in the neonate presents with abdominal distention and respiratory distress. However, even though massive, its recognition on supine roentgenograms can be elusive. This is true even though the entire abdomen is filled with air. On upright or decubitus films, the problem is not as difficult, but on supine view, massive volumes of free air can be missed entirely (Fig. 4.256). In such cases, the abdomen is distended and appears extremely radiolucent, indeed, almost diagrammatic.

In addition to these findings, with pneumoperitoneum, the walls of the individual loops of bowel are more discretely visualized becasue air is present both in and outside the intestine. One also may see the falciform ligament (2), as an opaque stripe in the right upper quadrant or upper mid-abdomen (Fig. 2.256A), and less often, a similar stripe, the urachus, in the mid-lower abdomen. In the lower abdomen, the umbilical arteries, passing from the umbilicus to the lower extremities in an inverted "V" configuration, also occasionally can be visualized. In a few cases, air may pass through the patent processus vaginalis and be seen in the scrotum.

With small collections of air, one must inspect the films with diligence (Fig. 4.257) and obtain one or more gravity-

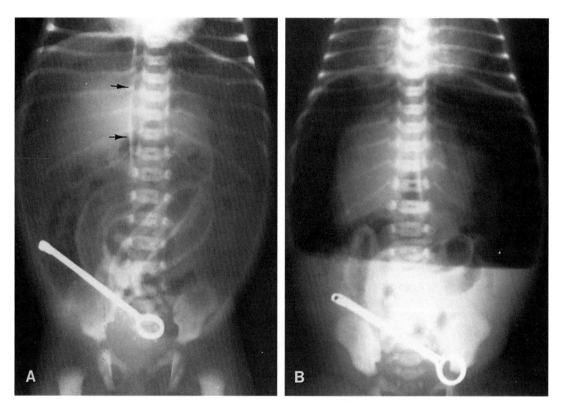

FIGURE 4.256. Massive pneumoperitoneum: gastric perforation. A. Note the extreme hyperlucency of entire abdomen resulting from massive accumulation of free air. Also note the falciform ligament (arrows) and discretely defined walls of the small bowel. **B.** Upright film confirms the massive amount of free air and demonstrates the typical central displacement of the abdominal viscera. Note the loops of small bowel floating in the fluid in the lower abdomen.

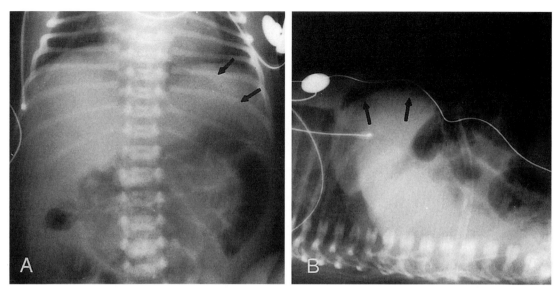

FIGURE 4.257. Pneumoperitoneum: subtle supine film findings. A. Note vague radiolucency over the left upper abdomen (arrows). This is the result of free air layering over the left lobe of the liver. **B.** Cross-table lateral view demonstrates the free air (arrows).

dependent views (e.g., lateral decubitus, cross-table lateral, upright).

In many cases, it is not until these views are obtained that the free air is visualized. On cross-table lateral views, a small triangle of air can serve to alert one to the presence of a perforation (Fig. 4.258). This "telltale" triangle (3) of air usually lies just below the liver edge.

In older children, free peritoneal air is an uncommon finding except for that seen with blunt abdominal trauma, after abdominal surgery, and with peritoneal dialysis. Occasionally, one can see free air from a perforated ulcer, appendix, or other portion of the GI tract, and the findings can be misleading (Fig. 4.259), just as they are in the neonate.

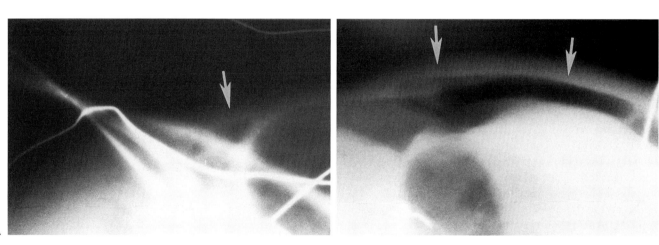

FIGURE 4.258. Telltale triangle of pneumoperitoneum. A. Note the small triangular collection of gas (arrow) just below the liver edge on this cross-table lateral view of an infant with necrotizing enterocolitis and early perforation. **B.** A few hours later, note the massive pneumoperitoneum (arrows) in the same infant.

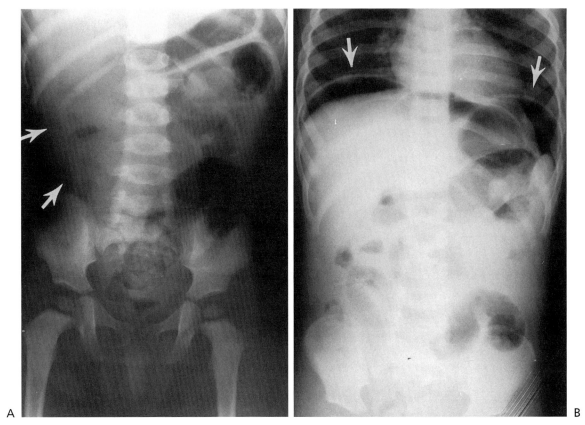

A

B

FIGURE 4.259. Occult pneumoperitoneum. A. Older patient with perforated Meckel's diverticulum demonstrates a vague lucency over the liver (arrows). This is a subtle, but important, plain film finding of free air. **B.** Upright film demonstrates a large volume of free air under both diaphragmatic leaflets (arrows).

REFERENCES

1. Lloyd JR. The etiology of gastrointestinal perforations in the newborn. J Pediatr Surg 1969;4:77–84.
2. Cronen PW, Nagaraj HS, Janik JS, et al. Effect of indomethacin on mesenteric circulation in mongrel dogs. J Pediatr Surg 1982; 17:474–478.
3. Seibert JJ, Parvey LS. The telltale triangle: use of the supine cross table lateral radiograph of the abdomen in early detection of pneumoperitoneum. Pediatr Radiol 1977;5:209–210.

Pneumatosis Cystoides Intestinalis

This lengthy term is used to denote the presence of air in the bowel wall. Most commonly, the air is seen in the colon but it can occur in the small bowel, and even in the stomach. Characteristically, one notes linear, curvilinear, or bubbly collections of gas within the wall of the intestine (Fig. 4.157) and in the newborn and preterm infant, most cases of pneumatosis cystoides intestinalis are seen as a complication of necrotizing enterocolitis. However, in any age group pneumatosis can be seen with any cause of intestinal schemia where there is mucosal necrosis, loss of mucosal integrity and bacterial overgrowth. It is the gas formed by the bacterial overgrowth that accounts for the pneumatosis. On the other hand, when pneumatosis cystoides intestinalis is secondary to prolonged intestinal overdistention (i.e., obstruction, profound paralytic ileus) mucosal tears occur and allow bowel gas to enter the bowel wall. This form of pneumatosis is referred to as **"benign pneumatosis" and also can occur in the colon** of older infants and children with cystic fibrosis (1), collagen vascular disease, leukemia, and the immunodeficiency states (2–4). Benign pneumatosis cystoides intestinales also can be associated with rotavirus infection (5) and milk intolerance.

REFERENCES

1. Hernanz-Schulman M, Kirkpatrick J Jr, Schwachman H, et al. Pneumatosis intestinalis in cystic fibrosis. Radiology 1986;160: 497–499.
2. Burton EM, Mercado-Deane MG, Patel K. Pneumatosis intestinalis in a child with AIDS and pseudomembranous colitis. Pediatr Radiol 1994;24:609–610.

3. Sivit CJ, Josephs SH, Taylor GA, et al. Case report: pneumatosis intestinalis in children with AIDS. AJR 1990;155:133–134.
4. Tang MLK, Williams LW. Pneumatosis intestinale in children with primary combined immunodeficiency. J Pediatr 1998;132: 546–549.
5. Capitanio MA, Greenberg SB. Pneumatosis intestinalis in two infants with rotavirus gastroenteritis. Pediatr Radiol 1991;21: 361–362.

PERITONITIS, ASCITES, AND HEMOPERITONEUM

Meconium Peritonitis

Meconium peritonitis usually results from intrauterine GI perforation. Initially, it is a sterile chemical peritonitis, but if perforation of the GI tract persists after birth, complicating bacterial infection supervenes and the prognosis becomes more serious. Perforation usually is due to come type of intrauterine obstruction or volvulus. Often, meconium ileus as part of cystic fibrosis is the underlying problem (1). In any case, if the perforation seals off in utero, the extruded, calcified meconium is noted as an incidental finding (Fig. 4.260). No further investigation or treatment is usually required in these cases, but in those infants where active peritonitis, intestinal obstruction, and/or pneumoperitoneum are noted, immediate surgical intervention is required.

The extruded meconium may or may not calcify, and when no calcifications are present, the roentgenogram merely suggests fluid in the abdomen. When calcifications are seen, one can be more specific about the diagnosis. These calcifications can be amorphous, irregular, clumpy, or curvilinear, the latter suggesting cystic loculation or coating of the peritoneum (Fig. 4.261). The term cystic or pseudocystic meconium peritonitis is used to describe this configuration.

A few infants with meconium peritonitis may present with swelling of, or masses in the scrotum (2). These result from passage of meconium into the scrotum through the patent processus vaginalis. In such instances one may at first believe that hydroceles are present, but calcifications within the scrotum provide an almost foolproof sign of meconium peritonitis (Fig. 4.262). Eventually, most of the calcifications in meconium peritonitis slowly disappear, and it is uncommon to encounter an older child with residual calcifications. In some cases, fluid and meconium can pass into the chest, presumably through normal congenital communications, and manifest as so-called meconium thorax (2) (Fig. 4.262).

Calcified meconium is readily demonstrable on plain films and also can be seen in utero with ultrasound (Fig. 4.263, A and B). Fluid (sonolucent areas) may be seen within the cyst, but usually echogenicity, resulting from debris and calcifications, is seen. The wall of the cyst may

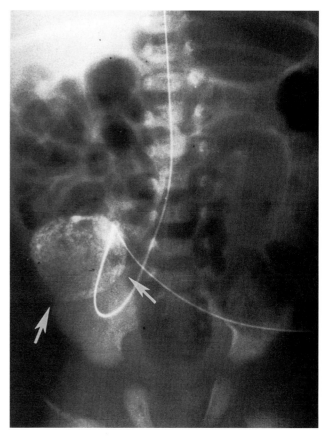

FIGURE 4.260. Meconium peritonitis: incidental finding. Note the calcified mass in the right lower quadrant (arrows). This was an incidental finding in a premature infant with respiratory distress.

be thin or thick, and one may even note loops of fluid-filled bowel bound into the matrix of the associated adhesions. With free-floating meconium in the abdomen, multiple, floating speckled echoes are seen and result in the "snowstorm" configuration (3) (Fig. 4.263 C). Peritoneal calcification mimicking meconium peritonitis can be seen with hydrometrocolpos where the inspissated uterine contents are forced into the peritoneal cavity through the fallopian tubes (4).

REFERENCES

1. Lang I, Daneman A, Cutz E, et al. abdominal calcification in cystic fibrosis with meconium ileus. Radiologic pathologic correlation. Pediatr Radiol 1997;27:523–527.
2. Salman AB, Karaoglanoglu N, Suma S. Abdominal, scrotal, and thoracic calcifications owing to healed meconium peritonitis. J Pediatr Surg 1999;34:1415–1416.
3. Lawrence PW, Chrispin A. Sonographic appearance of two neonates with generalized meconium peritonitis: the snowstorm sign. Br J Radiol 1984;57:340–342.

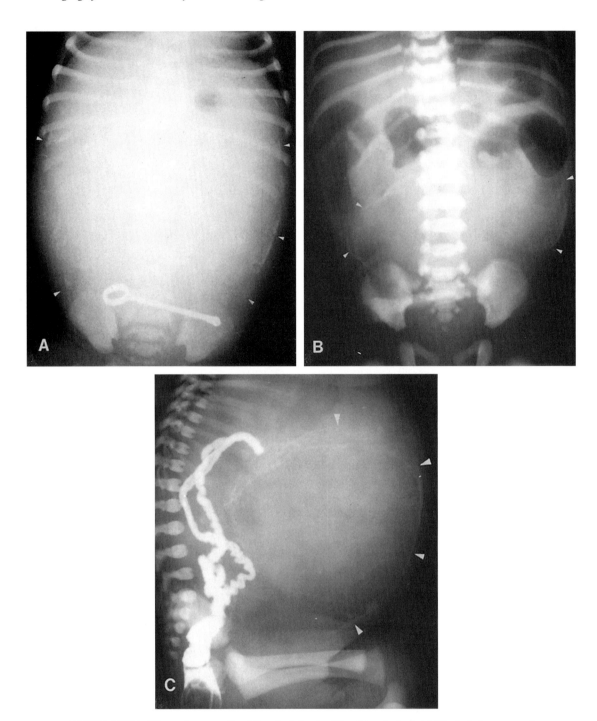

FIGURE 4.261. Meconium peritonitis. A. Infant with distended, fluid-filled abdomen and irregular peripheral calcification of meconium (arrows). **B.** Curvilinear configuration of calcified meconium peritonitis (arrows). At laparotomy, numerous loculated compartments were present. **C.** Another infant with pseudocystic-appearing meconium peritonitis (arrows). Also note the microcolon in this infant with meconium ileus.

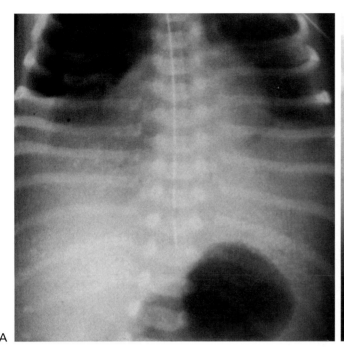
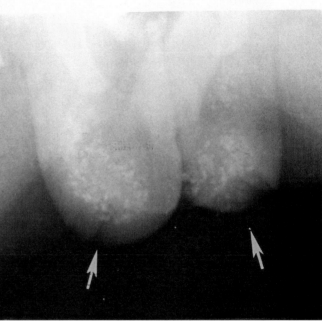

A   B

FIGURE 4.262. Meconium peritonitis: unusual locations of calcifications. A. Calcifications in pleural cavities. Note the stippled calcification located throughout the upper abdomen and over the lower thorax. Fluid is present in both pleural spaces, and bilateral pneumothoraces are present. The calcifications were secondary to meconium peritonitis, and most were located in the pleural cavities, deep in the posterior costophrenic sulci. Presumably, fluid entered the pleural space from the abdomen through congenital communications. **B.** Scrotal calcifications. Note calcified meconium masses (arrows) in the scrotum, having entered through a patent processus vaginalis. ((**A** courtesy of B. Gay, M.D.; **B** reproduced with permission from Ellis K. Residents' corner. Med Radiogr Photogr 1971;47:83.)

4. Hu MX, Methratta S. An unusual case of neonatal peritoneal calcifications associated with hydrometrocolpos. Pediatr Radiol 2001;31:742–744.

Bacterial Peritonitis

Childhood bacterial peritonitis can result from appendiceal perforation, other perforations of the GI tract, omphalitis, generalized sepsis, or in association with meconium peritonitis. Primary peritonitis in the neonate is rare and primarily is a disease of older children (1). In addition, primary peritonitis, usually pneumococcal in origin, also is a common problem in the nephrotic syndrome. Abdominal distention is usually present and abdominal roentgenograms demonstrate the presence of abdominal fluid. The findings are not specific because they can be seen with any fluid accumulation. Ultrasonography is the best method with which to detect the fluid, but CT also is useful.

REFERENCE

1. Freji BJ, Votteler TP, McCracken GH Jr. Primary peritonitis in previously healthy children. Am J Dis Child 1984;138:1058–1061.

Ascites and Abdominal Fluid

Massive ascites is a common problem throughout the pediatric group and in older children often is secondary to renal disease (i.e., nephrotic syndrome), or primary liver disease, such as cirrhosis or portal vein obstruction. It also can be seen with abdominal lymphoma and any type of protein-losing enteropathy. Ascites secondary to urinary tract obstruction, producing so-called "urine ascites," occurs after bladder rupture or rupture of a previously hydronephrotic and often occult upper collecting system (i.e., occult ureteropelvic junction obstruction).

Bile ascites occurs after rupture or tear of the biliary tract, either after a blunt abdominal trauma or in neonates on an unexplained basis. Chylous ascites also can be seen and results from congenital hypoplasia or obstruction of the lymphatic system. As with chylothorax, if the infant has not been on milk feedings, the ascitic fluid is clear. It is only after fat has been introduced into the diet that the characteristic chylous appearance is seen. Most of these infants recover spontaneously but a few have persistent ascites and hypoproteinemia. Medium chain triglycerides and total parenteral nutrition can be used in treating these infants. Occasionally, direct ligation of the lymphatic ducts may be required.

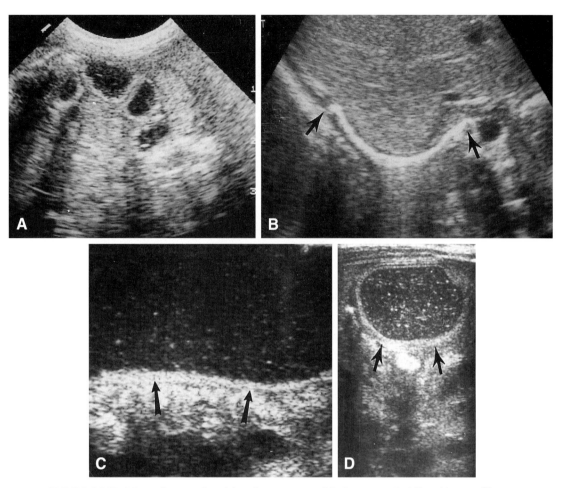

FIGURE 4.263. Meconium peritonitis: ultrasonographic features. A. Dilated loops of intestine are seen in echogenic fluid, which filled the abdomen. **B.** Another patient with echogenic fluid (arrows). **C.** In this patient, the fluid is hypoechoic (arrows), but scattered flecks of echogenic meconium are seen drifting through the fluid (i.e., "snowstorm" effect). **D.** Another patient demonstrating a cystic collection (arrows) of fluid with meconium debris, once again demonstrating the snowstorm effect.

Chylous ascites also can be seen with mesenteric venous obstruction resulting from intestinal volvulus. In addition, it can be seen with intestinal lymphangiectasia, hypoproteinemia, pancreatitis, and with ovarian cysts that rupture. Ascites also can be seen with erythroblastosis fetalis and cardiac conditions where dysrhythmias lead to right-side cardiac decompensation. A very rare cause of ascites is lysosome storage disease (1, 2). Ascites can be mimicked by large, flaccid, mesenteric or omental cysts. In these cases the cyst wall is so thin that free fluid is suggested. Finally, if ascites is massive, fluid may pass through the processus vaginalis, and large communicating hydroceles may be palpable in the scrotum.

Roentgenographically, a uniform density to the abdomen is noted and floating air-filled loops of bowel tend to cluster in the center of the abdomen (Fig. 4.264A). However, as with any abdominal fluid, its presence is most read-

ily demonstrated with ultrasound (Fig. 4.264B), although it can also be readily visualized with CT and MR imaging.

Small amounts of free fluid can be seen in the abdomen with perforated appendicitis, bleeding ovarian cysts, bowel schemia or necrosis, intussusception, and gastroenteritis (3). In addition, many cases are unexplained, and in a series by Sivit et al. (3), 40% were unexplained and 40% resulted from gastroenteritis. Therefore, one must treat small amounts of fluid in the abdomen with caution.

REFERENCES

1. Daneman A, Stringer D, Reilly BJ. Neonatal ascites due to lysosomal storage disease. Radiology 1983;149:463–467.
2. Gillan JE, Lowden JA, Gaskin K, et al. Congenital ascites as a presenting sign of lysosomal storage disease. J Pediatr 1984;104:225–231.

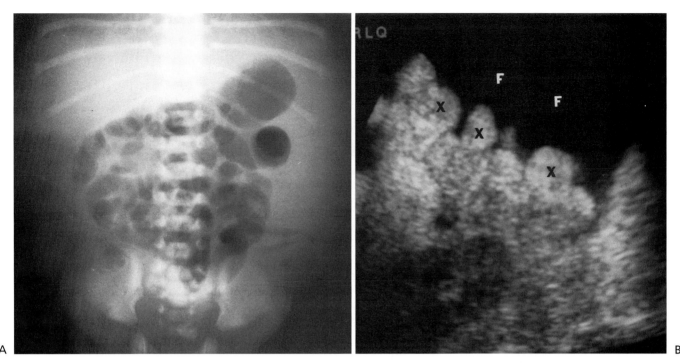

A   B

FIGURE 4.264. Ascites. A. Note the large volume of fluid in the abdomen causing the loops of air-filled intestine to float in the center of the abdomen of this infant in supine position. **B.** Ultrasonogram demonstrates loops of intestine (X) floating in free ascitic fluid (F).

3. Sivit CJ. Significance of peritoneal fluid identified by ultrasonographic examination in children with acute abdominal pain. J Ultrasound Med 1993;12:743–746.

Hemoperitoneum

In the older child hemoperitoneum is most commonly seen after abdominal trauma, either accidental or intentional. Occasionally, it can be seen with bleeding disorders or as a complication of umbilical vessel catheterization. In the neonate, hemoperitoneum often results from birth trauma and injury to the liver or spleen. Less commonly hemoperitoneum is iatrogenic, resulting from umbilical artery catheterization. In terms of imaging, the findings are the same as for any type of fluid in the abdomen except that, with MRI, old blood produces high signal on both T1- and T2-weighted images.

THE APPENDIX

Acute Appendicitis

Acute appendicitis is a very common condition both in infancy and childhood and even can be seen in the neonate (1). It is more difficult to diagnose in infants than in children, and consequently perforation in infants under 2 years of age is much more common. As far as plain film findings are concerned, with nonperforated appendicitis the abdomen often is airless secondary to vomiting and diarrhea. On the other hand, many times the abdominal films may be normal. More specific findings include scoliosis with concavity to the right and air-fluid levels in the right lower quadrant or pelvis (2), both in the cecum and terminal small bowel (Fig. 4.265). These become especially important when the abdomen also is relatively airless (Fig. 4.265). Another finding of value is the presence of a calcified fecalith (Fig. 4.265D). However, now that imaging with ultrasound and CT is available, fecaliths frequently can be seen as incidental findings (3).

When perforation occurs, the patient's clinical condition often temporarily improves. After all, what happens is that the inflamed appendix, acting as an abscess, drains itself spontaneously. Unless diffuse peritonitis results, physical findings, although somewhat localized to the right lower quadrant, are less definite. In addition, since these patients now begin to swallow air and even eat, air accumulates within the intestine and a so-called functional obstruction develops (2, 4). In most cases there is no definite abscess present, but the post perforation inflammatory changes produce a partial, functional obstruction of the small bowel as it impedes the passage of air and intestinal contents into the colon (Fig. 4.266). In some of these cases the transverse colon is dilated and filled with air while the ascending colon is spastic and airless. This results in the "right-side colon

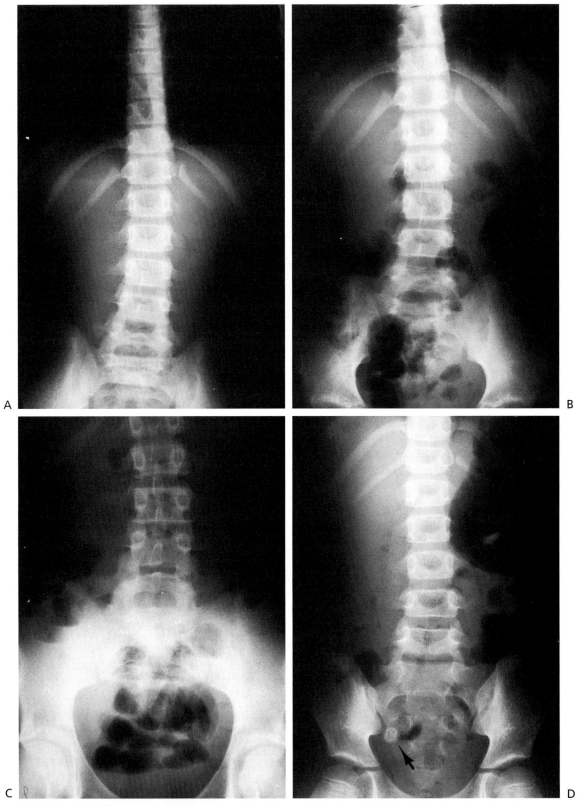

FIGURE 4.265. Acute appendicitis: nonperforated, on plain films. A. Note scoliosis and an airless abdomen. **B.** Scoliosis is present, but the gas pattern is relatively normal. **C.** In this patient, scoliosis is present, but there also are air-fluid levels in the right flank (arrows). In addition, note the dilated loops of bowel in the pelvis. The latter is not an uncommon finding with appendicitis. **D.** Another patient has a normal gas pattern, minimal scoliosis, and a calcified fecalith (arrow) in the right lower quadrant.

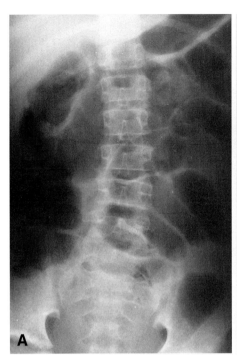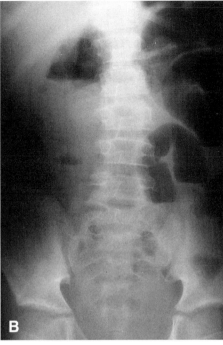

FIGURE 4.266. Appendicitis: perforated, on plain films. A. Note gas scattered throughout the GI tract. There are a number of obstructed-appearing small bowel loops in the left mid-abdomen, but there is a paucity of gas in the pelvis and right lower quadrant. Gas is present in the colon. **B.** Upright view demonstrates inverted U-shaped loops of small intestine consistent with an obstruction.

cutoff sign" (5). The finding is valuable (Fig. 4.267), although not overly common. It can be mimicked by normal air in the transverse colon in the supine position, and if there is doubt as to its presence, one can obtain decubitus films with the right side up. If a true colon cutoff sign is present, the ascending colon, because it is spastic, will not fill with air.

Ultrasound has made great inroads into the investigation of the acute abdomen in children. In addition, not only is it a very productive imaging modality but it also allows one to perform a transducer-guided physical examination. To be sure, ultrasound is the "ultimate physical examination" (6) and is the premiere imaging modality for the investigation of patients with suspected appendicitis (7–11). The study is best performed with linear 10- to13-MHz transducers and the appendix can be searched for by scanning the right lower quadrant from side to side and then top to bottom. What one is looking for is an **abnormal finding which should not be there and does not go away**. In terms of the appendix, what one is looking for is a fluid-filled, distended, swollen appendix or, **if you like, "a small sausage."** This is most common configuration of the inflamed appendix but in other cases the appendix can be larger or longer.

The normal appendix is not fluid-filled and not distended, but collapsed. It has a diameter of less than 4 mm (Fig. 4.268, A and B), and **often is difficult to find**. In this regard, it is not **absolutely essential that one find a normal appendix in**

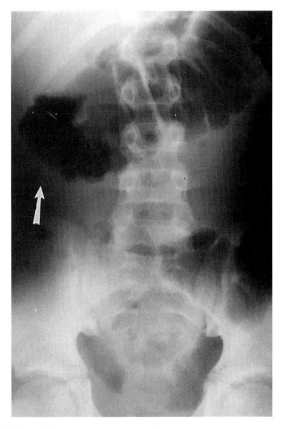

FIGURE 4.267. Acute appendicitis: perforated, colon cut-off sign. The transverse colon is dilated, but a cut-off is present in the hepatic flexure (arrow).

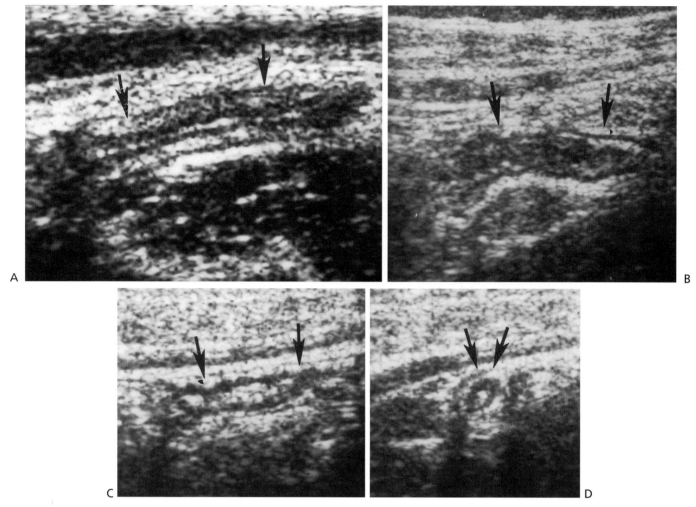

FIGURE 4.268. Normal appendix. A. Note the collapsed normal appendix (arrows). **B.** Another case with an irregular but collapsed-appearing appendix (arrows). **C.** Another small, collapsed appendix (arrows). **D.** On cross-section, the appendix has a more oval than round appearance (arrows).

every case. What one is looking for is an abnormal appendix. If one does not find an abnormal appendix and no other findings to support appendicitis, spending a lot of time trying to find a normal appendix is counterproductive. Occasionally, a normal appendix contains fluid (Fig. 4.269) but is not distended or tender. In such cases, paralytic ileus of the appendix, along with the intestines is present for some unrelated reason and the appendix just happens to contain some fluid. In such cases, it is helpful to apply color-flow Doppler, because such appendices do not demonstrate increased blood flow. In addition, on cross-section, these appendices appear a little more oval than round and this is important because an inflamed appendix is round on cross-section. Finally, an appendix floating, **and bouncing** in fluid is not abnormal (Fig. 4.270). The fluid in these cases is the result of some other disease process and usually is clear. However, it does outline the appendix very vividly but the appendix is collapsed, measures below pathologic diameter measurements and does "bounce." If it bounces, it is normal.

Once the abnormal appendix is identified, graded compression can be used to determine whether it is non-compressible and painful. However, this is not always necessary, because if one easily defines the inflamed appendix, compression will merely make the patient uncomfortable and probably is not required (12). It is worthwhile to ask the patient where he or she hurts, because self-localization (13) has been shown to be of considerable value in pinpointing the site of the inflamed appendix. In this regard, most appendices are located just under the abdominal wall and that is why ultrasound is so successful in detecting them. To be sure, the ultrasonographic investigation of appendicitis definitely has led to better patient selection for surgery and use of hospital resources (7, 8, 11). However, ultrasound is better for nonperforated, than perforated appendicitis, but still in one series a 92% identification rate of perforated appendicitis was documented (14). Our own success rate for appendicitis overall, is at least 98% (10).

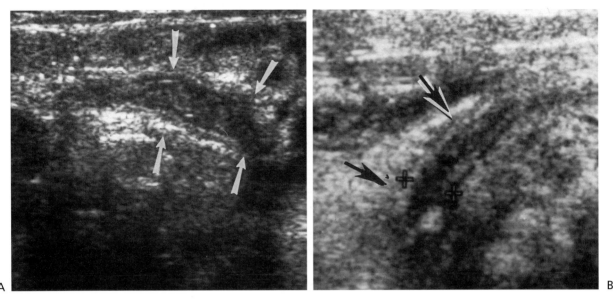

FIGURE 4.269. Normal appendix with fluid. A. Note the fluid-filled, slightly distended appendix (arrows). There is no significant echogenic mesentery surrounding the appendix. This patient had sickle cell disease, and the appendix was fluid-filled as part of generalized paralytic ileus of the intestines. **B.** Fluid-filled appendix with paralytic ileus. In this patient, with pelvic inflammatory disease (PID), secondary inflammation of the appendix caused it to dilate slightly and become fluid-filled (arrows).

The usual ultrasonographic criteria for the identification of acute, nonperforated appendicitis include the identification of a fixed, tender, and noncompressible fluid-filled tubular structure measuring 6 mm or more in diameter (Fig. 4.271). In addition, a fecalith may be present (Fig. 4.272). In the early stages, mucosa is intact, and color flow Doppler (15) is very helpful (Fig. 4.272). Later, the mucosa becomes destroyed, usually in association with gangrenous appendicitis (Fig. 4.273). Other findings include presence of debris within the lumen, and in some cases, a small amount of fluid around the appendix.

Echogenic, thickened mesentery surrounding the appendix is a common and useful adjunctive finding with acute appendicitis and corresponds to fat stranding as seen on CT. However, it is easier to identify with ultrasound. Adenopathy in acute nonperforated appendicitis is not as common as originally believed. The reason for this is that it does take some time for lymph nodes to reactively enlarge after an inflammatory process begins. This being the case, it would not be surprising to see less adenopathy with nonperforated appendicitis, and more adenopathy with perforated appendicitis where a longer period of time passes from the onset of symptoms to the detection of the disease process. In addition, in some children lymph nodes, from a previous infection are present and are not inflamed. They just happen to incidentally be there.

Variations and pitfalls in the ultrasonographic diagnosis of appendicitis are few and include inflammation of the tip of the appendix only (Fig. 4.274), a gas-filled appendix, a large appendix, and a dilated fallopian tube mimicking a distended appendix.

Retrocecal appendicitis often is difficult to detect, and one has to search for the inflammatory process for a longer period of time. Often, these appendices have perforated before they are discovered, and since the inflammatory process usually is present for longer than usual, adjacent inflammation of the cecum and terminal ileum can be seen (Fig. 4.275). In addition reactive adenopathy is more common (Fig. 4.275D). Otherwise, in most cases of acute appendicitis, adenopathy is not a predominant feature.

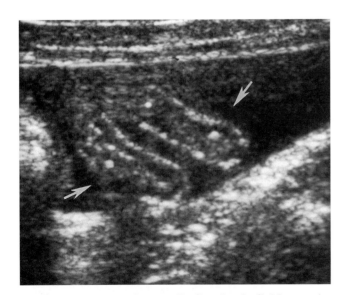

FIGURE 4.270. Normal appendix floating in fluid. Note the normal, collapsed appendix (arrows) floating in acitic fluid secondary to peritonitis.

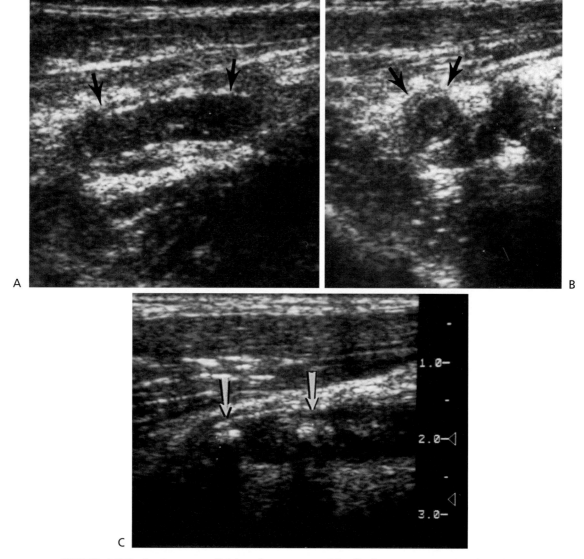

FIGURE 4.271. Acute appendicitis: ultrasonographic findings. A. Note the fluid-filled appendix (arrows) resembling a small sausage. There is some echogenic mesentery around the appendix, and the mucosal lining still is present. **B.** Cross-sectional view demonstrates the typical concentric ring configuration (arrows). Note surrounding echogenic mesentery. **C.** In this patient, two echogenic fecaliths (arrows) are present in the fluid-filled, distended appendix.

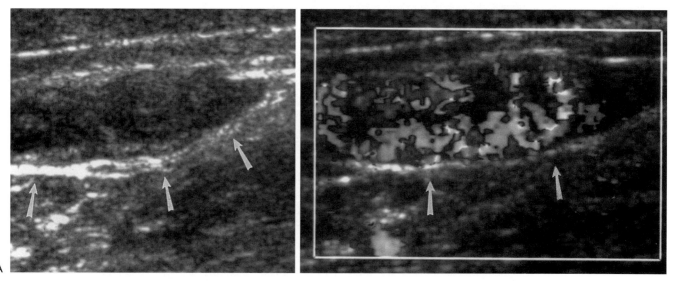

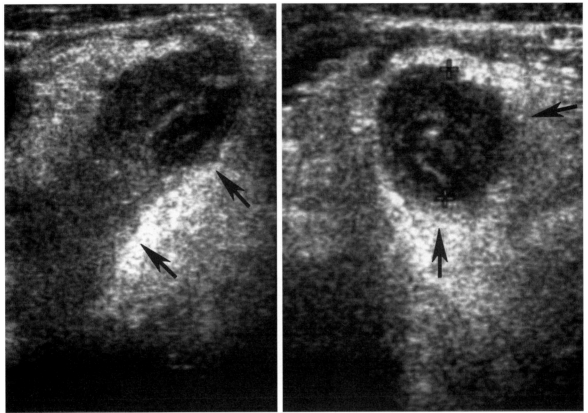

FIGURE 4.273. Gangrenous appendicitis: ultrasonographic findings. A. Note the enlarged, hypoechoic, ill-defined appendix (arrows). No mucosal lining is seen. There is intense echogenic mesentery all around the appendix. **B.** Similar findings on cross-section. Note the hypoechoic appendix (arrows) with ill-defined edges. It is surrounded by intensely echogenic mesentery.

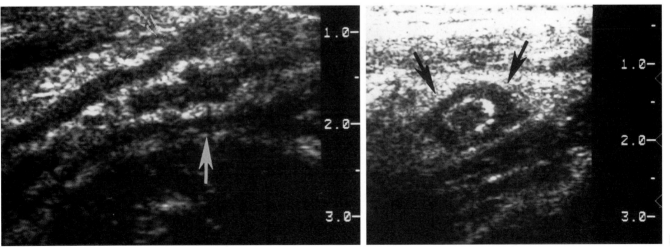

FIGURE 4.274. Acute appendicitis: tip of appendix. A. Note the slightly distended, fluid-filled appendiceal tip (arrow). The proximal appendix appears relatively normal. **B.** Cross-sectional view of the tip of the appendix demonstrates a typical concentric ring configuration (arrows).

FIGURE 4.272. Acute appendicitis: value of color Doppler. A. Note the fluid-filled appendix (arrows) just beneath the abdominal wall. There is no thickening of the wall, and there is no echogenic mesentery. **B.** Color Doppler, however, demonstrates extensive hyperemia (arrows) of the appendix substantiating acute appendicitis.

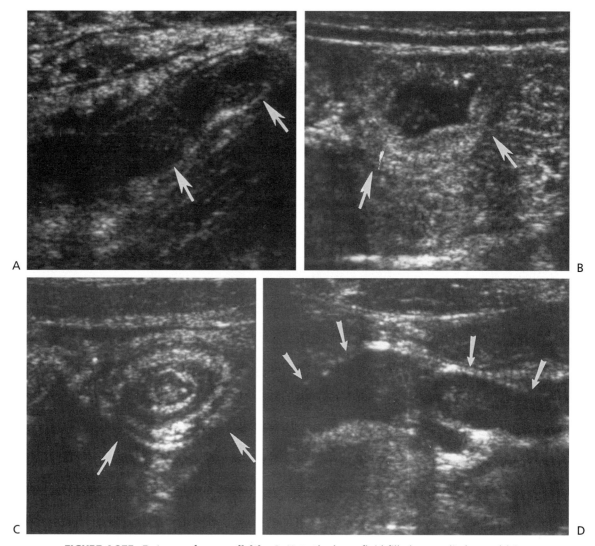

FIGURE 4.275. Retrocecal appendicitis. A. Note the large fluid-filled appendix (arrows) lying deep against the psoas muscle. **B.** Thickened mucosa is present in adjacent small bowel (arrows). **C.** Concentric rings of thickened mucosa are seen in the cecum (arrows). **D.** Enlarged inflamed lymph nodes are present (arrows).

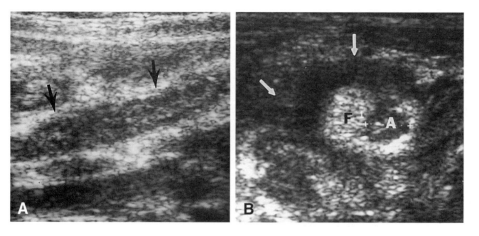

FIGURE 4.276. Acute appendicitis: perforated, ultrasonographic findings. A. The appendix (arrows) is more difficult to identify because it is collapsed and empty. It is surrounded by echogenic fat. **B.** Another patient, whose appendix (A) is seen on cross-section. It is surrounded by echogenic mesenteric fat (F) and an early hypoechoic peripheral fluid collection (arrows).

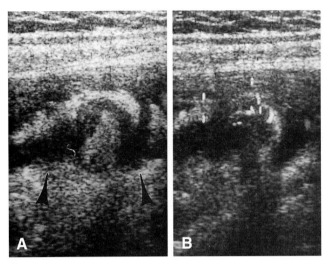

FIGURE 4.277. Appendicitis: perforation with phlegmon. A. Note the nonspecific mixed echo pattern of a mass (arrows) representative of a phlegmon. **B.** Color-flow Doppler demonstrates increased blood flow (white speckled areas) to the lesion.

In terms of perforated appendicitis, ultrasound evaluation usually is more difficult because the appendix is no longer fluid-filled, but instead it is drained and collapsed (Fig. 4.276A). However, other findings may be helpful and include the presence of small amounts of fluid around the appendix and increased thickness and echogenicity of periappendiceal mesenteric fat (Fig. 4.276B).

In other cases, of perforated appendicitis, the inflammatory process may be even more nondescript and as such manifest as a phlegmon (Fig. 4.277). In these cases one clearly realizes that some abnormality is present, but yet a definite abscess or inflamed appendix cannot be identified, only a nonspecific

inflammatory mass, **the phlegmon. This is the only way to define a phlegmon—a phlegmon is a phlegmon—it is inflammation of the soft tissues without a defined border.** In other cases, frank abscesses can be identified with ultrasound (Fig. 4.278A), but most often are finally delineated with CT (Fig. 4.278B). Although these abscesses can be localized to the right lower quadrant they frequently extend anywhere into the abdomen, and even into the chest.

CT of the abdomen, with a focused study over the right lower quadrant currently is in common use in adults and is becoming more popular in children (16–22). This study often is augmented by the use of oral and rectal contrast. In addition, CT does deliver ionizing radiation to the patient. Nonetheless, in some patients it is quite valuable, especially heavier, older patients and any patient where the disease is suspected and the ultrasonographic findings are less than satisfactory (19–22). With CT one looks for the same findings as with ultrasound (i.e., a fluid-filled appendix which on cross-section is round (Fig. 4.279). In addition, stranding due to edema of the surrounding mesenteric fat is the equivalent of the echogenic mesenteric fat seen around the inflamed appendix on ultrasound. In the end, no matter what the age, if the patient is thin, appendicitis is easily found with ultrasound while if the patient is heavier or obese, CT is more productive (Fig. 4.280).

A few interesting peculiarities of appendicitis include location of the appendix in an inguinal hernia (23, 24), appendicitis secondary to a foreign body (25) and urinary tract involvement with ureteral obstruction (26). In addition, it should be remembered that small amounts of fluid postoperatively are not uncommon and should not be misinterpreted for abscesses (27). Spontaneously resolving appendicitis also should be remembered (28, 29) and in one

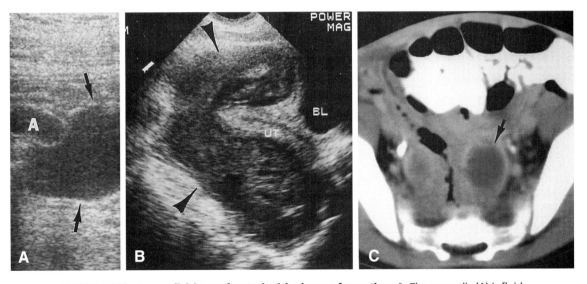

FIGURE 4.278. Appendicitis: perforated with abscess formation. A. The appendix (A) is fluid-filled and in this case still a little distended, but a large fluid collection, representing an abscess, (arrows) also is seen. **B.** Another patient with a large abscess (arrows) surrounding the uterus (UT) and rising above the urinary bladder (BL). **C.** Abscess in the pelvis (arrow) with a low-density center and a slightly enhancing peripheral wall. Another smaller one is present on the right.

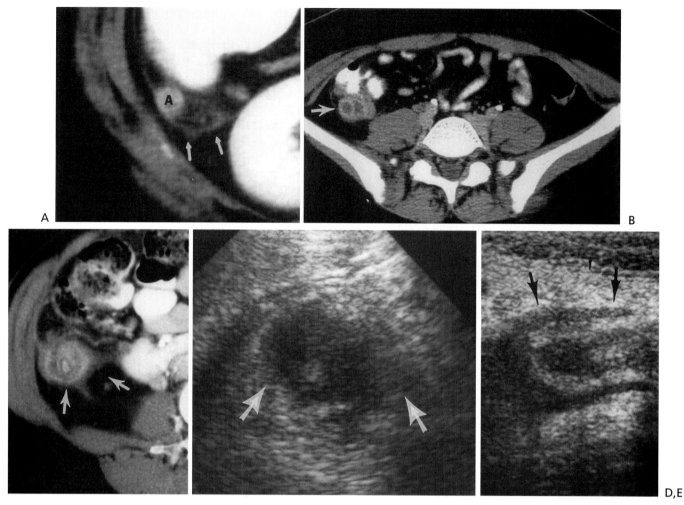

FIGURE 4.279. Acute appendicitis: CT findings. A. Note the inflamed appendix (A), surrounded by mesenteric fat stranding (arrows). **B.** In this patient, a larger fluid-filled, round, and distended appendix (arrow) is seen. **C.** Note the large, inflamed appendix (arrows) with surrounding fat stranding and a central fecalith. **D.** Ultrasound study demonstrates the same findings (arrows) but less vividly. **E.** High-resolution ultrasound study, however, clearly demonstrates the inflamed fluid-filled appendix (arrows).

series (28) this occurred in 1 out of 13 patients, and the overall recurrence rate was 38%. Most cases recurred within 1 year. Partially treated (antibiotics) appendicitis also can be a dilemma. In these cases, the appendix and periappendiceal mesenteric fat appears inflamed, but all of the attendant findings, such as it being fluid-filled, tender, and noncompressible, are not present.

Acute appendicitis also can be imaged with MRI, which is quite accurate (30, 31). However, it probably never will be the first imaging modality to be used, but it may have a place in confusing cases. Finally, appendiceal abscesses can be successfully drained percutaneously but antibiotic coverage is important (32).

REFERENCES

1. Ruff ME, Soughgate WM, Wood BP. Radiological case of the month. Neonatal appendicitis with perforation. Am J Dis Child 1991;145:111–112.
2. Phillpott JW, Swischuk LE, John SD. Appendicitis in the era of ultrasound: are plain radiographs still useful? Emerg Radiol 1997;4:68–71.
3. Lowe LH, Penney MW, Scheker LE, et al. Appendicolith revealed on CT in children with suspected appendicitis: how specific is it in the diagnosis of appendicitis? AJR 2000;175:981–984.
4. Riggs W, Parvey LS. Perforated appendix presenting with disproportionate jejunal distension. Pediatr Radiol 1976;5:47–49.
5. Swischuk LE, Hayden CK Jr. Appendicitis with perforation: the dilated transverse colon sign. AJR 1980;135:687–689.
6. Swischuk LE. Ultrasonography, the ultimate physical exam of the acute abdomen in pediatrics. Emerg Radiol 2000;7:324–325.
7. Carrico CW, Fenton LZ, Taylor GA, et al. Impact of sonography on the diagnosis and treatment of acute lower abdominal pain in children and young adults. AJR 1999;172:513–516.
8. Dilley A, Wesson D, Munden M, et al. The impact of ultrasound examinations on the management of children with suspected appendicitis: a 3-year analysis. J Pediatr Surg 2001;36:303–308.
9. Fuhi Y, Hata J, Futagami K, et al. Ultrasonography improves

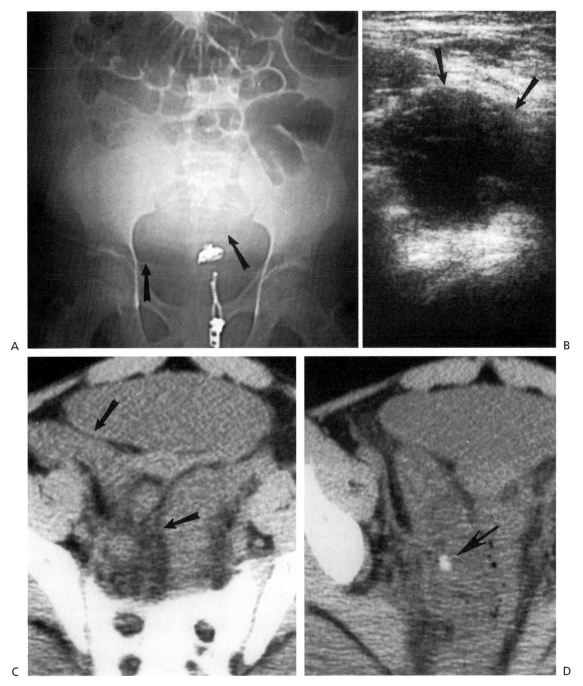

FIGURE 4.280. Value of CT in large patient. A. CT topogram demonstrates a colon cut-off sign, some air in small bowel, and a paucity of air-filled intestine in the lower abdomen. **B.** Ultrasound study demonstrates a nonspecific hypoechoic area (arrows) in the right lower quadrant. The appendix could not be visualized. **C.** CT study through the pelvis demonstrates the appendix (upper arrow) and considerable secondary fat stranding (lower arrow). **D.** A slightly lower CT slice demonstrates similar findings and a calcified fecalith (arrow).

diagnostic accuracy of acute appendicitis and provides cost savings to hospitals in Japan. J Ultrasound Med 2000;19:409–414.

10. Hendrick EP, Chong-Han C, Swischuk LE, et al. Accuracy of ultrasonography in acute right lower quadrant problems in children. Emerg Radiol 1999;6:350–354.

11. Rice HE, Arbesman M, Martin DJ, et al. Does early ultrasonography affect management of pediatric appendicitis? A prospective analysis. J Pediatr Surg 1999;34:754–759.

12. Baldisserotto M, Marchiori E. Accuracy of non-compressive sonography of children with appendicitis according to the potential positions of the appendix. AJR 2000;175:1387–1392.

13. Chesbrough RM, Burkhard TK, Balsara ZN, et al. Self-localization in US of appendicitis: an addition to graded compression. Radiology 1993;187:349–351.

14. Ceres L, Alonso I, Lopez P, et al. Ultrasound study of acute

appendicitis in children with emphasis for the diagnosis of retro-cecal appendicitis. Pediatr Radiol 1990;20:258–261.

15. Lim HK, Lee WJ, Kim TH, et al. Appendicitis: usefulness of color Doppler US. Radiology 1996;201:221–225.

16. Quillin SP, Siegel MJ. Diagnosis of appendiceal abscess in children with acute appendicitis: value of color Doppler sonography. AJR 1995;164:1251–1254.

17. Garcia BM, Mandl KD, Kraus SJ, et al. Ultrasonography and limited computed tomography in the diagnosis and management of appendicitis in children. JAMA 1999;282:1041–1046.

18. Garcia BM, Taylor GA, Lund DP, et al. Effect of computed tomography on patient management and costs in children with suspected appendicitis. Pediatrics 1999;104:440–446.

19. Grayson DE, Wettlaufer JR, Dalrymple NC, et al. Appendiceal CT in pediatric patients: relationship of visualization to amount of peritoneal fat. AJR 2001;176:497–500.

20. John SD. The use of advanced imaging for appendicitis in children. Emerg Radiol 2001;7:331–338.

21. Sivit CJ, Dudgeon DL, Applegate KE, et al. Evaluation of suspected appendicitis in children and young adults: helical CT. Radiology 2000;216:430–433.

22. Sivit CJ, Applegate KE, Stallion A, et al. Imaging evaluation of suspected appendicitis in a pediatric population: effectiveness of sonography versus CT. AJR 2000;175:977–980.

23. Friedman SC, Sheynkin YR. Acute scrotal symptoms due to perforated appendix in children: case report and review of the literature. Pediatr Emerg Care 1995;11:181–182.

24. Mendez R, Tallado M, Montero M, et al. Acute scrotum: an exceptional presentation of acute nonperforated appendicitis in childhood. J Pediatr Surg 1998;33:1435–1436.

25. Sukhotnik I, Klin B, Siplovich L. Foreign-body appendicitis. J Pediatr Surg 1995;30:1515–1516.

26. Buckley K, Buonoma C. Bilateral ureteral obstruction and renal failure due to a perforated appendix. Pediatr Radiol 1994;24:308–309.

27. Aveline B, Guimaraes R, Bely N, et al. Intraabdominal serous fluid collections after appendectomy: a normal sonographic finding. AJR 1993;161:71–73.

28. Cobben LPJ, van Otterloss ADEM, Puylaert JBCM. Spontaneously resolving appendicitis. Frequency and natural history in 60 patients. Radiology 2000;215:349–352.

29. Migraine S, Atri M, Bret PM, et al. Spontaneously resolving

acute appendicitis. Clinical and sonographic documentation. Radiology 1997;205:55–58.

30. Hormann M, Paya K, Eibenberger K, et al. MR imaging in children with non-perforated acute appendicitis: value of unenhanced MR imaging in sonographically selected cases. AJR 1998;171:467–470.

31. Incesu L, Coskun A, Selcuk MB, et al. Acute appendicitis: MR imaging and sonographic correlation. AJR 1997;168:669–674.

32. Jamieson DH, Chait PG, Fillelr R. Interventional drainage of appendiceal abscesses in children. AJR 1997;169:1619–1622.

Other Appendiceal Problems

Mucoceles of the appendix are rare (1), as are tumors such as carcinoid tumors of the appendix (2). Inspissated mucoceles can be seen with cystic fibrosis (3), and the appendix also can be a lead point for intussusception. In addition, Crohn's disease has been noted to occasionally be confined to the appendix (4, 5). Adenocarcinoma of the appendix in childhood is rare (6).

REFERENCES

1. Madwed D, Mindelzun R, Jeffrey RB Jr. Pictorial essay. Mucocele of the appendix: imaging findings. AJR 1992;159:69–72.

2. Moertel CL, Weiland LH, Telander RL. Carcinoid tumor of the appendix in the first two decades of life. J Pediatr Surg 1990;25:1073–1075.

3. Coughlin JP, Gauderer MWL, Stern RC, et al. The spectrum of appendiceal disease in cystic fibrosis. J Pediatr Surg 1990;25:838–839.

4. Cohen WN, Denbesten L. Crohn's disease with predominant involvement of the appendix. AJR 1970;113:361–363.

5. Threatt B, Appelman H. Crohn's disease of the appendix presenting as acute appendicitis: report of 3 cases with a review of the literature. Radiology 1974;110:313–317.

6. Driver CP, Bowen J, Bruce J. Adenocarcinoma of the appendix in a child. J Pediatr Surg 1998;33:1437–1438.

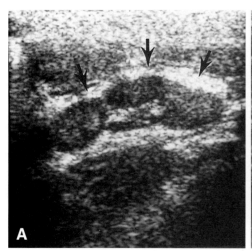
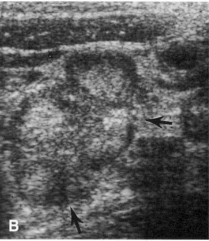

FIGURE 4.281. Mesenteric adenitis. A. Note a cluster of inflamed lymph nodes (arrows) surrounded by some echogenic inflamed mesenteric fat. **B.** Another patient with a cluster of large lymph nodes (arrows).

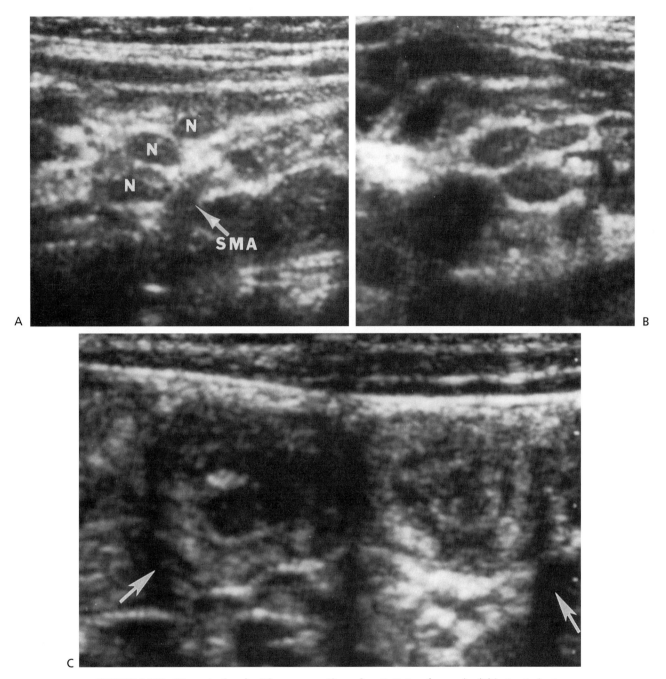

FIGURE 4.282. Mesenteric adenitis: para-aortic nodes. A. Note a few nodes (N) just anterior to the superior mesenteric artery (SMA). **B.** Just a little laterally, more nodes are seen embedded in mesentery. **C.** Slightly lateral to this, note two loops of jejunum (arrows) with thickened mucosa.

Mesenteric Adenitis and Enteritis

Mesenteric adenitis usually is viral in origin but also can be seen with *Yersinia enterocolitica* infections (1) and *Salmonella* infections (2, 3). The hallmark of this condition is the presence of inflamed, tender, and enlarged lymph nodes in the right lower quadrant (Fig. 4.281), but the problem usually is seen in association with inflammation the terminal ileum (ileitis) and even the cecum (4–6). The entire small bowel can be involved, usually segmentally, and it is not uncommon to encounter involvement of the jejunum (5). Furthermore, adenopathy frequently also is present in the small bowel mesentery, often best seen at its root in the para-aortic region. For this reason we have, for some years, referred to the condition not merely as

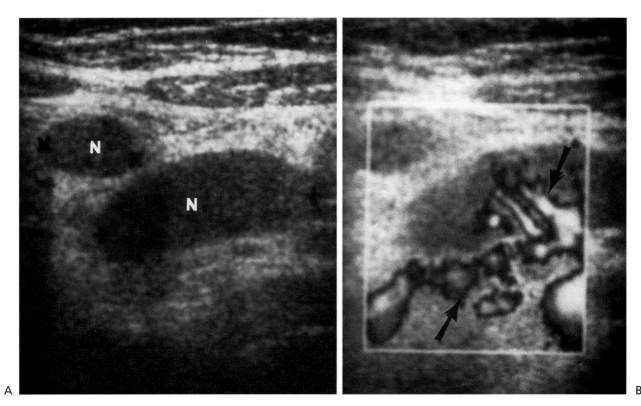

A   B

FIGURE 4.283. Mesenteric adenitis: color-flow Doppler. A. Note the enlarged lymph nodes
(N). **B.** Color-flow Doppler demonstrates marked increase blood flow (arrows) to the lymph nodes
and the surrounding soft tissues.

mesenteric adenitis, but **"mesenteric adenitis-enteritis."**
Pathophysiologically, although lymph node inflammation and
enlargement can be primary, they usually are secondary to
small bowel inflammation. **Therefore in the early stages
small bowel findings may predominate.** In a day or so,
lymph node involvement is seen. Lymph node involvement
and clinical findings are variable, just as they are with inflammatory adenopathy anywhere. Overall, lymph node enlargement is more prominent in infants and young children than in
older children and teenagers. Indeed, in the latter group symptoms may be striking and yet lymph node involvement often
is minimal, and small bowel changes subtle.

The hallmark of mesenteric adenitis, as noted earlier, is
the presence of enlarged and tender lymph nodes in the
right lower quadrant (Fig. 4.281) and in the root of the
mesentery in the paraaortic area (Fig. 4.282). At either site,
but more often in the paraaortic area, the lymph nodes may
show considerable clustering. The lymph nodes in the
mesentery are best seen through a left anterior flank
approach. Increased blood flow to the lymph nodes and
surrounding soft tissues (important) can be demonstrated
with color-flow Doppler (5) (Fig. 4.283). In this regard, the
enlarged lymph nodes often are surrounded by echogenic,
inflamed, and thickened, fatty mesentery (Fig. 4.282). The

lymph nodes can measure up to 2 cm in diameter, but most
often they are smaller and often are no more than 0.5–1 cm
in diameter (5). This is important to appreciate for lymph
nodes this small also can be normal (7). Therefore, size
alone cannot be used for diagnosis; the nodes also must be
tender and show increased blood flow. In this regard,
another CT study (8) indicated that enlarged mesenteric
lymph nodes in the patients without abdominal pain,
specifically a group of patients with blunt abdominal
trauma, were not found. In addition, it was indicated that
mesenteric adenitis can be primary (viral-induced mesenteric adenitis-enteritis) or secondary to some other GI
inflammatory problem such as Crohn's disease.

Mucosal changes in the terminal ileum, small bowel, and
at times the cecum, consist of circumferential smooth or
nodular mucosal thickening. In addition, with color-flow
Doppler hyperemia of the bowel wall will be seen. In the
terminal ileum nodular thickening of the mucosa is more
common (Fig. 4.284) but in the more proximal small bowel
both circumferential thickening and nodular thickening of
the intestinal mucosa are common (Figs. 4.285 and 4.286).
In most of these cases the bowel is hyperperistaltic and the
segments demonstrating mucosal thickening may be interspersed with dilated, hyperperistaltic fluid-filled segments

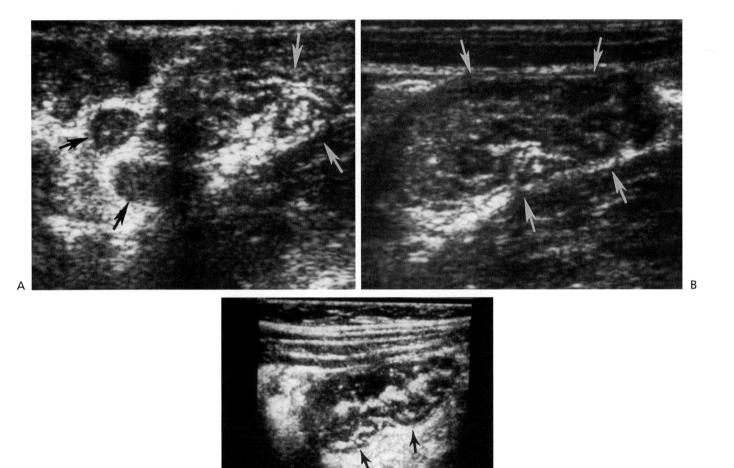

FIGURE 4.284. Mesenteric adenitis; terminal ileum. A. Note the enlarged lymph nodes (black arrows) embedded within echogenic mesentery. Just adjacent is intestine (terminal ileum) with mucosal thickening (white arrows). This represents a tangential view of the terminal ileum. **B.** Longitudinal view of the terminal ileum demonstrates enlargement (arrows), mucosal thickening, and some intramural lymph node enlargement. **C.** Another patient with nodular thickening of the mucosa of the terminal ileum (arrows). It is surrounded by echogenic, inflamed mesentery.

demonstrating no mucosal thickening (Fig. 4.286A). Hyperperistalsis of the segments of intestine demonstrating nodular or tortuous mucosal thickening (Fig. 4.286C) causes the peristalting intestine to resemble a churning bag of worms. Hence, the **"bag of worm sign"** (5). Transient intussusceptions also are common in these patients (Fig. 4.285E).

In some cases, the terminal ileum and surrounding lymph nodes are wrapped within thickened, echogenic mesentery, and an inflammatory mass develops, often resembling a phlegmon (Fig. 4.287). This pseudophlegmon can be become quite large and in the past has been referred to as **"giant" mesenteric adenitis**. However, in any of these

cases the inflammatory mass is not nearly as tender as the one produced by a true postappendiceal perforation phlegmon. In addition the normal appendix may be trapped within this inflammatory pseudomass (Fig. 4.287). At first, the appendix may appear to be the primary problem (Fig. 4.288). However, when there many lymph nodes present and the small bowel and terminal ileal mucosal changes are present, one will come to the conclusion that the appendix is secondarily involved. With color-flow Doppler, the inflamed appendix is not hyperemic. In addition, these appendices are compressible without significant pain.

The findings of mesenteric adenitis ileitis although demonstrable with CT (6, 8) are often not as clearly

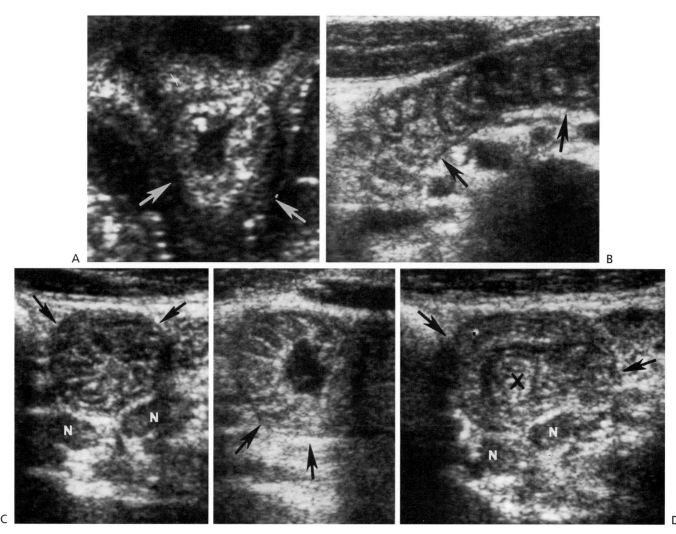

FIGURE 4.285. Mesenteric adenitis: small bowel findings. A. In this patient, a segment of distal jejunum demonstrates circumferential mucosal thickening (white arrows). **B.** A segment of jejunum (arrows) in the left upper quadrant of another patient demonstrates nodular mucosal thickening. **C.** Cross-sectional view of the same loop of jejunum demonstrates a nodular, "bag of worms" configuration (arrows). Note the enlarged lymph nodes (N) just below the loop. Echogenic mesentery surrounds the area. **D.** Moments later, the segment of jejunum opens (arrows). Note the nodular thickening of the mucosa and some hypoechoic fluid within the lumen. **E.** Moments later, a transient intussusception (X) is seen within the loop of jejunum (arrows). Note the enlarged lymph nodes (N).

depicted as with ultrasound. This is especially true of the fine detail mucosal changes seen in the terminal ileum and jejunum. Nonetheless the enlarged lymph nodes can be demonstrated, especially in obese patients (Fig. 4.289). **Nonetheless, as with appendicitis, ultrasound is our primary imaging tool for the evaluation of mesenteric adenitis-enteritis in children.**

REFERENCES

1. Sue K, Nishimi T, Yamada T, et al. A right lower abdominal mass due to *Yersinia* mesenteric lymphadenitis. Pediatr Radiol 1994;24: 70–71.
2. Arda IS, Ergin F, Varan B, et al. Acute abdomen caused by *Salmonella typhisuis* infection in children. J Pediatr Surg 2001;36: 1849–1852.

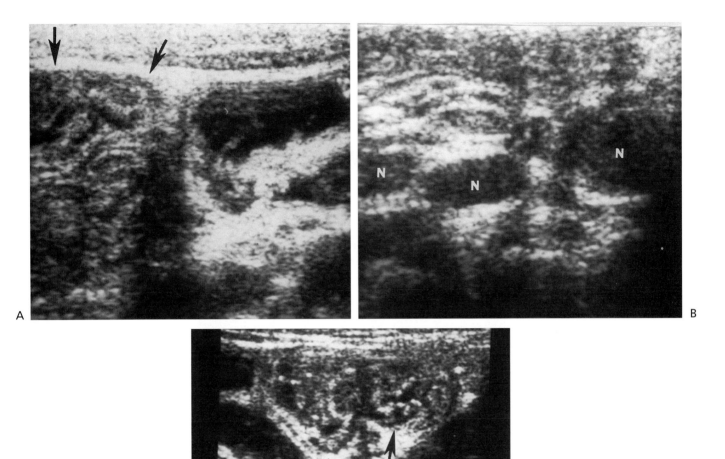

FIGURE 4.286. Nodular, tortuous mucosal fold thickening and "bag of worms" sign.
A. Note the nodular thickening of the mucosa in a loop of jejunum (arrows) in the left upper quadrant. Adjacent to it is a fluid-filled loop with no mucosal thickening. **B.** Just adjacent to this area is echogenic mesentery in which are embedded a number of enlarged lymph nodes (N). **C.** Another patient with two loops of jejunum showing nodular, tortuous thickening of the mucosa (arrows). When these loops are hyperperistaltic, they produce a constantly changing, kaleidoscopic picture resembling a "bag of worms."

3. Martin HCO, Goon HK. *Salmonella* ileocecal lymphadenitis masquerading as appendicitis. J Pediatr Surg 1986;21:377–378.
4. Puylaert JB. Mesenteric adenitis and acute terminal ileitis: ultrasound evaluation using graded compression. Radiology 1986;161:691–695.
5. Swischuk LE, John SD. Mesenteric adenitis-acute ileitis: a constellation of findings definable with ultrasound. Emerg Radiol 1998;5:210–218.
6. Rao PM, Rhea JT, Novelline RA. CT diagnosis of mesenteric adenitis. Radiology 1997;202:145–149.
7. Sivit CJ, Newman KD, Chandra RS. Visualization of enlarged mesenteric lymph nodes at US examination: clinical significance. Pediatr Radiol 1993;23:471–475.
8. Macari M, Hines J, Bathazar E, et al. Mesenteric adenitis CT diagnosis of primary versus secondary causes, incidence, and clinical significance in pediatric and adult patients. AJR 2002;178:853–858.

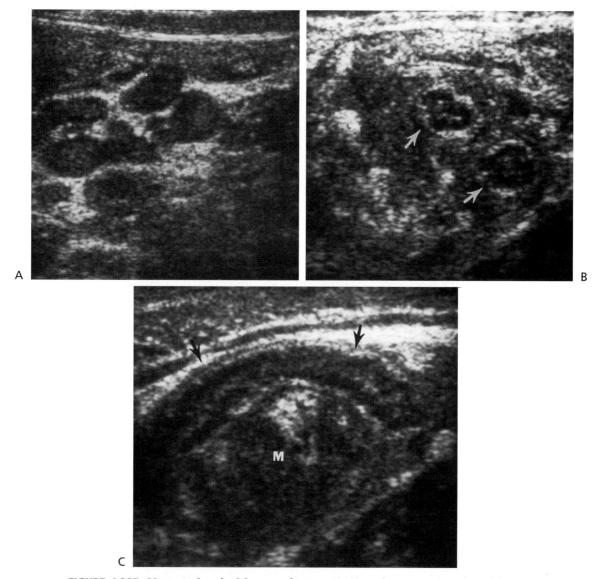

FIGURE 4.287. Mesenteric adenitis: pseudomass. A. Note the numerous enlarged hypoechoic lymph nodes in the right lower quadrant. **B.** Just adjacent is an inflammatory mass in which was embedded the appendix (arrows). The appendix is U-shaped and therefore seen on end twice. **C.** Longitudinal view through the area demonstrates the pseudomass (M) and the appendix (arrows) layered over it. There is no fluid in the appendix, but there is edema of the mucosa.

FIGURE 4.289. Mesenteric adenitis: CT findings. A. Note the enlarged nodes in the mesentery (arrows). **B.** In this patient, a number of enlarged nodes (arrows) are seen in the right lower quadrant. They are easy to see because of abundant fat.

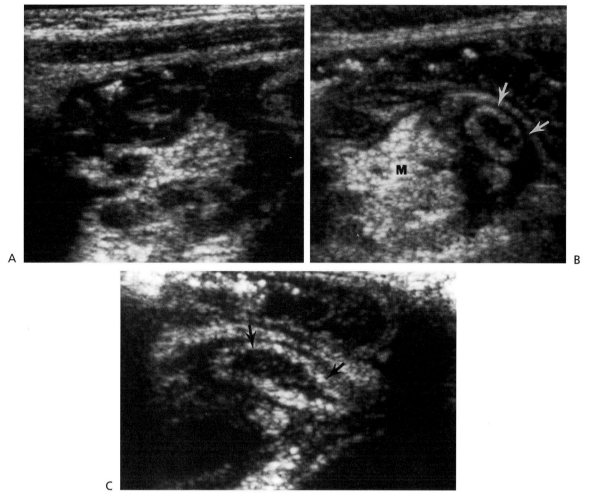

FIGURE 4.288. Mesenteric adenitis, appendiceal involvement. A. Note numerous hypoechoic lymph nodes embedded in echogenic mesentery in the right lower quadrant. **B.** The echogenic, inflamed mesentery (M) is again seen on this view. However, the appendix (arrows) is slightly enlarged and is seen adjacent to the inflamed mesentery. **C.** Longitudinal view through the appendix demonstrates slight thickening of the mucosa (arrows). The hypoechoic center is not due to fluid but rather edema of the mucosa. Such appendices are silent on color-flow Doppler and minimally or not tender and compressible on physical examination.

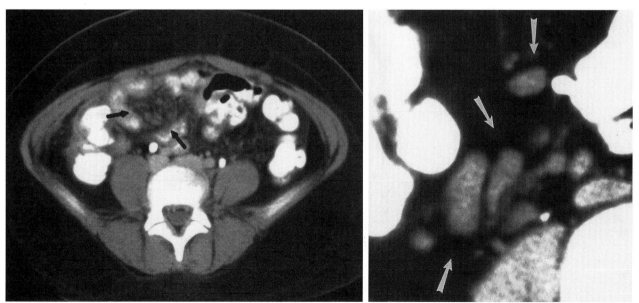

OTHER MISCELLANEOUS ABDOMINAL AND GASTROINTESTINAL ABNORMALITIES

Abdominal Abscess

Abdominal abscesses in infants and children most commonly occur after perforated appendicitis and overall abdominal abscess without preceding intestinal perforation or abdominal surgery, is uncommon. However, they can occur in immunosuppressed patients, patients with AIDS, and with chronic granulomatous disease (neutrophil dysfunction) of childhood. On plain films an intraabdominal abscess may present either as a solid mass or an area of amorphous gas and solid material (Fig. 4.290). In searching for an occult abscess, ultrasonography probably is one's best initial imaging modality. Abscesses usually are hypoechoic, but if they contain debris they are variably echogenic (Fig. 4.278A), and some may demonstrate debris-fluid levels. In assessing abscesses with ultrasound , one must be careful not to misinterpret a paralyzed loop of intestine for an abscess.

Other modalities used for detecting abscesses include CT (contrast enhanced), and gallium-67 and indium-111 white blood cell labeled scintigraphy. With CT studies the abscess presents as a mass, and if it contains air, the air is clearly visualized within the abscess. With contrast a rim of enhancement around the abscess frequently is seen. The center of the abscess does not enhance.

Abdominal Tuberculosis

The most common finding in abdominal tuberculosis in children is mesenteric adenopathy (1). This is followed by solid organ involvement where multiple granulomas can be seen, especially in the liver and spleen. Ascites also is relatively common (1).

REFERENCE

1. Andronikou S, Welman CJ, Kader E. The CT features of abdominal tuberculosis in children. Pediatr Radiol 2002;32:75–81.

Psoas Abscess

The psoas muscle can become abscessed (1–3) and although usually believed to be tuberculous in origin, most childhood abscesses on this continent are pyogenic. They can be drained percutaneously (4, 5). On plain films one usually sees nothing more than scoliosis resulting from psoas spasm, but on ultrasound and CT, the abscess is readily demonstrated within the psoas muscle. The findings are not very different from those seen with psoas muscle hematomas (Fig. 4.291).

REFERENCES

1. Parbhoo A, Govender S. Acute pyogenic psoas abscess in children. J Pediatr Orthop 1992;12;663–666.
2. Kleiner O, Cohen Z, Barki Y, et al. Unusual presentation of psoas abscess in a child. J Pediatr Surg 2001;36:1859–1860.
3. Prassopoulos PK, Giannakopoulou CA, Apostolaki EG, et al. Primary ilio-psoas abscess extending to the thigh in a neonate: US, CT and MR findings. Pediatr Radiol 1998;28:605–607.
4. Dib M, Bedu A, Garel C, et al. Ilio psoas abscess in neonates: treatment by ultrasound-guided percutaneous drainage. Pediatr Radiol 2000;30:677–680.
5. Kang M, Gupta S, Gulati M, et al. Ilio-psoas abscess in the paediatric population: treatment by US-guided percutaneous drainage. Pediatr Radiol 1998;28:478–481.

Psoas Hematoma

Psoas hematoma can occur after trauma or in patients with bleeding disorders. Psoas muscle spasm leads to scoliosis on plain films, and with ultrasound, during the early stages of the bleed, an echogenic mass is seen within the psoas muscle. Later, with liquefaction of the clot, a sonolucent abscess-like appearance develops (Fig. 4.291A). The findings also are demonstrable with CT (Fig. 4.291B).

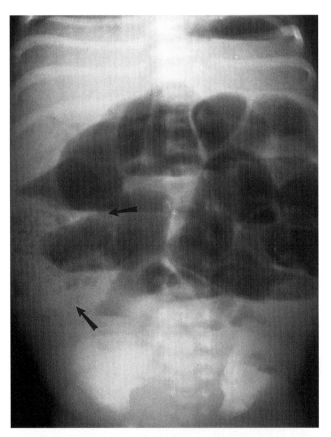

FIGURE 4.290. Abdominal abscess. Note the granular material in this right lower quadrant abscess (arrows) secondary to spontaneous small bowel perforation. Numerous distended loops of small bowel indicate partial functional obstruction.

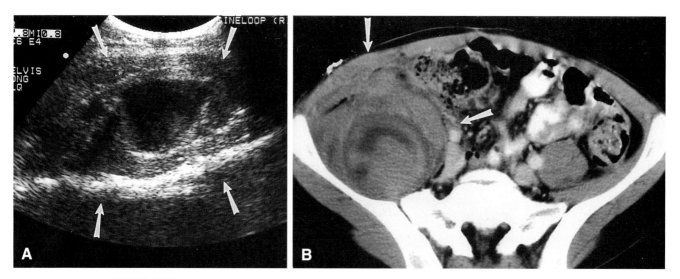

FIGURE 4.291. Psoas hematoma. A. Ultrasound demonstrates the expanded psoas muscle (arrows), which contains a hypoechoic fluid collection (blood). **B.** CT study demonstrates the typical concentric appearance of the hematoma (arrows).

Intestinal Infarction

Intestinal infarction usually is secondary to some mechanical problem such as volvulus, intussusception, or strangulated hernias. Occasionally, infarction can be seen secondary to arterial stenotic or occlusive disease or severe intestinal hypoperfusion (i.e., splanchnic shock). It also can be seen with sickle cell crisis. Focal schemia and infarction occurring in the fetus can lead to intestinal stenosis, atresia, or pseudocyst formation. The underlying problem in these cases is believed to be mesenteric vascular compromise secondary to arterial spasm, thrombosis, or embolism. If the problem occurs in the immediate postnatal period, perforation is the rule. In these cases schemia is believed to result from hypoperfusion, which often results from diversion of blood from the splanchnic circulation during episodes of perinatal hypoxia or anoxia (diving reflex). In older infants and children when mesenteric vessel thrombosis occurs, dehydration and/or sepsis are the common underlying problems. In addition, vascular thrombosis frequently is seen in infants delivered of diabetic mothers and also in patients with periarteritis nodosa (1).

Intestinal schemia and perforation of the GI tract also can occur following exchange transfusion and umbilical vessel catheterization. The etiology of such perforations is not certain, but reflex vascular spasm with subsequent intestinal schemia is most likely the problem.

REFERENCE

1. Oguzkurt P, Senocak ME, Ciftci AO, et al. Mesenteric vascular occlusion resulting in intestinal necrosis in children. J Pediatr Surg 2000;35:1161–1164.

Neonatal Sepsis

Neonatal sepsis usually is bacterial in origin, but viral sepsis also occurs. Clinically, infants with sepsis can present with lethargy, apneic spells, thrombocytopenia, abdominal distention, and feeding difficulties such as spitting up or vomiting. These findings are similar to those seen in infants with necrotizing enterocolitis except that pneumatosis does not usually develop. Radiographically, one of the first findings of sepsis is abdominal distention resulting from paralytic ileus of the intestines (Fig. 4.292A). This finding is nonspecific, but in the proper context, it is very suggestive. Another roentgenographic finding seen in sepsis is enlargement of the liver. This usually is readily apparent on plain films (Fig. 4.292, B and C).

Intraabdominal Calcifications

There are numerous causes of calcifications in the abdomen of newborn and young infants. Table 4.4 summarizes these conditions and many are illustrated in other parts of this book. Calcifications are relatively easy to identify on plain films or, better still, with CT. Their configurations and locations serve to differentiate them, one from another.

Fine curvilinear calcifications are seen with cysts, cystic tumors, pseudocysts of various abdominal organs, longstanding hydronephrotic kidneys, renal cortical necrosis, and meconium or plastic (hydrometrocolpos) peritonitis. In these latter cases, calcification of material extruded from the obstructed uterus through the fallopian tubes occurs. Irregular calcifications are seen with meconium or plastic peritonitis and with malignant tumors, inflamed lymph nodes, thromboemboli of various intraabdominal vessels, renal papillary necrosis, intestinal infarction and atresia, meco-

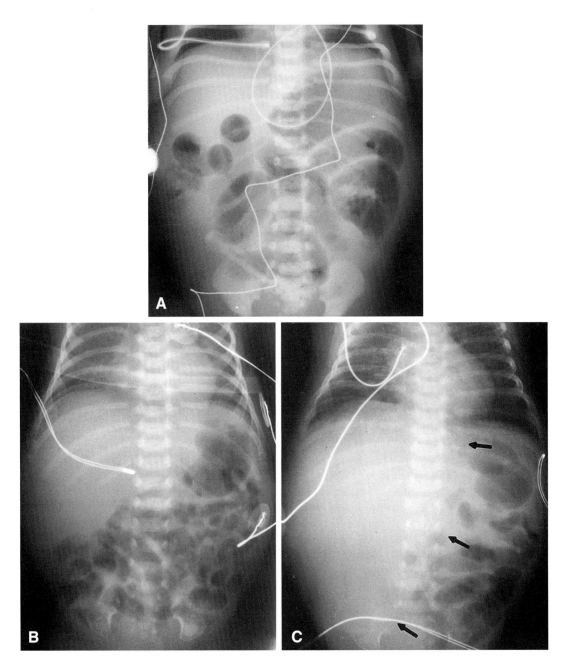

FIGURE 4.292. Neonatal sepsis. A. Note the marked distention of the small bowel, suggesting an obstruction in this patient with sepsis. The findings are the result of profound paralytic ileus. **B.** Another infant, not septic at the time, demonstrates a normal abdomen with a normal liver. **C.** With the development of sepsis, the liver shows marked enlargement (arrows).

nium peritonitis, and on a posthemorrhagic basis, in the adrenal gland. The latter also may be curvilinear and seen to outline the edge of the gland. Long, linear calcifications, located in the intestinal wall, can be seen with intestinal atresia, and pellet-like calcifications are seen with intraluminal meconium concretions. Most often, this occurs with imperforate anus where there is an associated urinary tract fistula, for it would appear that the presence of urine within the intestine enhances the calcifications to develop (1, 2).

Liver calcifications in the neonate can be the result of neonatal infections such as toxoplasmosis, herpes, and cytomegalic inclusion disease, or with thromboemboli associated with umbilical vein catheterization. The calcifications can be solitary or generalized in their distribution, and

TABLE 4.4. CAUSES OF NEONATAL ABDOMINAL CALCIFICATION

Abdominal wall
Fat necrosis
Calcium salt injection
Generalized fibromatosis
Peritoneal
Meconium peritonitis
Plastic peritonitis resulting from hydrometrocolpos
Hepatic
Primary tumor
Hemangioma
Hemangioendothelioma
Hepatoblastoma
Hamartoma
Metastatic tumor
Neuroblastoma
Portal vein thromboemboli
Vascular
Idiopathic arterial calcification
Portal vein thromboemboli
Inferior vena cava thrombus
Renal rein thrombosis
Retroperitoneal
Adrenal
Adrenal hemorrhage
Neuroblastoma
Wolman's disease
Renal
Cortical necrosis
Papillary necrosis
Renal vein thrombosis
Cystic disease
Hydronephrosis
Teratoma
Scrotal
Meconium peritonitis
Teratoma
Fat necrosis
Miscellaneous
Teratoma, fetus-in-fetu
Ovarian dermoid
Prune belly syndrome

Adapted from Kirks CR, Taybi H. Prune belly syndrome: of an unusual cause of neonatal abdominal calcification. *AJR* 1975;123:778–782, with permission.

some are incidentally discovered. Inflammatory calcifications in lymph nodes are not generally encountered in the neonate, but in older children such calcifications are more common. For the most part, they appear irregular or flocculent. Renal calculi and calcified gallstones are occasionally encountered in young infants but are rare in the neonate. They are, however, not uncommon in older children. Oval or tubular calcifications occur around thrombi of the portal or renal vein, or the inferior vena cava. Calcifications of the colon, bladder, and urachus due to stasis in the prune belly syndrome also have been reported (3). Most of these calcifications are demonstrated in the various sections of this

book pertaining to the specific diseases in which these calcifications occur.

REFERENCES

1. Selke AC Jr, Cowley CE. Calcified intraluminal meconium in a female infant with imperforate anus. AJR 1978;130:786–788.
2. Berdon WD, Baker DH, Wigger HJ, et al. Calcified intraluminal meconium in newborn males with imperforate anus: enterolithiasis in the newborn. AJR 1975;125:449–455.
3. Kirks DR, Taybi H. Prune belly syndrome: an unusual cause of neonatal abdominal calcification. AJR 1975;123:778–782.

Abdominal Foreign Bodies and Foreign Material

Children swallow and eat many things. Those that are opaque are generally readily visible on plain films and include a variety of metallic foreign bodies, dirt, pebbles, and clay (Fig. 4.293, A and B). Opacities, scattered throughout the intestine, also are commonly seen with medications such as Pepto-Bismol. In addition, lead ingestion results in dense, white-speckled material in the GI tract (Fig. 4.293C). Other heavy metals also produce dense, white foreign material in the GI tract, including mercury, which shows up as small, opaque globules. Iron tablets also can be seen (Fig. 4.293D), but often they are difficult to detect for they are faint and dissolve quickly (1).

As far as solitary foreign bodies are concerned, if they are round or oval and not too large, and have passed into the stomach, there is little problem with passage through the remainder of the GI tract. However, if they are long, straight, or pointed, they are likely to become impacted in the duodenum (Fig. 4.293, E and F). In the odd case, where an intraluminal obstructing lesion is present but unsuspected, cessation of progress of the foreign body through the GI tract may be the first finding to alert one to the presence of the underlying lesion (2) (Fig. 4.294). For this reason, once a foreign body is seen in the stomach or GI tract, it should be followed with x-rays until it passes, or is seen to pass, clinically.

Other manifestations of foreign bodies include visualization of bubble gum as a foreign body (3), and the fact that increased lead levels have been demonstrated in patients who ingest other foreign materials (4). This probably reflects the fact that infants who tend to ingest foreign bodies tend to ingest a variety of foreign bodies including lead flakes. Metallic foreign bodies can be removed with magnetic orogastric tubes (5).

REFERENCES

1. Everson GW, Oudjhane K, Young LW, et al. Effectiveness of abdominal radiographs in visualizing chewable iron supplements following overdose. Am J Emerg Med 1989;7:459–463.

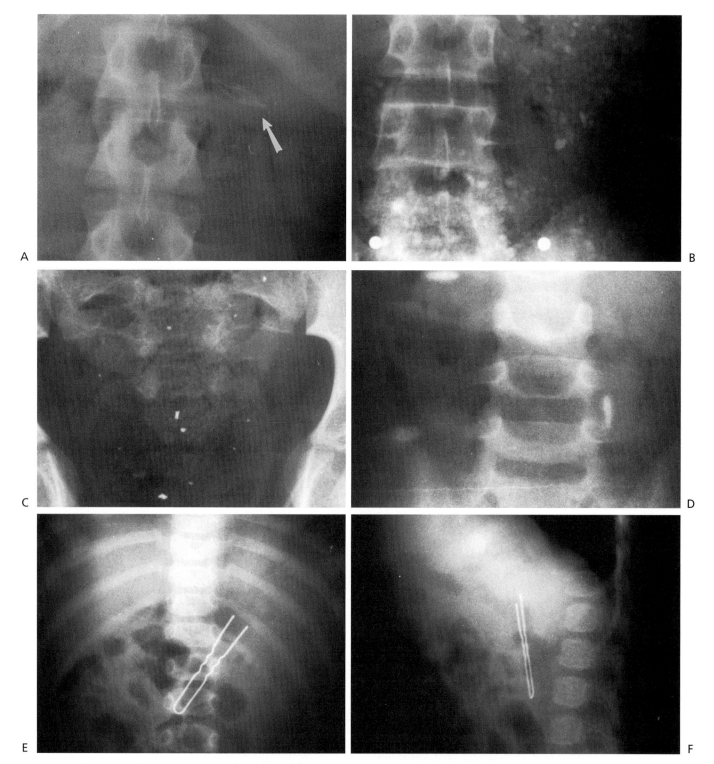

FIGURE 4.293. Foreign material in intestine. A. Note the aluminum pop-top (arrow) in the stomach. **B.** Scattered opacities in a clay eater. **C.** Dense, scattered flecks of lead. **D.** Note the numerous oval opacities resulting from ingestion of iron tablets. **E.** Metallic hairpin in the duodenal-jejunal junction region. **F.** Lateral view confirms posterior position of the hairpin.

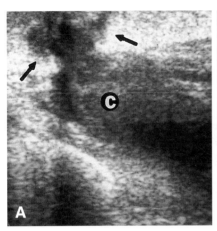 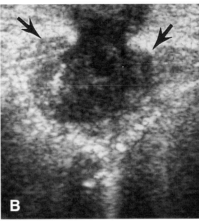

FIGURE 4.294. Infected urachal cyst remnant. A. On sagittal imaging, the debris-laden cyst (C) shows a small portion of it extending into the umbilical region (arrows). **B.** Cross-sectional view demonstrates the extension of the cyst (arrows) into the umbilical region.

2. Swischuk LE. Fever, cough and irritability. Pediatr Emerg Care 1999;15:280–282.
3. Geller E, Smergel EM. Bubble gum simulating abdominal calcifications. Pediatr Radiol 1992;22:298–299.
4. Wiley JF II, Henretig FM, Selbst SM. Blood lead levels in children with foreign bodies. Pediatrics 1992;89:593–596.
5. Paulson EK, Jaffe RB. Metallic foreign bodies in the stomach: fluoroscopic removal with a magnetic orogastric tube. Radiology 1990;174:191–194.

Abdominal Wall and Umbilical Abnormalities

Most abdominal wall and umbilical abnormalities are investigated with ultrasound or CT (1). In other cases, contrast material can be injected into fistulous communications between the umbilicus and incompletely involuted omphalomesenteric or urachal ducts and cysts. Umbilical hernia and omphalocele are, for the most part, not radiologic problems except that, in many cases of large omphalocele, small bowel malrotation and volvulus occur. Occasionally, umbilical hernias can strangulate and cause intestinal obstruction. Omphaloceles or umbilical hernias also commonly occur with the Beckwith-Wiedemann syndrome.

Gastroschisis is a condition in which there is herniation of the abdominal contents through a **focal, nonmidline defect** of the abdominal musculature. It is generally considered to be separate from omphalocele, and in terms of etiology it has been suggested that the problem results from intrauterine interruption of the omphalomesenteric artery blood supply (2). However, no one really knows why the defect occurs, and in both gastroschisis and omphalocele, postoperative intestinal problems include adhesions, malrotation, decreased intestinal motility, and chylous ascites (3). Occasional cases of familial gastroschisis occur (4).

Defects of the midabdominal wall associated with diaphragmatic, sternal, cardiac, and pericardial midline defects constitute a syndrome of mesodermal midline defects (5, 6).

Aneurysm of the paraumbilical vein is rare (7) but can be demonstrated with ultrasound. Spigelian hernias (8) can be demonstrated with ultrasound or CT.

REFERENCES

1. Nagasaki A, Handa N, Kawanami T. Diagnosis of urachal anomalies in infancy and childhood by contrast fistulography, ultrasound and CT. Pediatr Radiol 1991;21:321–323
2. Hoyme HE, Higginbottom MC, Jones KL. The vascular pathogenesis of gastroschisis: intrauterine interruption of the omphalomesenteric artery. J Pediatr 1981;98:228–231.
3. Lloyd DA. Gastroschisis, malrotation, and chylous ascites. J Pediatr Surg 1991;26:106–107.
4. Nelson TC, Toyama WM. Familial gastroschisis. A case of mother-and-son occurrence. J Pediatr Surg 1995;30:1706–1708.
5. Casey BM, Neiman H, Gallagher T, et al. Syndrome of mesodermal defects involving the abdominal wall, diaphragm, sternum, heart and pericardium. Br J Radiol 1975;48:52–54.
6. Spitz L, Bloom KR, Milner S, et al. Combined anterior abdominal wall, sternal diaphragmatic, pericardial, and intracardiac defects: a report of five cases and their management. J Pediatr Surg 1975;10:491–496.
7. Goktay AY, Secil M, Kovanlikaya A, et al. Aneurysmal dilatation of the paraumbilical vein in an infant. Pediatr Radiol 2000;30:604–606.
8. Iuchtman M, Kessel B, Kirshon M. Trauma-related acute spigelian hernia in a child. Pediatr Emerg Care 1997;13:404–405.

Retroperitoneal Fibrosis

Retroperitoneal fibrosis is uncommon in children and virtually unheard of in infants. Characteristically, it produces obstruction of the urinary tract and is of unknown etiology (1, 2).

REFERENCES

1. Snow BW, Garrett RA. Retroperitoneal fibrosis in children (eosinophilic and idiopathic). Urology 1984;23:569–572.

2. Sherman C, Winchester P, Brill PW, et al. Childhood retroperitoneal fibrosis. Pediatr Radiol 1988;18:245–247.

Retroperitoneal Fascitis

Retroperitoneal fascitis, a diffuse necrotizing infection, is uncommon but can be seen in infants and children (1). The findings can be demonstrated with ultrasound or CT (1) and consist of thickening of the retroperitoneal fascia with areas of fluid collection. The abdominal wall also can be involved.

REFERENCE

1. Retroperitoneal necrotizing fasciitis in a 4-year-old girl. J Pediatr Surg 1998;33:778–780.

Omental Torsion and Infarction

Primary omental torsion in children is rare (1–3), but can present as an acute abdominal problem. The abnormality can be imaged with CT or ultrasound, or even MR. The findings are those of a nonspecific mass. Similar findings can be seen with omental infarction (4, 5). In both instances. a heterogenous mass is identified between the abdominal wall and the colon (5)

REFERENCES

1. Chew DKW, Holgersen L-Ol, Friedman D. Primary omental torsion in children. J Pediatr Surg 1995;30:816–817.
2. Oguzhurt P, Kotilouglu E, Tanyel FC, et al. Primary omental torsion in a 6-year-old girl. J Pediatr Surg 1995;30:1700–1701.
3. Phillips BJ, Mazaheri MK, Matthews MR, et al. Imitation appendicitis: primary omental torsion. Pediatr Emerg Care 1999;15:271–273.
4. Myers MT, Grisoni ER, Sivit CJ. Segmental omental infarction in a 9-year-old girl. Emerg Radiol 1997;4:112–114.
5. Gratton-Smith JD, Blews DE, Brand T. Omental infarction in pediatric patients: sonographic and CT findings. AJR 2002;178:1537–1539.

Abdominal Findings with Immunosuppression (AIDS)

A number of abdominal findings can be seen in immunosuppressed patients, especially those with AIDS (1–4). Candidiasis is one of the most common infections of the esophagus, but herpes simplex virus and cytomegalovirus also can involve the esophagus. For the most part, changes consist of ulcerations or nodular (cobblestone) mucosal thickening. As far as the stomach and small bowel are concerned, cytomegalovirus is usually the underlying problem and results in mucosal ulcerations secondary to a vasculitis. All of these conditions can produce granulomas in the liver and spleen.

Thickening of the mucosal folds of the stomach can be seen with *Helicobacter* infections, cryptosporidiosis, and lymphoproliferative disorders, some of which are associated with Epstein-Barr virus infection. *Mycobacterium avium-intracellulare* complex and *Mycobacterium tuberculosis* infections tend to produce large mesenteric lymph nodes. *M. avium-intracellulare* complex infections also can produce thickening or nodularity of the intestinal mucosal folds. AIDS-related lymphoma can appear almost anywhere in the abdomen and involve almost any organ.

Obviously the pathologic changes associated with immunosuppression are varied and extensive. Their complete discussion is beyond the scope of this book, and an excellent review of the subject is present in the article by Haller and Cohen (3).

REFERENCES

1. Day DL, Carpenter BLM. Abdominal complications in pediatric bone marrow transplant recipients. Radiographics 1993;13:1101–1112.
2. Haller JO. Imaging the gastrointestinal tract of children with AIDS. Pediatr Radiol 1995;25:94–96.
3. Haller JO, Cohen HL. Review: gastrointestinal manifestations of AIDS in children. AJR 1994;162:387–393.
4. Siskin GP, Haller JO, Miller S, et al. AIDS-related lymphoma: radiologic features in pediatric patients. Radiology 1995;196:63–66.

Abdominal Complications from Various Tubes in the Abdomen

With the advent of prolonged intubation of infants for feeding and the use of long-term intravenous hyperalimentation, a variety of complications secondary to tubes going astray or perforating various organs (1) have become commonplace. Abdominal complications associated with ventriculoperitoneal shunts include pseudocyst accumulations of cerebral spinal fluid, scrotal migration of the catheter (2), migration of catheters elsewhere, and intestinal perforation. The most common problem, however, is pseudocyst formation, and although these cysts can be visualized on plain films, they are more readily detected with ultrasonography or CT (Fig. 4.252). Nasoduodenal or jejunal tubes most commonly lead to perforation as a complication, and perforation can occur into the peritoneal cavity (3, 7, 9) or into another organ such as the kidney (1, 2).

REFERENCES

1. McAlister WH, Siegel MJ, Shackelford GD, et al. Intestinal perforations by tube feedings in small infants: clinical and experimental studies. AJR 1985;145:687–692.
2. Crofford MJ, Balsam D. Scrotal migration of ventriculoperitoneal shunts. AJR 1983;141:369–371.

Blunt Abdominal Trauma

Injury to the various organs in blunt abdominal trauma has been covered in sections dealing with these organs throughout Chapters 4 and 5. At this point, however, one might appreciate that both ultrasound and CT are often used in the investigation of blunt abdominal trauma. However, more and more it has been determined that ultrasound is not adequate (1, 2). It can miss many injuries. Ultrasound probably has its most usefulness in the detection of massive collections of peritoneal fluid (blood), a finding that would mitigate toward immediate surgical intervention (3, 4). Otherwise, ultrasound can be misleading for it has been determined that if no fluid is demonstrated (5), it does not necessarily mean that there is no underlying organ injury. **Overall, CT is best for the evaluation of blunt abdominal trauma to the abdomen in the pediatric age group (6) and indeed, probably across the entire population. It provides most information about most organs and in addition can demonstrate the presence of free fluid and free air.** It is not necessary that oral contrast be used; in fact, it probably delays the study (7–10).

Gastrointestinal perforations secondary to blunt trauma often are occult and are best detected with CT (6, 11, 12). The findings may be subtle but consist of increased enhancement of thickened bowel wall in the area of injury and the presence of free air and fluid (13). The findings of increased enhancement of the bowel wall are due to hypoperfusion and must be differentiated from similar findings seen on a diffuse basis with hypovolemic shock (14). In the latter cases, although the small bowel wall becomes hyperintense after the administration of intravenous contrast material, it is not thickened. A similar phenomenon has been noted with the adrenal gland (15).

Seat belt injuries are not as common in childhood as they are in adulthood. Nonetheless they do occur. Very often they are associated with "Chance" fractures of the lumbar spine and when this fracture is detected, one should be alerted to the possible presence of underlying intestinal injury. The findings can be quite subtle, and it therefore behooves close inspection of the intestines and abdomen. Strictures after such injuries can be a complication (16). Chylous ascites, resulting from blunt abdominal trauma, is a rare complication (17).

REFERENCES

1. Benya EC, Lim-Dunham JE, Landrum O, et al. Abdominal sonography in examination of children with blunt abdominal trauma. AJR 2000;174:1613–1616.
2. Mutabagani KH, Coley BD, Zumbewrge N, et al. Preliminary experience with focused abdominal sonography for trauma (FAST) in children: is it useful? J Pediatr Surg 1999;34:48–54.
3. Bode PJ, Edwards, MJR, Kruit MC, et al. Sonography in a clinical algorithm for early evaluation of 1671 patients with blunt abdominal trauma. AJR 1999;172:905–911.
4. Lentz KA, McKenney MG, Nunez DB Jr, et al. Evaluating blunt abdominal trauma: role for ultrasonography. J Ultrasound Med 1996;15:447–451.
5. Shanmuganathan K, Mirvis SE, Sherbourne CD, et al. Hemoperitoneum as the sole indicator of abdominal visceral injuries: a potential limitation of screening abdominal US for trauma. Radiology 1999;212:423–430.
6. Sivit CJ, Frazier AA, Eichelberger MR. Computed tomography of pediatric blunt abdominal trauma. Emerg Radiol 1997;4:150–166.
7. Ryan SP, Gaisie G, Kraus RA. CT scanning of children with blunt abdominal trauma—is oral contrast useful? Emerg Radiol 2000;7:212–217.
8. Shanker KR, Lloyd DA, Kitteringham L, et al. Oral contrast with computed tomography in the evaluation of blunt abdominal trauma in children. Br J Surg 1999;86:1073–1077.
9. Beierle EA, Chen MK, Whalen TV, et al. Free fluid on abdominal computed tomography scan after blunt trauma does not mandate exploratory laparotomy in children. J Pediatr Surg 2000;35:990–993.
10. Taylor CA, Sivit CJ. Posttraumatic peritoneal fluid: is it a reliable indicator of intraabdominal injury in children? J Pediatr Surg 1995;30:1644–1648.
11. Ciftci AO, Tanyel AB, Salman, et al. Gastrointestinal tract perforation due to blunt abdominal trauma. Pediatr Surg Int 1998;13: 259–264.
12. Strouse PJ, Close BJ, Marshall KW, et al. CT of bowel and mesenteric trauma in children. Radiographics 1999;19:1237–1250.
13. Sivit CJ, Eichelberger MR, Taylor GA. CT in children with rupture of the bowel caused by blunt trauma: diagnostic efficacy and comparison with hypoperfusion complex. AJR 1994;163: 1195–1198.
14. Sivit CJ, Taylor GA, Bulas DI, et al. Post-traumatic shock in children: CT findings associated with hemodynamic instability. Radiology 1992;182:723–726.
15. O'Hara SM, Donnelly LF. Intense contrast enhancement of the adrenal glands: another abdominal CT finding associated with hypoperfusion complex in children. AJR 1999;173:995–997.
16. Lynch JM, Albanese CT, Meza MP, et al. Intestinal stricture following seat belt injury in children. J Pediatr Surg 1996;31: 1354–1357.
17. Beal AL, Gormley CM, Gordon DL, et al. Chylous ascites: a manifestation of blunt abdominal trauma in an infant. J Pediatr Surg 1998;33:650–652.

5

GENITOURINARY TRACT AND ADRENAL GLANDS

Ultrasonography is the primary imaging modality used in the investigation of urinary tract disease in infants and children. It has taken the place of intravenous pyelography, and even computed tomography (CT) and magnetic resonance imaging (MRI) have failed to make a significant dent in its use. Radionuclide studies, on the other hand, have remained intact. The most useful agent for nuclear scintigraphy studies is technetium-99m diethylenetriaminepentaacetic acid (DTPA) because it affords physiologic (excretory) and anatomic data. However, for focused cortical imaging, agents such as glucoheptonate and dimercaptosuccinic acid (DMSA) are required. With these agents, an image is obtained comparable to the nephrogram obtained during the early stage of an intravenous pyelogram or arteriogram, and as a result, these agents have become extremely useful in the detection of renal scars or areas of focal inflammation.

The voiding cystourethrogram remains the most important study with which to evaluate the lower urinary tract, especially in males, in whom evaluation of the urethra is most important. Although nuclear cystography also is useful for the detection of ureterovesicular reflux, it provides no information regarding urethral anatomy in males. This is not a problem in females, and the nuclear cystogram can, and often does, serve as the initial imaging study of the lower urinary tract in females. It also is liberally used to follow reflux in both sexes but cannot replace the voiding cystourethrogram for grading reflux.

UPPER URINARY TRACT

Normal Anatomy

There are certain differences in the appearance of the kidneys in the neonate and young infant as compared with the appearance of the kidneys in older children. In neonates and infants, the renal cortex is much thinner, fetal lobulations can be quite marked, and the medullary pyramids are prominent and, on ultrasonography, often hypoechoic (Fig. 5.1). This latter configuration of the medullary pyramids should not be misinterpreted as renal cysts. Neonatal kidneys often are more spherical than those seen in older children, but as far as the neonatal and infantile bladder is concerned, there are no real differences from findings in older children. There are any number of methods for determining renal size or volume from ultrasound studies (1–3), a summary of which is presented in Figure 5.2.

In the neonate and up to the age of 2–3 months, normal kidneys are sonographically more echogenic than are those of older infants and children. Echogenicity is equal to or greater than that of the liver, but after 2–3 months, the renal cortex assumes the adult appearance and becomes less echogenic than the liver (Fig. 5.3). It has been suggested that the increase in cortical echogenicity in neonates and young infants is secondary to the fact that there are more glomeruli in the renal cortex in neonates and that 20% of the loops of Henle lie within the cortex rather than the medulla (4). It is presumed that all of this results in an increased number of acoustical interfaces and increased echogenicity. However, if echogenicity of the neonatal kidney parenchyma greatly surpasses that of liver, one should suspect underlying renal parenchymal disease. This finding, even though nonspecific, still is a sensitive marker for the presence of parenchymal disease. The same holds true for older infants and children, when parenchymal echogenicity equals or surpasses that of the liver.

In the neonate, a transient increase in echogenicity of the papillae of the medullary pyramids can be seen with lower nephron nephrosis (5–8). This phenomenon results from the precipitation of Tamm-Horsfall proteinuria and, on intravenous urography, is manifested by a markedly prolonged nephrogram. Dehydration and the injection of hyperosmolar contrast agents aggravate the problem. However, the phenomenon is temporary and self-limiting, and the kidneys shortly return to normal echogenicity (Fig. 5.4). On CT, the renal pyramids appear hypodense (9).

Central echoes in the normal kidney result from a conglomeration of normal structures, primarily the collapsed renal pelvis and parapelvic (sinusoidal) fat. In some instances, the renal pelvis may show a small amount of fluid (urine) in it; this occurs if the patient is undergoing diure-

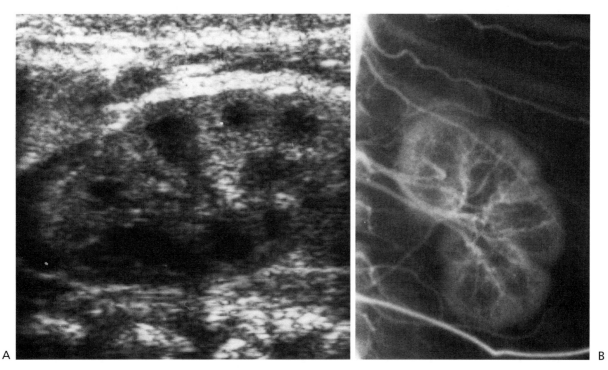

FIGURE 5.1. A. Normal kidneys. Ultrasonogram demonstrates prominent medullary pyramids in the neonate producing sonolucencies that can be misinterpreted for cysts. **B.** Nephrographic stage of aortogram demonstrates the same prominent medullary pyramids and the relatively thin cortex.

Average Age*	Interval*	Mean Renal Length (cm)	SD	n
0 mo	0–1 wk	4.48	0.31	10
2 mo	1 wk–4 mo	5.28	.66	54
6 mo	4–8 mo	6.15	.67	20
10 mo	8 mo–1 yr	6.23	.63	8
1½	1–2	6.65	.54	28
2½	2–3	7.36	.54	12
3½	3–4	7.36	.64	30
4½	4–5	7.87	.50	26
5½	5–6	8.09	.54	30
6½	6–7	7.83	.72	14
7½	7–8	8.33	.51	18
8½	8–9	8.90	.88	18
9½	9–10	9.20	.90	14
10½	10–11	9.17	.82	28
11½	11–12	9.60	.64	22
12½	12–13	10.42	.87	18
13½	13–14	9.79	.75	14
14½	14–15	10.05	.62	14
15½	15–16	10.93	.76	6
16½	16–17	10.04	.86	10
17½	17–18	10.53	.29	4
18½	18–19	10.81	1.13	8

*Years unless specified otherwise.

FIGURE 5.2. Renal size: ultrasonographic measurements. Normal measurements. (From Rosenbaum DM, Korngold E, Teele RL. Sonographic assessment of renal length in normal children. AJR 1984;142:467–469, with permission.)

sis or if the bladder is full and causing backpressure on the upper tracks. The problem is temporary and of no particular consequence, but it is worth reexamining the patient after voiding to determine whether dilation persists.

Finally, consideration of one or two other normal variations that mimic pathology is in order. One of these configurations results because the kidney fuses from two primitive masses. In some cases, a residual, oblique, echodense stripe of nonrenal, fatty tissue can be seen to cross the kidney through its upper pole. This stripe is called the parenchymal or interrenicular junction line (10) or Odonno's sulcus (11). If it is only partially seen, it is referred to as the interrenicular ridge (Figs. 5.5 and 5.6) or junctional parenchymal defect (Fig. 5.6). It is important that one not misinterpret the junctional parenchymal defect or the junction line for a renal scar. More commonly, fusion of these masses is more complete, and only a wedge-like echogenic triangle of fibrous tissue along the outer aspect of the kidney, the so-called junctional parenchymal defect (12, 13), is seen (Fig. 5.6). This finding should not be misinterpreted as a renal scar.

The resistive index is higher in infants younger than 6 months of age than in adults. We do not use it very often, although others find it more useful. Usually, however, there is too much overlap between normal and abnormal for it to be of value. It measures resistance to intrarenal blood flow. Ultrasound is also useful for recording Doppler waveforms (14), which are illustrated in Figure 5.7. Column of Bertin

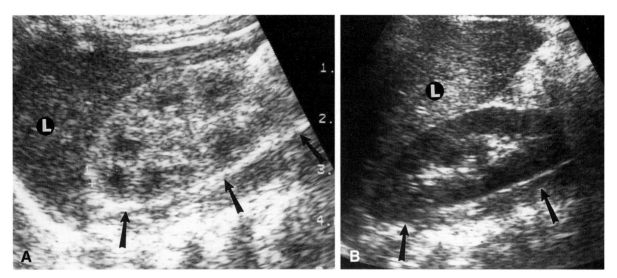

FIGURE 5.3. Normal kidney, ultrasonographic findings. A. In this neonatal kidney (arrows), note the prominent sonolucent medullary pyramids and echogenic cortex. Cortical echogenicity is greater than that of the liver (L). **B.** Older infant demonstrates the typical adult pattern with central echoes and a sonolucent outer parenchyma (arrows). The parenchyma is much more sonolucent than the adjacent liver (L).

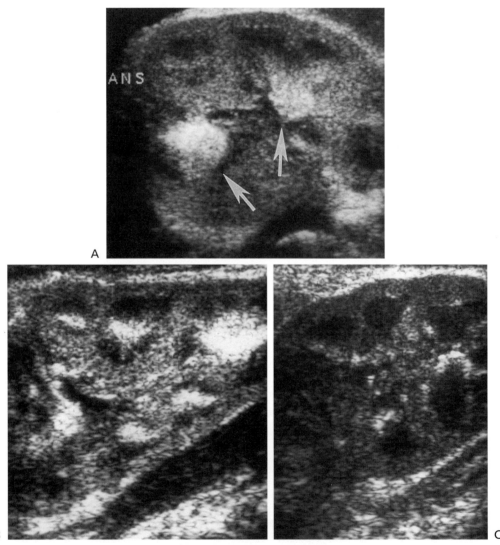

FIGURE 5.4. Lower nephron nephrosis. A. Note the hyperechogenic medullary pyramids (arrows) in this neonate with lower nephron nephrosis. **B.** Another patient with similar findings. **C.** One week later the kidney has a normal appearance. The medullary pyramids are now sonolucent.

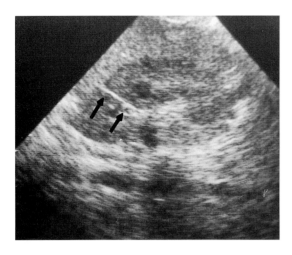

FIGURE 5.5. Interrenicular ridge. Note the echogenic band (arrows) through the upper pole of the kidney.

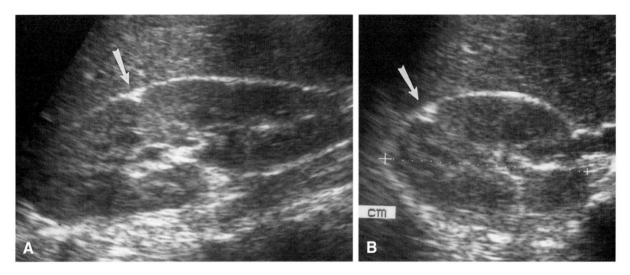

FIGURE 5.6. Junctional parenchymal defect. A. Note a small, but characteristic, triangular echogenicity in the upper pole of the kidney (arrow). **B.** Same defect (arrow) on cross-section.

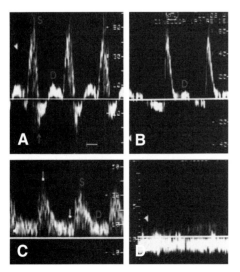

FIGURE 5.7. Normal Doppler tracings of the aorta, renal artery, and its branches. A. Characteristic aortic tracing demonstrates a high systolic peak (S), a rapid drop-off, slight inversion below the baseline (arrow), and then flat diastolic flow (D). **B.** Main renal artery demonstrates a prominent systolic peak, rapid drop-off, no inversion below the baseline, and a flat configuration of the diastolic runoff (D). **C.** Intrarenal artery demonstrates a less pronounced systolic peak (S) and a sloping diastolic (D) runoff pattern. **D.** Venous tracing demonstrates a flat, uniform flow pattern.

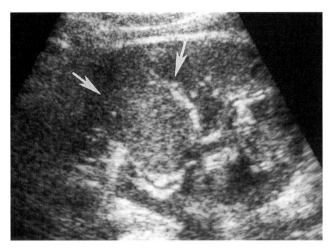

FIGURE 5.8. Column of Bertin. Note the prominent column of Bertin (arrows) between calyces. A mass could be erroneously suggested.

hypertrophy also needs to be addressed. This finding represents a column of normal renal parenchyma that can hypertrophy between medullary pyramids and mimic an intrarenal tumor (Fig. 5.8).

The kidney also is readily identified with MRI and CT. CT scanning, however, requires the injection of contrast agents, and with ultrasound being so productive, there is a minimal role for CT and MRI in the investigation of renal problems other than those associated with trauma, tumors, and chronic obstruction.

REFERENCES

1. Blane CE, Bockstein F, DiPietro M, et al. Sonographic standards of normal infant kidney length. AJR 1985;145:1289–1292.
2. Han BK, Babcock DS. Sonographic measurements and appearance of normal kidneys in children. AJR 1985;145:611–616.
3. Zerin JM, Blane CE. Sonographic assessment of renal length in children: a reappraisal. Pediatr Radiol 1994;24:101–106.
4. Hricak H, Slovis TL, Callen CW, et al. Neonatal kidneys: sonographic-anatomic correlation. Radiology 1983;147:699–702.
5. Avni EF, Robberecht MS, Lebrun D, et al. transient acute tubular disease in the newborn: characteristic ultrasound pattern. Ann Radiol 1983;26:175–182.
6. Nakamura M, Yokota K, Chen C, et al. Hyperechoic renal papillae as a physiological finding in neonates. Clin Radiol 1999;54:233–236.
7. Riebel TW, Abraham K, Wartner P, et al. Transient renal medullary hyperechogenicity in ultrasound studies of neonates: is it a normal phenomenon and what are the causes? J Clin Ultrasound 1993;21:25–31.
8. Starinsky R, Vardi O, Batasch D, et al. Increased renal medullary echogenicity in neonates. Pediatr Radiol 1995;25:S43–S45.
9. McLaughlin MG, Swayne LC, Rubenstein JB, et al. Transient acute tubular dysfunction in the newborn: CT findings. Pediatr Radiol 1990;20:363–364.
10. Kenney IJ, Wild RS. The renal parenchymal junctional line in children: ultrasonic frequency and appearances. Br J Radiol 1987;60:865–868.
11. Currarino G, Lowichik A. The Oddono's sulcus and its relation to the renal "junctional parenchymal defect" and the "interrenicular septum." Pediatr Radiol 1997;27:6–10.
12. Hoffer FA, Hanabergh AM, Teele RL. The interrenicular junction: a mimic of renal scarring on normal pediatric sonograms. AJR 1985;145:1075–1078.
13. Yeh H-C, Halton KP, Shapiro RS, et al. Junctional parenchyma: revised definition of hypertrophic column of Bertin. Radiology 1992;185:725–732.
14. Friedman DM, Schacht RG. Doppler waveforms in the renal arteries of normal children. J Clin Ultrasound 1991;19:387–392.

ANOMALIES OF THE UPPER URINARY TRACT

Many anomalies, some significant and some insignificant, are encountered in the upper urinary tract, and the following brief review of the embryologic development of the kidneys and ureters can aid in understanding them. The renal parenchyma is derived, for the most part, from the primitive metanephros, which arises from mesenchymal tissue in the presacral area. This primitive tissue is often referred to as the nephrogenic blastema, and it eventually contributes to the development of nearly all of the renal parenchyma. As the primitive metanephros migrates upward and matures, it takes the form of the normal kidney. A specific rotation also occurs, and whereas the renal pelvis originally points ventrally, a gradual inward and medial turning takes place. Any arrest along this line results in an abnormal orientation of the kidney and some degree of malrotation.

The ureteric bud develops as an outpouching from the metanephric or wolffian duct at a site near the cloaca. It soon separates from the wolffian duct and opens into the portion of the cloaca destined to become the urinary bladder. Thereafter, the ureteric bud grows upward and eventually meets with the primitive renal parenchymal tissue. At its upper end, it forms the renal pelvis and then divides to form the renal calyces, straight renal collecting tubules, and the papillary ducts. The cloaca eventually forms the larger portion of the bladder and urethra, and the wolffian duct descends and helps to form the epididymis, ejaculatory duct, and vas deferens in the male. In the female, the wolffian duct system all but disappears, and the mullerian ducts give rise to the female internal genitalia. All of this is very complicated, and so it should be no surprise that complex anomalies related to these structures often arise.

Associated vascular changes occur with ascent of the kidney, and although the blood supply originally is derived primarily from pelvic vessels, as the kidney rises, these old vessels disappear, and new vessels appear at progressively higher levels. For this reason, an abnormally arrested kidney usually has an anomalous blood supply.

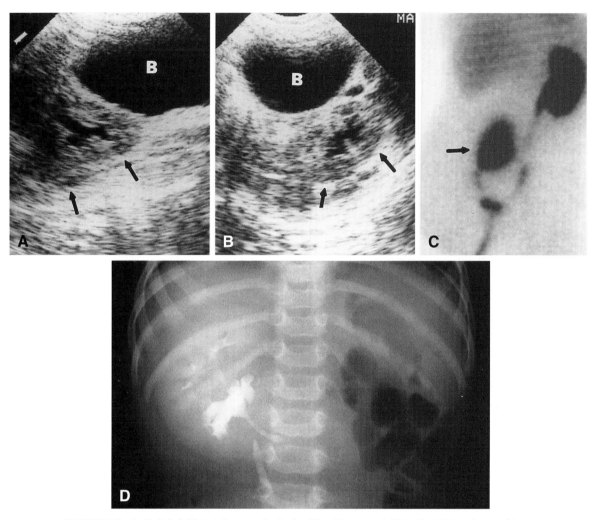

FIGURE 5.9. A. Pelvic kidney demonstrated with ultrasound. Note the kidney (arrows) just next to the urinary bladder (B). **B.** Transverse sonogram demonstrates the pelvic kidney (arrows). B, bladder. **C.** Nuclear scintigraphy demonstrating an ectopic right pelvic kidney (arrow). **D.** Intravenous pyelogram demonstrates crossed, fused ectopia in which both kidneys are on the right and fused.

Anomalies of Renal Position and Fusion

Anomalies of renal position range from minor degrees of unilateral malposition to totally abnormal positioning of both kidneys. Perhaps the most common variation is one in which the kidney is just a little lower in position than usual. However, when there is virtually no ascent of the kidney, and the kidney remains in the pelvis, often in proximity to the bladder, the so-called pelvic kidney results. In other instances, one kidney may lie across midline and be fused to the other kidney, producing the so-called crossed fused ectopy (Fig. 5.9). When both kidneys are low in position and fused across their lower poles, the typical horseshoe kidney results (Fig. 5.10).

None of these anomalies is particularly difficult to identify, and once one notes the absence of a kidney from its normal position, one should begin looking throughout the abdomen to determine whether it is truly absent or just ectopic. Ectopic kidneys, in addition being out of their normal place, tend to show lack of echogenic sinus fat (1). With horseshoe kidneys, the first clue to their presence may be that the right kidney (usually the first kidney to be imaged) lies more toward midline than usual. The horseshoe configuration is most clearly visible on cross-sectional images with any imaging modality (Fig. 5.10).

REFERENCE

1. Barnewolt CE, Lebowitz RL. Absence of a renal sinus echo complex in the ectopic kidney of a child: a normal finding. Pediatr Radiol 1996;26:318–323.

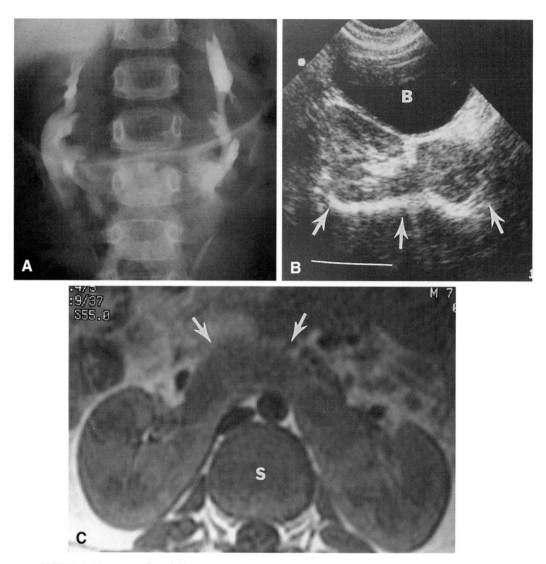

FIGURE 5.10. Horseshoe kidney. A. Intravenous pyelogram demonstrates the typical configuration of a horseshoe kidney. The kidneys are malrotated and their lower poles fused as they lie over the spine. **B.** Ultrasonogram in another patient demonstrates the characteristically fused lower poles (arrows) of a horseshoe kidney. B, urinary bladder. **C.** T1-weighted MR image in another patient demonstrates a fused, horseshoe kidney (arrows). S, spine.

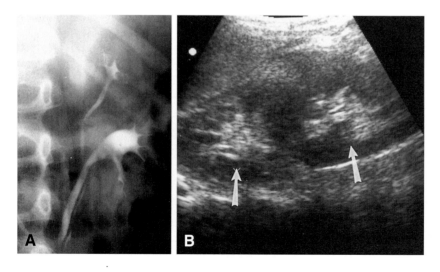

FIGURE 5.11. Renal duplication. A. Typical urographic findings of bilateral duplicated kidneys. **B.** Ultrasonogram of the left kidney demonstrates double central echoes (arrows) originating from the duplicated renal sinuses, pelves, and calyces. They are separated by normal hypoechoic renal parenchyma.

Renal Duplication

Complete duplication of the kidney, so that a separate ureter is present for each portion, may not be readily apparent with ultrasound. In these cases, the ureter may be duplicated throughout its course or may join the other ureter somewhere along the way. Furthermore, the ureter from the upper kidney may terminate ectopically and be associated with an ectopic ureterocele. These ureters, if not dilated, generally are not detected with ultrasound. Simple renal duplication, in which duplication is confined to the kidney, is of no particular consequence (Fig. 5.11).

Localized Upper Pole Caliceal Dilation

Localized upper pole caliceal dilation occurs most often in older children (Fig. 5.12) but can be seen in infancy. Usually, it is the right upper pole calyceal system that is involved, and it is usually an insignificant finding resulting from vascular compression of the infundibulum. On the other hand, a few children may experience pain with the condition, but this is a tenuous association, and for the most part, in the right upper pole or, rarely, the left upper pole, localized calyceal dilation should be evaluated with caution and probably considered normal.

Renal Hypoplasia and Agenesis

Hypoplasia or agenesis of one kidney is not uncommon and is believed to result from loss of vascular supply in utero. With renal agenesis, in addition to the kidney being absent, the ipsilateral ureter and hemitrigone also usually are absent. With renal hypoplasia, the kidney is a miniature of itself, and angiographically, the renal artery is small. When both kidneys are hypoplastic, renal insufficiency may ensue, and with both unilateral and bilateral disease, hypertension can occur.

With unilateral renal agenesis, anomalies of the contralateral kidney (1), maybe, and compensatory hypertrophy of the other kidney usually are evident (1–3). It has been determined that this represents true hypertrophy with an increase of nephrons (4), and with unilateral renal agenesis, there very frequently is duplication of the mullerian duct system (5). In such cases, unilateral hydrometrocolpos, on the side of renal agenesis of a duplicated uterus, is common (6, 7).

When a kidney is absent on either side, the hepatic or splenic flexures of the colon (depending on the side) occupy the space of the corresponding renal fossa and become displaced and distorted in their configuration (5, 8). Such malposition of these flexures may herald the presence of unsuspected unilateral renal agenesis.

Bilateral renal agenesis is rare in general but much more common in males. However, it does occur in females (9) and can be seen in families. Both unilateral and bilateral renal agenesis have been documented in a single family (10). Potter (11) described a characteristic facial appearance in infants with bilateral renal agenesis consisting of large, low-set, cartilage-deficient ears; prominent epicanthal folds; hypertelorism; nasal flattening; and micrognathia. Many of these infants are stillborn, and others remain alive for only a short time. Renal agenesis is clearly just one facet of this abnormality, because along with the other problems described, bilateral pulmonary hypoplasia is common. This associated abnormality can lead to severe respiratory distress and often to complicating pneumothorax and pneumomediastinum. Other anomalies of the genitourinary tract and gastrointestinal system are common. The condition also has been referred to as the fetal compression syndrome, because most of the abnormalities are believed to result from com-

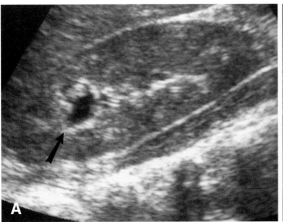
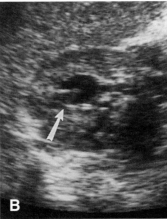

FIGURE 5.12. Upper pole calyceal dilation. A. Note the dilated right upper pole calyx (arrow). **B.** Another patient demonstrating a similar finding (arrow), but in this case, the echogenic renal papilla is seen projecting into the calyx.

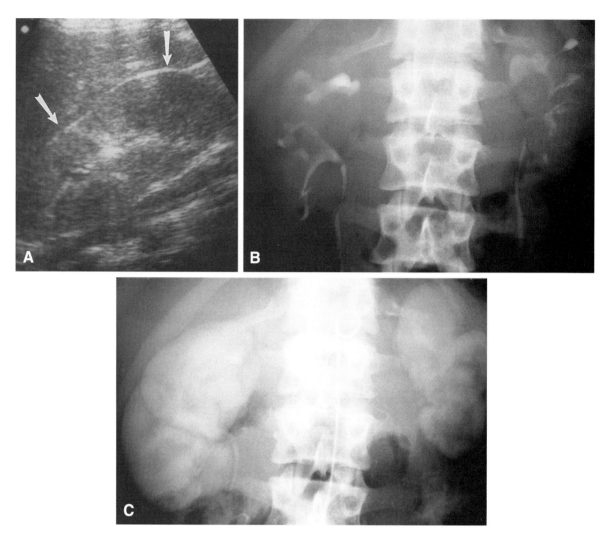

FIGURE 5.13. Ask-Upmark kidney. A. Ultrasonogram demonstrates the left kidney (arrows) to be echogenic without normal architecture. Peculiar echogenic bands coursing through the kidney also are seen. **B.** Intravenous pyelogram demonstrates the characteristic calyceal deformity. **C.** Nephrogram showing the deformed, lumpy kidneys. The left kidney is smaller than the right.

pression of the fetus secondary to oligohydramnios as the result of decreased urine output.

A rare cause of bilateral renal hypoplasia is renal hypoplasia with oligonephronia (12). Histologically, there is hypertrophy of the nephrons, and radiographically, the only significant finding is that of small kidneys, which eventually become nonfunctional. Segmental renal hypoplasia-dysplasia is seen in the Ask-Upmark kidney (Fig. 5.13) and is associated with hypertension. It is seen in older children and occasionally in infants (13). After birth, renal hypoplasia, or perhaps more accurately, atrophy, can result from renal vein thrombosis, renal artery obstruction, chronic infection, and reflux.

If a patient is suspected of having renal agenesis or hypoplasia, the best diagnostic tool is the ultrasonogram.

With this examination one can readily determine whether a kidney is present and, if so, whether it demonstrates abnormal echogenicity (Fig. 5.14). Thereafter, there is very little need for any other imaging modality. However, in cases of renal agenesis or renal hypoplasia, the adrenal gland may hypertrophy to the point where it erroneously suggests that a kidney is present (14, 15) (Fig. 5.15).

REFERENCES

1. Atiyeh B, Husmann D, Baum M. Contralateral renal abnormalities in patients with renal agenesis and noncystic renal dysplasia. Pediatrics 1993;91:812–815.
2. O'Sullivan DC, Dewan PA, Guiney EJ. Compensatory hyper-

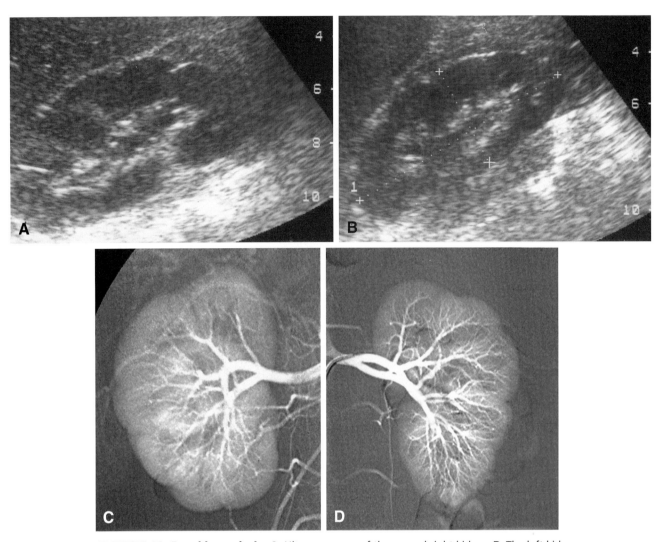

FIGURE 5.14. Renal hypoplasia. A. Ultrasonogram of the normal right kidney. **B.** The left kidney at first glance also might appear normal. However, it is smaller than the right kidney. **C.** Renal arteriogram on the right demonstrates a normal right kidney with normal intrarenal branches. **D.** On the left, the kidney is smaller, as is its supplying renal artery. The intrarenal branches, however, appear normal. This patient had systemic hypertension.

trophy effectively assesses the degree of impaired renal function in unilateral renal disease. Br J Urol 1992;69:346–350.

3. Glazabrook KN, McGrath FP, Steele BT. Prenatal compensatory renal growth: documentation with US. Radiology 1993;189: 733–735.

4. Maluf NSR. On the enlargement of the normal congenitally solitary kidney. Br J Urol 1997;79:836–841.

5. McDermott V, Orr JD, Wild SR. Duplicated mullerian duct remnants associated with unilateral renal agenesis. Abdom Imaging 1993;18:193–195.

6. Cohen RC, Davey RB, LeQuesne GW. Ultrasonography in the diagnosis and management of unilateral hematometrocolpos and associated renal agenesis. Aust Paediatr J 1982;18:287–290.

7. Radhakrishnan J, Reyes HM. Unilateral renal agenesis with hematometrocolpos: report of two cases. J Pediatr Surg 1982; 17:749–750.

8. Mascatello V, Lebowitz RL. Malposition of the colon in left renal agenesis and ectopia. Radiology 1976;120:371–376.

9. Rizza JN, Downing SE. Bilateral renal agenesis in two female siblings. Am J Dis Child 1971;121:60–63.

10. Kohn G, Borns PF. The association of bilateral and unilateral renal aplasia in the same family. J Pediatr 1973;83:95–97.

11. Potter EL. Bilateral absence of ureters and kidneys, report of fifty cases. Obstet Gynecol 1965;25:3–12.

12. Carter JE, Lirenman DS. Bilateral renal hypoplasia with oligomeganephronia. Am J Dis Child 1970;120:537–542.

13. Benz G, Willich E, Scharer K. Segmental renal hypoplasia in childhood. Pediatr Radiol 1976;5:86–92.

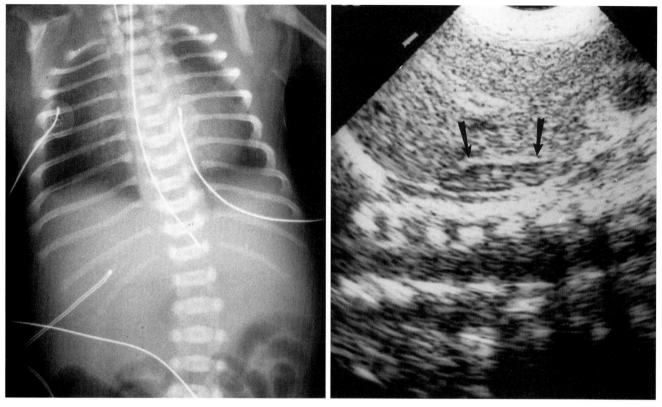

A B

FIGURE 5.15. Renal agenesis: Potter's syndrome. A. In this patient with Potter's syndrome, note that the lungs, although clear, are small. The heart is a little enlarged secondary to pulmonary hypertension. **B.** Sonogram demonstrates absence of the right kidney. The visible structure (arrows) is the adrenal gland.

14. McGahan JP, Myracle MR. Adrenal hypertrophy; possible pitfall in the sonographic diagnosis of renal agenesis. J Ultrasound Med 1986;5:265–268.
15. Silverman PM, Carroll BA, Moskowitz PS. Adrenal sonography in renal agenesis and dysplasia. AJR 1980;134:600–602.

URINARY TRACT INFECTION

Urinary tract infection in the neonate is not as common as that in older children and adults, and in the neonatal period, it is believed to be associated with neonatal sepsis. In this age group, very few infections result from urinary tract obstruction, and although there is a definite preponderance of females to males after the age of 3–6 months, males predominate in the neonatal period.

Urinary tract infections acquired after the neonatal period usually result from contamination of the urinary tract by organisms inhabiting the perineum. This is particularly true in girls, in whom contamination of the urethra with perineal organisms occurs quite readily. In boys, urinary tract infections more often are related to obstructive uropathy, but they also can be related to contamination by perineal organisms, especially those growing under the pre-

puce in uncircumcised individuals (1, 2). Whatever the cause and whether it is a male or female, after the first documented infection, ultrasonography (3, 4) should be performed. This imaging modality provides instant information regarding size, shape, and echotexture of the kidneys and about whether hydronephrosis or hydroureter is present. It also provides information related to the urinary bladder.

In a few cases of infection, the kidneys may show increased size (i.e., edema) and echogenicity (5) (Fig. 5.16), but our experience is that most are normal. Color flow Doppler also can be used in the evaluation of urinary tract infections and, in cases of pyelonephritis, shows increased flow to the kidney (6–8). It is not necessary in every case but is helpful when unilateral disease is present and when areas of lobar nephronia or abscesses are seen, because these areas demonstrate decreased flow. In terms of lobar nephronia, a focal area of hematogenous bacterial nephritis produces inflammation and small vein thrombosis (9, 10). Depending on the degree of associated hemorrhaging and thrombosis, the involved area is variably hyperechoic (Fig. 5.17). With DMSA cortical scintigraphy, lobar nephronia produces an area of photon deficiency (i.e., cold spot in the kidney).

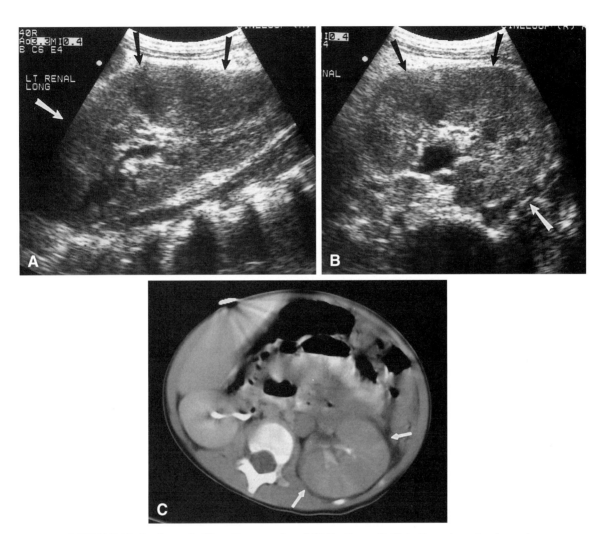

FIGURE 5.16. Pyelonephritis: ultrasound and CT findings. A. Note the enlarged, echogenic left kidney (arrows). It has, for the most part, lost its normal corticomedullary differentiation. **B.** Transverse view through the kidney (arrows) demonstrates the degree to which the kidney had enlarged and its abnormal parenchymal pattern. **C.** CT study demonstrates the left kidney to be enlarged (arrows), and although it shows function, function is less than on the right.

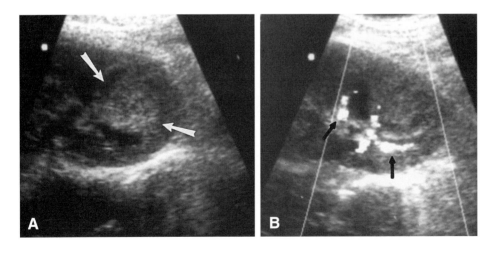

FIGURE 5.17. Lobar nephronia. A. Note the echogenic area (arrows) in the lower pole of the right kidney. **B.** Color flow Doppler demonstrates blood flow to the kidney (arrows) but none to the area of the lobar nephronia.

During the past decade, nuclear scintigraphy using cortical imaging agents such as DMSA and glucoheptonate has been advocated as the first study to be obtained (11, 12). The studies obtained when these imaging agents are used are quite sensitive in detecting areas of focal nephritis and possible eventual scarring (Fig. 5.18). However, these studies have not replaced the sonogram as the initial imaging procedure. One of the reasons is that it is not certain at this stage whether one must have the information provided by the cortical agents to adequately treat the patient. This information is probably unnecessary, because if scarring is going to occur, it will occur whether the initial insult is demonstrated or not. A scar in itself is not the real problem; it is whether enough scarring is present to result in complications such as hypertension, and hypertension is best evaluated clinically.

Renal scarring can be focal or diffuse and involve the entire kidney (Fig. 5.19). The latter condition is easier to detect with ultrasound. The kidneys are small and show loss of cortex with an abnormal corticorenal sinus ratio (Fig. 5.20). The outline of the kidney may be irregular. Focal scarring is much more difficult to detect with ultrasonography and is more readily detected with nuclear scintigraphy using cortical imaging agents (13). MRI also can detect areas of focal nephritis and scarring but is not in common use (14). When advanced scarring of one kidney occurs, the other kidney exhibits compensatory hypertrophy.

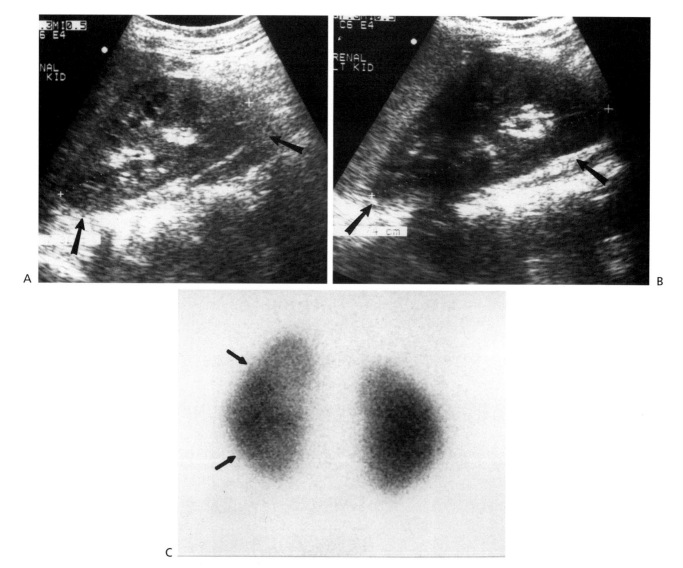

FIGURE 5.18. Acute pyelonephritis: value of cortical imaging. A. The right kidney is normal (arrows). **B.** The left kidney is a little enlarged and slightly hypoechoic (arrows). **C.** Glucoheptonate study demonstrates uneven uptake in the left kidney, which also is larger than the right. Uptake in the right kidney is uniform and normal.

A word about pyonephrosis is in order. Pyonephrosis exists when the collecting systems are hydronephrotic and full of purulent (bacterial) exudate. The problem also is common with *Candida* or other fungal infections, and in cases of pyogenic origin, urine-pus fluid levels can be seen in the dilated pelvis and calyces (Fig. 5.20).

Voiding cystourethrography also must be performed when investigating urinary tract infection and, in males, should be obtained early in the course of the disease (i.e., after the first documented infection). It is necessary to exclude lower urinary tract obstructive uropathy, primarily from posterior urethral valves. Otherwise, cystourethrography often is postponed until the urinary tract infection is under control and treated because acute infection alone can temporarily alter the ureterovesicular junction configuration and allow reflux to occur. As a result, one cannot decide whether reflux is temporary or permanent. However, not all agree with this stance. We usually postpone performance of the study until the infection subsides (i.e., after 6–8 weeks of antibiotic therapy).

For girls, because there is such a low incidence of obstructive urethral pathology, there is a greater tendency to perform scintigraphic cystography instead of the formal voiding cystourethrogram. The scintigraphic cystogram is sensitive in demonstrating high grades of reflux but not as effective in demonstrating minimal degrees of reflux. However, such reflux is of questionable clinical significance, and in favor of the scintigraphic cystogram, there is less radiation delivered to the patient. It has not universally replaced the voiding cystourethrogram and certainly cannot replace the initial study in males when urethral obstructive pathology is being sought. Because it is not possible to adequately

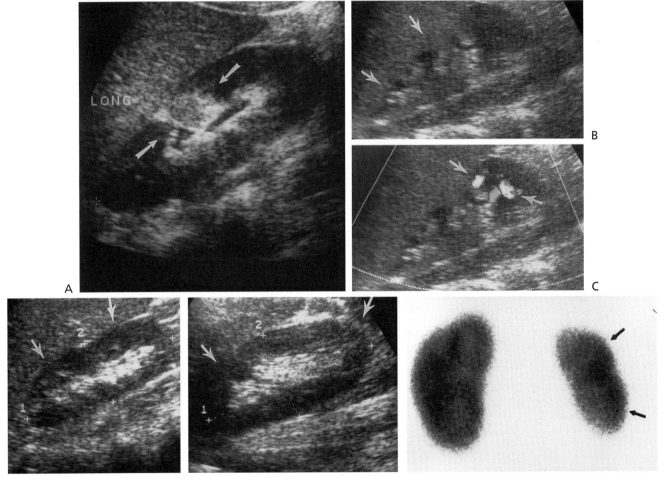

FIGURE 5.19. Renal scarring. A. Note the focal renal scar (arrows). The remainder of the kidney is unremarkable. **B.** In this patient, the upper two thirds of the right kidney are scarred and atrophic (arrows). **C.** With color flow Doppler, blood flow is seen only to the residual normal lower pole (arrows). **D.** In this patient, the right kidney is smaller than normal but still has surrounding parenchyma (arrows). **E.** The left kidney is larger and more normal appearing (arrows). **F.** Glucoheptonate study demonstrates a normal left kidney but a small right kidney (arrows).

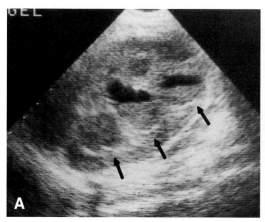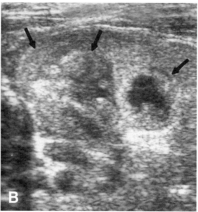

FIGURE 5.20. Pyonephrosis. A. In this patient, the calyces (arrows) are full of debris and demonstrate debris-urine levels. **B.** Another patient with dilated calyces full of debris (arrows).

grade reflux with the scintigraphic cystogram, there is no uniform policy on this issue.

REFERENCES

1. Wiswell TE, Smith FR, Bass JW. Decreased incidence of urinary tract infections in circumcised male infants. Pediatrics 1985;75: 901–903.
2. Wiswell TE, Enzenauer RW, Holton ME, et al. Declining frequency of circumcision: implications for changes in the absolute incidence and male to female sex ratio of urinary tract infections in early infancy. Pediatrics 1987;79:338–342.
3. Hayden CK Jr, Swischuk LE, Fawcett HD, et al. Urinary tract infections in childhood: a current imaging approach. Radiographics 1986;6:1023–1038.
4. Jequier S, Forbes PA, Nogrady MB. The value of ultrasonography as a screening procedure in a first-documented urinary tract infection in children. J Ultrasound Med 1985;4:393–400.
5. Winkler P, Altrogge H. Sonographic signs of nephritis in children. A comparison of renal echography with clinical evaluation, laboratory data and biopsy. Pediatr Radiol 1985;15:231–237.
6. Eggli KD, Eggli D. Color Doppler sonography in pyelonephritis. Pediatr Radiol 1992;22:422–425.
7. Dacher J-N, Pfister C, Monroc M, et al. Power Doppler sonographic pattern of acute pyelonephritis in children: comparison with CT. AJR 1996;166:1451–1455.
8. Winters WD. Power Doppler sonographic evaluation of acute pyelonephritis in children. J Ultrasound Med 1996;15:91–96.
9. Rathmore MH. Barton LL, Luisiri A. Acute lobar nephronia: a review. Pediatrics 1991;87:728–734.
10. Rigsby CM, Rosenfield AT, Glickman MG, et al. Hemorrhagic focal bacterial nephritis: findings on gray-scale sonography and CT. AJR 1986;146:1173–1177.
11. Benador N, Slosman DO, et al. Cortical scintigraphy in the evaluation of renal parenchymal changes in children with pyelonephritis. J Pediatr 1994;124:17–20.
12. Conwaty JJ, Cohn RA. Evolving role of nuclear medicine for the diagnosis and management of urinary tract infection. J Pediatr 1994;124:87–90.
13. Lavocat MP, Granjon D, Allard D, et al. Imaging of pyelonephritis. Pediatr Radiol 1997;27:159–165.
14. Lonergan GJ, Pennington DJ, Morrison JC, et al. Childhood pyelonephritis: comparison of Gadolinium-enhanced MR imag-

ing and renal cortical scintigraphy for diagnosis. Radiology 1998;207:377–384.

Candida Pyelonephritis

Candida renal infection of the premature infant is not uncommon (1–3). It also is a cause of sepsis and subsequent osteomyelitis in these patients. In terms of urinary tract infection, the collecting systems become impacted with *Candida* fungus balls, and obstruction can be so complete that anuria can result. Ultrasonographically, the debris within the collecting systems produces areas of focal increased echogenicity (i.e., fungal balls) in the calyces (Fig. 5.21A). In more aggressive cases, destruction of the parenchyma occurs (1). To alleviate the hydronephrosis caused by the impaction of the collecting system, one may need to resort to percutaneous nephrostomy drainage (4). *Candida* renal infection also is commonly seen in immunocompromised patients. One also can see fungus balls in the urinary bladder (Fig. 5.21 B).

REFERENCES

1. Berman LH, Stringer DA, St. Onge O, et al. An assessment of sonography in the diagnosis and management of neonatal renal candidiasis. Clin Radiol 1989;40:577–581.
2. Cohen HL, Haller JO, Schechter S, et al. Renal candidiasis of the infant: ultrasound evaluation. Urol Radiol 1986;8:17–21.
3. Kintanar C, Cramer BC, Reid WD, et al. Neonatal renal candidiasis: sonographic diagnosis. AJR 1980;135:1205–1210.
4. Matsumoto AH, Dejter SW Jr, Barth KH, et al. Percutaneous nephrostomy drainage in the management of neonatal anuria secondary to renal candidiasis. J Pediatr Surg 1990;25:1295–1297.

Tuberculous Urinary Tract Infection

Renal tuberculosis is not as common in children as it adults. Initially, the lesion is not visible radiographically (1) and

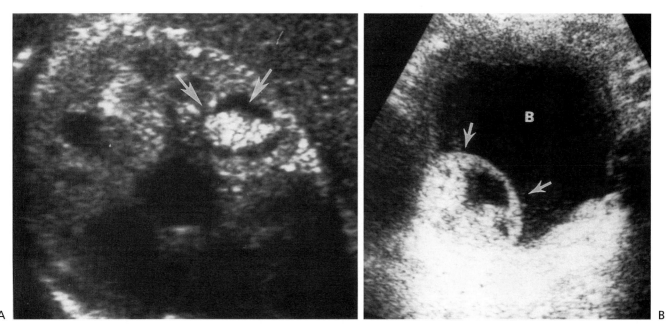

FIGURE 5.21. *Candida infection.* **A.** Note an echogenic fungus ball (arrows) in a dilated calyx. Debris fills other calyces **B.** A large fungus ball (arrows) is present in the bladder.

occurs in the cortical glomerular arterioles. Eventually, it passes down the nephrons to form papillary granulomas. The papillae are destroyed, the calyces become dilated, and parenchyma is involved.

REFERENCE

1. Cremin B. Radiological imaging of urogenital tuberculosis in children with emphasis on ultrasound. Pediatr Radiol 1987;17:34–38.

Xanthogranulomatous Pyelonephritis

This entity is much less common in children than in adults. It results from longstanding chronic, refractory renal infections, with xanthomatous debris accumulating in markedly dilated collecting systems (1–5). As a result, virtually no cortex remains, and when the thin layer of cortex is seen to outline the markedly dilated renal pelvis and calyces, the so-called "bear claw" sign is seen (Fig. 5.22). Some cases may present as an abdominal mass (6).

REFERENCES

1. Cousins C, Soners J, Broderick N, et al. Xanthogranulomatous pyelonephritis in childhood: ultrasound and CT diagnosis. Pediatr Radiol 1994;24:210–212.
2. Hughes PM, Gupta SC, Thomas NB. Xanthogranulomatous pyelonephritis in childhood. Clin Radiol 1990;41:360–362.
3. Hugosson C, Ahmed S, Sackey K, et al. Focal xanthogranuloma-
tous pyelonephritis in a young child. Pediatr Radiol 1994;24: 213–215.
4. Takamizawa S, Yamataka A, Kaneko K, et al. Xanthogranulomatous pyelonephritis in childhood. A rare but important clinical entity. J Pediatr Surg 2000;35:1554–1555.
5. Youngson GG, Gray ES. Neonatal xanthogranulomatous pyelonephritis. Br J Urol 1990;65:541–542.
6. Zia-ul-Miraj M, Cheema MA. Xanthogranulomatous pyelonephritis presenting as a pseudotumor in a 2-month-old boy. J Pediatr Surg 2000;35:1256–1258.

Sarcoid Nephritis

Sarcoid involvement of the kidney in childhood is rare but does occur. In one report (1), ultrasound demonstrated echogenic masses while CT demonstrated low-density lesions with mottled contrast enhancement.

REFERENCE

1. Herman TE, Shackelford GD, McAlister WH. Pseudotumoral sarcoid granulomatous nephritis in a child: case presentation with sonographic and CT findings. Pediatr Radiol 1997;27:752–754.

Renal Abscess

Renal abscess is an uncommon problem in the neonate and young infant and is uncommon in the pediatric age group in general. It can be demonstrated with ultrasonography, CT scanning, and MRI (Fig. 5.23). Ultrasonography is most expedient. In some cases, the findings may represent infected calyceal diverticula.

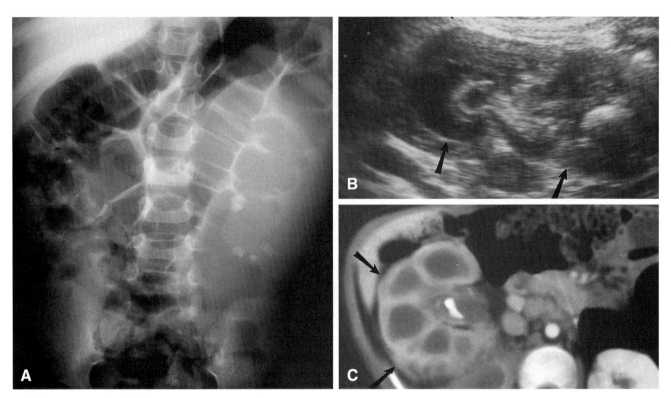

FIGURE 5.22. Xanthogranulomatous pyelonephritis. A. Plain films demonstrate a large, left flank mass with calcifications. **B**. Sonogram in another patient demonstrates a kidney (arrows) that has lost all of its normal architecture. Echogenic areas represent calculi. **C.** CT in another patient demonstrates dilated urine-filled calyces in the right kidney (arrows). There is peripheral enhancement of the cortex and a central echogenic obstructing stone. The overall pattern constitutes the "bear paw" sign. (From Cousins C, Sommers J, Broderick N, et al. Xanthogranuloma-tous pyelonephritis is childhood; ultrasound and CT diagnosis. Pediatr Radiol 1994;24:210–212, with permission.)

URETERAL REFLUX

Ureteral reflux is a common problem in North America and Europe but, interestingly enough, is not as great a problem in other parts of the world where black populations predominate (1, 2). Despite some disagreement (3, 4), it does seem that reflux is less common in blacks, even with obstructive uropathy (5). It has been suggested that all of this is due to earlier maturation of the ureterovesicular anti-reflux mechanism in blacks (1).

Ureteral reflux usually is first demonstrated with standard voiding cystourethrography, but recently, the scintigraphic cystogram also has become useful. The voiding cystourethrogram has the advantage of being able to delineate bladder and urethral anatomy and the physiology of bladder emptying. For this reason, it is indispensable as the first study in males, but in females, in whom obstructing urethral lesions are rare, the nuclear scintigraphic study can serve as the first study. It should be remembered, however, that this study is not as effective as standard voiding cystourethrography in precisely documenting the degree and grade of reflux. Ultrasonographic cystography with contrast enhancement also can demonstrate reflux (6–8), but as with

nuclear scintigraphy, it does not do well with milder degrees of reflux and does not accurately grade reflux. For this reason, it has not replaced the standard voiding cystourethrogram. Ureteral reflux also can co-exist with distal ureteral obstruction (9) and commonly is seen with urethral obstruction such as posterior urethral valves in males.

Further complicating philosophies about reflux is that it can be primary and even familial (10, 11). Reflux has been shown to be present in asymptomatic siblings of children with urinary tract infection and reflux (12–14). Incidence of this category of reflux has been demonstrated to be 30% overall and slightly higher in girls (14). In most such cases and with reflux in general (12), the problem tends to undergo spontaneous resolution, with only 5% or less of patients developing scarring (14, 15). Scarring tends to occur in the early years, usually before the age of 2 (13, 14), and the most damaging reflux most likely occurs before 2 years of age. Nonetheless, many believe that siblings who demonstrate silent reflux should be evaluated with ultrasound yearly throughout childhood. Although reflux occurs most commonly with infection and urinary tract obstruction, it also occurs on a silent basis in siblings of patients with pathologic reflux. It is not possible to draw a firm con-

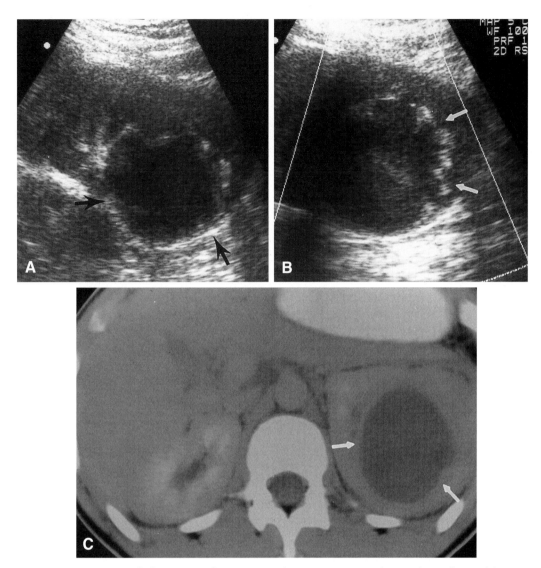

FIGURE 5.23. Renal abscess. A. Ultrasonogram demonstrates a sonolucent abscess (arrows) in the lower pole of the left kidney. **B.** Color flow Doppler demonstrates increased blood flow (arrows) around the periphery of the abscess. **C.** Another patient with renal abscess (arrows) demonstrated on CT.

clusion about this. It also should be appreciated that a normal sonogram does not exclude reflux (15), and that reflux has been demonstrated in normal children (16).

In the end, whatever one's disposition toward the cause of reflux, most feel that the problem lies in an anatomically altered ureterovesicular junction. Normally, the ureters enter the bladder at a slant, and as the bladder distends with urine, the slanted distal ureteral segment is squeezed shut. In effect, this is a pressure valve, and in neonates and very young infants, the "valve" is immature, and reflux is common. However, it is usually mild and dissipates as soon as the infant grows a little older. By 6 months to 1 year, one would not expect this phenomenon to occur. Later, if for some reason (e.g., infection, neurogenic bladder) the bladder wall becomes thickened, the distal ureteral segment is rendered horizontal in position (Fig. 5.24). Under such circumstances, the compressive valve-like action of the distended bladder is not accomplished, and reflux occurs. The same problem arises with the **"golf-hole" ureteral orifice.** In these cases, the ureter enters the bladder horizontally on a congenital basis, and the orifice of the ureter is gaping; hence the term golf-hole ureteral orifice. With infection, reflux is reversible after the infection clears, but this does not occur with the golf-hole orifice. In other cases, reflux may be associated with a "Hutch," or periureteral diverticulum. This usually occurs with bladder outlet or urethral obstruction and for the most part it is seen with posterior urethral valves and spastic, high-pressure neurogenic bladder.

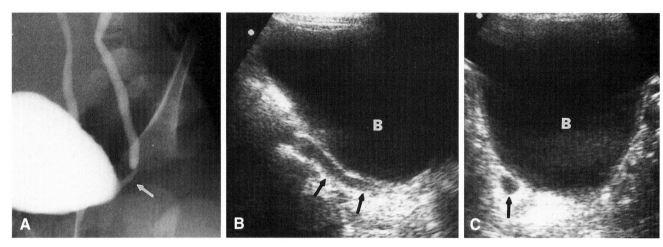

FIGURE 5.24. Reflux. A. Bilateral reflux. Note the almost horizontal insertion of the distal left ureter (arrow). **B.** Ultrasonogram in another patient with a dilated, refluxing ureter (arrows) inserting into the bladder (B). **C.** Cross-sectional view demonstrates the dilated left ureter (arrow). B, urinary bladder.

Reflux can be divided into two broad groups: low-pressure and high-pressure reflux. Low-pressure reflux occurs with early filling of the bladder and often is gross. High-pressure reflux occurs only when the bladder is fully distended and/or the patient is voiding. Reflux generally is graded according to the length of retrograde ureteral filling and upper tract dilatation. This grading is helpful in determining whether surgical correction (i.e., reimplantation of the ureters) is required. To meet this end, an international classification of reflux has been proposed (17) (Fig. 5.25). In this classification, grade V reflux is the only reflux that

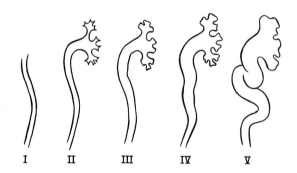

FIGURE 5.25. International classification of reflux. Grade I reflux; ureter only. Grade II reflux outlines the ureter, pelvis, and calyces, but no dilation is present. Grade III reflux demonstrates ureteral dilation and slight blunting of the calyceal fornices. Grade IV reflux demonstrates more pronounced dilation, tortuosity of the ureter, and marked blunting of the calyceal fornices. Grade V reflux demonstrates marked dilation and tortuosity of the ureter. The upper system is grossly hydronephrotic and the calyces are dilated. (Modified from Levitt SB. Medical versus surgical treatment of primary vesicoureteral reflux, report of the International Reflux Study Committee. Pediatrics 1981;67: 392–400.)

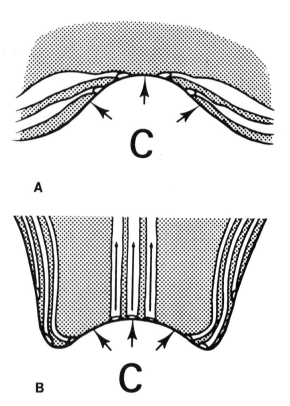

FIGURE 5.26. Intrarenal reflux in compound papilla. A. Simple papilla. Note that all the tubules are compressed and occluded by the distended calyx (C). Under such conditions reflux is less likely. **B. Compound papilla.** The tubules in the center are not compressed by the calyx (C), and reflux can occur readily (arrows). (Adapted from Ransley PG. Opacification of the renal parenchyma in obstruction and reflux. Pediatr Radiol 1976;4: 226–232, with permission.)

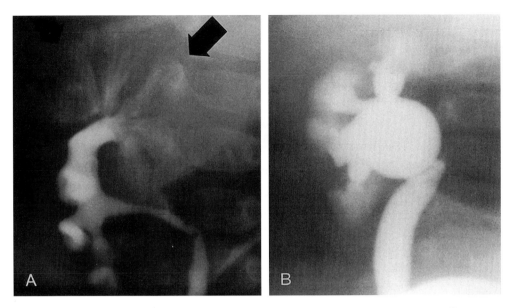

FIGURE 5.27. Intrarenal reflux. A. Two-month-old infant demonstrating intrarenal reflux confined primarily to the upper pole (arrow), an area where compound papillae predominate. **B.** Another infant, somewhat younger, demonstrating uniform intrarenal reflux. Such uniform reflux is more likely to occur in the neonate.

almost routinely comes to surgical correction. For the other grades, surgical intervention depends on the presence of associated refractory infection. Grades I and II reflux often are difficult to demonstrate with nuclear scintigraphy and ultrasound cystography, and overall, grade I reflux is of questionable clinical significance. Perhaps the one drawback to the classification outlined in Fig. 5.25 is that it does not include intrarenal reflux (i.e., reflux into the renal tubules themselves). Such reflux has a propensity to occur in infancy and is the type most often associated with subse-

quent renal scarring. In this regard, it has been demonstrated that compound renal papillae are more prone to this type of reflux (18, 19), because the central tubules are not easily compressed and occluded by the distended calyx (Fig. 5.26). Compound papillae in humans predominate in the upper and, to lesser extent, lower poles of the kidney (20), and reflux often occurs preferentially in these areas (Fig. 5.27). The nuclear scintigraphic findings with reflux are rather straightforward (Fig. 5.28), but grading is not as accurate as with the standard voiding cystourethrogram,

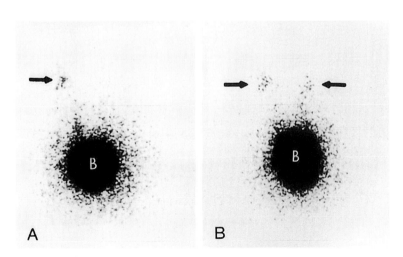

FIGURE 5.28. Reflux: radionuclide study. A. Note the reflux on the right (arrow). B, bladder. **B.** A little later, reflux is seen bilaterally (arrows).

and renal scarring is more likely to occur with high-grade reflux (Fig. 5.29).

Debate also continues as to whether sterile reflux can cause damage to the kidney (21). Although it is commonly held that infection also must be present to cause parenchymal damage, there is evidence that this is not necessarily true (22–25). These studies have demonstrated that sterile reflux can cause scarring. Another important point to remember regarding parenchymal damage leading to scarring is that the kidney is most vulnerable under the age of 2 years. After that, scarring tends not to occur and scarring tends not to progress unless reflux was initially very severe and refractory.

A note regarding the appearance of the ureterovesicular junction after the injection of collagen or Teflon (26) is in order. In these cases, there is deformity and thickening around the distal ureter as it enters the bladder. In some cases, hydronephrosis can be seen and diverticulum formation has been described.

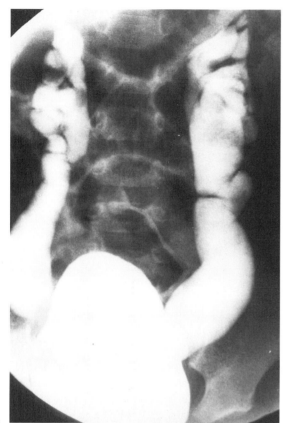

A

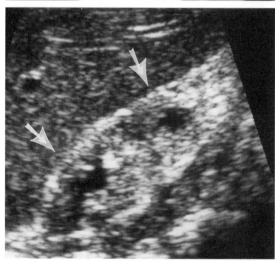

B

FIGURE 5.29. Severe grade V reflux with renal atrophy. A. Note the severe grade V reflux bilaterally. The ureters are markedly dilated but the kidneys are small. **B.** Ultrasound demonstrates a small echogenic atrophic kidney (arrows).

REFERENCES

1. West W, Venugopal S. The low frequency of reflux in Jamaican children. Pediatr Radiol 1993;23;591–593.
2. Melhem RE, Harpen MD. Ethnic factors in the variability of primary vesico-ureteral reflux with age. Pediatr Radiol 1997;27:750–751.
3. Askari A, Belman AB. Vesicoureteral reflux in black girls. J Urol 1982;127:747–750.
4. Skoog SJ, Belman AB. Primary vesico-ureteral reflux in the black child. Pediatrics 1991;87:538–543.
5. Nancarrow PA, Lebowitz RL. Primary vesico-ureteral reflux in blacks with posterior urethral valves: does it occur? Pediatr Radiol 1988;19:31–33.
6. Bosio M. Cystosonography with echocontrast: a new imaging modality to detect vesicoureteric reflux in children. Pediatr Radiol 1998;28:250–255.
7. Darge K, Troeger J, Duetting T, et al. Reflux in young patient. Comparison of voiding US of the bladder and retrovesical space with echo enhancement versus voiding cystourethrography for diagnosis. Radiology 1999;210:201–207.
8. Mentzel H-J, Vogt S, Patzer L, et al. Contrast-enhanced sonography of vesicoureterorenal reflux in children: preliminary results. AJR 1999;173:737–740.
9. Leighton DM, Mayne V. Obstruction in the refluxing urinary tract—a common phenomenon. Clin Radiol 1989;40:271–273.
10. Noe HN, Wyatt RJ, Peeden JN Jr, et al. The transmission of vesicoureteral reflux from parent to child. J Urol 1992;148:1869–1871.
11. Peeden JN Jr, Noe YHN. Screening for familial vesicoureteral reflux. Pediatrics 1992;89:758–760.
12. Connolly LP, Treves ST, Zurakowski D, et al. Natural history of vesicoureteral reflux in siblings. J Urol 1996;156:1805–1807.
13. Connolly LP, Treves SA, Connolly SA, et al. Vesicoureteral reflux in children: incidence and severity in siblings. J Urol 1997;157:2287–2290.
14. Wan J, Greenfield SP, Ng M, et al. Sibling reflux: a dual center retrospective study. J Urol 1996;156:677–679.
15. DePietro MA, Blane CE, Zerin JM. Vesicoureteral reflux in older children: concordance of US and voiding cystourethrographic findings. Radiology 1997;205:821–822.
16. Sargent MA. Opinion. What is the normal prevalence of vesicoureteral reflux? Pediatr Radiol 2000;30:587–593.
17. Levitt SB. Medical versus surgical treatment of primary vesicoureteral reflux: report of the International Reflux Study Committee. Pediatrics 1981;67:392–400.

18. Maling TMJ, Rolleston GL. Intra-renal reflux in children demonstrated by micturating cystography. Clin Radiol 1974;25: 81–85.

19. Ransley PG. Opacification of the renal parenchyma in obstruction and reflux. Pediatr Radiol 1976;4:226–232.

20. Funston MR, Cremin BJ. Intrarenal reflux–papillary morphology and pressure relationships in children's necropsy kidneys. Br J Radiol 1978;51:665–670.

21. Rushton HG, Majd M, Jantausch B, et al. Renal scarring following reflux and nonreflux pyelonephritis in children: evaluation with 99m technetium-dimercaptosuccinic acid scintigraphy. J Urol 1992;147:1327–1332.

22. Buonomo C, Treves T, Jones B, et al. Silent renal damage in symptom-free siblings of children with vesicoureteral reflux: assessment with technetium Tc 99m dimercaptosuccinic acid scintigraphy. J Pediatr 1993;122:721–723.

23. Kenda RB, Fettich JJ. Vesicoureteric reflux and renal scars in symptomatic siblings of children with reflux. Arch Dis Child 1992;67:506–508.

24. Marra G, Barbieri G, Dell'Agnola CA, et al. Congenital renal damage associated with primary vesicoureteral reflux detected prenatally in male infants. J Pediatr 1994;124:727–730.

25. Najmaldin A, Burge DM, Atwell JD. Reflux nephropathy secondary to intrauterine vesicoureteric reflux. J Pediatr Surg 1990; 25:387–390.

26. Rypens F, Avni EF, Bank WO, et al. The ureterovesical junction in children: sonographic findings after surgical or endoscopic treatment. AJR 1992;158:837–842.

RENAL VASCULAR DISEASE

Renal Vein Thrombosis

Renal vein thrombosis is the most common renal vascular abnormality in the neonate. It most often results from hemoconcentration with polycythemia, dehydration, and sepsis. In older infants, dehydration due to diarrhea or excessive vomiting also is a cause. In the neonate, renal vein thrombosis is especially prone to develop in infants delivered of diabetic mothers, because it is well known that such infants are "normally" relatively water depleted. Renal vein thrombosis due to hypercoagulability can occur in association with the nephrotic syndrome. There is, however, debate as to whether the syndrome results from the renal vein thrombosis or the syndrome causes it. Most likely, both situations exist.

Most cases of neonatal renal vein thrombosis are unilateral, but bilateral involvement does occur, and because emboli can be a problem, anticoagulation usually is required. The inferior vena cava also can be thrombosed, especially in cases of bilateral renal vein thrombosis. In these cases, the initial thrombosis is intrarenal in the small veins and then there is extension of the thrombus into the renal vein and, in some cases, the inferior vena cava.

Typically, infants with renal vein thrombosis present with abdominal distention, a rapidly enlarging kidney, vomiting, and fever. Hematuria, either microscopic or gross, is usually present but can be absent. Proteinuria and the presence of white blood cells in the urine frequently are seen, and the blood urea nitrogen usually is elevated. Hypertension is occasionally encountered, but it is not nearly as common as in renal artery thrombosis.

The kidney is not usually enlarged enough to be clearly seen on plain abdominal roentgenograms. When suspected clinically, renal vein thrombosis usually is first imaged with ultrasound. The enlarged kidney tends to be hyperechoic and has disorganized renal architecture. In other words, the normal corticomedullary differentiation is lost. The collecting systems are compressed by the extensive edema present, and the findings are rather homogeneous throughout the kidney (Fig. 5.30A). Seldom is one able to define the renal vein thrombi, but one may detect the echogenic thrombus extending into the inferior vena cava (Fig. 5.30B). Ultrasound can document the presence of small, thrombosed, interlobar and arcuate vessels as echogenic linear or curvilinear streaks (1). Color flow Doppler also is useful in detecting blood flow to the kidney.

CT and MRI are seldom necessary, and although nuclear scintigraphy can provide some information regarding function, it generally is not required. However, if performed, it will show decreased uptake of isotope and virtual nonfunction of the kidney. With recovery, the extensive edema of the kidney subsides rather briskly because blood flow returns quickly (2), but this should not be misinterpreted for total improvement. Many of these kidneys eventually become hypoplastic or atrophic.

Later, as the patient recovers from the initial insult, one may be able to define calcified thrombi in the large veins or even in the intrarenal small veins (Fig. 5.31). The intrarenal calcifications are typical, because they assume a lace-like configuration that radiates outward from the renal pelvis (3). In terms of treatment, nephrectomy or thrombectomy can be performed in more severe cases, but over the past decade or so, the trend has been to more conservative treatment (4). This is true even with bilateral involvement.

Renal vein thrombosis in the neonate can co-exist with adrenal hemorrhage. Most often, the association occurs on the left (5, 6), but it also has been described on the right. The ultrasonographic findings are typical (Fig. 5.30, C and D), and the association of the two conditions probably is more than coincidental. On the left, because the adrenal and renal veins have a common origin, it is easy for thrombus to extend from one to another. This phenomenon is more difficult to explain on the right, where separate drainage pathways usually exist. Another possible explanation, applicable to either side, is that the sheer size of the adrenal hemorrhage in some cases may compress the involved renal vein and cause stasis and thrombosis. Whatever the cause, there seems to be a more than passing association between the two conditions.

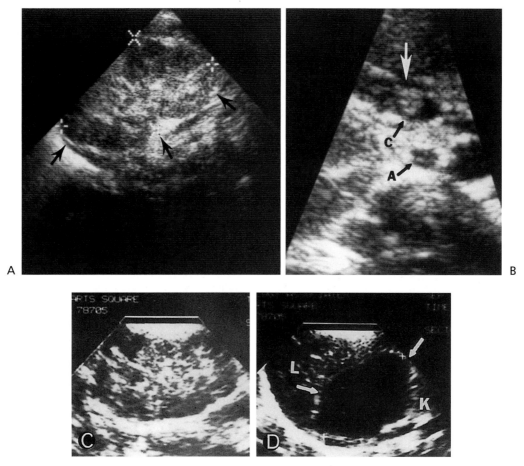

FIGURE 5.30. Renal vein thrombosis: sonographic findings. A. Note the enlarged kidney with increased echogenicity and altered architecture (arrows). **B.** Transverse sonogram demonstrates the normal aorta (A), the inferior vena cava (C), and the echogenic thrombus (arrow) within. **C. Renal vein thrombosis with adrenal hemorrhage.** Note the echogenic, enlarged kidney with abnormal architecture. **D.** Large sonolucent adrenal hemorrhage (arrows) above the kidney (K). L, liver. (**A** and **B** courtesy of Deborah Ahrendt; **D** courtesy of the late Sue Jacobi, M.D.)

REFERENCES

1. Wright NB, Blanch G, Walkinshaw S, et al. Antenatal and neonatal renal vein thrombosis: new ultrasonic features with high frequency transducers. Pediatr Radiol 1996;26:686–689.
2. Laplante S, Patriquin HB, Robitaille P, et al. Renal vein thrombosis in children: evidence of early flow recovery with Doppler US. Radiology 1993;189:37–42.
3. Brill PW, Mitty HA, Strauss L. Renal vein thrombosis: a cause of intrarenal calcification in the newborn. Pediatr Radiol 6:172–175.
4. Ricci MA, Lloyd DA. Renal venous thrombosis in infants and children. Arch Surg 1990;125:1195–1199.
5. Bennett WG, Wood BP. Radiological case of the month—left renal vein thrombosis and left adrenal hemorrhage. Am J Dis Child 1991;145:1299–1300.
6. Lebowitz JM, Belman AB. Simultaneous idiopathic adrenal hemorrhage and renal vein thrombosis in the newborn. J Urol 1983; 3:574–576.

Renal Artery Thrombosis and Embolism

Renal artery thrombosis is much less common than renal vein thrombosis. It is more common in infants delivered of diabetic mothers, and sepsis, dehydration, and hemoconcentration are predisposing factors. In other cases, thrombotic emboli from a closing ductus arteriosus or retrograde extension of the thrombus obliterating the umbilical arteries can cause occlusion of the renal arteries. Thromboembolic disease as a complication of umbilical artery catheterization is a common cause of thrombosis and embolus formation (1).

In its early stages, renal artery thrombosis frequently is misdiagnosed as renal vein thrombosis, but with renal artery thrombosis, the kidney does not enlarge. Unlike renal vein thrombosis, hypertension and congestive heart failure

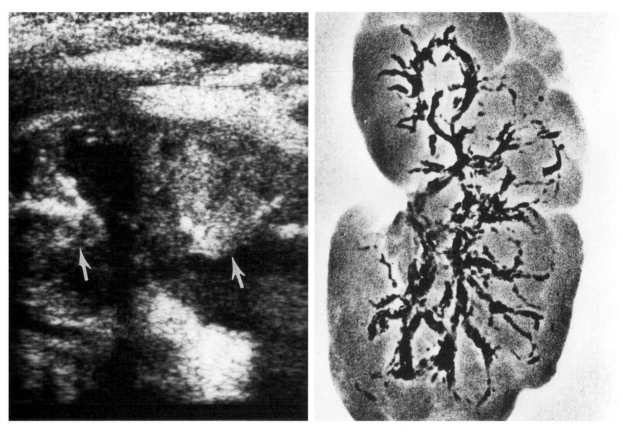

A   B

FIGURE 5.31. Renal vein thrombosis with small vessel calcification. A. Note the linear, echogenic calcifications (arrows) within the renal pyramids. **B.** Another patient whose post-mortem xeroradiograph demonstrates the typical distribution of the intravascular calcifications. (From Brill PW, Mitty HA, Strauss L. Renal vein thrombosis: a cause of intrarenal calcification in the newborn. Pediatr Radiol 1977;6:172–175, with permission.)

are common. Occlusion of the renal artery frequently is associated with thrombosis of the aorta and other vessels; unlike renal vein thrombosis, neonatal renal artery thrombosis usually is part of a more widespread intravascular thrombotic process. If thrombosis is bilateral, death usually ensues, but prompt nephrectomy can cure the infant with unilateral obstruction (1).

Ultrasonographic evaluation of renal artery thrombosis centers on demonstration of lack of renal arterial blood flow to the involved kidney. This is usually initially accomplished with color flow Doppler, but it is often difficult to identify these findings with clarity, and it may be necessary to go on to some form of arteriography. The kidney usually is of normal size and normal echotexture. Nuclear scintigraphy also can be helpful and demonstrates decreased flow and renal function. CT scans show no contrast entering the kidney, and MRI generally is not employed.

REFERENCE

1. Wilson DI, Appleton RE, Coulthard MG, et al. Fetal and infantile hypertension caused by unilateral renal arterial disease. Arch Dis Child 1990;65:881–884.

Miscellaneous Arterial Lesions

Renal arterial stenoses are occasionally encountered in children and may be focal or involve longer segments. In an excellent review of the subject (1), small vessel disease was the problem in 76% of all cases, and fibromuscular dysplasia was the cause of large vessel disease in 46% of cases. Fibromuscular dysplasia consists of a typical corrugated configuration of the renal artery (Fig. 5.32A). In other cases, discrete narrowings (Fig. 5.32, B and C) may be associated with hypertension. Stenoses of the renal arteries also can occur in association with conditions such as neurofi-

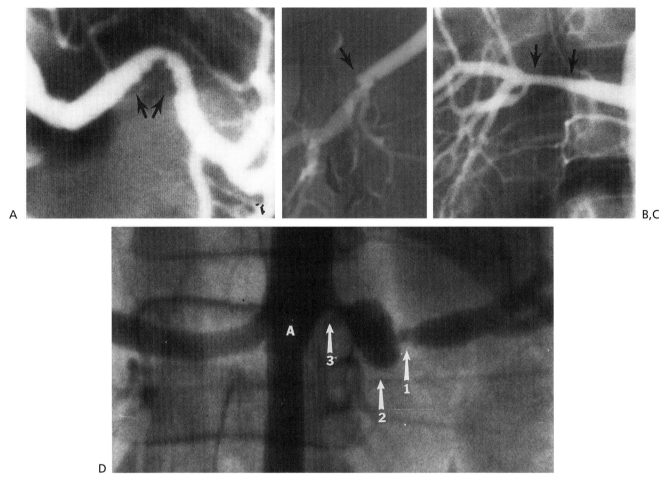

FIGURE 5.32. Renal artery stenosis. A. Typical corrugated appearance of fibromuscular hyperplasia (arrows). **B.** Focal area of corrugated stenosis (arrow) in another patient. **C.** Focal stenosis (arrows) in a patient with hypertension. **D.** Neurofibromatosis. Note the stenosis (l) of the right renal artery. There is prestenotic dilatation of the artery (2), and the takeoff (3) of the renal artery from the aorta (A) also is narrowed.

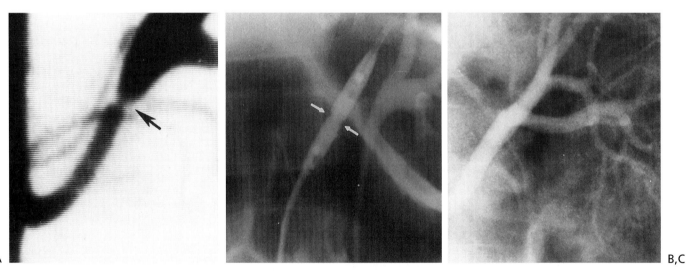

FIGURE 5.33. Renal artery stenosis, balloon angioplasty. A. Note the focal area of stenosis (arrow) in the left renal artery. **B.** Balloon angioplasty with area of stenosis demarcated by subtle indentation of the balloon (arrows) is performed. **C.** After angioplasty, the area of narrowing is no longer present.

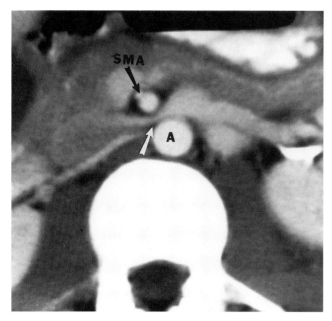

FIGURE 5.34. Nutcracker syndrome. Note the compression of the left renal vein (arrow) by the aorta (A) and the superior mesenteric artery (SMA).

bromatosis (Fig. 5.32D) (1), homocystinuria, and periarteritis nodosa. Aneurysms are more common with the latter condition, and aneurysms also are a common feature of Takayasu's arteritis. Congenital and mycotic aneurysms or arteriovenous malformations (2–4) are rare. The latter are readily demonstrated with ultrasound and color flow Doppler. All of these lesions can be, and frequently are, associated with systemic hypertension. Renal artery stenoses commonly are treated with percutaneous, transluminal, balloon angioplasty (5) (Fig. 5.33). The contralateral kidney, usually hypertrophied in patients with unilateral renal artery stenosis may show hyperechogenicity on ultrasound examination (6). It is believed that this is secondary to compensatory hyperfiltration (6).

The nutcracker syndrome is an only recently understood entity. In this condition, the left renal vein is compressed by the aorta and superior mesenteric artery (Fig. 5.34). As a result, there is increased venous pressure transmitted to the left kidney and hematuria results (7–10). The hematuria is painless, and the problem may be more common than generally realized. Stenting of the left renal vein has been attempted (8).

REFERENCES

1. Deal JE, Snell MF, Barratt TM, et al. Renovascular disease in childhood. J Pediatr 1992;121:378–384.
2. Bunchman TE, Walker HSJ III, Joyce PF, et al. Sonographic evaluation of renal artery aneurysm in childhood. Pediatr Radiol 1991;21:312–313.
3. Derchi LE, Saffioti S, De Caro G, et al. Arteriovenous fistula of the native kidney: diagnosis by duplex Doppler US. J Ultrasound Med 1991;10:595–597.
4. Macpherson RI, Fyfe D, Aaronson I A. Congenital renal arteriovenous malformations in infancy. The imaging features in two infants with hypertension. Pediatr Radiol 1991;21:108–110.
5. Courtel JV, Soto B, Niaudet P, et al. Percutaneous transluminal angioplasty of renal artery stenosis in children. Pediatr Radiol 1998;28:59–63.
6. Enriquez G, Castello F, Sousa P, et al. Increased cortical echogenicity of the normal kidney in infants with unilateral renal artery stenosis: report of two cases. J Ultrasound Med 1997; 16:59–63.
7. Park YB, Lim SH, Ahn JH, et al. Nutcracker syndrome: intravascular stenting approach. Nephrol Dial Transplant 2000;15: 99–101.
8. Russo D, Minutolo R, Laccarino V, et al. Gross hematuria of uncommon origin: the nutcracker syndrome. Am J Kidney Dis 1998;32:E3.
9. Weiner SN, Bernstein RG, Morehouse H, et al. Hematuria secondary to left peripelvic and gonadal vein varices. Urology 1983;22:81–84.
10. Kaneko K, Kiya K, Nishimura K, et al. Nutcracker phenomenon demonstrated by three-dimensional computed tomography. Pediatr Nephrol 2001;16:745–747.

RENAL MASSES

In the neonate, renal masses usually are nonmalignant. The most commonly encountered entities include hydronephrosis and renal cystic disease. In older infants, however, Wilms' tumor becomes a significant lesion, but solid masses of the kidney are much less common in neonates. Renal enlargement, usually unilateral, also occurs with renal vein thrombosis, and bilateral renal enlargement occurs in conditions such as the Beckwith-Wiedemann syndrome, infants of diabetic mothers, glycogen storage disease, lipoatrophic diabetes, hereditary tyrosinosis, sickle cell disease, thalassemia, amyloidosis, the reticuloendothelioses, and in the lymphoma-leukemia group of diseases. Ultrasonography is the primary diagnostic imaging modality for investigating renal masses. Its greatest advantage is that it can, in a totally noninvasive manner, immediately determine whether the mass is cystic or solid.

Hydronephrosis

Hydronephrosis can result from urinary tract obstruction or prolonged massive reflux. In terms of the imaging of hydronephrosis, ultrasonography is the primary screening imaging modality employed. With careful examination, the site of obstruction and cause of hydronephrosis almost always can be determined. However, it is most important that, once a dilated upper system is identified, one search for the ureter to determine whether it also is dilated. Only in this way will one be able to determine whether the obstruction is high or low.

The ultrasonographic findings of hydronephrosis are straightforward, and the degree of hydronephrosis is readily documented (Fig. 5.35). Ultrasound, however, does not provide any information regarding renal function, and although in the past intravenous pyelography provided crude information regarding function, it is the renal scintigram that is most useful today. Using technetium-99m–labeled DTPA or MAG-3, the scintigraphic study should be obtained to confirm the degree of obstruction and remaining renal function. A diuretic washout phase should be obtained to provide further information about the severity of obstruction (Fig. 5.36). As a result, in only very few cases is retrograde pyelography required. Diuretic ultrasonography (1) and resistive indices (2, 3) also have been proposed for studying hydronephrosis but are not in common use. In regard to the latter, it should be recalled that the normal resistive indices in infants younger than 1 year are a little higher than in older infants and children.

Detailed dissertations on the various obstructive lesions leading to hydronephrosis are presented later in this chapter. However, it should be noted that in the neonate hydronephrosis may erroneously be masked if ultrasound is

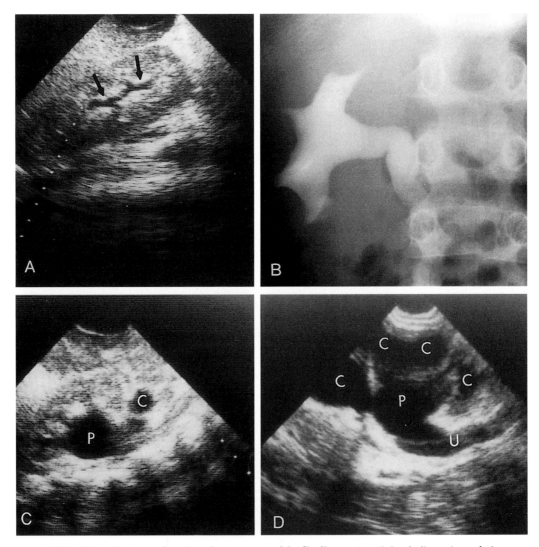

FIGURE 5.35. Hydronephrosis, ultrasonographic findings. A. Minimal distention of the renal pelvis (arrows). Note the early contiguous distention of the calyces. **B.** Intravenous pyelogram in the same patient. **C.** Another patient with more pronounced hydronephrosis resulting in dilation of the renal pelvis (P) and the calyces (C). **D.** Profound hydronephrosis demonstrating marked dilation of the renal pelvis (P), calyces (C), and proximal ureter (U).

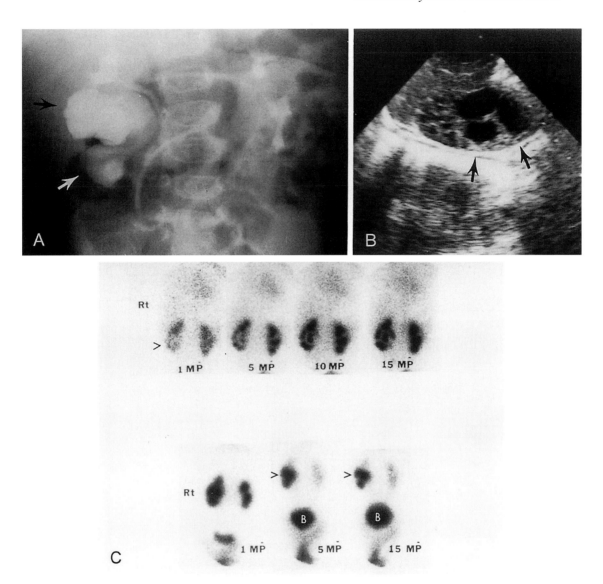

FIGURE 5.36. Hydronephrosis with diuretic washout. A. An intravenous pyelogram demonstrates a hydronephrotic (uteropelvic junction obstruction) lower right renal segment (arrows). There is minimal dilation of the upper segment on the right, and the left kidney is normal. **B.** Sonogram demonstrating the hydronephrotic lower segment (arrows). Minimal dilation of the calyces of the upper segment is seen. **C.** Technetium-99m DTPA study demonstrates delayed excretion of contrast material in the right lower pole at 1 minute (upper arrow). Excretion evens out by 15 minutes, but in the lower scan series, after diuretic washout there is marked retention of isotope (arrows) in the hydronephrotic lower segment on the right. B, urinary bladder.

performed immediately after birth (Fig. 5.37). This occurs because of the relatively dehydrated state of the neonate. With subsequent hydration, the true degree of hydronephrosis becomes apparent (4, 5) and can be surprisingly pronounced. This explains the cases in which hydronephrosis is

seen in utero, but immediately after birth, no hydronephrosis is detected. Another interesting aspect of hydronephrosis is that, if discovered in utero, it has been demonstrated that 50% of these infants improve spontaneously (6). A conservative approach to the problem is suggested.

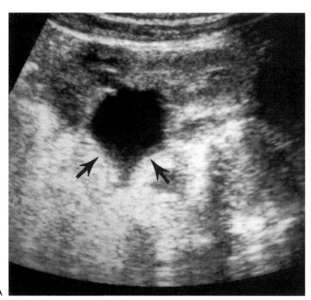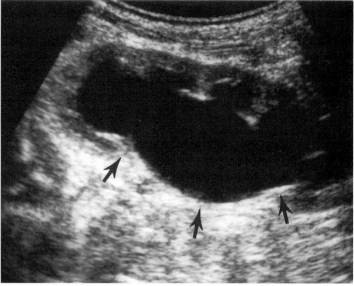

A   B

FIGURE 5.37. Delayed imaging for hydronephrosis in neonates. A. On the first day of life note the minimal pelvic dilatation (arrows). **B.** Later, gross hydronephrosis (arrows) due to ureteropelvic junction obstruction is present.

REFERENCES

1. Rosi P, Virgili G, Di Stasi SM, et al. Diuretic ultrasound: a non-invasive technique for the assessment of upper tract obstruction. Br J Urol 1990;65:566–569.
2. Blane CE, Barr M, DiPietro MA, et al. Renal obstructive dysplasia: ultrasound diagnosis and therapeutic implications. Pediatr Radiol 1991;21:274–277.
3. Kessler RM, Quevedo H, Lankau CA, et al. Obstructive vs. nonobstructive dilatation of the renal collecting system in children: distinction with duplex sonography. AJR 1993;160:353–357.
4. Clautice-Engle T, Anderson NG, Allan RB, et al. Diagnosis of obstructive hydronephrosis in infants: comparison sonograms obtained 6 days and 6 weeks after birth. AJR 1995;164:963–967.
5. Laing FC, Burke VD, Wing VW, et al. Post-partum evaluation of fetal hydronephrosis: optimal timing for follow-up sonography. Radiology 1981;152:423–424.
6. Kletscher B, de Badiola F, Gonzalez R. Outcome of hydronephrosis diagnosed antenatally. J Pediatr Surg 1991;26:455–460.

Congenital Megacalyces

This condition is a form of renal dysplasia in which there is enlargement of the calyces and hypoplasia or flattening of the medullary pyramids (1). Renal function often is completely normal, but the findings can be misinterpreted for those of advanced hydronephrosis (Fig. 5.38). The deformity can be unilateral or bilateral, and the infundibula are short and broad, but the pelves and ureters are normal.

There is no evidence of obstruction or significant reflux. Often, the kidneys are larger than one would expect for the age, and fetal lobulation is prominent (1). More than the normal number of calyces is present.

REFERENCE

1. Garcia CJ, Taylor KJW, Weiss RM. Congenital megacalyces: ultrasound appearance. J Ultrasound Med 1987;6:163–165.

Cystic Disease of the Kidney

Classification of cystic disease of the kidney still usually starts with the work of Osathanondh and Potter (1). Their classification divides polycystic disease of the kidney into four types and is based on microdissection studies of pathologic specimens: type I, infantile polycystic disease; type II, multicystic dysplastic kidney; type III, adult polycystic disease; and type IV, cortical cysts associated with massive obstructive hydronephrosis. Unfortunately, this classification does not include all forms of cystic kidney disease, but because it does deal with the major types, it still is the one used most often. An overall classification of cystic disease in childhood is presented in Table 5.1, and the data are obtained from a summary of the numerous classifications available in the literature (2). Over the years, ultrasound has

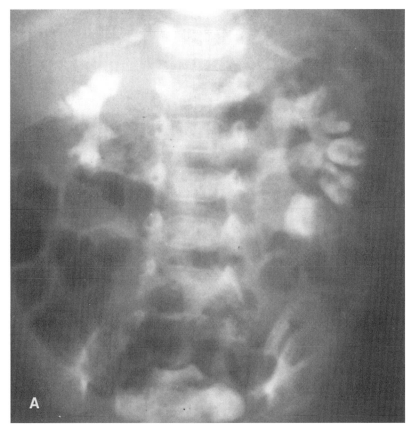

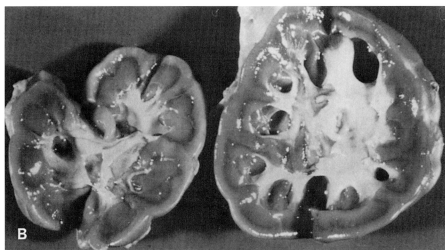

FIGURE 5.38. Congenital megacalyces. A. Note the typical appearance of the dilated calyces on the left. The renal pelvis and ureter are normal. Slight dilation of the upper calyces on the right also is noted. Note the flattened medullary pyramids. Both kidneys are enlarged, but the left is larger than the right. **B.** Pathologic specimen demonstrating the large dilated calyces, but normal cortical thickness. (From Kozakewich H, Lebowitz R. Congenital megacalyces. Pediatr Radiol 1974;2:251–257, with permission.)

TABLE 5.1. RENAL CYSTIC DISEASE IN CHILDHOOD

Polycystic disease
Infantile (Potter type I, autosomal recessive)
Juvenile (same as infantile)
Adult (Potter type III, autosomal dominant)
Multicystic disease
Multicystic-dysplastic kidney (Potter type II)
Multilocular cyst (benign cystic nephroblastoma, cystic Wilms' tumor, polycystic nephroma)
Medullary cysts
Medullary sponge kidney
Medullary cystic disease; uremic (juvenile nephrophthisis)
Solitary cyst
Simple cyst
Hydrocalycosis, pelvicalyceal cyst, calyceal diverticulum
Miscellaneous cysts (cortical)
Conradi's disease, Zellweger syndrome, trisomies, Turner's syndrome
Tuberous sclerosis
Cortical with obstructive hydronephrosis (Potter type IV)
Cortical without obstructive hydronephrosis

come to play a key role in the imaging investigation of cystic disease of the kidney, and it alone should strongly suggest the diagnosis in most cases. There is little place for CT or MR.

REFERENCES

1. Osathanondh V, Potter EL. Pathogenesis of polycystic kidneys; historical survey; type I due to hyperplasia of interstitial portions of collecting tubules; type II due to inhibition of ampullary activity; type III due to multiple abnormalities of development; type IV due to urethral obstruction: survey of results of microdissection. Arch Pathol 1964;77:459–512.
2. Hayden CK Jr, Swischuk LE, Smith TH, et al. Renal cystic disease in childhood. Radiographics 1986;6:97–116.

Infantile (Recessive) Polycystic Kidney Disease (Potter Type I: RPKD)

This form of polycystic disease is inherited as an autosomal recessive condition. It is said by some to be more common in females, but others do not record such a sex predilection. Hepatic fibrosis is a common associated feature, and overall, a spectrum of the cystic renal disease and associated hepatic fibrosis exists (1). Of interest, however, is that these two aspects of the disease vary inversely. Whereas the kidney problems bring the patient to the attention of the physician in infancy, in later childhood, portal hypertension and gastrointestinal bleeding secondary to hepatic fibrosis are the problems. Often, this form of the disease is called juvenile polycystic disease or tubular ectasia with hepatic fibrosis. Renal involvement usually is less pronounced in these patients.

Infants presenting in the immediate neonatal period usually have a poor prognosis and demonstrate large kidneys with poor renal function. Azotemia is pronounced, and the blood pressure usually is elevated. Liver problems are not a prominent feature at this time, but respiratory distress secondary to bilateral pulmonary hypoplasia can be severe. Hypoplasia of the lungs results from the so-called fetal compression syndrome secondary to oligohydramnios, which results from decreased urine output. Ultrasonographically, the kidneys characteristically are large and show increased echogenicity (Fig. 5.39). There is complete distortion of normal renal architecture, and corticomedullary differentiation is lost. The pyramids are not clearly visualized, and the calyces are compressed, separated, splayed, and generally not well seen. In the past, it was generally held that no discrete cysts were present, but it has become apparent (2) that some of these infants may demonstrate ultrasonographically visible small cysts from the beginning (Fig. 5.39).

Increased echogenicity in these patients probably is the result of the numerous dilated, outwardly radiating tubules (Fig. 5.39), presenting the transducer with many acoustical interfaces. In the past, the radiating pattern of the dilated tubules was seen on delayed roentgenograms of the intravenous pyelogram, but with high-resolution linear transducers, the dilated radiating tubules are readily detected (2, 3, 5) (Fig. 5.39). The cysts in this condition do not involve the subcortical region and therefore the periphery is free of cysts and in some cases hypoechoic (3–5). The dilated tubules also can be demonstrated with MRI (6). In patients with the juvenile form of the disease, increased echoes from the liver may be seen as a result of associated hepatic fibrosis, and the kidneys become even more echogenic and may show larger, more discrete cysts (Fig. 5.40).

Ancillary findings in these patients include asymmetric involvement (7), calcifications (8), increased echogenicity of the medullary pyramids (9), associated Caroli's disease of the liver (10–12), and the Ivemark's syndrome (13). In Caroli's disease, the dilated biliary ducts are readily demonstrated with any imaging modality, including MRI (12), which is excellent for evaluation of the bile ducts in any condition. In Caroli's disease, the biliary system shows marked and extreme non-uniform dilatation.

REFERENCES

1. Premkumar A, Berdon WE, Levy J, et al. The emergence of hepatic fibrosis and portal hypertension in infants and children with autosomal recessive polycystic kidney disease. Initial and follow-up sonographic and radiographic findings. Ped Rad 1988;18:123–129.
2. Worthington JL, Shackelford GD, Cole BR, et al. Sonographically detectable cysts in polycystic kidney disease in newborn and young infants. Pediatr Radiol 1988;18:287–293.

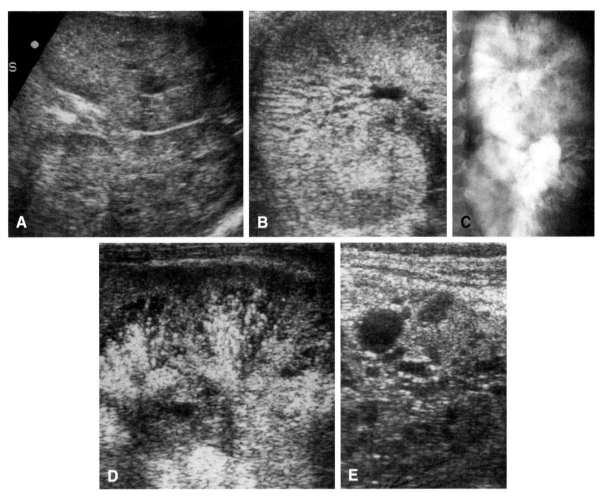

FIGURE 5.39. Infantile (autosomal recessive) polycystic kidney disease: ultrasonographic findings. A. Both kidneys are large and echogenic and have completely lost their normal internal architecture. **B.** High-resolution linear scan in another patient demonstrates the elongated tubules radiating outward from the center of the kidney. **C.** Intravenous pyelogram in another patient demonstrating large kidneys, altered architecture, and the radiating tubules. **D.** In this patient, the medullary pyramids are echogenic resulting from stasis of protein in the dilated tubules. **E.** This patient demonstrates more spherical cysts of various sizes.

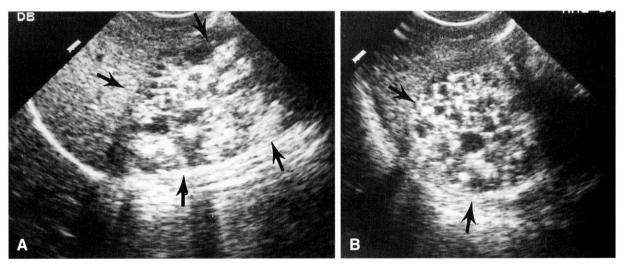

FIGURE 5.40. Autosomal recessive polycystic kidney disease: juvenile form. A. In this patient, note the marked echogenicity of the enlarged kidney (arrows). Small cysts also are present. **B.** Cross-sectional view demonstrates the same findings (arrows).

3. Hayden CK Jr, Swischuk LE, Smith TH, et al. Renal cystic disease in childhood. Radiographics 1986;6:97–116.
4. Currarino G, Stannard MW, Rutledge JC. The sonolucent cortical rim in infantile polycystic kidneys: histologic correlation. J Ultrasound Med 1989;8:571–574.
5. Jain M, LeQuesne GW, Bourne AJ, et al. High-resolution ultrasonography in the differential diagnosis of cystic diseases of the kidney in infancy and childhood: preliminary experience. J Ultrasound Med 1997;16:235–240.
6. Kern S, Zimmerhackl LB, Hildebrandt F, et al. Appearance of autosomal recessive polycystic kidney disease in magnetic resonance imaging and RARE-MR-urography. Pediatr Radiol 2000; 30:156–160.
7. Kogutt MS, Robichaux WH, Boineau FG, et al. Case report. Asymmetric renal size in autosomal recessive polycystic kidney disease: a unique presentation. AJR 1993;160:835–836.
8. Lucaya J, Enriquez G, Nieto J, et al. Renal calcifications in patients with autosomal recessive polycystic kidney disease: prevalence and cause. AJR 1993;160:359–362.
9. Herman TE, Siegel MJ. Pyramidal hyperechogenicity in autosomal recessive polycystic kidney disease resembling medullary nephrocalcinosis. Pediatr Radiol 1991;21:270–271.
10. Davies CH, Stringer DA, Whyte H, et al. Congenital hepatic fibrosis with saccular dilatation of intrahepatic bile ducts and infantile polycystic kidneys. Pediatr Radiol 1986;16:302–305.
11. Hussman KL, Friedwald JP, Gollub MJ, et al. Caroli's disease associated with infantile polycystic kidney disease: prenatal sonographic appearance. J Ultrasound Med 1991;10:235–237.
12. Jung G, Benz-Bohm G, Kugel H, et al. MR cholangiography in children with autosomal recessive polycystic kidney disease. Pediatr Radiol 1999;29:463–466.
13. Krull F, Schulze-Neick I, Luhmer I. Polycystic kidneys in Ivemark's syndrome. Acta Paediatr 1992;81:562–563.

Adult (Autosomal Dominant) Polycystic Disease (ADPK: Potter Type III)

Adult-type polycystic disease of the kidneys is inherited as an autosomal dominant condition and is usually referred to as autosomal dominant polycystic kidney disease. The abnormality in this condition involves the ampullary and interstitial portions of the collecting tubules and the nephrons. Symptoms usually become apparent in older children and young adults, but renal enlargement can be detected in some neonates. In these cases, however, renal insufficiency and hypertension as seen with the infantile form of polycystic disease is not a problem. When adult polycystic disease is suspected in an infant or child, it is worthwhile to ultrasonographically examine the parents and siblings (1), but it also should be noted that cysts that later become apparent may be too small to see in infants (2).

In the older child and adult, the large, sonolucent cysts in this condition are readily demonstrable with ultrasound (Fig. 5.41). The findings are rather characteristic, consisting of various sizes and numbers of cysts scattered throughout the kidney, including the subcortical region (3). Further imaging generally is not required even though these and associated hepatic cysts can be demonstrated with CT (Fig. 5.42), and MRI. The changes may be more pronounced in

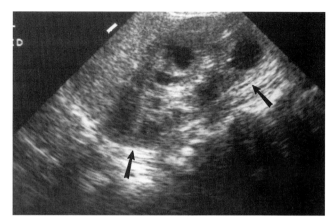

FIGURE 5.41. Adult (autosomal dominant) polycystic kidney disease. Note the multiple cysts in a slightly echogenic kidney (arrows).

one kidney than the other or even unilateral (4), but bilateral involvement generally is the rule. When adult polycystic kidney disease presents in infancy, cyst development is minimal, and the enlarged kidneys are echogenic (Fig. 5.43) and easily mistaken for those of infantile polycystic kidney disease. However, with high-resolution linear transducers, distinction between the types of cysts seen with the two conditions usually can be accomplished. With the infantile form of the disease, the cysts have a linear, tubular configuration, while with adult polycystic disease, the cysts are small and spherical. Because there are so many of them, a multitude of acoustical interfaces are present and lead to the characteristic echogenicity of the kidneys.

Calcification of these cysts can occur with time and the cysts can grow in size. Cysts also can be present in other organs, including the liver and pancreas, but as opposed to infantile polycystic disease, hepatic fibrosis rarely occurs (5). Occult intracranial arterial aneurysms also occur (6, 7), and it has been suggested that it probably is worthwhile to screen these patients with cranial MRA for occult aneurysms (7). Seminal vesicle cysts (8) have been seen with the condition.

REFERENCES

1. Gabow PA, Kimberling WJ, Strain JD, et al. Utility of ultrasonography in the diagnosis of autosomal dominant polycystic kidney disease in children. J Am Soc Nephrol 1997;8:105–110.
2. Nicolau C, Torra R, Badenas C, et al. Autosomal dominant polycystic kidney disease types 1 and 2: assessment of US sensitivity for diagnosis. Radiology 1999;213:273–276.
3. Jain M, LeQuesne GW, Bourne AJ, Henning P. High resolution ultrasonography in the differential diagnosis of cystic diseases of the kidney in infancy and childhood. Preliminary experience. J Ultrasound Med 1997;16:235–240.
4. Porch P, Noe HN, Stapleton FB. Unilateral presentation of adult-type polycystic kidney disease in children. J Urol 1986;135: 744–746.

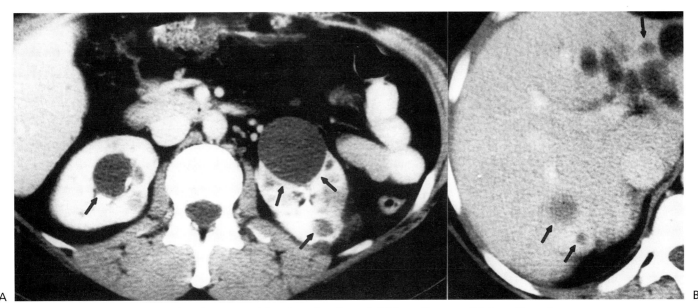

FIGURE 5.42. Adult (autosomal dominant) polycystic kidney disease with hepatic cysts. **A.** On this CT study, note the bilateral renal cysts (arrow). **B.** Cysts (arrows) also are present in the liver.

5. Lipschitz B, Berdon WE, Defelice AR, et al. Association of congenital hepatic fibrosis with autosomal dominant polycystic kidney disease. Report of a family with review of literature. Pediatr Radiol 1993;23:131–133.
6. Ruggieri PM, Poulos N, Masaryk TJ, et al. Occult intracranial aneurysms in polycystic kidney disease: screening with MR angiography. Radiology 1994;191:33–39.
7. Butler WE, Barker FG II, Crowell RM. Patients with polycystic kidney disease would benefit from routine magnetic resonance angiographic screening for intracerebral aneurysms: a decision analysis. Neurosurgery 1996;38:506–516.
8. Weingardt JP, Townsend RR, Russ PD, et al. Seminal vesicle cysts associated with autosomal dominant polycystic kidney disease detected by sonography. J Ultrasound Med 1995;14:475–477.

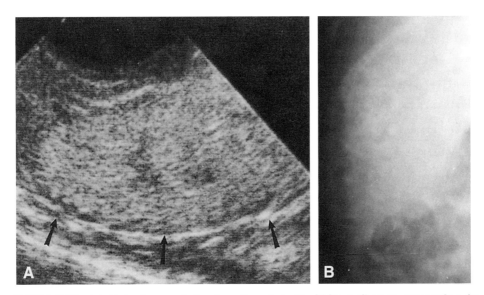

FIGURE 5.43. Adult (autosomal dominant) polycystic kidney disease presenting in infancy. Ultrasonogram demonstrates a large kidney (arrows) with a rather homogeneous pattern of increased echogenicity. Corticomedullary differentiation is lost, and scattered small cysts are seen in the kidney.

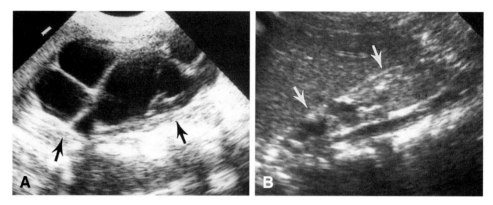

FIGURE 5.44. Multicystic dysplastic kidney with regression. A. The kidney is totally replaced by large cysts (arrows). Intervening septa are characteristically thin. **B.** Some months later, the cystic kidney has involuted and all that remains is a small echogenic, atrophic kidney (arrows) with a few cysts in the upper pole.

Multicystic Dysplastic Kidney Disease (MDKD: Potter Type II)

Multicystic dysplastic kidney is the most common form of cystic disease of the kidney in infants and children. It probably is the most common cause of a renal mass in the first week of life. Involvement usually is unilateral although bilateral disease can occur (1), and in some cases, segmental involvement of one kidney is seen (2, 3). In the latter cases, it usually is the upper pole that is involved. Overall, left side involvement is more common, and the condition is more common in males. Renal duplication and abnormalities such as ureteroceles can be associated (2, 4).

Typically, infants with multicystic dysplastic kidney disease present with a unilateral abdominal mass, and since only one kidney is involved, overall renal function is normal. In the past, these kidneys were routinely removed, but currently, they more often are left in situ (5). In support of this are data that have shown that some of these cysts decrease in size and regress spontaneously (5, 6). However, some may continue to enlarge, and if there is any doubt about the correct diagnosis (i.e., multilocular, cystic Wilms' tumor), surgical removal is advised (7). Differentiation of the two conditions can be accomplished on the basis of the fact that multilocular cystic kidneys demonstrate cysts within the intervening septa (8). Multicystic dysplastic kidneys that regress may regress to the point where the kidney is virtually gone or is small and dysplastic (Fig. 5.44).

When bilateral involvement occurs (rare), renal function is markedly impaired, and death soon ensues. These latter infants, similar to infants with infantile polycystic kidney disease, tend to have hypoplastic lungs secondary to the oligohydramnios-induced fetal compression syndrome. In cases proceeding to adulthood, calcifications in the rims of the cysts may develop. Wilms' tumor has been documented in association with multicystic dysplastic kidney (9, 10). If

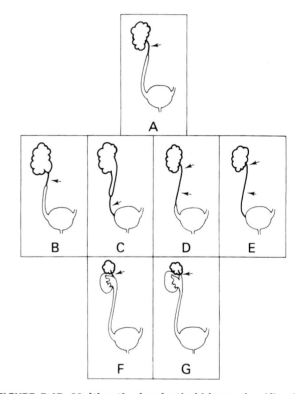

FIGURE 5.45. Multicystic dysplastic kidney: classification of types according to site and extent of ureteral atresia. A. High pelvoinfundibular atresia. This is the most common form and usually is not associated with a contralateral abnormality. **B–E. Lower ureteral atresia. All of these forms demonstrate variable degrees of atresia of the ureter below the renal pelvis. In B and C**, a dilated renal pelvis can be seen. All of these forms frequently are associated with contralateral ureteropelvic junction obstructions or multicystic dysplastic kidneys. **F. and G. Segmental atresia.** Usually, the upper pole is involved—either the upper part of a partially duplicated pole and adjacent infundibulum of a single kidney (F) or the upper part of a partially duplicated kidney (G). (Adapted from DeKlerk DP, Marshall FF, Jeffs RD. Multicystic dysplastic kidney. J Urol 1977;118:306–308.)

this is documented more often, it could lead to a reversal of the current trend of conservative, observational therapy.

The cause of multicystic dysplastic kidney is incompletely understood, but there is general belief that a multicystic dysplastic kidney is an end-stage hydronephrotic kidney. Although it has been known for some time that severe degrees of hydronephrosis can result in a multiloculated, completely destroyed kidney, only relatively recently has the theory that multicystic dysplastic kidney is an end-stage, hydronephrotic kidney gained popularity. It is postulated that a vascular insult to the upper ureter and/or renal pelvis occurs in utero; if this occurs early, a completely dysplastic kidney results, and if later, a hydronephrotic (ureteropelvic junction obstruction) kidney is seen.

Multicystic dysplastic kidney is associated with atresia of a variable length of the ureter and/or renal pelvis and with hypoplasia or atresia of the renal artery and vein (Fig. 5.45). In the most common form, high pelvoinfundibular atresia occurs. When atresia involves the ureter at lower levels, 40% of contralateral kidneys show abnormality, most often ureteropelvic junction obstruction (11, 12). These latter patients tend to do poorly.

Ultrasonographically, multicystic dysplastic kidneys present with a characteristic pattern, in which numerous spherical cysts of various sizes are seen scattered throughout the kidney. Virtually all of the kidney is replaced by the cysts, but intervening echogenic tissue remains (Fig. 5.46). These cysts may be large and numerous or small and not so

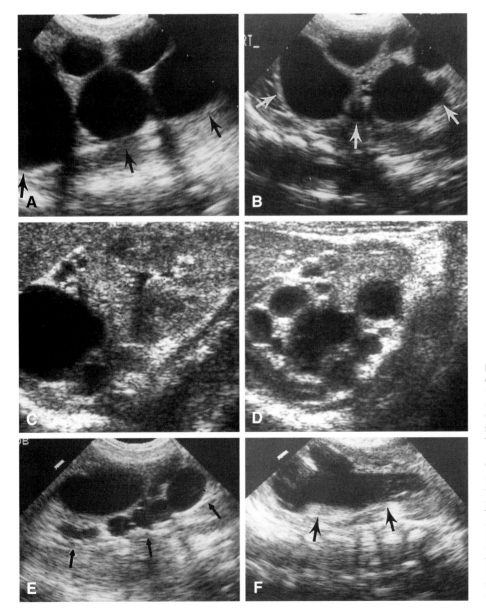

FIGURE 5.46. Spectrum of multicystic dysplastic kidney. A. Typical large, multiple cysts (arrows). No normal renal parenchyma remains. **B.** Cross-sectional view demonstrates the same findings (arrows). However, a few smaller cysts are seen between the large cysts. **C.** In this patient, cystic changes are confined to the upper pole. However, the kidney is enlarged and echogenic and has lost its normal architecture. **D.** Cross-sectional view of the upper pole demonstrates numerous cysts of various sizes. **E.** In this patient, a characteristic multicystic dysplastic kidney (arrows) is present on the right. **F.** On the left, a dilated renal pelvis and calyces are seen (arrows) secondary to a ureteropelvic junction obstruction.

numerous. Although most multicystic dysplastic kidneys are large and cystic, a few are atrophic and cystic (Fig. 5.46). It also is important that a multicystic dysplastic kidney be differentiated from a grossly hydronephrotic kidney. For the most part, this is accomplished by noting whether an identifiable renal pelvis is present and whether the cystic structures communicate with it. If the cystic structures communicate with the renal pelvis, they will be dilated calyces, and hydronephrosis will be the problem. If the cystic structures do not communicate and there is no identifiable renal pelvis, the diagnosis is multicystic dysplastic kidney. Most of these kidneys demonstrate associated dysplasia in the involved kidney and the contralateral, noninvolved kidney (13). ***This latter kidney may appear echogenic and without normal corticomedullary differentiation.***

REFERENCES

1. Schifter T, Heller RM. Bilateral multicystic dysplastic kidneys. Pediatr Radiol 1988;18:242–244.
2. Corrales JG, Elder JS. Segmental multicystic kidney and ipsilateral duplication anomalies. J Urol 1996;155:1398–1401.
3. Jeon A, Cramer BC, Walsh E, et al. A spectrum of segmental multicystic renal dysplasia. Pediatr Radiol 1999;29:309–315.
4. Karmazyn B, Zerin JM. Lower urinary tract abnormalities in children with multicystic dysplastic kidney. Radiology 1997;203:223–226.
5. Gordon AC, Thomas DFM, Arthur RJ, et al. Multicystic dysplastic kidney. Is nephrectomy still appropriate? J Urol 1988;140:1231–1234.
6. Strife JL, Souza AS, Kirks DR, et al. Multicystic dysplastic kidney in children: US follow-up. Radiology 1993;186:785–788.
7. Minevich E, Wacksman J, Phipps L, et al. The importance of accurate diagnosis and early close followup in patients with suspected multicystic dysplastic kidney. J Urol 1997;158:1301–1304.
8. Duncan AW, Charles AK, Berry PJ. Cysts within septa. An ultrasound feature distinguishing neoplastic renal lesion in children. Pediatr Radiol 1996;26:315—317.
9. Homsy YL, Anderson JH, Oudjhane K, et al. Wilms' tumor and multicystic dysplastic kidney disease. J Urol 1997;158:2256–2260.
10. Oddone M, Marino C, Sergi C, et al. Wilms' tumor arising in a multicystic kidney. Pediatr Radiol 1994;24:236–238.
11. Kaneko K, Suzuki Y, Fukuda Y, et al. Abnormal contralateral kidney in unilateral multicystic dysplastic kidney disease. Pediatr Radiol 1995;25:275–277
12. Sheih C-P, Hung C-S, Wei C-F, et al. Cystic dilatation within the pelvis in patients with ipsilateral renal agenesis or dysplasia. J Urol 1990;144:324–327.
13. Atiyeh B, Husmann D, Baum M. Contralateral renal abnormalities in multicystic-dysplastic kidney disease. J Pediatr 1992;121:65–67.

Multilocular Cyst

Although this condition generally is discussed with cystic disease of the kidney, multilocular cyst is in reality a tumor.

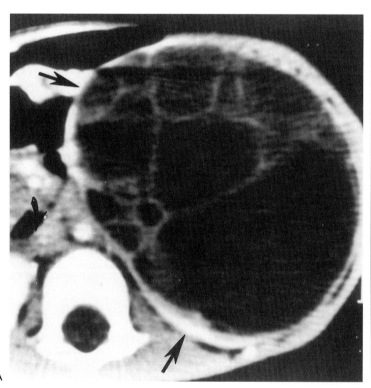
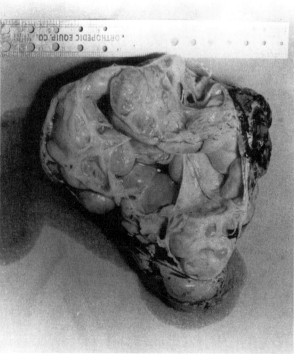

FIGURE 5.47. Multilocular cyst of the kidney: polycystic nephroma, cystic Wilms' tumor. **A.** Typical CT findings consisting of a multiseptate cystic lesion (arrows). **B.** Specimen from another patient demonstrating the multilocular nature of this lesion.

Most authorities feel that it is a form of epithelial nephroblastoma (i.e., precursor of Wilms' tumor). Renal multilocular cyst also is known as polycystic nephroma, cystic Wilms' tumor, or multilocular cystic nephroblastoma (1). The cysts in this condition are lined with epithelium, and the intervening stroma is fibromyxomatous. No renal elements, except for a few deformed nephrons, are present within the cysts, and the compressed, remaining portion of the kidney and the contralateral kidney are normal. Only occasionally is bilateral involvement seen.

Ultrasonography readily differentiates this cystic abnormality from solid Wilms' tumor. Characteristically, the multiseptated, cystic lesion is seen to compress the remaining, normal kidney in a curved, or crescentic "claw sign" manner. These findings are virtually diagnostic, although imaging with modalities such as CT (Fig. 5.47) and MR also usually is performed.

Differentiation from segmental multicystic dysplastic kidney may be difficult. However, in multicystic dysplastic kidney, no cysts are seen within the intervening septa (2).

REFERENCES

1. Agrons GA, Wagner BJ, Davidson AJ, et al. From the archives of the AFIP multilocular cystic renal tumor in children: radiologic-pathologic correlation. Radiographics 1995;15:653–669.
2. Duncan AW, Charles AK, Berry PJ. Cysts within septa. An ultrasound feature distinguishing neoplastic renal lesion in children. Pediatr Radiol 1996;26:315–317.

Medullary Cystic Disease

There are two forms of medullary cystic disease, medullary sponge kidney and medullary cystic disease. Medullary sponge kidney is uncommon in the newborn and young infant. It is a congenital abnormality of the collecting tubules confined to the medullary zone. No cysts appear in the cortical portion of the kidney. The abnormality in itself does not alter renal function, but its complications of stone formation and infection eventually bring these patients to the attention of a physician. As it is, however, they usually do not present with these problems until late childhood or adulthood. In older patients, the typical oval, radially aligned, intratubular calcifications and dilated distal tubules seen just along the edge of the renal papillae are characteristic. Ultrasonographically, the kidneys usually are normal, although some increase in echogenicity of the medullary pyramids can be seen (1) (Fig. 5.48). Most likely, this results from the development of early calcifications.

Medullary cystic disease with profound azotemia is another form of collecting tubule abnormality confined to the medullary zone of the kidneys. The kidneys in these patients are small and show considerable fibrosis. No cases have been reported in the neonate, and most consider the condition to be the same as juvenile hereditary nephronophthisis (1, 2). Many of these patients also have skeletal dysplasia (3, 4), short stature, cerebellar ataxia, retinal pigmentary dystrophy, and hepatic fibrosis (3). With ultrasound, the small, echogenic kidney with small

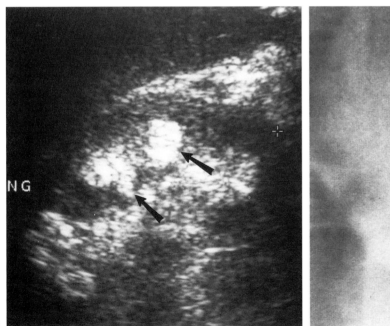
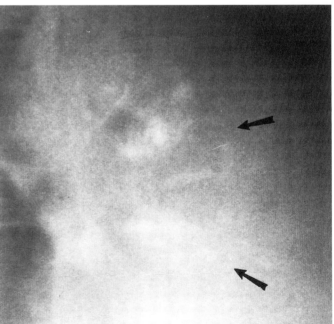

A

B

FIGURE 5.48. Sponge kidney. A. Ultrasonographic findings demonstrate echogenic renal papillae (arrows). **B.** On the intravenous pyelogram, note the puddling of contrast in the tubules (arrows).

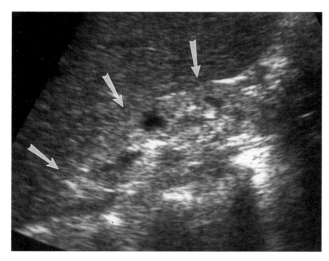

FIGURE 5.49. Familial nephronophthisis (azotemic medullary cystic disease). Note the small hyperechoic kidneys with a few scattered cysts (arrows).

medullary or corticomedullary cysts is highly suggestive of the condition (2) (Fig. 5.49). However, the cysts may not be present early in the course of this disease (1).

REFERENCES

1. Blowey DL, Querfeld U, Geary D, et al. Ultrasound findings in juvenile nephronophthisis. Pediatr Nephrol 1996;10:22–24.
2. Garel LA, Habib R, Pariente D, et al. Juvenile nephronophthisis:

sonographic appearance in children with severe uremia. Radiology 1984;15:93–96.
3. Popovic-Rolovic M, Calic-Perisic N, Bunjevacki G, et al. Juvenile nephronophthisis associated with retinal pigmentary dystrophy, cerebellar ataxia, and skeletal abnormalities. Arch Dis Child 1976;51:801–803.
4. Robins DG, French TA, Chakera TM. Juvenile nephronophthisis associated with skeletal abnormalities and hepatic fibrosis. Arch Dis Child 1976;51:799–801.

Solitary Renal Cysts

Solitary or simple renal cysts are not as common in children as in adults (1, 2) and are rare in neonates. However, with the increased use of ultrasonography, incidental, simple cysts are being discovered more often. These cysts, no matter when encountered, usually are purely sonolucent (Fig. 5.50), although some may contain a little debris and some may become infected (3). There usually is little problem in differentiating uncomplicated cysts from other lesions, but direct cyst puncture with contrast material injection can be used to outline the cysts in difficult cases (1, 2). Most often, ultrasonography provides a clear-cut answer.

The so-called pelvicalyceal cyst, or congenital hydrocalycosis, is by many considered a calyceal diverticulum. It is uncommonly encountered in infancy and childhood and differs from the other cysts in that it communicates with a calyx (Fig. 5.51). These cysts are rare, as are acquired calyceal cysts or diverticula.

REFERENCES

1. McHugh K, Stringer DA, Hebert D, et al. Simple renal cysts in

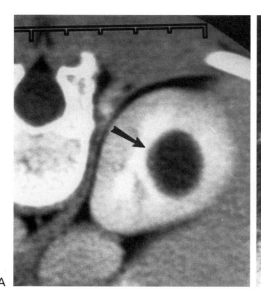
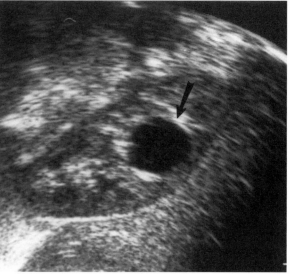

FIGURE 5.50. Simple renal cyst. A. Note the solitary cyst (arrow) in the upper pole of the right kidney. **B.** CT study shows a similar cyst (arrow).

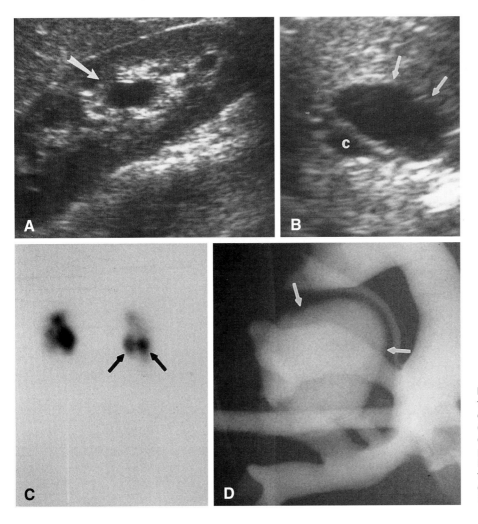

FIGURE 5.51. Calyceal cyst. A. Longitudinal sonogram demonstrates a renal cyst (arrow). **B.** Cross-sectional view demonstrates the cyst (arrows) adjacent to a calyx (C). **C.** Nuclear scintigraphy shows the cyst and calyx (arrows), both filled with isotope. **D.** Nephrostogram showing that the cyst (arrows) connects with the contrast-filled collecting system.

children: diagnosis and follow-up with US. Radiology 1991;178:383–385.

2. Steinhardt GF, Slovis TL, Perimutter AD. Simple renal cysts in infants. Radiology 1985;155:349–350.

3. Frishman E, Orron DE, Heiman Z, et al. Infected renal cysts: sonographic diagnosis and management. J Ultrasound Med 1994; 12:7–10.

Miscellaneous Cysts and Cystic Disease

A number of syndromes such as Conradi's disease, Zellweger syndrome, and Turner's syndrome can be associated with small cortical cysts. The kidneys in these patients often are small and hyperechoic. The small cysts may be numerous or sparse (Fig. 5.52). Small cortical cysts also occur in some trisomies, and cysts also can be seen in infants with tuberous sclerosis (1). In adults, the characteristic renal lesion in tuberous sclerosis is the angiomyolipoma, but in children, cysts are more likely to bring the disease to one's attention (Fig. 5.53).

Small cortical cysts also can be seen with severe obstructive hydronephrosis, such as occurs with posterior urethral

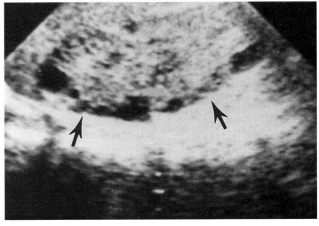

FIGURE 5.52. Cortical cysts in Zellweger syndrome. Note the small, hyperechoic kidney with numerous cysts scattered throughout its periphery (arrows).

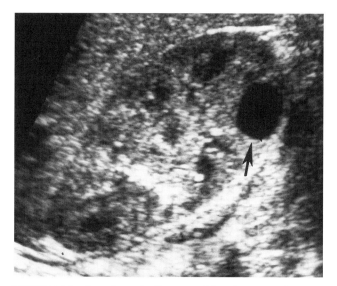

FIGURE 5.53. Renal cystic disease with tuberous sclerosis. Note the generally echogenic kidney parenchyma and the presence of simple renal cysts (arrows).

valves and results in the Potter's type IV cyst (Fig. 5.54). A relatively rare problem is "glomerulocystic disease" of the kidney. This is a rare form of polycystic kidney disease that occurs in infants (2–4). The kidneys characteristically are large and hyperechoic (Fig. 5.55). They can be confused with autosomal recessive polycystic kidney disease, but the underlying problem is different in that cystic dilation involves Bowman's space of the glomerulus and not the tubules, and cysts can be seen in the subcortical region (5).

The ultrasonographic findings are reasonably characteristic, and while renal function is normal at the onset, it deteriorates as the patient grows older (2).

REFERENCES

1. Mitnick JS, Bosniak MA, Hilton S, et al. Cystic renal disease in tuberous sclerosis. Radiology 1983;147:85–87.
2. Cachero S, Montgomery P, Seidel FG, et al. Glomerulocystic kidney disease: case report. Pediatr Radiol 1990;20:491–493.
3. Fitsch SJ, Stapleton FB. Ultrasonographic features of glomerulocystic disease in infancy: similarity to infantile polycystic kidney disease. Pediatr Radiol 1986;16:400–402.
4. Greer M-LC, Danin J, Lamont AC. Glomerulocystic disease with hepatoblastoma in a neonate: a case report. Pediatr Radiol 1998; 28:703–705.
5. Duncan AW, Charles AK, Berry PJ. Cysts within septa. An ultrasound feature distinguishing neoplastic renal lesions in children. Pediatr Radiol 1996;26:315–317.

Wilms' Tumor

Wilms' tumor of the kidney is the most common renal neoplasm in childhood. It arises from the nephrogenic epithelium, and its histologic picture can range from the relatively benign renal blastema or Wilms' tumor in situ to the highly malignant, sarcomatous, rhabdoid form of Wilms' tumor. In terms of the renal blastema, it is a relatively common necropsy finding in "normal" neonates and very young infants. As with neuroblastoma in situ, most of these lesions regress and seldom are they found after 4 months of age. When they do not regress, they may continue to grow and

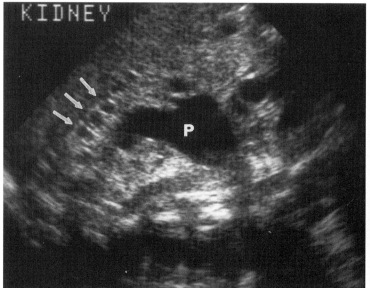

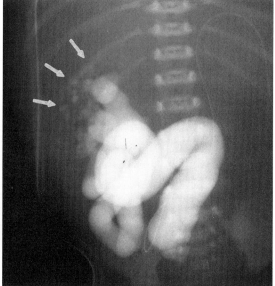

A   B

FIGURE 5.54. Type IV cyst. A. Note dilation of the renal pelvis (P) and numerous small peripheral cysts (arrows). **B.** Reflux into the right ureter as a result of posterior urethral valves demonstrates the small cysts (arrows) and the dilated collecting tubules resulting from backpressure. (Courtesy of C. Keith Hayden, M.D.)

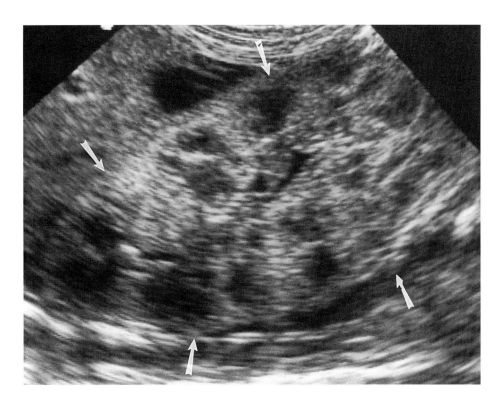

FIGURE 5.55. Glomerulocystic disease. The kidney (arrows) is enlarged and echogenic, and although a few medullary pyramids are seen, overall architecture is abnormal.

produce a true neoplasm, but in any given patient, one cannot predict when this will happen. Furthermore, a case has been reported in which diffuse nephroblastomatosis in an infant regressed, and a Wilms' tumor developed later (1).

Most often, Wilms' tumor presents as a nontender, rapidly growing, unilateral abdominal mass in older infants and children. The tumor in neonates is rare (2). If the tumor ruptures, or if intratumoral hemorrhage occurs, rapid enlargement and more acute symptoms develop. Microscopic hematuria can be seen with Wilms' tumor, but gross hematuria is rare. Associated hypertension also is rare but can occur and generally is caused by disruption of the blood flow to or from the kidney by vascular tumor involvement. This can occur by direct extension of the tumor into the vessel or by vascular compression, and it is more common with more malignant tumors (3). Hypertension also can result from actual production of renin by the tumor (4).

Aniridia is frequently associated with Wilms' tumor (5), and Wilms' tumor has been demonstrated in the so-called Drash or Denys-Drash syndrome (6–8). This condition, characterized by male pseudohermaphrodism, nephritis, and Wilms' tumor, is an uncommon but distinct entity. Not all of the features of the syndrome need be present, and in two of our patients, male pseudohermaphrodism was not present. Ultrasonographically, the kidneys in these patients demonstrate markedly increased echogenicity, but their size may be normal (Fig. 5.56). The associated Wilms' tumor appears no different from that seen in other patients, but because of the foregoing associations and others such as the

Beckwith-Wiedemann syndrome (9), there is strong belief that chromosomal abnormality (10) is at play in Wilms' tumor.

Hemihypertrophy of the extremities also occurs with Wilms' tumor and predominantly manifests in the lower extremities. This phenomenon also can be seen with other abdominal tumors and can occur before or after the tumor is discovered. Wilms' tumor also has been described on a familial basis (11) and in older children and young adults (12). However, peak incidence is in infants and children younger than 6 years.

Wilms' tumor generally is staged on the basis of local extent of the lesion and the presence or absence of metastases (Fig. 5.57). On the basis of such staging, therapy is prescribed and usually consists of surgery, chemotherapy, and in some cases, radiation therapy. Prognosis depends on the degree of sarcomatous and anaplastic change and on whether capsular or vascular invasion is present. When the capsule is invaded, local recurrences are more common, and when the renal vein, inferior vena cava, and right atrium are invaded (13–15), distant metastases are more common. Metastatic disease most commonly occurs to the lungs, but metastases to the bones and other organs also occur (16). Rarely, pulmonary metastases can cavitate (17), and overall, pulmonary metastases are best assessed with CT.

Bilateral Wilms' tumor poses a special problem and is variably estimated to occur in about 10% of cases. Bilateral disease can present simultaneously or asynchronously. Other peculiarities of Wilms' tumor include an increased

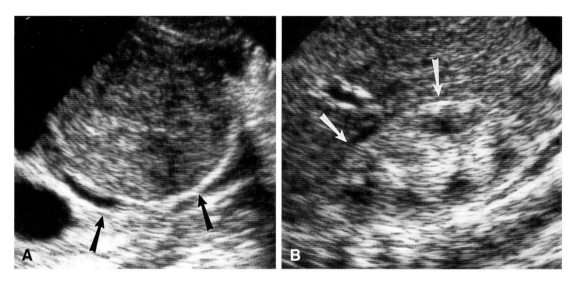

FIGURE 5.56. Wilms' tumor and nephritis (Drash syndrome). A. Note the large Wilms' tumor in the left kidney (arrows). Hydronephrosis of the upper pole exists. **B.** Contralateral right kidney shows marked increased echogenicity and smallness (arrows) consistent with nephritis.

incidence of the tumor in horseshoe kidneys and crossed renal ectopy. Wilms' tumor can arise from extrarenal sites, ranging from the mediastinum down to the groin (18, 19). Intrapelvic (renal pelvis) Wilms' tumor is relatively rare (20, 21), but in such cases, as the tumor invades the pelvis it can mimic neuroblastoma (Fig. 5.58) or some other problem such as xanthogranulomatous nephritis (20).

In terms of imaging, Wilms' tumor is a "clean" lesion, because in most cases, it is confined by the renal capsule and presents as a well-defined mass. Any imaging modality can demonstrate this aspect of the tumor, but in uncommon cases in which the tumor bursts through the capsule, the mass may not be as clearly defined. All of this is different from neuroblastoma, which usually demonstrates extension

beyond its original site at an early stage. Calcification is uncommon in Wilms' tumor but does occur, and when it does, it is irregular and indistinguishable from that seen with other malignant tumors. Ultrasonography, CT scanning, and MRI are commonplace in the investigation of Wilms' tumor, but even with these modalities, confusion between Wilms' tumor and neuroblastoma still occurs.

Ultrasonography is useful for initial diagnosis and in obtaining important additional information such as extent of the tumor into the inferior vena cava and tumor in the other kidney. On ultrasound, Wilms' tumor generally is solid and echogenic (Fig. 5.59A), although with tumor necrosis, cyst-like areas frequently can be encountered (Fig. 5.59, C–E). Hydronephrosis (often focal) is commonly present, and overall determination of renal origin of the tumor usually is readily accomplished. This is done by looking for normal renal tissue cupping the tumor in the "claw sign" configuration (Fig. 5.59C). Subcapsular hemorrhage (Fig. 5.59F) is rare but is said to be more common in and even diagnostic of rhabdoid tumors (22–24). In the right upper quadrant, it often is difficult to determine whether a tumor is arising from the liver or kidney. In these cases, the ultrasonographic sliding sign (25) can be used, and the uninvolved organ (i.e., organ from which the tumor is not arising) is seen to slide over the tumor. If one is fortunate enough to detect a Wilms' tumor in its early stages, an echogenic mass can be seen in the kidney (Fig. 5.60).

As far as MR examinations are concerned, on this study the tumor produces medium signal on T1-weighted images. On T2-weighted images, signal increases markedly, but it also becomes more difficult to separate tumor from kidney, because kidney parenchyma also shows increase in signal

Stage	Description
I	Tumor limited to kidney; capsule intact
II	Tumor extends beyond kidney or into blood vessels, including vena cava, but does not involve adjacent organs or regional lymph nodes; completely resectable
III	Residual nonhematogenous tumor confined to abdomen but does not involve liver; includes those that rupture during operation; completely resectable
IV	Hematogenous metastases (lung, liver, bone, or brain)
V	Bilateral renal involvement

FIGURE 5.57. Wilms' tumor, staging. Wilms' tumor is staged on the basis of local extent and metastatic spread. Stage V deals with bilateral disease.

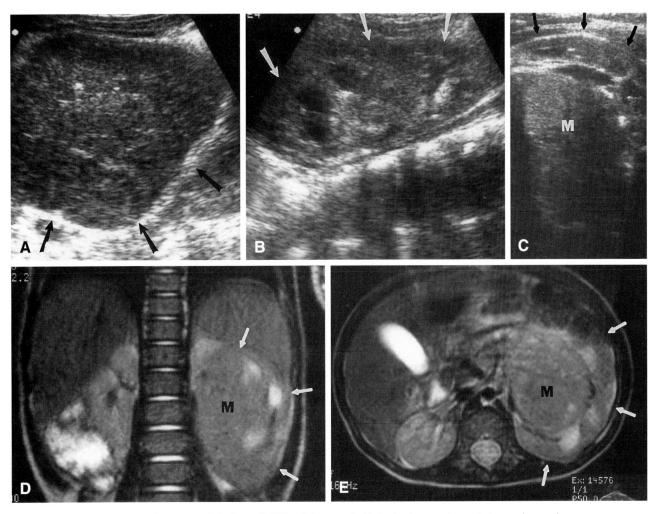

FIGURE 5.58. Intrapelvic (renal) Wilms' tumor. A. Note the large echogenic tumor (arrows). **B.** The ipsilateral kidney (arrows) is a little distorted and shows slightly dilated calyces. It was located lateral to the mass. **C.** Cross-sectional view demonstrates the mass (M) displacing the apparently compressed kidney (arrows) outwardly. **D.** Coronal, proton-density image demonstrates the central location of the tumor mass (M). Hydronephrosis of the surrounding calyces is seen (arrows). **E.** Cross-sectional image demonstrates the central, intrapelvic location of the tumor mass (M). The kidney (arrows) appears to surround the mass.

(Fig. 5.61). On T1-weighted images, focal areas of increased signal intensity represent hemorrhage, but we prefer CT over MRI for evaluating Wilms' tumor after initial investigation with ultrasound.

Intracaval and intracardiac tumor thrombus extension also can be identified with ultrasound, CT, or MRI (Fig. 5.62), but MRI may be best for mapping extensive thrombi. With ultrasound, it may be difficult to differentiate simple compression of the inferior vena cava from true intraluminal thrombus extension (Fig. 5.63). Contrast-enhanced CT and MRI are more useful in this regard, and as far as the rare problem of metastases to bones is concerned, they are best evaluated with nuclear scintigraphy and plain film radiography. With nuclear scintigraphy the metastatic lesions appear "hot," and on plain radiography, they appear lytic and aggressive.

REFERENCES

1. Rosenfield NS, Shimkin P, Berdon W, et al. Wilms tumor arising from spontaneously regressing nephroblastomatosis. AJR 1980; 135:381–384.
2. Ritchey ML, Azizkhan RG, Beckwith JB, et al. Neonatal Wilms' tumor. J Pediatr Surg 1995;30:856–859.
3. Steinbrecher HA, Malone PSJ. Wilms' tumour and hypertension: incidence and outcome. Br J Urol 1996;76:241–243.
4. Spahr J, Demers LM, Shochat SJ. Renin producing Wilms' tumor. J Pediatr Surg 1981;16:32–34.
5. Yunis JJ, Ramsay NKC. Familial occurrence of the aniridia-Wilms' tumor syndrome with deletion 11p13-14.1. J Pediatr 1980;96:1027–1030.
6. Coppes MJ, Huff V, Pellerier J. Denys-Drash syndrome: relating a clinical disorder to genetic alterations in the tumor suppressor gene WT1. J Pediatr 1993;123:673–678.
7. Jadresic L, Leake J, Gordon I, et al. Clinicopathologic review of

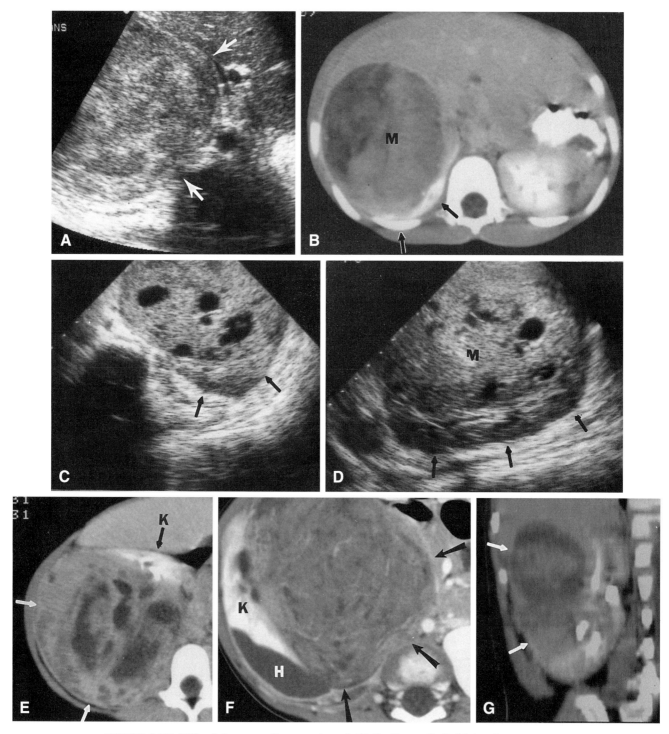

FIGURE 5.59. Wilms' tumor: ultrasound and CT findings. A. Solid but heterogeneous-appearing tumor (arrows) on the cross-sectional view. Echogenic areas probably represent foci of hemorrhage. **B.** CT study demonstrates a heterogeneous intrarenal mass (M) compressing the ipsilateral kidney (arrows). **C.** Another patient with a solid mass demonstrating numerous fluid-filled cyst-like areas (areas of necrosis) compressing the remainder of the kidney (arrows) into a typical "claw" sign configuration. **D.** Longitudinal view demonstrates the solid mass (M) compressing the kidney (arrows). **E.** Cystic-appearing Wilms' tumor on CT (arrows) compressing and displacing the residual kidney (K) anteriorly. **F.** Another basically solid tumor (arrows) compressing the remaining kidney (K). Also note an area of subcapsular hemorrhage (H). **G.** Reconstructed computed tomogram in this patient demonstrates the large mass (arrows) displacing the remaining kidney medially.

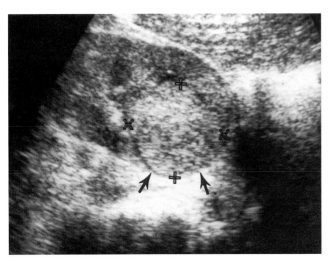

FIGURE 5.60. Early Wilms' tumor seen on ultrasound as an echogenic mass (arrows).

twelve children with nephropathy, Wilms' tumor, and genital abnormalities (Drash syndrome). J Pediatr 1990;117:717–725.

8. Tank ES, Melvin T. The association of Wilms' tumor with nephrologic disease. J Pediatr Surg 1990;25:724–725.
9. Andrews MW, Amparo EG. Case report. Wilms' tumor in a patient with Beckwith-Wiedemann syndrome: onset detected with 3-month serial sonography. AJR 1992;159:835–836.
10. Walton JM, Lee CLY, Mikhail E, et al. Unbalanced translocation of chromosome 3p in Wilms' tumor. Pediatr Surg 1992;27: 1311–1314.
11. Cordero JF, Li FP, Holmes LB, et al. Wilms' tumor in five cousins. Pediatrics 1980;66:716–719.
12. Kumar R, Amparo EG, David R, et al. Adult Wilms' tumor: clinical and radiographic features. Urol Radiol 1984;6:164–169.
13. Arens R, Frand M, Rechavi G, et al. Radiological cases of the month. Intracardiac extension of Wilms' tumor-related thrombus via the inferior vena cava. Am J Dis Child 1992;146: 1091–1092.
14. Crankson S, Ahmed S, Kumar N, et al. Rhabdoid tumour of the kidney with caval and cardiac extension. Pediatr Surg Int 1992;7: 225–228.
15. Weese DL, Applebaum H, Taber P. Mapping intravascular extension of Wilms' tumor with magnetic resonance imaging. J Pediatr Surg 1991;26:64–67.
16. Gururangan S, Wilimas JA, Fletcher BD. Bone metastases in Wilms' tumor–report of three cases and review of the literature. Pediatr Radiol 1994;24:85–87.
17. Kassner EG, Goldman HS, Elquezabal A. Cavitating lung nodules and pneumothorax in children with metastatic Wilms' tumor. AJR 1976;126:728–733.
18. Arkovitz MS, Ginsburg HB, Eidelman J, et al. Primary extrarenal Wilms' tumor in the inguinal canal: case report and review of the literature. J Pediatr Surg 1996;31:957–959.
19. Fahner JB, Switzer R, Freyer DR, et al. Extrarenal Wilms' tumor. Am J Pediatr Hematol Oncol 1993;15:117–119.
20. Groeneveld D, Robben SGF, Meradji M, et al. Intrapelvic Wilms: tumor simulating xanthogranulomatous pyelonephritis. Pediatr Radiol 1995;25:S68–S69.
21. Niu C-K, Chen WF, Chuang J-H, et al. Intrapelvic Wilms tumor: report of 2 cases and review of the literature. J Urol 1993; 150:936–939.
22. Chung CJ, Lorenzo R, Rayder D, et al. Rhabdoid tumor of the kidney in children: CT findings. AJR 1995;164:697–700.
23. Agrons GA, Kingsman KD, Wagner BJ, et al. Rhabdoid tumor of the kidney in children: a comparative study of 21 cases. AJR 1997;168:447–451.
24. Han TI, Kim M-J, Yoon H-K, et al. Rhabdoid tumour of the kidney: imaging findings. Pediatr Radiol 2001;31:233–237.

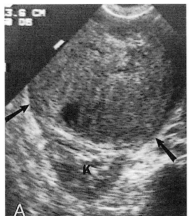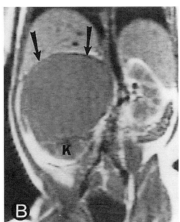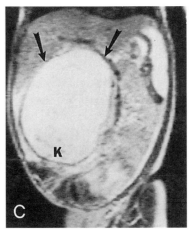

FIGURE 5.61. Wilms' tumor: MR characteristics. A. Transverse sonogram demonstrates a large echogenic tumor (arrows) compressing the ipsilateral kidney (K) into a typical "claw" sign configuration. **B.** T1-weighted MR image demonstrates moderate signal from the tumor (arrows) and poor separation from the kidney (K). **C.** T2-weighted image demonstrates marked increase in signal of the tumor mass (arrows) and extremely poor distinction from the kidney (K).

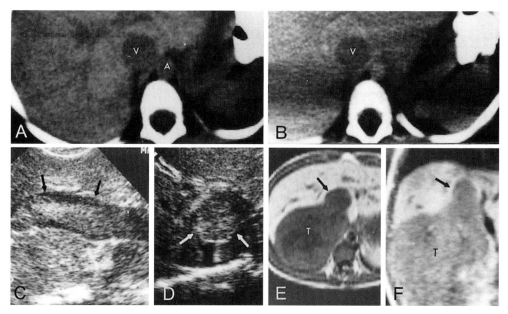

FIGURE 5.62. Wilms' tumor: CT, MR, and ultrasound demonstration of thrombus. A. Note on this precontrast CT study that both the aorta (A) and inferior vena cava (V) are visible. The inferior vena cava appears large. **B.** With contrast enhancement, contrast is seen in the aorta. The inferior vena cava (V), however, did not opacify because of tumor thrombus. **C.** Ultrasonogram in another patient demonstrates a large tumor thrombus (arrows) in the inferior vena cava. **D.** Cross-section in the same infant shows the thrombus (arrows). **E.** Axial MR scan shows the tumor (T) with extension through the renal vein into the IVC (arrow). **F.** Coronal slice shows the tumor (T) and its extension into the IVC (arrow). (**B** courtesy of Deborah Albin, M.D.)

25. Lim JH, Ko YT, Lee DH. Sonographic sliding sign in localization of right upper quadrant mass. J Ultrasound Med 1990;9: 455–459.

Nephroblastomatosis (Nodular Renal Blastema)

Nephroblastomatosis, or nodular renal blastema, is directly related to classic Wilms' tumor (1–3). Wilms' tumor is believed to originate from primitive metanephric epithelium, and in the fetus and newborn infant, small islands of such tumor tissue commonly occur. The situation is much the same as with neuroblastoma in situ, where most such lesions regress. On the other hand, in some infants, the tumors grow to form a classic Wilms' tumor or its relative, the multilocular cystic nephroma. In other cases, multiple such rests persist and result in nephroblastomatosis, a diffuse, bilateral disease usually occurring before the age of 4 months. It also can be seen with the Beckwith-Wiedemann syndrome.

Ultrasonographically, the kidneys afflicted with nephroblastomatosis appear large and show disorganized architecture with increased echogenicity (Fig. 5.64). On CT scanning and MRI, the large kidneys, with their associated splayed and compressed calyces, also are readily identified (Fig. 5.64). Nephroblastomatosis generally results in a uniform texture of the enlarged kidneys on all imaging modalities (3, 4), and with MRI, enhancement with gadolinium is seen. Nephroblastomatosis is quite amenable to chemotherapy.

REFERENCES

1. Lonergan GJ, Martinez-Leon MI, Agrons GA, et al. From the archives of the AFIP nephrogenic rests, nephroblastomatosis, and associated lesions of the kidney. Radiographics 1998;947–968.
2. Stone MM, Beaver BL, Sun C-CJ, et al. The nephroblastomatosis complex and its relationship to Wilms' tumor. J Pediatr Surg 1990;25:933–938.
3. Gylys-Morin V, Hoffer FA, Kozakewich H, et al. Wilms' tumor and nephroblastomatosis: imaging characteristics at gadolinium-enhanced MR imaging. Radiology 1993;188:517–521.
4. Rohrschneider WK, Weirich A, Rieden K, et al. US, CT and MR imaging characteristics of nephroblastomatosis. Pediatr Radiol 1998;28:435–443.

Benign Fetal Mesoblastic Nephroma (Hamartoma, Mesenchymoma, or Fibroma)

This tumor, also called Bolandes tumor, is the most common renal tumor of the neonate (1, 2), but a basic contro-

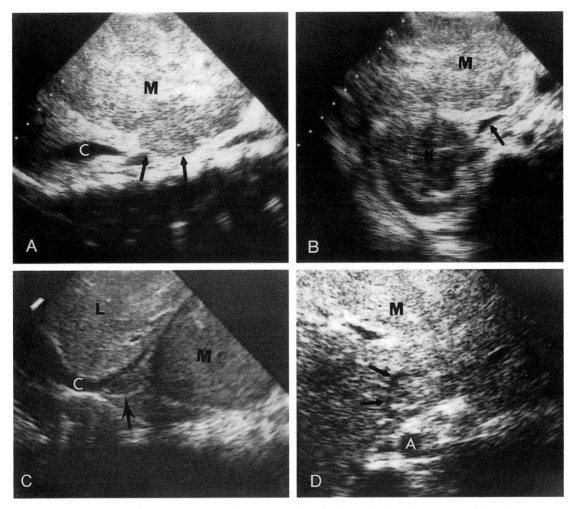

FIGURE 5.63. Wilms' tumor: caval compression. A. Note the large tumor mass (M) and a nodule of tumor (arrows) compressing the inferior vena cava (C). **B.** Transverse sonogram demonstrates the large mass (M) and the compressed inferior vena cava (arrow). K, kidney. **C.** Another patient with a large tumor mass (M) on the right. The inferior vena cava (C) appears to contain an intraluminal tumor thrombus (arrow). L, liver. **D.** Transverse sonogram in the same patient demonstrates the large tumor mass (M) and the aorta (A). Between is what appears to be a tumor-filled inferior vena cava with only a thin rim of sonolucent lumen remaining (arrows). A subsequent inferior vena cavagram in this patient demonstrated that the apparent intracaval tumor was actually extracaval.

versy still centers on whether it is a lesion totally separate from Wilms' tumor or just a peculiar variant. It probably is just a variant. In the past, however, many of these tumors were considered to be congenital Wilms' tumor, and their inclusion with Wilms' tumor probably contributed to the notion that neonatal Wilms' tumor had a better prognosis than it did when it occurred later.

To further complicate matters, the roentgenographic findings with ultrasound, CT, and MRI are still not typical enough to allow one to always differentiate the two tumors. For the most part, mesoblastic nephroma is solid and echogenic on ultrasonography, but some cases may show cystic components (3) (Fig. 5.65). Some of these tumors may bleed and present as a hemorrhagic cyst (4) or rupture

and cause hemoperitoneum and shock (5). Another variation of this tumor consists of the presence of dense calcifications (Fig. 5.65D), which has led to the term "ossifying renal tumor of infancy" (6–9). Congenital mesoblastic nephroma also can produce rennin, leading to hypertension (10), and can metastasize (11, 12) (Fig. 5.66).

REFERENCES

1. Gerber A, Gold JH, Bustamante S, et al. Congenital mesoblastic nephroma. J Pediatr Surg 1981;16:758–759.
2. Hartman DS, Lesar MSL, Madewell JE, et al. Mesoblastic nephroma: radiologic-pathologic correlation of 20 cases. AJR 1981;136:69–74.

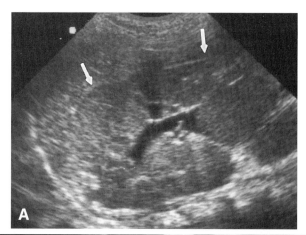

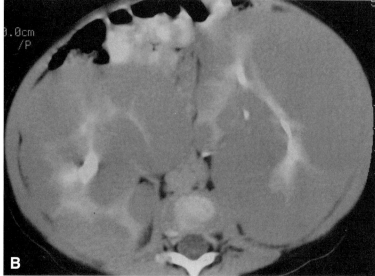

FIGURE 5.64. Nephroblastomatosis. A. Note the enlarged lumpy kidney (arrows). The fluid-filled calyces are compressed and splayed. **B.** CT demonstrates bilateral large kidneys virtually filling the entire abdomen. The calyces are compressed and splayed.

3. Grider RD, Wolverson MK, Jagannadharao B, et al. Congenital mesoblastic nephroma with cystic component. J Clin Ultrasound 1981;9:43–45.

4. Christmann D, Becmeur F, Marcellin L, et al. Mesoblastic nephroma presenting as a haemorrhagic cyst. Pediatr Radiol 1990;20:553.

5. Goldberg J, Liu P, Smith C. Congenital mesoblastic nephroma presenting with hemoperitoneum and shock. Pediatr Radiol 1994;24:54–55.

6. Steffens J, Kraus J, Misho B, et al. Ossifying renal tumor of infancy. J Urol 1993;149:1080–1081.

7. Sostre G, Johnson JF III, Cho M. Ossifying renal cell carcinoma. Pediatr Radiol 1998;28:458–460.

8. Vazquez JL, Barnewolt CE, Shamberger RC, et al. Ossifying renal tumor of infancy presenting as a palpable abdominal mass. Pediatr Radiol 1998;28:454–457.

9. Wheeler RA, Moore IE, Atwell JD. An infantile ossifying renal tumour. Pediatr Surg Int 1994;9:135–136.

10. Malone PS, Duffy PG, Ransley PG, et al. Congenital mesoblastic nephroma, renin production and hypertension. J Pediatr Surg 1989;24:599–600.

11. Schlesinger AE, Rosenfield NS, Castle VP, et al. Congenital mesoblastic nephroma metastatic to the brain: a report of two cases. Pediatr Radiol 1997;25:73S–75S.

12. Bell MG, Goodman TR. Perinephric cystic mesoblastic nephroma complicated by hepatic metastases: a case report. Pediatr Radiol 2002;32:829.

Other Renal Tumors

Renal cell carcinoma is not common in infancy but can be encountered in childhood (1–3). It can also arise after radiation therapy for neuroblastoma (4). It is not possible to histologically identify this tumor with any imaging modality, and it behaves just as do renal cell carcinomas in adults. Extension into the inferior vena cava and right atrium and pulmonary metastases are common (5). Overall the findings are similar to those of Wilms' tumor, especially the more malignant rhabdoid type. Primary renal lymphoma is rare (6–8), and as with lymphoma anywhere, the lesion is hypoechoic on ultrasonography. A rare tumor is the renal hemangiopericytoma (9), a tumor that originates from the capillaries and shows a mixture of solid and cystic components. Other tumors encountered include adenomas (10),

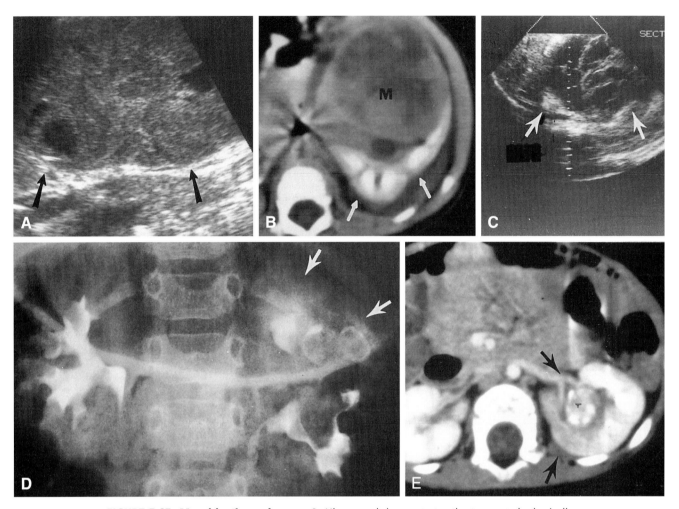

FIGURE 5.65. Mesoblastic nephroma. A. Ultrasound demonstrates the tumor to be basically solid (arrows). A few cystic areas are seen. **B.** CT demonstrates the heterogeneous appearance of the mass (M). It is characteristically intrarenal, and the compressed remaining kidney (arrows) is seen. **C.** Sonogram in another patient demonstrates a multicystic-appearing mesoblastic nephroma (arrows). **D.** Ossifying tumor of infancy, mesoblastic nephroma variant. Note the extensive calcification within the tumor (arrows), which itself is displacing the remainder of the kidney downward. **E.** CT study demonstrates the central tumor with calcification (arrows) and surrounding displaced renal parenchyma. (C courtesy of T. A. Smith; **D** and **E** from Steffens J, Kraus J, Misho B, et al. Ossifying renal tumor of infancy. J Urol 1993;149:1080–1081, with permission.)

intrarenal teratomas (11), and neuroectodermal tumors (12, 13).

REFERENCES

1. Aronson DC, Medary I, Finlay JL, et al. Renal cell carcinoma in childhood and adolescence: a retrospective survey for prognostic factors in 22 cases. J Pediatr Surg 1996;31:183–186.
2. Kabala JE, Shield J, Duncan A. Renal cell carcinoma in childhood. Pediatr Radiol 1992;22:203–205.
3. Kalyanpur A, Schwartz DS, Fields JM, et al. Case report. Renal medulla carcinoma in a white adolescent. AJR 1997;169:1037–1038.
4. Donnelly LF, Rencken IO, Shandell K, et al. Renal cell carcinoma after therapy for neuroblastoma. AJR 1996;167:915–917.
5. Roubidoux MA, Dunnick NR, Sostman HD, et al. Renal carcinoma: detection of venous extension with gradient-echo MR imaging. Radiology 1992;182:169–172.
6. Dobkin SF, Brem AS, Caldamone AA. Primary renal lymphoma. J Urol 1992;146:1588–1590.
7. Hugosson C, Mahr MA, Sabbah R. Primary unilateral renal lymphoblastic lymphoma. Pediatr Radiol 1997;27:23–25.
8. McGuire PM, Merritt CRB, Ducos RS. Ultrasonography of primary renal lymphoma in a child. J Ultrasound Med 1996;15:479–481.
9. Wan Y-L, Chen W-J, Chen W-F, et al. Renal hemangiopericytoma in childhood: noninvasive imaging. J Ultrasound Med 1992;11:237–239.
10. Navarro O, Conolly B, Taylor G, et al. Metanephric adenoma of the kidney: a case report. Pediatr Radiol 1999;29:100–103.
11. Ishii I, Okabe I, Hirose H, et al. Intrarenal teratoma in childhood. J Jpn Soc Pediatr Surg 1989;25:290–295.

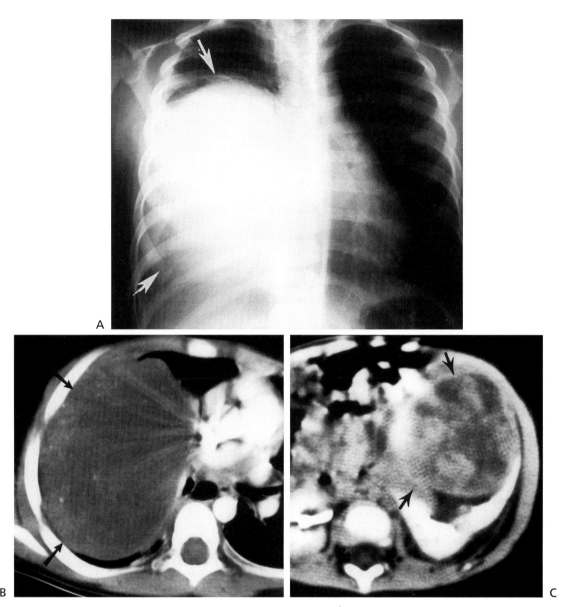

FIGURE 5.66. Mesoblastic nephroma with metastases. A. Note the large right lung mass (arrows). **B.** CT demonstrates the same mass (arrows). **C.** Previous perinatal CT demonstrates a large renal mass (arrows) on left.

12. Doerfler O, Reittner P, Groell R, et al. Peripheral primitive neuroectodermal tumour of the kidney: CT findings. Pediatr Radiol 2001;31:117–119.
13. Herman TE, McAlister WH, Dehner LP. Peripheral primitive neuroectodermal tumor: report of a case arising in the kidney. Pediatr Radiol 1997;27:620–621.

URETERAL ABNORMALITIES

Ectopic Ureter, Simple Ureterocele, and Ectopic Ureterocele

Ectopic insertion of the ureter stems from abnormal ureteral bud migration. Normally, the primitive ureteral bud travels cephalad, while the wolffian duct, from which it originates, travels caudad. However, if the ureteral bud fails to separate from the wolffian duct, the bud may be carried into a more caudal position than normal. As a consequence, the opening of the ureter becomes ectopic and in the female inserts into the lower bladder, urethra, vestibule, or vagina. Rarely, it can empty into the uterus or a wolffian duct remnant such as Gartner's duct or cyst. In males, it empties into the lower bladder, posterior urethra, seminal vesicle, vas deferens, or ejaculatory duct. In rare instances, it can empty into the rectum in either sex. In girls, if insertion of the ureter is below the urethral sphincter, dribbling is a chronic problem (1–4). This is important to appreciate, because these ureters may be occult, and only a high degree of suspicion may push one to cystography. In addition to the ectopic insertion of the ureter in these cases, the kidney also may be malpositioned or dysplastic, or both.

An ectopic ureter also can enter the bladder at a point above where it normally would insert. Faulty ureteral bud migration probably also accounts for these cases, and it has been demonstrated that the precise site of ectopia governs the degree of renal atrophy or dysplasia in the involved kidney (5). It appears that, if the ureter enters the bladder above its normal location, atrophy of the kidney is minimal, but if it inserts a little lower but still in a relatively normal position, a little more atrophy occurs. If, however, the ureter inserts distal to its normal site, severe renal dysplasia occurs.

A ureterocele can be seen with single kidneys with a normally inserting ureter and then it is referred to as a simple, single system, or orthoptic ureterocele (6, 7). This condition is more common in males, and the kidney frequently is ectopic and/or dysplastic. When a ureterocele develops in an ectopic ureter, it is called an ectopic ureterocele and is more common than simple ureterocele. It is more common in females. Urinary tract infection is common in these patients, especially in girls, as the ectopic ureter frequently inserts below the external ureteral sphincter or the vagina allowing for the retrograde introduction of perineal bacteria. With ectopic ureterocele, ectopic ureter drains the upper segment (moiety) of the kidney (i.e., Weigert-Meyer law).

All ureteroceles develop secondary to stenosis of the distal end of the ureter, leading to sac-like distal dilatation of the segment of ureter immediately above the stenotic segment (i.e., the ureterocele). The ureterocele presents with variable bulging or herniation into the bladder and can be unilateral or bilateral (Fig. 5.67). On voiding cystourethrography, the ureterocele produces a negative filling

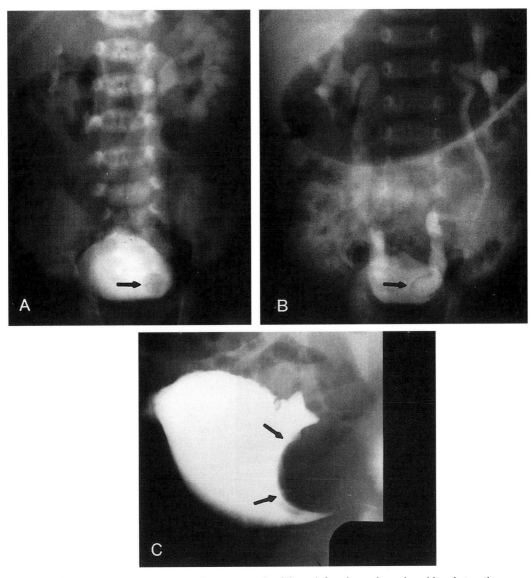

FIGURE 5.67. Simple ureterocele. A. Note the filling defect (arrow) produced by obstructing simple ureterocele. The left ureter and calyces are dilated. **B.** Bilateral obstructing simple ureteroceles producing bilateral hydroureter and hydronephrosis. The typical radiolucent halo (cobra head deformity) is best seen on the left (arrow). **C.** Another large filling defect produced by a simple ureterocele in a neonate (arrows).

defect in the contrast-filled bladder (Fig. 5.67A). Ureteroceles usually are detected initially with ultrasound, and the
round or oval wall of the ureterocele produces a cyst-like
structure protruding into the bladder (Fig. 5.68).
Hydroureter and hydronephrosis are variable, but not all
ureteroceles are associated with obstruction.

Ectopic ureteroceles usually are seen in association with
a nonfunctioning or poorly functioning duplicated upper
moiety. If the upper moiety is enlarged as a result of
hydronephrosis, it will displace the normal lower moiety
outwardly and inferiorly (Fig. 5.69). The large dilated collecting system of the upper moiety poses little difficulty in
differential diagnosis, except in the neonate, in whom a liquefying adrenal hemorrhage can produce similar findings.
Unfortunately, however, in some cases the upper moiety is
atrophic (8) and difficult to identify as being the upper
moiety of a duplicated kidney. This is important to appreciate for one can totally miss the finding (Fig. 5.70), except
that once one identifies a uterocele, especially in a female,
one should diligently search for the duplicated kidney and
expect the upper moiety to be very variable in its appearance. The ureter draining the duplicated kidney often is
dilated and can compress the other ureter. It also can alter
the insertion of the other ureter into the bladder and cause
reflux.

In any given case, on voiding cystourethrography, the
appearance of a ureterocele can be variable depending primarily on internal pressures in the ureterocele. If it is incarcerated and nonreducible, it is tense and presents as a persistent filling defect in the urinary bladder. If it is more
flaccid, it can be flattened during bladder filling and gives
rise to the disparity of having the ureterocele clearly visible

on ultrasound but invisible during voiding cystourethrography. In still other cases, the ureterocele herniates or pro-
lapses back into its ureter and results in an intraureteral
diverticulum (9). This also has been called the everting
ureterocele, and its presence can cause confusion (Figs. 5.71
and 5.72). Ureteroceles can prolapse into the urethra, and
this can be seen during voiding cystourethrography (Fig.
5.73). Such ureteroceles can present as perineal masses, and
although most commonly seen in females, they also occur
in males. Rarely, large ureteroceles can occlude the urethral
orifice during micturition and cause obstruction of the
bladder outlet (10).

REFERENCES

1. Braverman RM, Lebowitz RL. Case report. Occult ectopic ureter
   in girls with urinary incontinence: diagnosis by using CT. AJR
   1991;156:365–366.
2. Carrico C, Lebowitz RL. Incontinence due to an infrasphincteric
   ectopic ureter: why the delay in diagnosis and what the radiologist can do about it. Pediatr Radiol 1998;28:942–949.
3. Gharagozloo AM, Lebowitz RL. Detection of a poorly functioning malpositioned kidney with single ectopic ureter in girls with
   urinary dribbling: imaging evaluation in five patients. AJR 1995;
   164:957–961.
4. Borer JG, Bauer SB, Peters CA, et al. A single-system ectopic
   ureter draining an ectopic dysplastic kidney: delayed diagnosis in
   the young female with continuous urinary incontinence. Br J
   Urol 1998;81:474–478.
5. Mackie GG, Stephens FD. Duplex kidneys: a correlation of renal
   dysplasia with position of the ureteral orifice. J Urol 1975;114:
   274–280.
6. Blane CE, Ritchey ML, DiPietro MA, et al. Single system ectopic

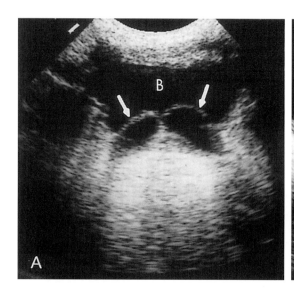
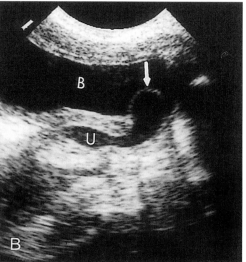

FIGURE 5.68. Simple ureterocele, ultrasonographic findings. A. Note the bilateral, spherical, simple ureteroceles (arrows) in this neonate. **B.** Lateral view demonstrates the ureterocele
(arrow) and its dilated ureter (U). B, bladder.

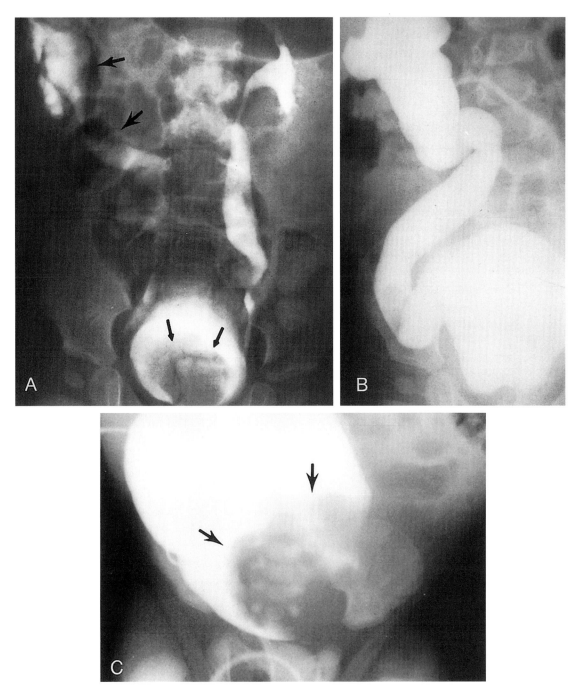

FIGURE 5.69. Ectopic ureterocele. A. Note the large oval filling defect resulting from the ureterocele in the contrast-filled bladder (lower arrows). Also note the inferolaterally displaced right kidney (upper arrows). Just above the right kidney, one can see a faint collection of contrast material in the poorly functioning, duplicated upper right kidney. Note the indentations along the right ureter produced by the dilated ectopic ureter. **B.** Cystogram with reflux into the ectopic system shows that the filling defect in the bladder and the indentations and deviations of the normal ureter on the right resulted from a massively dilated ureter from the upper kidney. **C.** Another patient with a lobulated filling defect (arrows) secondary to an ectopic ureterocele. (**B** courtesy of R. Macpherson, M.D.)

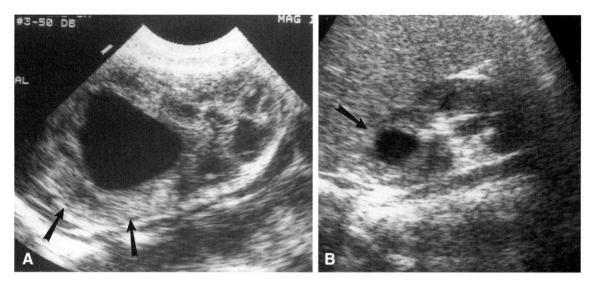

FIGURE 5.70. Ectopic ureterocele: various appearances of the upper moiety. A. In this patient, the duplicating upper system shows considerable hydronephrosis (arrows). **B.** In this case, the upper moiety is small and the hydronephrotic collecting system (arrow) could be misinterpreted for a simple cyst. Overall, the kidney appears normal.

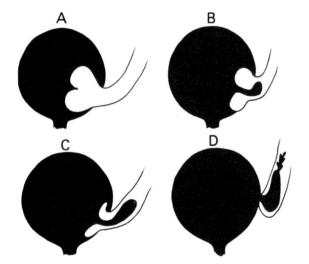

FIGURE 5.71. Ectopic ureterocele: mechanics of diverticulum formation. A. The ureterocele is protruding into the bladder. This produces a characteristic radiolucent filling defect. **B.** The ureterocele has emptied partially and is showing early prolapse into its own ureter. **C.** More prolapse produces a larger diverticulum located within the ureter. **D.** Still later, reflux from the prolapsed diverticular ureterocele occurs into the ureter. (Adapted from Cremin BJ, Funston MR, Aaronson IA. The intraureteric diverticulum, a manifestation of ureterocele intussusception. Pediatr Radiol 1977;6:92–96.)

ureters and ureteroceles associated with dysplastic kidney. Pediatr Radiol 1992;22:217–220.

7. Zerin JM, Baker DR, Casale JA. Single system ureteroceles in infants and children: imaging features. Pediatr Radiol 2000;30: 139–146.

8. Share JC, Lebowitz RL. The unsuspected double collecting system on imaging studies and at cystoscopy. AJR 1990;155: 561–564.

9. Bellah RD, Long FR, Canning DA. Ureterocele eversion with vesicoureteral reflux in duplex kidneys: findings at voiding cystourethrography. AJR 1997;165:409–413.

10. Shetty BP, John SD, Swischuk LE, et al. Bladder neck obstruction caused by a large simple ureterocele in a young male. Pediatr Radiol 1995;25:460–461.

Ureteropelvic Junction Obstruction

Ureteropelvic junction obstruction is a commonly occurring congenital abnormality that often is first diagnosed in the fetus. Interestingly, however, it has been found that many cases discovered in the fetus are self-limiting (1). Ureteropelvic junction obstruction is believed to be slightly more common on the left than on the right, but bilateral involvement is not unusual. It also is more common in males, and ectopic kidneys also are prone to ureteropelvic junction obstruction (2). Overall, the condition probably is one of the most common causes of obstructive hydronephrosis in children. The actual cause of obstruction usually is stenosis, probably resulting from an intrauterine segmental vascular insult to the ureter or pelvis. Extrinsic pressure from aberrant vessels (3) or fibrous bands also can cause obstruction, and even less common causes include valve-like flaps of tissue in the ureter, deficiency of the mus-

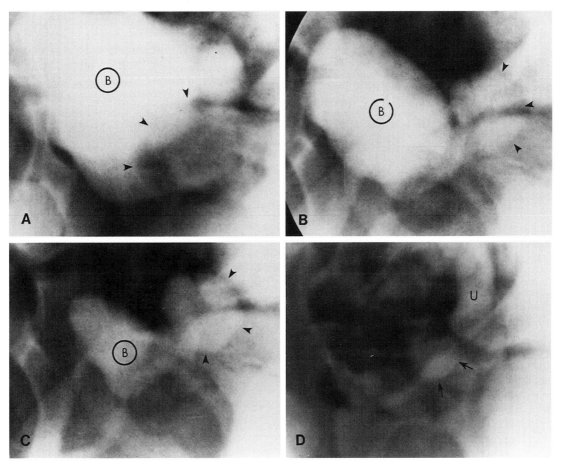

FIGURE 5.72. Everting or prolapsing ectopic ureterocele. A. With a bladder (B) full of contrast material, the ureterocele presents as a filling defect (arrows). **B.** Later, with voiding, the ureterocele has everted or prolapsed into the ureter to produce a diverticulum (arrows). **C.** The bladder has completely emptied and only the diverticulum (arrows) remains. **D.** Still later, the diverticulum has become smaller (arrows) because some of its contents have refluxed into the ureter (U).

cle at the ureteropelvic junction, and polyps (4). However, fetal schemia-induced stenosis is believed to be the most common cause of obstruction.

Roentgenographically, if hydronephrosis is advanced, a mass might be seen on plain films, but the entity generally is detected with ultrasound. After the hydronephrotic kidney is identified, one must make sure that obstruction truly is located at the ureteropelvic junction and that there is no dilated ureter below this level. Cases of giant hydronephrosis must be differentiated from multicystic dysplastic kidney and this is accomplished by noting that the dilated calyces communicate with the dilated pelvis (Fig. 5.74, A and B). The pelvis can be very large and elongated in some cases and may erroneously be interpreted for a dilated ureter (5) or large abdominal cyst (Fig 5.74C).

Not all cases of ureteropelvic junction obstruction result in marked dilation of the renal pelvis from the onset. Some cases, with equivocal obstruction, show minimal change

and may remain that way. The findings in these patients must be differentiated from the findings seen in patients with an extrarenal pelvis. It is in such cases that diuretic washout scintigraphy is most helpful, because there are no signs of obstruction with an extrarenal pelvis. With established uteropelvic junction obstruction, one sees delayed accumulation of isotope in the kidney and obstructed pelvis and lack of its washout from the pelvis during the diuretic phase of the study (Fig. 5.75). With equivocal obstruction, these findings are attenuated but still abnormal.

Clinically, patients with significant obstruction may present with intermittent pain (6) (which waxes and wanes with fluid load), infection, an abdominal mass, or hematuria. Hematuria is especially common after abdominal trauma, which in itself may be minor. In other cases, the patient is totally asymptomatic, and an abdominal mass is discovered on routine physical examination. Ureteropelvic junction obstruction can co-exist with ureterovesical junc-

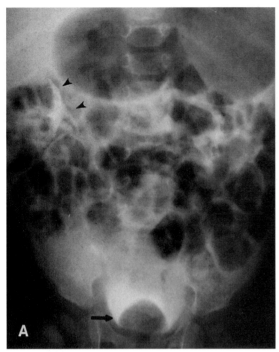

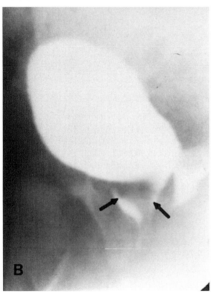

FIGURE 5.73. Prolapsing ectopic ureterocele. A. Note the characteristic displacement of the lower right kidney (upper arrows) and the classic filling defect in the bladder (lower arrow). **B.** Voiding cystourethrogram shows the ectopic ureterocele partially prolapsed into the urethra (arrows).

tion obstruction (7) and with reflux. For this reason, a voiding cystourethrogram should be performed in all cases (Fig. 5.76).

Ultrasound can be used to determine the degree of obstruction by measuring resistive indices before and after diuretic therapy (8). However, this procedure is not in gen-

eral use, because the information obtained with ordinary ultrasound and nuclear scintigraphy usually provides enough information for therapeutic decision-making. Postoperatively, dilatation as demonstrated with ultrasound is slow to clear, but this does not necessarily indicate persistent obstruction (9, 10). The possibility of persistent obstruction is best evaluated with nuclear scintigraphy. Parenchymal regrowth appears to occur more quickly (10), and balloon dilatation can be used to treat the condition (11).

REFERENCES

1. Freedman ER, Rickwood AM. Prenatally diagnosed pelviureteric junction obstruction: a benign condition? J Pediatr Surg 1994; 29:769–772.
2. Ulchaker J, Ross J, Alexander F, et al. The spectrum of uretero-pelvic junction obstructions occurring in duplicated collecting systems. J Pediatr Surg 1996;31:1221–1224.
3. Rooks VJ, Lebowitz RL. Extrinsic ureteropelvic junction obstruction from a crossing renal vessel: demography and imaging. Pediatr Radiol 2001;31:120–124.
4. Greig JD, Azmy AF. An unusual case of pelviureteric junction obstruction. J Pediatr Surg 1992;27:525–526.
5. Schlesinger AE, Shackelford GD, Colberg JW. Ureteropelvic junction obstruction in infants mimicking ureterovesical junction obstruction on sonography. Pediatr Radiol 1995;25:476–477.
6. Belman AB. Ureteropelvic junction obstruction as a cause for intermittent abdominal pain in children. Pediatrics 1991;88:1066–1069.
7. McGrath MA, Estroff J, Lebowitz RL. The coexistence of obstruction at the ureteropelvic and ureterovesical junctions. AJR 1987;149:403–406.
8. Kincaid AS, Hollman, Azmy AF. Doppler ultrasound in pelvi-ureteric junction obstruction in infants and children. J Pediatr Surg 1994;29:765–768.
9. Amling CL, O'Hara SM, Wiener JS, et al. Renal ultrasound changes after pyeloplasty in children with ureteropelvic junction obstruction: long-term outcome in 47 renal units. J Urol 1996; 156:2020–2040.
10. Kis E, Verebely T, Kovi R, et al. The role of ultrasound in the follow-up of postoperative changes after pyeloplasty. Pediatr Radiol 1998;28:247–249.
11. Wilkinson AG, Azmy A. Balloon dilatation of the pelviureteric junction in children. Early experience and pitfalls. Pediatr Radiol 1996;26:882–886.

Megaureter

Primary megaureter may be caused by distal ureteral obstruction or gross vesicoureteral reflux. With primary megaureter, the ureterovesical junction obstruction is functional, resulting from the distal most segment of the ureter being aperistaltic (1). In the past, the findings were demonstrable with intravenous pyelography (Fig. 5.77A), but ultrasonography is the imaging modality of choice when the persistently narrowed, aperistaltic segment suggests the

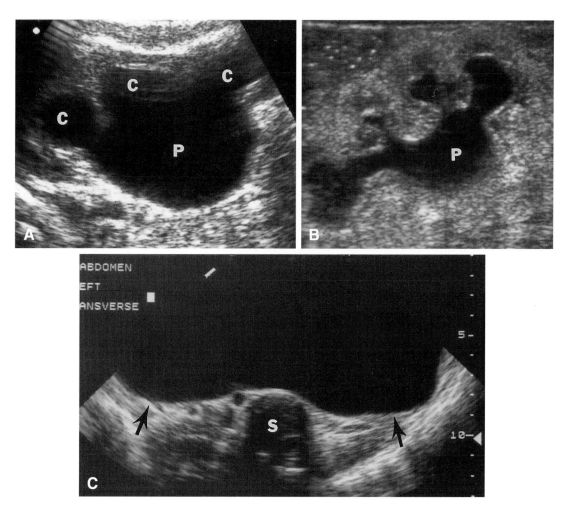

FIGURE 5.74. Ureteropelvic junction obstruction: ultrasonographic findings. A. Markedly distended renal pelvis (P) and calyces (C). **B.** Another patient with a distended renal pelvis (P) and calyces. **C.** In this patient, the markedly dilated renal pelvis (arrows) occupies most of the abdomen and is located to both sides of the spine (S).

diagnosis (Fig. 5.77B). Nuclear scintigraphy also can demonstrate the same findings (Fig. 5.77C). It is not known why this short segment of the ureter is aperistaltic, but comparisons to Hirschsprung's disease have been made. However, aganglionosis has not been proved to be the problem, and the cause of the condition remains unknown. In some cases, the ureter may become extremely large and virtually occupy the whole abdomen, and reflux can co-exist (2). Concomitant megacalyces also have been documented (3).

With chronic megaureter resulting from gross reflux, the distal end of the ureter is seen to be wide open (Fig. 5.78), but if the problem is distal ureteral obstruction resulting from a problem such as ureteral stenosis, a narrowed, fixed, distal ureteral segment is seen (Fig. 5.79). Bilateral large ureters not resulting from reflux or obstruction also can be

seen with hyperdiuretic states such as Bartter's syndrome and chronic water intoxication.

REFERENCES

1. Ramaswamy S, Bhatnagar V, Mitra DK, et al. Congenital segmental giant megaureter. J Pediatr Surg 1995;30:123–124.
2. Blickman JG, Lebowitz RL. The coexistence of primary megaureter and reflux. AJR 1984;143:1053–1058.
3. Vargas, B, Lebowitz, RL. The coexistence of congenital megacalyces and primary megaureter. AJR 1986;147:313–316.

Ureteral Atresia and Stenosis

Atresia of the ureter usually is seen with renal agenesis or dysplasia (i.e., multicystic, dysplastic kidney). A diagram-

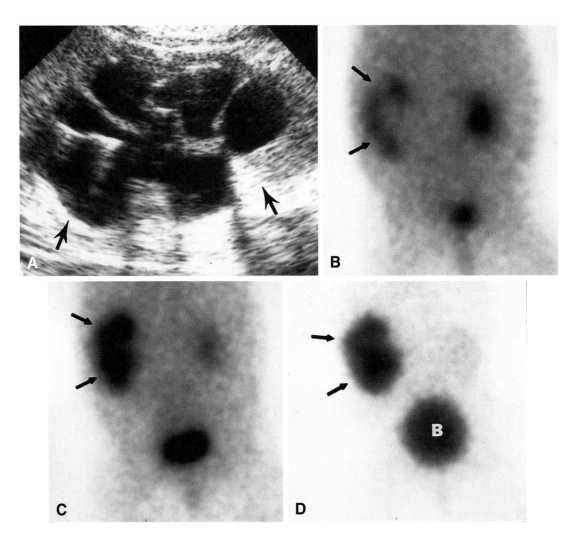

FIGURE 5.75. Ureteropelvic junction obstruction: scintigraphic evaluation. A. Marked hydronephrosis of the left kidney (arrows) is present. **B.** Early during renal scintigraphy, the cortex of the left kidney (arrows) is seen to function, but there is no filling of the pelvis. **C.** Later, the pelvis (arrows) fills but there is lack of passage of isotope into the ureter. The findings are typical of obstruction. **D.** Seventy-five minutes after Lasix injection, virtually none of the isotope has left the left kidney (arrows). All of the isotope has washed out of the normal right kidney. B, bladder.

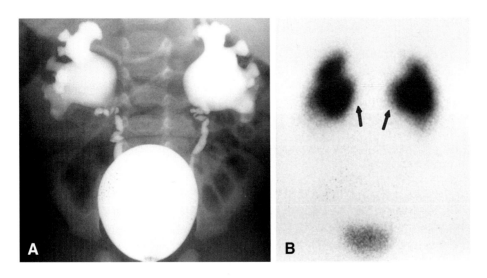

FIGURE 5.76. Ureteropelvic junction obstruction and reflux. A. Note the reflux into both collecting systems. The renal pelves and calyces are markedly dilated bilaterally. **B.** Nuclear scintigraphy demonstrates bilateral accumulation of isotope from both kidneys (arrows). The findings persisted on Lasix washout and are characteristic of bilateral ureteropelvic junction obstruction.

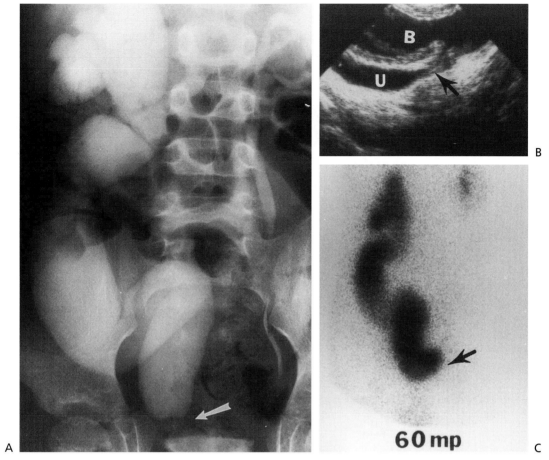

FIGURE 5.77. Primary megaureter. A. Postvoiding intravenous pyelogram demonstrates the massively dilated right ureter. Note the empty, stenotic distal segment (arrow). **B.** Sonogram in same patient demonstrates the dilated ureter (U) and the stenotic distal segment (arrow). B, urinary bladder. **C.** Nuclear scintigraphy at 60 minutes demonstrates accumulation of isotope in the dilated, obstructed (arrow) ureter.

matic representation of the different forms of ureteral atresia is shown in Figure 5.45. In some of these cases, the lower portion of the ureter may remain patent, but in others, the entire ureter and hemitrigone are absent. In cases of lower end patency, the ureter extends upward from the bladder and ends as a blind pouch (Fig. 5.80). If only the distal ureteral segment is atretic, hydroureter and hydronephrosis of the ureter and kidney above it result. Congenital stenoses of the ureter, other than those at the ureteropelvic or ureterovesicular junctions, are uncommon. The cause of ureteral atresias and stenoses is believed to lie in the realm of intrauterine vascular insult.

Acquired stenoses can occur after trauma, infection, and as an aftermath of Henoch-Schönlein purpura (1). Narrowing and obstruction of the ureter can result from secondary compression by pelvic masses and inflammatory processes in the right lower quadrant such as appendiceal abscess and regional enteritis.

REFERENCE

1. Smet M-H, Marchal G, Oyen R, et al. Stenosing hemorrhagic ureteritis in a child with Henoch-Schönlein purpura: CT appearance. J Comput Assist Tomogr 1991;15:326–328.

Ureteral Duplication

Duplication of the ureter is a commonly encountered anomaly of the urinary tract. Incomplete duplication is more common than complete duplication, and neither was difficult to identify with intravenous pyelography. Duplicated, nondilated ureters, however, are easily missed with ultrasound. CT is more productive. In most cases, the anomaly is associated with duplication of the renal pelvis and/or kidney, and if duplication is complete, two ureters can be traced down to their separate insertions into the bladder. On the other hand, if duplication is partial, two

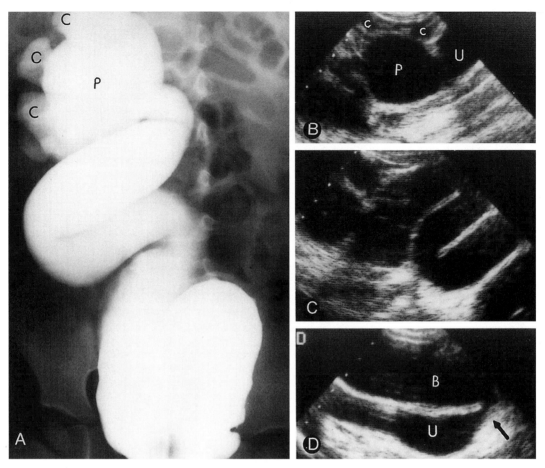

FIGURE 5.78. Refluxing megaureter. A. Note the massive hydronephrosis and megaureter on the right, secondary to reflux. C, calyces; P, pelvis. **B.** Longitudinal sonogram demonstrates the same findings. C, calyces; P, dilated pelvis; U, ureter. **C.** Sonogram (a little lower down) demonstrates the markedly dilated and tortuous ureter. **D.** Longitudinal sonogram at the level of the urinary bladder (B) demonstrates the dilated ureter (U) and its open distal end (arrow).

separate ureters leave the kidney, but before entering the bladder, both ureters unite and empty through a single orifice. When duplication is complete, the ureter from the upper kidney inserts lower than that from the lower kidney (i.e., Weigert-Meyer law).

In rare instances, a ureter may be duplicated in its lower portion only and, as a result, may appear as a blind-ending pouch during cystourethrography. In still other instances, also rare, triplication (1) or quadruplication (2) of the ureter may be seen. All of these ureteral anomalies probably result from abnormalities in division of the primitive ureteral buds. Ureteral and renal duplication also can be associated with ureteropelvic junction obstruction of the lower pole of the kidney, an entity that is more common in males. (3)

REFERENCES

1. Gopsalbez R Jr, Gosalbez R, Piro C, et al. Ureteral triplication and ureterocele: report of three cases and review of the literature. J Urol 1991;145:105–108.

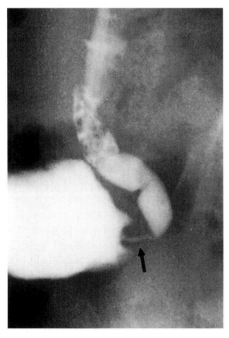

FIGURE 5.79. Ureteral stenosis. Note the stenotic distal ureter (arrow).

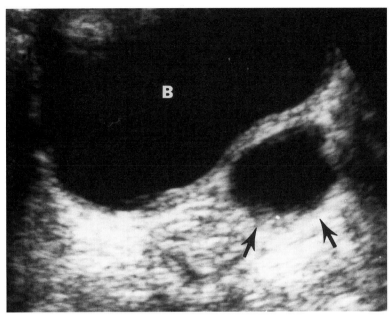

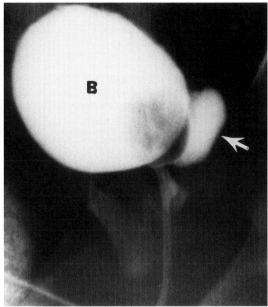

A

B

FIGURE 5.80. Ureteral atresia: remnant distal ureteral pouch. A. On this ultrasound study, note the hypoechoic pouch (arrows) extending from the bladder (B). **B.** Cystogram demonstrates the same ureteral remnant (arrow). B, bladder.

2. Sourtzis S, Damry N, Janssen F, et al. Ureteral quadruplication: the fourth case report. Pediatr Radiol 1994;24:604–605.
3. Fernbach SK, Zawin JK, Lebowitz RL. Complete duplication of the ureter with ureteropelvic junction obstruction of the lower pole of the kidney: imaging findings. AJR 1995;164:701–704.

Ureteral Valves, Diverticula, Polyps, and Tumors

Ureteral valves or membranes causing obstruction are uncommonly encountered in any age group (1) and are rare in the neonate. By the same token, ureteral diverticula are uncommon but, when present, can be large. Polyps of the ureter are rare (2), as are tumors (3).

REFERENCES

1. Maizels M, Stephens FD. Valves of the ureter as a cause of primary obstruction of the ureter: anatomic, embryologic and clinical aspects. J Urol 1980;123:472–474.
2. Liddell RM, Weinberger E, Schofield DE, et al. Case report. Fibroepithelial polyp of the ureter in a child. AJR 1991;157: 1273–1274.
3. Charny CK, Glick RD, Genega EM, et al. Ewing's sarcoma/primitive neuroectodermal tumor of the ureter: a case report and review of the literature. J Pediatr Surg 2000;35:1356–1358.

Ureteral Hernias

Ureteral hernias can be inguinal, femoral, or sciatic, but all are uncommon. The diagnosis often is made on an inci-

dental basis by noting the ureter being kinked and located in one of these abnormal areas. Often, no obstruction is present, but it can occur. One of the major problems with this unusual abnormality is that the ureter can be injured during repair of the hernia if its presence in the hernial sac is unsuspected.

LOWER URINARY TRACT

Normal Bladder and Urethra

Normal anatomic features of the male and female urinary bladder and urethra are demonstrated in Figure 5.81. In the male, the normal bladder neck may appear narrow, but it should not be misinterpreted as representing bladder neck contracture. Transient herniation of the bladder into the inguinal canal of infants is frequently encountered up to the age of 6 months (Fig. 5.82). The finding has been referred to as "bladder ears."

Ultrasonographically, the bladder should be examined when fully distended, because otherwise, the bladder wall often erroneously appears thickened (Fig. 5.83). With the bladder fully distended, one can identify the echogenic mucosal lining and the surrounding, thin, sonolucent smooth muscle layer. Normal bladder wall measurements are available, and it has been determined that, with the bladder distended, the wall is about 1.5 mm thick (1). Methods for measuring normal and abnormal bladder capacity are available (2–4), but most often, this judgment is made subjectively.

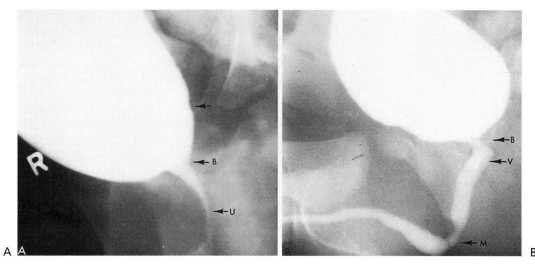

FIGURE 5.81. Normal bladder and urethra. A. Normal female bladder showing urethra (U), bladder neck (B), and posterior notch indicating site of insertion of the ureter (upper arrow). **B.** Male bladder showing normal bladder neck (B), oval radiolucency resulting from the verumontanum (V), and membranous urethra (M). The apparent narrowing at the bladder neck is normal and is usually present in newborn male infants. It should not be misinterpreted as representing bladder neck contracture.

In males, with angulation of the transducer toward the pelvis, one can outline the proximal portion of the posterior urethra and the surrounding prostate gland (Fig. 5.84). In other cases, one also can identify the normal distal ureter as it inserts into the bladder. It produces a thin, sonolucent, slanted, hypoechoic tubular structure (Fig. 5.85A) in the bladder wall. Because urine is normally squirted into the bladder by ureteral peristalsis, echogenic turbulence results in a hyperechoic ureteral jet (5) (Fig. 5.85C). The phenomenon is the same as the ureteral jet seen on intravenous pyelography (Fig. 5.85B).

REFERENCES

1. Jequier S, Rousseau O. Sonographic measurements of the normal bladder wall in children. AJR 1987;149:563–566.

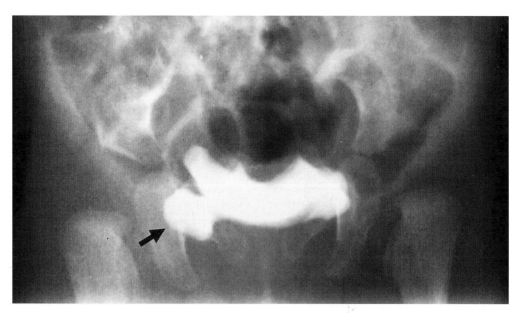

FIGURE 5.82. Bladder ears. Note the herniation of bladder through the right inguinal canal (arrow). A smaller herniation is present on the left.

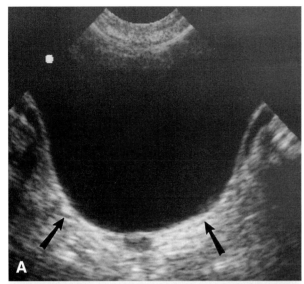

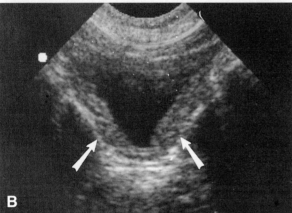

FIGURE 5.83. Normal bladder: ultrasonographic findings.
A. The bladder is distended (arrows) and the wall is clearly out-lined. **B.** With the bladder empty, the bladder wall (arrows) appears thickened. This is a pitfall that should be avoided. The bladder should be examined when it is full.

2. Bis KG, Slovis TL. Accuracy of ultrasonic bladder volume mea-surement in children. Pediatr Radiol 1990;20:457–460.
3. Fairhurst JJ, Rubin CME, Hyde I, et al. Bladder capacity in infants. J Pediatr Surg 1991;26:55–57.
4. Hiraoka M, Tsukahara H, Tsuchida S, et al. Ultrasonographic evaluation of bladder volume in children. Pediatr Nephrol 1993;7: 533–535.
5. Jequier S, Paltiel H, Lafortune M. Ureterovesical jets in infants and children: duplex and color Doppler US studies. Radiology 1990;175:349–353.

Voiding Cystourethrography

Voiding cystourethrography truly was one of the great advances in the radiologic investigation of urinary tract disease in children. When properly performed, it is a safe procedure, but it is not without the occasional complica-tion. Although these are relatively uncommon, they include bladder perforation and sepsis secondary to intrarenal reflux of infected urine. Most often, the study is performed by inserting a catheter into the bladder and then fluoroscopically observing the bladder fill by gravity drip. However, one can inject the contrast material directly into the bladder. I prefer this method because it is faster.

Getting the infant to void may be a problem. The bladder must be fully distended so that there is a definite urge to void. If, however, the infant is unable to void, one may try running the tap in the room or pouring warm water over the perineum. I have found that it is best to use water slightly warmer than lukewarm water. This seems to distract the infant, and then the infant can void. If the catheter remains in the urethra during voiding, it does not interfere with voiding or the interpretation of the cystogram. This is important, because the patient often begins to void with the catheter in the bladder, and

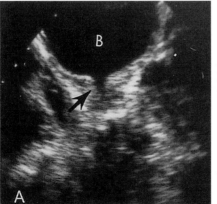
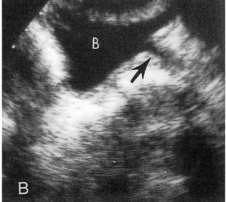

FIGURE 5.84. Normal bladder and urethra: ultrasonographic findings. A. Transverse view of the bladder (B) demonstrates a little urine in the proximal posterior urethra (arrow). Sur-rounding it is the moderately echogenic prostate gland. **B.** Longitudinal view of the bladder (B) demonstrates the echogenic mucosa and sonolucent, outer thin layer of muscle. These same find-ings are seen on transverse section in **A.** Note fluid in the proximal posterior urethra (arrow).

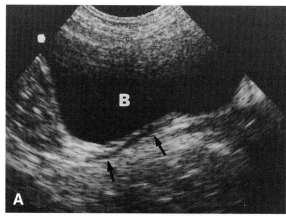

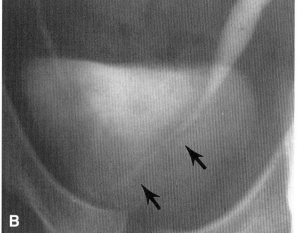
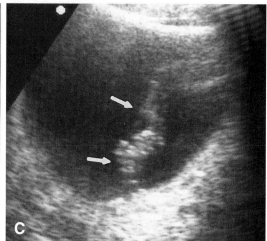

FIGURE 5.85. **A. Normal insertion of ureter**. Note the normal ureter (arrows) inserting into the bladder (B) on this sagittal view. **B. Ureteral jet**. Note the ureteral jet (arrows) on this intravenous pyelogram. **C.** Ultrasonographic demonstration of a ureteral jet (arrows).

then, as one removes the catheter, voiding ceases. The tricks used to induce voiding are endless, and all practitioners have their favorites.

Commonly, during voiding, female infants can fill their vagina by retrograde reflux. Usually, this is considered normal, although there is some feeling that such reflux may favor the development of urinary tract infections. In terms of patient comfort for the procedure, a topical anesthetic can be used to lubricate the catheter and mild sedation also has been advocated (1). However, we seldom sedate our patients and do not use topical anesthetic.

REFERENCE

1. Elder JS, Longenecker R. Premedication with oral midazolam for voiding cystourethrography in children: safety and efficacy. AJR 1995;164:1229–1232.

ABNORMALITIES OF THE BLADDER AND URETHRA

Agenesis of the Bladder

Agenesis of the bladder is rare (1). It produces urinary tract obstruction and may be associated with other urinary tract anomalies.

REFERENCE

1. Gopal SC, Gangopadhyay AN, Sharma P, et al. Agenesis of the bladder: a rare clinical entity in a male child. Pediatr Surg Int 1993;8:60–61.

Exstrophy of the Bladder

One of the most serious anomalies of the bladder is exstrophy. It is associated with marked diastasis of the pubic bones (Fig. 5.86) and is easily diagnosed both clinically and

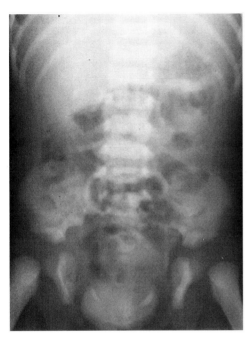

FIGURE 5.86. Bladder exstrophy. Note the widely separated pubic bones and the centrally placed, low-lying bladder.

roentgenographically. Radiologic investigation centers on evaluation of the upper urinary tract complications, and the whole complex can be evaluated with three-dimensional CT (1).

REFERENCE

1. Yazici M, Sozuibir S, Kilicoglu G, et al. Three-dimensional anatomy of the pelvis in bladder exstrophy: description of bone pathology by using three-dimensional computed tomography and its clinical relevance. J Pediatr Orthop 1998;18:132–135.

Bladder Diverticula

Congenital diverticula of the bladder in children are not particularly common (1), and whereas some can cause obstruction, recurrent infections, or hematuria, others are silent. Multiple bladder diverticula are a feature of Menkes' syndrome, congenital cutis laxa (i.e., Ehlers-Danlos syndrome), and William's syndrome (1–3). Spontaneous rupture of a diverticulum in the Ehlers-Danlos syndrome has recently been reported (3).

The diverticulum occurring at the ureterovesicular junction usually is called a Hutch diverticulum and often is associated with reflux. The reason for this is that the presence of the diverticulum alters the normal slanted insertion of the ureter into the bladder (Fig. 5.87A). This diverticulum is more common in older infants and children, and the diverticulum itself usually results from increased intravesicular pressure secondary to some type of lower tract obstruc-

tion, including neurogenic bladder. Any of these diverticula are readily demonstrable with voiding cystourethrography and ultrasonography (Fig. 5.87). Color Doppler jets can be used to differentiate bladder diverticula from pelvic cysts (3). The reason this is helpful is that very often bladder diverticula empty and fill from the bladder while pelvic cysts do not.

Persistent urachal remnants also may present as bladder diverticula, with or without persistent communication to the umbilical region. These blind-ending pouches arise off of the dome of the bladder (Fig. 5.88) and, although usually small, can become very large. This is especially true in the absent abdominal musculature syndrome where these diverticula are common. If such remnants are located near the umbilicus, bulging and enlargement of the umbilical cord in newborns or of the umbilicus in infants may be seen. When these remnants are closed at both ends, a urachal cyst results and can be tubular with a thin wall or fusiform with a thick wall (4). These cysts also can become infected.

REFERENCES

1. Blane CE, Zerin JM, Bloom DA. Bladder diverticula in children. Radiology 1994;190:695–697.
2. Harcke HT Jr, Capitanio MA, Grover WD, et al. Bladder diverticula and Menkes' syndrome. Radiology 1977;124:459–461.
3. Levine D, Filly RA. Using color Doppler jets to differentiate a pelvic cyst from a bladder diverticulum. J Ultrasound Med 1994; 13:575–577.
4. Leicher-Duber A, Schumacher R. Urachal remnants in asymptomatic children: sonographic morphology. Pediatr Radiol 1991;21: 200–202.

Septate Bladder or Duplicated Bladder and Urethra

This is an uncommon anomaly in which the bladder is completely or incompletely septate. The bladder is normal externally but may be divided into multiple chambers internally (1). Duplication of the bladder and urethra also are rare (Fig. 5.89).

REFERENCES

1. Berrocal T, Novak S, Arjonilla A, et al. Complete duplication of bladder and urethra in the coronal plane in a girl: case report and review of the literature. Pediatr Radiol 1999;29:171–173.

Neurogenic Bladder

A neurogenic bladder may be large and atonic (i.e., posterior nerve root lower motor neuron abnormality) or elongated, thick-walled and trabeculated (i.e., upper motor neuron lesion) (Fig. 5.90, A and C). The most common cause

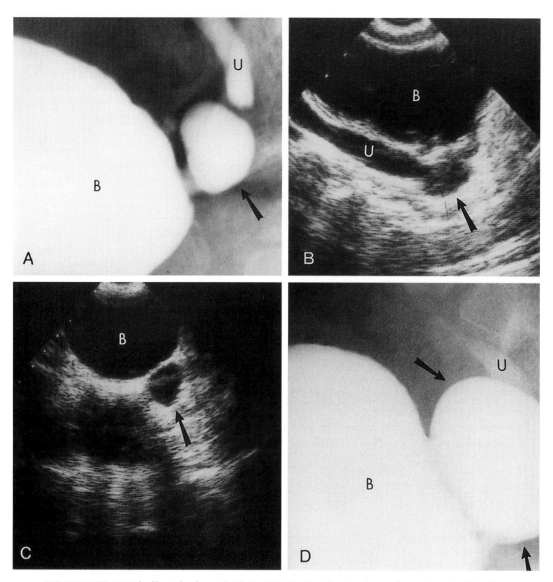

FIGURE 5.87. Hutch diverticulum. A. Typical Hutch diverticulum (arrow) associated with reflux into the ureter (U). B, bladder. **B.** Sonographic (longitudinal section) demonstration of a large Hutch diverticulum (arrow). Note the dilated ureter (U). B, bladder. **C.** Another Hutch diverticulum (arrow) demonstrated on transverse examination of the bladder (B). **D.** Cystogram in the same patient demonstrates the large diverticulum (arrows) with reflux into the ureter (U). B, bladder.

of neurogenic bladder is meningomyelocele, but it can also be seen with hypoplasia or absence of the sacrum, diastematomyelia, tethered cord, presacral teratomas, anterior sacral meningocele, and less commonly, intraspinal cysts and tumors.

The urethra in large, atonic, low-pressure, neurologically deficient bladders usually shows a low-flow (thin urethra) pattern on voiding. With a thick, trabeculated, high-pressure bladder, the urethral configuration consists of widening of the posterior urethra secondary to persistent spasm (or lack of relaxation), of the external sphincter, and in males, a low-flow pattern (i.e., narrow anterior urethra) (1) (Fig 5.90, B and C). In these patients, as the spastic bladder

tries to empty against a sphincter that will not open, it induces thickening and marked trabeculation of the bladder wall. In all cases of neurogenic bladder, emptying of the bladder is impaired and reflux is common (Fig. 5.90A).

Various surgical procedures can be used to circumvent and correct the neurogenic bladder. In the past, this included ileal diversion, which has the problems of reflux and, on a long-term basis, complicating malignancy. More recently, bladder augmentation has been preferred, especially with small, high-pressure spastic bladders. One can use small bowel, large bowel, or as currently preferred, the stomach (1) for such augmentation. However, there seems to be less mucosal damage and less stone formation when

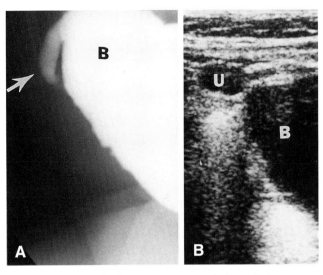

FIGURE 5.88. Urachal remnant. A. Typical urachal remnant (arrow) located at the dome of the bladder (B). **B.** Ultrasonogram demonstrating similar findings. B, bladder ; U, urachal remnant.

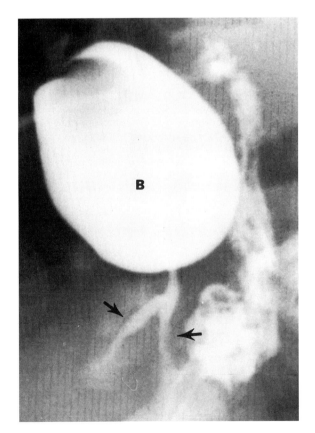

FIGURE 5.89. Double urethra. Note the double urethras (arrows). They originate from a single urethra. B, urinary bladder.

the stomach is used. The augmented bladder can rupture (2), and in these patients, this is a serious problem, because their neurologic impairment includes defective sensory neuronal function, and they do not appreciate or complain about the symptoms caused by perforation. Another interesting feature of augmentation is that the staples used for the procedure can eventually calcify and so can the bladder (1).

REFERENCES

1. Zawin JK, Lebowitz RL. Neurogenic dysfunction of the bladder in infants and children: recent advances and the role of radiology. Radiology 1992;182:297–304.
2. Glass RB, Rushton HG. Delayed spontaneous rupture of augmented bladder in children: diagnosis with sonography and CT. AJR 1992;158:833–835.

Nonneurogenic Neurogenic Bladder and Bladder Instability: Hinman Syndrome

In the Hinman syndrome, the problem is functionally the same as spastic neurogenic bladder. Many refer to the problem as bladder instability, because when the bladder contracts, the external sphincter does not open and the posterior urethra widens. The configuration is similar to that seen with a spastic neurogenic bladder, but because there is no underlying neurogenic disease, the term "nonneurogenic neurogenic bladder" is used (1, 2).

REFERENCES

1. Johnson JF III, Hedden RJ, Piccolello ML, et al. Distention of the posterior urethra: associated with nonneurogenic neurogenic bladder (Hinman syndrome). Radiology 1992;185:113–117.
2. Sacton HM, Borzyskowski M, Robinson LB. Nonobstructive posterior urethral widening (spinning top urethra) in boys with bladder instability. Radiology 1992;182:81–85.

Cystitis

Cystitis in the newborn infant usually is part of a generalized urinary tract infection secondary to sepsis. However, in older infants and children, cystitis can occur in association with ascending urinary tract infection or as a primary infection. Generally, it is caused by bacterial infection, but viral cystitis also can occur. Viral cystitis frequently leads to a hemorrhagic cystitis (1, 2), and presents with hematuria. Cystitis also occurs in immunosuppressed patients and is a complication of Cytoxan therapy in oncology patients (1). Cystitis also can be seen in association with granulomatous disease of childhood (2, 3), eosinophilic cystitis, and secondary to adjacent inflammatory disease such as regional enteritis, chronic perforated appendicitis, and pelvic inflammatory disease.

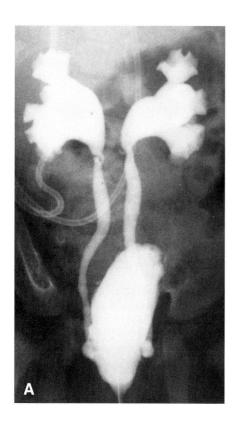

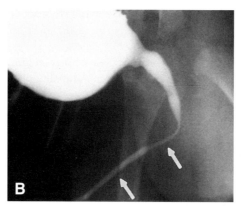

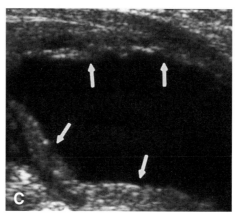

FIGURE 5.90. Neurogenic bladder. A. Elongated, trabeculated neurogenic bladder with bilateral diverticula. Massive bilateral reflux is present. **B.** Another patient with early changes consisting of mild trabeculation of the bladder along the posterior wall. However, note that the posterior urethra is slightly dilated while the anterior urethra (arrows) shows a low-flow pattern. This patient could not empty his bladder. **C.** Ultrasonogram of the bladder demonstrates thickening of the bladder wall (arrows).

Radiographically, the acute changes of cystitis consist of mucosal irregularity and thickening. Later, bladder wall trabeculation with cellule formation can be seen (Fig. 5.91). In other cases, the thickened bladder wall, especially if focal, can erroneously suggest the presence of a bladder tumor (4). Multiple filling defects in the bladder usually are blood clots or congregations of purulent exudate. Fungal infection, primarily of the Monilia class, leads to cystitis in immunocompromised patients, and in some of these patients, mobile fungus balls can be seen within the bladder (Fig. 5.92). Fungus balls also can occur in the upper collecting system.

Cystitis often is first and best demonstrated with ultrasound where the bladder mucosa is circumferentially or focally thickened (Fig. 5.93). It should be cautioned, however, that thickening of the urinary bladder mucosa can be erroneously suggested if the bladder is insufficiently distended with urine. However, with cystitis, the bladder often is irritable, spastic, and small, and so a problem can arise. In such cases, one must make a decision as to whether mucosal thickening is pathologic or fortuitous because of a poorly filled bladder. Color flow Doppler is helpful, because if the mucosa is thickened on the basis of inflammation, increased blood flow to the mucosa usually occurs.

REFERENCES

1. McCarville MB, Hoffer FA, Gingrich JR, et al. Imaging findings of hemorrhagic cystitis in pediatric oncology patients. Pediatr Radiol 2000;30:131–138.
2. Bauer SB, Kogan SJ. Vesical manifestations of chronic granulomatous disease in children: its relation to eosinophilic cystitis. Urology 1991;37:463–466.
3. Heffel JC, Drews K, Gassner I, et al. Pseudotumoral cystitis. Pediatr Radiol 1993;23:510–514.
4. Rosenberg HK, Eggli KD, Zerin M, et al. Benign cystitis in children mimicking rhabdomyosarcoma. J Ultrasound Med 1994;13:921–932.

Bladder Perforation or Rupture

Bladder perforation and bladder rupture are discussed with urine ascites.

Bladder Tumors

Tumors of the bladder generally are uncommon in children, and although a few benign lesions such as hemangioma, inverted papilloma (1), and inflammatory pseudotumor (2) occasionally can be encountered, the problem most often is rhabdomyosarcoma. Other malignant tumors such as squa-

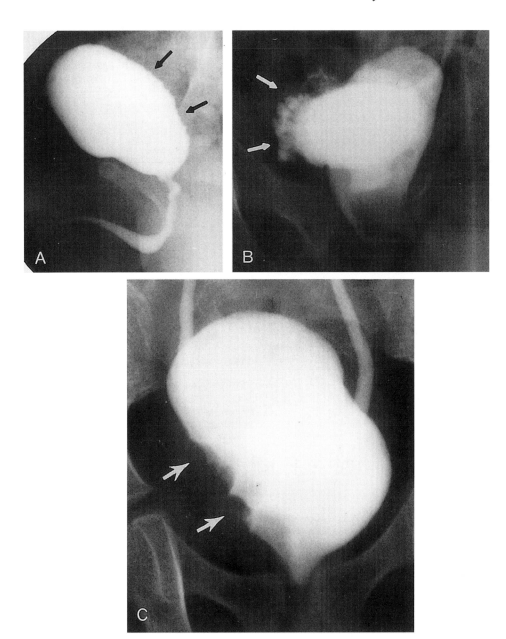

FIGURE 5.91. Cystitis. A. Male infant with cystitis. Note irregularity of the posterior bladder wall (arrows). Such irregularity must persist with the fully distended bladder, because it can be mimicked by early bladder contraction during voiding. **B.** Female infant with extensive local bladder wall thickening and cellule formation secondary to cystitis (arrows). Contrast material also is present in the vagina. **C.** Marked deformity and edema of the bladder resulting from Cytoxan cystitis (arrows).

mous cell and transitional cell carcinoma of the bladder are rare (3–6). Neurofibromatosis also can involve the urinary bladder in children, and in such cases, the neurofibromas can become quite large and produce considerable deformity of the bladder.

Rhabdomyosarcoma of the bladder tends to occur around the trigone and produces variable defects on the contrast cystogram and echogenic masses protruding into the bladder on ultrasonography (Fig. 5.94). Because these tumors tend to arise around the trigone, they may be difficult to differentiate from prostate rhabdomyosarcomas. Occasionally, a rhabdomyosarcoma may arise in the dome of the bladder (7). Associated hydronephrosis is readily demonstrable with any imaging modality but the tumor itself, although readily detected with ultrasonography, probably is best defined with MRI.

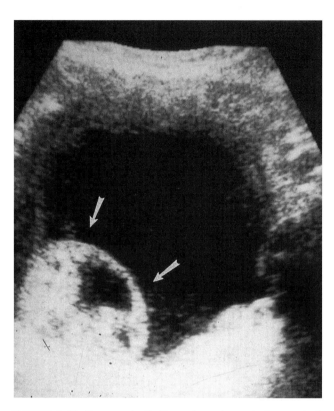

FIGURE 5.92. Fungus ball. Note the echogenic fungus ball (arrows) in the bladder.

REFERENCES

1. Tamsen A, Casas V, Patil UB, et al. Inverted papilloma of the urinary bladder in a boy. J Pediatr Surg 1993;28:1601–1602.
2. Gardner MP, Lowichik A, Cartwright PC. Inflammatory (pseudosarcomatous) myofibroblastic tumor of the urinary bladder causing acute abdominal pain. J Pediatr Surg 1999;34:1417–1419.
3. Hoenig DM, McRae S, Chen SC, et al. Transitional cell carcinoma of the bladder in the pediatric patient. J Urol 1996;156:203–205.
4. Suan JD, Koyle MA. Squamous cell carcinoma of the bladder in a pediatric patient. J Pediatr Surg 2000;35:1838–1839.
5. Wilson-Storey D, Allen AE, Variend S. Transitional cell papillary ladder neoplasm in a girl: an unusual presentation. J Pediatr Surg 1992;27:113–114.
6. Williams JL, Cumming WA, Walker RD III, et al. Transitional cell papilloma of the bladder. Pediatr Radiol 1986;16:322–323.
7. Royal SA, Hedlund GL, Galliani CA. Case report. Rhabdomyosarcoma of the dome of the urinary bladder: a difficult imaging diagnosis. AJR 1996;167:524–525.

Megacystis-Microcolon Intestinal Hypoperistalsis Syndrome

Megacystis-microcolon intestinal hypoperistalsis syndrome is an uncommon condition, usually occurring in females who present with a large bladder and a microcolon (1). The condition is discussed in Chapter 4.

REFERENCE

1. Srikanth MS, Ford EG, Isaacs H Jr, et al. Megacystis microcolon intestinal hypoperistalsis syndrome: late sequelae and possible pathogenesis. J Pediatr Surg 1993;28:957–959.

Calcification of the Bladder

Calcification of the bladder in infancy is very uncommon but has been noted on the basis of urine stasis, in the prune belly syndrome (1). In older infants and children, Cytoxan cystitis can lead to bladder calcification, and calcification of the bladder also occurs in older children with hemorrhagic cystitis and schistosomiasis.

REFERENCE

1. Kirks DR, Taybi H. Prune belly syndromes: an unusual cause of neonatal abdominal calcification. AJR 1975;123:778–782.

Posterior Urethral Valves

This serious urethral abnormality occurs in males, and the diagnosis must be made early, because many infants have marked reflux and impaired renal function even at birth. Many cases are detected prenatally, but thereafter, the best clinical clue for the diagnosis of the condition is the absence of a good, powerful urinary stream. Unfortunately, however, this early and valuable finding may evade the inexperienced parent or unwary physician. In the past, many infants first came to the attention of a physician because of palpably enlarged kidneys (i.e., hydronephrosis) or failure to thrive resulting from decreased renal function. Currently, however, with the widespread use of prenatal ultrasound, most severe cases are detected before birth.

Posterior urethral valves usually are classified into three types, a classification originally proposed by Young et al. (1). In this classification, type I refers to valves occurring below the verumontanum, type II to similar valves occurring above the verumontanum, and type III to a diaphragm below the verumontanum. Over the years, however, there has been serious question as to whether type II valves actually exist.

The type I valve is the most common by far (5, 12, 15) and results from abnormal migration and insertion of the urethrovaginal folds. These folds are distal remnants of the wolffian or mesonephric ducts and, in early embryonic life, are located anteriorly in the urogenital sinus. Under normal circumstances, they migrate laterally and posteriorly to attach to the posterior urethral wall, under the verumontanum, as the normal plicae colliculi. Occasionally, these structures can be seen during voiding cystourethrography (Fig. 5.95). When these folds fail to migrate posterolaterally, they insert anteriorly, fuse along

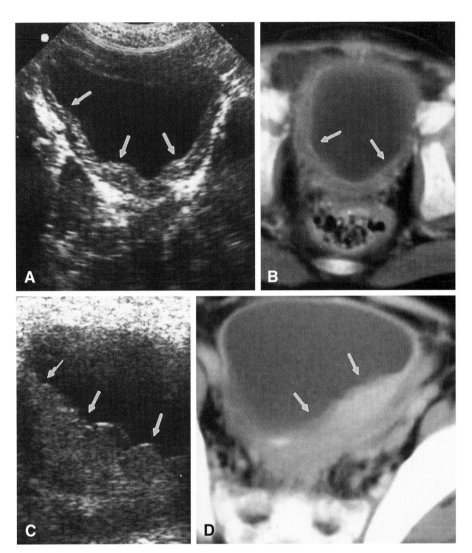

FIGURE 5.93. Cystitis: ultrasonographic and CT findings. A. Note circumferential thickening of the bladder mucosa (arrows). **B.** In this patient with Cytoxan cystitis, similar mucosal thickening (arrows) is seen on CT. **C.** Focal area of mucosal thickening (arrows) is seen in this patient. **D.** Corresponding CT study demonstrates the same area of mucosal thickening (arrows).

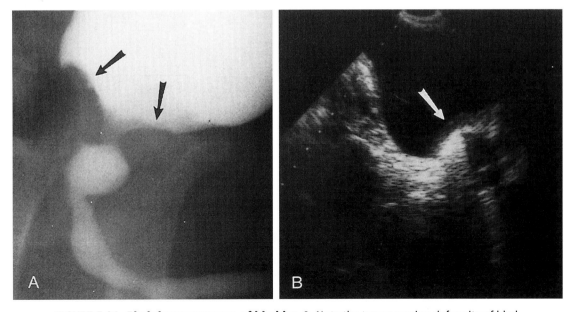

FIGURE 5.94. Rhabdomyosarcoma of bladder. A. Note the tumor causing deformity of bladder neck (arrows). **B.** Ultrasonogram demonstrates tumor arising from the bladder wall (arrow).

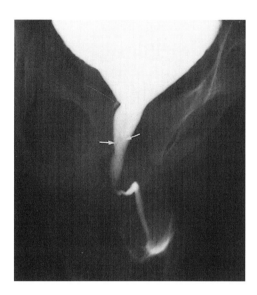

FIGURE 5.95. Plicae colliculi. Normal mucosal folds (plicae colliculi) extending downwardly (arrows) from the verumontanum. These should not be misinterpreted as obstructing posterior urethral valves.

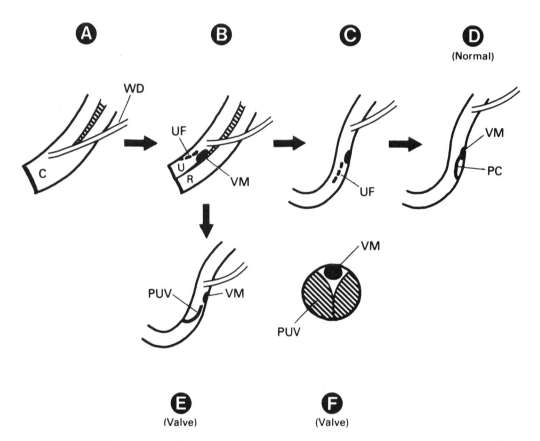

FIGURE 5.96. Posterior urethral valve, type I: embryology. A. Note the anterior position of the wolffian or mesonephric duct (WD) as it enters the cloaca (C). The urorectal septum (shaded area) is beginning to divide the cloaca into the anterior urogenital sinus and posterior rectum. **B.** The wolffian duct has migrated upwardly, but the residual urethrovaginal folds (UF) remain anterior. Note the position of the verumontanum (VM). The urorectal septum (shaded area) has divided the cloaca into the anterior urogenital sinus (U) and posterior rectum (R). **C.** During the next stage, there is posterolateral migration of the urovaginal folds (UF). **D.** Normally, the urovaginal folds migrate posteriorly and extend downward from the verumontanum (VM) as the plicae colliculi (PC). **E.** Posterior urethral valve (PUV) results from persistent anterior positioning of the urethrogenital folds. Note the posterior opening in the valve **F.** Overhead view demonstrating the position of the posterior opening in the PUV. Note the position of the verumontanum (VM).

the midline, leave an opening posteriorly, and produce the type I posterior urethral valve (Fig. 5.96). In essence, the valve is a diaphragm, but since it is more rigid along its line of fusion, progressive distention during voiding causes it to become bilobed or sail-like in appearance. These valves are best demonstrated with voiding cystourethrography (Fig. 5.97), but they can be variable in their configuration. Their appearance can be different from film to film in the same patient, because the degree of distention of the valve directly influences its overall configuration, and the degree of distention depends on the volume of urine flow. In most cases, the valve itself is not visualized but merely inferred to be present by noting the characteristic appearance of the obstructed posterior urethra. Mild type I valves produce little obstruction and can mimic the appearance of type III valves (2).

The type III valve is a membrane with a central or eccentric opening and, as such, is a true diaphragm. In

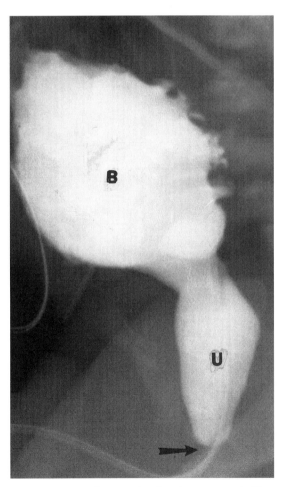

FIGURE 5.97. Posterior urethral valves, type I. Note the dilated posterior urethra (U) and the obstructing valve (arrow). The bladder (B) is small and trabeculated.

some cases, the membrane occupies only one half of the urethral lumen, and when such a membrane is distended, a windsock configuration can result. Embryologically, the type III valve is believed to result from incomplete eradication of the urogenital membrane (Fig. 5.98). This membrane covers the opening of the urogenital sinus and, normally, spontaneously perforates and then is totally obliterated. If it persists, it produces a transverse diaphragm located above the membranous portion of the urethra but below the verumontanum (Fig. 5.98). Roentgenographically, the findings are different from those seen in the more common type I valve. For the most part, a transverse radiolucent diaphragm is seen in the middle-to-lower posterior urethra (Fig. 5.99A). There usually is a little dilation of the posterior urethra, and the bladder usually is smooth and not heavily trabeculated (3). However, in some cases, the bladder may show hypertrophy and may be the first finding seen in these patients (Fig. 5.99B). This form of urethral valve can, and frequently does, manifest in later childhood.

The bladder with type I valves usually is markedly thickened and grossly trabeculated (Fig. 5.97), and gross hydronephrosis also frequently is present. Most of these infants show abnormal upper tract findings at the time of presentation. Ureterovesicular reflux into the dilated, tortuous ureters is common, and perforation of the bladder or upper tracts can lead to urine ascites. Posterior urethral valves probably are the most common cause of urine ascites in the neonate. The high-grade obstruction often causes reflux of contrast material into the seminal vesicles and prostatic ducts (Fig. 5.100). With the marked degree of hydronephrosis present in these patients, it should be no surprise that the kidneys often show poor function, reflux (Fig. 5.101A), and cystic dysplastic changes.

In terms of imaging, the voiding cystourethrogram is ultimately the procedure of choice in demonstrating valves, but ultrasound can demonstrate the associated hydronephrosis, thickened bladder, and even the dilated posterior urethra (8). The latter finding is nonspecific, but in the proper clinical setting (i.e., a male with hydronephrosis), presence of this dilated posterior urethra should be taken as strong presumptive evidence that one is dealing with posterior urethral valves (Fig. 5.101, B and C). The dilated posterior urethra can be demonstrated on both longitudinal and transverse sections, and inferior angulation of the transducer under the pubic bone enhances visualization on cross-section. Transperineal imaging also is helpful (4), and imaging during voiding can enhance visualization of the dilated urethra (5). In terms of treatment, the valves usually are obliterated surgically, currently with laser surgery. With successful surgery, the urethral obstruction can be alleviated, and then one must concentrate on salvaging the upper tracts and kidneys.

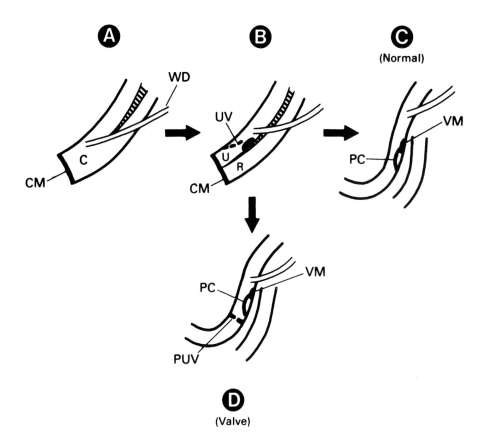

FIGURE 5.98. Type III posterior urethral valve: embryology. A. Note the cloacal membrane (CM) occluding the cloaca (C). The wolffian duct (WD) and urorectal septum (shaded area) are indicated. **B.** The urorectal septum has divided the cloaca into the anterior urogenital sinus (U) and posterior rectum (R). The wolffian duct has migrated upward and the residual urethrovaginal (UV) folds remain anterior. However, they are not involved in the formation of this type of valve. The cloacal membrane (CM) is the important structure and, at this point, occludes the urogenital sinus and rectum. The portion covering the urogenital sinus is the urogenital membrane. **C.** The urogenital membrane has been obliterated and a free channel connects the posterior urethra with the anterior urethra. Note the position of the normal verumontanum (VM) and plicae colliculi (PC). **D.** Type III posterior urethral valve (PUV) results from persistence of the urogenital membrane. It is located below the verumontanum (VM) and plicae colliculi (PC) and produces obstruction between the posterior and anterior portions of the urethra.

REFERENCES

1. Young HH, Frontz WA, Baldwin JC. Congenital obstruction of the posterior urethra. J Urol 1919;3:289–354.
2. Peiretti R. The mild end of the clinical spectrum of posterior urethral valves. J Pediatr Surg 1993;28:701–706.
3. Rosenfeld B, Greenfield SP, Springate JE, et al. Type III posterior urethral valves: presentation and management. J Pediatr Surg 1994;29:81–85.
4. Cohen HL, Susman M, Haller JO, et al. Posterior urethral valve: transperineal US for imaging and diagnosis in male infants. Radiology 1994;192:261–264.
5. Good CD, Vinnicombe SJ, Minty IL, et al. Posterior urethral valves in male infants and newborns: detection with US of the urethra before and during voiding. Radiology 1996;198:387–391.

"Spinning Top" Urethra in Females

Originally, much was made of the "cone-shaped" or "spinning top" urethra in female children. The lesion was considered to be a form of "distal meatal stenosis," but distal meatal stenosis in the female infant is exceptionally uncommon. We have encountered an odd case in which calibration of the distal urethra proved it to be definitely stenotic, but most often, the cause of the cone-shaped, or spinning top, urethra is distal sphincter spasm (Fig. 5.102). In my experience and that of others (1, 2), it is seen most fre-

quently in females with recurrent urinary tract infections. Overall, however, it has little clinical significance. An excellent review of all forms of urethral obstructions in females has been presented by Walker and Richard (3), and their conclusions serve to underscore these feelings regarding the spinning top urethra.

REFERENCES

1. Tanagho EA, Miller ER, Lyon RP, et al. Spastic striated external sphincter and urinary tract infection in girls. Br J Urol 1971;43:69–82.
2. Sacton HM, Borzyskowski M, Mundy AR, et al. Spinning top urethra: not a normal variant. Radiology 1988;168:147–150.
3. Walker D, Richard GA. A critical evaluation of urethral obstruction in female children. Pediatrics 1973;51:272–277.

Miscellaneous Urethral Abnormalities

Occasionally, one can encounter urethral polyps (1–3), urethral diverticula (4), and duplications of the urethra (5). By and large, these abnormalities produce obstruction and are readily demonstrable with cystourethrography. **Polyps** manifest as filling defects and **diverticula** as abnormal outpouchings of the urethra. These latter structures probably represent

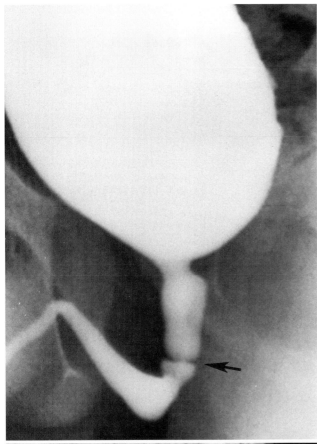

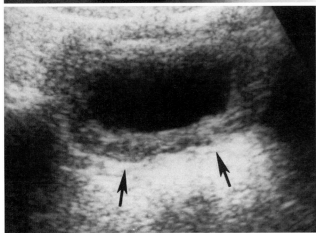

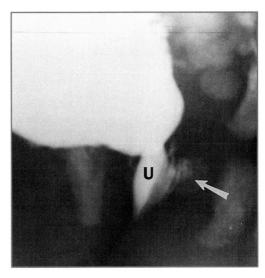

FIGURE 5.100. Posterior urethral valve and reflux into prostatic ducts. Note the dilated urethra (U). Reflux of contrast material has occurred into the prostatic ducts and seminal vesicles (arrow).

FIGURE 5.99. Type III posterior urethral valve. A. Note the transverse diaphragm (arrow) located just below the verumontanum. **B.** Ultrasound study in this patient demonstrates a thickened bladder wall (arrows), the first positive finding noted in this patient.

variations of urethra duplication, which in itself can range from the rare complete duplication of the urethra and double penis to simple blind-ending pouches. Urethral diverticula also are not uncommonly seen in the prune belly syndrome.

In most instances, urethral diverticula are saccular and arise from the ventral aspect of the urethra. A lip of tissue may be seen around the diverticulum (Fig. 5.103A), and with distention of the diverticulum, the lip of tissue is pressed against the urethral wall, and a valve-like obstruction results. In the past, this flap of tissue probably had been misinterpreted as an anterior urethral valve. Another diverticulum, although uncommon, is that which occurs with retention cysts of Cowper's ducts. While the cyst is intact, it lies along the dorsal surface of the urethra and produces a localized filling defect in its bulbous portion. However, it evidently can erode spontaneously or after surgery into the bulbous urethra (6), and then the cyst fills during voiding, and a diverticulum results (Fig. 5.103B). Flaps of tissue associated with this form of diverticulum also can be misinterpreted for anterior urethral valves, but it should be remembered that true anterior urethral valves are rare (7).

In some cases, urethral diverticula can become so large that they produce one form of so-called megalourethra. In the other form, absence of the corpora cavernosa and/or the corpus spongiosum leads to lack of normal support of the urethra and its dilation to enormous proportions (8, 9). The findings usually are striking (Fig. 5.104).

Distal meatal stenosis is common in the male infant and primarily is a problem for clinical diagnosis. Radiographically, the entire urethra, but especially the anterior portion, shows dilation on micturition. There is

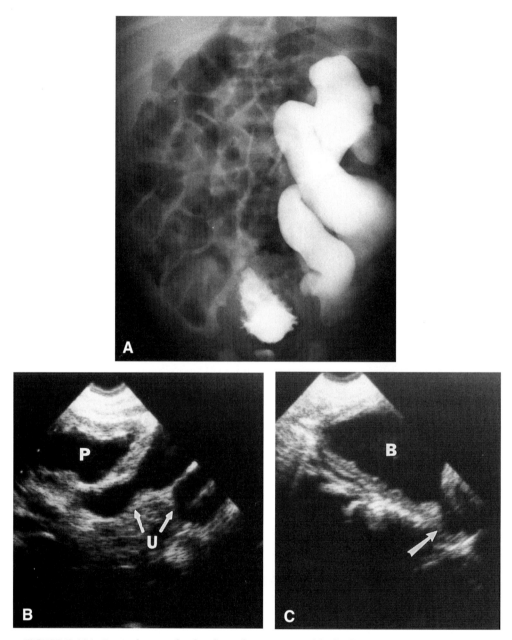

FIGURE 5.101. Posterior urethral valve, ultrasonographic findings. A. Cystogram demonstrates the trabeculated bladder and the markedly tortuous, dilated left ureter and hydronephrotic kidney. **B.** Sonogram of the kidneys demonstrates marked dilation of the renal pelvis (P) and a tortuous dilated ureter (U). **C.** Ultrasonographic study of the bladder demonstrates the dilated posterior urethra (arrow) and urinary bladder (B). The inferior wall of the bladder shows thickening.

impedance of urine flow through the distal meatus and, occasionally, abnormalities in the upper urinary tracts can be seen. The same problem occasionally arises with severely obstructing phimosis (10). However, in either of these conditions, the urethra, bladder, and upper tracts usually are normal. Distal meatal stenosis is a rare lesion in females. Hypertrophy of the median bar of the prostate gland occasionally can produce obstruction in the neonate, but it also is a rare lesion. Acquired strictures, after infection or trauma or for iatrogenic reasons, also occur, primarily in older children, and urethral calculi also can lead to obstruction (11, 12).

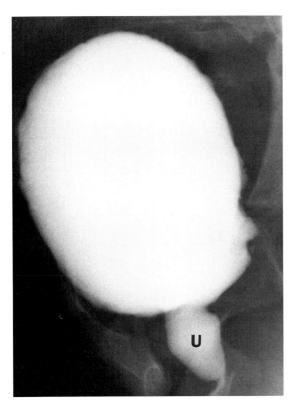

FIGURE 5.102. Spinning top urethra: distal urethral spasm in females. In this patient with longstanding cystitis, note that the bladder is slightly trabeculated and that the urethra (U) is markedly dilated in the so-called "spinning top" configuration.

REFERENCES

1. Caro PA, Rosenberg HK, Snyder HM III. Case report. Congenital urethral polyp. AJR 1986;147:1041–1042.
2. Crankson SJ, Abdul-Aaly M, Hugosson C, et al. Haemangiomatous polyp of the posterior urethra in a boy. Pediatr Radiol 1992;22:74–75.
3. De Castro R, Campobasso P, Belloli G, et al. Solitary polyp of posterior urethra in children: report on seventeen cases. Eur J Pediatr Surg 1993;3:92–96.
4. Kirks DR, Grossman H. Congenital saccular anterior urethral diverticulum. Radiology 1981;140:367–372.
5. Lorenzo RL, Turner WR, Bradford BF, et al. Duplication of the male urethra with posterior urethral valves. Pediatr Radiol 1981; 11:39–41.
6. Moskowitz PS, Newton NA, Lebowitz RL. Retention cysts of Cowper's duct. Radiology 1976;120:377–380.
7. Zia JL, Miraj M. Anterior urethral valves: a rare cause of infravesical obstruction in children. J Pediatr Surg 35:556–558, 2000.
8. Appel RA, Kaplan GW, Brock WA, et al. Megalourethra. J Urol 1986;21:1012.
9. Wakhlu AK, Wakhlu A, Tandon RK, et al. Congenital megalourethra. J Pediatr Surg 1996;31:441–443.
10. Angtuaco EE, Klein SG, Wood BP. Radiological case of the month–pathologic phimosis. Am J Dis Child 1992;146: 763–764.
11. Kessler A, Rosenberg HK, Smoyer WE, et al. Urethral stones: US for identification in boys with hematuria and dysuria. Radiology 1992;185:767–768.
12. Seltzer LG, Fischer WW, Miller SZ. Pediatric bladder outlet obstruction due to urethral calculus. Case report and review of the literature. Pediatr Radiol 1993;23:549–550.

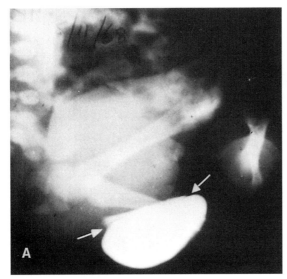
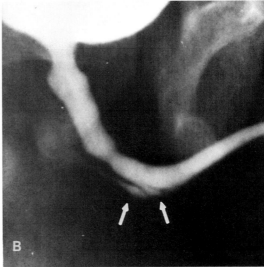

FIGURE 5.103. Urethral diverticula. A. Note the large urethral diverticulum with thin flaps of tissue at the edges (arrows). These flaps are often obstructing and are frequently misinterpreted as representing anterior urethral valves. **B.** Diverticulum resulting from spontaneous perforation of a Cowper's duct cyst into the urethra. The diverticulum is rather long (arrows), and the two flap-like structures above it often are misinterpreted for anterior urethral valves. (**A** from Meiraz D, Dolberg L, Dolberg M, et al. Diverticulum of the urethra in two boys. Am J Dis Child 1971;122:271–273, with permission; **B** courtesy of Virgil Graves, M.D.)

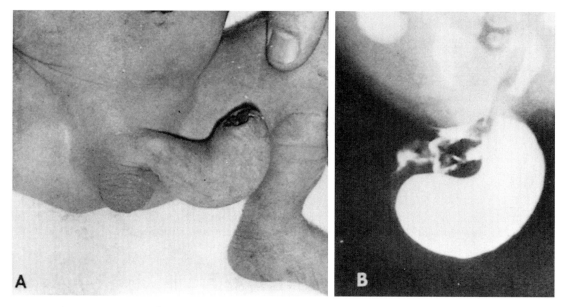

FIGURE 5.104. Megalourethra. A. Note the markedly enlarged penis with pronounced ventral bulging. **B.** Urethrogram demonstrating the megalourethra. In this infant, the corpora cavernosa was present, but the corpus spongiosum was absent. (From Johnston JH, Coimbra JAM. Megalourethra. J Pediatr Surg 1970;5:304–308, with permission.)

MISCELLANEOUS URINARY TRACT ABNORMALITIES

Urolithiasis and Nephrocalcinosis

Any type of renal calcification is unusual in the newborn, except for nephrolithiasis and nephrocalcinosis in premature infants when it is associated with furosemide therapy (1, 2). On long-term follow-up of these infants, the calcifications tend to regress (1). In older infants and children, nephrocalcinosis and renal calculi are more common and usually are calcium phosphate or calcium oxalate deposits. Most often, the underlying problem is some metabolic dis-

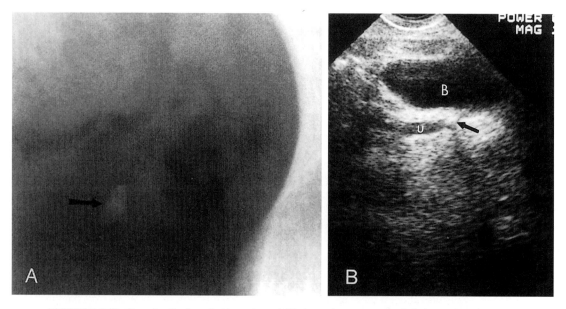

FIGURE 5.105. Renal calculus. A. Note the calcified renal stone on the left (arrow). **B.** Sagittal sonogram through the urinary bladder (B) and ureterovesical junction demonstrates an echogenic stone (arrow) with distal acoustical shadowing. Note the dilated ureter (U) proximally.

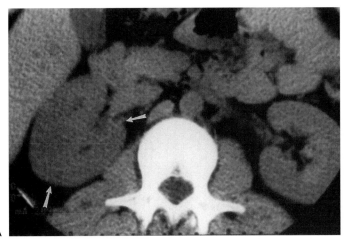

A

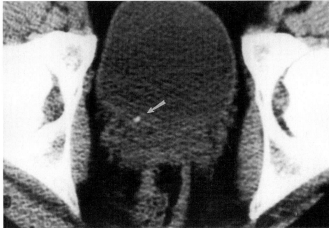

B

FIGURE 5.106. Renal calculus: CT imaging. A. Note the large right kidney (arrows). It demonstrates decreased profusion by being less dense than the normal contralateral kidney. **B.** Axial CT image through the lower pelvis demonstrates the obstructing renal stone (arrow), located at the ureterovesicular junction. The bladder is full of urine.

turbance such as cystinosis, oxalosis, renal tubular acidosis, idiopathic hypercalcemia, or hyperparathyroidism. However, idiopathic stone formation also occurs and is more common than generally appreciated in the past. Renal stone formation and nephrocalcinosis also are more common with other hypercalcemic states such as steroid therapy, William's syndrome, Cushing's syndrome, sarcoidosis (3), hypercalcemia-inducing tumors (4), and in older children, Bartter's syndrome (5). Nephrocalcinosis also has been documented in a case of glycogen storage disease type IA (6), and uric acid lithiasis is seen in cyanotic congenital heart disease associated with polycythemia. Uric acid stones can be seen in the Lesch-Nyhan syndrome (7). Renal stones also occur after chronic infections, especially *Candida* infections (8), and around staples used for bladder augmentation procedures (9). The latter finding is characteristic, because the staple can be seen inside the stone.

Renal calculi can be seen on plain films (Fig. 5.105A) and are demonstrable with ultrasound where they appear as echogenic foci with distal shadowing (Fig. 5.105B). Currently, however, noncontrast, high-resolution helical CT is best for identifying renal calculi (10–12). If a soft tissue rim or halo is seen around a calcification, one can be certain that it is a renal calculus with the rim representing the edematour ureteral wall (13). This is helpful in distinguishing renal calculi from other stones, especially in older female patients. CT is very sensitive in identifying renal calculi (Fig. 5.106).

Diffuse parenchymal renal calcification is seen with oxalosis (Fig. 5.107A) in which medullary calcification also occurs, and the latter also is seen with renal tubular acidosis (Fig. 5.107, B and C). These findings are characteristic both on plain films and ultrasound, because they follow the distribution of the renal pyramids and can be seen in the

tubules (Fig. 5.108A). On ultrasound, the medullary pyramids are very echogenic. These calcifications also are vividly demonstrable with CT (Fig. 5.108B). However, plain films and ultrasonography usually suffice.

Regarding renal lithotripsy in children, generally a conservative approach was advocated (14, 15). The reason for this was that no one really knew the long-term effects on renal growth after renal lithotripsy. However, it has been demonstrated that there is very little detrimental effect on a long-term basis. Nonetheless, it still probably is best to treat patients with small stones (16). It also has been noted that there is a slight decrease in renal function just after lithotripsy (17). However, this does not appear to be a long-term risk.

REFERENCES

1. Downing GJ, Egelhoff JC, Daily DK, et al. Furosemide-related renal calcifications in the premature infant. A longitudinal ultrasonographic study. Pediatr Radiol 1991;21:563–565.
2. Katz ME, Karlowicz G, Adelman RD, et al. Nephrocalcinosis in very low birth weight neonates: sonographic patterns, histologic characteristics, and clinical risk factors. J Ultrasound Med 1994; 13:777–782.
3. Nocton JJ, Stork JE, Jacobs G, et al. Sarcoidosis associated with nephrocalcinosis in young children. J Pediatr 1992;121: 937–940.
4. Allbery SM, Swischuk LE, John JD. Hypercalcemia associated with dysgerminoma: case report and imaging findings. Pediatr Radiol 1998;28:183–185
5. Matsumoto J, Han BK, Restrepo de Rovetto C, et al. Hypercalciuric Bartter syndrome: resolution of nephrocalcinosis with indomethacin. AJR 1989;152:1251–1253.
6. Fick JJ, Baeek FJ. Echogenic kidneys and medullary calcium deposition in a young child with glycogen storage disease type IA. Pediatr Radiol 1992;22:72–73.
7. Rosenfeld DL, Preston MP, Salvaggi-Fadden K. Serial renal sono-

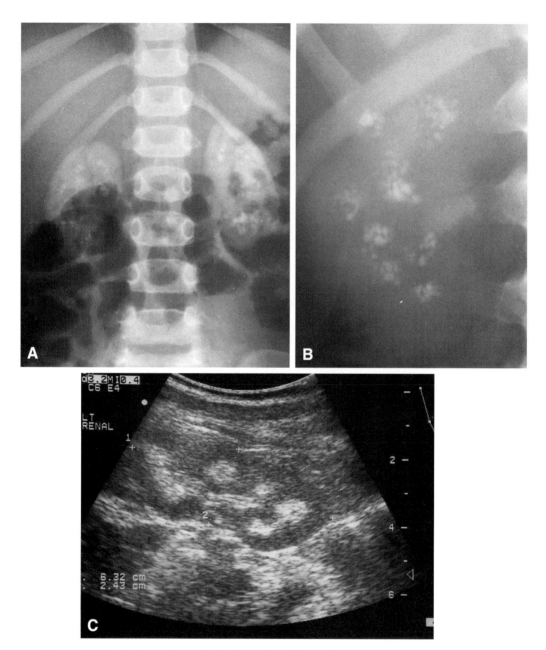

Figure 5.107. Nephrocalcinosis. A. Note the diffuse bilateral parenchymal and punctate medullary calcifications in a patient with oxalosis. **B.** Typical irregular-punctate calcifications conforming to the medullary pyramids in renal tubular acidosis. **C.** Corresponding findings on ultrasound demonstrating echogenic medullary pyramids.

graphic evaluation of patients with Lesch-Nyhan syndrome. Pediatr Radiol 1995;24:509–512.

8. Cramer BC, Ozere R, Andrews W. Renal stone formation following medical treatment of renal candidiasis. Pediatr Radiol 1990;21:43–44.

9. Dangman BC, Lebowitz RL. Urinary tract calculi that form on surgical staples: a characteristic radiologic appearance. AJR 1991; 157:115–117.

10. Catalano O, Nunziata A, Altei F, et al. Suspected ureteral colic: primary helical CT versus selective helical CT after unenhanced radiography and sonography. AJR 2002;178:379–387.

11. Sommer FG, Jeffrey RB Jr, Rubin GD, et al. Detection of ureteral calculi in patients with suspected renal colic: value of reformatted noncontrast helical CT. AJR 1995;165:509–513.

12. Strouse PJ, Bates DG, Bloom DA, et al. Non-contrast thin-section helical CT of urinary tract calculi in children. Pediatr Radiol 2002;32:326–332.

13. Heneghan Jr, Dairymple NC, Verga M, et al. Soft-tissue "rim sign in the diagnosis of ureteral calculi with use of unenhanced helical CT. Radiology 1997;202:709–711.

14. Moazam F, Nazir Z, Jafarey A. Pediatric urolithiasis: to cut or not to cut. J Pediatr Surg 1994;29:761–764.

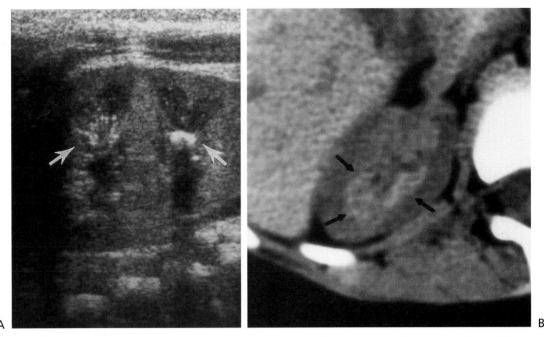

FIGURE 5.108. Nephrocalcinosis: ultrasound and CT findings. A. In this patient with renal tubular acidosis, note bronching echogenicity of the tubules (arrows) in the medullary pyramids. This represents calcium within the tubules. **B.** CT study of another patient demonstrates vague densities (arrows) over the same region of the kidney.

15. Farsi HM, Mosli HA, Alzemaity M, et al. In situ extracorporeal shock wave lithotripsy (ESWL) for the management of primary ureteric calculi in children. J Pediatr Surg 1994;29:1315–1316.

16. Goel MC, Basrge NS, Babu RVR, et al. Pediatric kidney: functional outcome after extracorporeal shock wave lithotripsy. J Urol 1996;155:2044–2046.

17. Corbally MT, Ryan J, FitzPatrick J, et al. Renal function following extracorporeal lithotripsy in children. J Pediatr Surg 1991;26:539–540.

Absent Abdominal Musculature (Prune Belly Syndrome, Eagle-Barrett Syndrome)

In this condition, the abdominal musculature is deficient, and gross urinary tract anomalies are present (1). One theory about the development of this condition is that there is a mesenchymal insult to the fetus at about 6 weeks' gestational age (2). As part of this insult, there is deficient abdominal muscular development and associated urinary tract anomalies. It also has been suggested that the abdominal muscular problem might be secondary to chronic intrauterine abdominal distention and pressure atrophy of the abdominal muscles (3). In other words, any entity leading to chronic abdominal distention (e.g., mass, ascites) could produce deficient abdominal musculature, or so-called pseudo-prune belly syndrome (4) (Fig. 5.109). The former situation, however, is much more common.

As far as the usual type of absent abdominal musculature problem (i.e., associated with urinary tract abnormalities) is concerned, there is evidence to suggest that two separate subgroups of infants can be encountered. The first group has, as part of the problem, an obstructing lesion of the urethra, and the second group has a functional abnormality of bladder emptying but no mechanical urethral obstruction. The first group generally does poorly, and most of these infants die shortly after birth. The second group survives the neonatal period but develops chronic urinary tract problems later on. This grouping of patients with the prune belly syndrome also explains why, in the past, some investigators reported urethral obstruction to be common, while others spoke to the contrary.

When a definite urethral obstruction exists, the problem usually is frank urethral atresia (5) or a posterior urethral valve. Because of this, the bladder is hypertrophied, and the kidneys are usually severely hydronephrotic. They often become multicystic and dysplastic. These patients demonstrate decreased urine output in utero and subsequent oligohydramnios. Because of this, they develop all of the features of the Potter syndrome, including severely hypoplastic lungs. This is one reason that most of these infants die shortly after birth. Other congenital anomalies also occur and include malrotation of the intestine, intestinal atresia, imperforate anus, genital anomalies (6), skeletal abnormalities, and congenital heart disease.

In the second group of infants, associated congenital anomalies do not occur, no obstructing lesion of the urethra is defined, but bladder emptying is definitely abnormal.

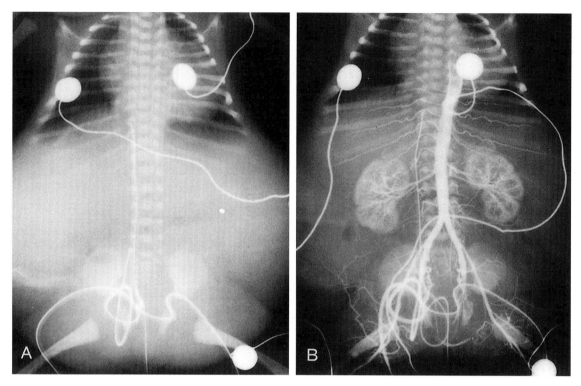

FIGURE 5.109. Prune belly syndrome: normal urinary tract. A. Note the massive distention of the abdomen. The lungs are clear, but probably hypoplastic. At autopsy they were hypoplastic. Also note cardiomegaly. **B.** Aortogram demonstrates normal renal arteries and normal kidneys. This patient had portal vein thrombosis and massive ascites, leading to a prune belly.

There may be deficiency in the autonomic innervation of the urinary tract in these patients, but whatever the underlying cause, there does seem to be a serious bladder-emptying problem in these patients. Unlike patients with obstructing urethral lesions, the urinary bladder in these infants usually is large and floppy, and large urachal remnants (diverticula) are common. Severe hydronephrosis usually is present (Fig. 5.110), and the urethra, although not demonstrating a definite obstruction, has a bizarre configuration (Fig. 5.111). Pulmonary hypoplasia also occurs in many of these patients, and in most cases of prune belly syndrome with hydronephrosis, dilatation of the ureters is greater than dilatation of the renal pelvis and calyces.

With hydronephrosis, ureteral dilation usually is greater than is dilation of the renal pelvis and calyces. Urethral diverticula can be associated (7) and may become so large that they mimic the findings of megalourethra. In longstanding cases, calcification of the urachus and bladder from urine stasis leading to fibrosis can be seen (8).

The prune belly syndrome occurs almost exclusively in males, with only the occasional female being recorded (8). Clinically, in the well-developed case, the abdominal wall is very thin, a sagging potbelly is present, and associated findings include undescended testicles, clubfoot deformity, and dislocated hips. The undescended testicles probably have their origin in decreased intraabdominal pressure, and the

clubfoot deformity and dislocated hips probably result from the fetal compression syndrome. In the milder cases, abdominal wall deficiency may be more difficult to detect, and the abdomen may pass for normal.

REFERENCES

1. Woodhouse CRJ, Ransley PG, Innes-Williams D. Prune belly syndrome—report of 47 cases. Arch Dis Child 1982;57:856–859.
2. Loder RT, Guiboux J-P, Bloom DA, et al. Musculoskeletal aspects of prune-belly syndrome: description and pathogenesis. Am J Dis Child 1992;146:1224–1229.
3. Nakayama DK, Harrison MR, Chinn DH, et al. The pathogenesis of prune belly. Am J Dis Child 1984;138:834–836.
4. Bellah RD, States LJ, Ducker JW. Pseudoprune-belly syndrome: imaging findings and clinical outcome. AJR 1996;167:1389–1399.
5. Kuga T, Esato K, Sase M, et al. Prune belly syndrome with penile and urethral agenesis: report of a case. J Pediatr Surg 1998;33:1825–1828.
6. Reinberg Y, Shapiro E, Manivel JC, et al. Prune belly syndrome in females: a triad of abdominal musculature deficiency and anomalies of the urinary and genital systems. J Pediatr 1991;118:395–398.
7. Kirchner SG, Kirchner FK Jr, Jolles H, et al. Bladder calcifications in the prune-belly syndrome. Radiology 1981;138:597–600.
8. Aaronson IA, Cremin BJ. Prune belly syndrome in young females. Urol Radiol 1979/1980;1:151–155.

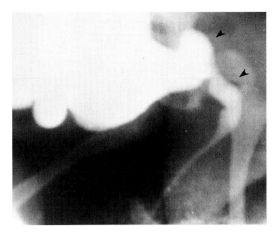

FIGURE 5.111. Prune belly syndrome: posterior urethra. Note the typical, dilated appearance of the posterior urethra and bladder neck (arrows). No obstructing lesions are defined in this type of patient, but bladder emptying and urethral function obviously are abnormal.

Urine Ascites

Most infants with urine ascites are males and have some form of bladder outlet or urethral obstruction, but the most common problem is posterior urethral valves. However, extrinsic masses compressing the bladder outlet and neurogenic bladder also can result in upper tract distention and urine ascites. Finally, there are cases where no obstruction is present, and ascites results from perforation of the urinary bladder, either spontaneous (1) or iatrogenic. Urine ascites can be secondary to perforation of the bladder from acute urinary retention and with trauma, both accidental and nonaccidental.

In terms of the pathophysiology of urine ascites developing from upper track distention, once perforation occurs, there is escape of urine into the space defined by the perirenal fascia and then through a peritoneal defect or tear, into the free peritoneal space. A discrete communication is not always demonstrated, and with bladder rupture, extravasation of urine can be extraperitoneal or intraperitoneal.

Ultrasonography or CT can demonstrate the presence of urine around the kidney, and extravasation of urine and contrast material can be seen on the voiding cystourethrogram if reflux occurs (Fig. 5.112). With bladder rupture, cystography is more informative. If CT is employed, delayed images are necessary (2), because the extravasation may not be immediately apparent (Fig. 5.113).

REFERENCES

1. Zerin JM, Lebowitz RL. Spontaneous extraperitoneal rupture of the urinary bladder in children. Radiology 1989;170:487–488.
2. Sivit CJ, Cutting JP, Eichelberger MR. CT diagnosis and localization of ruptured bladder in children with blunt abdominal

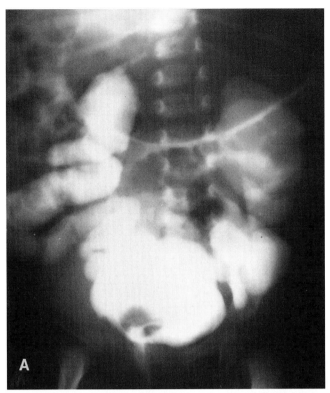

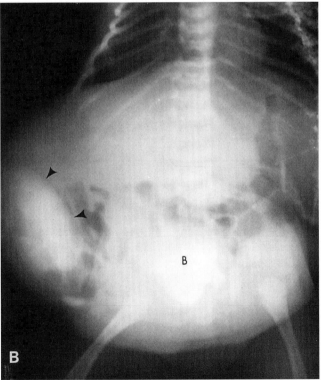

FIGURE 5.110. Prune belly syndrome. A. Characteristic large, floppy bladder and marked bilateral hydronephrosis and hydroureter. **B.** Another infant with a large, floppy abdomen. There is contrast material in the bladder (B) and a large anteriorly extending urachus (arrows).

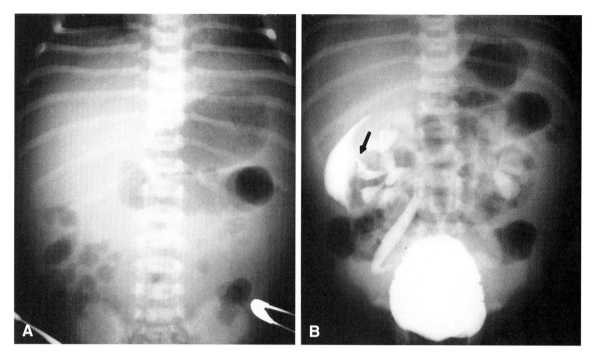

FIGURE 5.112. Urine ascites. A. Note abdominal distention, some separation of the air-filled loops of intestine, and lack of visualization of the liver edge. All of these findings are consistent with fluid in the abdomen. **B.** Cystogram demonstrates reflux into both ureters, bilateral hydroureter and hydronephrosis, and a leak from the middle right calyx (arrow) into the perirenal space.

trauma: significance of contrast material extravasation in the pelvis. Am J Roentgenol 1995;164:1243–1246.

Urinoma

Urinomas in the neonatal period are uncommon but have been recorded with obstructions secondary to posterior urethral valves (1) and ureteropelvic junction obstruction. The mechanics of upper tract perforation are the same as those of urine ascites. In urinoma, however, the urine and contrast material do not enter the peritoneal cavity; rather they remain in their perinephric location and produce a pseudocyst or urinoma. With cystourethrography or retrograde pyelography, reflux into the affected ureter causes the urinoma to become opacified, but ultrasonography and CT also are explicit in demonstrating this lesion. Some urinomas may be multiseptate, and calcification of the periphery of a urinoma occasionally occurs (2). Urinomas in older children are more common and are seen with urinary tract obstruction and after trauma to the urinary tract.

REFERENCES

1. Hoffer FA, Winters WD, Retik AB, et al. Urinoma drainage for neonatal respiratory insufficiency. Pediatr Radiol 1990;20: 270–271.
2. Kirchner SG, Braren V, Heller RM, et al. Uriniferous perirenal

pseudocyst. An unusual cause of a calcified abdominal mass in the neonate. Pediatr Radiol 1980;9:43–44.

Nephritis, Nephrosis, and the Nephrotic Syndrome

None of these conditions is common in the newborn infant, but all are commonly seen in the older infant and child. In terms of nephritis, most often the problem is acute glomerulonephritis secondary to the acute immune-complex mediated problem resulting from streptococcal infection in older children. The condition is most prevalent during the school-age years and seldom seen in infancy, but in infants, the so-called nonspecific membranoproliferative glomerulonephritis occurs. Renal parenchymal abnormalities consisting of increased renal echogenicity and loss of cortical medullary differentiation also occur in sickle cell disease (1) and Henoch-Schönlein purpura (2) (Fig. 5.114). Evaluating renal echogenicity is easier with the right kidney than with the left kidney because one has the liver for comparison on the right.

The nephrotic syndrome presents through all pediatric age groups and can result from a number of renal or nonrenal, systemic conditions. In neonates and young infants in the United States, the nephrotic syndrome most commonly results from syphilitic infection, but it also can be seen with other torch infections such as rubella (2), toxoplasmosis,

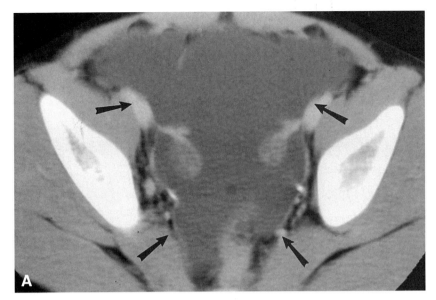

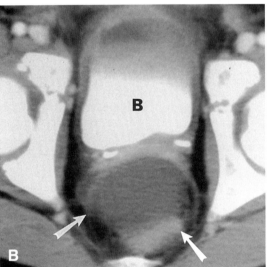
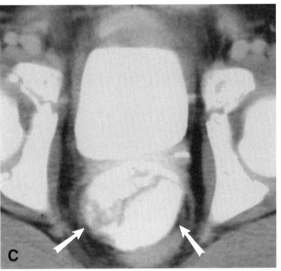

FIGURE 5.113. Urine ascites demonstrated with CT: value of delayed films. A. This patient had blunt abdominal trauma and demonstrated a large volume of fluid (arrows) in the pelvis. The oval structures floating in the peritoneal fluid are the ovaries. **B.** Lower in the pelvis the urinary bladder (B) is seen to contain contrast material. A peculiar structure is seen behind the bladder (arrows). **C.** With delayed films this structure opacifies (arrows), demonstrating that it represents fluid in the cul-de-sac and that bladder rupture has occurred. (From Swischuk LE. Vomiting and anuria after bicycle accident. Pediatr Emerg Care 1996;12:137–139, with permission.)

and cytomegalic inclusion disease. In the Scandinavian countries and in some other parts of the world, a congenital, familial form of the nephrotic syndrome (Finnish-type) is more common (3). This condition is inherited as an autosomal recessive trait and usually is lethal. Primary peritonitis usually pneumococcal in origin, is a common problem in the nephrotic syndrome (4).

Renal vein thrombosis also is a cause of the nephrotic syndrome in infancy, but it is interesting that the nephrotic syndrome also can cause renal vein thrombosis. The reason for this is that patients with the nephrotic syndrome are hypercoagulable, and renal vein thrombosis is common. Consequently, often it is difficult to determine whether the nephrotic syndrome or the renal vein thrombosis was the primary problem. Other causes of the nephrotic syndrome include lupus (5) and acquired immunodeficiency syndrome (AIDS) (6).

Ultrasound is the best way to demonstrate changes in any of these conditions, even though the changes are nonspecific and consist primarily of increased echogenicity of the kidney and loss of normal architecture (Fig. 5.114). It should be remembered, however, that in the neonate and up to about the age of 2–3 months, echogenicity of the normal kidney approaches that of liver and should not be misinterpreted as being abnormal. However, in the neonate, if renal echogenicity exceeds that of the liver, and in the older infant and child, if echogenicity of the kidney approaches that of liver, parenchymal disease should be suspected. However, even though these changes occur in many conditions, our experience is that most cases of acute glomerulonephritis and the nephrotic syndrome show normal renal echogenicity. On the other hand, patients with nephrotic syndrome can show large, plump kidneys (Fig. 5.115).

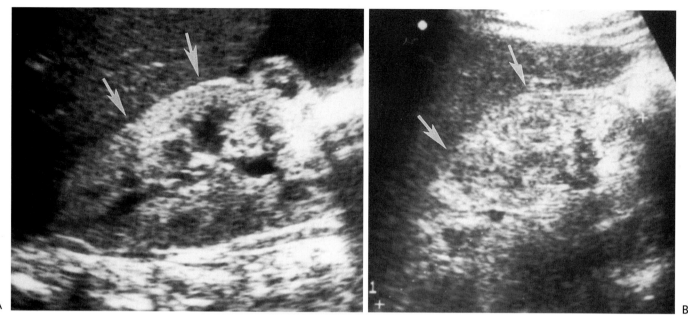

A
B

FIGURE 5.114. **Nephritis: other causes. A.** Echogenic kidney (arrows) in Henoch-Schölein Purpura. **B.** A similarly echogenic kidney (arrows) in sickle cell disease.

REFERENCES

1. Wigfall DR, Ware RE, Burchinal MR, et al. Prevalence and clinical correlates of glomerulopathy in children with sickle cell disease. J Pediatr 2000;136:749–753.
2. Patriquin HB, O'Regan S, Robitaille P, et al. Hemolytic-uremic syndrome: arterial Doppler patterns as a useful guide to therapy. Radiology 1989;172:625–628.
3. Huttunen NP. Congenital nephrotic syndrome of Finnish type: study of 75 patients. Arch Dis Child 1976;51:344–348.
4. Markenson DS, Levine D, Schacht R. Primary peritonitis is a presenting feature of nephritic syndrome. A case report and review of the literature. Pediatr Emerg Care 1999;15:407–409.
5. Massengill SF, Richard GA, Donnelly WH. Infantile systemic lupus erythematosus with onset simulating congenital nephrotic syndrome. J Pediatr 1994;124:27–31.

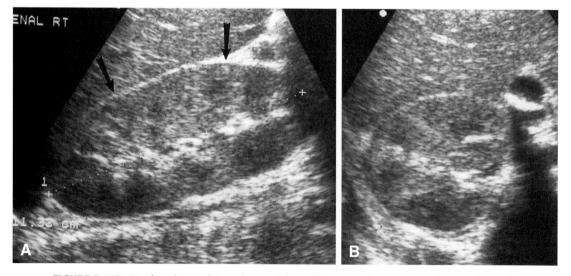

A
B

FIGURE 5.115. **Nephrotic syndrome in an older child with ultrasonographic findings. A.** The kidney is enlarged and plump appearing (arrows). Corticomedullary differentiation is poor. **B.** Cross-section demonstrates a round (plump), rather than oval, renal configuration.

6. Ingulli E, Tejani A, Fikrig S, et al. Nephrotic syndrome associated with acquired immunodeficiency syndrome in children. J Pediatr 1991;119:710–716.

Renal Cortical and Medullary (Papillary) Necrosis

Most often, these conditions result from severe dehydration, neonatal sepsis, massive blood loss, twin-to-twin transfusion, or severe hypoxia. In older children, papillary necrosis also can be seen with sickle cell disease (1), presumably resulting from capillary sludging and subsequent necrosis of the papillae.

With medullary (papillary) necrosis, initial ultrasonographic findings consist of increased echogenicity of the renal papillae (Fig. 5.116A). Later, as the papillae are destroyed, the calyces become blunted, or actual calyceal diverticula develop (Fig. 5.116B). Ultrasonographically, these areas appear as multiple cystic areas arranged in a pattern similar to that seen when the calyces are distended as a result of hydronephrosis. However, with medullary (papillary) necrosis, the renal pelvis usually is not dilated, and certainly not to a degree that would suggest severe hydronephrosis with marked calyceal dilation. With renal cortical necrosis, ultrasonography usually demonstrates nothing more than diffuse increase in echogenicity of the cortex of the kidneys (Fig. 5.117A). Eventually, a thin rim of peripheral calcification may be seen (Fig. 5.117B).

REFERENCE

1. Zinn D, Haller JO, Cohen HL. Focal and diffuse increased echogenicity in the renal parenchyma in patients with sickle hemoglobinopathies–an observation. J Ultrasound Med 1993;12: 211–214.

Hyperechoic Renal Papillae

There are numerous causes for echogenic renal papillae (1, 2), including nephrocalcinosis, hypercalcemia, papillary necrosis, vascular congestion, fibrosis, urate deposition, and protein deposition. With hypercalcemic states and renal tubular acidosis, plain film calcifications can be seen in the pyramids, and on ultrasonography, the pyramids are very echogenic (Fig. 5.108). Ultrasound is excellent in detecting echogenic papillae, even though the finding is nonspecific. Transient renal stasis, associated with Tamm-Horsfall proteinuria produces echogenic renal pyramids in the neonate (Fig. 5.4).

REFERENCES

1. Jequier S, Kaplan BS. Echogenic renal pyramids in children. J Clin Ultrasound 1991;19:85–92.
2. Schultz PK, Strife JL, Strife CF, et al. Hyperechoic renal medullary pyramids in infants and children. Radiology 1991;181:163–167.

Ask-Upmark Kidney

In this condition, the kidneys appear scarred and lobulated and often are considerably smaller than normal (1). There are segmental areas of hypoplasia or fibrosis, and the adjacent calyces are distorted and dilated. In the past, it was believed that the condition represented a developmental

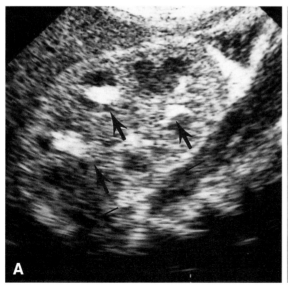
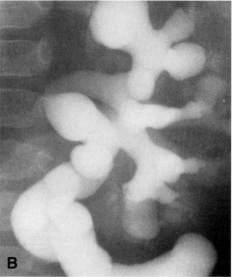

FIGURE 5.116. Papillary necrosis. A. Note the echogenic renal papillae (arrows). Echogenicity of the kidney in general is increased. **B.** Late stage. With reflux during cystourethrography, marked dilation and blunting of the calyces along with small diverticula and some pyelotubular backflow are seen.

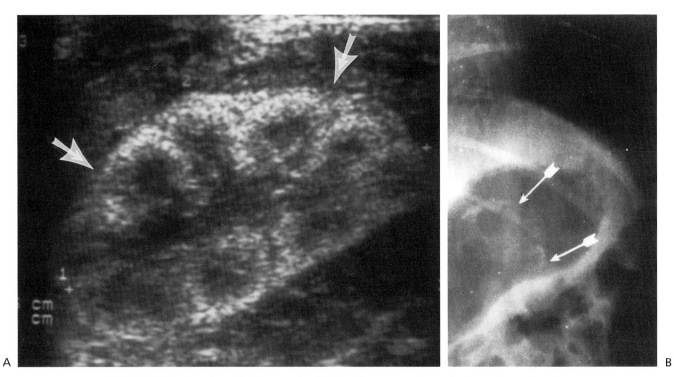

A   B

FIGURE 5.117. Renal cortical necrosis. **A.** On ultrasonography, note the echogenic cortex (arrows). **B.** Late changes demonstrating a fine rim of calcification outlining the renal cortex (arrows). (**B** from Leonidas JC, Berdon WE, Gribetz D. Bilateral renal cortical necrosis in the newborn infant; roentgenographic diagnosis. J Pediatr 1971;79:623–627, with permission.)

abnormality, but there is now growing feeling that the problem may result from chronic infection. The kidneys do appear much as those that are subject to chronic infection, reflux, and subsequent scarring. At any rate, clinical problems usually center on refractory hypertension and urinary tract infections. The characteristic lobulation and scarred appearance of the kidneys is readily demonstrable with CT (Fig. 5.13).

REFERENCE

1. Himmelfarb E, Rabinowitz JG, Parvey L, et al. The Ask-Upmark kidney. Am J Dis Child 1975;129:1440–1444.

Renal Transplant

Imaging of renal transplants generally centers on ultrasonography (1) and nuclear scintigraphy. Retrograde pyelography may be performed in selective cases, and the lesions generally sought for include lymphoceles (Fig. 5.118A), urinomas (Fig. 5.118B), hydronephrosis, renal artery or renal vein thrombosis, renal artery stenosis (2) (Fig. 5.118C), ureteral necrosis, ureteral stenosis (Fig. 5.118D), renal tubular necrosis, and both acute (Fig. 5.118E), and chronic rejection (1). Color flow Doppler is valuable for the evaluation of vascular abnormalities (3).

Ultrasound, including Doppler ultrasound, is not particularly reliable in detecting acute rejection (4, 5), and I personally have no confidence in renal index determinations in these kidneys. As far as scintigraphy is concerned, with rejection, using technetium-99m DTPA, there is tardy accumulation of the isotope in the kidney and markedly delayed excretion. However, even with all these studies, definitive diagnosis usually relies on renal biopsy. The most important ultrasound finding is a complete lack of blood flow to the kidney, because if the main renal artery and vein are open in such cases, one can be confident that the kidney is in the final stages of rejection. On the other hand, ultrasound is extremely useful when it comes to detecting pararenal fluid collections such as lymphoceles and urinomas, hydronephrosis, and renal vein thrombosis. With renal artery obstruction, arteriography often is finally required and these lesions now can be treated with balloon dilation (6). When renal vein thrombosis is the problem, the kidney enlarges and the internal architecture becomes disorganized. We noticed the appearance of focal hypoechoic cortical lesions in one patient, supporting the concept that with renal vein thrombosis the problem first starts in the small intrarenal veins and then extends retrograde into the renal vein and inferior vena cava. Urine leaks often are best substantiated with delayed nuclear scintigraphy (Fig. 5.118F).

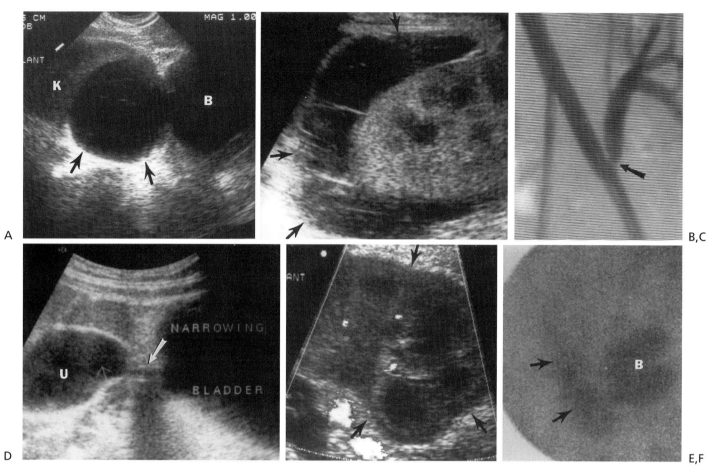

FIGURE 5.118. Renal transplant complications. A. Lymphocele. Note the hypoechoic, cyst-like structure (arrows). The kidney (K) is just adjacent to the lymphocele. B, bladder. **B.** Perinephric urinoma (arrows). **C.** Renal artery stenosis. **D.** Ureteral stenosis. Note the dilated ureter (U) and the stenotic (arrow) distal end. BLADDER, urinary bladder. **E.** Rejection; poor renal perfusion. On this color flow Doppler study, note that, although there is considerable blood flow in the renal pedicle (arrows), virtually none is seen in the kidney itself. This kidney went on to total rejection. **F.** Urine leak. Nuclear scintigraphy at 30 minutes demonstrates isotope accumulation outside the kidney (arrows). K, kidney.

REFERENCES

1. Sheldon CA, Churchill BM, Khoury AE, et al. Complications of surgical significance in pediatric renal transplantation. J Pediatr Surg 1992;27:485–490.
2. Stanley P, Malekzadeh M, Diament MJ. Post-transplant renal artery stenosis: angiographic study in 32 children. AJR 1987;148:487–490.
3. Mutze S, Turk I, Schonberger B, et al. Colour-coded duplex sonography in the diagnostic assessment of vascular complications after kidney transplantation in children. Pediatr Radiol 1997;27:898–902.
4. Briscoe DM, Hoffer FA, Tu N, et al. Duplex Doppler examination of renal allografts in children: correlation between renal blood flow and clinical findings. Pediatr Radiol 1993;23:365–368.
5. Kelcz F, Pozniak MA, Pirsch JD, et al. Pyramidal appearance and resistive index: insensitive and nonspecific sonographic indicators of renal transplant rejection. AJR 1990;155:531–535.
6. Spijkerboer AM, Mali WP, Donckerwolcke RA. Renal transplant artery stenosis in children: treatment with percutaneous transluminal angioplasty. Pediatr Radiol 1992;22:519.

Postrenal Biopsy Complications

Complications seen with renal biopsy include intrarenal or subcapsular hematoma, extravasation of blood beyond the renal capsule, and AV fistula formation (1). Most often, these abnormalities are first detected with ultrasound (Fig. 5.119). AV fistulas often are clearly visualized with color Doppler sonography (1).

REFERENCE

1. Riccabona M, Schwinger W, Ring F. Arteriovenous fistula after renal biopsy in children. J Ultrasound Med 1998;17:505–508.

Urinary Tract Trauma

Although trauma to the urinary tract can be iatrogenic most often it is secondary to blunt abdominal trauma such as sus-

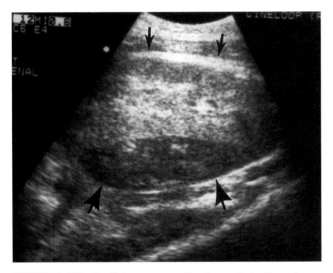

FIGURE 5.119. Postbiopsy complications. Note the subcapsular hematoma (lower arrows). The kidney itself (upper arrows) is echogenic.

tained motor vehicle accident. As far as the kidney is concerned, the findings are best evaluated with CT, because ultrasound can miss significant contusions. However, patients can be followed with ultrasound (1). Intravenous pyelogram is seldom now used (2). Lacerations of the kidney can be confined within the capsule or can involve the capsule and result in extravasation of blood into the perirenal space (Fig. 5.120). Trauma to the ureter is less frequently encountered, but trauma to the bladder is common. With trauma to the bladder, one can encounter both intraperitoneal and extraperitoneal bladder leaks. Urethral injuries are more common in males than in females and suspected urethral injuries usually are first imaged with retrograde urethrography. In this regard, one should not pass a catheter through a urethra that is suspected of being injured until it has been determined with retrograde urethrography that an injury is or is not present.

REFERENCES

1. Abdalati H, Bula DI, Sivit CJ, et al. Blunt renal trauma in children: healing of renal injuries and recommendations for imaging follow-up. Pediatr Radiol 1994;24:573–576.

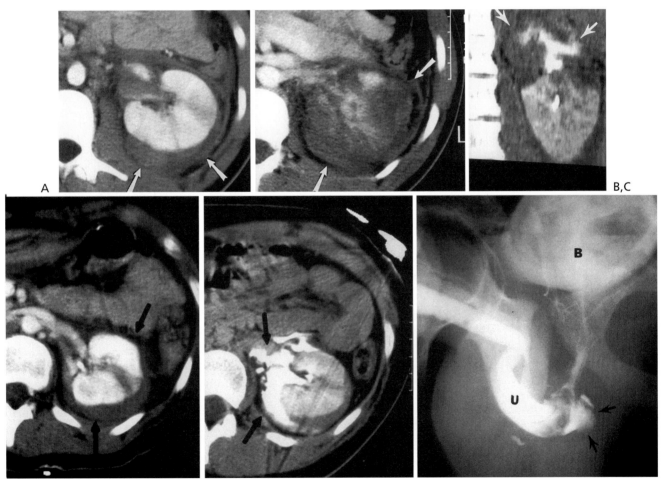

2. Mayor B, Gudincher F, Wicky S, et al. Imaging evaluation of blunt renal trauma in children: diagnostic accuracy of intravenous pyelography and ultrasonography. Pediatr Radiol 1995;25: 214–218.

GENITAL TRACT

With the advent of CT, MR, and especially ultrasonographic imaging (1) of the genital tract, delineation of normal anatomy and detection of abnormalities has become relatively commonplace. In the neonate, because of maternal hormonal influences, the uterus often is more prominent than expected (Fig. 5.121). Thereafter, it decreases in size and remains about the same until about 11–13 years, when a rapid increase in size occurs (2), and in the adolescent, it assumes near adult size. The vagina and ovaries grow correspondingly, but it should be noted that in the neonate during the first month of life the ovaries can appear a little larger than expected (3). Follicular cysts also can be seen on a normal basis in the first 2 years of life. Ovarian size measurements throughout the pediatric age group have been documented by Cohen et al. (3).

The normal testicle has a uniform granular texture ultrasonographically and offers no problem in imaging (Fig. 5.122). The epididymis, however, is larger than expected in neonates and young infants (Fig. 5.122C), but later becomes smaller and is identified as an echogenic focus along the posterior aspect of the upper pole of the testis. The prostate gland is best imaged with CT or MR, but generally, imaging of the prostate gland is important primarily when tumors of the gland are present. Normal seminal vesicles can appear large in the adolescent male and can be visualized with any imaging modality (Fig. 5.123).

REFERENCES

1. Siegel MJ. Pediatric gynecologic sonography. Radiology 1991;179: 593–600.
2. Haber HP, Mayer EI. Ultrasound evaluation of uterine and ovarian size from birth to puberty. Pediatr Radiol 1994;24:11–13.
3. Cohen HL, Shapiro MA, Mandel FS, et al. Normal ovaries in neonates and infants: a sonographic study of 77 patients 1 day to 24 months old. AJR 1993;160:583–586.

Absent and Ectopic Gonads (Cryptorchidism)

Absence of the ovaries most commonly occurs with Turner's syndrome. Ectopic ovaries can be located in the inguinal canal (1) and are readily identified with ultrasound. These ovaries can undergo torsion or can become incarcerated. If gonads are in an ectopic position in the abdomen (including testes) they usually are detected during exploratory laparotomy, because it is difficult to detect them with any imaging modality. However, if in the inguinal canal, testes can be identified with ultrasound, but thereafter one may need to resort to MRI (Fig. 5.124).

In terms of investigating male cryptorchidism, one first relies on the clinical examination and then on ultrasonography. MRI (2–4) should be employed if ultrasound fails. However, our experience suggests that it is not easy to identify intraabdominal testicles even with MRI. For this reason, some suggest that one finally resort to laparoscopy (5). CT also can be used but is not as rewarding as MRI. Urinary tract anomalies can be associated with cryptorchidism (6), but the incidence probably is not much greater than that in the general population.

REFERENCES

1. Goske MJ, Emmens RW, Rabinowitz R. Inguinal ovaries in children demonstrated by high resolution real-time ultrasound. Radiology 1984;151:635–636.
2. Myano T, Kobayashi H, Shimomura H, et al. Magnetic resonance imaging for localizing the nonpalpable undescended testis. J Pediatr Surg 1991;26:607–609.
3. Maghnie M, Vanzulli A, Paesano P, et al. The accuracy of magnetic resonance imaging and ultrasonography compared with surgical findings in the localization of the undescended testis. Arch Pediatr Adolesc Med 1994;148:699–703.
4. Troughton AH, Waring J, Longstaff A, et al. The role of magnetic resonance imaging in the investigation of undescended testes. Clin Radiol 199041:178–181.
5. Fritzche PJ, Hricak H, Kogan BA, et al. Undescended testis: value of MR imaging. Radiology 1987;164:169–173.
6. Pappis CH, Argianas SA, Bousgas D, et al. Unsuspected urological anomalies in asymptomatic cryptorchid boys. Pediatr Radiol 1988;18:51–53.

FIGURE 5.120. Urinary tract trauma. A–C. Renal fracture with devitalized kidney. In **A,** note a normal nephrogram in the lower pole. It is surrounded by perinephric blood (arrows). **B.** The upper pole fails to demonstrate contrast material within it and is surrounded by a hematoma (arrows). **C.** Coronal reconstructed view demonstrates the viable lower pole, the renal fracture (arrow), and the nonviable upper pole. **D.** Renal contusion fracture with delayed demonstration of extravasation. This kidney demonstrates a fracture line (arrow) and a contusion. **E.** Later, with a second run through the kidneys, extravasation of contrast material (arrows) is noted. **F.** Urethral injury. Retrograde urethrogram demonstrates extravasation of contrast (arrows). U, urethra; B, bladder.

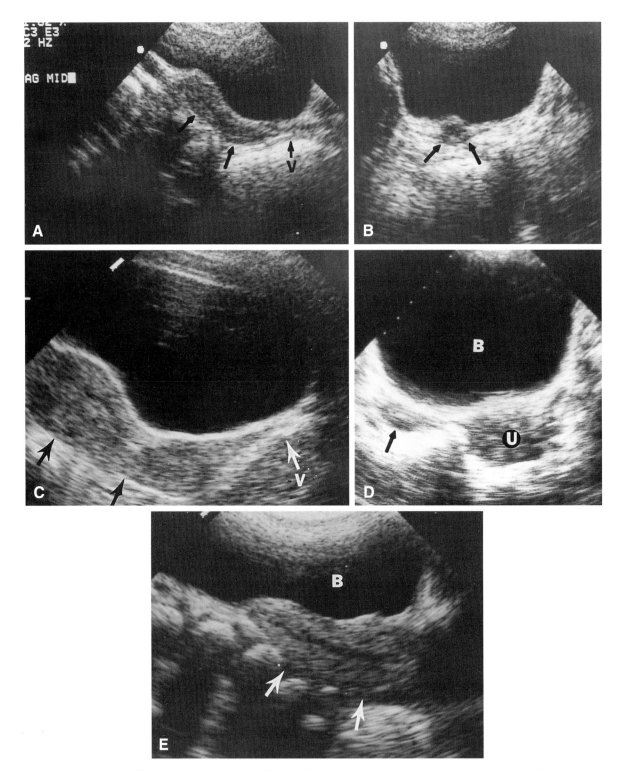

FIGURE 5.121. Normal female genital tract. A. Normal uterus (arrows) in a 4-year-old girl. Vagina (V). **B.** Cross-sectional view through the fundus of the uterus (arrows). The thin lines on either side represent the broad ligaments. **C.** Adolescent with a larger, but normal, uterus (arrows). Vagina (V). **D.** Cross-sectional view demonstrates the uterus (U) and the right ovary (arrow). **E.** Large, normal uterus (arrows) in a newborn. B, bladder.

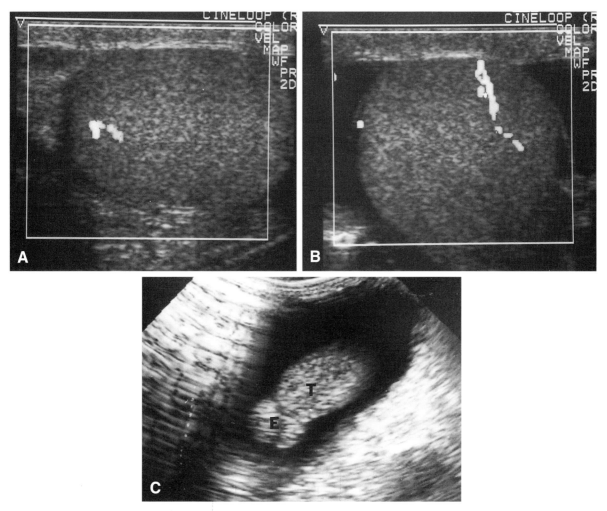

FIGURE 5.122. Normal testicle. A. Sagittal view demonstrates the normal texture of the testicle. Intratesticular blood flow (white areas) is seen with color flow Doppler. **B.** Cross-sectional view demonstrates the round testicle, and intratesticular blood flow is seen. **C.** In the neonate, the epididymis (E) is larger than that in older children. The testicle (T) is surrounded by a hydrocele.

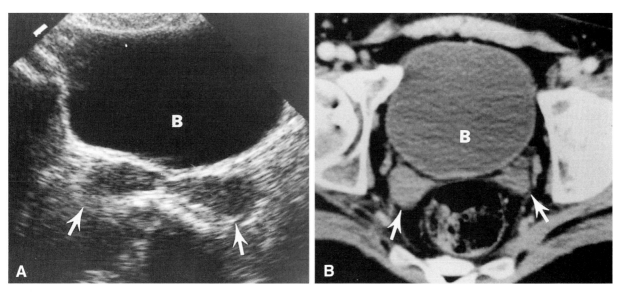

FIGURE 5.123. Normal seminal vesicles. A. On this cross-sectional view, note the appearance of the normal seminal vesicles. B, bladder. **B.** CT study in another patient demonstrates the seminal vesicles (arrows). B, urinary bladder.

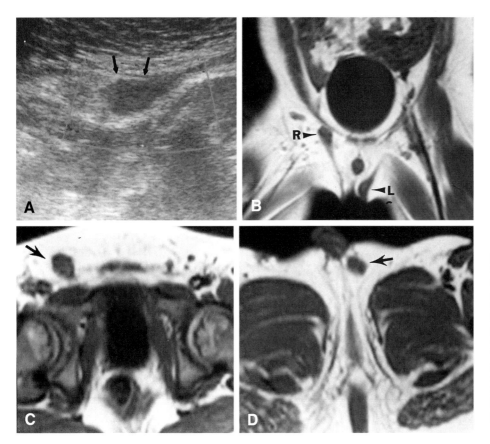

FIGURE 5.124. Undescended testicles. A. Ultrasound detects a testicle (arrows) in the inguinal canal just above the inguinal ligament. **B.** T1-weighted magnetic resonance image of another patient demonstrates the right testicle (R) to be located high in the inguinal canal. The left testicle (L) is in a more normal position. **C.** Cross-sectional view demonstrates the right testicle (arrow) high in the inguinal canal. **D.** A slightly lower image demonstrates the left testicle (arrow) in a lower position.

Anomalies of the Uterus and Vagina

Absence of the uterus is uncommon but can be seen in the Mayer-Rokitansky-Kuster-Hauser syndrome (1). Other anomalies of the uterus also can be seen in this syndrome, and the vagina also may be absent or hypoplastic. Skeletal anomalies, primarily of the vertebral bodies, also occur. Other, sporadic, uterine anomalies usually result from failure of fusion of the mullerian ducts and consist of a wide variety of uterine duplications. Anomalies of the uterus also are seen in the so-called hand-foot-uterine syndrome, and a small uterus occurs in Turner's syndrome. However, the *most problematic anomaly of the vagina and uterus, especially in the neonate and then later in the adolescent, is hydrometrocolpos or hematometrocolpos.* If only the vagina is filled with fluid, the term hydrocolpos is used, but if both the uterus and vagina are fluid-filled, the term hydrometrocolpos is used. If the fluid is bloody, the term is changed to hematometrocolpos. In any case, it is the mass produced by the dilated vagina and/or uterus that calls attention to the problem and, if large enough, can cause obstruction of the venous and lymphatic return from the lower extremities. Displacement of the ureters and bladder leads to associated hydronephrosis, and an adhesive peri-

tonitis secondary to retrograde passage of the secretions through the fallopian tubes also can occur.

Simple vaginal hypersecretion and slight enlargement of the vagina are not uncommon in normal neonatal female infants and are believed to result from the effects of maternal estrogens. However, if there is hypersecretion and the vagina is obstructed, excessive accumulation of these secretions produces a large mass and hydrometrocolpos develops. Obstruction of the vagina results from either an imperforate membrane (hymen) or vaginal atresia (2, 3). When obstruction results from an imperforate hymen, there is no increased incidence of associated anomalies, and the condition is benign. It is easily treated by simple incision of the hymen. This type of vaginal obstruction can present in the neonatal period, or early in adolescence when menses begin. When the vagina is atretic, the condition presents in the neonatal period and usually is serious. The area of atresia is segmental and usually consists of a thick transverse vaginal septum that occludes the upper third of the vagina.

Other anomalies of the genitourinary commonly occur with atretic vaginal obstruction and include persistence of a cloaca or urogenital sinus, communications between these structures and the rectum, vaginourethral communications, and bicornuate uterus. Anomalies of other systems commonly occur and include imperforate anus, sacral dysplasia or agenesis, esophageal or duodenal atresia, malrotation of the intestines, and congenital heart disease. When these anomalies are accompanied by polydactyly, chances are that one is dealing with the McKusick-Kaufman syndrome, a recessively inherited syndrome that includes vaginal atresia (1).

All these findings, in addition to the dilated vagina and uterus, are readily demonstrated with ultrasound or MRI (4) (Figs. 5.125 and 5.126). If a rectovaginal fistula is present, air may be seen in the enlarged vagina and/or uterus (Fig. 5.127), and with cystourethrography or vaginography, contrast material can pass into the vagina and uterus, either through a vesicovaginal fistula or by reflux through the vaginal orifice if stenosis, rather than atresia, is present. In those cases where associated plastic peritonitis occurs, irregular or curvilinear peritoneal calcifications can be seen (Fig.

5.128), and when imperforate anus is present, meconium calcification within the obstructed colon can occur (Fig. 5.129).

REFERENCES

1. Strubbe EH, Willemsen WN, Lemmens JA, et al. Mayer-Rokitansky-Kuster-Hauser syndrome: distinction between two forms based on excretory urographic, sonographic, and laparoscopic findings. AJR 1993;160:331–334.
2. Blask ARN, Sanders RC, Gearhart JP. Obstructed uterovaginal anomalies: demonstration with sonography. Part I. Neonates and infants. Radiology 1991;179:79–83, Apr.
3. Blask ARN, Sanders RC, Rock JA. Obstructed uterovaginal anomalies: demonstration with sonography. Part II. Teenagers. Radiology 1991;179:84–88.
4. Hugosson C, Jorulf H, Bakri Y. MRI in distal vaginal atresia. Pediatr Radiol 1991;21:281–283.

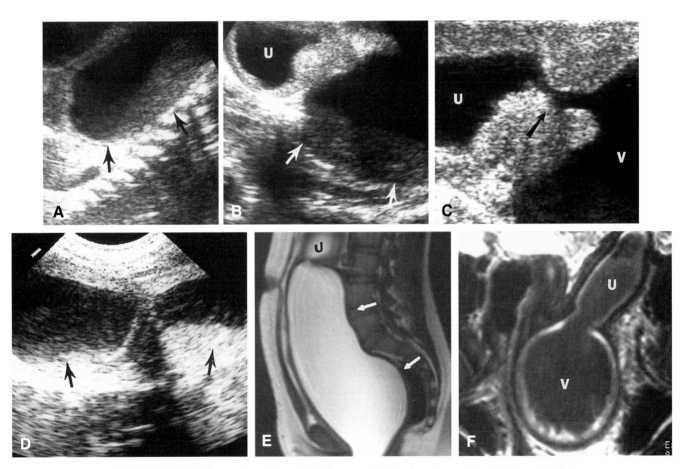

FIGURE 5.125. Hydrometrocolpos. A. A large cystic structure (arrows) containing debris is identified anterior to the sacrum. **B.** More cephalad, the same structure is identified (arrows), but another structure, the dilated uterus (U), also is identified. **C.** With high-resolution ultrasonography, the uterus (U) and vagina (V) are identified, as is the communication (arrow) through the cervical os. **D.** Another patient with hydrometrocolpos in a duplicated uterus (arrows). **E.** Sagittal, T2-weighted MR study demonstrates the large fluid-filled vagina (arrows) above which sits a smaller and slightly dilated uterus (U). **F.** Another patient whose MR, T1-weighted study demonstrates unilateral hydrometrocolpos in a duplicated uterus. U, uterus; V, vagina.

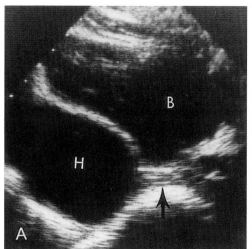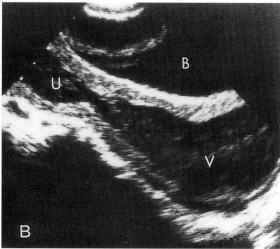

FIGURE 5.126. Hydrometrocolpos: ultrasonographic findings. A. Vaginal atresia. Note the large fluid-filled structure representing hydrometrocolpos (H). Above it lies the bladder (B), and the arrow points to the vaginal segment distal to the point of atresia. **B.** Imperforate hymen. The uterus (U) and vagina (V) are dilated. There is no evidence of a distal vaginal segment past the site of atresia. The narrowing between the uterus and vagina represents the cervical os.

Ovarian Cysts

Ovarian cysts are relatively common in childhood and in general are simple, follicular, or corpus luteal cysts. Such cysts are especially common in adolescent girls after menses begins, but follicular cysts also can be seen in younger girls, and even in the neonate and young infant (1–3) (Fig. 5.130). They are, however, more common in adolescents.

In the neonate, ovarian cysts can become quite large (Fig. 5.131, D–F) and case can be single or multiple and bilateral. In addition, some may rupture, undergo torsion, or even regress (1, 4–8). As a result of the latter, treatment now often is conservative (1, 6, 7). However, torsion can be a complication and immediate surgical correction is required once discovered (3, 6, 9, 10). In this regard, because of the propensity of these cystic ovaries to undergo torsion, some advocate prenatal decompression of the cyst (11).

Any ovarian cyst is readily demonstrable with ultrasound, CT, or MRI (Fig. 5.131). Simple cysts usually appear as smooth-walled, hypoechoic structures (Fig. 5.131A). Occasionally, they may contain debris resulting from bleeding (Fig. 5.131B), and when bleeding occurs, an echogenic fibrin rim may be detected with ultrasound (Fig. 5.132 A). The fibrin rim mimics the echogenic mucosal layer seen with duplication cysts. Corpus luteal cysts that bleed present as a heterogeneous round or oval mass with fluid collections mixed with solid tissue (Fig. 5.131 C). The appearance usually cannot be differentiated from that of torsion of the ovary, torsion of a dermoid or teratoma, or even a teratoma that has not undergone torsion. When an ovarian cyst ruptures, it can lead to accumulation of fluid in the peritoneal cavity and to ascites.

Cysts also are a component of two ovarian tumor groups: dermoids or teratomas and cystadenomas or cystadenocarcinomas. Multiple cysts also are seen in the Stein-Leventhal syndrome, or polycystic ovary syndrome (Fig. 5.132, C and D), and in the McCune-Albright syndrome (12).

REFERENCES

1. Campbell BA, Garg RS, Garg K, et al. Perinatal ovarian cyst: a nonsurgical approach. J Pediatr Surg 1992;27:1618–1619.
2. Cohen HL, Eisenberg P, Mandel F, et al. Ovarian cysts are common in premenarchal girls: a sonographic study of 101 children 2–12 years old. AJR 1992;159:89–91.
3. Croitoru DP, Aaron LE, Laberge J-M, et al. Management of complex ovarian cysts presenting in the first year of life. J Pediatr Surg 1991;26:1366–1368.
4. Amodio J, Abramson S, Berdon W, et al. Postnatal resolution of large ovarian cysts detected in utero: report of two cases. Pediatr Radiol 1987;17:467–469.
5. Nussbaum AR, Sanders RC, Benator RM, et al. Case report. Spontaneous resolution of neonatal ovarian cysts AJR 1987;148: 175–176.
6. Garel L, Filiatrault D, Brandt M, et al. Antenatal diagnosis of ovarian cysts: natural history and therapeutic implications. Pediatr Radiol 1991;21:182–184.
7. Zachariou Z, Roth H, Boos R, et al. Three years' experience with large ovarian cysts diagnosed in utero. J Pediatr Surg 1989;24: 478–482.
8. Muller-Leisse C, Bick U, Paulussen K, et al. Ovarian cysts in the fetus and neonate–changes in sonographic pattern in the follow-up and their management. Pediatr Radiol 1992;22:395–400.
9. Godfrey H, Abernatrhy L, Boothroyd A. Torsion of an ovarian cyst mimicking enteric duplication cyst on transabdominal ultrasound: two cases. Pediatr Radiol 1998;28:171–173.
10. Schmahmann S, Haller JO. Neonatal ovarian cysts: pathogenesis, diagnosis and management. Pediatr Radiol 1997;27:101–105.

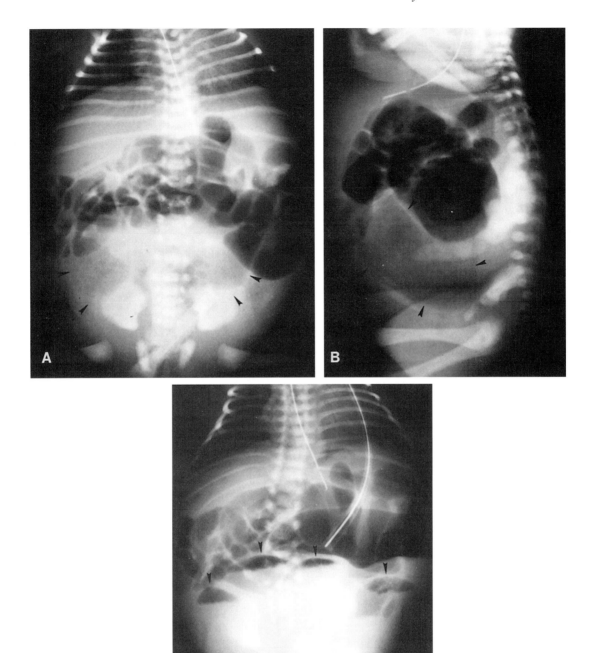

FIGURE 5.127. Hydrometrocolpos with air in the vagina. A. Note the distended abdomen, elevated intestines, and bubbly collection of air and fluid in the lower midabdomen (arrows). **B.** Lateral view demonstrating the same bubbly collection of air mixed with fluid in the distended, obstructed vagina and uterus (arrows). **C.** Upright film demonstrating air-fluid levels in four compartments of the duplicated uterus and vagina (arrows).

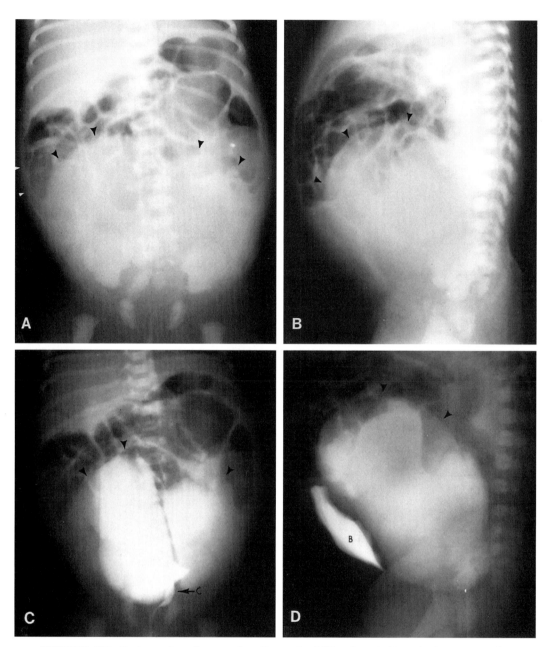

FIGURE 5.128. Hydrometrocolpos and peritoneal calcification. A. Note the large mass arising out of the pelvis and displacing the intestines upward (black arrows). A fine rim of calcification is seen along the right lateral abdominal wall (white arrows). This represented calcific peritonitis secondary to spillover of secretions from the fallopian tubes. **B.** Lateral view demonstrates the large mass (arrows). **C and D.** Anteroposterior and lateral views showing a large, dilated, bicornuate uterus filled after retrograde injection of contrast material into a cloaca (C). Note how the bladder (B) is displaced anterosuperiorly by the large mass in **D.** At surgery, this infant had severe vaginal stenosis, a vesicovaginal fistula, and imperforate anus.

11. Crombleholme TM, Craigo SD, Garmel S, et al. Fetal ovarian cyst decompression to prevent torsion. J Pediatr Surg 1997; 32:1447–1449.
12. Rieth KG, Comite F, Shawker TH, et al. Pituitary and ovarian abnormalities demonstrated by CT and ultrasound in children with features of the McCune-Albright syndrome. Radiology 1984;153:389–393.

Genital Tract Tumors

Tumors of the genital tract in the neonate and young infant are rare but they are a little more common in older children, primarily in girls. In terms of malignant ovarian tumors, the most common are the various germ cell tumors (1) (Fig.

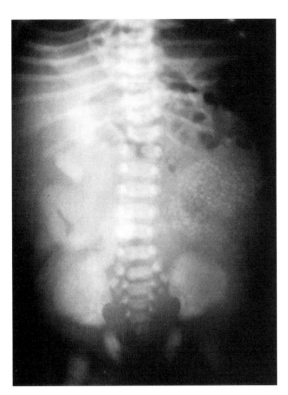

FIGURE 5.129. Hydrometrocolpos, hydronephrosis, imperforate anus, and meconium calcifications. Note the severe hydronephrosis on the right. Also note the stippled calcified meconium in the obstructed (imperforate anus) colon on the left.

5.133). In infants, however, the most common malignant tumor of the genital tract is rhabdomyosarcoma. It arises from the vagina in girls and the prostate or bladder in boys. In females it is also referred to as sarcoma botryoides. Ovarian dermoids are common in female infants and children

and present as tumors of mixed tissue intermingled with cysts and calcifications (Fig. 5.134). In some cases, the calcifications are formed and take the configuration of teeth or bony structures. Other tumors of the female genital tract include cystadenomas of the ovary (Fig. 5.135), granulosa cell ovarian tumors (2, 3) (Fig. 5.136), and ovarian fibromas (4). All of these tumors are rare and so is massive edema of the ovary resulting from chronic, partial ovarian torsion (5).

Testicular tumors in male infants and young children also are rare. In this regard, although seminoma is the commonest neoplasm of the testes in adults, in infants and young children the most common tumor is embryonal cell carcinoma (yolk cell carcinoma). All of these tumors usually are first imaged with ultrasound, but while it is generally believed that these tumors produce uniform hypodensity, in our experience they may be hypoechoic, hyperechoic, or normally echogenic (Fig. 5.137).

Fibrous hamartoma of the genital tract is a rare tumor occurring mostly in female infants. It often is rather extensive and at first suggests malignancy but usually, it is benign (6) on imaging. It can involve both the internal genital and the external tract (i.e., vulva, perineum) and, on imaging, frequently erroneously suggests a serious malignancy (Fig. 5.138). With rhabdomyosarcomas of the genital tract, mixed ultrasonographic echogenicity is seen, but final definition of the lesion is best accomplished with MRI or CT scanning. With rhabdomyosarcoma of the prostate, voiding cystourethrography may erroneously suggest normality, because these tumors often grow around the urethra rather than invade it (Fig. 5.139). On the other hand, if they invade the base of the bladder, it may be difficult to determine whether the tumor is arising from the prostate or urinary bladder.

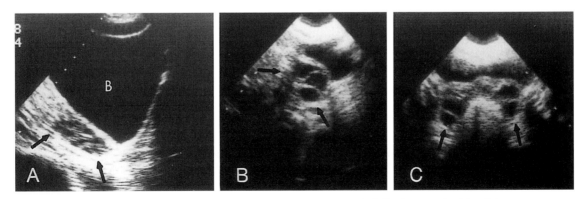

FIGURE 5.130. Follicular cysts. A. Note the numerous small follicular cysts in this adolescent female (arrows). B, bladder. **B.** Three-month-old infant with large, multiple cysts in the ovary (arrows). **C.** Both ovaries are similarly involved (arrows) and the findings were incidental.

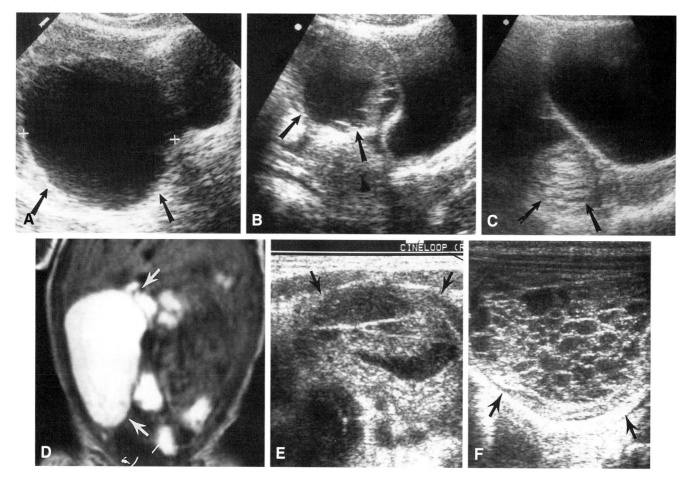

FIGURE 5.131. Ovarian cysts: variable appearance. A. A predominantly clear, fluid-filled cyst (arrows). **B.** This cyst (arrows) contains debris secondary to bleeding. **C.** Hemorrhagic corpus luteal cyst (arrows) is almost completely solid. **D.** Large ovarian cyst in a neonate (arrows) is demonstrated on a T2-weighted, coronal MR study. **E.** Ultrasonographically, the cyst contains considerable debris (arrows). **F.** In one area, a multicystic appearance (arrows) probably results from fibrinous exudate.

REFERENCES

1. Gribbon M, Ein SH, Mancer K. Pediatric malignant ovarian tumors: a 43-year review. J Pediatr Surg 1992;27:480–484.
2. Bouffet E, Basset T, Chetail N, et al. Juvenile granulose cell tumor of the ovary in infants: a clinicopathologic study of three cases and review of the literature. J Pediatr Surg 1997;32:762–765.
3. Chan YF, Restall P, Kimble R. Juvenile granulose cell tumor of the testis: report of two cases in newborns. J Pediatr Surg 1997;32:752–753.
4. Laufer L, Barki Y, Mordechai Y, et al. Ovarian fibroma in a prepubertal girl. Pediatr Radiol 1996;26:40–42.
5. Heiss KF, Zwiren GT, Winn K. Massive ovarian edema in the pediatric patient: a rare solid tumor. J Pediatr Surg 1994;29:1392–1394.
6. Popek EJ, Montgomery EA, Fourcroy JL. Fibrous hamartoma of infancy in the genital region: findings in 15 cases. J Urol 1994;152:990–993.

Intersex Problems in the Neonate

Primordial gonadal structures differentiate into ovaries and testes at an early fetal stage of development. Absence or maldevelopment of these structures occurs in conditions such as Turner's syndrome (Bonnevie-Ullrich syndrome in the neonate), Klinefelter's syndrome, and true hermaphrodism. In true hermaphrodism both ovaries and testes are present, often combined into a single structure called the ovotestes.

If a testis develops, it induces the development of male external genitalia. It is the androgens from the testes and from the adrenal glands that induce the development of the male external genitalia. If for some reason there is an excessive production of these androgens, as in the adrenogenital syndrome, virilization effects are noted. In females, female

(Text continues on page 694.)

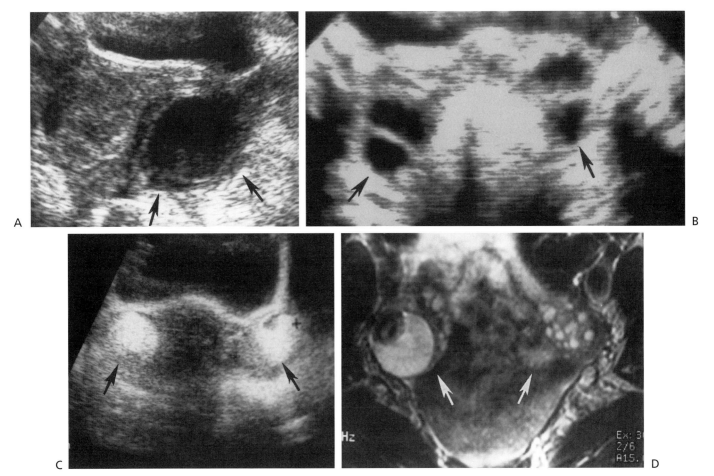

FIGURE 5.132. Ovarian cysts: other configuration. A. Not the hypoechoic cyst (arrows). It has an echogenic lining. **B.** Bilateral cysts (arrows) in three month old infant. **C.** Stein-Leventhal syndrome. Note the echogenic ovaries (arrows) on ultrasound examination. Echogenicity is due to multiple acoustical interfaces produced by the numerous cysts. **D.** MR study demonstrates numerous cysts on both sides (arrows). A dominant, large cyst is present on the right.

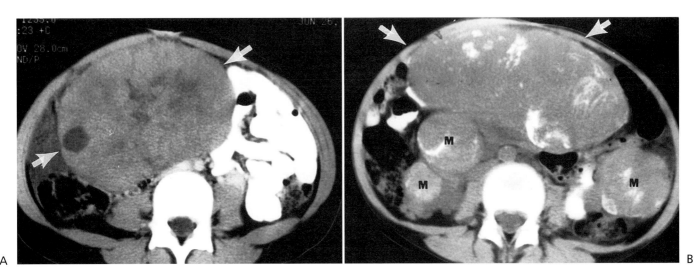

FIGURE 5.133. Germ cell tumors. A. Dysgerminoma. Note the large tumor (arrow) with some areas of low signal intensity and a cystic area. **B.** Malignant teratoma. Note the large tumor (arrows) with scattered irregular calcifications. At least three metastatic (M) lesions also are present.

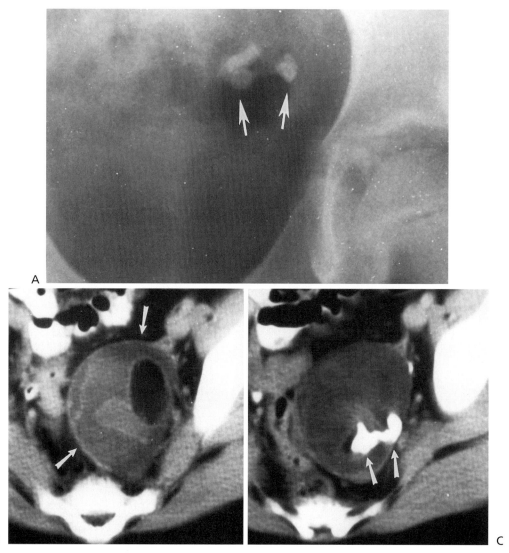

FIGURE 5.134. Ovarian dermoid. A. Note the teeth (arrows) in the dermoid. **B.** CT study demonstrates a mass with multiple tissues present. These include fat, fluid, and solid tissue. **C.** Another image demonstrates the presence of teeth (arrows).

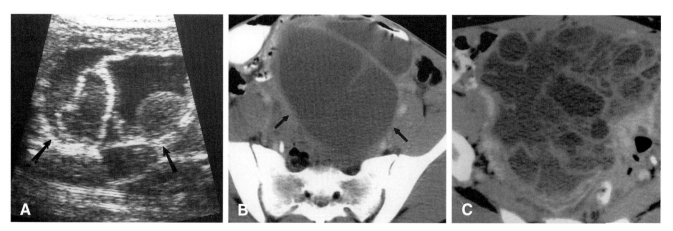

FIGURE 5.135. Female genital tumors. A. Multiloculated ovarian cystadenoma (arrows). Some of the loculi of fluid contain echogenic debris. **B.** Another patient with CT demonstration of a multicystic fluid-filled cystadenoma (arrows). **C.** Unusual appearance of cystoadenoma mimicking a lymphangioma. (Courtesy of Jean-Claude Hoeffel, M.D.)

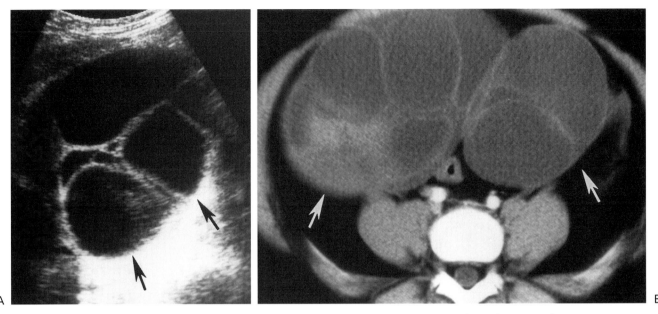

FIGURE 5.136. Granulosa cell tumor. A. Note the large, multicystic tumor (arrow). **B.** CT study demonstrates the extensive size of the tumor, which is multicystic (arrows). Only a small amount of solid tissue is seen on the right.

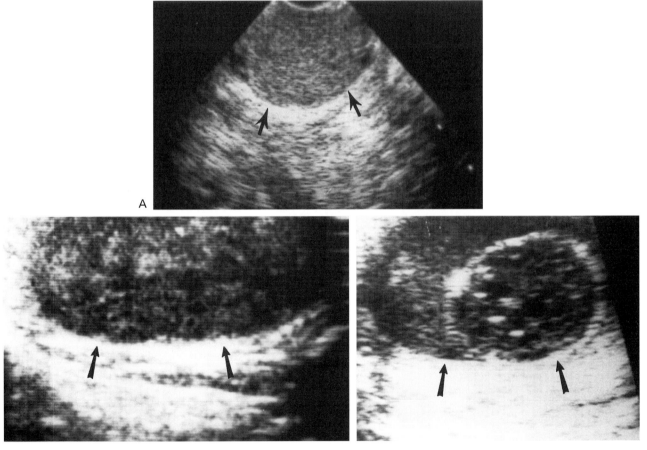

FIGURE 5.137. Testicular tumors. A. Testicular yoke sac tumor with uniform coarse echogenicity. **B.** Teratoma (arrows) manifesting with heterogeneous echogenicity and multiple cyst-like structures. **C.** Seminoma demonstrating a heterogeneous echogenic pattern (arrows).

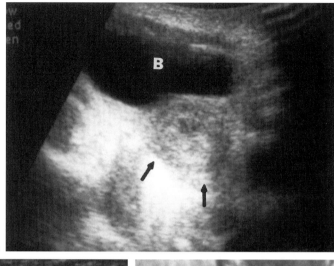

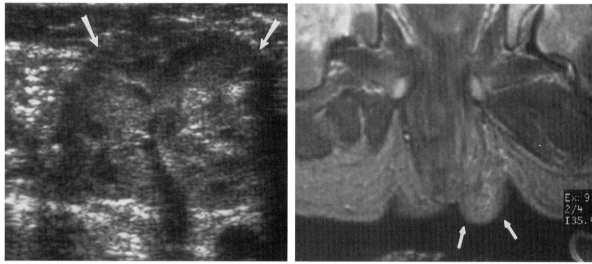

FIGURE 5.138. Benign hamartoma. A. Note the solid and nonspecific tumor (arrow). This was a hamartoma of the vagina. B, bladder. **B.** In this patient with a vulvar mass, ultrasound demonstrates a nonspecific heterogenous solid tumor (arrows). **C.** MR study demonstrates the vulvar mass (arrows).

pseudohermaphrodism results, and in males, large external genitalia are seen. The radiologist's role in the case of a female infant with intersex problems (more the problem) lies in the demonstration of the anatomy of the genital and urinary tracts. In this regard, the genitographically oriented classification originally proposed by Shopfner (1) still is useful (Fig. 5.140).

In the past, investigation of the abnormal anatomy in these patients was relegated almost solely to retrograde flushing or selective catheterization of the various genital

FIGURE 5.140. Intersex anatomy classification. Classification based on genitographic delineation of the various anatomic configurations seen in the intersex states. 1, penis; 2, urethral orifice; 3, scrotum; 4, bladder; 5, urethra; 6, utriculus masculinus; 7, phallus; 8, vestibule orifice; 9, hypoplastic vagina; 10, normal-size vagina; 11, uterus; 12, orifice of urogenital sinus; 13, urogenital sinus; 14, hypertrophied clitoris. Type I represents a normal female with slight clitoral hypertrophy. Type II represents the anatomy seen in female pseudohermaphrodism. Types III through VI represent increasing degrees of masculinization. In the type III anomaly, there is only a small urogenital sinus and elongation of the urethra to a more male-like configuration. However, the uterus is still present. In the type IV anomaly, the vagina and uterus are underdeveloped, and the urethra shows a verumontanum (male urethra). In the type V anomaly, the vagina fails to descend and forms the utriculus masculinus. In this type, the opening of the male urethra is often hypospadiac. The type VI anomaly represents simple hypospadias, often associated with a rudimentary utriculus masculinus. (From Shopfner CE. Genitography in intersexual states. Radiology 1964;82:664–674, with permission.)

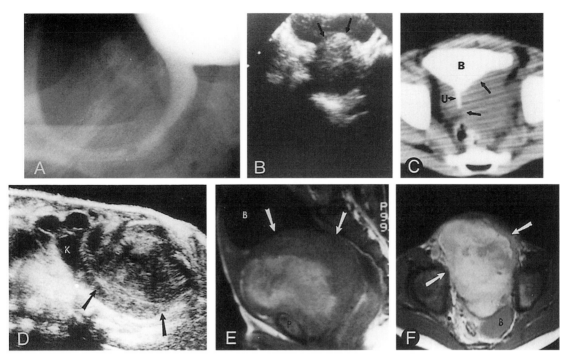

FIGURE 5.139. Prostatic rhabdomyosarcoma. A. Voiding cystogram erroneously might suggest that the urethra is normal. However, it is being stretched and curved in a diffuse arc by the surrounding prostatic tumor. **B.** Ultrasonogram demonstrating the echogenic tumor (arrows) projecting into the base of the bladder. **C.** CT study demonstrates the tumor (arrows), indenting the base of the bladder (B). Note how the urethra (U) is surrounded by tumor. **D.** Another patient with a large tumor producing heterogeneous echogenicity on this longitudinal ultrasound study. The kidney (K) above it is hydronephrotic. **E.** Sagittal T1-weighted MR study demonstrates the large tumor (arrows) with a large area of increased signal intensity representing bleeding into the tumor. B, bladder. **F.** Axial, T2-weighted MR image demonstrates generally increased signal intensity in the large tumor (arrows). Note the compressed bladder (B). (**E** and **F** courtesy of D. Albin, M.D.)

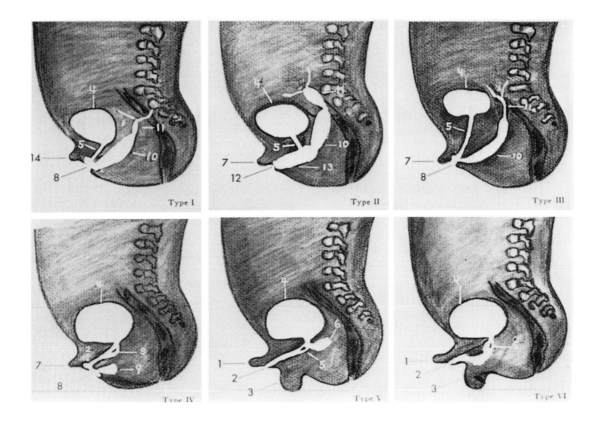

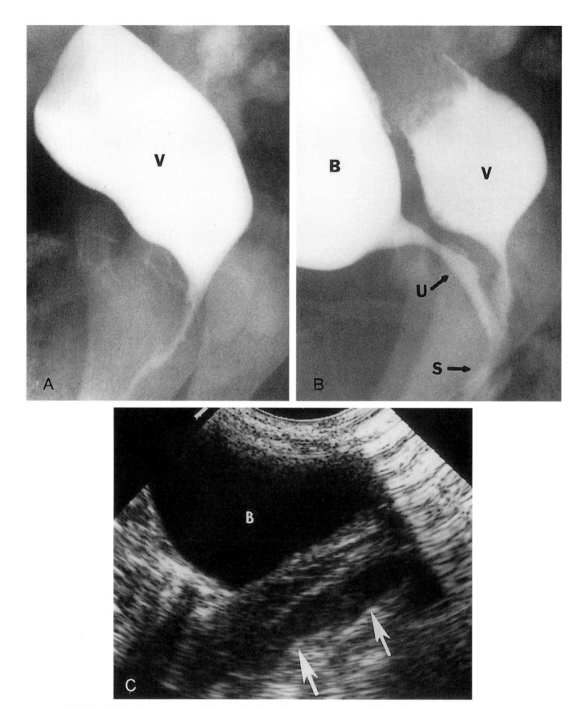

FIGURE 5.141. Intersex problems. A. Note the large vagina (V) in this female with an intersex problem. The dimple of the cervix is just barely visible. **B.** Cystogram demonstrates the bladder (B), vagina (V), urethra (U), and the urogenital sinus (S). **C.** Longitudinal sonogram demonstrates the bladder (B) and, behind it, a large uterus (arrows).

openings available (Fig. 5.141). Currently, however, this may be complemented or preceded by ultrasound and MRI (2, 3). In any case, one's efforts are directed primarily toward the demonstration of the size of the vagina, presence of a uterus, and whether the urethra opens separately into the vestibule or into a common urogenital sinus. These are most important considerations for later sex determination and possible reconstructive surgery.

REFERENCES

1. Shopfner CE. Genitography in intersexual states. Radiology 1964; 82:664–674.
2. Gambino J, Caldwell B, Dietrich R, et al. Pictorial essay. Congenital disorders of sexual differentiation. MR findings. AJR 1992; 158:363–367.
3. Secaf E, Hricak H, Gooding CA, et al. Role of MRI in the evaluation of ambiguous genitalia. Pediatr Radiol 1994;24:231–235.

MISCELLANEOUS GENITAL ABNORMALITIES

Hypospadias

Hypospadias usually is considered an isolated problem, but in some ways, it is an intersex problem at the far end of the male spectrum of abnormality. With hypospadias, the incidence of significant associated upper urinary tract anom-

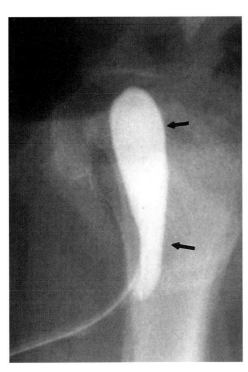

FIGURE 5.142. Large utriculus. Note the large, contrast-filled utriculus (arrows) in this patient with hypospadias. During catheterization of the urethra, the catheter preferentially entered the utriculus.

alies is frequent enough that ultrasound evaluation of the urinary tract is advised (1, 2). With voiding cystourethrography, the urethra often appears deformed, and a prominent utriculus may be demonstrated. This structure is a vestigial utricle, arising from the mullerian system and in some cases may be quite large (Fig. 5.142).

Other Anomalies of the Testicles and Seminal Vesicles

Polyorchidism is a rare anomaly (1) in which testicular rests are seen all along the route of descent of the normal testicle. Other anomalies can co-exist and these anomalous testicles can undergo torsion. A somewhat related anomaly consists of splenogonadal or hepatogonadal fusion (2, 3). These conditions usually are diagnosed intraoperatively and consist of persistent fusion of the gonads to either the spleen or the liver.

Ectopic insertion of the vas deferens into the bladder neck or urethra of males is uncommon but can be demonstrated with voiding cystourethrography. In such cases, there is retrograde filling of the ectopically inserting vas, and the condition results from failure of reabsorption of the terminal portion of the mesonephric ducts (4). As a result, the vas deferens communicates with the ureter and, as such, comes to insert ectopically into the bladder neck or urethra.

Congenital cystic disease of the seminal vesicles is uncommon (5). It often is associated with other renal abnormalities, including renal agenesis (6), ectopic ureter, and anomalies of the vas deferens. Acquired cysts of the seminal vesicles are rare, and similarly, congenital testicular cysts are uncommon (7–9).

REFERENCES

1. Kale N, Basaklar AC. Polyorchidism. J Pediatr Surg 1991;26: 1432–1434.
2. Ferro F, Lais A, Boldrini R, et al. Hepatogonadal fusion. J Pediatr Surg 1996;31:435–436.
3. Patel RV. Splenogonadal fusion. J Pediatr Surg 1995;30:873–874.
4. Pereira JKM, Chait PG, Daneman A. Case report. Bilateral persisting mesonephric ducts. AJR 1993;160:367–369.
5. King BF, Hattery RR, Lieber MM, et al. Congenital cystic disease of the seminal vesicle. Radiology 1991;178:207–211.
6. Ngai RLC, Yeung BKF, Tsui WMS, et al. Cystic dysplasia of the testis associated with ipsilateral renal agenesis and high anorectal anomalies.
7. Grunert RT, Van Every MJ, Uehling DT. Bilateral epidermoid cysts of the testicle. J Urol 1992;147:1599–1601.
8. Neumann DP, Abrams GS, Hight DW. Testicular epidermoid cysts in prepubertal children: case report and review of the world literature. J Pediatr Surg 32:1786–1789.
9. Slaughenhoupt B, Klauber GT. Simple testicular cyst in the neonate. J Pediatr Surg 1995;30:636–637.

Hydroceles

Hydroceles can be communicating or noncommunicating and are common in the infant male. They are also seen in

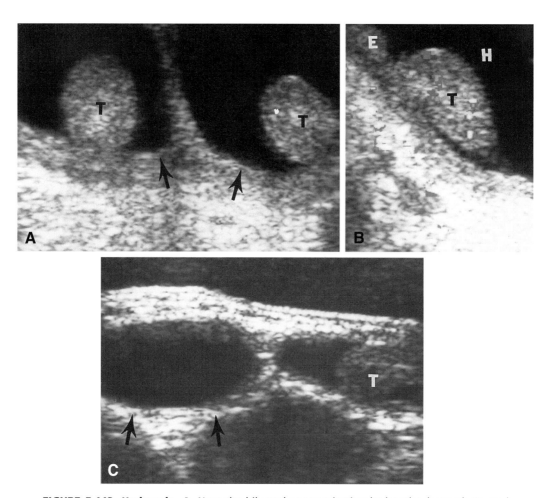

FIGURE 5.143. Hydrocele. A. Note the bilateral communicating hydroceles (arrows). Normal testicles (T) are seen within the hydroceles. **B.** Sagittal view on one side demonstrates the hydrocele (H) and the normal testicle (T) along with the prominent but normal epididymis (E). **C.** Noncommunicating hydrocele in the inguinal canal (arrows). The testicle (T) is associated with a small intrascrotal hydrocele.

utero (1). Those that communicate can readily be reduced, but noncommunicating hydroceles present as scrotal masses. Ultrasonography is exceptionally useful in delineating these hypoechoic lesions (Fig. 5.143). Hydroceles of the spermatic cord also can be encountered (2).

REFERENCES

1.Pretorius DH, Halsted MJ, Abels W, et al. Hydroceles identified prenatally. Common physiologic phenomenon? J Ultrasound Med 1998;17:49–52.
2. Martin LC, Share JC, Peters C, et al. Hydrocele of the spermatic cord: embryology and ultrasonographic appearance. Pediatr Radiol 1996;26:528–530.

Pelvic Inflammatory Disease

The findings in pelvic inflammatory disease in children are the same as in adults. Transvaginal ultrasonography (1) often is helpful in demonstrating dilated fallopian tubes, frank abscesses, and fluid in the pelvis (Fig. 5.144). However, the findings often are nonspecific.

REFERENCE

1. Bulas DI, Ahlstrom PA, Sivit CJ, et al. Pelvic inflammatory disease in the adolescent: comparison of transabdominal and transvaginal sonographic evaluation. Radiology 1992;183:435–439.

Ovarian Torsion

Torsion of the normal ovary (1–3) occasionally can be associated with fallopian tube torsion , and fallopian tube torsion also can occur as an isolated phenomenon (4). Regardless, the ultrasonographic findings in these patients are nonspecific and basically demonstrate an enlarged, heterogeneous, and echogenic ovarian mass. In neonates, the mass

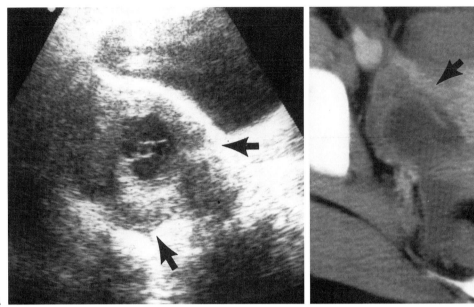

FIGURE 5.144. Tuboovarian abscess. A. Note the nonspecific configuration of this tuboovarian abscess (arrows) demonstrated on ultrasound. **B.** CT study demonstrating a large tuboovarian abscess (arrows). It is located above the uterus and is displacing and indenting the bladder to the left.

tends to be extraadnexal and manifests more as an abdominal mass (3). In older girls, however, an adnexal mass is the usual presentation. Ovaries undergoing torsion eventually can become calcified (5).

REFERENCES

1. Alrabeeah A, Galliani CA, Giacomantonio M, et al. Neonatal ovarian torsion: report of three cases and review of the literature. Pediatr Pathol 1988;8:143–149.
2. Meyer JS, Harmon CM, Harty MP, et al. Ovarian torsion: clinical and imaging presentation in children. J Pediatr Surg 1995;30: 1433–1436.
3. Stark JE, Siegel MJ. Ovarian torsion in prepubertal and pubertal girls: sonographic findings. AJR 1995;163:1479–1482.
4. Kurzbart E, Mares AJ, Cohen Z, et al. Isolated torsion of the fallopian tube in premenarcheal girls. J Pediatr Surg 1994;29: 1384–1385.
5. Currarino G, Rutledge JC. Ovarian torsion and amputation resulting in partially calcified pedunculated cystic mass. Pediatr Radiol 1989;19:395–399.

Acute Scrotal Problems

The main imaging modalities used in the investigation of acute scrotal problems are ultrasound and nuclear scintigraphy (1–5). They both are equally productive, but neither is foolproof. ***Ultrasonography, however, is faster.*** In regard to ultrasonographically demonstrated testicular blood flow, it needs to be realized that prepubertal testicular blood flow may be difficult to demonstrate in normal testicles. This is not so important on a practical basis because one generally is not concerned with the normal testicle. A testicle undergoing torsion usually enlarges and shows change in echotexture, and if no blood flow is demonstrated in such a testicle, then one can assume that torsion has occurred. Power Doppler (6, 7) is more sensitive than ordinary color flow Doppler for the demonstration of blood flow to a testicle.

Conditions presenting as acute scrotal problems include epididymitis, orchitis, testicular torsion, torsion of the appendix testis, trauma, post-inguinal hernia repair, and conditions such as Henoch-Schönlein purpura. In one series (3), 16% of patients presented with torsion; 46% with torsion of the appendix testis; 35% with epididymitis-orchitis; and 3% with miscellaneous problems. In the end, however, whether one uses nuclear scintigraphy or color flow Doppler to demonstrate these problems, the only testicle that one can safely not surgically explore ***is the one that is large, tender, inflamed and shows exuberant blood flow to the epididymis and testicle.*** No matter what else one sees, ***as long as blood flow to the involved testicle is not demonstrable or is markedly less than that in the epididymis, surgical exploration should be undertaken (8).*** The reason for this is that the latter can be seen with partial torsion.

REFERENCES

1. Atkinson GO Jr, Patrick LE, Ball TI Jr, et al. The normal and abnormal scrotum in children: evaluation with color Doppler sonography. AJR 1992;158:613–617.

2. Hollman AS, Ingram S, Carachi R, et al. Colour Doppler imaging of the acute paediatric scrotum. Pediatr Radiol 1993;23:83–87.
3. Lewis AG, Bukowski TP, Jarvis PD, et al. Evaluation of acute scrotum in the emergency department. J Pediatr Surg 1995;30: 277–282.
4. Paltiel HJ, Connolly LP, Atala A, et al. Acute scrotal symptoms in boys with an indeterminate clinical presentation: comparison of color Doppler sonography and scintigraphy. Radiology 1998;207: 223–231.
5. Middleton WD, Siegel BA, Melson GL, et al. Acute scrotal disorders: prospective comparison of color Doppler US and testicular scintigraphy. Radiology 1990;177:177–181.
6. Bader TR, Kammerhuber F, Herneth AM. Testicular blood flow in boys as assessed at color Doppler and power Doppler sonography. Radiology 1997;202:559–564.
7. Barth RA, Shortliffe LD. Normal pediatric testis: comparison of power Doppler and color Doppler US in the detection of blood flow. Radiology 1997;204:389–393.
8. Hendrick EP, Aldridge M, Swischuk LE. Acute testicular problems: simplified ultrasound approach. Emerg Radiol 2000;7: 326–330.

Epididymitis and Orchitis

These inflammatory conditions often co-exist, although epididymitis can exist without orchitis. When they co-exist, both the testicle and epididymis are enlarged and show increased blood flow with color flow Doppler and nuclear scintigraphy (Fig. 5.145, A–D). In such cases, one can be confident that infection only is present (1). If blood flow is increased to the epididymis but absent in the testicle, one cannot differentiate the findings from missed testicular torsion, torsion of the appendix testes, and epididymitis without orchitis.

REFERENCE

1. Horstman WG, Middleton WD, Melson GL. Scrotal inflammatory disease: color flow Doppler US findings. Radiology 1991; 179:55–59.

Testicular Torsion

Generally, one has 6 hours to make the diagnosis of testicular torsion, because after this period, recovery of a viable testicle is unlikely. Therefore, the diagnosis of testicular torsion must be accomplished promptly. Most cases of testicular torsion are unilateral for bilateral torsion is rare (1).

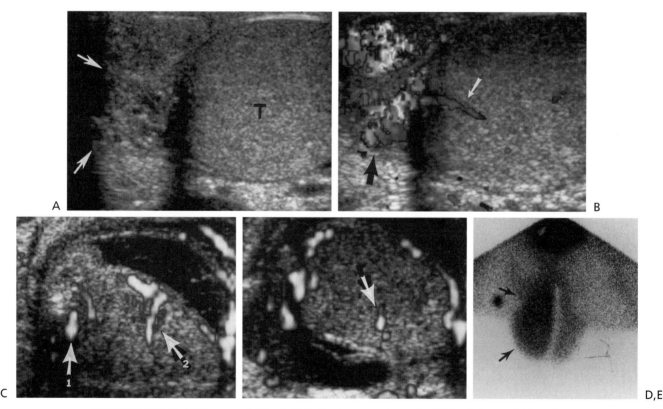

FIGURE 5.145. Epididymo-orchitis. A. Note the large, congested epididymis (arrows). T, testicle. **B.** Color flow Doppler shows increased flow to the epididymis (black arrows) and also to the testicle (white arrows). **C.** Color flow Doppler in this patient demonstrates increased blood flow to the epididymis (1) and testicle (2). **D.** Another image from the same patient demonstrates increased paratesticular blood flow, and blood flow to the testicle (arrow). **E.** Nuclear scintigraphy in epididymo-orchitis demonstrates typical increased activity in the inflamed and enlarged hemiscrotum (arrows).

In the acute phase of testicular torsion, blood flow will not be seen in the variably enlarged, tender testicle. The testicle itself will show increased echogenicity and often a heterogenous echotexture (2). The epididymis is displaced (not always easy to see) out of its normal position (i.e., Bell-Clapper deformity) (3). Whether one uses color Doppler or nuclear scintigraphy, the absence of blood flow to the enlarged, tender testicle should be considered diagnostic of testicular torsion (Fig. 5.146). However, pitfalls can arise with incomplete torsion or when detorsion occurs. In either case, blood flow to the testicle can be present. This can be a real problem, and therefore, *if there is any question whatsoever on a clinical basis that torsion is present, the patient should undergo surgical exploration (4).*

In cases of late presenting testicular torsion, blood flow in the involved testicle usually is absent, but there is thickening of the epididymis and increased blood flow to the epididymis (Fig. 5.146 D–F). The findings in such cases cannot be differentiated from epididymitis without orchitis

or torsion of the appendix testis, *and all these testicles must be surgically explored.* Manual or spontaneous detorsion of the testicle under ultrasonographic visualization and/or guidance has been reported (5). In such cases, one can see blood flow, often exuberant, returning to the testicle after it has been detorsed (Fig. 5.147). *Partial torsion, when it occurs, can produce misleading findings.* The reason for this is that often there still is some blood flow to the testicle, and one will then assume that the testicle still is viable and did not undergo torsion. It may be viable, but it is at risk, and if one detects considerable blood flow to the surrounding epididymis and little flow to the testicle itself, partial torsion should be considered, among other entities. *This is especially true if the history is very suggestive of torsion.*

With prenatal testicular torsion, the entire spermatic cord undergoes torsion along with the testicle (6, 7). The testicle is nonviable by the time it is discovered postnatally and very often is firm or hard and, on ultrasonography, very

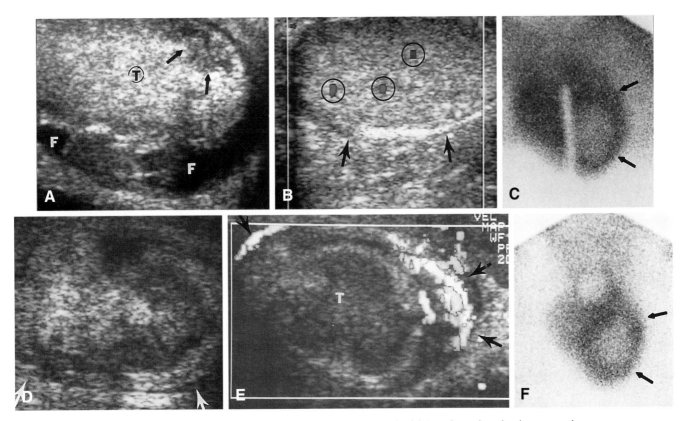

FIGURE 5.146. Acute testicular torsion. A. The testicle (T) is enlarged and echotexture is nonuniform with scattered hypoechoic areas (arrows). No internal blood flow was seen with color flow Doppler. Fluid (F) surrounds the testicle. **B.** Normal testicle for comparison. Note the uniform normal testicle (arrows) for comparison and the uniform echotexture and areas of internal blood flow (circles). **C.** Nuclear scintigraphy with acute torsion demonstrates a photopenic area (torsed testicle) in the left hemiscrotum (arrows). **D.** Missed torsion. The testicle is enlarged, heterogeneous in texture, and surrounded by a thickened epididymis (arrows). **E.** Color flow Doppler demonstrates increased blood flow (arrows) to the epididymis and periventricular soft tissues but no flow to the testicle (T). **F.** Nuclear scintigraphy in missed torsion demonstrates a photopenic area (torsed testicle) surrounded by a hyperemic rim (arrows).

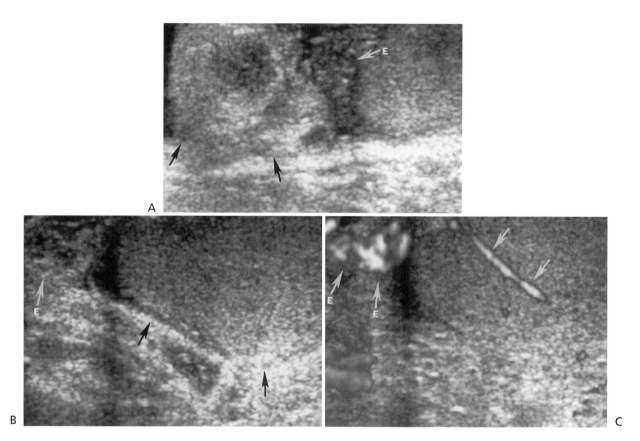

FIGURE 5.147. Testicular torsion and detorsion. A. Note the enlarged right testical (black arrows). Its orientation is abnormal on this cross-sectional image. Also note that the epididymis (E) is medially placed. **B.** Moments later the testice assumes a more normal configuration (black arrows). The epididymis (E) now is laterally placed. The patient's symptoms resolved. **C.** Color flow Doppler demonstrates blood flow to the epididymis (E) and brisk blood flow returning to the testicle (white arrows). Prior to this there was no testicular flow.

echogenic (Fig. 5.148). Calcifications frequently are present, and the testicle usually should be removed (6).

REFERENCES

1. Benge BN, Eure GR, Winslow BH. Acute bilateral testicular torsion in the adolescent. J Urol 1992;148:134.
2. Middleton WD, Middleton MA, Dierks M, et al. Sonographic prediction of viability in testicular torsion. Preliminary observations. J Ultrasound Med 1997;16:23–27.
3. Luker GD, Siegel MJ. Pictorial essay. Color Doppler sonography of the scrotum in children. AJR 1994;163:649–655.
4. Hendrick EP, Aldridge M, Swischuk LE. Acute testicular problems. Simplified ultrasound approach. Emerg Radiol 2000;7: 326–330.
5. Cannon ML, Finger MJ, Blas DI. Manual testicular detorsion aided by color Doppler ultrasonography. J Ultrasound Med 1995; 14:407–409.
6. Brandt MT, Sheldon CA, Wacksman J, et al. Prenatal testicular torsion: principles of management. J Urol 1992;147:670–672.
7. Hernanz-Schulman M, Yenicesu F, Heller RM. Sonographic identification of perinatal testicular torsion. J Ultrasound Med 1997; 16:65–67.

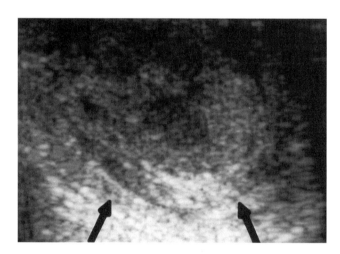

FIGURE 5.148. Prenatal testicular torsion. Note the heterogenous echotexture of this hard, firm testicle (arrows). On this color flow study, no blood flow was demonstrated to the testicle.

Torsion of Appendix Testis

Torsion of the appendix testis is much more common than testicular torsion (1–3). On ultrasonography, the appendix testis becomes echogenic and is located between the head of the epididymis and the upper pole of the testis (3). However, it is not always easy to detect, and while blood flow to the inflamed epididymis is increased, testicular blood flow usually is normal or even absent. As a result, most cases of torsion of the appendix testis will undergo surgical exploration *(i.e., no flow to the testicle–torsion is possible–explore).* If, on the other hand, the torsed appendix testis is clearly visualized (rare cases), the diagnosis can be made with more confidence (Fig. 5.149). Clinically, the torsed appendix testis presents as the so-called "palpable blue dot" sign.

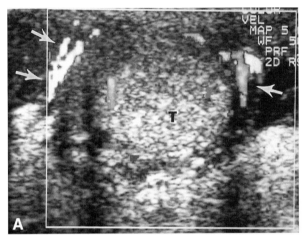

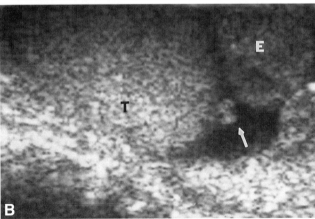

FIGURE 5.149. Torsion appendix testis. A. Cross-sectional view. The testicle (T) is enlarged. There is peritesticular blood flow (arrows), but none is seen in the testicle. The findings are difficult to differentiate from missed torsion of the testicle. **B.** Sagittal view in another patient demonstrates the testicle (T), enlarged epididymis (E), and the torsed appendix testis (arrow). It is more clearly visible because of the presence of associated fluid.

REFERENCES

1. Cohen HL, Shapiro MA, Haller JO, et al. Torsion of the testicular appendage. J Ultrasound Med 1992;11:81–83.
2. Hesser U, Rosenborg M, Gierup J, et al. Gray-scale sonography in torsion of the testicular appendages. Pediatr Radiol 1993;23:529–532.
3. Strauss S, Faingold R, Manor H. Torsion of the testicular appendages: sonographic appearance. J Ultrasound Med 1997;16:189–192.

Miscellaneous Acute Scrotal Problems

The scrotum can become swollen; and so can the intrascrotal contents *after inguinal hernia repair* (1). Testicular infarction also can be a rare complication (Fig. 5.150). Furthermore, there may be recurrence of the hernia, and then the hernia itself can be identified with ultrasonography. *Acute scrotal infection (cellulites)* results in a markedly thickened and hyperemic scrotal sac while the intrascrotal contents remain normal. Bleeding into a testicle can occur in patients with *Henoch-Schönlein purpura,* in which increased flow to the epididymis is seen in addition to hematoma (2–4). These findings may arise before the characteristic rash appears.

REFERENCES

1. Kilkenny TE. Acute scrotum in an infant post-herniorrhaphy complication. Sonographic evaluation. Pediatr Radiol 1993;23:481–482.
2. Ben-Chaim J, Korat E, Shenfeld O, et al. Acute scrotum caused by Henoch-Schönlein Purpura, with immediate response to short-term steroid therapy. J Pediatr Surg 1995;30:1509–1510.
3. Ben-Sira L, Laor T. Severe scrotal pain in boys with Henoch-Schönlein purpura: incidence and sonography. Pediatr Radiol 2000;30:125–128.

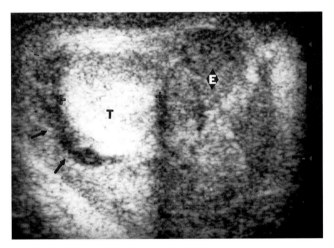

FIGURE 5.150. Infarction of testis after hernia repair. Note the echogenic, infarcted testicle (T). The epididymis (E) is enlarged. A small amount of fluid (arrows) surrounds the testicle.

4. Laor T, Atala A, Teele RL. Scrotal ultrasonography in Henoch-Schönlein purpura. Pediatr Radiol 1992;22:505–506.

Trauma to the Testicle

Trauma to the testicle can result in simple contusion, epididymal and testicular hemorrhage, or fracture of the testicle (Fig. 5.151). The findings are relatively easy to demonstrate with ultrasound, and intratesticular hematomas also may be encountered. In the early phase, the hematoma is echogenic, but later, as it liquefies, it becomes hypoechoic.

Epididymal Cysts, Varicoceles, and Microlithiasis

Epididymal cysts can be small or large and incidental or symptomatic (Fig. 5.152 A). Similarly, *varicoceles* may be symptomatic or asymptomatic. Often, they present only with scrotal enlargement. They are readily demonstrable with color flow Doppler ultrasound, and their blood flow can be exaggerated with a Valsalva maneuver (Fig. 5.152, B and C). In the pediatric age group, varicoceles are not necessarily associated with intraabdominal tumors.

Microlithiasis does not occur in infants and children with the same frequency that it occurs in adults. However, it can be seen and the findings are rather characteristic. There is a certain association between microlithiasis and eventual development of malignancy in adults, and although it is generally considered that this is not as common in childhood, a recent publication suggests the contrary (1).

REFERENCE

1.Leenan AS, Riebel TW. Testicular microlithiasis in children: sonographic features and clinical implications. Pediatr Radiol 2002; 32:575–579.

Spermatic Cord Torsion

This is an uncommon problem but can be detected with ultrasound when it is noted that the spermatic cord is rotated and twisted (1). It has been suggested that, if one is examining a patient for suspected testicular torsion and the testicle demonstrates normal blood flow, one should look up along the spermatic cord to see if it is twisted (1).

REFERENCE

1. Arce JD, Cortes M, Vargas JC. Sonographic diagnosis of acute spermatic cord torsion. Rotation of the cord: a key to the diagnosis. Pediatr Radiol 2002;32:485–491.

ADRENAL GLANDS

Normal Adrenal Glands

In the neonate, the adrenal gland is plump and readily demonstrable with ultrasound. Typically, the gland is characterized by a thin, echogenic core (medulla) surrounded by a thick sonolucent cortex (Fig. 5.153A). Normal glands are up to 3.5 cm long and 0.5 cm wide. However, a rapid decrease in size of the adrenal gland occurs by the age of 2 months (1). With renal agenesis, the adrenal gland can become large, lose its characteristic V-shaped configuration, and erroneously mimic the configuration of a kidney (Fig. 5.153B).

REFERENCE

1. Scott EM, Thomas A, McGarrigle HG, et al. Serial adrenal ultrasonography in normal neonates. J Ultrasound Med 1990;9: 279–283.

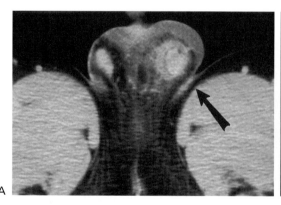 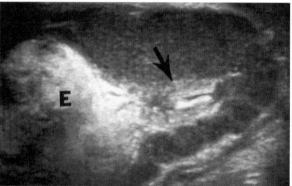

FIGURE 5.151. Trauma to the testicle. A. Traumatic epididymis. Note the echogenic hemorrhage in the epididymis (arrow). **B.** Another view demonstrates the same enlarged, hemorrhagic epididymis (E) and a small hematoma (arrow) in the testicle.

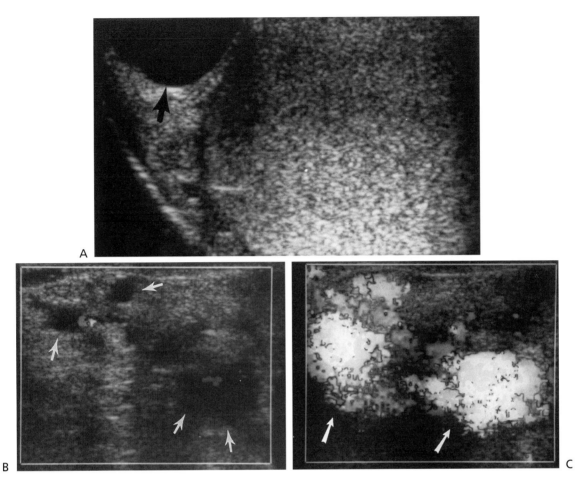

FIGURE 5.152. Miscellaneous testicular problems. A. Epididymal cyst. Note the large cyst (arrow) in the epididymis. The testicle is normal. **B**. **Varicocele.** Note the numerous hypoechoic areas (arrows) representing blood vessels. **C.** With a Valsalva maneuver and color flow Doppler, there is marked increase in signal over these areas.

ANOMALIES OF THE ADRENAL GLAND

Anomalies of the adrenal gland are uncommon, and a review of the subject, including adrenal agenesis, ectopia, and malpositioning of the adrenal gland, is available in a publication by Burton et al. (1). In this communication, the authors bring specific attention to the so-called circumrenal and horseshoe adrenal glands. The circumrenal adrenal gland is one where the two limbs of the normal V- or Y-shaped adrenal gland fuse and form a circular gland (Fig. 5.154A). In the other anomaly, the horseshoe adrenal gland (2, 3), the adrenal gland lies behind the aorta, and both the right and left glands are fused much the same as with a horseshoe kidney (Fig. 5.154B).

REFERENCES

1. Burton EM, Strange ME, Edmonds DB. Sonography of the circumrenal and horseshoe adrenal gland in the newborn. Pediatr Radiol 1993;23:362–364.

FIGURE 5.153. Normal adrenal gland. A and B. Note the typical configuration of the normal gland (arrows) in a neonate.

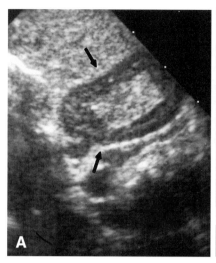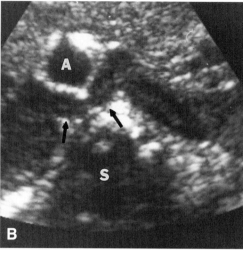

FIGURE 5.154. Adrenal gland anomalies. A. Typical circumrenal renal gland (arrows). **B.** Horseshoe adrenal gland. The transverse sonogram demonstrates fusion between the medial limbs of the right and left adrenal gland, producing an isthmus (arrows) posterior to the aorta (A). S, spine. (From Burton EM, Strange ME, Edmonds DB. Sonography of the circumrenal and horseshoe adrenal gland in the newborn. Pediatr Radiol 1993;23:362–364, with permission.)

2. Shafaie FF, Katz ME, Hannaway CD. A horseshoe adrenal gland in an infant with asplenia. Pediatr Radiol. 1997;27:591–593.
3. Strouse PJ, Haller JO, Berdon WE, et al. Horseshoe adrenal gland in association with asplenia: presentation of six new cases and review of the literature. Pediatr Radiol 2002;32:778.

Adrenal Hemorrhage

The adrenal glands normally are large in newborn infants, and most show evidence of small hemorrhages at birth. In most cases, these hemorrhages go unnoticed, but when they are massive, complete exsanguination of the infant can occur. More commonly, however, the problem is an infant presenting with an abdominal mass, jaundice, or anemia. Most of these infants are not particularly ill, and adrenal insufficiency is a rare complication. As the hemorrhages resolve, they can produce pseudocysts of the adrenal gland (1).

Various postulated mechanisms and predisposing causes for adrenal hemorrhage have been considered and as with all visceral injuries in the neonate, it has been noted that large babies such as those seen in diabetic mothers or the Beckwith-Wiedemann syndrome are especially predisposed to adrenal hemorrhage. However, other factors also are invoked, including obstetric trauma, neonatal sepsis, and neonatal hypoxia. In many cases, more than one factor is at play and can be operative in utero. Adrenal hemorrhage also has been documented with steroid therapy (2), the battered child syndrome (3), and after liver transplantation (4). With ultrasound, if adrenal hemorrhage is examined early (i.e., within the first day or two of life), it appears echogenic and solid (Fig. 5.155, A and B). Shortly thereafter, liquefaction of the hematoma occurs and a cystic or multicystic appearance develops (Fig. 5.155, C and D). If this does not occur, underlying neuroblastoma should be considered.

In most instances, the enlarged, hemorrhagic adrenal gland quickly subsides in size, but calcifications may become apparent within a few weeks or months. The calcifications are typical and usually outline the adrenal gland in a rim-like fashion. With time, as the adrenal gland becomes smaller, the calcifications become more compact, but still most often conform to the triangular configuration of the normal adrenal gland (Fig. 5.155E). Such calcifications may be seen as incidental findings in older infants without previous documentation of adrenal hemorrhage. However, it is assumed that prior adrenal hemorrhage had occurred. With ultrasound, old hemorrhages are echogenic, and associated calcifications are readily demonstrable with CT imaging. Renal vein thrombosis (4) also is seen in association with some of the cases, especially on the left. The reason for this is that the left adrenal gland, more than the right adrenal gland, shares its renal drainage with the ipsilateral kidney, and thrombosis in the kidney can extend into the adrenal gland.

REFERENCES

1. Wagner AC. Bilateral hemorrhagic pseudocysts of the adrenal glands in a newborn. AJR 1961;86:540–544.
2. Levin TL, Morton E. Adrenal hemorrhage complicating ACTH therapy in Crohn's disease. Pediatr Radiol 1993;123:457–458.
3. Nimkin K, Teeger S, Wallach NT, et al. Adrenal hemorrhage in abused children: imaging and postmortem findings. AJR 1994;162:661–663.
4. Brill PW, Jagannath A, Winchester P, et al. Adrenal hemorrhage and renal vein thrombosis in the newborn: MR imaging. Radiology 1989;170:95–98.

Neuroblastoma and Ganglioneuroma

Neuroblastoma and ganglioneuroma are the same tumor; ganglioneuroma is a mature neuroblastoma. In the fetus or neonate, neuroblastoma is more likely to present with a

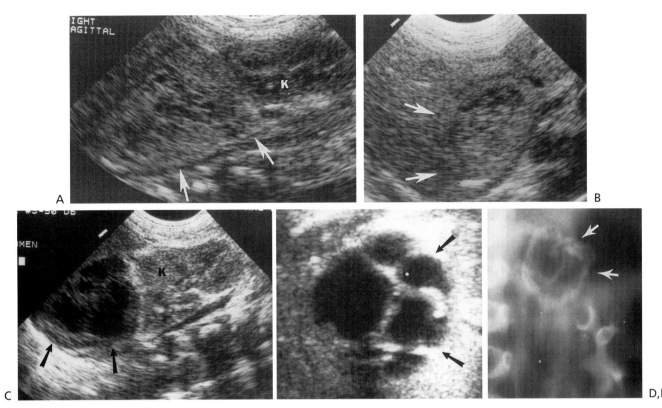

FIGURE 5.155. Adrenal hemorrhage. A. Note the echogenic suprarenal hematoma (arrows). It blends with the kidney (K) and the whole complex could be misinterpreted for that of a kidney. **B.** Cross sectional view through the hematoma demonstrates the increased echogenicity (arrows). **C.** In this patient, a similar hematoma has liquified (arrows). K, kidney. **D.** In this patient, the degenerating liquifying hematoma is multicystic in appearance (arrows). **E.** Long-term sequelae. Note the peripheral calcification (arrows) in the periphery of an old adrenal hematoma.

large liver resulting from metastatic disease (Fig. 5.156) than a primary tumor (1). Neuroblastoma also can be identified in utero, when the tumor often has favorable outcome (2). Neuroblastoma in situ (Fig. 5.157), or incidental neuroblastoma also occurs, and is documented in up to 1.5% of cases in neonates and young infants (3, 4). However, most of these tumors probably are insignificant and regress.

In the older infant and child, the most common presentation of neuroblastoma is that of an adrenal mass (50–60%), but it should be noted that these tumors can also arise from the sympathetic ganglia in the lower abdomen, the presacral region from the gland of Zukerkandl (5), the chest, the gonads (6), and even the neck and nasopharynx. Occasionally, in the neonate, massive hemorrhage into the tumor can occur, and then the findings may be difficult to differentiate from simple adrenal hemorrhage (Fig. 5.158). If the tumor is cystic, it can mimic other cystic tumors and pose problems with diagnosis (7–9).

Neuroblastoma usually is staged on the basis of local extent and presence or absence of metastases (Fig. 5.159). There is, however, a special group of infants in whom the tumor is disseminated (e.g., liver, skin nodules), but bony metastases are absent. For some reason, the tumors in these patients seem less aggressive, and spontaneous maturation or regression is relatively common (10). As a result, this group of patients has been designated as having stage IV-S disease. These patients are similar to, but should be differentiated from, those with another peculiar form of neuroblastoma, that is, multifocal neuroblastoma (11). This form of the tumor is familial and most likely inherited on an autosomal dominant basis. Although these tumors are multifocal, the disease is not disseminated, and there is some suggestion that prognosis may be better in these patients. Prognosis also is better for intrathoracic neuroblastoma and that occurring on a primary basis in the neck (12). Another variation of neuroblastoma is neuroblastoma arising in an adrenal gland in a young infant and metastasizing into the chest and neck to manifest with lymph node enlargement as Virchow's nodes. This form of neuroblastoma has been designated type IV-N (13). Neuroblastoma also can spontaneously mature into a ganglioneuroma and even disappear. Inherited genetic factors are believed to be at play in these patients (14, 15).

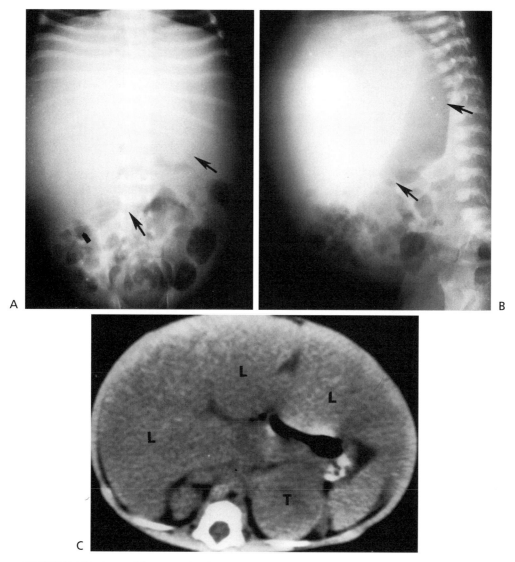

FIGURE 5.156. Neuroblastoma in the neonate. A. Note the large liver (arrows). **B.** Lateral view demonstrates similar enlargement (arrows). **C.** Another patient with an adrenal neuroblastoma (T) and widespread metastases to the large liver (L).

Clinically, patients with neuroblastoma usually present with well-developed disease, often with signs of metastases and elevated blood vanillylmandelic acid (VMA) levels. Unlike Wilms' tumor, most neuroblastomas are not "clean" lesions, because they usually spread beyond the confines of the adrenal gland, frequently cross the abdomen, and commonly extend into the chest. Tumors developing in the pelvis may mimic presacral teratoma, while aggressive neuroblastomas may invade the kidney (2, 29) and mimic the findings of Wilms' tumor (Fig. 5.160).

On plain films, because neuroblastoma quickly extends beyond its initial site, visualization of the tumor crossing the abdomen and extending into the chest in the form of paraspinal soft tissue thickening is common (Fig. 5.161A).

After plain films ultrasonography usually is the first imaging modality in the investigation of suspected neuroblastoma where most neuroblastomas are echogenic (Fig. 5.161B). A few cases may demonstrate hypoechoic areas representing sites of necrosis, but this finding is not as common as it is with Wilms' tumor. In still other cases, echogenic nodules within the tumor occur, and are believed to represent areas of hemorrhage and thrombosis, and possibly early calcification. This latter finding is relatively characteristic of neuroblastoma (16) and (Fig. 5.161C).

Because neuroblastomas often are large tumors that spread throughout the abdomen and even into the chest, ultrasound may not be able to define their precise extent. For this reason, CT or MRI become useful (Fig. 5.161, E

(Text continues on page 712.)

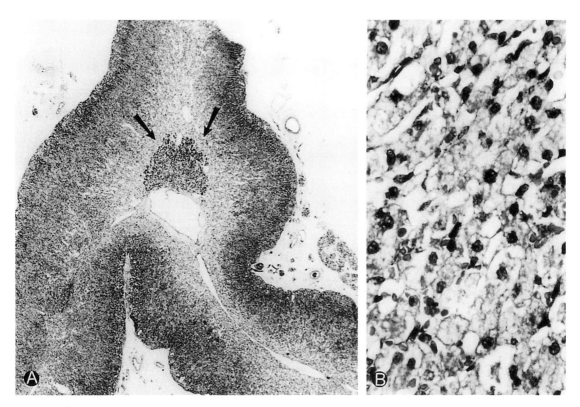

FIGURE 5.157. Neuroblastoma in situ. A. Note the incidental cluster of cells (arrows) found in this otherwise normal adrenal gland. **B.** Magnified view of the cells demonstrates them to be neuroblastoma cells (i.e., neuroblastoma in situ). (Courtesy of M. Nichols, M.D.)

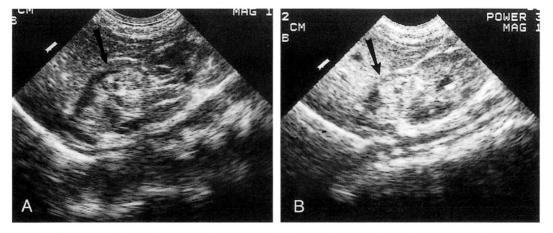

FIGURE 5.158. Neonatal neuroblastoma with hemorrhage. A. Note the enlarged adrenal gland (arrow) with mixed echoes and areas of sonolucent fluid (blood). **B.** A few days later, the mass has decreased in size (arrow) but has not become sonolucent, as would a liquefying hematoma. The mass was surgically removed and histologically proved to be a neuroblastoma with hemorrhage.

STAGING OF NEUROBLASTOMA

Stage I   Tumor confined to organ or structure of origin.

Stage II   Tumor extending in continuity beyond the organ or structure of origin but not crossing the midline. Regional lympth nodes on the homolateral side may be involved.

Stage III   Tumor extending in continuity beyond the midline. Regional lymph nodes may be involved bilaterally.

Stage IV   Remote disease involving skeleton, organs, soft tissues, or distant lympth nodes.

Stage IVS   Patients who would otherwise be stage I or II but who have remote disease confined only to one or more of the following sites: liver, skin, but without radiographic evidence of bone metastases.

FIGURE 5.159. Staging of neuroblastoma. Staging is accomplished on the basis of local extent of the tumor, regional lymph node involvement, and distant metastases. Stage IV-S represents a peculiar group who demonstrate remote disease in many organs but not in the bones. This group of patients has a better prognosis.

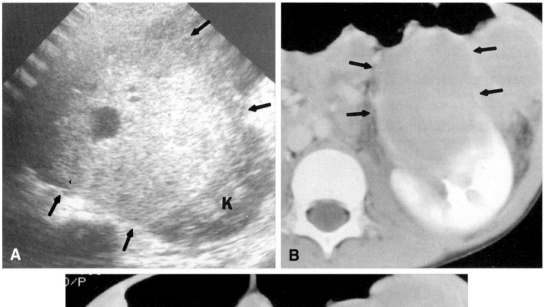

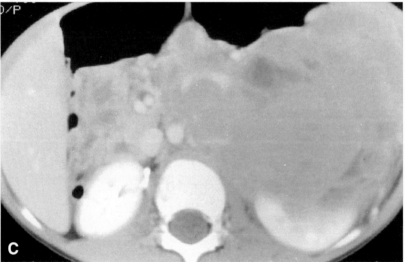

FIGURE 5.160. Neuroblastoma mimicking Wilms' tumor. A. Cross-sectional sonogram demonstrates a large solid tumor (arrows) with some cystic degeneration deforming the kidney (K) in a typical "claw" sign fashion. An intrarenal tumor is suggested. **B.** CT study with contrast demonstrates the tumor (arrows), which appears to originate from the kidney. **C.** A lower slice demonstrates a large tumor, which appears to be arising from the kidney. The aorta and inferior vena cava are displaced to the right, and the tumor does cross the midline.

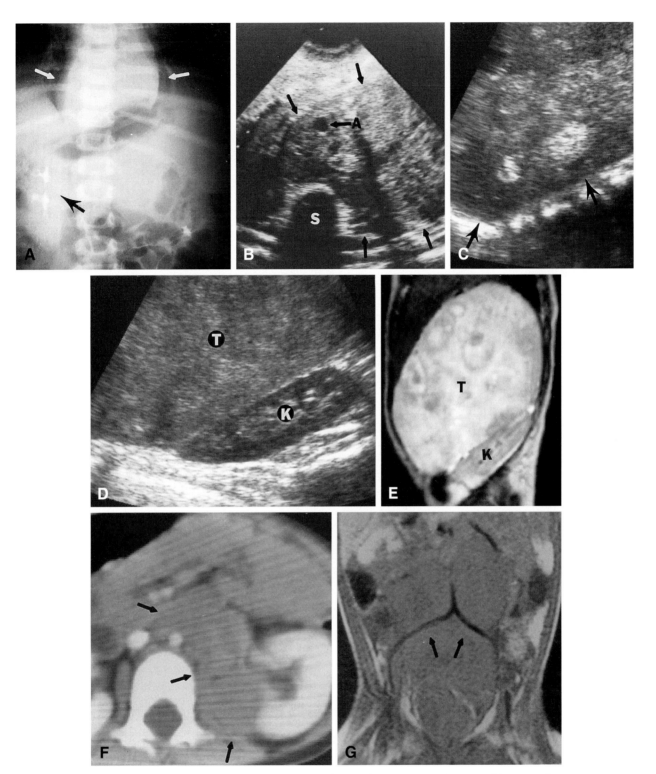

FIGURE 5.161. Neuroblastoma: various configurations. A. Extensive neuroblastoma displacing the left kidney downward (arrow) and extending along the paraspinal regions (upper arrows) into the chest. **B.** Ultrasonogram in the same patient demonstrates the echogenic tumor (arrows) and the aorta (A), which is displaced away from the spine (S) by the interposed tumor. An echogenic area of hemorrhage is seen just above and to the left of the spine. **C.** A large echogenic tumor (arrows) with multiple hyperechoic foci. **D.** Another slice demonstrates that the tumor (T) is clearly separated from the kidney (K). **E.** T2-weighted MR study also demonstrates the large tumor (T), which is clearly separated from the kidney (K). **F.** CT study in another patient demonstrates a paraspinal neuroblastoma (arrows) displacing the kidney outward. **G.** Large neuroblastoma occupying the entire abdomen and elevating and displacing the aorta and common iliac vessel (arrows).

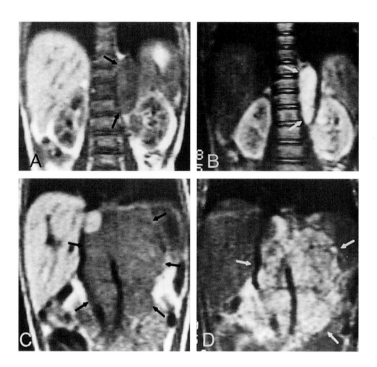

FIGURE 5.162. Neuroblastoma: MR findings. A. T1-weighted MR image demonstrates the left suprarenal tumor (arrows). It is of low to medium signal and displaces the kidney outward. **B.** T2-weighted image demonstrates high signal intensity in the tumor (arrows). **C.** A more anterior coronal T1-weighted image demonstrates the main bulk of the tumor (arrows). **D.** T2-weighted image shows heterogeneously increased signal intensity in the tumor (arrows).

and F), and these imaging modalities play a significant role in locating occult tumors. The main advantage of MRI is that it provides the surgeon or oncologist with a more definitive, triplanar location, configuration, and extent of the tumor (Figs. 5.162 and 5.163). MRI also is excellent in detecting dumbbell tumors that extend into the spinal canal (Fig. 5.164). However, helical CT with reconstruction can provide images in multiple planes and has become more competitive with MRI.

Calcification of neuroblastoma also is common; although a 50–75% incidence on plain films has often been quoted, our experience is that it is far less. With CT scanning, one can detect more of these calcifications, but in any case they are finally speckled or irregular (Fig. 5.165).

Neuroblastoma tends to metastasize to the bones and liver and not so often to the lungs. However, in a recent CT study of the chest in neuroblastoma (17) it was noted that lung spread was more common than generally believed. It was suggested that the prognosis was less favorable when lung metastases were seen at time of presentation. Metastases also can occur almost anywhere, including the brain (18), and gonads (19). However, liver and bone metastases remain the most common. In terms of bone metastases, one of the more common presentations is extremity pain, which very often is localized to the hip and attendant with limping. This should not be such a surprise, because the hip is a weight-bearing joint and one that is exercised very frequently, even by ordinary daily activities. In cases of metastatic disease, there usually is evidence of permeative destruction (aggressive) of the involved bone (Fig. 5.166A), and in many cases reactive periosteal new bone formation.

Involvement of the ribs may present with thoracic cage pain and pleural thickening while skull metastases present as lytic bone lesions and spreading of the sutures, especially the coronal suture (Fig. 5.166C). Spreading in part is due to increased intracranial pressure and part to destruction of bone along the suture line.

Nuclear scintigraphy is extremely useful in detecting and demonstrating the distribution of bone and liver metastases. Liver metastases also may be detected with ultrasound, CT, and MR, but bony metastases usually are detected with plain films and nuclear scintigraphy (Fig. 5.166). On technetium-99m phosphate bone scans, areas of increased scintigraphic activity correspond to the metastatic tumor sites. This imaging modality is especially useful when plain films are subtle or absent (Fig. 5.166, A and B). However, in regard to the nuclear scintigram, while in some cases the positive areas are easy to detect, in others, where there is lack of clear distinction between the normally "hot" epiphyseal line and the abnormally "hot" metaphysis, metastases can be missed. This is especially likely to occur when tumor spread is widespread and all of the metaphyses are involved. Nuclear scintigraphy, using technetium-99 pyrophosphate scans also can demonstrate activity in the tumor itself (Fig. 5.167).

The permeative bone destruction seen with metastatic neuroblastoma is no different from that which is seen with osteomyelitis. For this reason, the two entities can be confused, especially on initial presentation. However, with metastatic neuroblastoma, soft tissue changes around the involved bone are minimal or nonexistent. On the other hand, with osteomyelitis, soft tissue edema and thickening

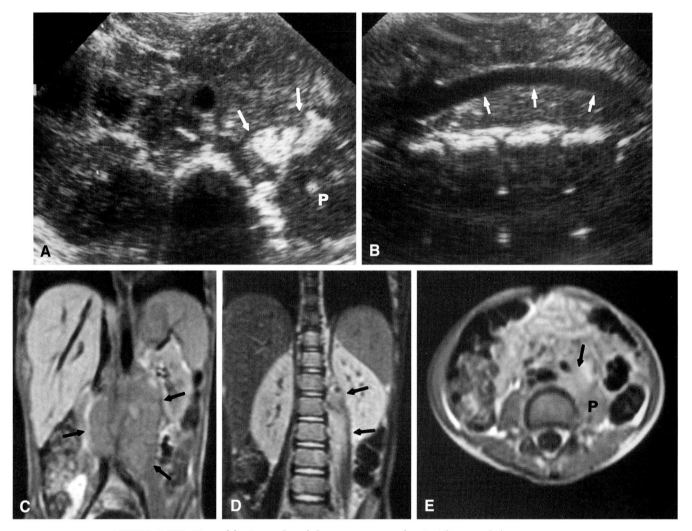

FIGURE 5.163. Neuroblastoma involving psoas muscle. A. Ultrasound demonstrates an echogenic mass (arrows) that is immediately adjacent to the psoas muscle (P). The aorta is displaced from the spine because of interposed tumor. **B.** Lateral view demonstrates the aorta (arrows) being displaced forward by the tumor lying between it and the spine. **C.** T2-weighted MR study demonstrates the tumor (arrows) in the paraaortic region. **D.** A slightly more posterior slice demonstrates invasion of the left psoas muscle (arrows). **E.** T1-weighted, cross-sectional image demonstrates the tumor (arrow) invading the ipsilateral psoas muscle (P).

of the tissues usually is present. On nuclear scintigraphy, because there is not a major inflammatory response evoked by metastatic neuroblastoma, the blood flow phase of a nuclear scintigraphy study does not demonstrate the markedly increased blood flow seen with osteomyelitis (20).

Metaiodobenzylguanidine (MIBG) scans can be used for visualization and evaluation of tumor and bone marrow involvement (Fig. 5.167D). Many times, they are used in combination with regular bone scans (24–26) and can be used for follow-up after therapy. In addition, they are useful with bone marrow transplantation (27), but it should be remembered that regular bone scintigraphy may produce false-positive foci at the sites of bone marrow harvest (28).

Patients with neuroblastoma usually are followed with ultrasound, CT, or MRI for the primary tumor and nuclear scintigraphy for metastatic lesions. With successful therapy, the main tumor will regress and become fibrotic, but it may be difficult to completely assure everyone that the tumor has completely disappeared. In these cases, it is important to perform imaging sequentially to demonstrate that the area of residual fibrotic tissue has not changed. MIBG scans, along with positron emission tomography (PET) scanning, are useful in these cases. With extensive adrenal tumors, the ipsilateral kidney may have its blood supply interrupted (29).

The foregoing comments have dealt primarily with the usual case of neuroblastoma, but there are many ***peculiar***

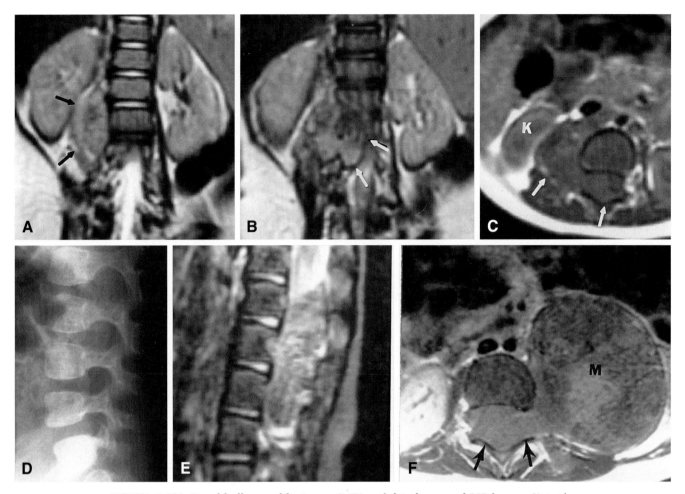

FIGURE. 5.164. Dumbbell neuroblastoma. A. T1-weighted, coronal MR image. Note the small adrenal tumor (arrows) just medial to the ipsilateral kidney. **B.** A slightly more posterior cut demonstrates the tumor extending into the spinal canal (arrows). **C.** Axial image also demonstrates the tumor (arrows) extending into the spinal canal. The kidney (K) is displaced outward. **D.** Another case where the lateral spine demonstrates multiple enlarged intravertebral foramina. **E.** Sagittal, T1-weighted MR study demonstrates the intraspinal component of the tumor which at multiple levels is seen extending into the vertebral bodies. **F.** Axial view demonstrates the large tumor (M) extending into the spinal canal (arrows). (**D–F** courtesy of C. Keith Hayden, Jr., M.D.)

presentations of neuroblastoma, and one must be aware of all of them so as not to delay or miss the diagnosis. In this regard, aggressive neuroblastoma can mimic Wilms' tumor (21–23) (Fig. 5.168). Another peculiar presentation is the one of bizarre myoclonic seizures, cerebellar symptoms (i.e., ataxia), and opsoclonus, or "dancing eyes" (30). Paraneoplastic encephalitis also has been documented with neuroblastoma (31) and another peculiar manifestation of unknown etiology is heel cord shortening (32, 33). Some neuroblastomas can manifest as dumbbell tumors of the spine, and this initial problem may be one of paraplegia or bowel or bladder dysfunction (34). In these cases, the diagnosis should be suspected when, in addition to the tumor mass, there is plain film evidence of rib erosion, scoliosis, enlargement of the intervertebral foramina, widening of the spinal canal, or posterior scal-

loping of the vertebral bodies. These tumors are best studied with MRI (Fig. 5.169).

Some neuroblastomas produce a vasoactive intestinal peptide, and this can lead to intractable diarrhea (35). One study has shown that the vasoactive peptide also may serve as an inhibitor factor to tumor growth (36). Neuroblastoma also has an association with the fetal hydantoin and alcohol syndromes where greater than usual incidence of the tumor has been noted. Another peculiar association of neuroblastoma is that of neuroblastoma, Hirschsprung's disease, and Ondine's curse (37, 38), all believed to represent a neurocristopathy. Hypertension also can be a presentation of neuroblastoma (39), as can the so-called "raccoon eyes," in which there are dark, even black, circles around the eyes on physical examination. Often, the first consideration is trauma as part of the battered child syndrome (40), but it

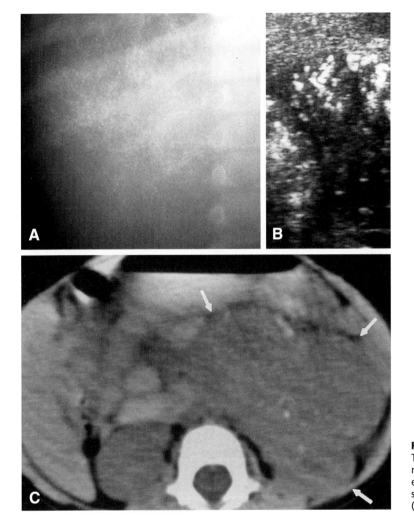

FIGURE 5.165. Neuroblastoma: calcifications. A. Typical granular calcifications in the right upper quadrant. **B.** Ultrasonography demonstrates characteristic echogenic foci representing the calcifications. **C.** CT study in another patient with a large neuroblastoma (arrows) showing a few stippled calcifications.

should be remembered **that faint to moderately intense discoloration around the orbits is not an uncommon presentation of neuroblastoma.**

REFERENCES

1. Jennings RW, LaQuaglia MP, Leong K, et al. Fetal neuroblastoma: prenatal diagnosis and natural history. J Pediatr Surg 1993;28:1168–1174.
2. Granata C, Fagnani AM, Gambini C, et al. Features and outcome of neuroblastoma detected before birth. J Pediatr Surg 2000;35:88–91.
3. Beckwith JB, Perrin EV. In situ neuroblastoma; a contribution to the natural life history of neural chest tumors. Am J Pathol 1963; 43:1089–1104.
4. Ikeda Y, Lister J, Bouton JM, et al. Congenital neuroblastoma, neuroblastoma in situ, and the normal fetal development of the adrenal. J Pediatr Surg 1981;16:636–644.
5. Berdon WE, Stylianos S, Ruzal-Shapiro C, et al. Neuroblastoma arising from the organ of Zuckerkandl: an unusual site with a favorable biologic outcome. Pediatr Radiol 1999;29:497–502.
6. Encinas A, Matute JA, Gmez A, et al. Primary neuroblastoma presenting as a paratesticular tumor. J Pediatr Surg 1997;32: 624–626.
7. Cassady C, Winters WD. Bilateral cystic neuroblastoma: imaging features and differential diagnoses. Pediatr Radiol 1997;27: 758–759.
8. Croitoru DP, Sinsky AB, Laberge J-M. Cystic neuroblastoma. J Pediatr Surg 1992;27:1320–1321.
9. Zaizen Y, Suita S, Yamanaka K, et al. Bilateral adrenal neuroblastoma. Eur J Pediatr Surg 1998;33:806.
10. Haas D, Ablin AR, Miller C, et al. Complete pathologic maturation and regression of stage IVS neuroblastoma without treatment. Cancer 1988;62:818–825.
11. Cohen MD, Auringer ST, Grosfeld JL, et al. Multifocal primary neuroblastoma. Pediatr Radiol 1993;23:463–466.
12. Abramson SJ, Berdon WE, Ruzal-Shapiro C, et al. Cervical neuroblastoma in eleven infants–a tumor with favorable prognosis. Clinical and radiologic (US, CT, MRI) findings. Pediatr Radiol 1993;23:253–257.
13. Abramson SJ, Berdon WE, Stolar C, et al. Stage IVN neuroblastoma: MRI diagnosis of left supraclavicular "Virchow's nodal spread" Pediatr Radiol 1996;26:717–719.
14. Iwata M, Koshinaga T, Okabe I, et al. Biological characteristics of neuroblastoma with spontaneous tumor reduction: a case report. J Pediatr Surg 1995;30:722–723.

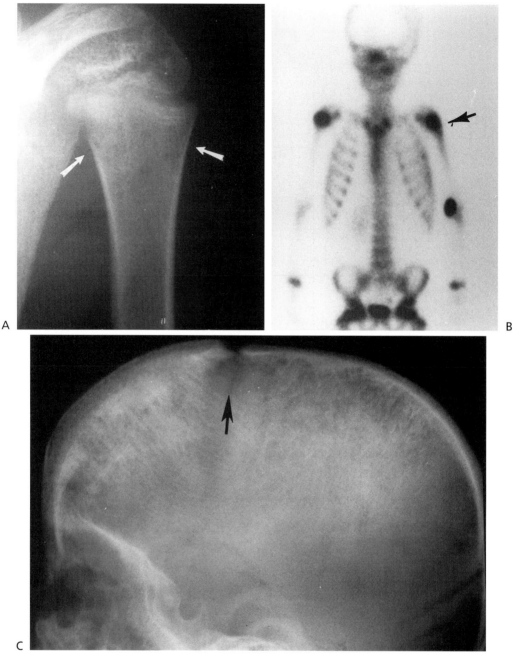

FIGURE 5.166. Metastatic neuroblastoma. A. Note the subtle, permeated, moth-eaten appearance of the proximal humerus (arrows). **B.** Technetium-99m pyrophosphate scan demonstrates increased uptake in the proximal left humerus (arrow). **C.** Metastatic disease to the calvarium demonstrates mottled bony destruction and spread of the coronal suture (arrow).

15. Nakagawara A, Arima NM, Scavarda NJ, et al. Association between high levels of expression of the Trk gene and favorable outcome in human neuroblastoma. N Engl J Med 1993;328: 847–853.

16. Amundson GM, Trevenen CL, Mueller DL, et al. Neuroblastoma: a specific sonographic tissue pattern. AJR 1987;148: 943–945.

17. Kammen BF, Matthay KK, Pacharn P, et al. Pulmonary metas-

tases at diagnosis of neuroblastoma in pediatric patients: CT findings and prognosis. AJR 2001;176:755–759.

18. Kenny BJ, Pizer BL, Duncan AW, et al. Cystic metastatic cerebral neuroblastoma. Pediatr Radiol 1995;25:S97–S98.

19. McHugh K, Pritchard J, Dicks-Mireaux C. Bilateral ovaria involvement at presentation in metastatic (stage 4) neuroblastoma. Pediatr Radiol 1999;29:741.

20. Applegate K, Connolly LP, Treves ST. Neuroblastoma presenting

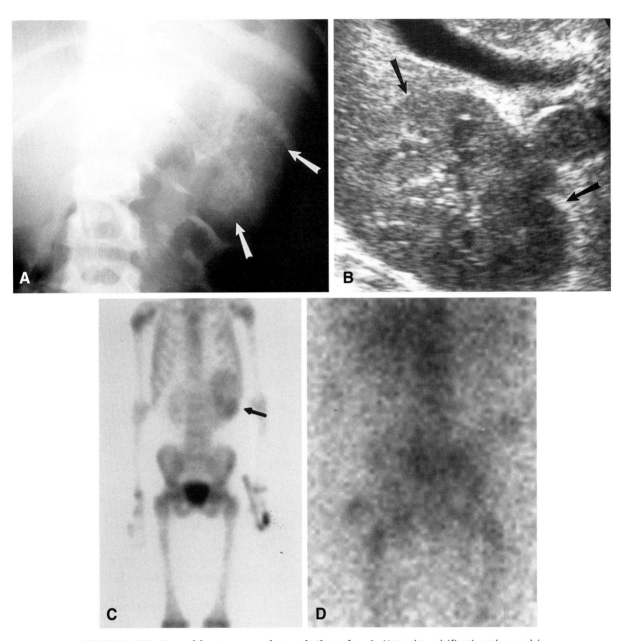

FIGURE 5.167. Neuroblastoma: nuclear scintigraphy. A. Note the calcifications (arrows) in the tumor. **B.** Ultrasonogram demonstrates the large echogenic tumor (arrows) with stippled echogenic areas representing the calcifications. **C.** Technetium-99m pyrophosphate scan demonstrates uptake of isotope in the tumor (arrow). The rest of the study is normal with no evidence of bony involvement. **D.** The MIBG scintigram, however, demonstrates widespread bone marrow involvement.

clinically as hip osteomyelitis: a "signature" diagnosis on skeletal scintigraphy. Pediatr Radiol 1995;25:S93–S96.

21. Albregts AE, Cohen MD, Galliani CA. Neuroblastoma invading the kidney. J Pediatr Surg 1994;29:930–933.

22. Day DL, Johnson R, Cohen MD. Abdominal neuroblastoma with inferior vena caval tumor thrombus: report of three cases (one with right atrial extension). Pediatr Radiol 1991;21:205–207.

23. Rosenfield NS, Leonidas JC, Barwick KW. Aggressive neurob-

lastoma simulating Wilms' tumor. Radiology 1988;166:165–167.

24. Najaen DB, Siles S, Panuel M, et al. Value of MRI and MIBG-^{123}I scintigraphy in the diagnosis of spinal bone marrow involvement in neuroblastoma in children. Pediatr Radiol 1992;22:443–446.

25. Clapuyt P, Saint-Martin C, DeBatselier P, et al. Urachal neuroblastoma: first case report. Pediatr Radiol 1999;29:320–321.

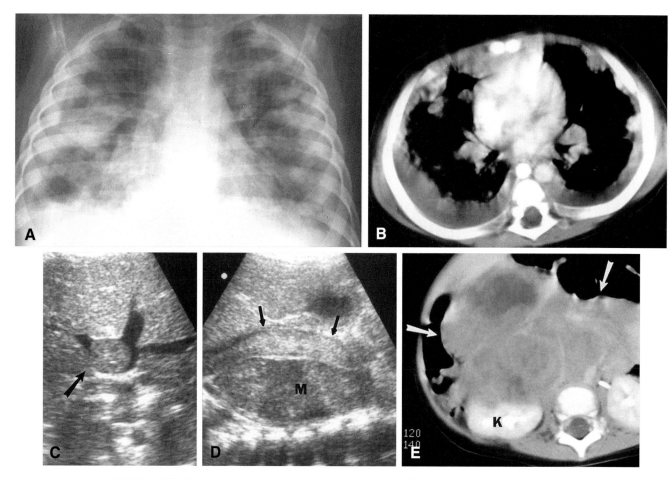

FIGURE 5.168. Aggressive neuroblastoma. A. Note the widespread metastatic disease to the lungs. **B.** Axial CT demonstrates numerous pleural implants in addition to parenchymal nodules. **C.** Cross-sectional ultrasonogram demonstrates tumor extension into the inferior vena cava (arrow). **D.** Sagittal view demonstrates the large echogenic mass (M) displacing the inferior vena cava forward (arrows). The inferior vena cava also is shown to contain echogenic tumor thrombus. **E.** CT demonstrates the large tumor (arrows) invading the kidney (K).

26. Shulkin BL, Shapiro B, Hutchinson RJ. Iodine-131-metaiodo-benzylguanidine and bone scintigraphy for the detection of neuroblastoma. J Nucl Med 1992;33:1735–1740.

27. Englaro EE, Gelfand MJ, Harris RE, et al. I-131 MIBG imaging after bone marrow transplantation for neuroblastoma. Radiology 1992;182:515–520.

28. Ortiz SS, Miller JH, Villablanca JG, et al. Bone abnormalities detected with skeletal scintigraphy after bone marrow harvest in patients with childhood neuroblastoma. Radiology 1994;192:755–758.

29. Day DL, Johnson RT, Odrezin GT, et al. Renal atrophy or infarction in children with neuroblastoma. Radiology 1991;180:493–495.

30. Kinast M, Levin HS, Rothner AD, et al. Cerebellar ataxia, opsoclonus, and occult neural crest tumor. Am J Dis Child 1980;134:1057–1059.

31. Meyer JJ, Bulteau C, Adamsbaum C, et al. Paraneoplastic encephalomyelitis in a child with neuroblastoma. Pediatr Radiol 1995;25:S99–S101.

32. Burns WW, Brownlee RC Jr, Bomar WE Jr. Heel cord shortening with ganglioneuroblastoma. Am J Dis Child 1975;129:750.

33. Martin LW, Kosloske AM. Heel cord shortening with ganglioneuroblastoma. Am J Dis Child 1975;129:254–255.

34. Holgersen LO, Santulli TV, Schullinger JN, et al. Neuroblastoma with intraspinal (dumbbell) extension. J Pediatr Surg 1983;18:406–411.

35. El Shafie M, Samuel D, Klippel CH, et al. Intractable diarrhea in children with VIP-secreting ganglioneuroblastomas. J Pediatr Surg 1983;18:34–36.

36. Pence JC, Shorter NA. Autoregulation of neuroblastoma growth by vasoactive intestinal peptide. J Pediatr Surg 1992;27:935–944.

37. Roshkow JE, Haller JO, Berdon WE, et al. Hirschsprung's disease, Ondine's curse, neuroblastoma-manifestations of neurocristopathy. Pediatr Radiol 1988;19:45–49.

38. Stovroff M, Dykes F, Teague WG. The complete spectrum of neurocristopathy in an infant with congenital hypoventilation, Hirschsprung's disease, and neuroblastoma. J Pediatr Surg 1995;30:1218–1221.

39. Sendo D, Katsura M, Akiba K, et al. Severe hypertension and cardiac failure associated with neuroblastoma. A case report. J Pediatr Surg 1996;31:1688–1690.

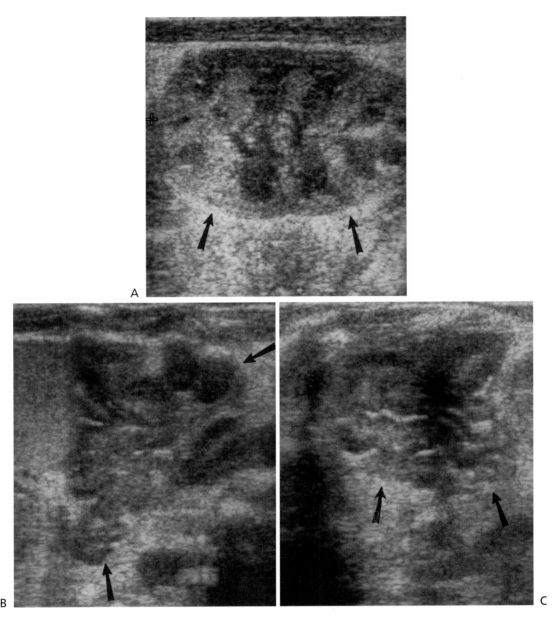

FIGURE 5.169. Adrenal hyperplasia: cerebriform pattern. A. Note the enlarged adrenal gland (arrow) demonstrating a classic cerebriform pattern. **B.** Cross-sectional view of one of the adrenal glands demonstrates the same (arrows). **C.** Cross-sectional view of the other adrenal gland (arrows).

40. Bohdiewicz PJ, Gallegos E, Fink-Bennett D. Raccoon eyes and MIBG super scan: scintigraphic signs of neuroblastoma in a case of suspected child abuse. Pediatr Radiol 1995;25:S90-S92.

Adrenogenital Syndrome

Most often, the problem in patients with adrenogenital syndrome is simple adrenal hyperplasia, but occasionally, an adenoma can be encountered. The condition is characterized by excessive secretion of androgenic hormones, and there is a familial tendency. Both males and females are affected, and it is believed that the problem is the result of a deficiency of 21-hydroxylase enzyme (1). The problem also has been induced by ACTH therapy (2).

In males, virilizing effects produce enlargement of the external genitalia, and in females, virilization produces various degrees of female pseudohermaphrodism. The changes may be mild, consisting only of hypertrophy of the clitoris, or so marked that the external genitalia appear like those of a male. Internally the urethra and vagina may open into a common urogenital sinus or separately into the vestibule. If these infants are not recognized early, problems in sex assignment can arise. Roentgenographically, the prime consideration lies in the determination of the size of the vagina and whether it opens into the vestibule or with the urethra into a urogenital sinus. Ultrasound can be used to evaluate the adrenal glands for size and morphology. Normal adrenal size is approximately 14×2 mm, but in patients with the adrenogenital syndrome and hyperplasia, the average measurement in one series was 24×5 mm (1). These authors suggest that abnormality exists if the adrenal gland measures more than 20×4 mm. This also has been confirmed by others (3).

On ultrasonography, the hyperplastic adrenal gland may appear structurally normal (1) or demonstrate the so-called cerebriform pattern (4), in which irregular striations result in an appearance resembling cerebral cortex (Fig. 5.169). In addition to these findings, adrenal rests have been demonstrated in the testicles of these patients, and this "syndrome" has been referred to as the "testicular adrenal-like tissue" syndrome (TALT) (5–7). In some infants—and there is indication that it is more common in males—adrenal insufficiency may also be present. Such infants often die in adrenal crisis, and the entire syndrome is characterized by excessive salt and water loss, peripheral vascular collapse, and rapid death. It is most important that this condition be recognized early, and an important clue to the early diagnosis of these infants may lie in noting virilization of the external genitalia. Such early recognition is invaluable, because with proper supportive fluids, electrolytes, and hormonal therapy these infants can be saved and nurtured into adult life.

REFERENCES

1. Sivit CJ, Hung W, Taylor GA, et al. Sonography in neonatal congenital adrenal hyperplasia. AJR 1991;156:141–143.
2. Liebling MS, Starc TJ, McAlister WH, et al. ACTH induced adrenal enlargement in infants treated for infantile spasms and acute cerebellar encephalopathy. Pediatr Radiol 1993;23:454–456.
3. Al-Alwan I, Navarro O, Daneman D, et al. Clinical utility of adrenal ultrasonography in the diagnosis of congenital adrenal hyperplasia. J Pediatr 1999;135:71–75.
4. Avni EF, Rypens F, Smet MH, et al. Sonographic demonstration of congenital adrenal hyperplasia in the neonate: the cerebriform pattern. Pediatr Radiol 1993;23:88–90.
5. Avila NA, Shawker TS, Jones JV, et al. Testicular adrenal rest tissue in congenital adrenal hyperplasia: serial sonographic and clinical findings. AJR 1999;172:1235–1238.
6. Vanzulli A, DelMaschio A, Paesano P, et al. Testicular masses in association with adrenogenital syndrome: US findings. Radiology 1992;183:425–429.
7. Willi U, Atares M, Prader A, et al. Testicular adrenal-like tissue (TALT) in congenital adrenal hyperplasia: detection by ultrasonography. Pediatr Radiol 1991;21:284–287.

Aldosteronism and Cushing's Disease

Occasionally, both aldosteronism and Cushing's disease can be produced by an adenoma (1), but most often, the problem is adrenal hyperplasia (2). Ultrasonography can be used along with CT and MRI to detect any adrenal tumors present, and it is interesting that nephrocalcinosis has been noted in association with hyperaldosteronism. Calcification of the tumor itself also can be seen. Clinical findings include refractory hypertension, polydipsia, polyuria, headaches, and muscle weakness. Treatment usually is conservative with the administration of spironolactone, although when adenomas are identified they are removed surgically (2). With Cushing's syndrome, radiographic findings consist primarily of widespread bone demineralization and pathologic fractures, especially compression fractures of the spine.

REFERENCES

1. Abasiyanik A, Oran B, Kaymakci A, et al. Conn syndrome in a child, caused by adrenal adenoma. J Pediatr Surg 1996;31:430–431.
2. Agarwala S, Mitra DK, Bhatnagar V, et al. Aldosteronoma in childhood: a review of clinical features of management. J Pediatr Surg 1994;29:1388–1391.

MISCELLANEOUS ADRENAL GLAND ABNORMALITIES

Wolman's Disease

Wolman's disease is a peculiar lipidosis in which the most significant radiographic finding is the presence of dense calcification in enlarged adrenal glands (1, 2). There is a familial tendency, and the infants tend to die at an early age. Hepatosplenomegaly also is usually present, and the densely calcified adrenal glands are vividly demonstrated with plain films, ultrasound, and CT (Fig. 5.170).

REFERENCES

1. Dutton RV. Wolman's disease. Ultrasound and CT diagnosis. Pediatr Radiol 1985;15:144–146.
2. Ozmen MN, Aygun N, Kilic I, et al. Wolman's disease: ultrasonographic and computed tomographic findings. Pediatr Radiol 1992;22:541–542.

Adrenal Abscess

Adrenal abscess can occur in the neonate and most likely is the result of neonatal sepsis (1–3). Although usually unilateral, bilateral abscesses have been documented (3). The findings may be difficult to differentiate from adrenal hemorrhage or adrenal tumor.

REFERENCES

1. Atkinson GO Jr, Kodroff MB, Gay BB Jr, et al. Adrenal abscess in the neonate. Radiology 1985;155:101–104.

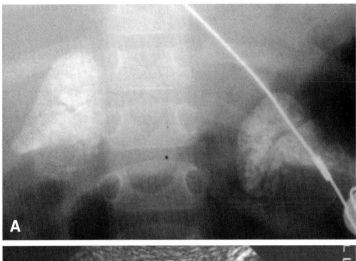

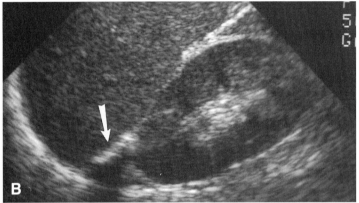

FIGURE 5.170. Wolman's disease. A. Characteristic bilateral, dense triangular calcifications of the adrenal glands. **B.** Ultrasonogram demonstrates the echogenic adrenal gland (arrow) above the kidney. (Courtesy of Deborah Day, M.D.)

2. Rajani K, Shapiro SR, Goestzman BW. Adrenal abscess: complication of supportive therapy of adrenal hemorrhage in the newborn. J Pediatr Surg 1980;15:676–678.
3. Steffens J, Zaubitzer T, Kirsch W, et al. Neonatal adrenal abscesses. Eur Urol 1997;31:347–349.

Miscellaneous Adrenal Tumors and Cysts

Congenital adrenal cysts are rare and often are misdiagnosed for some other lesion such as adrenal hemorrhage. Spontaneous resolution of these cysts can occur in the neonate (1). These cysts also can occur in older children, usually girls (2). Their appearance, no matter what the imaging modality, is that of a cyst (Fig. 5.171). Bilateral multicystic adrenal glands also have been demonstrated in the Beckwith-Wiedemann syndrome (3).

Tumors other than neuroblastoma of the adrenal glands are rare. The most common of these in infancy, however, is adrenal cortical carcinoma (2–7), a tumor that can produce virilizing symptoms. Calcification of the periphery of these tumors are common (Fig. 5.172). Ultrasonography usually demonstrates the tumor to be solid (8), and the tumor may extend into the inferior vena cava and right atrium (9). There also is an association of this tumor with the fetal alcohol syndrome (10) and congenital hemihypertrophy (11).

Pheochromocytomas are rare in children, especially in infancy (12–14). Hypertension is one of the foremost symptoms and the tumors tend to be bilateral in children, although they may not be present at the same time. Pheochromocytomas also are a part of the multiple

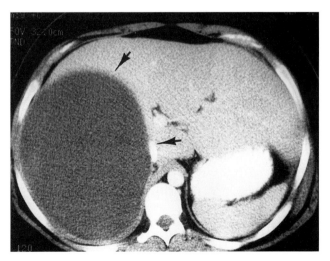

FIGURE 5.171. Adrenal cyst. Note the large, hypodense adrenal cyst (arrows).

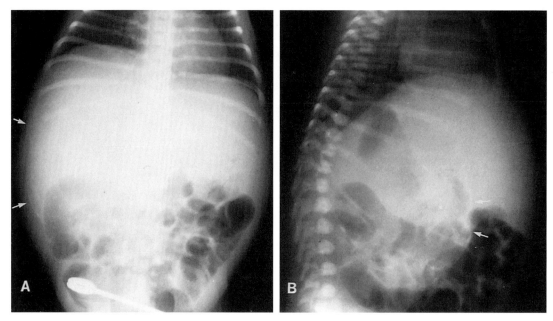

FIGURE 5.172. Adrenal cortical carcinoma. A and B. Unusual case of large right adrenal cortical carcinoma presenting as abdominal mass with peripheral curvilinear calcification (arrows) in a neonate. (Courtesy of C. K. Hendrick, M.D.)

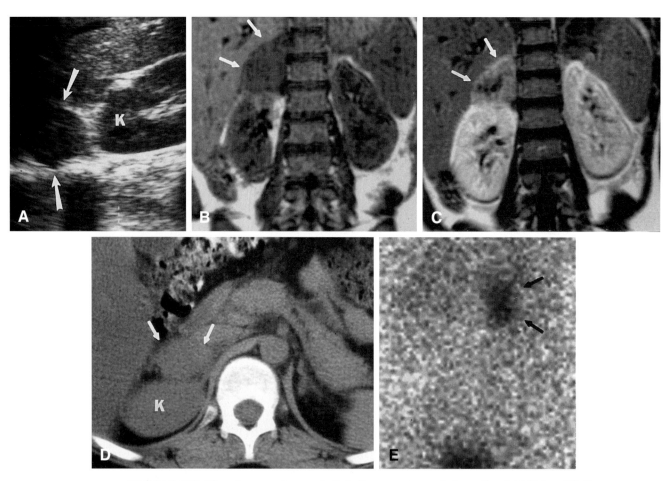

FIGURE 5.173. Pheochromocytoma. A. Note the mass (arrows) above the right kidney (K). **B.** Coronal, T1-weighted MR image demonstrates the suprarenal mass (arrows). **C.** T2-weighted image shows increased signal intensity in the mass (arrows). **D.** Another patient with a pheochromocytoma (arrows) located just anterior to the upper pole of the right kidney (K). **E.** MIBG study, posterior view, demonstrates uptake in the tumor (arrows). (**A–C** courtesy of C. Keith Hayden, Jr., M.D.)

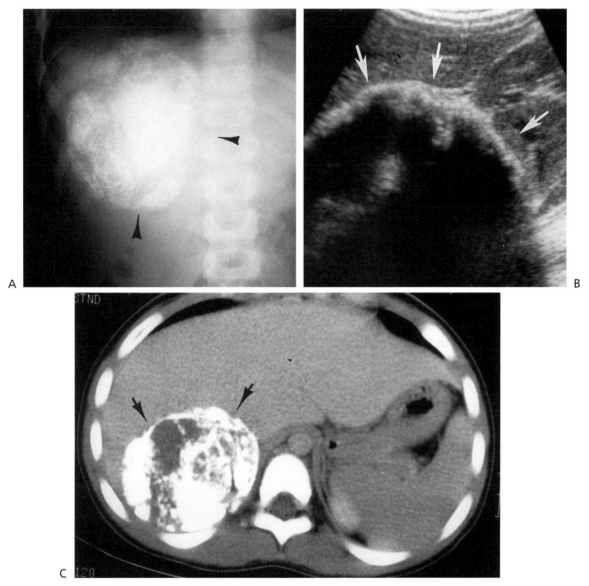

FIGURE 5.174. Adrenal adenoma. A. Note the large, heavily calcified tumor (arrows). **B.** Ultrasonography demonstrates a typical echogenic rim (arrows). **C.** CT study demonstrates the large, heavily calcified tumor (arrows).

endocrine neoplasia syndrome (12) and biochemically are characterized by increased catecholamines in the urine. Ultrasonography may miss the tumors, because they do not have to be very large (14). The tumor is often best demonstrated with MRI, CT, and MIBG scintigraphy (Fig. 5.173). Angiography also still is useful in identifying these tumors, and interestingly enough, brachydactyly occurring as a late complication can be seen, supposedly secondary to ischemia (15).

Adrenal adenoma and adrenocorticoadenoma are rare tumors. However, they can occur (16) and in some cases may appear heavily calcified (Fig. 5.174). Rarely, hemangioendothelioma of the adrenal gland can occur (17).

REFERENCES

1. Morganti VJ, Anderson NG. Simple adrenal cysts in fetus, resolving spontaneously in neonate. J Ultrasound Med 1991;10: 521–524.
2. Broadley P, Daneman A, Wesson D, et al. Large adrenal cysts in teenage girls: diagnosis and management. Pediatr Radiol 1997; 27:550–552.
3. Akata D, Haliloglu M, Ozmen MN, et al. Bilateral cystic adrenal masses in the neonate associated with the incomplete form of Beckwith-Wiedemann syndrome. Pediatr Radiol 1997;27:1–2.
4. Hanson JA, Weber A, Reznek RH, et al. Magnetic resonance imaging of adrenocortical adenomas in childhood: correlation with computed tomography and ultrasound. Pediatr Radiol 1996;26:794–799.

5. Mayer SK, Oligny LL, Deal C, et al. Childhood adrenocortical tumors: case series and reevaluation of prognosis—a 24-year experience. J Pediatr Surg 1997;32:911–915.

6. Morales L, Rovira J, Rottermann M, et al. Adrenocortical tumors in childhood: a report of four cases. J Pediatr Surg 1989;24: 276–281.

7. Ribeiro J, Ribeiro RC, Fletcher BD. Imaging findings in pediatric adrenocortical carcinoma. Pediatr Radiol 2000;30:45–51.

8. Smets A, Mortele K, DeWever N, et al. Coexistence of an adrenocortical carcinoma with an abdominal ganglioneuroma in a child. Pediatr Radiol 1998;28:329–331.

9. Godine LB, Berdon WE, Brasch RC, et al. Adrenocortical carcinoma with extension into inferior vena cava and right atrium: report of 3 cases in children. Pediatr Radiol 1990;20:166–168.

10. Hornstein L, Crowe C, Gruppo R. Adrenal carcinoma in a child with history of fetal alcohol syndrome. Lancet 1977;2:1292.

11. Haicken BN, Schulman NH, Schneider KM. Adrenocortical carcinoma and congenital hemihypertrophy. J Pediatr 1973;83: 284–285.

12. Caty MG, Coran AG, Geagen M, et al. Current diagnosis and treatment of pheochromocytoma in children: experience with 22 consecutive tumors in 14 patients. Arch Surg 1990;125: 978–981.

13. Deal JE, Sever PS, Barratt TM, et al. Phaeochromocytoma–investigation and management of 10 cases. Arch Dis Child 1990; 65:269–274.

14. Revillon Y, Daher P, Jan D, et al. Pheochromocytoma in children: 15 cases. J Pediatr Surg 1992;27:910–911.

15. Hoeffel JC, Galloy MA, Worms AM, et al. Brachydactyly secondary to pheochromocytoma. Am J Dis Child 1993;147: 260–261.

16. Hanson JA, Weber A, Reznek RH, et al. Magnetic resonance imaging of adrenocortical adenomas in childhood: correlation with computed tomography and ultrasound. Pediatr Radiol 1996;26:794–799.

17. Soboleski D, Mehta S, Kamal I, et al. Case report. Hemangioendothelioma of the adrenal gland in a 4-month-old male infant. AJR 172:235–237.

SKELETAL SYSTEM AND SOFT TISSUES

NORMAL ANATOMY AND VARIATIONS

Bone Age

The primary ossification centers for most of the bones of the skeleton develop early in fetal life. The center for the clavicle is first to appear, and by the end of 2–3 gestational months, all primary ossification centers are well developed. The only secondary ossification centers routinely seen in full-term infants are those in the distal ends of the femurs and proximal ends of the tibiae (Fig. 6.1A). These centers generally are used in the determination of fetal and neonatal bone age, with the distal femoral epiphysis appearing at approximately 36 weeks of gestation and the proximal tibial epiphysis at 38 weeks. It also has been noted that the proximal humeral head is ossified in 40–50% of full-term infants (1), and in many full-term infants, early ossification of the coracoid process of the scapula can be seen (Fig. 6.1B).

The carpal bones are not ossified at birth, but in the foot, one almost always sees ossification centers for the calcaneus (23 weeks) and talus (27 weeks), the calcaneus being slightly more consistent. For a more detailed study of fetal and neonatal ossification centers and rates of growth, one can refer to the article by Kuhns and Finnstrom (2). These authors demonstrated that the sequence of ossification of certain key centers in the fetal and neonatal skeleton was as follows: The calcaneus was first, then the talus, and then the distal femoral epiphysis. Thereafter, the proximal tibial epiphysis, epiphysis of the humeral head, and ossification center for the cuboid bone appeared, more or less together (Table 6.1).

After birth, in the wrist, the capitate and hamate are the first bones to ossify and usually appear at approximately 3 months. The head of the femur usually appears somewhere between 2 and 6 months of age. Other early ossification centers include that for the capitellum, becoming visible at approximately 3 months of age, and that for the body of the hyoid. This latter ossification center is present in more than half of normal newborn infants.

Generally speaking, female infants and children show a slightly advanced degree of maturity compared with males,

and it has been shown that blacks, Asians, and Hispanics often show earlier appearance of ossification centers than do whites (3, 4). These discrepant results have been cited (3, 4) as a major drawback to the Greulich-Pyle bone age tables. These tables, the most widely used for determination of bone age, were constructed for middle class white children and therefore are not uniformly applicable to all races. However, they still are the best and most readily available tables used.

More recently, more sophisticated and even computer-driven programs for determining bone age have been designed (5, 6), but these may be too complicated. Another method of estimating bone age is the Elgenmark method (7). With this method, all ossification centers of the epiphyses, apophyses, and tarsal and carpal bones on one side of the body are added together and the total count applied to a table yielding the appropriate bone age (Fig. 6.2). This method is believed to be more accurate than the Greulich-Pyle tables but is useful only up to the age of 5 years. However, I have not found it to be particularly more reliable than other methods. With the Greulich-Pyle tables, morphology of each of the centers and appearance of the bone in general are also used. This is important because counting centers alone is not always accurate. In addition, one should place more emphasis on the epiphyses of the small bones of the hands than on the carpal bones (8).

Finally, and in addition to the foregoing methods of determining bone age, a simple scheme I constructed years ago for convenience's sake also can be used. **This scheme is based on the fact that certain centers are extremely reliable in their appearance and that their temporal spacing is close enough that a reasonably accurate and educated estimate of the bone age can be made (Fig. 6.3).** The advantage of this scheme is that if one is performing a large number of bone age determinations, the data provided basically can be memorized. Delayed, advanced, and disharmonic bone age in newborns has been studied by Kuhns and Finnstrom (2) and the data summarized in Table 6.2.

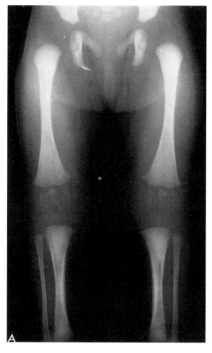
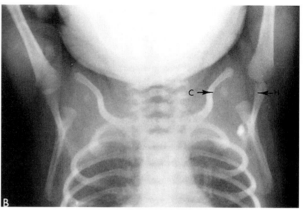

FIGURE 6.1. Normal extremities. A. Lower extremity showing small distal femoral epiphyses (approximately 36-week centers) and very early ossification centers for the proximal tibial epiphyses (38-week centers). Also note the normal striated appearance of the metaphyses and the small nutrient foramina in the center of both femurs. **B.** Upper extremities showing normal clavicles, scapulae, and proximal humeri. Note the small secondary ossification center of the coracoid process of the scapula (C) and, just barely visible, the ossification center of the humeral head (H). Both are not infrequently seen in the neonate.

REFERENCES

1. Kuhns LR, Sherman MP, Poznanski AK, et al. Humeral head and coracoid ossification in the newborn. Radiology 1973;107:145–149.
2. Kuhns LR, Finnstrom O. New standards of ossification of the newborn. Radiology 1976;119:655–660.
3. Loder RT, Estle DT, Morrison K, et al. Applicability of the Greulich and Pyle skeletal age standards to black and white children of today. Am J Dis Child 1993;147:1329–1333.
4. Ontell FK, Ivanovic M, Ablin DS, et al. Bone age in children of diverse ethnicity. AJR 1996;167:1395–1398.
5. Hernandez M, Sanchez E, Sobradillo B, et al. A new method for assessment of skeletal maturity in the first 2 years of life. Pediatr Radiol 1988;18:484–489.
6. Frisch H, Riedl S, Waldhor T. Computer-aided estimation of skeletal age and comparison with bone age evaluations by the method of Gruelich-Pyle and Tanner-Whitehouse. Pediatr Radiol 1996;26:226–231.
7. Elgenmark O. Normal development of the ossific centers during infancy and childhood: clinical, roentgenologic and statistical study. Acta Paediatr Scand 1946;33(suppl 1):1–79.
8. Carpenter CT, Lester EL. Skeletal age determination in young children: analysis of three regions of the hand/wrist. J Pediatr Orthop 1993;13:76–79.

TABLE 6.1. FIFTH AND NINETY-FIFTH PERCENTILES OF EPIPHYSEAL OSSIFICATION OF THE NEONATE

Center	5th Percentile	95th Percentile
Humeral head	37th wk	16 postnatal wk
Distal femoral	31st wk	39th wk (female)
Proximal tibial (female)	34th wk	2 postnatal wk
		5 postnatal wk (male)
Calcaneus	22nd wk	25th wk
Talus	25th wk	31st wk
Cuboid (female)	37th wk	8 postnatal wk
		16 postnatal wk (male)

Source: From Kuhns LR, Finnstrom O. New standards of ossification of the newborn. Radiology 1976;119:655–660, with permission.

Normal Bone Marrow Imaging

With the advent of magnetic resonance imaging (MRI), it has become possible to routinely image normal bone marrow. This is important in the pediatric age group because hemopoietic bone marrow is present originally and later converts to fatty bone marrow. Fat produces high signal on T1-weighted images, while hemopoietic bone marrow produces low signal. These data are important when one wishes to determine whether bone marrow is involved with tumor,

BOYS		GIRLS	
Age, Mo	Av. No. * Centers	Age, Mo	Av. No. * Centers
1	4.8	**1**	4.7
2	5.7	**2**	6.2
3	6.5	**3**	7.6
4	8.9	**4**	8.5
5	9.8	**5**	10.4
6	11.2	**6**	11.5
7	12.5	**7**	12.9
8	13.0	**8**	14.6
9	13.6	**9**	16.3
10	15.2	**10**	18.1
11	15.8	**11**	22.7
12	16.5	**12**	25.1
13-15	19.9	**13-15**	28.6
16-18	23.5	**16-18**	32.9
19-21	25.5	**19-21**	41.3
22-24	32.3	**22-24**	47.2
25-27	36.8	**25-27**	50.8
28-30	39.8	**28-30**	53.2
31-33	44.1	**31-33**	55.8
34-36	48.5	**34-36**	60.5
37-42	49.5	**37-42**	59.5
43-48	56.6	**43-48**	61.4
49-54	59.3	**49-54**	63.5
55-60	61.8	**55-60**	64.2

*NUMBER OF OSSIFICATION CENTERS AT DIFFERENT MONTHS OF AGE

FIGURE 6.2. Bone age determination: Elgenmark method. With this method, all the visible epiphyseal tarsal and carpal ossification centers are counted on one side of the body and the total is applied to the table. [Modified from Elgenmark O. Normal development of the ossific centers during infancy and childhood: clinical, roentgenologic, and statistical study. Acta Paediatr Scand 1946;33(suppl 1):33].

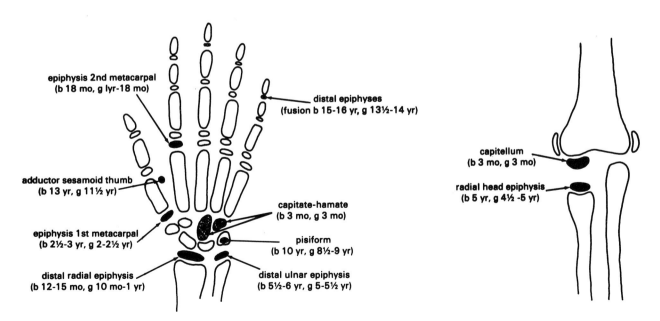

FIGURE 6.3. Bone age: key marker method. With this method, certain reliable ossification centers can be used to establish a rough estimate of the bone age. b, boy; g, girl. (Reproduced with permission from Swischuk LE, John SD. Differential diagnosis in pediatric radiology. 2nd ed. Baltimore: Williams & Wilkins, 1995).

TABLE 6.2. DELAYED, ACCELERATED, AND DYSHARMONIC OSSIFICATION IN THE NEWBORN

A. Retarded osseous maturation of the neonate
  Achondrogenesis
  Achondroplasia
  Camptomelic syndrome
  Carpenter's syndrome (acrocephalopolysyndactyly)
  Cephaloskeletal dysplasia (Taybi-Linder syndrome)
  Cerebrohepatorenal syndrome
  Chondrodysplasia punctata
  Chondroectodermal dysplasia
  Cloverleaf skull
  Cornelia de Lange syndrome
  Diastrophic dwarfism
  Generalized gangliosidosis
  Hypothyroidism
  Infants of toxemic mothers
  Leprechaunism
  Mesomelic dwarfism, Nievergelt type
  Metatropic dwarfism
  Pierre-Robin syndrome
  Rubella, congenital
  Short limb-polydactyly syndromes
  Small-for-gestational-age neonate
  Spondyloepiphyseal dysplasia
  Thanatophoric dwarfism
  Trisomy 18
  Trisomy 21
B. Accelerated osseous maturation in the neonate
  Asphyxiating thoracic dysplasia
  Beckwith-Wiedeman syndrome
  Chondroectodermal dysplasia
  Diastrophic dwarfism
  Hyperthyroidism
  Marshall syndrome
  Typus edinburgenesis
  Weaver syndrome
C. Dysharmonic osseous maturation in the neonate
  Asphyxiating thoracic dystrophy
  Chondroectodermal dysplasia
  Diastrophic dwarfism
  Short limb-polydactyly syndromes

Source: From Kuhns LR, Finnstrom O. New standards of ossification of the newborn. Radiology 1976;119:655–660, with permission.

infection, etc., and in this regard, it has been demonstrated that hemopoietic bone marrow begins to change to fatty bone marrow at approximately 3 months of age (1, 2). This change occurs in the epiphyses first, next in the diaphyses, and then in the proximal and distal metaphyses of the long bones. Detailed dissertations on the normal appearance of bone marrow in the long bones are available in a number of articles on the subject (1–6).

REFERENCES

1. Waitches G, Zawin JK, Posnanski AK. Sequence and rate of bone marrow conversion in the femora of children as seen on MR imaging: are accepted standards accurate? AJR 1994;162:1399–1406.
2. Zawin JK, Jaramillo D. Conversion of bone marrow in the humerus, sternum, and clavicle: changes with age on MR images. Radiology 1993;188:159–164.
3. Jaramillo D, Laor T, Hoffer FA, et al. Epiphyseal marrow in infancy: MR imaging. Radiology 1991;180:809–812.
4. Sebag GH, Dubois J, Tabet M, et al. Pediatric spinal bone marrow: assessment of normal age-related changes in the MRI appearance. Pediatr Radiol 1993;23:515–518.
5. Taccone A, Oddone M, Dell'Acqua A, et al. MRI "road-map" of normal age-related bone marrow. II. Thorax, pelvis, and extremities. Pediatr Radiol 1995;25:596–606.
6. Taccone A, Oddone M, Occhi M, et al. MRI "road-map" of normal age-related bone marrow. I. Cranial bone and spine. Pediatr Radiol 1995;25:588–595.

Long Bones

Ossified portions of the long bones in neonates represent a miniature configuration of the corresponding bones in the older child. Most epiphyseal centers are not fully ossified, and thus wide areas of cartilage separate the ends of the long bones at the various joints. Nutrient foramina and grooves

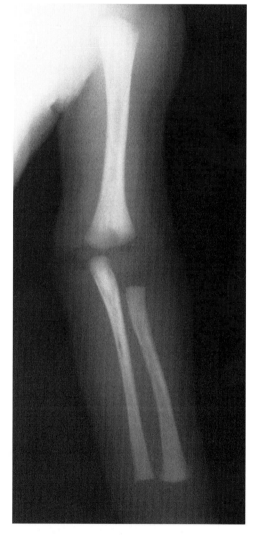

FIGURE 6.4. Normal upper extremity. Note that no ossification centers are present in the wrist or elbow. This is usual in the neonate. The oblique radiolucent line in the middle of the humerus is a vascular groove.

are often prominent, especially in the femurs, tibiae, and humeri (Figs. 6.1 and 6.4). These grooves should not be misinterpreted for fractures or other lesions. In addition, the radius and ulna in some infants tend to have a somewhat wavy and undulating configuration (Fig. 6.5A). This is an entirely normal appearance in the newborn and young infant and disappears with age. In many infants, with extension of the arms, the normal bicipital groove on the inner aspect of the proximal humerus can be seen (Fig. 6.5B).

Some infants may show minimal beaking or fragmentation at the edge of the metaphyses (Fig. 6.6). This finding also is considered a normal variation and may be difficult to differentiate from the beaking seen with child abuse (1). The distinction, however, is important, and distinction can be made on the basis of no other findings of child abuse, no abnormality on nuclear scintigraphy, and simply being aware of the phenomenon. The long bones also are frequently used in evaluating bone dysplasias and growth disturbances; in this regard, standards for normal long bone length ratios in children are available (2).

As the long bones and other bones of the body grow from infancy through older childhood, considerable change in their configuration occurs. Generally, this poses little problem in diagnosis of disease entities, but still one should be familiar with these changes in configuration. The subject is too extensive to be included in this text but is amply dealt with in the textbook on normal development by Keats and Smith (3).

Evaluation of the joints can be accomplished with plain films and ultrasonography, and ultrasound is used extensively in the evaluation of the hip joint. Ultrasonography also is used to analyze other joints. MRI is also useful in evaluating joint disease and is used most extensively in the knees. It is excellent for soft tissue assessment and, as mentioned earlier, for evaluation of the bone marrow. Specific points relating to these findings are discussed throughout this chapter.

Pelvis and Hips

The pelvic bones are well ossified at birth, and the iliac bones often show a normal, stellate-like radiating configuration of

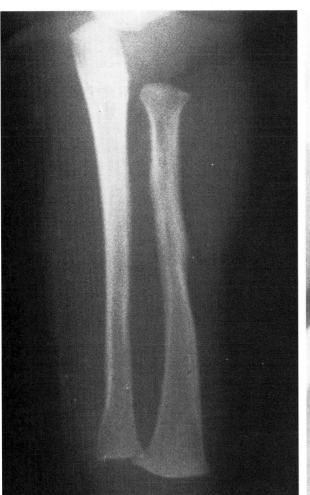
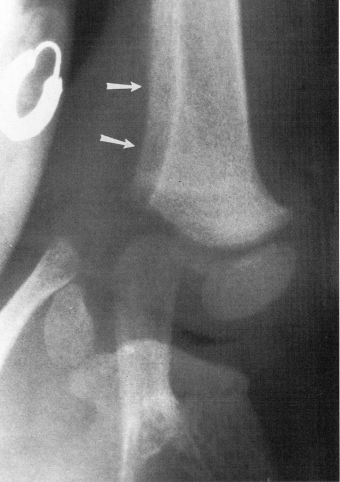

A

B

FIGURE 6.5. A. Normal forearm. Note that the cortex of the radius has a wavy appearance, a normal configuration not uncommonly seen in the neonate. **B. Normal humeral groove.** Note the normal groove (arrow) for the insertion of the biceps muscle. It is the site of muscle attachment. Often, it is best seen in this extended position of the humerus.

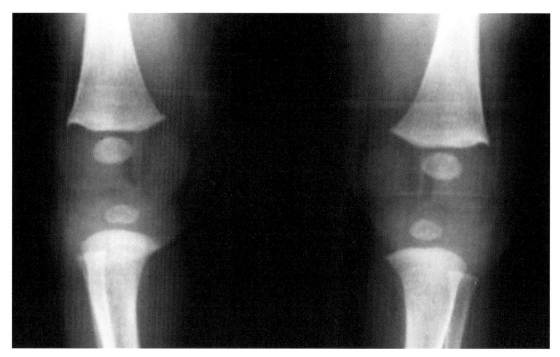

FIGURE 6.6. Normal metaphyseal beaking. Note pronounced beaks at the distal end of the femurs. These are within normal variation. Also note the well-developed distal femoral and proximal tibial epiphyses.

trabecular markings (Fig. 6.7A). The acetabular roofs also are well developed, and normal acetabular angles range from 20 to 30°. The cartilage bands between the incompletely ossified iliac, pubic, and ischial bones are prominent. Femoral head ossification centers are absent in the neonate but appear at approximately 2–6 months. The secondary ossification centers for the greater and lesser trochanters are not visualized in the neonate. In addition, premature infants frequently show failure of ossification of the pubic bones (Fig. 6.7B). In older patients, the symphysis pubis also often appears wider than expected because ossification is incomplete and cartilage is present (Fig. 6.8, A and B). In addition to this normal varia-

tion, the ischiopubic synchondrosis can normally appear quite bulky and suggest disease (Fig. 6.8, C and D).

The Clavicle

On many chest roentgenograms of newborn infants, the clavicle "appears" abnormal because it is relatively easy to distort its normal configuration by rotation of the chest or elevation of the shoulder. In many such cases, a midclavicular fracture or congenital pseudoarthrosis is erroneously suggested (Fig. 6.9). Familiarity with this phenomenon and a repeat roentgenogram readily clear any confusion.

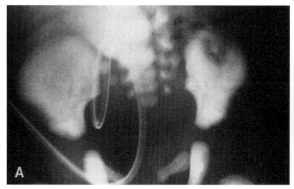
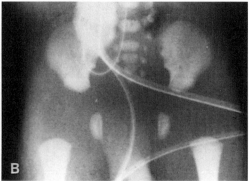

FIGURE 6.7. Pelvis. A. Normal pelvis. Note the stellate appearance of the iliac wings. Also note the ossification pattern of the ischia and pubic bones. **B. Premature infant.** Note that, in general, the bones are smaller. Also note that the pubic bones have not ossified. Only the ischia show ossification.

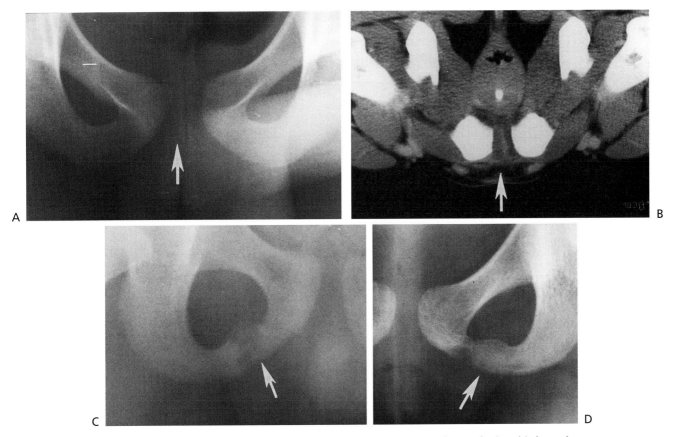

FIGURE 6.8. Pelvis: normal variations. A. Note the apparently wide symphysis pubis (arrow). This is normal. **B.** Another patient whose computed tomography demonstrates a normal wide symphysis pubis (arrow). Note the hypodense cartilage caps over the ossified pubic bones. **C.** Normal irregular ischiopubic synchondroses (arrows). **D.** Normal, lumpy-appearing ischiopubic synchondrosis (arrow) on the left.

The Sternum

The sternal segments are well ossified at birth and are best seen on lateral projection. They are rarely seen on frontal projection, except when the chest is rotated. In such cases, they appear as round bony structures (Fig. 6.10A) and are occasionally misinterpreted as representing pulmonary nodules. Normally, there are five sternal segments including the manubrium and xiphoid process; however, in many cases, the xiphoid process is incompletely ossified and only four centers are visualized. Bifid centers also are common (Fig. 6.10B).

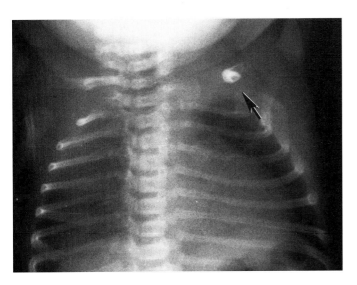

FIGURE 6.9. Clavicle pseudofracture. Left-sided rotation of the chest projects the left clavicle to suggest fracture or deformity (arrow). Also note how it distorts the ribs.

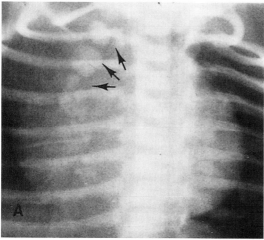

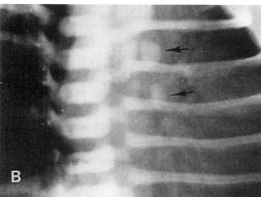

FIGURE 6.10. Normal sternal segments. A. Right-sided rotation of the chest projects the normal round sternal segments over the right lung (arrows). When this occurs, the configuration may suggest pulmonary nodules. **B.** The same phenomenon has occurred with rotation to the left, but, in addition, note the bifid sternal segments (arrows).

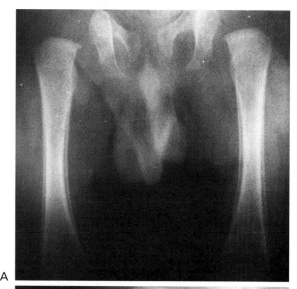

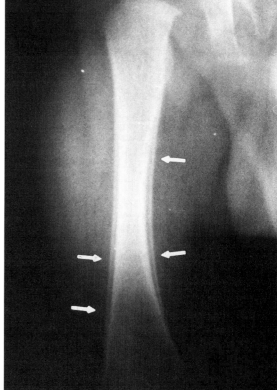

FIGURE 6.12. Normal periosteal new bone. A. Note characteristic normal periosteal new bone being layered along the femurs. Such periosteal new bone usually is most pronounced in the femurs, tibiae, and humeri. It is most commonly seen at approximately 3 months of age. **B.** Magnified view of the periosteal new bone deposition (arrows). Note that it lies along the diaphysis and stops short of the metaphysis.

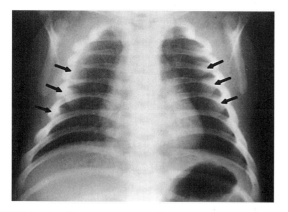

FIGURE 6.11. Ribs: exaggerated cupping. Note exaggerated cupping of the anterior aspect of the ribs (arrows). Such cupping is normal and should not be misinterpreted for pathologic cupping seen with a variety of metabolic and bony dysplastic conditions.

The Ribs

In premature infants, the ribs often are extremely thin and fragile, and thinning may be more pronounced posteriorly. Anteriorly, normal cupping of the ribs often is marked (Fig. 6.11) in both premature and full-term infants and should not be misinterpreted for that seen with conditions such as rickets or certain bony dysplasias.

Osteosclerosis of the Newborn

Some newborn infants demonstrate extremely dense and sclerotic bones. Neonatal bones are composed of more spongiosa than those of older infants; in some cases, this causes the bones to become denser and the cortices thicker than in the usual neonate. The changes usually are widespread but disappear within a few weeks; overall, the findings usually are considered normal. The uninitiated, however, often will first consider osteopetrosis or intrauterine infection in these infants.

Normal Periosteal New Bone Formation

Many infants, especially prematures, show normal periosteal new bone formation along the long bones of the extremities (Fig. 6.12). **This is the only time in life that periosteal new bone formation is normal, and its formation is most pronounced in the second and third months of life.** Thereafter, it slowly becomes incorporated into the diaphysis. It has been documented in 35–50% of infants in this age group (4) and is generally considered a reflection of exuberant bone growth at this age.

Characteristically, this normal periosteal new bone layers along the inner (more common) and outer aspects of the midshafts of the long bones and most frequently involves the femurs, humeri, and tibiae. It is less commonly seen in the bones of the forearm. Progressive films show normal incorporation of the periosteal bone into the existing cortex. It is most important not to mistake these changes for those of infantile cortical hyperostosis (Caffey's disease), congenital lues, trauma, battered child syndrome, or vitamin deficiency or excess. This is accomplished by noting that when normal new bone deposition is present, it stops short of the metaphysis (Fig. 6.12). When it is pathologic, there is usually some destructive or traumatic abnormality involving the metaphysis, and the periosteal new bone extends down to the epiphyseal line.

Vacuum Joint

A vacuum joint phenomenon can be produced in various joints when excessive stress is applied to the extremity (Fig. 6.13A). This is an entirely normal finding and can also be seen in hypotonic infants (Fig. 6.13B). The airspace is believed by some to represent a vacuum, while others favor nitrogen or water vapor.

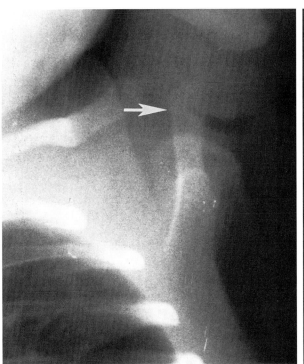 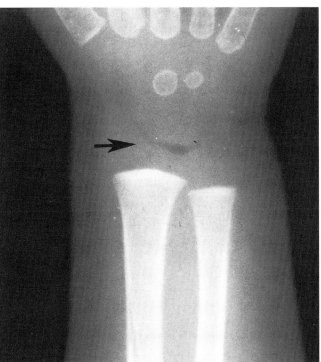

A   B

FIGURE 6.13. Vacuum joint phenomenon. A. Traction of humerus produces a crescent-shaped vacuum joint in the shoulder (arrow). **B.** Infant with trisomy 21, somewhat hypotonic, showing vacuum joint phenomenon in the wrist (arrow).

REFERENCES

1. Kleinman PK, Belanger PL, Karellas A, et al. Pictorial essay. Normal metaphyseal radiologic variants not to be confused with findings of infant abuse. AJR 1991;156:781–783.
2. Robinow M, Chumlea WC. Standards for limb bone length ratios in children. Radiology 1982;143:433–436.
3. Keats TE, Smith TH. An atlas of normal developmental roentgen anatomy. 2nd ed. Chicago: Year Book Medical Publishers, 1988.
4. Shopfner CE. Periosteal bone growth in normal infants: a preliminary report. AJR 1966;97:154–163.

CONGENITAL ABNORMALITIES

Hypoplasia and Aplasia

One or more of the bones of the extremities can be hypoplastic or entirely absent. The general term "phocomelia" is applied to the condition, and thalidomide-induced malformation was the classic example of this type of bony abnormality. In terms of these abnormalities, McCredie (1) suggested that the problem lies in an insult to the neural crest early in fetal life. This produces a peripheral neuropathy, which subsequently leads to underdevelopment of the involved bones and soft tissues. Supporting this hypothesis is the fact that one can correlate the various patterns of hypoplasia or aplasia with sensory nerve distribution (1).

The femur and radius are the most commonly involved bones; thereafter, in decreasing order, one can see involvement of the fibula (2), ulna, humerus, and tibia. Multiple involvement is not uncommon, and absence of the radius, or at least hypoplasia of the radius, and the first and second digits often occurs in Holt-Oram syndrome, Poland's syndrome, and Fanconi's anemia. Hypoplasia of this portion of the forearm is often referred to as the "radial ray syndrome." Underdevelopment of the lower extremities is seen in the caudal regression syndrome. Isolated hypoplasia of the glenoid fossa also can occur (3), and although absence or hypoplasia of the patella is characteristic of nail-patella syndrome, absence can occur as an isolated phenomenon on a familial basis (4).

Roentgenographically, these hypoplastic bones also often show abnormal curvature (bowing) and thickening of the cortex along the inner aspect of the curve. When the **fibula is absent or hypoplastic, associated anterior bowing**

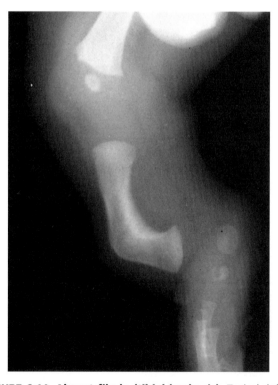

FIGURE 6.14. Absent fibula (tibial kyphosis). Typical deformity of the tibia associated with absence of the fibula. A vestige of the fibula, in the form of a fibrous band, attaches to the angulated portion of the tibia. Note the overlying soft tissue bulge.

Type	Radiological Description
1a	• Tibia not seen • Hypoplastic lower femoral epiphysis
1b	• Tibia not seen • Normal lower femoral epiphysis
2	• Distal tibia not seen
3	• Proximal tibia not seen
4	• Diastasis

FIGURE 6.15. Absent tibia with intact fibula: various types. Four types of deformity are identifiable radiographically. This typing facilitates the type of surgical treatment to be undertaken. (Modified from Jones D, Barnes J, Lloyd-Roberts GC. Congenital aplasia and dysplasia of the tibia with intact fibula. J Bone Joint Surg 1978;60:31–39).

(kyphosis) and dysplasia of the tibia occur. With tibial kyphosis, dimpling or pitting of the skin over the bowed tibia, clubfoot deformity, and absence of the lateral ray of the foot also are party to the problem (Fig. 6.14). The ipsilateral femur often also is underdeveloped, and a fibrous band, replacing the fibula, extends to the point of tibial kyphosis. Resection of this band is believed to retard further deformity.

Dysplasia or aplasia of the tibia also can occur with an intact fibula. Furthermore, tibiofibular diastasis (5–7) can occur as part of this anomaly. Associated claw hand deformity has also been documented (8). Diagrammatic representations of these abnormalities are presented in Fig. 6.15, and some of them are illustrated in Fig. 6.16.

REFERENCES

1. McCredie J. Segmental embryonic peripheral neuropathy. Pediatr Radiol 1975;3:163–168.
2. Gupta AK, Berry M, Verma IC. Congenital absence of both fibulae in four siblings. Pediatr Radiol 1994;24:220–221.
3. Kozlowski K, Scougall J. Congenital bilateral glenoid hypoplasia: a report of four cases. Br J Radiol 1987;60:705–706.
4. St. Braun H. Familial aplasia or hypoplasia of the patella. Clin Genet 1978;13:350.
5. Adamsbaum C, Kalifa G, Seringe R, et al. Minor tibial duplication: a new cause of congenital bowing of the tibia. Pediatr Radiol 1991;21:185–188.
6. Garbarino JL, Clancy M, Jarcke HT, et al. Congenital diastasis of the inferior tibiofibular joint: a review of the literature and report of two cases. J Pediatr Orthop 1985;5:225–228.

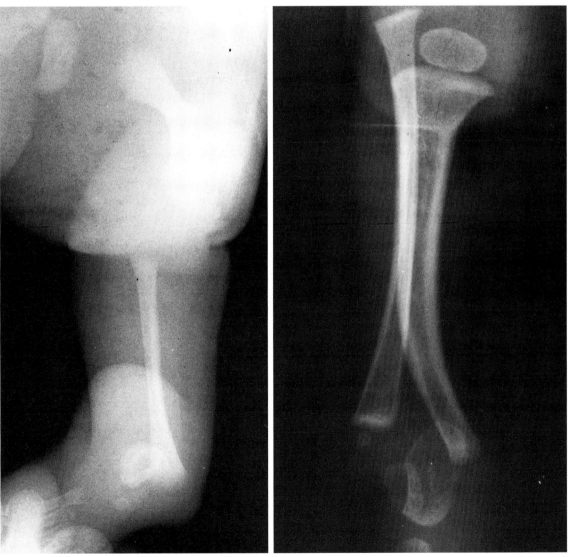

A   B

FIGURE 6.16. Absent tibia with intact fibula. A. Type 1A. Note absence of the tibia but presence of the fibula. A clubfoot deformity is present, and there is underdevelopment of the bones of the foot. The femur also is hypoplastic, thickened, and bowed. The distal femoral epiphysis is not visualized. **B. Type 4.** Another patient with hypoplasia and dysplasia of the tibia associated with diastasis of the distal tibia and fibula. This patient also had a clubfoot deformity.

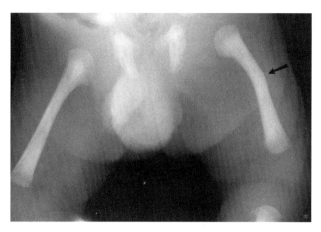

FIGURE 6.17. Bowing of femur. Note the bowed, slightly angulated, and kyphotic (arrow) right femur.

7. Onimus M, Laurain JM, Picard F. Congenital diastasis of the inferior tibiofibular joint. J Pediatr Orthop 1990;10:172–176.
8. Sener RN, Isikan E, Diren HB, et al. Bilateral split-hand with bilateral tibial aplasia. Pediatr Radiol 1989;19:258–260.

Bowing of Long Bones in Neonates

Long bones can be bowed as a result of faulty intrauterine positioning. Eventually, these straighten. However, in other cases, focal bowing with angulation or kyphosis of a long

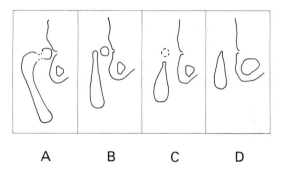

FIGURE 6.18. Proximal focal femoral deficiency: various types. Type A. Even though ossification of the femoral neck may not be visible in the neonate, eventual ossification occurs. The femoral head develops relatively normally, and the acetabular roof is well formed. A coxa vara deformity is present. **Type B.** A femoral head is present, and the acetabular roof is reasonably well formed. A defect between the shaft of the femur and femoral neck persists, however, and the hip is unstable. The upper femoral shaft usually is bulbous. **Type C.** A femoral head does not develop or is vestigial. The proximal end of the underdeveloped femur is bulbous or clubbed, and the acetabular roof is poorly developed. The hip is extremely unstable. **Type D.** A "pencil-sharpened" type of deformity of the femur is present. There is no femoral head, the acetabular roof is totally dysplastic, and the hip is completely unstable. Types C and D are variations of one another. (Modified from Aitken GT. Proximal femoral focal deficiency. Definition, classification, and management. In: Aitken GT, ed. Proximal femoral focal deficiency, a congenital anomaly: a symposium. Washington, D.C.: National Academy of Sciences, 1968).

bone such as the femur can be seen (Fig. 6.17). In these cases, the bone tends to remain short.

Proximal Focal Femoral Deficiency

Hypoplasia or underdevelopment of the upper femur is referred to as "proximal focal femoral deficiency" (1, 2). In this condition, a variable portion of the upper part of the femur is underdeveloped (Fig. 6.18), and often there is associated hypoplasia or absence of the fibula and undergrowth of the tibia. In more severe cases, the proximal end of the remaining femoral shaft has a "pencil-sharpened" appearance (Fig. 6.19A). The femoral head does not develop in the more severe cases, but some indication of whether it is present can be inferred by the degree of development of the acetabular roof (Fig. 6.19). In some cases, however, arthrography is required to demonstrate its presence, but currently, ultrasonography (Fig. 6.20) or MRI (3) is preferred.

In its mildest form, proximal focal femoral deficiency is manifest in a condition referred to as "congenital infantile coxa vara" (4). In such cases, the femoral neck is underdeveloped and fibrous union is present between the head and shaft (Fig. 6.21). The coxa vara deformity is profound, and early identification is necessary for proper surgical correction. The condition often goes undetected, however, until the patient begins to walk.

Distal femoral deficiency also can occur (5) but usually is associated with hypoplasias and anomalies of the bones below the knee. For a complete dissertation and classification of femoral and associated lower limb hypoplasias, refer to the work by Pappas (6).

REFERENCES

1. Levinson ED, Ozonoff MB, Royen PM. Proximal femoral focal deficiency (PFFD). Radiology 1977;125:197–204.
2. Sanpera I Jr, Sparks LT. Proximal femoral focal deficiency: does a radiologic classification exist? J Pediatr Orthop 1994;14:34–38.
3. Grissom LE, Harcke HT. Sonography in congenital deficiency of the femur. J Pediatr Orthop 1994;14:29–33.
4. Pavlov H, Goldman AB, Freiberger RH. Infantile coxa vara. Radiology 1980;135:631–640.
5. Kalamchi A, Cowell HR, Kim KI. Congenital deficiency of the femur. J Pediatr Orthop 1985;5:129–134.
6. Pappas AM. Congenital abnormalities of the femur and related lower extremity malformations: classification and treatment. J Pediatr Orthop 1983;3:45–60.

Supernumerary and Duplicated Digits and Symphalangism

Supernumerary digits most often occur sporadically, while duplicated digits (polydactyly) characteristically are seen in the Ellis-van Creveld and asphyxiating thoracic dystrophy syndromes. Symphalangism can be seen as an isolated anomaly or as part of Poland's syndrome, Apert's syndrome, and other forms of acrocephalosyndactyly.

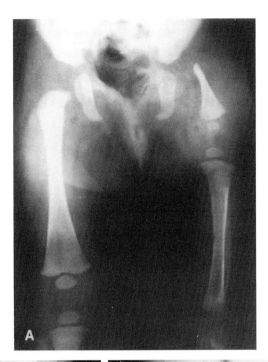

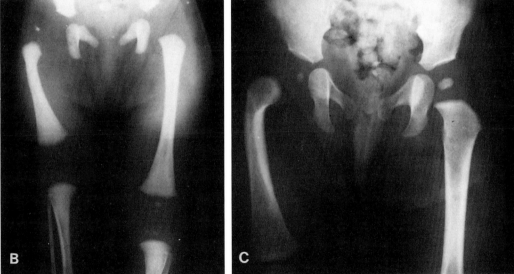

FIGURE 6.19. Proximal focal femoral deficiency. A. Type D. Note the extremely short left femur and typical "pencil-sharpened" deformity. The acetabular roof is poorly developed, and there appears to be a pseudoacetabulum. Note that the fibula is absent and that the tibia is slightly underdeveloped. **B. Type B.** The right femur in this newborn infant is short and appears dislocated. The upper end is bulbous. Note, however, that the acetabular roof is reasonably well developed. This should suggest the presence of an unossified femoral capital epiphysis. Also note that the fibula, although present, is thin and underdeveloped. The tibia also is underdeveloped, and there is delayed appearance of the epiphyseal ossification centers around the knee. **C.** A few months later, note that the femoral head on the right is ossifying and is well within the acetabulum. Also note a pronounced coxa vara deformity and marked thickening along the inner aspect of the femur.

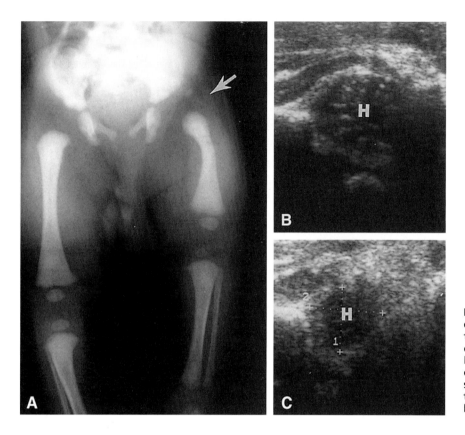

FIGURE 6.20. Proximal focal femoral deficiency: use of ultrasound. A. Note typical changes of proximal focal femoral deficiency on the left (arrow). The cartilaginous femoral head is not visible on either side. **B.** Normal right side demonstrates a normal femoral head (H). **C.** On the left side, a femoral head (H) is present, but it is small and underdeveloped.

Synostoses and Coalitions

Synostoses most commonly occur in the forearm and foot, and some can produce significant limitation of motion. Ankyloses were common in the thalidomide era, and it was suggested that, as with bony aplasia in general, the underlying problem was an embryonic peripheral

neuropathy (1). Radioulnar synostoses (Fig. 6.22) commonly are seen with many syndromes, including sex chromatin abnormalities. Fusion of the various carpal bones, often in massive form, occurs in the Ellis-van Creveld syndrome. Coalition of the carpal bones is much more common on an isolated basis, however, and in this regard, the most commonly involved bones are the tri-

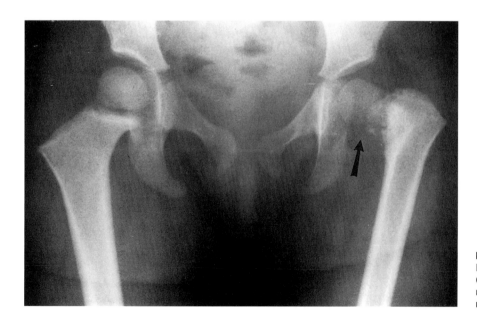

FIGURE 6.21. Congenital coxa vara. Note the defect in the left femoral neck (arrow). It results in shortening of the neck and an associated coxa vara deformity.

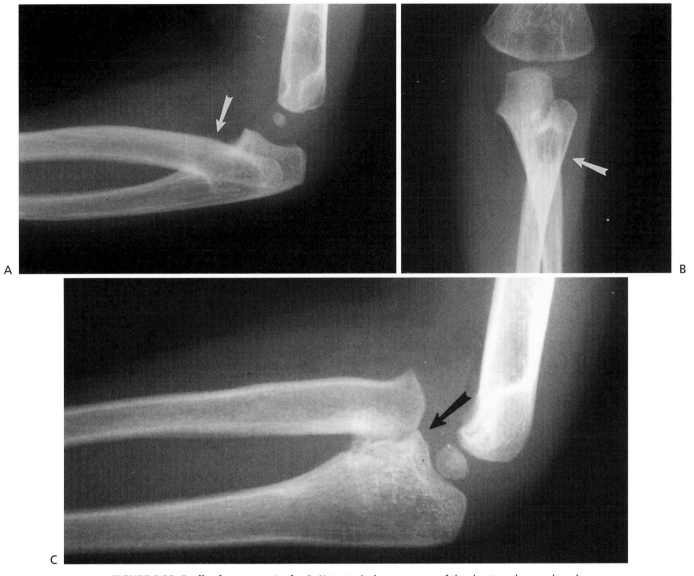

FIGURE 6.22. Radioulnar synostosis. A. Note typical appearance of the shortened, curved, and fused proximal radius (arrow) on lateral view. **B.** On frontal view, similar findings (arrow) are seen. **C.** Lesser degree of synostosis (arrow) in another patient.

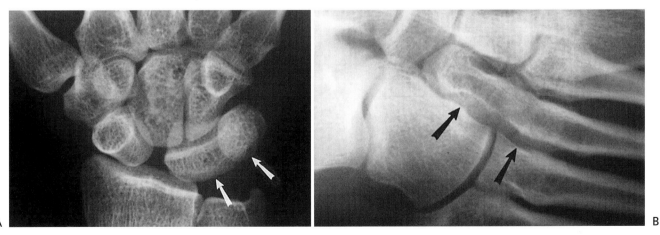

FIGURE 6.23. Carpal and tarsal coalition. A. Note coalition of the lunate and triquetral bones (arrows). The space between the lunate and navicular bone has increased, and the navicular bone appears rotated. **B. Tarsal-metacarpal coalition.** Note coalition of the third metatarsal and lateral cuneiform (arrows). The middle and medial cuneiform bones also have fused into a single cuboid block.

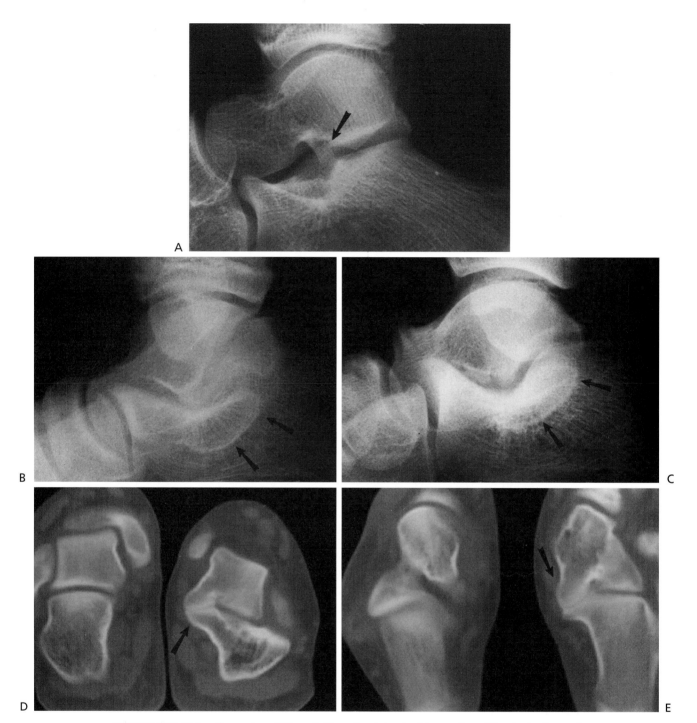

FIGURE 6.24. Talocalcaneal coalition. A. There is minimal evidence of coalition in the form of a small bony bar (arrow). **B.** In this patient, more advanced coalition results in disruption of the talocalcaneal joint and an early "C sign" (arrows). **C.** Another patient with a more profound "C sign" (arrows). **D.** Computed tomography study demonstrates typical talocalcaneal bony coalition (arrow). Compare with the normal side. **E.** Sagittal plane demonstrates the same bony coalition (arrow).

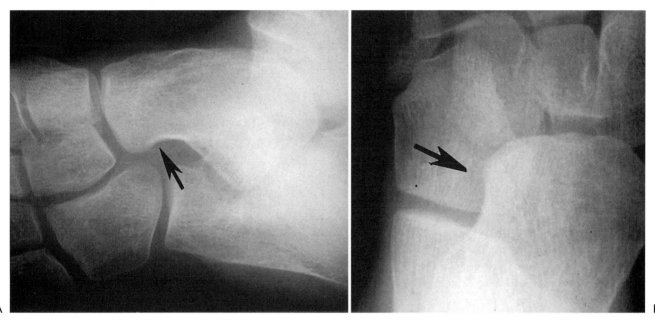

A

B

FIGURE 6.25. Talonavicular coalition. A. Note the elongated talus, which has united with the navicular bone (arrow). The cuneiforms are seen anterior to the coalition. **B.** Anteroposterior view demonstrates the same talonavicular coalition (arrow) into a single bone. The cuneiforms are seen more distally.

quetral and lunate (Fig. 6.23A). Fusion of these two bones often results in an unusually wide space between the scaphoid and lunate bones (2). Depending on the specific bones involved, limitation of motion may or may not be present. Carpometacarpal and tarsometatarsal coalitions also can occur (Fig. 6.23B).

In the foot, fusion most commonly occurs between the calcaneus and talus (Fig. 6.24) and the calcaneus and navicular (Fig. 6.25). However, symptomatic talonavicular fusion also can occur (3) (Fig. 6.26). Often, tarsal coalitions lead to congenital spastic flatfoot. Computed tomography (CT) (4) is best for the demonstration of these conditions, but they also can be seen on plain films where deformed tarsal bones provide clues for the diagnosis. With talocalcaneal or so-called "subtalar" coalition, an early bar often can be visualized (Fig. 6.24A); later on, a so-called "C sign" (5) is seen (Fig. 6.24, B and C). CT studies, as with all coalitions, more vividly demonstrate the abnormality (Fig. 6.24, D and E). With calcaneonavicular coalitions, the anterior end of the calcaneus becomes tapered (Fig. 6.26A), resulting in the so-called "anteater sign" (6). Other findings consist of medial wedging of the navicular bone (Fig. 6.26C), and the abnormality is usually clearly seen on oblique views (Fig. 6.26D). CT, of course, also can be employed.

Finally, when fusion of bones occurs across a joint, for example, elbow ankylosis (7), the deformity can be profound

and limitation of motion severe (Fig. 6.27). In addition, multiple coalitions in the hands and feet (8) also can occur.

REFERENCES

1. McCredie J. Congenital fusion of bones: radiology, embryology, and pathogenesis. Clin Radiol 1975;26:47–51.
2. Metz VM, Schimmerl SM, Gilula LA, et al. Wide scapholunate joint space in lunotriquetral coalition: a normal variant? Radiology 1993;188:557–559.
3. Doyle SM, Kumar SJ. Symptomatic talonavicular coalition. J Pediatr Orthop 1999;19:508–510.
4. Wechsler RJ, Schweitzer ME, Deely DM, et al. Tarsal coalition: depiction and characterization with CT and MR imaging. Radiology 1994;193:447–452.
5. Lateur LM, Van Hoe LR, Van Ghillewe KV, et al. Subtalar coalition: diagnosis with the C sign on lateral radiographs of the ankle. Radiology 1994;193:847–851.
6. Oestreich AE, Mize WA, Crawford AH, et al. The "anteater nose": a direct sign of calcaneonavicular coalition on the lateral radiograph. J Pediatr Orthop 1987;7:709–711.
7. Jocobsen ST, Crawford AH. Humeroradial synostosis. J Pediatr Orthop 1983;3:96–98.
8. Clark DM. Multiple tarsal coalitions in the same foot. Pediatr Orthop 1997;17:777–780.

Accessory Limb with Spina Bifida

In this condition, an accessory limb extends from the back of the infant and frequently is associated with spina bifida

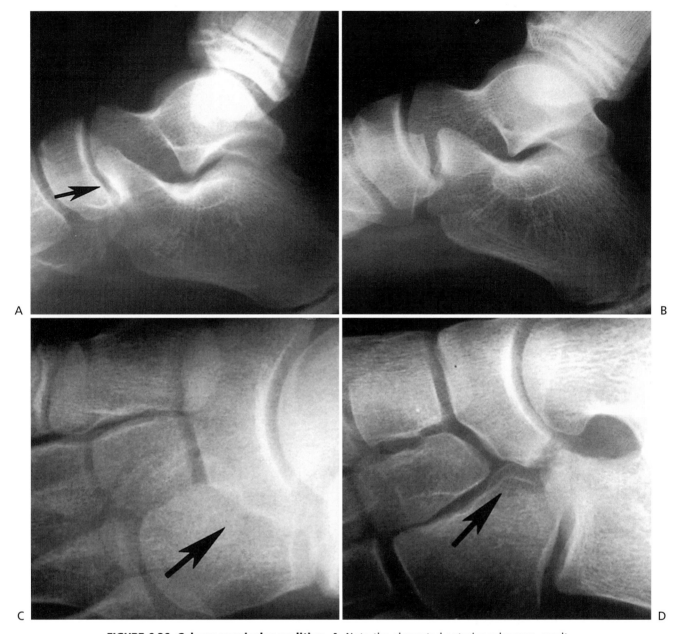

FIGURE 6.26. Calcaneonavicular coalition. A. Note the elongated anterior calcaneus, resulting in the so-called "anteater sign" (arrow). **B.** Normal side for comparison. **C.** Anteroposterior view demonstrates lateral wedging (arrow) of the navicular bone. **D.** Oblique view demonstrates fibrous and bony calcaneal navicular coalition (arrow).

(1, 2). The condition is rare and believed to represent aborted twinning.

REFERENCES

1. Krisha A, Chadna S, Mishra NK, et al. Accessory limb associated with spina bifida. J Pediatr Surg 1989;24:604–606.
2. Chadha R, Bagga D, Malhoira CJ, et al. Accessory limb attached to the back. J Pediatr Surg 1993;28:1615–1617.

Congenital Kyphoscoliosis and Pseudoarthrosis of the Tibia and Fibula

There are two entities under this broad umbrella, and they often are somewhat erroneously intertwined. It is important to differentiate congenital kyphoscoliosis and pseudoarthrosis of the tibia and fibula because only one condition is predisposed to development of congenital pseudoarthrosis of the tibia and fibula. In those patients with pseudoarthrosis, the problem often is very refractory (1) and gen-

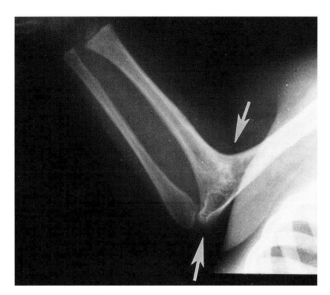

FIGURE 6.27. Ankylosis of the elbow. Note fusion of the humerus and radius (arrows).

erally part of the problem of neurofibromatosis. Bone grafting may be attempted (2) but has had borderline success. More recently, treatment with the Ilizarov device has been advocated (3–5).

In differentiating these conditions, one should note the direction of curvature of the involved bones. In pseudoarthrosis, there is anterolateral bending, while in nonpseudoarthrosis, bending is posteromedial. In some infants, rare anteromedial bowing is self-limiting (6) (Fig. 6.28). In the other infants, however, there seems to be an actual growth aberration, leading to more persistent curvature and, unfortunately, shortening of the involved leg (7). The roentgenographic findings are rather characteristic and show thickening of the cortex along the inner aspect and widening and shortening of the involved bones (Fig. 6.29, A and B). Clubfoot deformity commonly is associated, but no dysplastic changes in the long bone shafts are seen. This is important to note because lack of dysplasia signifies that pseudoarthrosis will not develop.

When anterolateral bending of the fibula and tibia is seen (Fig. 6.29, C–E), one should think of neurofibromatosis. It is this type of kyphoscoliosis that results in pseudoarthrosis. In these patients, there is a basic mes-

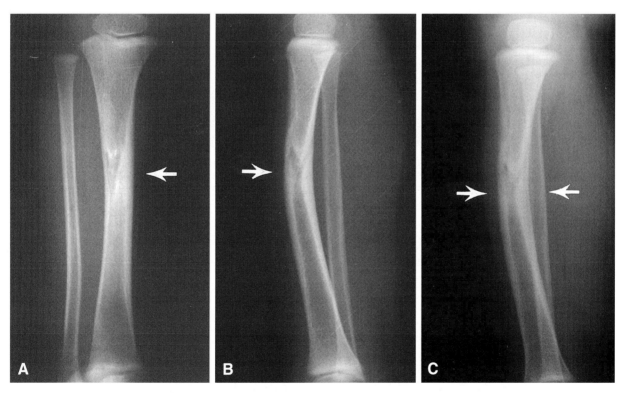

FIGURE 6.28. Self-limiting kyphoscoliosis of the tibia. A. Note dysplastic changes on frontal view (arrow). **B.** Lateral view demonstrates anterior bowing of the tibia. Dysplastic changes (arrow) also are present. **C.** Six months later, the degree of bowing is less and remodeling is occurring at the site of bending (arrows).

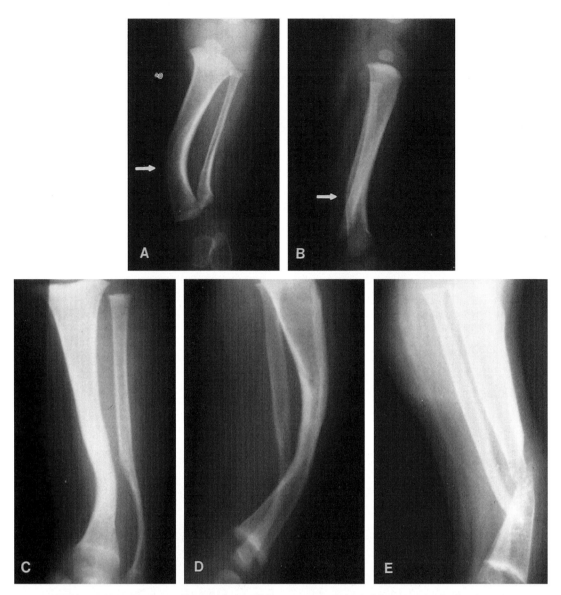

FIGURE 6.29. A. Kyphoscoliosis of the tibia: nonpseudoarthritic type. Typically, there is medial angulation of the tibia and fibula (arrow). These bones also are shortened, and the cortex along the inner aspect of the curve is thickened. The medullary canals show no dysplastic changes, however. **B.** Lateral view demonstrating typical posterior angulation (arrow). Asymmetric thickening of the cortex is caused by abnormal stresses. **C. Kyphoscoliosis of the tibia: pseudoarthritic type.** Typical lateral angulation and dysplastic changes in the distal tibia and fibula. Note that the bones are thin and abnormally formed at the site of curvature. **D.** Classic anterior bowing deformity and dysplastic changes in the same bones. **E.** Same patient when older. Note the development of characteristic pseudoarthrosis of the tibia and fibula. This patient had neurofibromatosis.

enchymal defect in the formation of the tibia and fibula, and dysplastic changes, in association with curvature abnormalities, are seen. These changes consist of thinning of the diaphysis of the bone and eventual resorption of the bone to produce a pseudoarthrosis (Fig. 6.29E).

Anterior bending of the tibia (kyphosis) with thickening and shortening of the shaft also occurs with absence of the fibula (see Fig. 6.14). Although some include this condition with congenital kyphoscoliosis of the tibia, its only resemblance is that the tibia is bent.

REFERENCES

1. Traub JA, O'Connor Q, Masso PD. Congenital pseudoarthrosis of the tibia: a retrospective review. J Pediatr Orthop 1999;19:735–738.

2. Coleman SS, Coleman DA. Congenital pseudoarthrosis of the tibia: treatment by transfer of the ipsilateral fibula with vascular pedicle. J Pediatr Orthop 1994;14:156–160.

3. Boero S, Catagni M, Donzelli O, et al. Congenital pseudoarthrosis of the tibia associated with neurofibromatosis—1: treatment with Ilizarov's device. J Pediatr Orthop 1997;17:675–684.

4. Ghanem I, Damsin JP, Carlioz H. Ilizarov technique in the treatment of congenital pseudoarthrosis of the tibia. J Pediatr Orthop 1997;17:685–690.

5. Guidera KJ, Raney EM, Ganey T, et al. Ilizarov treatment of congenital pseudoarthroses of the tibia. J Pediatr Orthop 1997;17: 668–674.

6. Tuncay IC, Johnston CE II, Birch JG. Spontaneous resolution of congenital anterolateral bowing of the tibia. J Pediatr Orthop 1994;14:599–602.

7. Pappas AM. Congenital posteromedial bowing of the tibia and fibula. J Pediatr Orthop 1984;4:525–531.

Congenital Pseudoarthrosis of the Radius and Ulna

Although uncommon, pseudoarthroses of both the radius and ulna occurs (1–3). The roentgenographic appearance is similar to that seen with congenital pseudoarthrosis of the tibia and fibula, and these cases also may represent cases of neurofibromatosis (2). Roentgenographically, the bone is dysplastic and thinned in the area where frank pseudoarthrosis develops (Fig. 6.30).

REFERENCES

1. Bell DF. Congenital forearm pseudoarthrosis: report of six cases and review of the literature. J Pediatr Orthop 1989;9:438–443.

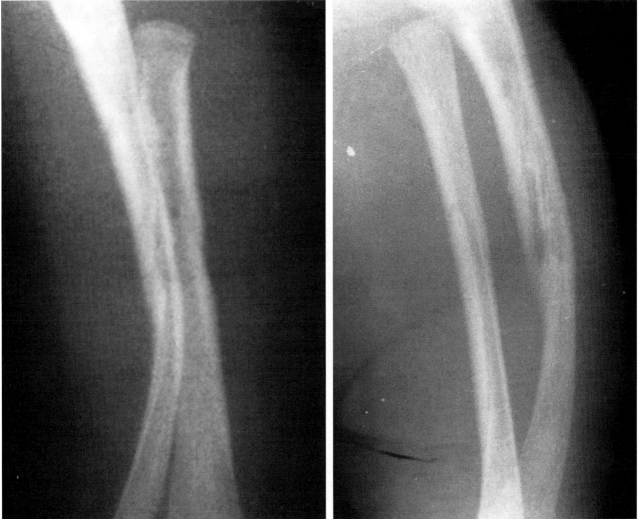

A   B

FIGURE 6.30. Congenital pseudoarthrosis of the forearm. A and B. Note dysplasia and thinning of the midshaft of the ulna. Later, as in the tibia, pseudoarthrosis may develop.

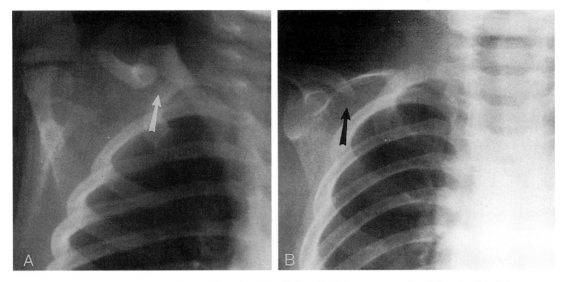

FIGURE 6.31. Congenital pseudoarthrosis of the clavicle. A. Note the defect in the right clavicle (arrow). The residual bony fragments show smooth, bulbous ends. **B.** Another patient with a bony defect (arrow) but with more pointed clavicular ends.

2. Herring JA, Roach JW. Congenital pseudoarthrosis of the radius. J Pediatr Orthop 1985;5:367–369.
3. Ostrowski DM, Filert RE, Waldstein G. Congenital pseudoarthrosis of the ulna: a report of two cases and a review of the literature. J Pediatr Orthop 1985;5:463–467.

Congenital Pseudoarthrosis of the Clavicle

Congenital pseudoarthrosis of the clavicle is rather uncommon and can be mistaken for the much more common

neonatal fracture of the clavicle. In congenital pseudoarthrosis, however, the opposing ends of the bony fragments are smooth, and there is no suggestion of callus formation (Fig. 6.31). Congenital pseudoarthrosis of the clavicle occurs almost exclusively on the right (1) but also can be seen bilaterally.

REFERENCE

1. Schnall SB, King JD, Marrero G. Congenital pseudoarthrosis of

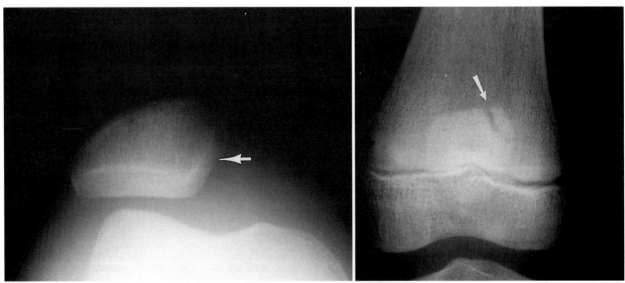

FIGURE 6.32. Patellar abnormalities. A. Dislocating patella. On this skyline view, note that the patella is laterally displaced (arrow). The intracondylar groove is shallow. **B. Bipartite patella.** Note the typical location of the bipartite patellar fragment (arrow).

the clavicle: a review of the literature and surgical results of six cases. J Pediatr Orthop 1988;8:316–321.

Congenital Pseudoarthrosis of the Fibula

Congenital pseudoarthrosis of the fibula usually occurs in conjunction with the same problem in the tibia. It also can occur alone but is a rare lesion (1).

REFERENCE

1. Monte AD, Donzelli O, Sudanese A, et al. Congenital pseudoarthrosis of the fibula. J Pediatr Orthop 1987;7:14–18.

Congenital Abnormalities of the Patella

The patella can be congenitally dislocated, often on an isolated basis. However, dislocation also is common in Larsen's syndrome and with underlying neurogenic disease. On an isolated congenital basis, congenital dislocation of the patella is associated with a tracking problem of the patella in the intercondylar groove. In such cases, the intercondylar groove is shallow, and the best way to demonstrate this abnormality is with skyline views of the patella (Fig. 6.32A). The patella also can be bipartite, with the second fragment usually being located in the upper outer quadrant (Fig. 6.32B). Tripartite patella is also seen but relatively uncommon.

Congenital absence of the patella can occur as an isolated phenomenon, but it is also part of the nail-patella syndrome. In the neonate and young infant, before patellar ossification occurs, absence of the patella can be determined with ultrasonography (Fig. 6.33) (1).

REFERENCE

1. Walker J, Rang M, Daneman A. Ultrasonography of the unossified patella in young children. J Pediatr Orthop 1991;11: 100–102.

Developmental Dysplasia of the Hip

Currently, the term "developmental dysplasia of the hip" is preferred over "congenital dislocation of the hip," although the two conditions are the same. This abnormality afflicts female infants at least five times as frequently as it does males. It is also much more common in breech-delivered infants (probably related to intrauterine position), but in this group, the female-to-male ratio is considerably reduced. Congenital dislocation of the hip also appears to be more common in certain Indian populations of North America and in other cultures where infant swaddling is common (1). With swaddling, the hips are bound in adduction, and this predisposes to dislocation.

Although in the past, acetabular dysplasia was considered the primary lesion in congenital dislocating hip, it is now believed to be secondary to dislocation. Dislocation is thought to be part of a generalized pelvic instability, secondary to excessive circulating maternal estrogens. In some infants, these hormones are evidently not metabolized at a normal rate, and their excessive accumulation leads to ligament and joint instability, most commonly manifesting in

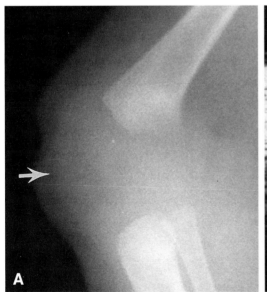
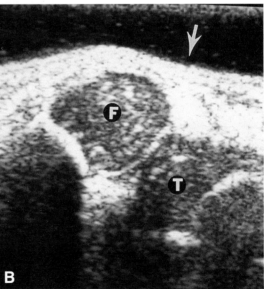

FIGURE 6.33. Absent patella. A. Note homogenicity of the soft tissues of the knee (arrow) and no suggestion of a cartilaginous primordium of the patella in this newborn infant. **B.** Ultrasonogram substantiates absence of the patella (arrow). The distal femoral epiphysis (F) is slightly anteriorly subluxed on the proximal tibial epiphysis (T).

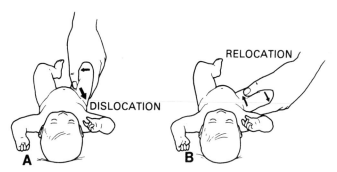

FIGURE 6.34. Ortolani maneuver (Barlow modification). A. First, the hip is dislocated by flexion and adduction of the hip. **B.** The leg then is abducted and internally rotated. This will cause the femoral head to ride over the acetabular roof and produce the jerk or click.

some degree of dislocation of the hips. Faulty intrauterine positioning that is, breech presentation, stretches the ligaments to produce a similar joint instability.

It is crucial to diagnose congenital dislocating hips as early as possible, for the earlier the diagnosis, the better the chance of a cure. Indeed, examination of the hips for possible dislocation should be a routine part of the physical examination in all newborn infants. Unfortunately, however, the findings of this examination frequently are unclear or confusing, primarily because of misinterpretation of benign tendon snaps (2) for the so-called "click of Ortolani." This "click" actually is a "clunk" that occurs when a dislocated hip is pulled back into the acetabulum. The Barlow maneuver (3), on the other hand, is designed to induce dislocation of the hip by abducting the flexed hip. At the same time, pressure is applied to the femur along its long axis so that if the hip is dislocatable, it will dislocate posterior to the acetabulum (Fig. 6.34A). The click or clunk actually occurs when the hip is reduced back into the acetabulum by the Ortolani maneuver (Fig. 6.34B). It results from the femoral head sliding over the acetabular edge. It should be recalled, however, that the click (clunk) generally does not develop until after 3 months of age because its presence depends on soft tissue contractures developing around the hip. Before this age, as alluded to earlier, most clicks are the result of fascial-tendon snaps and have nothing to do with dislocation. They are, in fact, benign (2).

Much has been written regarding the roentgenographic findings in congenital dislocating hip, but most of it deals with the well-established case. In such instances, the diag-

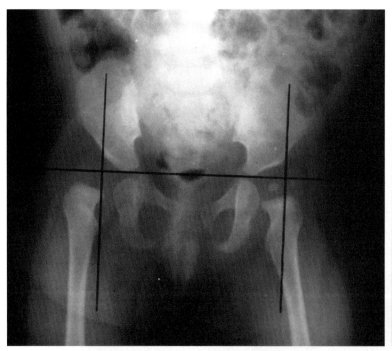

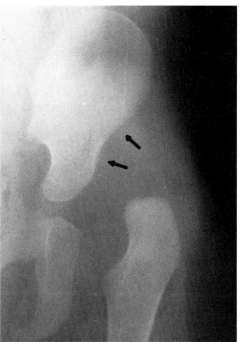

FIGURE 6.35. Congenital dislocating hip (developmental dysplasia of the hip). A. Infant beyond neonatal period. Classic findings show lateral displacement of the right femur, delayed ossification of the right femoral head, and increased angulation and underdevelopment of the right acetabular roof. On the left (normal side), the vertical line (Perkins line) runs through the center of the femur. On the right, the femur is displaced lateral to the line. **B. Chronic dislocating hip with pseudoacetabulum.** In this infant, note gross dislocation of the hip with outward and upward displacement. The femoral head is articulating with a pseudoacetabulum (arrows) above the true acetabulum.

nosis is not difficult to accomplish (Fig. 6.35A) because the femoral head shows delayed ossification, the femur is displaced laterally and upwardly, and any line that one wishes to apply is abnormal. Furthermore, the acetabular roof is more slanted than usual, the acetabulum is less cupped, and in very longstanding cases, a pseudoacetabulum develops just above the true acetabulum (Fig. 6.35B). As far as lines are concerned, the only one that I have found to be of use in the neonate is the vertical line of Perkins. This line is drawn vertically from the lateral edge of the acetabulum, and if it passes through the center of the upper femoral metaphysis, it is normal. If it passes medial to the innermost beak of the femoral metaphysis, it is abnormal, while if it touches the metaphysis, it is borderline (Fig. 6.36). In the past, the 45° abduction view was obtained to confirm dislocation (Fig. 6.36). When obtaining this view, it was important to have the hips positioned in 45° abduction and not in the frog-leg position. **Frog-leg positioning reduces dislocated hips.** Other plain film findings include increased steepness of the acetabular roof and loss of the normal acetabular cup. Increased steepness of the roof,

however, is not necessarily always predictive of dislocation (3). Indeed, some of these hips are stable, a point easily confirmed with dynamic ultrasound (4, 5), the current dominant imaging study for evaluation of developmental hip dysplasia.

Originally, with ultrasound, elaborate methods with measurement of various angles were devised (6, 7), but these quickly proved to be less popular than expected because of overlap between normal and abnormal (8). As a result, most settled for a simpler evaluation of the hips, and all generally now use some form of a dynamic study, which largely consists of applying posterior and abductive stresses to the hip and noting whether it subluxates or frankly dislocates (9, 10). These methods vary some from institution to institution, but we have settled on a relatively simple method, with examination primarily in the coronal plane. With this method, the patient is placed on a firm board and the hip first examined in the neutral extended or neutral flexed position (Fig. 6.37A). Thereafter, an attempt is made to dislocate the hip with the Barlow maneuver (Fig. 6.37B). In the resting position, the iliac wing is identified as a

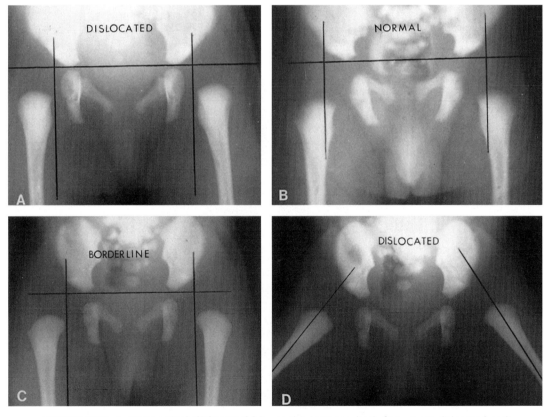

FIGURE 6.36. A. Congenital dislocated hip. In this instance, both femurs are dislocated and lie well lateral to the vertical line of Perkins. **B. Normal, for comparison.** Note that the inner thirds of the upper femurs are intersected by the vertical line of Perkins. **C. Congenital dislocated hip: borderline measurement.** Both upper femoral beaks are located just along the vertical line of Perkins. Clinically, these hips were dislocatable. **D. Andrén-von Rosen 45° abduction.** With abduction, the lines traveling through the midshaft of the femurs extend above the acetabular roofs. Normally, they would intersect the acetabular roofs.

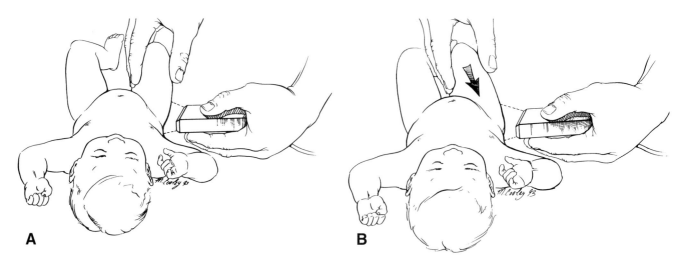

FIGURE 6.37. Ultrasonographic examination of the hip. A. With the patient recumbent and the hip flexed, the transducer is held in the coronal plane. **B.** With the Barlow maneuver (abduction and posterior pressure on the hip; arrow), an attempt is made to dislocate the hip. The transducer is still held in the coronal plane.

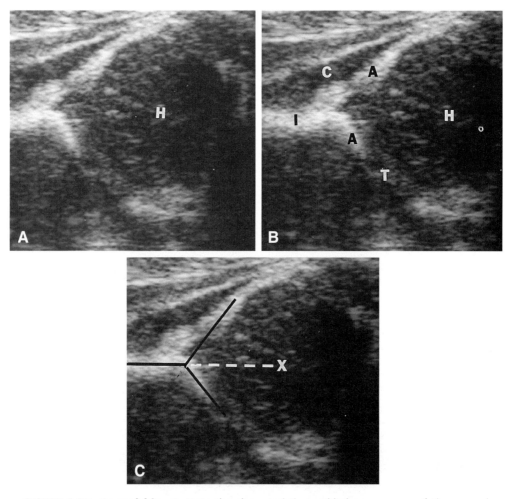

FIGURE 6.38. Normal hip. A. Note the characteristic speckled appearance of the normal femoral head (H). The iliac wing and acetabulum form an echogenic "Y" within which the femoral head is located. **B.** Same patient. Note the echogenic, straight line of the ischium (I). A, acetabulum; C, cartilaginous portion of the lateral acetabular roof; H, femoral head; T, triradiate cartilage. **C.** Black lines delineate the Y-shaped configuration of the iliac wing and acetabulum. A dashed white line extending the black line demarcating the iliac wing is seen to intersect the femoral head approximately through its center (X).

straight line joining the V-shaped lines of the acetabular roof. Together these structures assume a Y-shaped configuration (Fig. 6.38, A and B). No measurements are made, but note is made of where the white line of the iliac wing intersects the femoral head. Generally, it does so through, or near, the center of the head (Fig. 6.38C), and it has been suggested that if it intersects it lower, and less than 40% of the femoral head remains below the line (see Fig. 6.40D), abnormality should be suspected (10). However, over the years, these rigid criteria have been somewhat modified because in some patients, the acetabular roof may be steep (i.e., after breech positioning) and yet the femoral heads may be located within these steep acetabular roofs and be completely stable (Fig. 6.39).

The foregoing identifies lateral displacement of the femoral head. Thereafter, the Barlow maneuver (dynamic study), as illustrated in Fig. 6.37B, is applied. With this maneuver, note is made as to whether the head remains in the acetabulum, subluxes, or frankly dislocates out of the acetabulum (Figs. 6.40 and 6.41). This latter maneuver is designed to assess posterior and combined posterolateral dislocation. If the femoral head dislocates, it will come to lie posterior to the midcoronal plane of the acetabular roof (the "Y"-shaped acetabulum). At the same time, the arc of the femoral neck will come into view in this plane. In other words, the head will disappear and the femoral neck will take its place (Fig. 6.41, C and D). If, on the other hand, both the pelvis and the femur are fortuitously displaced downward as a unit, the femoral neck will come into view, but not in the midcoronal (acetabular "Y") plane. At this point, one should lower the transducer until the head is in view, and it will be in the normal acetabular "Y" plane (Fig. 6.41, E and F). Finally, if the femoral head is dislocated to begin with, it will not be visible in the standard midcoronal

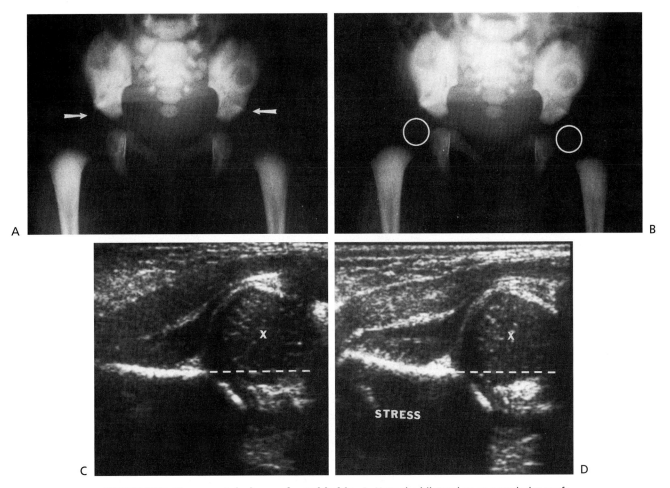

FIGURE 6.39. Steep acetabular roofs: stable hip. A. Note the bilateral steep acetabular roofs (arrows). **B.** With circles representing where the unossified femoral heads would be located, one can see that the femoral heads are still within the acetabular roofs. **C.** Resting ultrasound on the right demonstrates marked lateral displacement of the femoral head. The line from the iliac wing intersects the femoral head well below its midpoint (X). **D.** With stress applied, there is no significant change in the location of the femoral head (X). Similar findings were present on the left. Although one's first impression would be that both hips were unstable, they were stable.

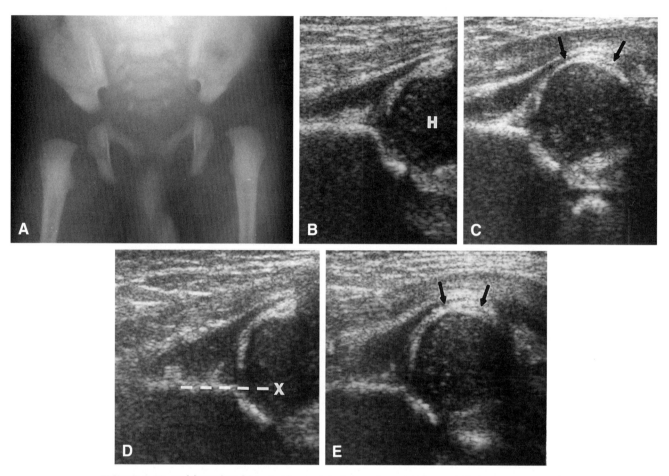

FIGURE 6.40. Subluxating hip. A. The acetabular roofs are steep, and their cups are poorly developed. Neither hip, however, is dislocated. **B.** The right femoral head (H) is in normal location. **C.** With pressure, there is slight lateral displacement of the femoral head (arrows) with associated bulging of the overlying capsule. **D.** Left hip, in the resting position, is laterally displaced. The line (dashed white) through the long axis of the iliac bone transects the femoral head through its lower third (X). Less than 40% of the head lies below this level. The femoral head is clearly abnormally positioned. **E.** With the Barlow maneuver, the femoral head can be displaced a little more laterally, and the capsule shows considerable bulging (arrows). Neither hip could be dislocated posteriorly with the Barlow maneuver. Both hips are markedly subluxed but were not dislocatable.

plane and the femoral neck will be seen in its place (Fig. 6.41C). However, as opposed to when this occurs if both these structures are fortuitously displaced (Fig. 6.41, E and F), when the hip is truly dislocated, the femoral head when ultimately located will be seen to be out of the acetabular "Y" (Fig. 6.41D). In addition, when the hip initially presents in a dislocated position, one can pull the hip back up into the acetabulum to substantiate that dislocation was present.

Ultrasound has proven extremely useful in the evaluation of congenital hip dysplasia, but, as noted earlier, **at times it can be too sensitive.** It can detect even minimal degrees of laxity in the joint, and in this regard, it should be noted that in the neonate, the normal left hip can move as much as 6 mm, while the right can move as much as 4 mm (11, 12). The discrepancy between the right and left sides is not completely understood, and on a practical basis, one could accept 6 mm for both sides. It is impor-

tant to be aware of these normal degrees of movement because such hips should not be misinterpreted for being pathologic. In between these two extremes are a large number of infants with mere hypermobility of the hip joints. They are neither dislocatable nor truly subluxable but are just slightly hypermobile. There is an entire spectrum of findings in the condition, a point that has come into sharper focus with the use of ultrasound. **Ultimately, it is important that one convey the following information to the clinician: (a) The hip is completely secure and does not move at all or movement is within normal range; (b) the hip is laterally displaced in the resting position and can be further laterally displaced with the Barlow maneuver (lateral subluxation), but no posterior or lateral dislocation occurs; and (c) the hip can be laterally or posteriorly dislocated with the Barlow maneuver, indicating frank dislocation.**

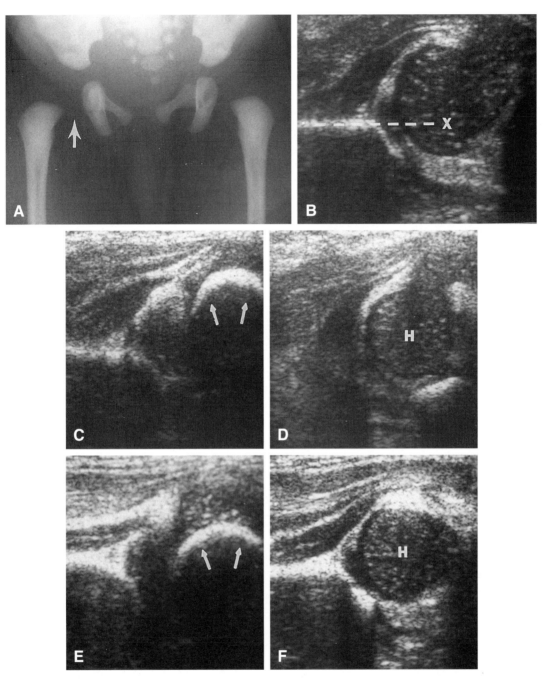

FIGURE 6.41. Classic dislocating hip. A. Anteroposterior view of the pelvis demonstrates lateral displacement of the right femur with widening of the joint space (arrow). **B.** In the resting position, the long axis of the iliac wing intersects the femoral head through its lower third (X). The femoral head is clearly laterally displaced. **C.** With the Barlow maneuver and posterior pressure on the hip, the femoral head disappears and the echogenic arc (arrows) of the femoral neck comes into view. Note that the Y-shaped configuration of the iliac wing-acetabular complex is still visible, although a little distorted. **D.** With the transducer still in the coronal plane but at a lower position, the femoral head (H) comes into view, but there is no visualization of the Y-shaped iliac wing-acetabular complex. The femoral head is posteriorly dislocated. **E.** Normal hip for comparison. In this patient with posterior pressure caused by the Barlow maneuver, the echogenic arc of the femoral neck (arrows) comes into view and the Y-shaped iliac wing-acetabular complex is basically lost. This might suggest that the femoral head has been displaced posteriorly. **F.** However, with the transducer still in the coronal plane but now at a lower level, there is confirmation that the femoral head (H) and Y-shaped iliac wing-acetabular complex still are in normal relationship and simply were displaced posteriorly as a unit.

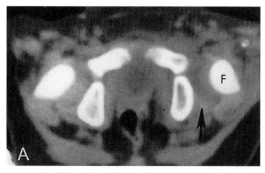

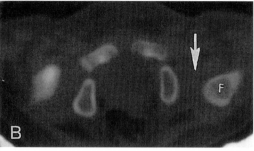

FIGURE 6.42. Congenital dislocating hip: computed tomography findings. A. The left joint space is wider (arrow), and there is lateral displacement of the left femur (F). **B.** Same infant (at a later date) demonstrates persistent lateral dislocation and a widened joint space (arrow), but, in addition, the femur (F) now has also moved posteriorly.

CT and MRI have little place in the initial evaluation of developmental hip dysplasia. They are used more often for postreduction evaluation, especially in casted infants (13, 14), where it may be more difficult to perform ultrasound. Ultrasound, however, can be used to evaluate the hips being treated with a Pavlik harness (15, 16), and CT is extremely effective in demonstrating persistent dislocation of the hip, especially posterior dislocation (Fig. 6.42). In addition, it will clearly demonstrate loss of the acetabular cup. Finally, preoperative three-dimensional imaging also has been used (17).

For the most part, congenital dislocating hip is treated conservatively, and complications are few. Occasionally, complicating aseptic necrosis of the femoral head results and is secondary to pressure on the head from the extreme frog-leg positioning required with the Pavlik harness or casting (18). Aseptic necrosis also can be evaluated with MR (19, 20), and in one study, 20% of the hips placed in greater than 55% abduction developed aseptic necrosis (20). In very severe or refractory cases (very few), surgery in the form of a Salter osteotomy of the iliac wing to contain the femoral head within the acetabulum is required. In such cases, dislocation is persistent and refractory because of spasticity secondary to contractures resulting from the chronic dislocation. After treatment, the acetabular roof may remain somewhat steep and the ipsilateral femoral

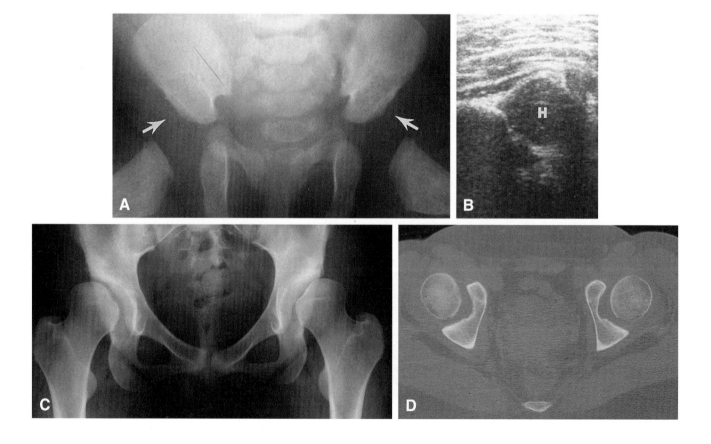

head ossification center may lag behind the normal head, in terms of both ossification and size. Patients with underlying neurologic disease or hypotonia (such as seen in hypothyroidism) often also develop dislocation of the hips. In these cases, however, the problem is not true congenital dislocation of the hip. With diagnosis of late-presenting chronic congenital dislocating hip, often a bilateral problem, it is probably better not to perform corrective surgery in these patients for they seem to do relatively well on their own (21).

In primary acetabular dysplasia, the acetabular roofs are dysplastic and there is no frank dislocation, but the femoral heads ride high in the acetabulum and actually extend laterally out of the acetabulum. The findings are vividly demonstrated on plain films but can also be demonstrated with CT (Fig. 6.43).

REFERENCES

1. Kutlu A, Memik R, Mutlu M, et al. Congenital dislocation of the hip and its relation to swaddling used in Turkey. J Pediatr Orthop 1992;12:598–602.
2. Bond CD, Henrikus WL, DellaMagglore ED. Prospective evaluation of newborn soft-tissue hip "clicks" with ultrasound. J Pediatr Orthop 1997;17:199–201.
3. Barlow TG. Early diagnosis and treatment of congenital dislocation of the hip. J Bone Joint Surg 1962;44:292–301.
4. Holen KJ, Terjesen T, Tegnander A, et al. Ultrasound screening for hip dysplasia in newborns. J Pediatr Orthop 1994;14:667–673.
5. Johnston CE II, Birch JG, Herring JA, et al. Outcome of ultrasonographic hip abnormalities in clinical stable hips. J Pediatr Orthop 1999;19:754–759.
6. Graf R. Fundamentals of sonographic diagnosis of infant hip dysplasia. J Pediatr Orthop 1984;4:735–740.
7. Harcke HT, Clarke NMP, Lee MS, et al. Examination of the infant hip with real-time ultrasonography. J Ultrasound Med 1984;3:131–138.
8. Castelein RM, Sauter AJM, de Vlieger M, et al. Natural history of ultrasound hip abnormalities in clinically normal newborns. J Pediatr Orthop 1992;12:423–427.
9. Andersson JE, Per-Ove F. Neonatal hip instability: screening with anterior-dynamic ultrasound method. J Pediatr Orthop 1995;15:322–324.
10. Nimityongskul P, Hudgens RA, Anderson LD, et al. Ultrasonography in the management of developmental dysplasia of the hip (DDH). J Pediatr Orthop 1995;15:741–746.
11. Andersson JE. Neonatal hip instability: normal values for physiological movement of the femoral head determined by an anterior-dynamic ultrasound method. J Pediatr Orthop 1995;15:736–740.
12. Keller MS, Weltin GG, Rattner Z, et al. Normal instability of the hip in the neonate: US standards. Radiology 1988;169:733–736.
13. Eggli KD, King SH, Boal DKB, et al. Technical note. Low-dose CT of developmental dysplasia of the hip after reduction: diagnostic accuracy and dosimetry. AJR 1994;163:1441–1443.
14. Helms CA, Goodman PC, Jeffrey RB. Use of computed tomography in congenital dislocation of the hip. CT 1983;7:363–365.
15. Harding MB, Hacke HT, Bowen JR, et al. Management of dislocated hips with Pavlik harness treatment and ultrasound monitoring. J Pediatr Orthop 1997;17:189–198.
16. Song KM, Lapinsky A. Determination of hip position in the Pavlik harness. J Pediatr Orthop 2000;20:317–319.
17. Kim HT, Wenger DR. The morphology of residual acetabular deficiency in childhood hip dysplasia: three-dimensional computed tomographic analysis. J Pediatr Orthop 1997;17:637–647.
18. Fogarty EE, Accardo NJ Jr. Incidence of avascular necrosis of the femoral head in congenital hip dislocation related to the degree of abduction during preliminary traction. J Pediatr Orthop 1981;1:307–311.
19. Jaramillo D, Villegas-Medina O, Laoi T, et al. Gadolinium-enhanced MR imaging of pediatric patients after reduction of dysplastic hips: assessment of femoral head position, factors impeding reduction, and femoral head schemia. AJR 1998;170:1633–1637.
20. Smith BG, Millis MB, Hey LA, et al. Postreduction computed tomography in developmental dislocation of the hip: part II: predictive value for outcome. J Pediatr Orthop 1997;1:631–636.
21. Crawford AH, Mehlman CT, Slovek RW. The fate of untreated developmental dislocation of the hip: long-term follow-up of eleven patients. J Pediatr Orthop 1999;19:641–644.

Congenital Dislocated Knee (Genu Recurvatum)

In congenital dislocated knee, the knee is hyperextended and the tibia displaced or dislocated anteriorly. It can occur as an isolated phenomenon and, in such cases, is secondary to faulty intrauterine positioning (1, 2). Treatment is conservative, consisting of splinting in a tubular cast. Bilateral genu recurvatum occurs in Larsen's syndrome, a condition characterized by multiple joint dislocations and other skeletal abnormalities. Roentgenographically, the knee appears bizarre because the foot appears to be pointing the wrong way (Fig. 6.44).

REFERENCES

1. Bensahel H, Dal Monte A, Hjelmstedt A, et al. Congenital dislocation of the knee. J Pediatr Orthop 1989;9:174–177.
2. Johnson E, Audell R, Oppenheim WL. Congenital dislocation of the knee. J Pediatr Orthop 1987;7:194–200.

FIGURE 6.43. Primary acetabular dysplasia. A. Note the dysplastic and poorly formed acetabular roofs (arrows). They are steep and lack their normal cups. **B.** Ultrasonography demonstrates that the femoral head (H) is present and within the Y-shaped iliac wing-acetabular complex. Neither hip could be dislocated. **C.** Older patient with bilateral acetabular dysplasia. The acetabulae again are poorly formed and somewhat shallow. There is associated lateral displacement of the femoral heads. **D.** Computed tomography study demonstrates the dysplastic acetabulae.

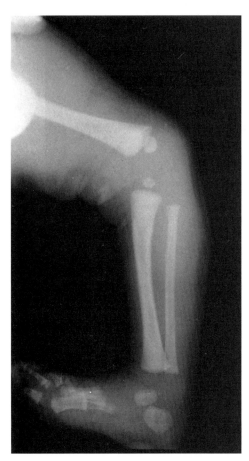

FIGURE 6.44. Genu recurvatum: dislocated knee. Note hyperextension of the knee and anterior displacement of the tibia.

Congenital Foot Deformities

Pes talipes equinovarus is the most common foot deformity in the neonate (1, 2). It is the classic clubfoot and can be seen as an isolated finding or in association with underlying neurologic or neuromuscular disease. Adduction (varus deformity) of the forefoot, equinus deformity of the foot at the ankle (plantar flexion), and inversion of the foot are present. The radiographic findings are illustrated and compared with those of a normal foot in Fig. 6.45 (A–C).

Pes talipes equinovalgus is a much less common deformity and can be considered the opposite of the common clubfoot. In these cases, the foot is everted, and there is a marked flatfoot deformity (Fig. 6.45, D and E). The talus is vertical in position, constituting the so-called "vertical talus" or "talonavicular dislocation."

In metatarsus varus, the forefoot primarily is deformed. There is marked varus deviation of the metatarsals and toes, but talocalcaneal relationships remain relatively normal (Fig. 6.46).

Pes calcaneovalgus is a condition in which the entire foot is dorsiflexed at the ankle. It is easily corrected, and there are no specific bony abnormalities, although it does resemble a flatfoot deformity. Usually, it is seen after prolonged intrauterine dorsiflexion of the foot. For other foot deformities, one can refer to the article by Condon (3). Finally, these foot deformities can be investigated with CT, MR, and ultrasound. In most cases, however, these supplemental imaging studies are not required.

REFERENCES

1. Chami M, Daoud A, Maestro M, et al. Ultrasound contribution in the analysis of the newborn and infant normal and club foot: a preliminary study. Pediatr Radiol 1996;26:298–302.
2. Downey DJ, Drennan JC, Garcia JF. Magnetic resonance image findings in congenital talipes equinovarus. J Pediatr Orthop 1992; 12:224–228.
3. Condon VR. Radiology of practical orthopedic problems. Radiol Clin North Am 1972;10:203–223.

Bowlegs, Knock-Knees, and Blount's Disease

Bowlegs commonly occur with bone-softening problems such as rickets, and bowing also is inherent in many chondrodystrophies. Physiologic bowing also occurs and is seen at approximately 2 years of age. Such bowing usually is seen in stocky infants showing early ambulation, and many of these patients also have some degree of tibial torsion. The bowing (Fig. 6.47A) generally resolves by the age of 3 or 4 years, but in a few instances, it may persist and take the form of infantile Blount's disease (Fig. 6.47B).

Physiologic knock-knees occur at approximately 4–6 years of age (1). They are especially prone to occur in girls and, again, generally resolve spontaneously. On the other hand, surgical intervention may be required in some cases of either bowleg or knock-knee deformity, by way of a femoral osteotomy or physeal stapling (2).

Blount's disease generally is considered a subclinical impaction injury of the medial upper tibial plateau. The growth plate also is involved, and there is impairment of linear medial growth. This leads to an acute bowing deformity through the upper tibia and with associated tibial beaking and fragmentation results in the typical Blount's disease (3). Blount's disease is seen in two age groups: in infancy, as just discussed, and in adolescents, where it is associated with obesity (3, 4). In these patients, there may be predisposition to bowing because of associated femoral anteversion, which is believed to place undue stresses on the medial aspect of the knee. The radiographic findings in adolescent Blount's disease are exactly the same as those in infantile Blount's disease (Fig. 6.48). The disease tends to be bilateral but asymmetric.

In many infants, Blount's disease can be treated conservatively (5), but in others with more pronounced deformity, the findings are refractory and require osteotomy for cor-

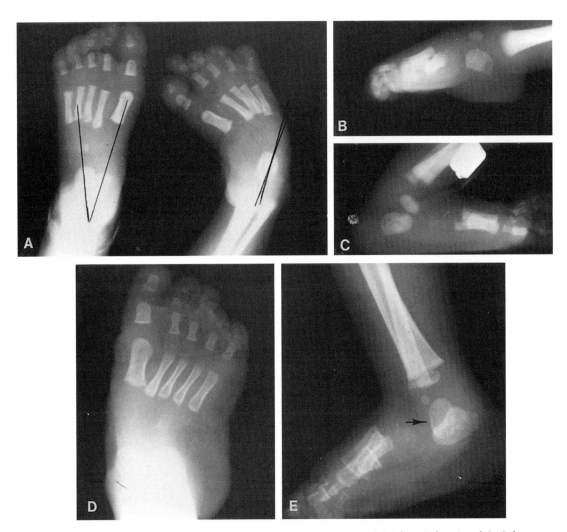

FIGURE 6.45. Typical clubfoot (talipes equinovarus). A. Typical clubfoot deformity of the left foot includes varus deviation of the metatarsals and rotation of the calcaneus so that it lies directly under the talus. The right foot is normal. The normal angle between the talus and calcaneus (approximately 30°) is lost in the clubfoot deformity on the left. In the normal foot, the longitudinal axis of the calcaneus passes through the fourth metatarsal, and the axis of the talus passes through the first metatarsal. **B.** Lateral view of clubbed left foot shows typical cavus deformity and loss of angle between the now parallel talus and calcaneus. **C.** Normal right foot for comparison showing normal talo-calacaneal angle (approximately 30–35°) and orientation of the talus and calcaneus. The foot was inadvertently positioned into a slight hyperflexion posture. **D and E. Talipes equinovalgus.** The less common clubfoot deformity shows valgus deformity of the metatarsals in **D,** and in **E,** the talus assumes a vertical position (arrow).

rection. In this regard, it is generally believed that the angle formed by the shaft of the tibia and epiphyseal-metaphyseal line should be no more than 11–12° for the findings to still be considered normal (6). Physeal bridging (premature closure) can occur in more severe cases, and resection of the bridge may be required (7). Evidence of such premature fusion of the medial aspect of the physeal plate is demonstrable with MR (8, 9), and overall the pathophysiology is the same as that seen with overt fractures of the extremities leading to premature closure of the epiphyseal plate. A final, interesting feature of Blount's disease is that there is widen-

ing of the opposite side of the epiphyseal plate, with separation of the epiphysis from the metaphysis. This further attests to the fact that while the problem medially is compression, laterally it is distraction.

When bowlegs are caused by tibial torsion, marked intoeing is seen, but in-toeing also occurs with **femoral anteversion.** In this condition, the femurs are anteverted at their necks, but regular radiography fails to show any abnormality. With CT, however, one can draw a line through the long axis of the femoral neck and another through the femoral condyles (10). The angle formed by

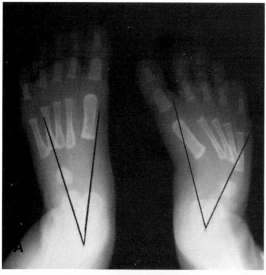

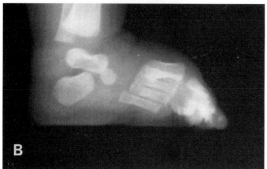

FIGURE 6.46. Metatarsus varus. A. Note the varus deformity of the metatarsals on the left. As opposed to the classic clubfoot (Fig. 6.45), the normal angle between the talus and calcaneus is retained or a little increased. The right foot is normal. **B.** Lateral view also shows that the angle between the talus and calcaneus is retained or slightly increased in the metatarsus varus deformity. Compare with classic clubfoot in Fig. 6.45.

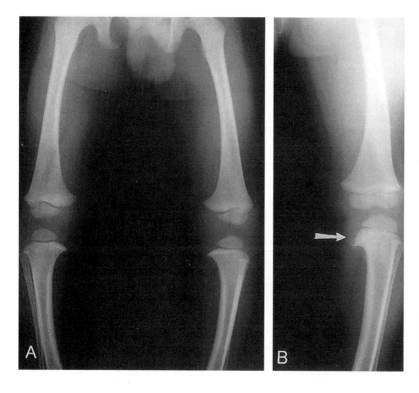

FIGURE 6.47. A. Physiologic bowing of lower extremities. Note typical appearance of bowed legs. There are no signs of rickets or any other metabolic disturbance. **B. Blount's disease.** Full-blown Blount's disease with medial beaking and fragmentation of the upper tibia (arrow).

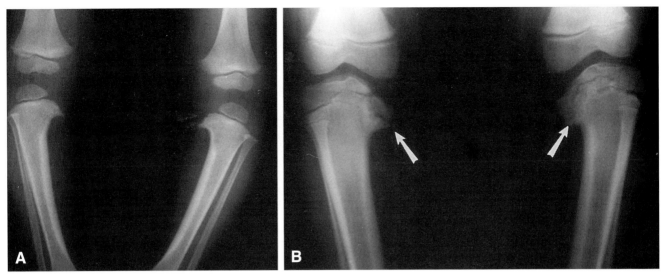

FIGURE 6.48. Blount's disease: infantile and adolescent forms. A. Infantile form. Note bilateral upper tibial beaking. On the right, bowleg deformity is minimal and still could correct itself spontaneously. On the left, the degree of bowing is much more marked and spontaneous correction is less likely. **B.** Adolescent with bilateral Blount's disease with severe beaking of the upper tibial metaphyses (arrows). On the left, the epiphyseal line appears to be closing medially. These changes will not spontaneously correct.

these two lines then can be measured and the degree of femoral (Fig. 6.49) anteversion determined.

REFERENCES

1. Lin C-J, Lin S-C, Huang W, et al. Physiologic knock-knee in preschool children: prevalence, correlating factors, gait analysis and clinical significance. J Pediatr Orthop 1999;19:650–654.
2. Stevens PM, Maguie M, Dales MD, et al. Physeal stapling for idiopathic genu valgum. J Pediatr Orthop 1999;19:645–649.
3. Thompson GH, Carter JR. Late-onset tibia vara (Blount's disease): current concepts. Clin Orthop 1990;255:24–35.
4. Henderson RC. Tibia vara: a complication of adolescent obesity. J Pediatr 1992;121:482–486.

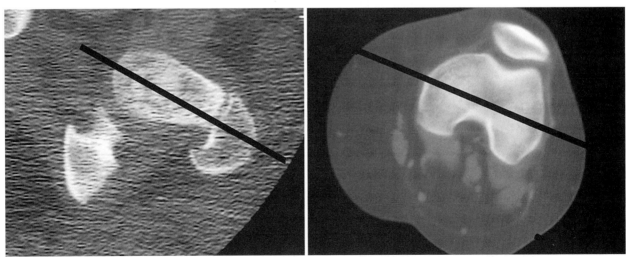

FIGURE 6.49. Femoral anteversion: radiographic measurements. A. Axial image of the femoral neck. Note the configuration and location of the long axis (line). **B.** Axial image through the femoral condyles. Again, note the configuration of the line through the long axis (line). When the lines are superimposed, the normal angle should measure near 15° in older children and adolescents. With femoral anteversion, it is greater.

5. Zionts LE, Shean CJ. Brace treatment of early infantile tibia vara. J Pediatr Orthop 1976;18:102–109.
6. Heath CH, Staheli LT. Normal limits of knee angle in white children—genu varum and genu valgum. J Pediatr Orthop 1993;13:259–262.
7. Beck CL, Burke SW, Roberts JM, et al. Physeal bridge resection in infantile Blount disease. J Pediatr Orthop 1987;7:161–163.
8. Ducou le Pointe H, Mousselard H, Rudelli A, et al. Blount's disease: magnetic imaging. Pediatr Radiol 1995;25:12–14.
9. Iwasawa T, Inaba Y, Nishiura G, et al. MR findings of bowlegs in toddlers. Pediatr Radiol 1999;29:826–834.
10. Hernandez RJ, Tachdijian MO, Poznanski AK, et al. CT determination of femoral torsion. AJR 1981;137:97–101.

Tibial and Femoral Fibrous Defect (Fibrocartilaginous Dysplasia) and Blount's Deformity

Some interesting cases of patients who demonstrate Blount-like changes have been sporadically identified. These patients have a fibrocartilaginous dysplasia involving the medial aspect of the upper tibia (1–4), and the ensuing growth disturbance resembles that of Blount's disease (Fig. 6.50). Some of these lesions resolve spontaneously. A simi-lar lesion has been described in the distal femur (5, 6) and even in the long bones of the upper extremity, primarily the ulna and humerus (4, 7).

REFERENCES

1. Bell SN, Campbell PE, Cole WG, et al. Tibia vara caused by focal fibrocartilaginous dysplasia: three case reports. J Bone Joint Surg 1985;67:780–784.
2. Herman TE, Siegel MJ, McAlister WH. Focal fibrocartilaginous dysplasia associated with tibia vara. Radiology 1990;177:767–768.
3. Kariya Y, Taniguchi K, Yagisawa H, et al. Focal fibrocartilaginous dysplasia: consideration of healing process. J Pediatr Orthop 1991;11:545–547.
4. Choi I, Kim C, Cho T, et al. Focal fibrocartilaginous dysplasia of long bones: report of eight additional cases and literature. J Pediatr Orthop 2000;20:421–427.
5. Berson L, Dormans JP, Drummond DS, et al. Fibrous lesion of the distal femur associated with angular deformity. J Pediatr Orthop 1999;19:527–530.
6. Vallcanera-Calatayud A, Sanguesa-Nebot C, Martinez-Fernandez M, et al. Varus deformity of the distal end of the femur secondary to a focal fibrous lesion. Pediatr Radiol 1994;24:74–75.
7. Lincoln TL, Birch JG. Focal fibrocartilaginous dysplasia in the upper extremity. J Pediatr Orthop 1997;17:528–532.

Trophic Lines

Trophic lines basically are either radiolucent or radiodense. The radiolucent lines are largely nonspecific and simply represent the aftermath of an insult to enchondral bone formation. They are seen after many illnesses which temporarily interfere with body growth and metabolism. Once the insult is removed, resurgence of growth occurs and rebound healing with formation of adjacent white lines is seen. Although these latter lines commonly are referred to as "growth arrest lines," they are actually growth spurt or recovery lines.

Many normal children show multiple such lines, but when they are excessive, one should begin to think of chronic illnesses such as asthma, diabetes, and malignancy (Fig. 6.51). Multiple such lines are also seen in deprivational dwarfism and can be seen at birth secondary to any number of intrauterine insults (1), including intrauterine infections (Fig. 6.52). In addition, these lines are common in premature infants (Fig. 6.52C), in whom the lines lead to a bone-within-bone appearance in the vertebra (Fig. 6.52E).

The initial radiolucent lines can be broad (Fig. 6.52B), but, generally speaking, the white recovery lines are thin. Dense, broader white lines not caused by physiologic rebound bone growth are seen on a pathologic basis in lead poisoning, other heavy metal poisoning, and vitamin D intoxication. However, it should be noted that the commonest cause of dense white lines in the metaphysis of children is the normal zone of provisional calcification that often becomes pronounced during the summer when there

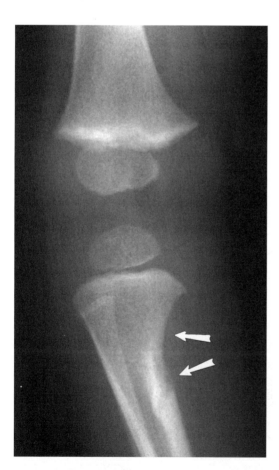

FIGURE 6.50. Fibrocartilaginous dysplasia with Blount's disease. Note characteristic defect (arrows) in the upper tibia with associated Blount-like changes.

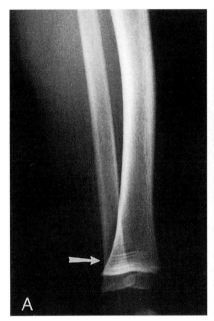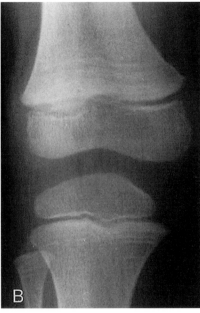

FIGURE 6.51. Trophic lines. A. Note numerous trophic, radiolucent lines with adjacent white recovery lines in this patient with asthma (arrow). **B.** Another patient with numerous growth arrest and recovery lines. The lines are more separated in the distal femurs because the distal femur grows faster than the proximal tibia.

is increased exposure to sunlight. These lines should not be confused with the lines of lead intoxication .

Finally, transverse radiolucent lines characteristically are seen in leukemia. They also can be seen with metastatic disease such as metastatic neuroblastoma but most often are seen with leukemia, or at times lymphoma. The findings again represent a trophic disturbance resulting from an insult to enchondral bone formation.

REFERENCE

1. Edwards DK III. Skeletal growth lines seen on radiographs of newborn infants: prevalence and possible association with obstetric abnormalities. AJR 1993;161:141–145.

TRAUMA

Birth Trauma

In the usual neonate with long bone fractures, difficult deliveries are the basic problem, and breech deliveries are the most problematic. In breech deliveries, fractures can be sustained in both the upper and the lower extremities, but the lower extremities are especially prone to injury. Overall, however, the clavicle is the bone most commonly fractured during delivery, and fractures most often are midclavicular (Fig. 6.53). In one study (1), clavicular fractures occurred in up to 3.5% of deliveries but, interestingly enough, were asymptomatic in 80% of cases. Fractures of the long bones are next most common and will be discussed later. Rib fractures also are occasionally seen (Fig. 6.53), but these fractures may go unnoticed or elude the examiner until fortu-

itous observation of callus at a later date. If many ribs are fractured, the infant may exhibit respiratory difficulties.

Fractures of the long bones can occur through the diaphysis or at the epiphyseal-metaphyseal junction. These latter fractures actually are Salter-Harris type I or II fractures and most commonly occur at either end of the humerus and the proximal femur (2–4). Because the epiphyses are not ossified in the neonate, the first study often shows nothing more than soft tissue swelling (Fig. 6.54). Under these circumstances, one should consider that an epiphyseal-metaphyseal fracture has occurred. Epiphyseal-metaphyseal fractures of the upper humerus can be associated with Erb's palsy (Fig. 6.55). In the upper femur, these fractures can falsely suggest dislocation (Fig. 6.56). True dislocation of a joint is an uncommon problem in the neonate. Epiphyseal-metaphyseal fractures can be identified with ultrasound (5, 6).

In other infants, small corner metaphyseal fractures are readily visible and serve to alert one to an underlying Salter-Harris type II injury. When any of these fractures heal, calcifying callus and subperiosteal new bone deposition often are profound (Fig. 6.57, A and B), and in some cases, there may be a tendency to first consider bone tumor. In addition, the findings are exactly the same as those seen in the typical epiphyseal-metaphyseal fractures of the battered child syndrome, but in this regard, it has been suggested that if a fracture is noted at 11 days of age and there are no signs of calcifying callus or subperiosteal bone deposition, one should consider the fracture to have occurred after birth (7). The reason for this is that birth injuries usually show calcified callus from 7 to 11 days after birth. In addition to these considerations, growth disturbances are common after neonatal injuries (3).

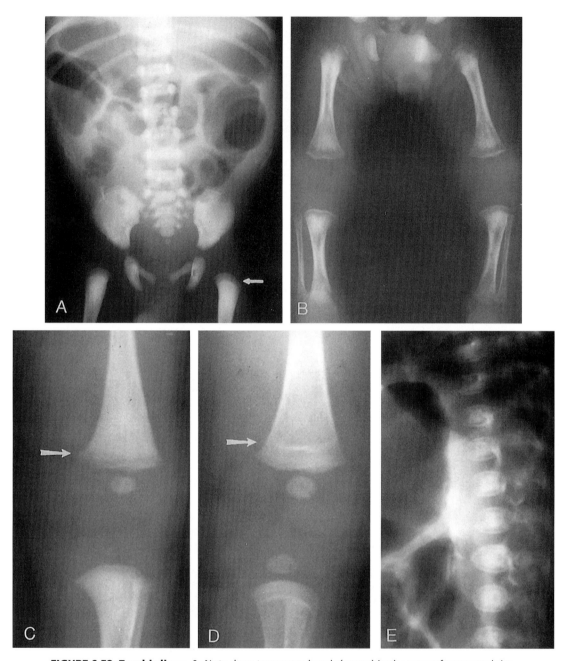

FIGURE 6.52. Trophic lines. A. Note deep transverse bands (arrow) in the upper femurs and similar bands in the iliac crests of this infant with intrauterine meconium peritonitis (note curvilinear calcifications in the abdomen and small bowel obstruction). **B.** Infant with congenital lues showing widespread broad transverse radiolucent bands. **C.** Normal premature infant with a transverse band through the distal femur (arrow). **D.** A few weeks later, a white line (recovery line) has formed in this infant (arrow). **E.** Another patient with bone-within-bone appearance of the vertebra caused by trophic lines.

Joint dislocation, as noted earlier, is rare in the neonatal period, although sternoclavicular dislocation due to birth trauma can occur (8). In addition, the shoulder joints can be dislocated after brachial plexus injury resulting in Erb's palsy. The plain film findings consist of widening of the involved joint space and some inferior positioning of the

involved extremity (Fig. 6.55B). Ultrasound has also been used to detect this abnormality (9).

Trauma to the soft tissues during delivery is less well appreciated but can pose a significant problem. Most often, such trauma occurs in breech deliveries, and many of these infants demonstrate features of the crush syndrome with

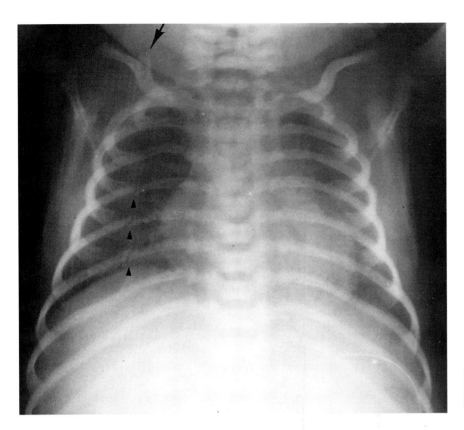

FIGURE 6.53. Clavicle and rib fractures. Note midshaft right clavicular fracture (arrow) and three posterior rib fractures on the right (arrowheads).

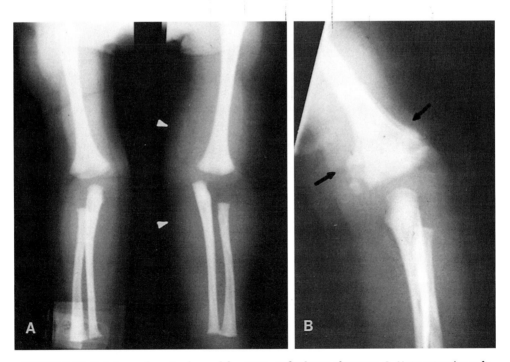

FIGURE 6.54. Epiphyseal-metaphyseal fracture: soft tissue changes. A. Note extensive soft tissue swelling around the right elbow (arrowheads). A clear-cut fracture is not visualized. **B.** Two weeks later, however, abundant callus formation and periosteal bone deposition attest (arrows) to the presence of an epiphyseal-metaphyseal injury.

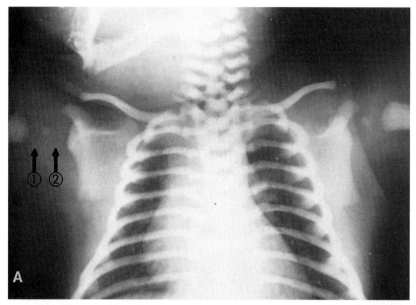

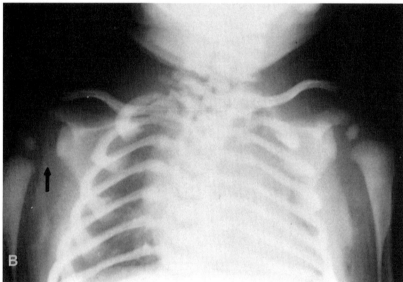

FIGURE 6.55. Shoulder epiphyseal-metaphyseal fracture and Erb's palsy. A. In this infant, note that the space between the right humerus and its epiphysis is increased (arrow 1). The space between the epiphysis and the glenoid fossa also is increased (arrow 2). Both of these findings should suggest an underlying epiphyseal-metaphyseal injury. This patient also had Erb's palsy. **B.** Another infant with Erb's palsy but no bony injury. Note the widened joint space on the right (arrow). Clinically, there was no swelling over the area, and widening is caused by laxity of the muscles. Note that the humerus is displaced downward.

evidence of intravascular coagulation. This obviously would be a problem with only the most severe injuries.

REFERENCES

1. Joseph PR, Rosenfeld W. Clavicular fractures in neonates. Am J Dis Child 1990;144:165–167.
2. Banagale RC, Kuhns LR. Traumatic separation of the distal femoral epiphysis in the newborn. J Pediatr Orthop 1983;3: 396–398.
3. Barrett WP, Almquist EA, Shaheli LT. Fracture separation of the distal humeral physis in the newborn. J Pediatr Orthop 1984;4: 617–619.
4. Ogden JA, Lee KE, Rudicel SA, et al. Proximal femoral epiphysiolysis in the neonate. J Pediatr Orthop 1984;4:285–292.
5. Diaz MJ, Hedlund GL. Sonographic diagnosis of traumatic separation of the proximal femoral epiphysis in the neonate. Pediatr Radiol 1991;21:238–240.
6. Ziv N, Litwin A, Katz K, et al. Definitive diagnosis of fracture-separation of the distal humeral epiphysis in neonates by ultrasonography. Pediatr Radiol 1996;26:493–496.
7. Cumming WA. Neonatal skeletal fractures: birth trauma or child abuse? J Can Assoc Radiol 1979;30:30–33.
8. Aretz S, Benz-Bohm G, Helling HJ, et al. Right sternoclavicular dislocation after traumatic delivery: a case report. J Pediatr Surg 1999;34:1872–1873.
9. Hunter JD, Franklin K, Hughes PM. The ultrasound diagnosis of posterior shoulder dislocation associated with Erb's palsy. Pediatr Radiol 1998;28:510–511.

Childhood Fractures

An extensive dissertation on childhood fractures will not be attempted because there are many good orthopaedic and

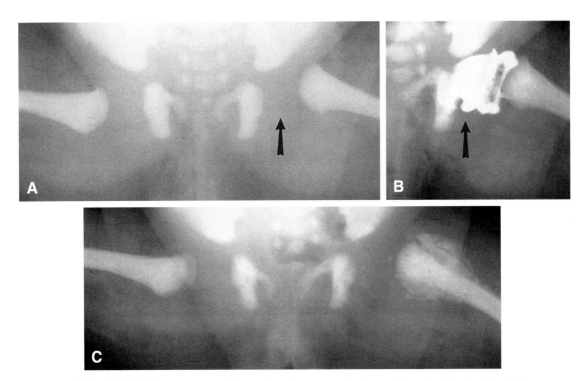

FIGURE 6.56. Epiphyseal-metaphyseal fracture: pseudodislocation. A. Note that the joint space on the left is slightly widened (arrow) and that there is upward displacement of the femur. **B.** Arthrogram demonstrates that the femoral head (arrow) is normally located within the acetabulum but is displaced on the femoral neck. **C.** Follow-up film demonstrating typical healing changes around the left hip. (Reproduced with permission from Towbin R, Crawford AH. Nontraumatic proximal femoral epiphysiolysis. Pediatrics 1979;63:456–459).

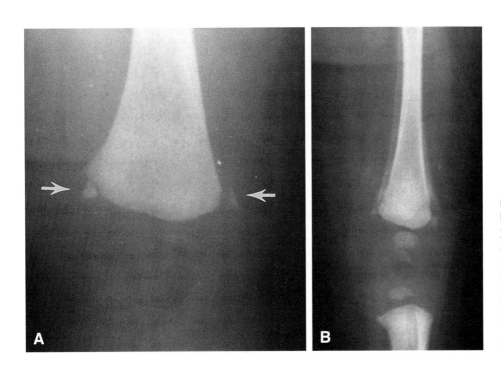

FIGURE 6.57. Birth trauma: epiphyseal-metaphyseal fractures. A. Typical metaphyseal fragmentation of distal femur secondary to fracture sustained during breech delivery (arrows). **B.** Another infant showing pronounced periosteal new bone proliferation along the femoral shaft (healing phase). Metaphyseal corner fractures are present in the distal femur, and there is residual beaking of the upper medial tibial metaphysis.

radiologic textbooks on the subject, and I have, in another publication (1), dealt with the more subtle aspects of these injuries. Overall, however, it should be remembered that because children's bones are soft and because the epiphyses are not fused, fractures in children are different from those seen in adults. Young infants and children are subject to buckle fractures of the cortex (torus fractures), epiphyseal-metaphyseal injuries of various types, greenstick fractures, and plastic bending fractures of the long bones. Bending fractures are most common in the forearm (2), next in the clavicle, and then in the lower extremity involving primar-

ily the fibula. It is important that one use comparative views liberally in all these cases because one will miss the more subtle of these fractures. Examples of these fractures are presented in Fig. 6.58, and a more thorough review is available in a series of articles by John and Phillips (3–5).

Stress fractures are not common in children, but the most common is that which occurs in the proximal tibia in older children. These are characterized by vague sclerosis along a transverse or oblique fracture line and periosteal new bone deposition (Fig. 6.59). The latter may at first appear sinister, but it is important that one not misinterpret

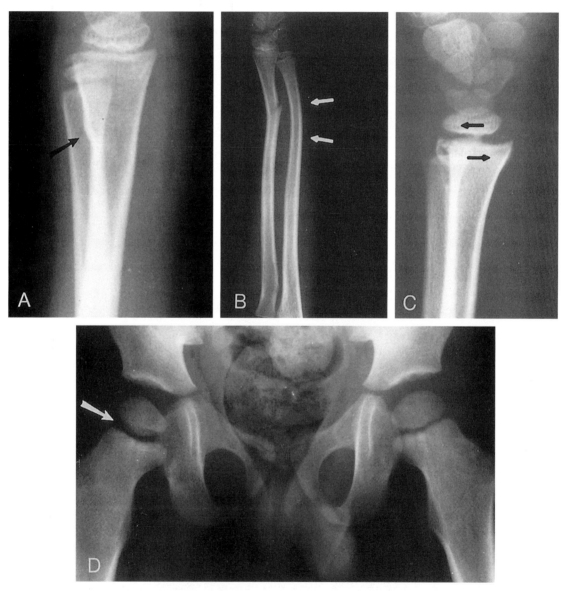

FIGURE 6.58. Typical childhood fractures. A. Note a typical cortical buckle, or torus, fracture (arrow). **B.** Typical greenstick fracture in the radius and an associated plastic bending fracture in the ulna (arrows). **C.** Epiphyseal-metaphyseal (Salter-Harris) fracture with epiphyseal displacement (arrows). There also is fragmentation of the metaphysis. **D.** Epiphyseal-metaphyseal fracture (Salter-Harris type I) of the right hip: subtle findings. Note that the epiphyseal line is wider and more radiolucent (arrow) on the right.

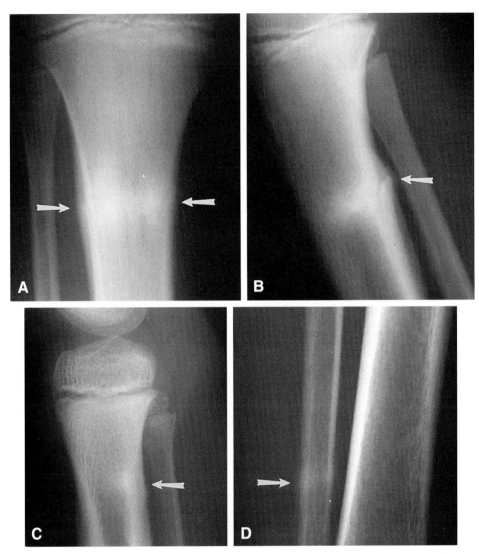

FIGURE 6.59. Stress fracture: upper tibia. A. Note sclerosis and periosteal new bone deposition through the upper tibia (arrows). **B.** Lateral view demonstrates characteristic healing appearance of a stress fracture (arrow). **C.** Another patient with a more subtle stress fracture (arrow). **D.** Stress fracture in the fibula (arrow).

the findings as evidence of an underlying malignancy. Stress fractures can occur in other bones, primarily the fibula (next most common) and femur (often the femoral neck) (6–10). Less commonly, stress fractures occur in the pelvic bones.

Stress fractures can be detected with nuclear scintigraphy and MRI, but usually by the time plain films are obtained in these patients, sclerosis is present and neither nuclear scintigraphy or MRI examination is required. With MRI, the area of sclerosis appears as a zone of low signal on T1-weighted images, while earlier these fractures appear as zones of decreased signal (bone bruises) on T2-weighted images. So-called "shin splints" probably are subclinical stress fractures (microfractures) (11).

In terms of **epiphyseal-metaphyseal fractures,** although more complex classification are available (12), epiphyseal-metaphyseal fractures are most often classified according to the standard Salter-Harris classification (Fig. 6.60). In the **type I fracture,** the epiphyseal line simply is widened; in the **type II injury,** a variable-size metaphyseal corner fracture occurs. In the **type III injury,** fractures occur through the epiphyseal plate and epiphysis; in the **type IV injury,** fractures occur in both the epiphysis and the metaphysis. **Type V fractures** show no radiographic changes and are impaction injuries of the epiphyseal-metaphyseal junction. Any of the fractures in the first four classifications may be displaced, while type IV and V fractures are most prone to go on to premature closure of the epiph-

SALTER-HARRIS CLASSIFICATION OF
EPIPHYSEAL-METAPHYSEAL FRACTURES

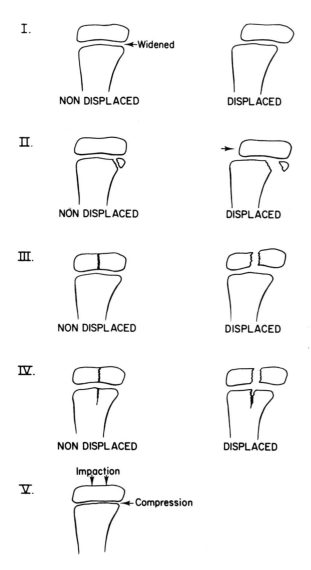

FIGURE 6.60. Salter-Harris classification of epiphyseal-metaphyseal fractures. Type I. The epiphyseal plate is widened, and there may or may not be displacement of the epiphysis. **Type II.** The epiphyseal plate is widened, and there is a corner fracture of the metaphysis. The fracture may or may not be displaced. **Type III.** Fractures exist through the epiphyseal line (widening) and the epiphysis. **Type IV.** Fractures exist through the epiphysis, epiphyseal line, and metaphysis. **Type V.** Axial compression causes compressive injury to the epiphyseal plate.

ysis. With premature closure of the epiphysis, one of the best early indications that this is occurring is the lack of development of a growth line in the involved metaphysis (13) (Fig. 6.61, A and B). Premature closure of the epiphysis caused by physeal bridging is best demonstrated with MRI or CT (14, 15). With CT, coronal and sagittal recon-

struction is beneficial, but MR is probably the premier imaging modality for final delineation of these bridges (Fig. 6.61C). MRI (15, 16) also has been used to detect epiphyseal-metaphyseal separation (Salter-Harris fractures), but if comparative views are obtained, there usually is little need for imaging beyond plain films.

When epiphyseal-metaphyseal fractures heal, they produce sclerosis along the epiphyseal plate and irregularity of the epiphyseal-metaphyseal junction (Fig. 6.62, A and B). In some cases, a bony dysplasia such as metaphyseal dysostosis might at first be suggested. This is a common problem in gymnasts who suffer repeated subclinical trauma to the wrists (17) (Fig. 6.62C). The same phenomena have been documented in older children in "Little Leaguer's shoulder" (18). In other cases, patients simply fail to communicate that they have injured themselves and may go for days or weeks before they come to radiographic examination. In all of these cases, it is important that one be familiar with the healing appearance of an epiphyseal-metaphyseal fracture.

Buckle (torus) fractures are perhaps the most common type of fracture, after epiphyseal-metaphyseal fractures, encountered in infancy and childhood. They occur most often in the wrist and ankle. In some cases, they are extremely subtle, and comparative views are almost mandatory for their detection (Fig. 6.63). The rule with buckle fractures is that the cortex of a normal bone is always smooth and gently curving; with buckle fractures, a variety of focal cortical slopes, angles, kinks, bumps, and breaks occur. Basically, however, there are two types of buckle fractures: the typical buckle fracture resulting from axial loading on the bone, where outward focal buckling of the cortex occurs, and the angled buckle fracture, where only angulation of the cortex is seen (19) (Fig. 6.64). In these latter cases, axial loading is accompanied by hyperextension, hyperflexion, valgus, or varus forces. A detailed dissertation on these two types of buckle fractures is available in an article by Hernandez (19). As buckle fractures heal, a zone of sclerosis develops along the fracture line.

Plastic bending fractures, as mentioned earlier (2), most commonly occur in the radius and ulna (Fig. 6.65A), but they are also common in the clavicle (Fig. 6.65B). Plastic bending fractures can be considered cousins of greenstick fractures for a greenstick fracture is merely an exaggerated plastic bending fracture, or vice versa (Fig. 6.65A). These fractures often are difficult to detect without comparative views. Plastic bending fractures usually produce no periosteal new bone deposition, but bone scintigraphy is positive. Scintigraphy, however, usually is not required if comparative views are obtained.

Hairline fractures are not as common in infants and children as they are in adults. The most classic hairline fracture in the infant is the toddler's (spiral) fracture of the tibia, but hairline fractures also occur transversely through the upper tibia and both longitudinally and transversely through the

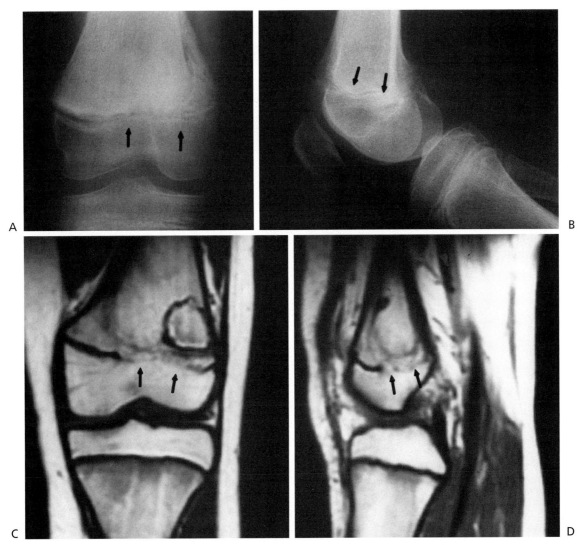

FIGURE 6.61. Premature closure of the epiphyseal plate. A. Note partial loss and indistinctness of the epiphyseal plate (arrows) of the distal femur. The white growth line is absent, but present laterally along the physis. **B.** Lateral view demonstrates similar changes (arrows). **C.** T1-weighted magnetic resonance study clearly demonstrates the obliterated epiphyseal plate (arrows) secondary to bony bridging. Also note the bone infarct (above). **D.** Lateral view demonstrates that the bridging (arrows) involves the posterior two-thirds of the epiphyseal plate.

proximal ulna (20, 21) (Fig. 6.66). They also can occur in other bones, especially the small bones of the hands and feet, and, as with hairline fractures anywhere, may be more detectable on one view than another. Hairline fractures occur through the scaphoid bone in older children, but in younger children, these fractures are more likely to be buckle-impaction fractures (22) (see Fig. 6.74).

Acute or chronic **avulsion fractures** usually are a problem of older children and adolescents who are active. These fractures are common in the pelvis (23) and are seen along the crest of the iliac wing, the superior and inferior iliac spines, the greater and lesser trochanters, and along the inferior aspect of the ischium (Fig. 6.67). The sites along

the inferior aspect of the ischium and inferior iliac spines are the most common (Fig. 6.68). With healing, a pseudomalignant appearance can result (24), especially with those injuries occurring through the inferior aspect of the ischium (Fig. 6.68E). During early stages, only underlying bony resorption may be seen (Fig. 6.68D). Another common site of avulsion injury is along the medial supracondylar ridge of the femur. On oblique views, this area of the bone can appear strikingly irregular (Fig. 6.69). Chronic avulsion injuries of the medial epicondyle are common in young children where excessive use of the arm leads to the so-called "Little Leaguer's elbow." The same injury occurs with tennis elbow.

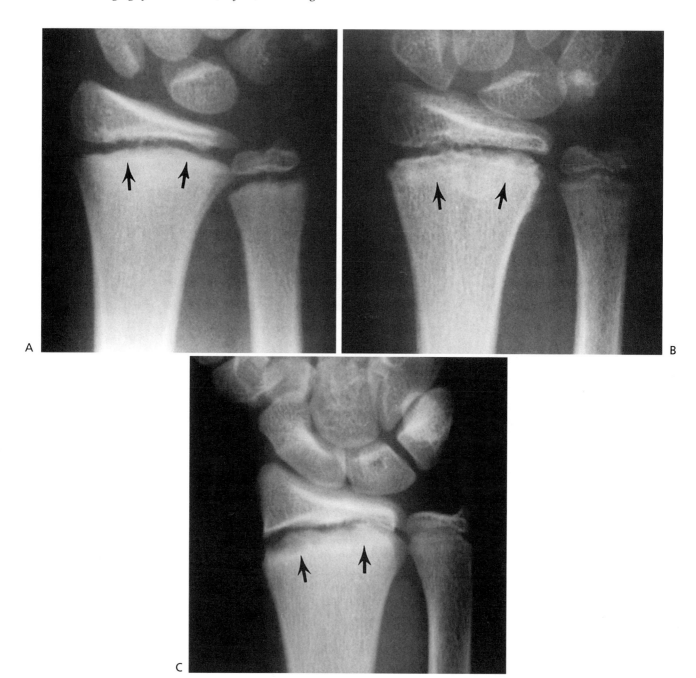

FIGURE 6.62. Healing epiphyseal-metaphyseal fracture. A. Note the widened epiphyseal line (arrows) through the radius. **B.** With healing, sclerosis along the metaphyseal edge (arrows) occurs. **C. Gymnast's wrist.** Note the widened epiphyseal line and adjacent metaphyseal sclerosis (arrows) in this gymnast.

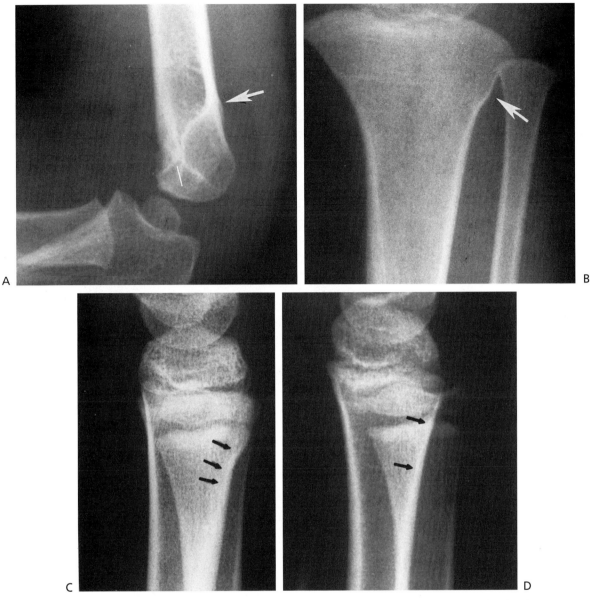

FIGURE 6.63. Subtle buckle fractures. A. Note the subtle buckle fracture through the distal humerus (arrow). This is a minimal supracondylar injury. Note that both the anterior and the posterior fat pads are elevated, indicating the presence of fluid in the joint. **B.** Subtle buckle fracture (arrow) in the upper tibia. **C.** Lateral view demonstrates a subtle buckle fracture in the distal radius (arrows). **D.** Normal side for comparison showing the normal smooth cortex (arrows).

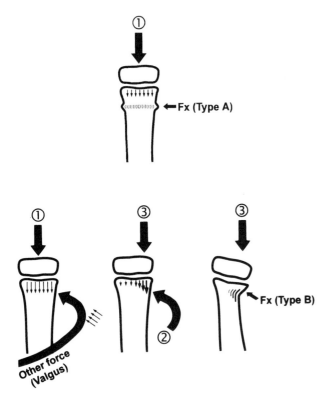

FIGURE 6.64. Buckle fractures: mechanics of injury. A. Typical buckle fracture, type A. Vertical forces (1) result in an even axial load on the metaphysis with resultant buckling and outward bulging of the cortex (FX). **B. Buckle fracture, type B.** Axial loading forces (1) again are present, but some other force, in this case a valgus force (2), also is present. This causes lateralization of the axial forces (3) and concentrates these forces along one edge of the metaphysis (2). This results in a type B angled buckle fracture (Fx type B).

Other locations of avulsion injuries include the upper tibial tubercle either acutely or chronically as Osgood-Schlatter disease and the inferior pole of the patella with similar findings in jumper's knee (25), the base of the fifth metatarsal (Iselin's disease) (26), and at the humeral insertion of the deltoid muscle (27). In any of these cases, the key to identifying these fractures correctly is to know where they occur and what they look like during their various stages of healing.

Acute elbow fractures are numerous and usually result from falling on the outstretched extremity with the elbow locked in extension (FOOSCH injury). Forces involved include hyperextension, rotation, and valgus and varus stresses. A detailed dissertation on the mechanisms of these fractures is available in the article by John et al. (20), and only a few examples will be demonstrated here. In the humerus, the most common fracture is the supracondylar fracture, followed by the lateral condylar fracture (Fig. 6.70). Overall, supracondylar fractures are most common

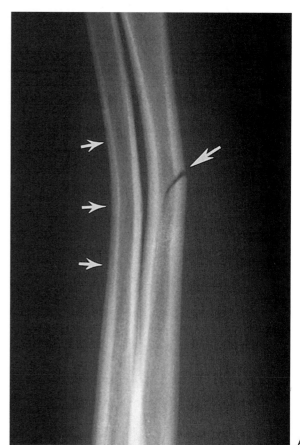

A

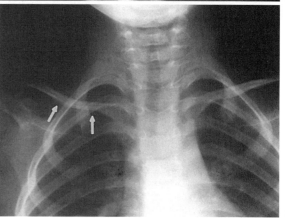

B

FIGURE 6.65. Greenstick and bending fractures. A. In this patient, there is a greenstick fracture of the radius (1) and a plastic bending fracture of the ulna (2). **B.** The right clavicle is bent (arrows), in keeping with a plastic bending fracture. Compare its configuration with a normal clavicle on the left.

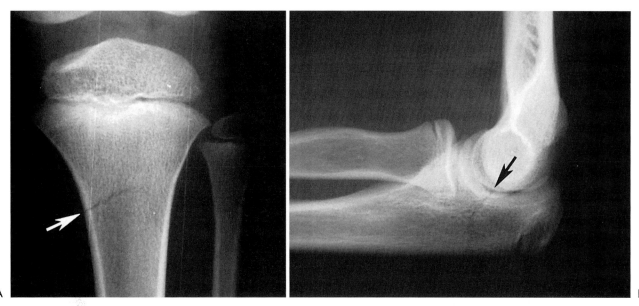

A   B

FIGURE 6.66. Hairline fractures. A. Typical hairline fracture (arrow) in the upper tibia. This fracture occurs as part of the hyperextension upper tibial injury (see Fig. 6.79). **B.** Transverse hairline fracture (arrow) through the proximal ulna. This fracture results from direct blows to the flexed elbow.

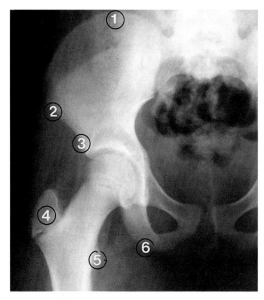

FIGURE 6.67. Common sites of pelvic avulsion fractures. Superior iliac wing (1), anterosuperior iliac spine (2), anteroinferior iliac spine (3), greater trochanter (4), lesser trochanter (5), and inferior aspect of ischium (6). The most common sites are 2, 3, and 6.

and subtle; most of these can be identified with use of the anterior humeral line (28). The radius tends to fracture by impaction, resulting in an impacted or buckled Salter-Harris type II injury (Fig. 6.71, A–C), while the ulna tends to demonstrate hairline fractures both in transverse and in longitudinal directions (Fig. 6.71E). Coronoid process avulsion fractures result from brachialis brevis muscle pull (Fig. 6.71F). In older children, acute avulsions of the medial epicondyle can occur (Fig. 6.70, G and H). Lateral epicondylar avulsions are much less common but lateral condylar avulsion fractures are common and often subtle (Fig. 6.71, E and F). Ultrasound also has been suggested in detection of these fractures (29) and when the radial head is dislocated in association with an ulnar fracture, a Monteggia fracture results (Fig. 6.71D).

The nursemaid's or pulled elbow is common in infants (30). In this condition, when the arm is pulled, the head of the radius slips out of the annular ligament and fails to return to normal position after the distracting forces stop. The injury is extremely painful; the infant usually will not move the arm at all, and the condition should be diagnosed and treated clinically. Treatment consists of supinating the forearm with the thumb over the head of the radius and feeling the head snap back into the annular ligament. Often, this maneuver is fortuitously performed while the patient is being x-rayed in an attempt to obtain a good lateral view of the elbow. After the radius has been reduced, in a few cases, displacement and elevation of the fat pads may be seen, but no fractures occur (31). Interestingly enough, most people who

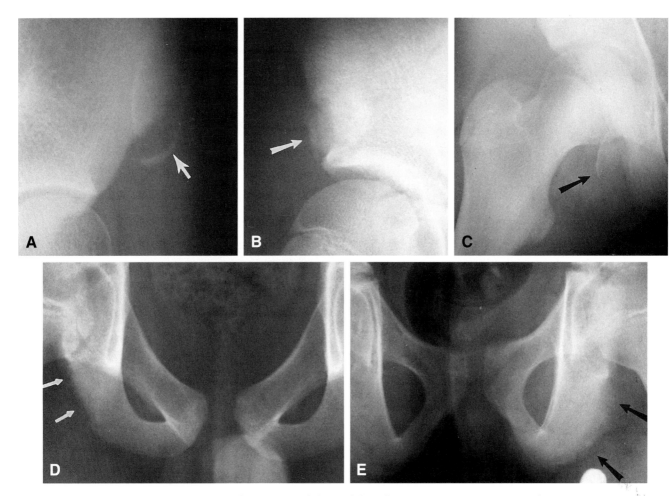

FIGURE 6.68. Acute and chronic pelvic avulsion fractures. A. Acute avulsion fracture (arrow) of the anterosuperior iliac spine. **B.** Chronic hypertrophic healing avulsion fracture (arrow) of the anteroinferior iliac spine. **C.** Acute avulsion of the ischium (arrow). **D.** Subacute (partially healed) avulsion fracture of the ischium (arrows). Only bone resorption is seen. **E.** Chronic hypertrophic avulsion fracture (arrow) of the ischium.

cause the pulled elbow believe that they have dislocated the shoulder or fail to tell the physician that the arm was pulled because they feel they will be accused of abuse of the infant.

In the wrist, buckle and epiphyseal-metaphyseal fractures are common. It is important to realize, however, that when an ulnar styloid fracture is seen, one is obligated to look for an occult, epiphyseal-metaphyseal, or buckle fracture if such a fracture, in overt form, is not present (32). The ulnar styloid process cannot fracture alone unless it sustains a direct blow; therefore, when an ulnar styloid fracture is seen, a radial fracture should be present and sought (Fig. 6.72). The other fracture to be considered in the wrist is the scaphoid fracture (Fig. 6.73). This fracture also is sustained from impaction when falling on an outstretched extremity, but it is important to realize that in young children, the fracture often is more of the buckle-compressive type than it is the typical

hairline fracture seen in adulthood (Fig. 6.74). Comparative views are important in the detection of these buckle-impacted fractures; however, if they are not detected radiographically, they will be positive on nuclear scintigraphy.

REFERENCES

1. Swischuk LE. Emergency radiology of the acutely ill or injured child. 2nd ed. Baltimore: Williams & Wilkins, 1995:361–547.
2. Crowe JE, Swischuk LE. Acute bowing fractures of the forearm in children. A frequently missed injury. AJR 1977;128:981–984.
3. John SD, Phillips WA. Imaging evaluation of pediatric extremity trauma, part I: injury patterns of the immature skeleton and imaging modalities. J Intens Care Med 1998;13:124–134.
4. John SD, Phillips WA. Imaging evaluation of pediatric extremity trauma, part II. J Intens Care Med 1998;13:184–194.
5. John SD, Phillips WA. Imaging evaluation of pediatric extremity

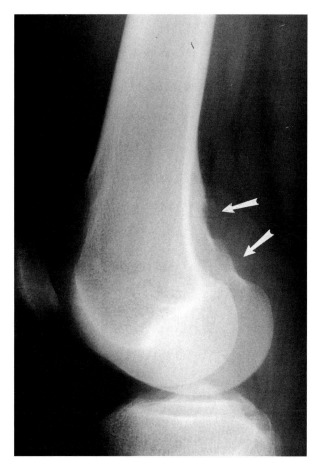

FIGURE 6.69. Medial femoral condylar ridge irregularity. Note normal irregularity (arrows) along the medial condylar ridge.

trauma, part III: lower extremity and soft tissues. J Intens Care Med 1998;13:241–252.

6. Horev G, Korenreich L, Ziv N, et al. The enigma of stress fractures in the pediatric age: clarification or confusion through the new imaging modalities. Pediatr Radiol 1990;20:469–471.

7. Kozlowski K, Azouz M, Hoff D. Stress fracture of the fibula in the first decade of life. Report of eight cases. Pediatr Radiol 1991; 21:381–382.

8. Walker RN, Green NE, Spindler KP. Stress fractures in skeletally immature patients. J Pediatr Orthop 1996;16:578–584.

9. Donnelly LF. Toddler's fracture (stress fracture) of the fibula. AJR 2000;175:922.

10. St. Pierre P, Staheli LT, Smith JB, et al. Femoral neck stress fractures in children and adolescents. J Pediatr Orthop 1995;15: 470–473.

11. Anderson MW, Ugalde V, Batt M, et al. Shin splints: MR appearance in a preliminary study. Radiology 1997;204:177–180.

12. Peterson HA. Physeal fractures: part 3 classification. J Pediatr Orthop 1994;14:439–448.

13. Hynes D, O'Brien T. Growth disturbance lines after injury of the distal tibial physis: their significance in prognosis. J Bone Joint Surg (Br) 1988;70:231–233.

14. Borsa JJ, Peterson HA, Ehman RL. MR imaging of the physeal bars. Radiology 1996;199:683–687.

15. Jarmillo D, Hoffer FA, Shapiro F, et al. NMR imaging of fractures of the growth plate. AJR 1990;155:1261–1265.

16. Smith BG, Rand F, Jaramillo D, et al. Early MR imaging of lower extremity physeal fracture separations: a preliminary report. J Pediatr Orthop 1994;14:526–533.

17. Liebling MS, Berdon WE, Ruzal-Shapiro C, et al. Case report. Gymnast's wrist (pseudorickets growth plate abnormality) in adolescent athletes: findings on plain films and MR imaging. AJR 1995;164:157–159.

18. Carson WG Jr, Gasser SI. Little Leaguer's shoulder: a report of 23 cases. Am J Sports Med 1998;26:575–580.

19. Hernandez JA, Alberto, Swischuk LE, Yagve DA, Carmichael KD. The angled buckle fracture in pediatrics. A frequently missed fracture. Emerg Radiol, 2004. In press.

20. John SD, Wherry K, Swischuk LE, et al. Improving detection of pediatric elbow fractures by understanding their mechanics. Radiographics 1996;16:1443–1460.

21. Wherry K, John SD, Swischuk LE, et al. Linear fractures in the proximal ulna (a frequently missed injury). Emerg Radiol 1995; 2:197–201.

22. Hernandez JA, Swischuk LE, Bathurst GJ, et al. Scaphoid (navicular) fractures of the wrist in children: attention to the plastic bending fracture. Emerg Radiol 2003;9:305–308.

23. Stevens MA, El-Khoury GY, Kathol MH, et al. Imaging features of avulsion injuries. Radiographics 1999;19:655–772.

24. Brandser EA, El-Khoury GY, Kathol MH. Adolescent hamstring avulsions that stimulate tumors. Emerg Radiol 1995;2: 273–278.

25. Khan KM, Bonar F, Desmond PM, et al. Patellar tendinosis (jumper's knee): findings at histopathologic examination, US, and MR imaging. Radiology 1996;200:821–827.

26. Canale ST, Williams KD. Iselin's disease. J Pediatr Orthop 1992; 12:90–93.

27. Donnelly LF, Helms CA, Bisset GS III. Chronic avulsion injury of the deltoid insertion in adolescents: imaging findings in three cases. Radiology 1999;211:233–236.

28. Rogers LF, Malave S Jr, White H, et al. Plastic bowing, torus and greenstick supracondylar fractures of the humerus: radiographic clues to obscure fractures of the elbow in children. Radiology 1978;128:145–150.

29. Connell D, Burke F, Combs P, et al. Sonographic examination of lateral epicondylitis. AJR 2001;176:777–782.

30. Choung W, Heinrich SD. Acute annular ligament interposition into the radiocapitellar joint in children (nursemaid's elbow). J Pediatr Orthop 1995;15:454–456.

31. Macias CG, Wiebe R, Bothner J. History and radiographic findings associated with clinically suspected radial head subluxations. Pediatr Emerg Care 2000;16:22–25.

32. Stansberry SD, Swischuk LE, Swischuk JL, et al Significance of ulnar styloid fractures in childhood. Pediatr Emerg Care 1990;6: 99–103.

Toddler's Fractures (The Toddler Fracture Expanded)

The original toddler's fracture described by Dunbar et al. (1) was a spiral fracture of the tibia resulting from torque or twisting applied to the lower leg (Fig. 6.75A). It often is a difficult fracture to detect. It is a true hairline fracture that

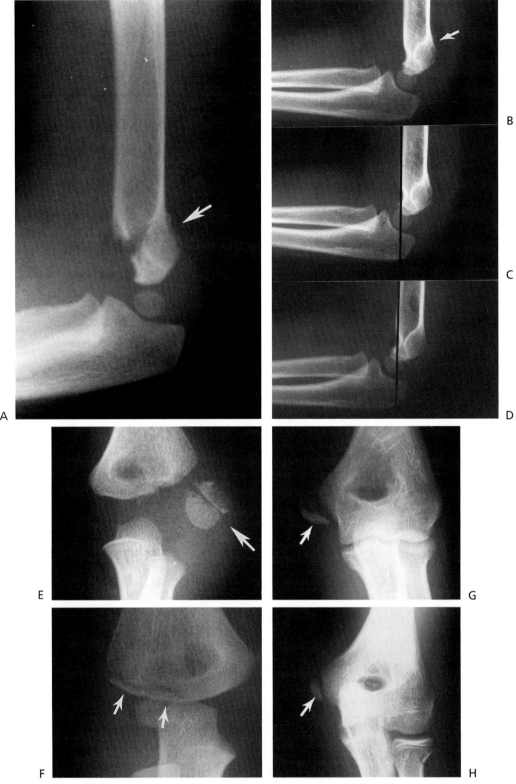

FIGURE 6.70. Elbow fractures: distal humerus. A. Typical supracondylar fracture (arrow) with posterior tilting of the distal fracture fragment. **B.** A more subtle bending fracture of the distal humerus is present. At first, the humerus might appear normal, but there is a slight buckle fracture present (arrow) and the posterior fracture fragment is posteriorly tilted to a slight degree. **C.** Confirmation with anterior humeral line. The anterior humeral line (black line) drawn along the anterior cortex of the humerus intersects the capitellum through its anterior third. It should intersect it through the middle to posterior thirds, and thus the findings suggest a posterior tilted distal fragment (i.e., plastic fracture). **D.** Normal side for comparison demonstrates the normal point of intersection of the capitellum by the anterior humeral line. This verifies that the distal segment in **B** and **C** is posteriorly tilted. **E.** Grossly avulsed and rotated capitellar fracture (arrow). **F.** More subtle, nondisplaced capitellar avulsion fracture (arrows). **G.** Medial epicondylar avulsion (arrow). **H.** More subtle medial epicondylar avulsion (arrow); soft tissue swelling over the fracture site. No swelling was present on the other side. Also note the compression fracture of the radial head.

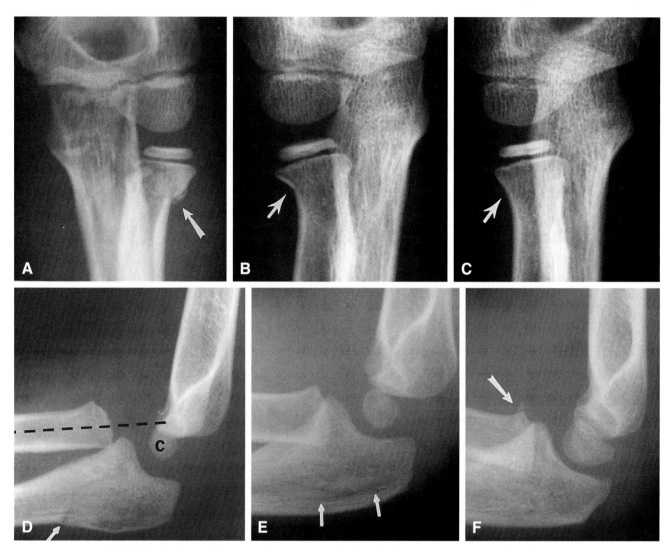

FIGURE 6.71. Elbow fractures (radius and ulna). A. Typical impacted, displaced radial head fracture (arrow). **B.** More subtle buckle-impaction fracture (arrow) manifest by a subtle cortical break and slight angulation of the cortex (arrow). **C.** Normal side for comparison. Note the smooth configuration of the radial cortex (arrow). **D.** Note the fracture in the proximal ulna (arrow). There is also some buckling of the cortex of the proximal fracture fragment. The radial head does not line up (dashed black line) with the capitellum (C). The radius is dislocated, constituting a Monteggia fracture. **E.** Subtle linear fracture in proximal ulna (arrows). **F.** Ulnar coronoid process avulsion fracture (arrow).

frequently is more readily visible on one view than another. Frequently, the fracture extends up the entire diaphysis of the tibia and is a common cause of **a mild to moderately painful limp in infancy.** Close scrutiny of the films is required for **clinically the problem often is believed to be in the ankle.** For this reason, ankle views usually are obtained, but fortunately the spiral fracture usually is seen on one of these views. If these fractures are missed, they evoke considerable periosteal new bone deposition with healing and, when detected at this stage, may erroneously suggest a tumor such as Ewing's sarcoma (Fig. 6.76). Overall, this fracture represents a spectrum (2) of subtle to overt spiral, torsion-induced injuries of the tibia.

Since the original toddler's fracture was described, a number of other fractures producing similar clinical findings have been encountered. For this reason, **the original toddler's fracture concept has been expanded** (3, 4) to include fractures through the base of the first metatarsal (Fig. 6.75, B and C), impaction cuboid bone fractures (Fig. 6.75B), buckle fractures of the distal tibia and fibula (Figs. 6.71, D and E), and impaction fractures of the calcaneus (5, 6). Fractures through the base of the first metatarsal often are buckle fractures and are attendant with adjacent soft tissue swelling. Cuboid fractures, however, are more difficult to detect and usually not seen until they start to heal and some sclerosis is visualized. Calcaneal fractures behave in

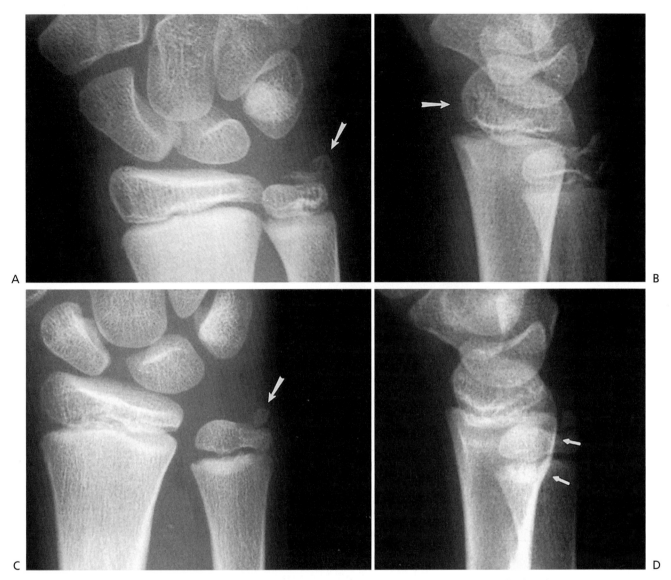

FIGURE 6.72. Ulnar styloid fracture with radial fracture. A. Note the ulnar styloid avulsion fracture (arrow). It may be difficult to appreciate that a radial epiphyseal-metaphyseal fracture is present. **B.** However, on lateral view, the distal radial epiphysis is posteriorly displaced (arrow). **C.** Another patient with an ulnar styloid avulsion fracture (arrow). **D.** Lateral view demonstrates a subtle buckle fracture (arrows) over the dorsal aspect of the distal radius.

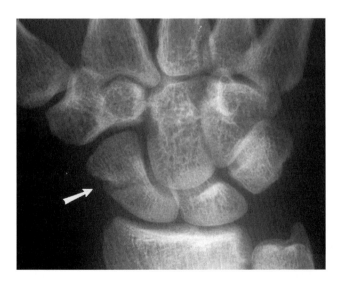

FIGURE 6.73. Classic navicular (scaphoid) fracture. Typical transverse fracture (arrow) through the scaphoid bone.

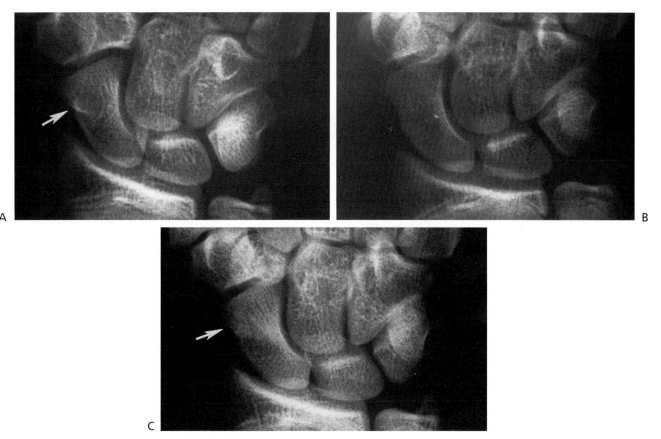

FIGURE 6.74. Navicular scaphoid fractures: buckle type. A. In this case, an impaction fracture with minimal buckling (arrow) is present. It might go unnoticed. **B.** Normal side demonstrates the normal configuration of the navicular bone. Note in **A** that in addition to the buckle fracture, the navicular bone is foreshortened because of impaction. **C.** With healing, sclerosis (arrow) is seen across the fracture site.

the same way and result from direct impaction of the calcaneus. These fractures usually are best demonstrated with tangential views, in which the calcaneus appears broader and fatter than on the normal side (Fig. 6.77). Cuboid and base of the first metatarsal fractures result from landing on the forefoot from a considerable height and therefore have been termed **bunkbed fractures.**

A recent addition to the expanded toddler's fracture concept is **the upper tibial hyperextension-induced injury** (7). In these cases, hyperextension of the knee results in impaction of the upper tibia and the following findings: a posterior distracting fracture, anterior compression with buckling of the cortex and deepening of the notch for the tibial tubercle, and anterior tilting of the epiphyseal plate (Fig. 6.78). These findings often are subtle, but important to recognize, and comparative views are indispensable (Fig. 6.79).

Finally, I have always used the following **physical examination to clinically detect the most likely site of injury**

(Fig. 6.80). Step 1. Take the knee in its flexed position and rotate it around the hip joint (hip problems). **Step 2.** Take the knee and ankle and twist in opposite directions (spiral toddler's fracture). **Step 3.** Take the lower extremity and hyperextend at the knee (hyperextension toddler's fracture). **Step 4.** Squeeze the distal ankle (buckle fractures of the distal tibia and fibula). **Step 5.** With the thumb, press over the cuboid bone and first metatarsal (cuboid and first metatarsal impaction fractures). **I have found these five steps extremely valuable in detecting the site of injury prior to imaging.**

REFERENCES

1. Dunbar JS, Owen HF, Nogrady MB, et al. Obscure tibial fracture of infants—the toddler's fracture. J Can Assoc Radiol 1964;15: 136–144.
2. Mellick LB, Miller L, Egsieker E. Childhood accidental spiral tibial (CAST) fractures. Pediatr Emerg Care 1999;15:307–309.

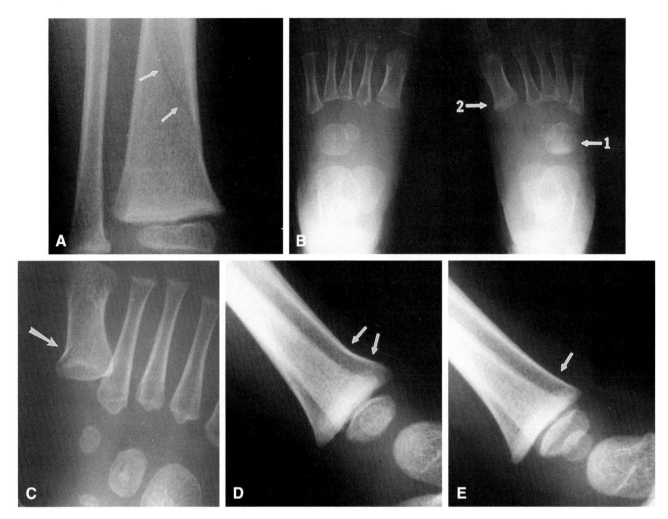

FIGURE 6.75. Toddler's fractures. A. Original toddler's fracture. Note the hairline spiral fracture (arrows) through the distal tibia. **B. Cuboid and first metatarsal fractures.** Note sclerosis of the left cuboid bone (1). In addition, there is a subtle buckle fracture of the base of the first metatarsal (2). Compare the configuration of the cortex with the cortex on the normal side. **C.** Another patient with a more clearly visible buckle fracture (arrow) of the base of the first metatarsal. **D. Subtle buckle fracture of the distal tibia (arrows).** Increased slope and angulation of the distal cortex are seen. **E.** Normal side for comparison. Note the smooth contour of the normal cortex (arrow).

3. John SD, Moorthy CS, Swischuk LE. Expanding the concept of the toddler's fracture. Radiographics 1997;17:367–376.
4. Tschoepe EJ, John SD, Swischuk LE. Tibial fractures in infants and children: emphasis on subtle injuries. Emerg Radiol 1998;5: 245–252.
5. Laliotis N, Pennie BH, Carty H, et al. Toddler's fracture of the calcaneum. Injury 1993;24:169–170.
6. Schindler A, Mason DE, Allington NJ. Occult fracture of the calcaneus in toddlers. J Pediatr Orthop 1996;16:201–205.
7. Swischuk LE, John SD, Tschoepe EJ. Upper tibial hyperextension fractures in infants: another occult toddler's fracture. Pediatr Radiol 1999;29:6–9.

Occult Skeletal Pain

Occult skeletal pain (i.e., pain without any radiographic evidence of bone abnormality) is a common problem in infants and young children. The underlying problem can be trauma, infection, or tumor, and when radiographs are negative and pain persists, one should go on to nuclear scintigraphy (1, 2). This study is sensitive but nonspecific (Fig. 6.81). In this regard, however, recently MRI (3–7) has come into play. MRI is more important in adults than in

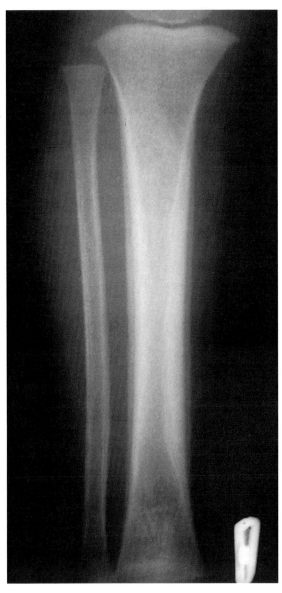

FIGURE 6.76. Healing toddler's fracture. Note abundant periosteal new bone around the tibia, often misinterpreted for that of an underlying tumor.

children, but still it is useful in cases that elude diagnosis. MRI also can detect chondral injuries (8), which, of course, are not detectable on plain films.

REFERENCES

1. Aronson J, Garvin K, Seibert J, et al. Efficiency of the bone scan for occult limping toddlers. J Pediatr Orthop 1992;12:38–44.
2. Englaro EE, Gelfand MJ, Paltiel HJ. Bone scintigraphy in preschool children with lower extremity pain of unknown origin. J Nucl Med 1992;33:351–354.
3. Griffith JF, Roebuck DJ, Cheng JY, et al. Acute elbow trauma in children: spectrum of injury revealed by MR imaging not apparent on radiographs. AJR 2001;176:53–60.
4. Hottya GA, Hackl FO, Iwasko NG, et al. Assessing radiographically occult upper extremity fractures with dedicated extremity MRI. Emerg Radiol 2000;7:339–348.
5. Johnson KJ, Haigh SF, Symonds KE. MRI in the management of scaphoid fractures in skeletally immature patients. Pediatr Radiol 2000;30:685–688.
6. Kamegaya M, Shinohara Y, Kurokawa M, et al. Assessment of stability in children's minimally displaced lateral humeral condyle fracture of magnetic resonance imaging. J Pediatr Orthop 1999; 19:570–572.
7. Naranja RJ Jr, Gregg JR, Dormans JP, et al. Pediatric fracture without radiographic abnormality: description and significance. Clin Orthop 1997;342:141–146.
8. Kim CW, Jaramillo D, Hresko MR. MRI demonstration of occult purely chondral fractures of the tibia: a potential mimic of meniscal tears. Pediatr Radiol 1997;27:765–766.

Joint Fluid

Joint fluid can be seen with trauma (blood), infections and inflammations, and, on a sympathetic basis, with extraarticular but adjacent inflammation or infection. The presence of abnormal amounts of joint fluid is readily detected with plain films in the elbow, ankle, and knee (1, 2). In the elbow, one should look for upward displacement of the anterior and posterior fat pads (Fig. 6.82, A and B). A similar finding is seen in the ankle (Fig. 6.82, C and D). In the knee, the suprapatellar bursa is the first to fill with fluid and is best visualized on lateral views as it distends and fills the space behind the quadriceps tendon (Fig. 6.83, A and B). Many times, especially in infants and with inflammations and infections, the bursa is not visualized as a discrete structure, but rather it blends in with the quadriceps tendon and the quadriceps tendon then appears thicker than normal (Fig. 6.83, C and D). In the shoulder and hip, the presence of joint fluid is manifest by lateral displacement of the humerus or femur and widening of the joint space (Fig. 6.84). Lesser volumes of fluid, however, may not cause displacement of the femur laterally; similarly, in older children in whom the joint capsule ligaments are stronger, displacement may not occur. For this reason, ultrasonography has become the imaging modality of choice for demonstrating fluid in the hip and, to some extent, the shoulder.

A final comment regarding the fat pads around the elbow might be in order. These fat pads have been useful for years for the detection of joint fluid in the elbow. However, there often is difference of opinion as to exactly what they convey. In our study (3), we determined that an occult fracture was present in only 15% of cases. This was confirmed by another study performed by Donnelly et al. (4), but recently another study on the subject (5) contradicted this and indicated that there was approximately a 75% incidence of occult fracture. However, upon examining this lat-

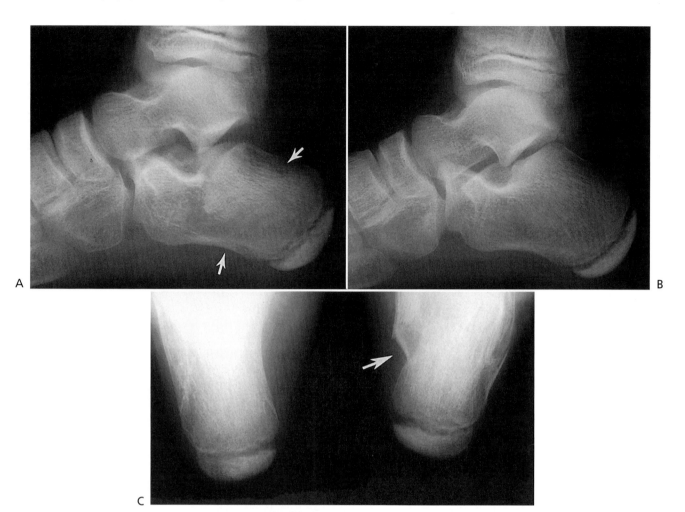

FIGURE 6.77. Calcaneal impaction fracture. A. On the lateral view, note that the calcaneus (arrows) shows some increased sclerosis and that Boehler's angle is reduced (i.e., the calcaneus is flattened). **B.** Normal side for comparison. Boehler's angle (lines) is normal, measuring approximately 140°. The calcaneus also is not flat. **C.** Tangential view demonstrates that the calcaneus is widened (arrows) because it is impacted. There also is some soft tissue swelling present.

ter communication, it was determined that comparative views were not obtained and that, in fact, the first illustrative case in the communication demonstrated a buckle fracture of the distal humerus. This fracture is subtle but with comparative views would probably have been picked up. Therefore, rather than concluding that three-quarters of the patients with initially abnormal fat pads have fractures subsequently detected, it might have been better to state that **if one does not obtain routine comparative views, then the incidence might be significantly higher than if one routinely obtained such views** (6).

REFERENCES

1. Hayden CK Jr, Swischuk LE. Para-articular soft tissue changes in infants and trauma of the lower extremity in children. AJR 1980; 134:307–311.
2. Towbin R, Dunbar JS, Towbin J, et al. Teardrop sign: plain film recognition of ankle effusion. AJR 1980;134:985–990.
3. Swischuk LE, Kupfer MC, Hayden CK. Intraarticular fluid with no visible fracture in children. (How often is an occult fracture present?) AJR 1984;142:1261.
4. Donnelly LF, Klostermeier TT, Klosterman LA. Traumatic elbow effusions in pediatric patients: are occult fractures the rule? AJR 1998;171:243–245.

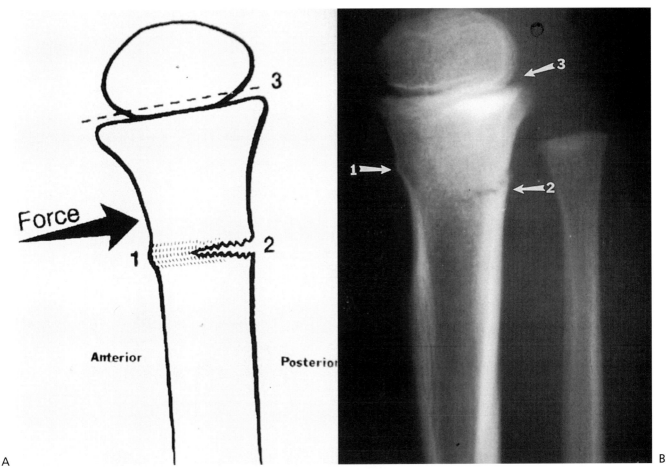

A

B

FIGURE 6.78. Toddler's fracture: tibial hyperextension type. A. With hyperextension, there is posterior cortical diastatic fracturing (1), anterior cortical buckling (2), and anterior tilting of the epiphyseal plate (3). In addition, the notch for the tibial tubercle becomes more concave. **B.** Radiographic demonstration of these findings.

5. Skaggs DL, Mirzayan R. The posterior fat pad sign in association with occult fracture of the elbow in children. J Bone Joint Surg (Am) 1999;81:1429–1433.
6. Swischuk LE. The posterior fat pad sign and use of comparison radiographs in the diagnosis of occult fractures. J Bone Joint Surg (Am) 2001;83:1435–1436.

Trauma to the Joints

Infants and children regularly sustain injuries that involve the large joints, but since the epiphyseal-metaphyseal junction is a weak zone, a Salter-Harris injury of the epiphysis occurs more often than does joint dislocation. As a consequence, joint dislocations are far less common in the early pediatric age group than in older children and adults. As for sprains, the ankle is the most common joint to be sprained, but often nothing more than joint fluid and paraarticular soft tissue swelling are seen. **If a sprain occurs in the wrist, however, an underlying fracture (albeit subtle in many cases) usually is present.**

The knee is commonly injured in older children and adolescents and is subject to many serious injuries. These include anterior cruciate ligament tears (1) with or without avulsion of the anterior tibial spine (Fig. 6.85, A–C), meniscal tears, and joint capsule tears with bursal herniation into the soft tissues, producing a false bursa or diverticulum. The latter injury is associated with swelling of the calf and, in some cases, associated venous stasis. The false bursa is readily detectible with ultrasound.

In terms of meniscal injury (Fig. 6.85, D and E), it is important to note whether the tear extends to the articular surface (2). In addition, it has been demonstrated that medial meniscus tears are more common than lateral

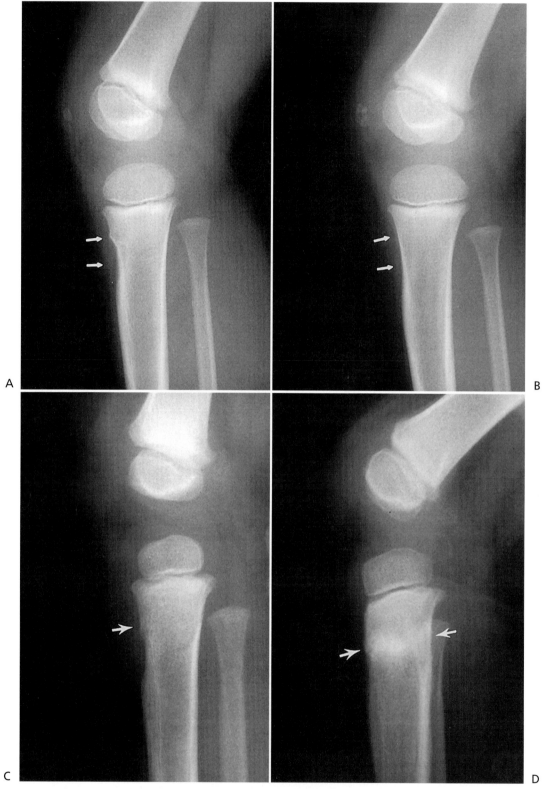

FIGURE 6.79. Toddler's fracture: tibial hyperextension type. A. Note the subtle anterior buckle (upper arrow) and increased concavity of the notch for the tibial tubercle (lower arrow). No posterior fracture is seen, but the epiphyseal plate is tilted anteriorly. **B.** Normal side for comparison. Note the smooth anterior tibial cortex (arrows). Also note that the epiphyseal plate is horizontal. **C.** Another patient with a subtle anterior buckle fracture (arrow). **D.** Healing phase demonstrates sclerosis (arrows) along the occult fracture line.

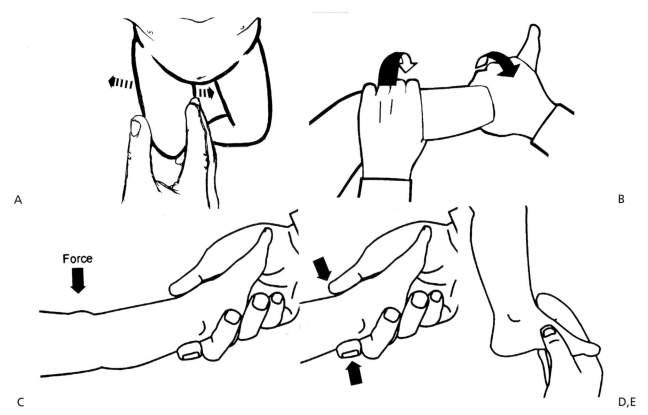

FIGURE 6.80. Toddler's fractures: physical examination. A. Rotate the hip for hip abnormalities. **B.** Twist the lower leg for detection of a spiral toddler's fracture of the tibia. **C.** Hyperextend the knee for the tibial hyperextension toddler's fracture. **D.** Squeeze the ankle through the tibia and fibula for buckle fractures in this region. **E.** Press and palpate over the base of the first metatarsal and the cuboid bone for bunkbed fractures.

meniscus tears (3). In children, one should be aware of the so-called "discoid meniscus." This meniscus, rather than being sickle shaped, is half-moon or discoid shaped, and thus the inner portion extends further into the joint than usual (Fig. 6.86C). As such, it is more subject to injury. It can be detected when a bowtie appearance of the disc, on sagittal views, is seen over more than two CT slices (Fig. 6.86, A and B).

Tears of the anterior cruciate ligament are readily identified with MRI (4, 5), but often the findings are more indirect than direct and consist of buckling of the posterior cruciate ligament, lack of clear visualization of the anterior cruciate ligament, and edema and hemorrhage in the area (Fig. 6.85, B and C). In addition, because there is instability of the knee, the tibia will be displaced anterior to the femur (6), constituting the so-called "drawer sign." Finally, Baker's cysts in the popliteal fossa can be a cause of chronic knee pain in children and are readily demonstrable with ultrasound (7) (Fig. 6.85, F and G). They, along with meniscal cysts, are also demonstrable with MR (8, 9). Bone bruises also accompany many of these injuries, especially anterior cruciate ligament tears (10).

REFERENCES

1. Chan WP, Peterfy C, Fritz RC, et al. MR diagnosis of complete tears of the anterior cruciate ligament of the knee: importance of anterior subluxation of the tibia. AJR 1994;162:355–360.
2. DeSmet AA, Norris MA, Yandow DR, et al. MR diagnosis of meniscal tears of the knee: importance of high signal in the meniscus that extends to the surface. AJR 1993;161:101–107.
3. Zobel MS, Borrello JA, Siegel MJ, et al. Pediatric knee MR imaging: pattern of injuries in the immature skeleton. Radiology 1994;190:397–401.
4. Gentili A, Seger LL, Yao L, et al. Anterior cruciate ligament tear: indirect signs at MR imaging. Radiology 1994;193:835–840.
5. McCauley TR, Moses M, Kier R, et al. MR diagnosis of tears of the anterior cruciate ligament of the knee: importance of ancillary findings. AJR 1994;162:115–119.
6. Vahey TN, Hunt JE, Shelbourne KD. Anterior translocation of the tibia at MR imaging. Secondary sign of anterior cruciate ligament tear. Radiology 1993;187:817–819.
7. Ward EE, Jacobson JA, Fessell DP, et al. Sonographic detection of Baker's cysts: comparison with MR imaging. AJR 2001;176: 373–380.
8. Lang IM, Hughes DG, Williamson JB, et al. MRI appearance of popliteal cysts in childhood. Pediatr Radiol 1997;27:130–132.
9. Ruten CM, Collins JP, van Kampen A, et al. Meniscal cysts: detection with high-resolution sonography. AJR 1998;171:491–496.

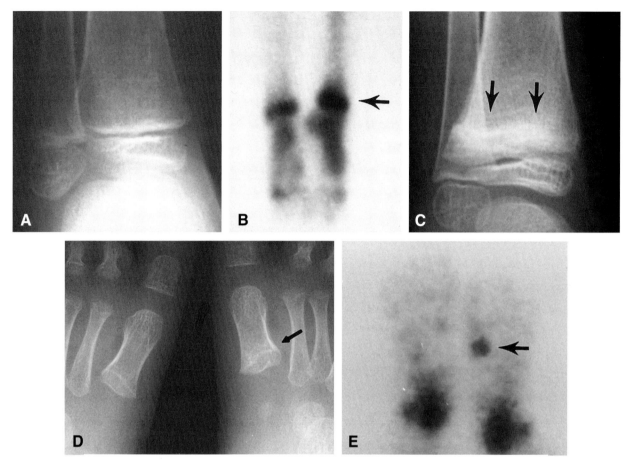

FIGURE 6.81. Use of nuclear scintigraphy with occult fractures. A. This patient had osteoporosis and ankle pain. No fracture is seen. **B.** Nuclear scintigram demonstrates increased activity in the distal right tibia (arrow). **C.** Two weeks later, there is evidence of healing (sclerotic area) of a distal tibial fracture (arrows). **D.** Patient with a subtle buckle fracture of the first metatarsal on the right (arrow). **E.** Nuclear scintigraphy more vividly demonstrates the fracture site (arrow).

10. Johnson DL, Urban WP Jr, Caborn DM, et al. Articular cartilage changes seen with magnetic resonance imaging-detected bone bruises associated with acute anterior cruciate ligament rupture. Am J Sports Med 1998;26:409–414.

Battered Child Syndrome and Deprivational Dwarfism

Since Caffey's original description of the battered infant in his communication entitled "Multiple fractures in long bones of a child suffering from chronic subdural hematoma" (1), much has been learned and written about the subject. Kempe et al. (2), however, eventually coined the term "battered child syndrome," and since many of the injuries were determined to be the result of violent shaking of the infant, the term "shaken infant syndrome" is now also used (3). Although skeletal injuries have always received the most attention, intracranial injuries are the more devastating ones, as are certain abdominal injuries.

The battered child syndrome is not usually a problem in the immediate postnatal period, but thereafter the incidence increases rapidly and remains about the same through early childhood, with most patients presenting before 3 or 4 years of age (4). In one study (5), the average age was 16 months. The importance of the roentgenogram in the detection of occult skeletal injuries in the battered child syndrome is well known, but it is less well known that as many as 50% of these children fail to show evidence of skeletal injury at the time of presentation (6, 7). They may show evidence only of cutaneous and soft tissue damage such as bruising, burns, and unexplained scars. In addition, skeletal injury is more common in infants and young children than it is in older battered children. For this reason, it has been suggested that positive clinical physical findings suggesting bony injury should be the major motivating factor toward obtaining general bone surveys in these latter patients (8). It probably is more appropriate to obtain bone scintigrams after the age of 5 years because it is too time consuming to x-ray all of the skeleton in an older child and results generally are unrewarding. Therefore, a simple total-body screening scintigram makes more sense.

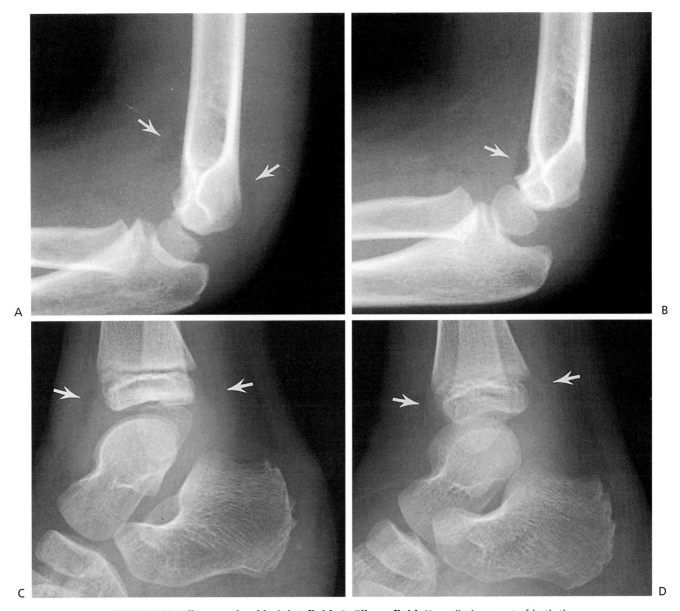

FIGURE 6.82. Elbow and ankle joint fluid. A. Elbow fluid. Note displacement of both the anterior and the posterior fat pads (arrows). **B.** Normally, the anterior fat pad (arrow) is visible against the anterior surface of the distal humerus and the posterior fat pad is not visible. **C. Ankle fluid.** Note elevation of the anterior and posterior fat pads (arrows), signifying the presence of fluid in the ankle. The bulging anterior capsule is referred to as the "teardrop sign." **D.** Normal side for comparison. Note the position of the fat pads.

In our institution, we obtain the roentgenographic bone survey in most other cases because it yields specific information about the type and site of fracture. The scintigraphic bone survey simply makes one aware of sites of bone abnormality, and thereafter one still must obtain radiographs of the suspicious areas. Our main use for the nuclear scintigram lies in the detection of occult injuries when an infant is strongly suspected of being abused and yet no radiographic evidence of skeletal injury is present. One can also obtain follow-up radiographic bone surveys in

these children (9), since healing fractures are easier to detect.

If one chooses the radiographic bone survey, one needs to decide how extensive it should be. In other words, there are those who favor that every joint be radiographed at least in two views and those who settle for a survey of the skeleton. Our survey for young infants consists of an anteroposterior view of the shoulders, upper extremities, and chest and another anteroposterior view that includes the pelvis and lower extremities. In larger infants, the pelvis is exam-

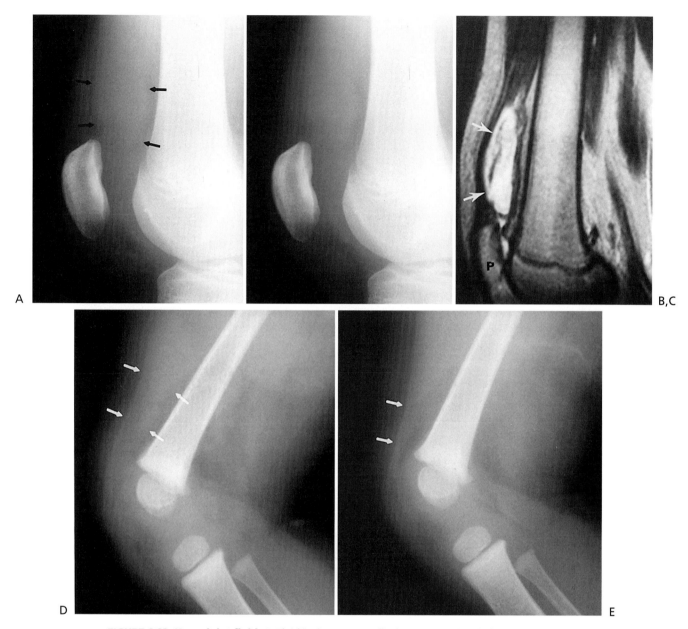

FIGURE 6.83. Knee: joint fluid. A. Fluid in the suprapatellar bursa causes it to bulge and compress (arrows) the prefemoral fat pad. **B.** Same patient without distracting arrows. **C.** Magnetic resonance image shows the location of the fluid (arrows). P, patella. **D.** In this patient, fluid in the suprapatellar bursa blends with the quadriceps tendon and makes the tendon appear thick (arrows). **E.** Normal side for comparison. Note the normal thin configuration of the quadriceps tendon (arrows).

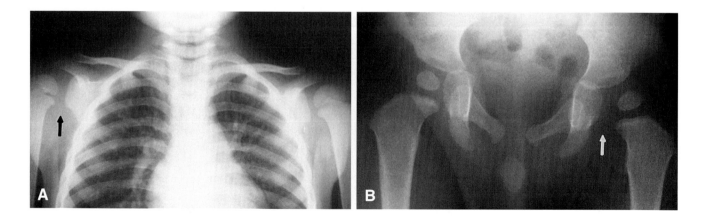

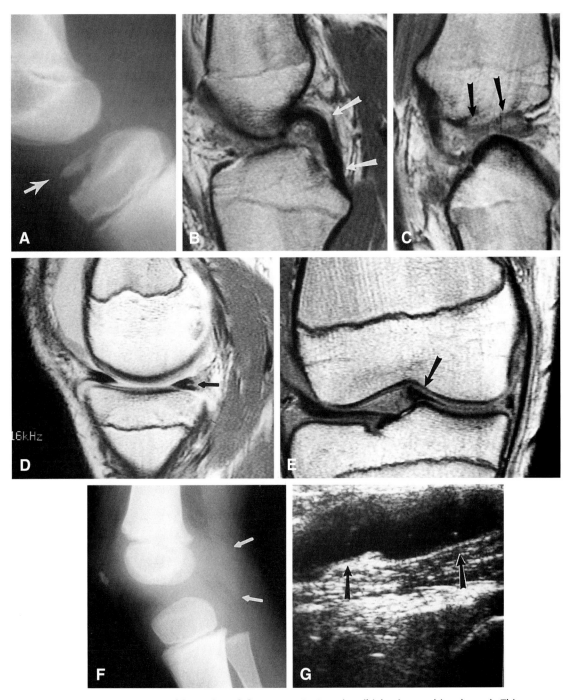

FIGURE 6.85. Knee problems in adolescence. A. Anterior tibial spine avulsion (arrow). This injury is associated with anterior cruciate ligament damage. **B.** Anterior cruciate ligament tear. Indirect findings are present in the form of buckling of the intact posterior cruciate ligament (arrows). **C.** There is poor visualization of the anterior cruciate ligament (arrows) where it normally would be visualized as an oblique line running in the opposite direction to that of the posterior cruciate ligament. **D.** Small tear (arrow) in the posterior limb of the meniscus. **E.** Bucket-handle tear with medial entrapment of the meniscus (arrow). **F.** Baker's cyst. Note fullness in the posterior popliteal region (arrows). **G.** Ultrasonogram clearly demonstrates that a hypoechoic cyst (arrows) is present.

FIGURE 6.84. Joint fluid. A. Shoulder. Note widening of the right shoulder joint (arrow). **B. Hip.** Note widening of the left hip joint (arrow).

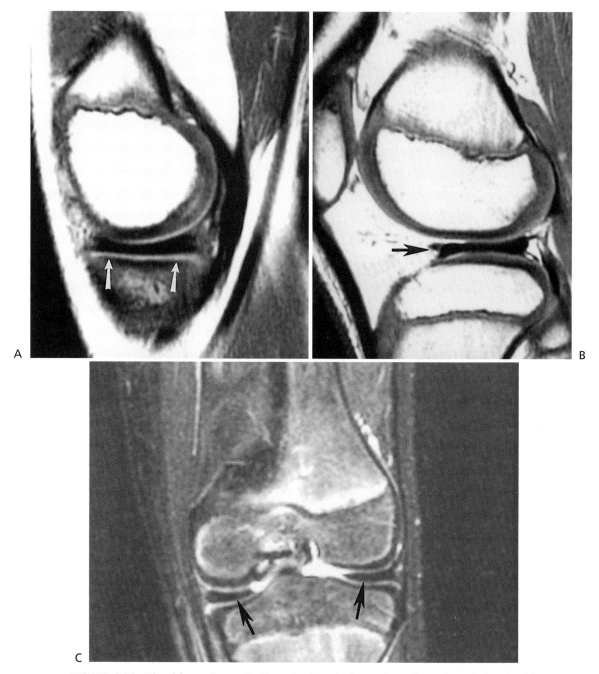

FIGURE 6.86. Discoid meniscus. A. Note the bowtie (arrows) configuration of the discoid meniscus. **B.** A similar configuration is seen on the third inward slice (arrows). This configuration was present bilaterally. **C.** Coronal magnetic resonance image shows that both menisci (arrows) extend further toward the center of the joint than normal.

ined alone, and, if needed, the wrists and ankles are examined alone. We also obtain a lateral view of the entire spine and an anteroposterior and lateral view of the skull. Proper positioning is critical, and if any suspicious areas arise, focused films of these areas are obtained. In addition, it has been suggested that digitized images are inferior in detecting fractures (10). This has been our experience with digitized images in general, but digital images obtained through a PACS system are very satisfactory and, in our opinion, superior.

In terms of skeletal injury in the battered child syndrome, the most typical and diagnostic fracture is the epiphyseal-metaphyseal injury (11), and when these fractures heal, callus formation, epiphyseal-metaphyseal irregularity, and periosteal new bone deposition can be profound (Figs. 6.87 and 6.88). Because of this, some underlying meta-

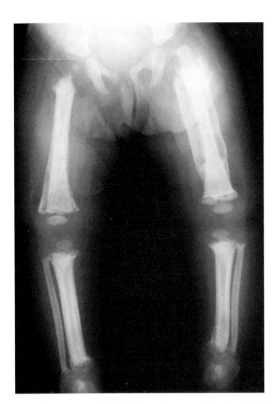

FIGURE 6.87. Battered child syndrome. Classic distribution and configuration of multiple healing fractures as seen in the battered child syndrome. Note widespread metaphyseal irregularity and fragmentation, sparing of the epiphyses, pronounced periosteal new bone deposition, and apparent dislocation of the left hip resulting from an epiphyseal-metaphyseal dislocation. These fractures are between 2 and 4 weeks old.

bolic, hematologic, dysplastic, or infective bone disorder often erroneously is first considered (11). In the battered child syndrome, however, bone architecture and mineralization usually are normal, while in the other conditions, they are not. That is, in the battered child syndrome, except for the fractures, the bones usually appear healthy, well mineralized, and corticated (Fig. 6.87). A problem also often arises in differentiating the battered child syndrome from osteogenesis imperfecta (12). This frequently is more a medicolegally induced problem than one of practicality because the legal profession is well aware that osteogenesis imperfecta can lead to excessive fracturing of the long bones, but it should be remembered that **in osteogenesis imperfecta, epiphyseal-metaphyseal fractures are not the rule.** Furthermore, except for the mildest form of osteogenesis imperfecta, the disease can basically be ruled out with plain x-rays when normal, rather than slender, demineralized, and thinly corticated, bones are seen. Nonetheless, the problem is real, and most often these patients are subject to skin biopsy in which a lack of type I collagen in the fibroblasts will be revealed if osteogenesis imperfecta is present (12).

Similarly, another entity known as "temporary brittle bone disease" often comes into play when dealing with bat-

tered children. This entity, however, is probably nonexistent, and, as has been suggested, it should remain a "hypothetical entity" (13) and a "nonacceptable clinical diagnosis" (14). I completely agree with this posture.

As far as the mechanism of injury in the typical epiphyseal-metaphyseal fracture is concerned, it usually consists of violent shaking or jiggling. The resulting fractures actually are modified Salter-Harris type I and II fractures, and as a consequence, one commonly sees small corner fractures. In the infant, however, the entire metaphyseal ring may be avulsed (11) (Fig. 6.89). Ordinary transverse and oblique fractures also are common, and probably just as common are the epiphyseal-metaphyseal injuries (6, 15–18). The most commonly involved bones are the femur and the humerus, and most fractures are transverse, spiral, or oblique (5, 16). These fractures, if occurring in an older infant or child, do not carry the same degree of suspiciousness as do they when they occur in the younger infant. The younger the infant, the more suspicious one should become (5, 8–23). In this regard, it is generally agreed that long bone fractures, especially if solitary and if not adequately explained, occurring in children under the age of 1 year should be considered the result of abuse until proven otherwise. Originally, this rule was applied to infants 2 years and younger, but this has been adjusted for femoral fractures for they are commonly seen with legitimate trauma, usually accidental, in the ambulating 2-year-old infant (20, 21). Therefore, it now is generally considered that a femoral fracture in a child under the age of 1 year be considered suspicious for the battered child syndrome and that a humeral fracture up to the age of 2 years be similarly considered suspicious. Other bones involved include the bones of the forearm and lower leg. Although tibial fractures are common in the battered child syndrome, there is considerable overlap between legitimate and illegitimate trauma with spiral fractures. For this reason, one must clearly substantiate the mechanism of injury when one sees an isolated spiral fracture of the tibia.

Most of the long bone fractures just discussed tend to occur through the diaphysis of the long bones, but fractures through the distal ends of the bones also occur (i.e., supracondylar, humeral fractures) (16–18). In addition, the typical spiral fracture of the tibia known as the "toddler's fracture" commonly seen on the basis of accidental trauma (24) is also frequently seen in the battered child syndrome. Many of the ordinary-appearing fractures occurring through the diaphyses of the long bones probably result from direct blows to the extremities. However, some may result from forceful leverage applied to the extremity. For example, if one abruptly, perhaps in anger, picks up an infant by the elbow or knee, leverage will be applied to the long bone so that it fractures through the midshaft and angles outward (Fig. 6.90). If angulation occurs inward, a direct blow or leverage applied in the opposite direction would explain the injury. We have noted this aspect of

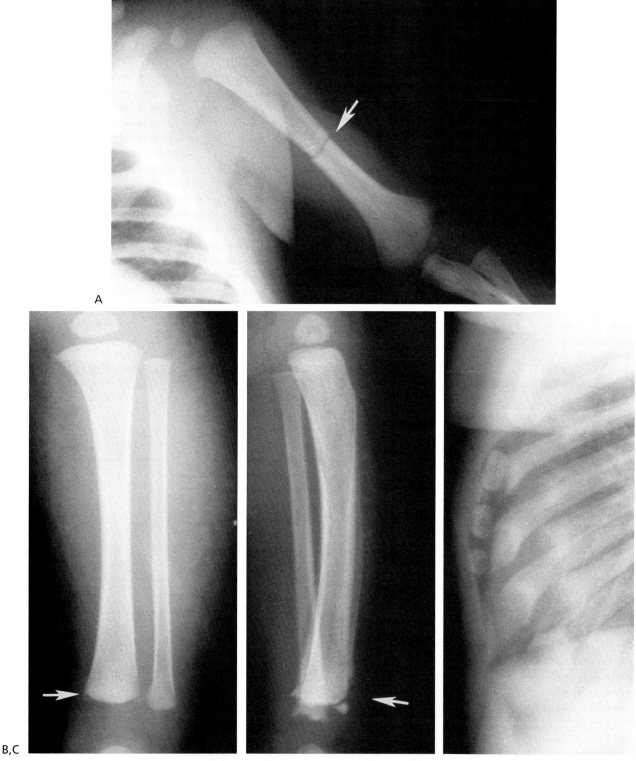

FIGURE 6.88. Battered child syndrome. A. Note an innocuous-appearing transverse fracture of the humerus (arrow). This was the only injury documented in this patient on the first admission. A bone survey was not obtained. **B.** The infant was readmitted 3 weeks later with another acute injury to the right lower leg. Note extensive soft tissue edema and an epiphyseal-metaphyseal injury at the distal end of the right (R) tibia (arrow). There is a subtle metaphyseal avulsion present. This injury is less than 10 days old. **C.** The other lower extremity demonstrates healing of an old epiphyseal-metaphyseal tibial injury (arrow) and periosteal new bone along the diaphysis. There also is an old injury of the metaphysis of the fibula. These injuries probably were sustained but not appreciated (roentgenograms were not obtained at that time) when the humeral fracture was sustained 3 weeks before. **D.** Lateral view of the chest demonstrating extensive cupping of the anterior ribs. This is the result of anterior costochondral injury.

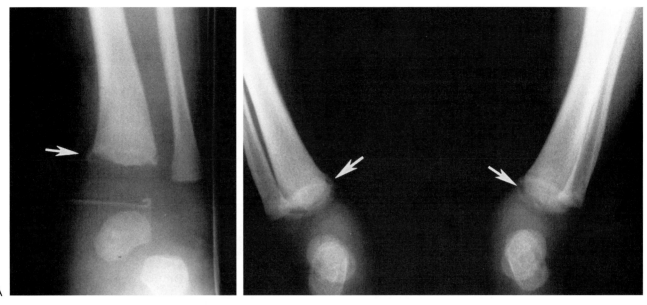

FIGURE 6.89. Epiphyseal-metaphyseal fracture: ring-like configuration. A. Note the ring-like appearance of this epiphyseal-metaphyseal fracture of the distal tibia (arrow). **B.** Another patient with healing ring-like epiphyseal-metaphyseal fractures (arrows).

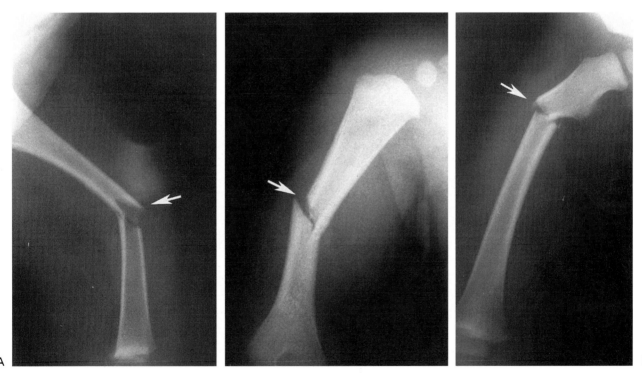

FIGURE 6.90. Long bone fractures. A. Angulated fracture of the femur (arrow). **B.** Similar fracture of the humerus (arrow). **C.** Another femoral fracture with outward angulation (arrow). In all these cases, it is unlikely that these fractures could have been sustained by direct blows or from falling. Leverage would have had to have been applied to these fractures by grabbing the involved bone through its lower end and lifting the child to produce forces that would crack the bone on the outer surface and leave a hinge on the inner surface.

humeral and femoral fractures and are now investigating the concept.

Epiphyseal-metaphyseal long bone injuries, as previously discussed, are the most pathognomonic of the battered child syndrome, but, not uncommonly, similar fractures occur at the distal end of the clavicle (Fig. 6.91A), at the anterior end of the ribs (see Fig. 6.88D), and even at the acromial process of the scapula (Fig. 6.91B). All of these latter fractures (6) are just as pathognomonic as are the classic long bone epiphyseal-metaphyseal fractures. Transverse scapular fractures are rare (Fig. 6.91C).

Rib fractures, in general, are common in the battered child syndrome and uncommon in infants on a legitimate basis. Therefore, their presence in infants should make one highly suspicious of intentionally inflicted trauma. It is difficult for infants and children to sustain rib fractures from ordinary activity and play; thus, there should be a history of a significant accident or direct blow to the ribs as might occur with automobile accidents or significant falls against a hard object. If such documentation is lacking and rib fractures are identified, pursue a diligent search for other evidence of bony injury. This is especially true when the fractures are bilateral.

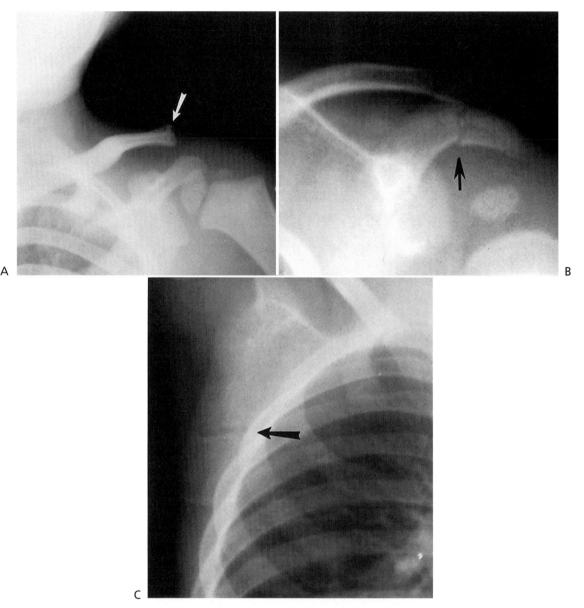

FIGURE 6.91. Battered child syndrome: clavicle and scapula fractures. A. Note a typical lateral and clavicular fracture with early callus formation (arrow). **B.** Linear fracture (arrow) of the acromion process of the scapula. This probably resulted from a shaking injury. **C.** Transverse fracture of the scapula (arrow), the probable result of a direct blow.

Rib fractures are believed to result from a combination of severe squeezing of the chest and shaking of the infant. The fractures occur posteriorly, laterally, and anteriorly at the costochondral junctions. The posterior and lateral fractures often demonstrate abundant callus in their healing phases (Fig. 6.92), while the anterior fractures show exaggerated cupping at the costochondral junction. Lateral fractures probably result primarily from squeezing, while anterior and posterior fractures likely result from squeezing and shaking (the latter probably being the more important). As

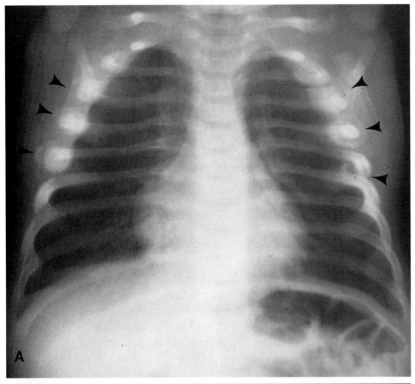

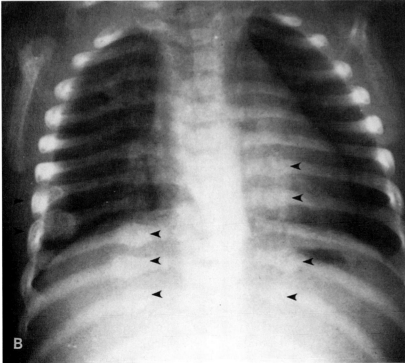

FIGURE 6.92. **Battered child syndrome: rib fractures. A.** Note bilateral healing rib fractures with abundant callus formation (arrowheads). **B.** Note numerous healing rib fractures on the right, both laterally and posteriorly (arrowheads). This patient also has bilateral scapular fractures.

for posterior rib fractures, the proximal portions of the ribs are levered against the transverse processes and thus are fractured (25). These fractures are notoriously occult in their early stages (26) and frequently difficult to detect even with early healing. It is in such cases that nuclear scintigraphy plays one of its most important roles. Finally, fractures of the first rib are not particularly common in the battered child syndrome, but, at the same time, they should be considered highly suspicious (27). Most often, rib fractures in the battered child syndrome occur over the lower two-thirds of the chest.

Skull fractures are common in the battered child syndrome and usually result from direct blows to the head. In terms of intracranial injury, parenchymal hemorrhage and subdural hematomas are most common, but subarachnoid, epidural, and intraventricular bleeds also can occur. Gray-white matter axonal shearing injuries also are common, and all of these abnormalities are readily demonstrable with CT and MR (28). They appear exactly the same as they do when trauma is purely accidental.

Intracranial bleeding also occurs with violent shaking (3), wherein tearing of veins over the surface of the brain leads to subdural hematomas. Shaking also leads to the axonal shearing injuries. Retinal hemorrhages in the form of Purtscher's retinopathy result from violent shaking (i.e., acceleration-deceleration) injuries and are considered pathognomonic of the battered child syndrome (29, 30).

Pelvic injuries are rare in the battered child syndrome (31, 32), as are spine and spinal cord injuries (33–37). The latter usually are seen with violent shaking or hyperflexion forces and may result in complete fracture-dislocation or a variety of compression and avulsion (corner) fractures. In addition, anterior compression (hyperflexion) may lead to notching of the vertebral bodies (37). Interestingly, with spine injuries in battered infants, especially cervical spine injuries, the fact that a fracture is present may be clinically silent (35, 36). A variety of spine and spinal cord injuries are illustrated in Fig. 6.93, but spinal cord injuries are, of course, best evaluated with MRI. Fractures of the hands and feet occur, but usually in older children (38). Most often, they are the result of hyperextension and twisting induced forces. In the immediate postneonatal period, it is important not to misinterpret obstetric trauma for that of the battered child syndrome. In this regard, if an infant presents with a fresh fracture 12–14 days after birth, the battered child syndrome should be suspected. The reason for this is that the first signs of healing in birth trauma usually become apparent somewhere between 10 and 14 days. Therefore, if a fresh fracture is seen toward the end of this time period, or definitely after this time period, birth trauma cannot be invoked as a causative factor.

Dating long bone and other skeletal fractures is very important in assessing the findings in battered infants. Long bone injuries under 10–14 days show soft tissue changes consisting of edema and thickening of the soft tis-

sues. It takes 10–14 days (usually 12–14 days) for periosteal new bone deposition and callus formation to manifest. Thereafter, periosteal new bone formation becomes thicker, and callus formation more evident. By 4 weeks, the findings are clearly evident, and thereafter, as resorption of the callus occurs, periosteal bone maturation and obliteration of the fracture line are seen (Fig. 6.94, A–C). After this point, solidification of the callus and periosteal new bone formation occur, and eventually by 8 weeks, the healing process is more or less complete (Fig. 6.94, D–G).

End of the clavicle and acromial fractures heal in the same way that epiphyseal-metaphyseal fractures of the long bones do. With rib fractures from 0 to 10 days, the fracture line may or may not be seen, and indeed, even with legitimate trauma, these fractures frequently are difficult to detect in their early stages. Between 10 days and 4 weeks, callus begins to form as an osseous "knot" around the fracture site (Fig. 6.95). Initially, an interior radiolucent ring is seen, producing a target sign, but eventually the callus becomes more uniform. This occurs somewhere between 4 and 8 weeks, and then the callus begins to remodel and blend with the rib. After 8 weeks, it often is difficult to find any residua except for slight thickening of the ribs at the fracture site (Fig. 6.95). It is not possible to date calvarial fractures except for the presence of soft tissue edema, which would be present with acute injuries. Overall, however, dating of fractures is important because it can, generally within a few days, give one a good idea of when the fracture occurred. This is even more important when multiple injuries at different stages of healing are seen.

Skull fracture resulting from head trauma is very common in the battered child syndrome and in one series was reported to be the most common fracture (5). When dealing with battered children, plain skull films are still important. CT studies of the calvarium do not detect all fractures for horizontal, linear fractures often are difficult to detect with CT studies. Thereafter, however, it is most important to proceed to CT and MR studies of the brain. However, it has been suggested (39) that if there are no significant clinical findings to suggest intracranial injury, CT of the brain and calvarium can be omitted.

Nonskeletal injury in the battered child syndrome also is common. Most often, it is the abdominal viscera that are involved, and in many cases, no skeletal injury is present. The abdominal viscera most commonly involved are the duodenum and jejunum (40, 41), with hematoma formation and, occasionally, perforation and stricture formation (40). The pancreas also is commonly involved, and pseudocyst formation is common. Gastric hematoma with perforation is less common (42). Ultrasound and CT are excellent at demonstrating these injuries, and the findings are no different than when they are sustained from legitimate trauma. Perforation of the urinary bladder also can occur, and injuries to the hypopharynx (43) and esophagus (44) with or without rupture of the pharyngeal or esophageal

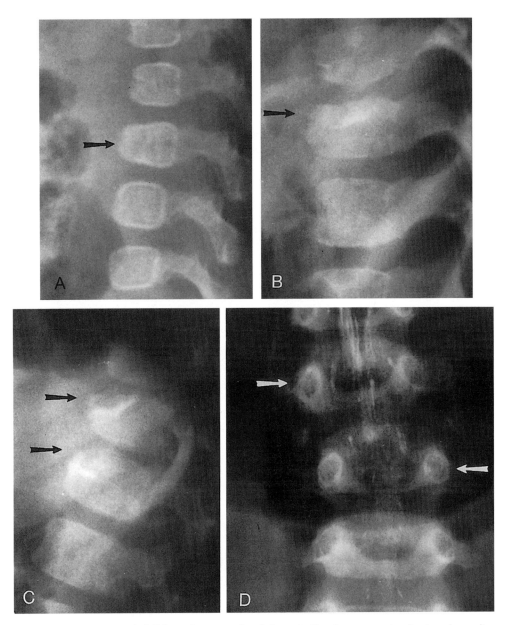

FIGURE 6.93. Battered child syndrome: spine injury. A. Simple compression fracture (arrow). **B.** Compression fracture with notching (arrow). **C.** More pronounced notching (arrows). **D.** Fracture dislocation with displaced vertebrae (arrows). Note residual contrast from a myelogram.

walls may be encountered. We encountered one such infant who presented with difficulties with feeding and transient aspiration into the trachea (Fig. 6.96). It was finally determined that this patient was a battered child.

Other nonskeletal traumatic lesions reported in the battered child syndrome are chylothorax (45) and arterial intraabdominal pseudoaneurysm (46). In addition, it has been noted that intraabdominal injury often is associated with anterior costochondral fractures of the ribs (47).

Sexual abuse is another form of the battered child syndrome. From the radiographic standpoint, there is usually little to demonstrate except when perirectal abscesses or for-

eign bodies inserted into the rectum or vagina are detected (48). Other forms of child abuse include strangulation (49), drowning (50), and burns, especially immersion burns (51). In my experience, however, most of these latter infants do not demonstrate skeletal injury.

Another feature of the battered child syndrome is the need for its differentiation from the sudden infant death syndrome (52, 53). In this regard, in one study (52), only 1 of 10 sudden infant deaths involved an abused infant. In the sudden infant death syndrome, the usual finding is brain edema resulting from asphyxia, but, of course, there are no physical or radiographic skeletal findings to say this

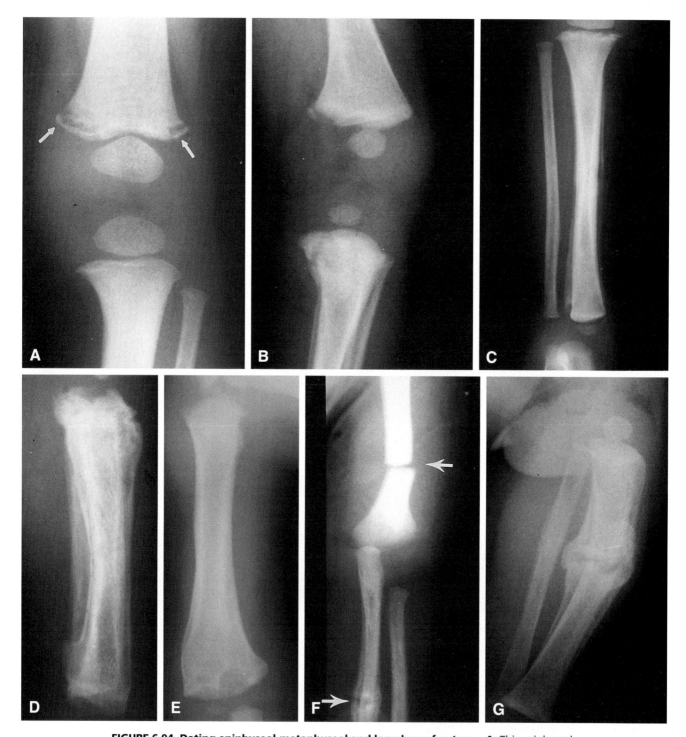

FIGURE 6.94. Dating epiphyseal-metaphyseal and long bone fractures. A. This epiphyseal-metaphyseal fracture (arrows), complete with ring and corner fractures (arrows), is less than 10 days old and probably closer to a week. **B.** The corner fracture in the distal femur is approximately 1 week old, while the upper tibial fracture shows healing and considerable periosteal new bone deposition, suggesting that it is approximately 2 weeks old. **C.** Extensive periosteal new bone on the tibia again suggests an approximately 14-day-old fracture. **D.** More extensive and mature-appearing periosteal new bone and metaphyseal irregularity are consistent with a fracture at least 3–4 weeks old and even up to 6 weeks. **E.** Well-healed fracture of the humerus undergoing remodeling, probably at least 8 weeks old and most likely a little older. **F.** Fresh humeral fracture (upper arrow). Abundant callus and periosteal new bone place the ulnar fracture (lower arrow) at at least 2 weeks of age and probably closer to 3 weeks. **G.** Abundant and mature callus around the fracture in the tibia along with mature periosteal new bone place this fracture at at least 4 weeks of age, but probably no more than 6 weeks.

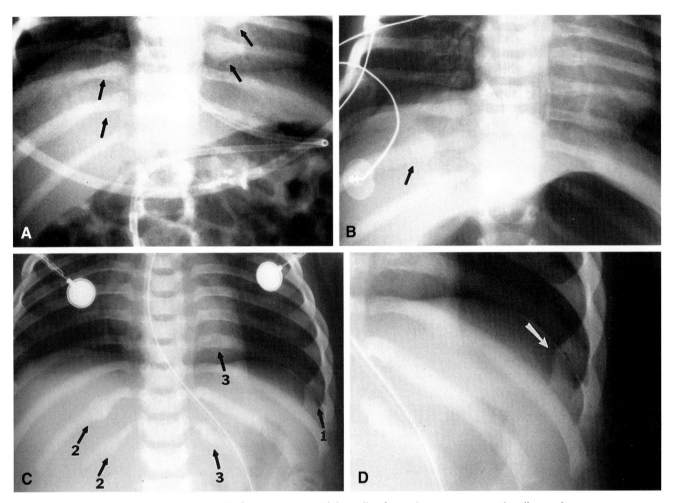

FIGURE 6.95. Dating rib fractures. A. Nodular callus formation on two posterior ribs on the left (arrows) dates the fractures as being approximately 2 weeks old. More mature, remodeled thickening of two posterior ribs on the right (arrows) signifies old fractures closer to 4 weeks of age. **B.** Two weeks later, the fractures on the left show similar remodeling, and only slight thickening of the ribs remains. On the right, a new fracture with nodular callus formation (arrow) has become visible. This fracture is approximately 2 weeks old. It was not seen on the initial chest film. On the other hand, the previously thickened posterior ribs on the right have almost completely remodeled and appear almost normal. **C.** This patient has evidence of rib fractures at different stages of healing. Along the left chest wall is a fresh bent fracture (1). Nodular callus suggests 2-week-old fractures on the right involving the eleventh and twelfth ribs (2). Posterior thickening of the ninth and twelfth ribs on the left (3) is consistent with 4-week-old fractures. **D.** Another view of the acutely fractured left rib (arrow).

has occurred. Finally, it has been noted that some battered infants also have increased blood lead levels (54). The most likely explanation for this is that these infants probably are not well attended, and as a result, there is a greater propensity for them to ingest materials containing lead.

In evaluating battered children, **it is of the utmost importance to obtain an accurate and detailed history.** Often, the diagnosis of the condition centers around a discrepancy between how the fracture is said to have occurred and how it must have occurred on the basis of its appearance and/or location. In other cases, the involved party may offer a time frame for an injury that cannot be correct

because of the findings seen on the roentgenograms. This is where dating of the fracture becomes most important. In addition, the more detail one requests, the less is forthcoming, and, in fact, many of the answers will be "I don't know" or "I don't remember," etc. With legitimate trauma, this does not occur. If the parent knows how the injury was sustained, he or she will tell you exactly how it was sustained. It is the lack of details or the changing story that becomes important in evaluating battered children.

In addition to the foregoing considerations, a history of cardiopulmonary resuscitation or falling from a bed often is given as a cause for unexplained fractures. Rib fractures sec-

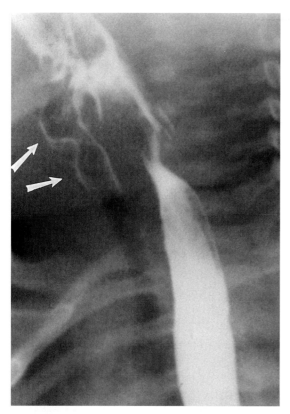

FIGURE 6.96. Dysphagia and aspiration with hypopharyngeal injury. Note aspiration into the trachea (arrows) in this patient who had difficulty swallowing because of posterior pharyngeal wall trauma. This patient presented with acute dysphagia.

ondary to cardiopulmonary resuscitation generally do not occur (55), and with regard to falling from a bed, unless it is from an upper-level bunkbed, injuries generally are minor and not to the skeleton (56–58). In fact, dropping an infant from one's arms is a more likely cause of fracturing (58). Finally, it must be remembered that certain metabolic and dysplastic bony conditions render the skeleton to fracturing, and in such cases, if the patient presents with a skeletal fracture, one must be cautious of the fact that the fracture may simply be part of the basic underlying condition.

Neglected infants can present with so-called **deprivational or psychosocial dwarfism.** Clinically, these patients may resemble those with hypopituitarism. Indeed, they have a temporary growth disturbance associated with decreased growth hormone production. The problem is transient, however, and readily reversible once the infant is removed from its deprived habitat. When this occurs, the patient grows rapidly and the brain participates in this catch-up phenomenon. Because of this, intracranial pressures increase and widening of the cranial sutures occurs. It is important that this be appreciated so that such spreading is not misinterpreted for pathologic spreading (Fig. 6.97A). Of course, one cannot make this distinction from the

roentgenographic appearance of the calvarium alone, but when considered with the overall clinical picture, a correct interpretation is possible. CT scans in these patients usually are normal, except that some may show smaller than normal ventricles as the brain mass increases. Because the infants resemble those with hypopituitarism, distinction between the two conditions can be made on the basis that deprivational dwarfs show numerous growth arrest lines, while those with idiopathic hypopituitarism do not (59). These growth lines often are striking and, in combination with other findings, should strongly suggest the diagnosis (Fig. 6.97B). Infants with deprivational dwarfism usually do not demonstrate evidence of skeletal trauma, but most often present as a failure-to-thrive problem.

Finally, it should be noted that not all patients with what appear to be nonaccidental fractures turn out to be battered children (60–62). Indeed, many metabolic bone diseases (Fig. 6.98), syphilis (63), and bleeding disorders (64) can be mistaken for a battered child problem. All of this is very important, and thus, once again, it is of the utmost necessity to obtain an adequate and accurate history in every case.

REFERENCES

1. Caffey J. Multiple fractures in long bones of a child suffering from chronic subdural hematoma. AJR 1946;56:163–173.
2. Kempe CH, Silverman FN, Steel J, et al. Battered child syndrome. JAMA 1962;181:17–24.
3. Caffey J. The whiplash shaken infant syndrome: manual shaking by the extremities with whiplash-induced intracranial and intraocular bleedings, linked with residual permanent brain damage and mental retardation. Pediatrics 1974;54:396–403.
4. Leventhal JM, Thomas SA, Rosenfield NS, et al. Fractures in young children distinguishing child abuse from unintentional injuries. Am J Dis Child 1993;147:87–92.
5. Loder RT, Bookout C. Fracture patterns in battered children. J Orthop Trauma 1991;5:428–433.
6. Kogutt MS, Swischuk LE, Fagan CJ. Patterns of injury and significance of uncommon fractures in the battered child syndrome. AJR 1974;121:143–149.
7. O'Neill J Jr, Meacham W, Griffin P, et al. Patterns of injury in the battered child syndrome. J Trauma 1973;13:332–339.
8. Ellerstein NS, Norris KJ. Value of radiologic skeletal survey in assessment of abused children. Pediatrics 1984;74:1075–1078.
9. Kleinman PK, Nimkin K, Spevak MR, et al. Follow-up skeletal surveys in suspected child abuse. AJR 1996;167:893–986.
10. Youmans DC, Don S, Hildebolt C, et al. Skeletal surveys for child abuse: comparison of interpretation using digitized images and screen-film radiographs. AJR 1998;171:1415–1419.
11. Kleinman PK, Marks SC, Blackbourne B. The metaphyseal lesion in abused infants: a radiologic-histopathologic study. AJR 1986;146:895–905.
12. Gahagan S, Rimsza E. Child abuse or osteogenesis imperfecta: how can we tell? Pediatrics 1991;88:987–992.
13. Chapman S, Hall CM. Non-accidental injury of brittle bones. Pediatr Radiol 1997;27:106–110.
14. Ablin DS, Sane SM. Non-accidental injury: confusion with temporary brittle bone disease and mild osteogenesis imperfecta. Pediatr Radiol 1997;27:111–113.

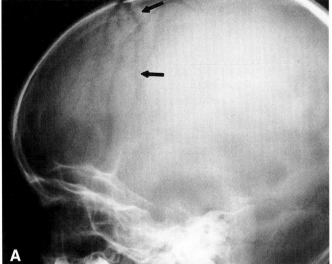
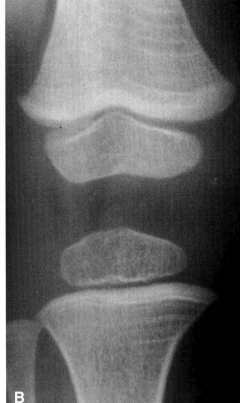

FIGURE 6.97. Deprivational dwarfism. A. Note that the sutures (arrows) are spread. **B.** Knee demonstrating numerous growth arrest lines.

15. Dalton HJ, Slovis T, Helfer RE, et al. Undiagnosed abuse in children younger than 3 years with femoral fracture. Am J Dis Child 1990;144:875–878.

16. King J, Diefendorf D, Apthorp J, et al. Analysis of 429 fractures in 189 battered children. J Pediatr Orthop 1988;8:585–589.

17. Strait RT, Siegel RM, Shapiro RA. Humeral fractures without

obvious etiologies in children less than 3 years of age: when is it abuse? Pediatrics 1995;96:667–671.

18. Thomas SA, Rosenfield NS, Leventhal JM, et al. Long-bone fractures in young children: distinguishing accidental injuries from child abuse. Pediatrics 1991;88:471–476.

19. Worlock P, Stower M, Barbor P. Patterns of fractures in acciden-

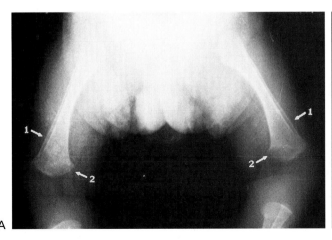
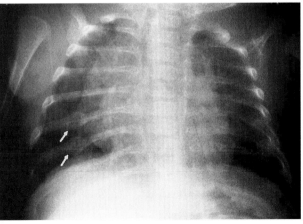

FIGURE 6.98. Metabolic bone disease mimicking a battered infant. A. Extensive periosteal new bone is seen on the femoral shafts, and there is some beaking of the metaphyses. The metaphyses, however, are indistinct because this patient had metabolic bone disease of the premature. The fractures were not intentionally inflicted. **B.** Note healing rib fractures (arrows).

tal and non-accidental injury in children: a comparative study. Br Med J Clin Res 1986;293:100–102.

20. Rex C, Kay PR. Features of femoral fractures in nonaccidental injury. J Pediatr Orthop 2000;20:411–413.

21. Schwend RM, Werth C, Johnston A. Femur shaft fractures in toddlers and young children: rarely from child abuse. J Pediatr Orthop 2000;20:475–481.

22. Shaw BA, Murphy KM, Shaw A, et al. Humerus shaft fractures in young children: accident or abuse? J Pediatr Orthop 1997;17:293–297.

23. Deleted in page proofs.

24. Mellick LB, Reesor K. Spiral tibial fractures of children: a commonly accidental spiral long bone fracture. Am J Emerg Med 1990;8:234–237.

25. Kleinman PK, Schlesinger AE. Mechanical factors associated with posterior rib fractures: laboratory and case studies. Pediatr Radiol 1997;27:87–91.

26. Kleinman PK, Marks SC, Adams VI, et al. Factors affecting visualization of posterior rib fractures in abused infants. AJR 1988;150:635–638.

27. Strouse PJ, Owings CL. Fractures of the first rib in child abuse. Radiology 1995;197:763–765.

28. Barlow KM, Gibson RJ, McPhillips M, et al. Magnetic resonance imaging in acute imaging in acute non-accidental head injury. Acta Paediatr 1999;88:734–740.

29. Tomasi LG, Rosman NP. Purtscher's retinopathy in the battered child syndrome. Am J Dis Child 1975;129:1335–1337.

30. Kapoor S, Schiffman J, Tang R, et al. The significance of white-centered retinal hemorrhages in the shaken baby syndrome. Pediatr Emerg Care 1997;13:183–185.

31. Ablin DS, Greenspan A, Reinhart MA. Pelvic injuries in child abuse. Pediatr Radiol 1992;22:454–457.

32. Predergast NC, Roux SJ de, Adsay NV. Non-accidental pediatric pelvic fracture: a case report. Pediatr Radiol 1998;28:344–346.

33. Carrion WV, Dormans JP, Drummond DS, et al. Circumferential growth plate fracture of the thoracolumbar spine from child abuse. J Pediatr Orthop 1996;16:210–214.

34. Kleinman PK, Marks SC. Vertebral body fractures in child abuse: radiologic histopathologic correlates. Invest Radiol 1992;27:715–722.

35. Kleinman PK, Shelton YA. Hangman's fracture in an abused infant. Imaging features. Pediatr Radiol 1997;27:776–777.

36. Rooks VJ, Sisler C, Burton B. Cervical spine injury in child abuse: report of two cases. Pediatr Radiol 1998;28:193–195.

37. Swischuk LE. Spine and spinal cord trauma in the battered child syndrome. Radiology 1969;92:733–738.

38. Nimkin K, Spevak MR, Kleinman PK. Fractures of the hands and feet in child abuse: imaging and pathologic features. Radiology 1997;203:233–236.

39. Mogbo KI, Slovis TL, Canady AI, et al. Appropriate imaging in children with skull fractures and suspicion of child abuse. Radiology 1998;208:521–524.

40. Shah P, Applegate KE, Buonomo C. Stricture of the duodenum and jejunum in an abused child. Pediatr Radiol 1997;27:281–283.

41. Orel SG, Nussbaum AR, Sheth S, et al. Case report: duodenal hematoma in child abuse: sonographic detection. AJR 1988;151:147–149.

42. Fulcher AS, Narla LD, Brewer WH. Case report. Gastric hematoma and pneumatosis in child abuse. AJR 1990;155:1283–1284.

43. Kleinman PK, Spevak MR, Hansen M. Case report. Mediastinal pseudocyst caused by pharyngeal perforation during child abuse. AJR 1992;158:1111–1113.

44. Morzaria S, Walton J, MacMillan A. Inflicted esophageal perforation. J Pediatr Surg 1998;33:871–873.

45. Geismar SL, Tilelli JA, Campbell JB, et al. Chylothorax as a manifestation of child abuse. Pediatr Emerg Care 1997;13:386–389.

46. Roche KJ, Genieser NB, Berger DK, et al. Traumatic abdominal pseudoaneurysm secondary to child abuse. Pediatr Radiol 1995;25:S247–S248.

47. Ng CS, Hall CM. Costochondral junction fractures and intra-abdominal trauma in non-accidental injury. Pediatr Radiol 1998;28:671–676.

48. McCann J, Voris J. Perianal injuries resulting from sexual abuse: a longitudinal study. Pediatrics 1993;91:390–397.

49. Bird CR, McMahan JR, Gilles FH, et al. Strangulation in child abuse: CT diagnosis. Radiology 1987;163:373–375.

50. Griest KH, Zumwalt RE. Child abuse by drowning. Pediatrics 1989;83:41–46.

51. Rosenberg NM, Marino D. Frequency of suspected abuse/neglect in burn patients. Pediatr Emerg Care 1989;5:219–221.

52. Emery JL. Child abuse, sudden infant death syndrome, and unexpected infant death. Am J Dis Child 1993;147:1097–1100.

53. Reece RM. Fatal child abuse and sudden infant death syndrome: a critical diagnostic decision. Pediatrics 1993;91:423–429.

54. Bithoney WG, Vandeven AM, Ryan A. Elevated lead levels in reportedly abused children. J Pediatr 1993;122:719–720.

55. Spevak MR, Kleinman PK, Belanger PL, et al. Cardiopulmonary resuscitation and rib fractures in infants: a post-mortem radiologic pathologic study. JAMA 1994;272:617–618.

56. Lyons TJ, Oates RK. Falling out of bed: a relatively benign occurrence. Pediatrics 1993;92:125–127.

57. Nimityongsku P, Anderson LD. The likelihood of injuries when children fall out of bed. J Pediatr Orthop 1987;7:184–186.

58. Tarantino CA, Dowd MD, Murdock TC. Short vertical falls in infants. Pediatr Emerg Care 1999;15:5–8.

59. Hernandez RJ, Poznanski AK, Hopwood NJ, et al. Incidence of growth lines in psychosocial dwarfs and idiopathic hypopituitarism. AJR 1978;131:477–479.

60. Swischuk LE. Not everything is child abuse. Emerg Radiol 2000;7:218–224.

61. Isaacman DJ, Poirier MP, Baxter AL, et al. Abuse or not abuse: that is the question. Pediatr Emerg Care 2002;18:203–208.

62. Stewart GM, Rosenbery NM. Conditions mistaken for child abuse: part I. Pediatr Emerg Care 1996;12:116–121.

63. Lim HK, Smith WL, Sato Y, et al. Congenital syphilis mimicking child abuse. Pediatr Radiol 1995;25:560–561.

64. Harles JR. Disorders of coagulation misdiagnosed as nonaccidental bruising. Pediatr Emerg Care 1997;13:347–349.

Trauma with Underlying Neurologic Disease

Many infants with underlying neurogenic or neuromuscular disease (e.g., meningomyelocele, arthrogryposis, amyotonia congenita) demonstrate diaphyseal or epiphyseal-metaphyseal fractures. Roentgenographically, they may resemble those seen in the battered child syndrome. These fractures often result from purposeful, therapeutic attempts at flexing and extending the spastic or contracted extremities. The osteoporotic, atrophic bones are quite susceptible to fracture, and because pain sensation usually is markedly reduced in these patients, lack of early immobilization leads to excessive callus formation and periosteal new bone deposition (Fig. 6.99A). Eventually, with repeated fracturing and healing, an Erlenmeyer flask deformity (widening) of the metaphysis can result (Fig. 6.99B).

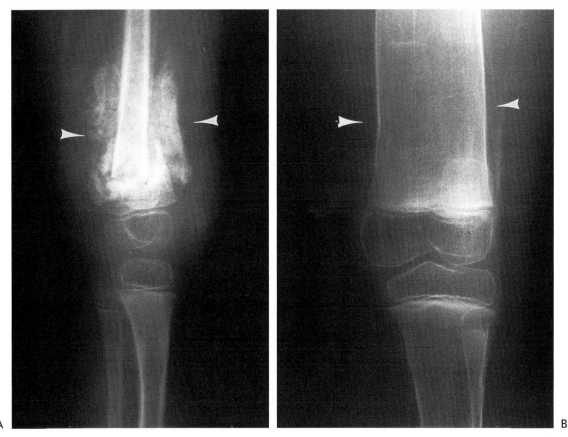

A   B

FIGURE 6.99. Trauma with neurogenic disease. A. Note pronounced callus formation (arrows) around the distal left femur. A pathologic fracture is present through the distal femoral metaphysis. The bones are markedly osteoporotic. **B.** With healing, residual widening of the osteoporotic distal femoral metaphysis (arrows) is seen.

Roentgenographically, clues to the proper diagnosis usually lie in the presence of wasted muscles, overabundant fatty tissue, and other evidence of associated neurologic disease, such as dislocated hips and the presence of meningomyelocele. In older infants, similar changes may be seen in the congenital insensitivity to pain syndrome.

Pathologic Fractures

Pathologic fractures can be seen with such conditions as osteogenesis imperfecta, hyperparathyroidism, progeria, hypophosphatasia, rickets, copper deficiency, and other conditions in which bony ossification is abnormal. Pathologic fracture through sites of bone tumor or infection can also occur.

Slipped Femoral Capital Epiphysis

Slipped femoral capital epiphysis generally is a condition of adolescence in which most of these children are somewhat obese or heavyset. There is a slight preponderance toward males, and overall the condition tends to occur in a narrow age window: approximately within 2 years of 12 years in females and 13 years in males (1). The condition usually is unilateral, although, in our study (2), 20% of the patients presented with synchronous bilateral slips. Another 20% presented with asynchronous sequential slips, and these patients usually did so within 2 years of the original slip. This is in keeping with other studies on the subject (3, 4). Because of this relatively low incidence of contralateral sequential slipping, a conservative approach to the problem is probably best (2, 5, 6). This consists of repeated clinical and radiographic evaluation of the hips at 6-month intervals or until epiphyseal closure occurs.

The basic problem in this condition is probably one of simple abnormal mechanics, where chronic subclinical shearing stresses are applied to the epiphyseal-metaphyseal junction (7–9). This evidently is aggravated by the lack of normal femoral anteversion (8, 9). In the early stages, the radiographic findings consist of smoothness and increased sclerosis of the white line (zone of provisional calcification) on the epiphyseal side and increased lucency and width of the epiphyseal plate itself (10, 11) (Fig. 6.100). Eventually, clear-cut slippage of the femoral head occurs and, since it often is more posterior than medial, is best visualized on frog-leg views (Fig. 6.101). More advanced cases demonstrate a coxa vara deformity with buttressing (thickening) of the cortex on the inner aspect of the femoral neck and clear-cut slippage of the femoral head (Fig. 6.102). CT can be used preoperatively to evaluate the degree of slippage and femoral neck angulation in severe cases (12) but in the ordinary case is not required. On the other hand, CT is invaluable in evaluating the postoperative hip in terms of determining the position of the fixating pin. In this regard, it is important that the pin be confined to the femoral head (i.e., under the femoral head cortex) and not enter the joint space (Fig. 6.103).

Postoperative chondrolysis (13) with resultant narrowing of the joint space probably is the result of an autoimmune phenomenon and has been shown to be more prevalent in blacks (14, 15). The characteristic roentgenographic feature is narrowing of the joint space (Fig. 6.103). Postoperative complicating avascular necrosis is not common and tends to occur in unstable hips (16). Preoperative bone scanning can aid in predicting the development of avascular necrosis, and in one study (16) utilizing this method, 0 of 63 stable hips demonstrated no avascular necrosis, while 5 of 10 unstable hips demonstrated avascular necrosis.

Femoral capital head slippage also occurs when bones are weakened by metabolic conditions such as rickets, renal osteodystrophy (17), hypothyroidism, and growth hor-

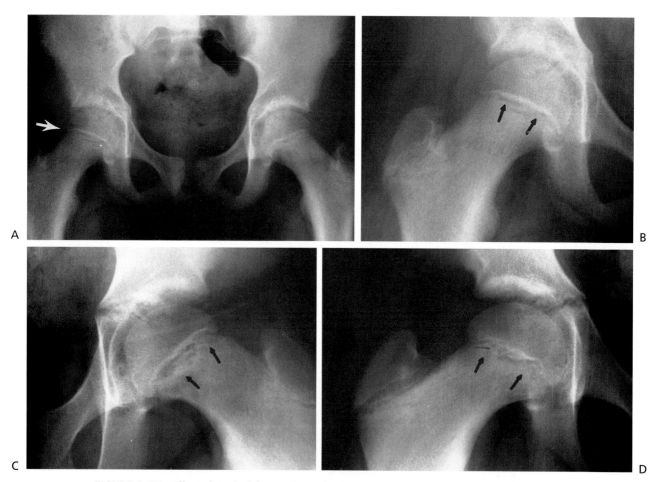

FIGURE 6.100. Slipped capital femoral epiphysis: early findings. A. On the right, note the smooth configuration of the epiphyseal line (arrows) with smooth sclerosis on the epiphyseal side. **B.** Magnified view demonstrates the findings more clearly (arrows). **C.** Another patient with more advanced changes. Note increased width and lucency of the epiphyseal plate (arrows). Also note the smooth sclerotic line on the epiphyseal side. **D.** Normal side for comparison. Note that the epiphyseal plate is not widened and that the sclerotic line on the epiphyseal side is indistinct and irregular. This is normal.

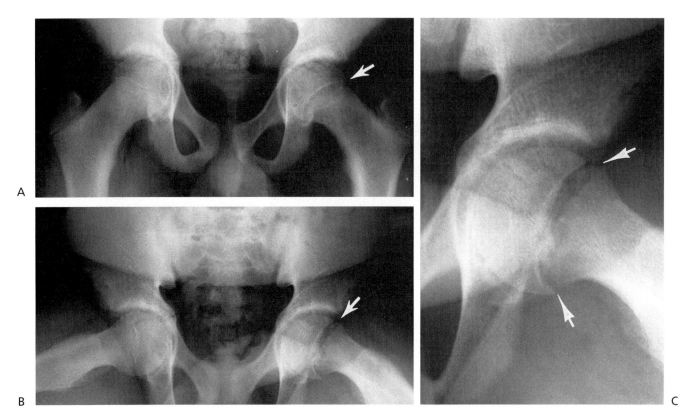

FIGURE 6.101. Slipped capital femoral epiphysis: value of frog-leg positioning. A. On this anteroposterior view, subtle changes of a slipped epiphysis (arrow) are present on the left. **B.** With frog-leg positioning, the widened epiphyseal plate (arrows) is more clearly visualized. **C.** Magnified view demonstrates the wide epiphyseal plate (arrows).

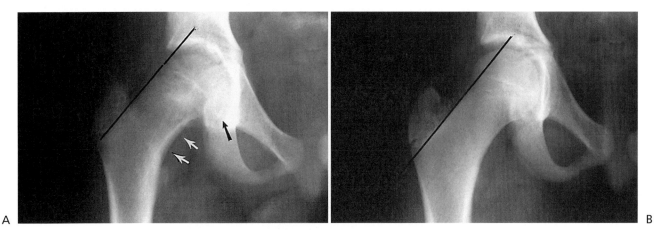

FIGURE 6.102. Slipped capital femoral epiphysis: longer-standing changes. A. Note that the femoral capital epiphysis has slipped medially (black arrow). In addition, there is some new bone formation along the inferior aspect of the femoral neck (white arrows), buttressing the slipped epiphysis. Finally, the line drawn along the outer femoral neck cortex does not intersect the femoral capital epiphysis. **B.** Normal side for comparison. Note that the line intersects the femoral lateral aspect of the femoral capital epiphysis.

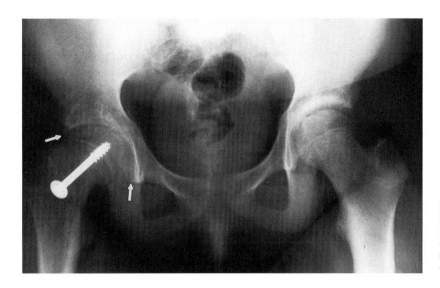

FIGURE 6.103. Slipped capital femoral epiphysis: chondrolysis. The right hip has been pinned. The bones are demineralized because of disuse atrophy. Note, however, that the joint space is narrowed (arrows), indicating the presence of chondrolysis.

mone deficiency (18–20). The latter two associated conditions, that is, hypothyroidism and growth hormone deficiency, are the most common predisposing problems (20). With metabolic problems, slippage usually is relatively symmetric and, of course, bilateral (Fig. 6.104). Radiation therapy is also a cause.

Finally, one should be aware that slipped capital femoral epiphysis as it occurs in adolescence is an insidious disease, even without hip pain in some patients (22). In other cases, the problem is one of knee pain (23, 24). In one study (23), knee pain was the presenting symptom in 15% of patients. This is not an uncommon problem with hip problems. In still other cases, an acute slip can occur on a superimposed insidious slip. Such patients have chronic slippage and few symptoms for weeks or months, and then, because of some

violent or semiviolent activity, the precariously "perched" femoral head undergoes superimposed acute slippage.

REFERENCES

1. Loder RT, Farley FA, Herzenberg JE, et al. Narrow window of bone age in children with slipped capital femoral epiphyses. J Pediatr Orthop 1993;13:290–293.
2. Hernandez, JA, Swischuk LE, Wallace J, et al. Slipped capital femoral epiphysis (SCFE) incidence of contralateral slip (submitted).
3. Loder RT, Arbor A, Aronson DD, et al. The epidemiology of bilateral slipped capital femoral epiphysis. J Bone Joint Surg (Am) 1993;75:1141–1147.
4. Jerre R, Billing L, Hanson G, et al. Bilaterality in slipped capital femoral epiphysis: importance of a reliable radiographic method. J Pediatr Orthop 1996;5:80–84.

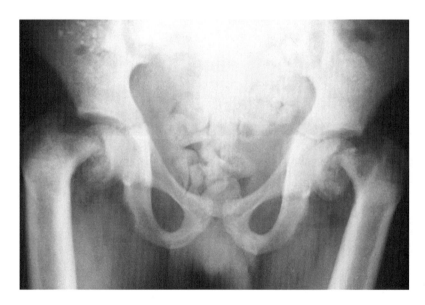

FIGURE 6.104. Slipped capital femoral epiphysis: renal osteodystrophy. Note marked bilateral slipped capital femoral epiphysis and resorption of the femoral necks.

5. Deleted in page proofs.

6. Castro FP Jr, Bennett JT, Doulens K. Epidemiological perspective on prophylactic pinning in patients with unilateral slipped capital femoral epiphysis. J Pediatr Orthop 2000;20: 745–748.

7. Loder RT. Slipped capital femoral epiphysis in children. Curr Opin Pediatr 1995;7:95–97.

8. Galbraith RT, Gelberman RH, Hajek PC, et al. Obesity and decreased femoral anteversion in adolescence. J Orthop Res 1987;5:523–528.

9. Gelberman RH, Cohen MS, Shaw BA, et al. The association of femoral retroversion with slipped capital femoral epiphysis. J Bone Joint Surg (Am) 1986;68:1000–1007.

10. Boles CA, El-Khoury GY. Slipped capital femoral epiphysis. Radiographics 1997;17:809–823.

11. Swischuk LE. Early findings in chronic hip problems in childhood. Postgrad Radiol 1995;15:77–94.

12. Guzzanti V, Falciglia F. Slipped capital femoral epiphysis: comparison of a roentgenographic method and computed tomography in determining slip severity. J Pediatr Orthop 1991;11:6–12.

13. Vrettos BC, Hoffman EB. Chondrolysis in slipped upper femoral epiphysis. J Bone Joint Surg (Br) 1993;75:956–961.

14. Aaronson DD, Loder RT. Slipped capital femoral epiphysis in black children. J Pediatr Orthop 1992;12:74–79.

15. Spero CR, Masciale JP, Tornetta P III, et al. Slipped capital femoral epiphysis in black children: incidence of chondrolysis. J Pediatr Orthop 1992;12:444–448.

16. Rhoad RC, Davidson RS, Heyman S, et al. Pretreatment bone scan in SCFE: a predictor of schemia and avascular necrosis. J Pediatr Orthop 1999;19:164–168.

17. Loder RT, Hensinger RN. Slipped capital femoral epiphysis associated with renal failure osteodystrophy. J Pediatr Orthop 1997;17:205–211.

18. Loder RT, Wittenberg B, DeSilva G. Slipped capital femoral epiphysis associated with endocrine disorders. J Pediatr Orthop 1995;15:349–356.

19. Wells D, King JD, Roe TF, et al. Review of slipped capital femoral epiphysis associated with endocrine disease. J Pediatr Orthop 1993;13:610–614.

20. Loder RT, Wittenberg B, DeSliva G. Slipped capital femoral epiphysis associated with endocrine disorders. J Pediatr Orthop 1995;15:349–356.

21. Loder RT, Hensinger RN, Alburger PD, et al. Slipped capital femoral epiphysis associated with radiation therapy. J Pediatr Orthop 1998;18:630–636.

22. Ledwith CA, Fleisher GR. Slipped capital femoral epiphysis without hip pain. Pediatrics 1992;89:660–662.

23. Matava MJ, Patton CM, Luhmann S, et al. Knee pain as the initial symptom of slipped capital femoral epiphysis: an analysis of initial presentation and treatment. J Pediatr Orthop 1999;19: 455–460.

24. Swischuk LE, Mild knee injury with prolonged problems. Pediatr Emerg Care 2001;17:301–302.

Osteochondritis Dissecans

Osteochondritis dissecans is a condition of adolescents that most often involves the medial femoral condyle. Characteristically, there is a subchondral avulsion fracture, with the bony fragment being variably displaced into the knee joint. The fragment usually comes from the anterior aspect of the medial condyle (Fig. 6.105A), and the condition is variably symptomatic. MRI is best for determining whether the fracture fragment is significantly displaced and likely to be sloughed into the joint space. On T2-weighted images, if a zone of high signal is seen around the bony fragment, separation can be predicted (1). The findings are the result of edema and bleeding around the avulsed bony fragment. When this high signal halo is absent (Fig. 6.105B), separation of the fracture fragment into the joint space is unlikely. Other relatively common sites of osteochondritis dissecans in children include the capitellum (2) (Fig. 5.106) and dome of the talus (3) (Fig. 6.105C). Rarer locations include the femoral and radial heads.

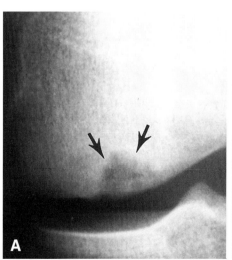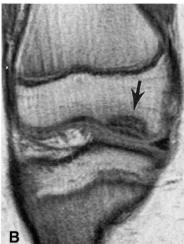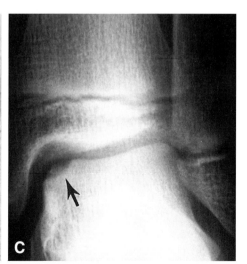

FIGURE 6.105. Osteochondritis dissecans. A. Typical defect (arrows) in the medial femoral condyle. **B.** Another patient with a T1-weighted magnetic resonance image demonstrating the bony defect (arrow). Absence of a high signal halo around the segment signifies that it is not loose. **C.** Similar small defect (arrow) representing osteochondritis dissecans of the talus.

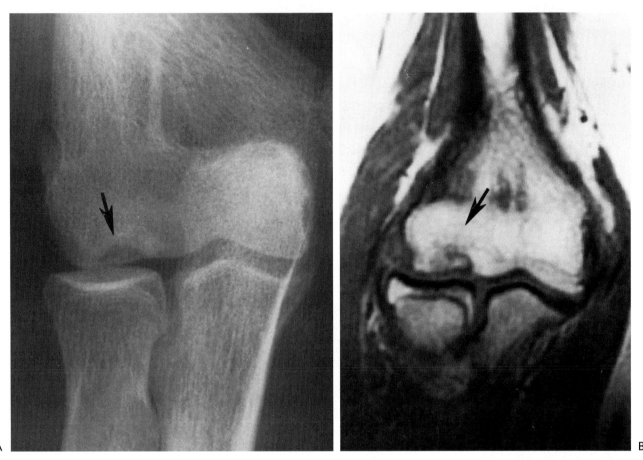

FIGURE 6.106. Osteochondritis dissecans: capitellum. A. Note the typical defect (arrow) in the capitellum. **B.** Magnetic resonance demonstrates the site of the defect (arrow) and that it has not detached itself from the bone.

REFERENCES

1. DeSmet AA, Fisher DR, Graf BK, et al. Osteochondritis dissecans of the knee: value of MR imaging in determining lesion stability and the presence of articular cartilage defects. AJR 1990;155: 549–553.
2. Clarke NMP, Blakemore ME, Thompson AG. Osteochondritis of the trochlear epiphysis. J Pediatr Orthop 1983;3:601–604.
3. Higuera J, Laguna R, Peral M, et al. Osteochondritis dissecans of the talus during childhood and adolescence. J Pediatr Orthop 1998;18:328–332.

INFECTIOUS AND INFLAMMATORY BONE DISEASE

Congenital Syphilis

Congenital syphilis on this continent is not as common a problem as in the past and results from transplacental infection transmitted from the mother to the fetus, usually in the second and third trimesters. Clinical manifestations include rhinorrhea, skin rash, anemia, hepatosplenomegaly, and, in some cases, the nephrotic syndrome. Skeletal involvement is common, and the lesions may produce enough pain to prevent the infant from moving his or her extremities, the so-called "pseudoparesis" or "paralysis of Parrot." Bony involvement is common in untreated cases, but with current policies of vigorous treatment of the mother (and hence the fetus), many infants are born with positive serology and yet never develop clinical symptoms or bony abnormalities. In those infants with skeletal involvement, a lag period of 6–8 weeks between the time of infection and the appearance of bony lesions is usual. Consequently, some infants may show roentgenographic stigmata of congenital lues at birth, while others may not develop them until 6 or 8 weeks later (1). In addition, if infection is acquired late in pregnancy, blood serology may be negative for the first week or two of postnatal life.

The bony changes are trophic (ischemic) in nature. The inflammatory process interferes with blood supply (small vessel) to the bone, and the bone undergoes necrosis. The changes are extremely symmetric and progress through a period of activity and healing regardless of when or whether treatment (penicillin) is instituted. In the majority of cases, healing is complete, and no residual deformities result.

Characteristically, widespread involvement of the skeleton occurs (2), but the lesions occurring in the long bones have become the best known. Occasionally, single-bone involvement occurs. In addition to the long bones, the ribs, calvarium, facial bones, flat bones, and even the spine can be involved.

In the long bones, the first changes occur in the metaphyseal regions. The epiphyses characteristically are spared. Metaphyseal changes vary from nonspecific radiolucent, transverse metaphyseal bands (trophic lines) to actual fragmentation and apparent rampant destruction of the metaphyses (Fig. 6.107). Whenever these destructive changes occur bilaterally in the upper medial tibiae, the term "Wimberger's sign" is applied (Fig. 6.107E). This finding is not totally pathognomonic of congenital luetic infection

because it can also be seen with osteomyelitis, infantile generalized fibromatosis, and hyperparathyroidism. Since most of these conditions are rare in the neonatal period, however, Wimberger's sign should still first suggest congenital lues.

Diaphyseal changes also occur and, in some cases, predominate. Primarily, they consist of periosteal new bone deposition or the so-called "luetic diaphysitis" (Fig. 6.107C). In addition, in some cases, the bones initially are very dense (Fig. 6.107A). The cause probably is the same as with rubella, wherein medullary bone is not absorbed at a proper rate. Skull and flat bone involvement usually manifest with discrete lytic lesions (Fig. 6.108A), and the same can be said for lesions occurring in the ribs. The small bones of the hands and feet can be involved and show nonspecific changes of dactylitis (Fig. 6.108B).

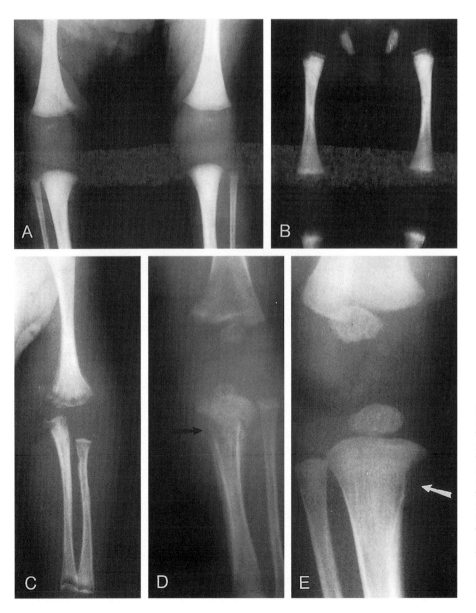

FIGURE 6.107. Congenital lues: various configurations. A. Note faint transverse bands in the distal femurs. Also note that the bones are denser than normal. **B.** Another infant with deeper and more pronounced transverse bands. The bones also are denser than usual. **C.** Another patient with dense bands and pathologic fractures with early periosteal new bone along the distal humerus. **D.** Wimberger's sign with fracture through the upper tibia (arrow) and periosteal new bone deposition. **E.** Classic Wimberger's sign (arrow) resulting in erosion of the upper medial tibial cortex.

Currently, there is ongoing debate regarding the value of long bone films in newborn infants with positive serology. Those who argue against obtaining such films say that they play no role in the decision making in terms of treatment (3). Others, however, believe that their presence is important in indicating active disease, especially in infants who are asymptomatic (4, 5). In our institution, the practice of obtaining long bone films in these cases has diminished over the years.

REFERENCES

1. Dorfman DH, Glaser JH. Congenital syphilis presenting in infants after the newborn period. N Engl J Med 1990;323: 1299–1302.
2. Rasool MN, Governder S. The skeletal manifestations of congenital syphilis: a review of 197 cases. J Bone Joint Surg (Br) 1989;71: 752–755.
3. Greenberg SB, Bernal DV. Are long bone radiographs necessary in neonates suspected of having congenital syphilis? Radiology 1991; 182:637–641.
4. Brion LP, Manuli M, Rai B, et al. Long bone radiographic abnormalities as a sign of active congenital syphilis in asymptomatic newborns. Pediatrics 1991;88:1037–1040.
5. Dunn RA, Zanker PN. Why radiographs are useful in evaluation of neonates suspected of having congenital syphilis. Radiology 1992;182:639–641.

Congenital Rubella Syndrome

The congenital rubella syndrome consists of intrauterine growth failure, thrombocytopenic purpura, eye defects, cataracts, deafness, anemia, hepatosplenomegaly, patent ductus arteriosus, bone changes, and aortic, systemic, and peripheral pulmonary artery stenoses. However, it is uncommon in the Western world. The roentgenographic changes in the bones are, as in congenital lues, trophic (vascular) in origin and consist of irregularity of the architecture of the metaphysis of the long bones. These changes often take the form of longitudinal radiolucent streaks (Fig. 6.109), but in some cases, the metaphyses may appear more ragged and even destroyed. The changes often are most pronounced around the knees, but metaphyseal irregularities can be seen in all of the long bones. In addition, the metaphyseal regions appear somewhat osteoporotic and are prone to pathologic fracture. In other cases, however, the bones are very dense throughout their diaphyses (Fig. 6.109). This probably reflects a degree of abnormal bone matrix development since it has been demonstrated that in rubella syndrome, bone next to the medullary canal is not resorbed at a normal rate (1). Because of this, more bone than normal is present, and the bones become dense. These changes usually disappear, as do the other lesions, by 6—8 weeks. Other bony changes seen in rubella syndrome include delayed epiphyseal development, defective

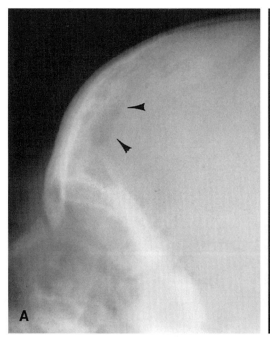
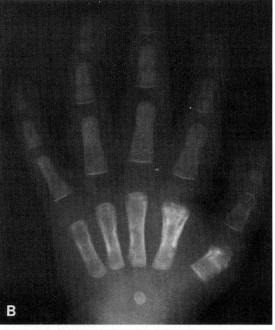

FIGURE 6.108. Congenital lues: other bone involvement. A. Note osteolytic lesions (arrowheads) in the frontal bone of this infant with congenital lues. **B.** Same infant demonstrating syphilitic dactylitis with destruction of the first and second metacarpals and periosteal new bone deposition along the shafts of the second and fourth metacarpals.

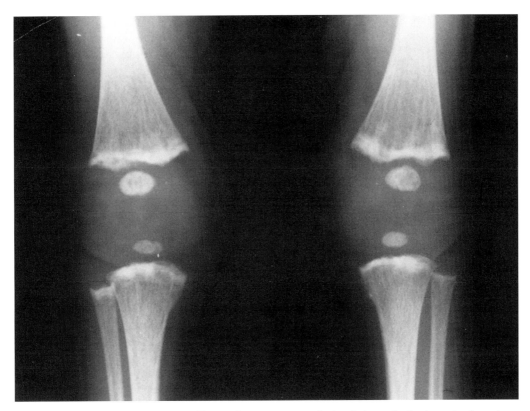

FIGURE 6.109. Congenital rubella syndrome. Note vertical radiolucencies in the metaphyseal regions producing the "celery stalk" appearance and pronounced sclerosis of the zone of provisional calcification in this infant with a refractory clinical course. Also note exaggerated cupping of the metaphyses, especially in the upper fibulae, and moderate metaphyseal beaking.

calvarial ossification with a large anterior fontanelle, and brain atrophy with a small skull.

REFERENCE

1. Whalen JP, Winchester P, Krook L, et al. Neonatal transplacental rubella syndrome: its effect on normal maturation of the diaphysis. AJR 1974;121:166–172.

Cytomegalic Inclusion Disease

The bony changes in cytomegalic inclusion disease or cytomegalic viral disease are the same as those in rubella syndrome. In addition, as with rubella and congenital lues, the bony changes represent a nonspecific trophic (vascular) disturbance of enchondral bone formation. Roentgenographically, the metaphyses of the long bones are poorly mineralized and irregular and often demonstrate the so-called "celery stalk configuration" also seen with rubella (Fig. 6.110).

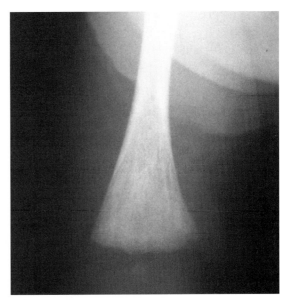

FIGURE 6.110. Cytomegalic inclusion disease: celery stalk appearance. Note typical celery stalk appearance of the metaphyses.

Varicella and Other Viral Syndromes

Although not as well appreciated, varicella prenatal infections can cause fetal deformities. These consist of cutaneous lesions, microphthalmia, cataracts, muscular underdevelopment, and extremity hypoplasia (1–3). It is likely that the findings are the results of a neuropathic embryonic injury caused by the virus.

REFERENCES

1. Savage MO, Moosa A, Gordon RR. Maternal varicella infection as a cause of fetal malformations. Lancet 1973;1:352–354.
2. Marion RW, Wiznia AA, Hutcheon RG, et al. Human T-cell lymphotrophic virus type III (HTLV-III) embryopathy. Am J Dis Child 1986;140:638–640.
3. Srabstein JC, Morris N, Larke RPB, et al. Is there a congenital varicella syndrome? J Pediatr 1974;84:239–243.

Osteomyelitis

In infancy, osteomyelitis and septic arthritis commonly occur together because, while in the older child, the blood supply to the epiphysis and metaphysis is separate, in the neonate and young infant, it is contiguous (1). Communicating vessels between the epiphysis and metaphysis transgress the growth plate (physis), and thus, it is not uncommon for infection to extend from its primary site in the metaphysis to the epiphysis and then out into the joint space (Fig. 6.111). In most cases, osteomyelitis is hematogenous in origin, but it can arise from penetrating injuries such as heel punctures in neonates, intraosseous infusions, and puncture wounds of the extremis in general. With the latter, and in the foot, pseudomonas infection is common and comes from wearing old sneakers (2). In addition, there is a propensity for hematogenous osteomyelitis to develop after fractures or other bony injury (3).

Roentgenographically, hematogenous osteomyelitis first manifests with deep soft tissue edema (Fig. 6.112) and then bone destruction. This is followed by periosteal new bone deposition, and in advanced cases, the findings are not difficult to detect (Fig. 6.113). Deep edema is present from the onset, but roentgenographically detectable bone changes (bone destruction and periosteal new bone elevation) are not seen before 10–14 days. It is during this time that if confirmation of osteomyelitis is required, the scintigraphic bone scan is useful. However, if deep edema is present and no soft tissue abscess or infection is present, osteomyelitis can be presumed and intravenous antibiotic therapy initiated. If clinical response is favorable, follow-up x-rays in 10–14 days are helpful, but if the disease process is treated early, it can be aborted and the follow-up roentgenograms will be normal. Otherwise, bony destruction and periosteal new bone deposition are seen and develop even though the patient is improving clinically. In severe cases, weakening of the bone may be so extensive that pathologic fractures may develop.

In terms of bone scintigraphy, if there is strong clinical and roentgenographic evidence that osteomyelitis is present, there is little need to rush into obtaining this study.

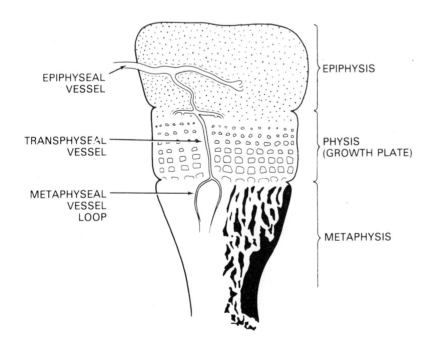

FIGURE 6.111. Blood supply to the neonatal epiphysis and metaphysis. In older children, there are two separate circulatory pathways: (a) the metaphyseal loops, which are derived from the diaphyseal nutrient artery; and (b) the epiphyseal vessels. No communication between the two circulations exists, but in the neonate and young infant, sinusoidal vessels (transphyseal vessels) connect the two systems. Because of this, osteomyelitis originating in the metaphysis easily spreads into the epiphysis and, subsequently, the joint space. (Modified and redrawn from Kaye JJ, et al. Neonatal septic "dislocation" of the hip. Radiology 1975;114:671–674).

EPIPHYSEAL VESSEL

TRANSPHYSEAL VESSEL

METAPHYSEAL VESSEL LOOP

EPIPHYSIS

PHYSIS (GROWTH PLATE)

METAPHYSIS

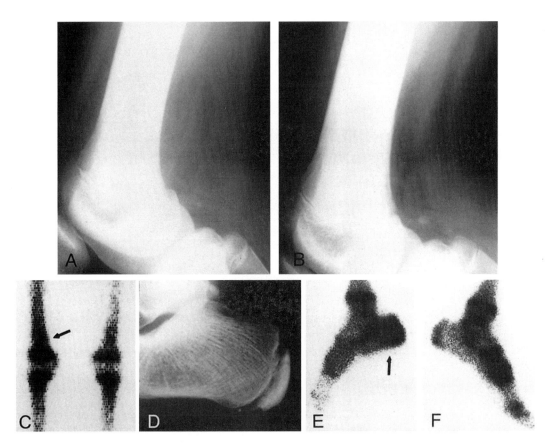

FIGURE 6.112. Osteomyelitis. A. Note indistinctness and expansion of the deep fat-muscle interfaces behind the femur. This is the result of deep edema and should signify the presence of osteomyelitis. **B.** Normal side for comparison. Note how clearly the fat planes are seen and that they are not displaced away from the bone. **C.** Technetium-99m scintigram demonstrates increased uptake in the distal femur (arrow). **D.** Patient with a painful heel. The calcaneus is normal. **E.** Technetium-99m scintigram, however, demonstrates increased uptake in the calcaneus (arrow). **F.** Normal other side for comparison. The increased activity in the calcaneal apophysis (posterior crescent-shaped structure) is normal.

The reason for this is that it is merely confirmatory, and furthermore, if it is obtained too soon, it can be falsely negative (i.e., in the first 24–48 hours). This occurs because the marrow cavity is so full of purulent exudate that there is inhibition of blood flow and, hence, no isotopic uptake. Usually, after 48 hours, the bone scan becomes positive (Fig. 6.112), and generally all that is required is the regular technetium-99m phosphate scan. Occasionally, indium-labeled white blood cell or gallium scans may be required, but in the pediatric age group, this is more the exception than the rule. The reason for this is that one generally is dealing with acute first-time osteomyelitis and not chronic, recurrent, or indolent osteomyelitis.

CT, MRI, and ultrasound can be used in the detection of osteomyelitis; however, plain films still are the most important and usually suffice. With CT, destruction of bone and periosteal new bone deposition are seen; with

MRI, bone marrow changes consisting of decreased signal on T1-weighted images and increased signal on T2-weighted images occur (Fig. 6.114). Unfortunately, MRI findings are nonspecific and generally not required. To be sure, they should not be obtained in lieu of, or before, nuclear scintigraphic studies. Ultrasonography can be helpful in demonstrating elevation of the periosteum (4, 5), either diffusely or in the form of a subperiosteal abscess (Fig. 6.114E) (6). Again, the study usually is not required, and actually we seldom use ultrasound in the investigation of osteomyelitis for by the time it is positive, it is too late.

Most cases of osteomyelitis in childhood are metaphyseal, but epiphyseal (7) and diaphyseal disease can also be seen. Diaphyseal involvement often is low grade and chronic, and the findings may be difficult to differentiate from malignant tumors such as Ewing's sarcoma (8). The plain film findings along with those seen on CT and MRI

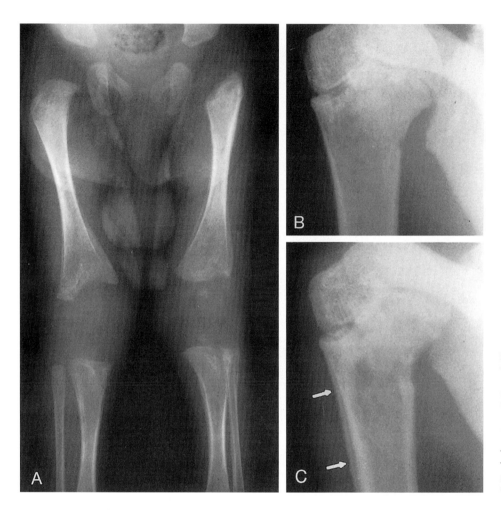

FIGURE 6.113 Osteomyelitis. A. Osteomyelitis with septic arthritis in a neonate. Note widespread metaphyseal destruction not unlike that seen with congenital lues. Also note periosteal new bone deposition. **B.** Older child. Note typical destructive changes in the proximal humerus. **C.** Later, there is evidence of associated periosteal new bone formation (arrows).

can be dramatic (Fig. 6.115). Such cases underscore the general and common problem of differentiating low-grade osteomyelitis from malignancy, no matter where in the skeleton it occurs.

Osteomyelitis in the neonate usually is just one manifestation of widespread bony and visceral infection (i.e., sepsis) and most often is caused by staphylococcal or streptococcal infections. Candida infections also are common (9). In addition, neonatal osteomyelitis often is multiple and clinically silent. It is not uncommon for physical findings to be focused around one joint, yet when roentgenograms are obtained, multiple areas of destruction are seen. In addition, the lesions often are silent with nuclear scintigraphy. Therefore, the nuclear scintigram is not favored when seeking sites of osteomyelitis in the neonate.

Osteomyelitis of the flat bones of the pelvis, clavicle, ribs, scapula, spine, etc., along with the sacroiliac joints (10) also can be seen with some degree of frequency. Infections in these areas often are low grade and indolent. Generally, destructive changes are similar to those seen in long bones, but periosteal new bone deposition is not nearly as preva-

lent. In the spine, osteomyelitis usually manifests as disc space infection with narrowing of the disc space and adjacent vertebral body destruction. In all of these cases, the bone scintigram can be invaluable (Fig. 6.116).

REFERENCES

1. Ogden JA, Lister G. The pathology of neonatal osteomyelitis. Pediatrics 1975;55:474–478.
2. Jarvis JG, Skipper J. Pseudomonas osteochondritis complicating puncture wounds in children. J Pediatr Orthop 1994;14: 755–759.
3. Morrissy RT, Haynes DW. Acute hematogenous osteomyelitis: a model with trauma as an etiology. J Pediatr Orthop 1989;9: 447–456.
4. Howard CB, Einhorn M, Dagan R, et al. Ultrasound in diagnosis and management of acute haematogenous osteomyelitis in children. J Bone Joint Surg (Br) 1993;75:79–82.
5. Larcos G, Antico VF, Cormick W, et al. How useful is ultrasonography in suspected acute osteomyelitis? J Ultrasound Med 1994;13:707–709.
6. Kaiser S, Rosenborg M. Early detection of subperiosteal abscesses

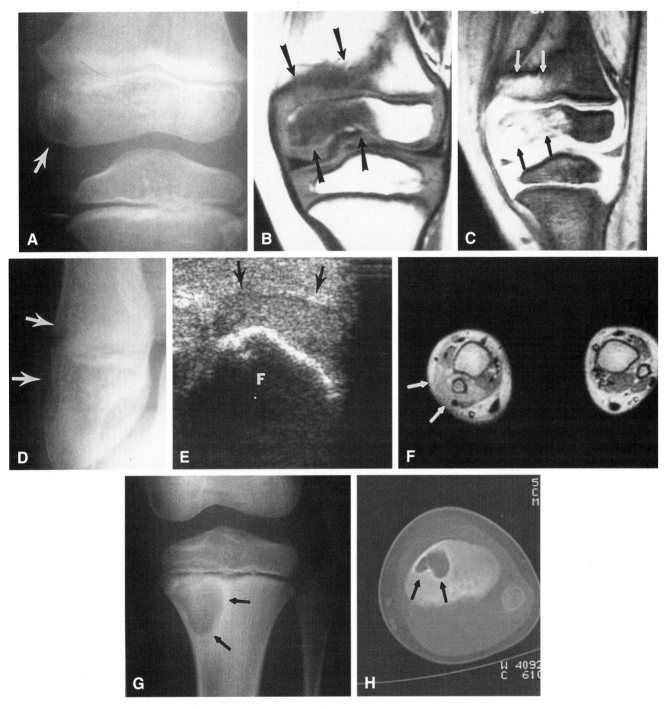

FIGURE 6.114. Osteomyelitis: computed tomography, magnetic resonance, and ultrasound. A. Note the destructive focus (arrow) in the distal femoral epiphysis. **B.** T1-weighted magnetic resonance study demonstrates more extensive involvement of the epiphysis (lower arrows) and previously unsuspected involvement of the metaphysis (upper arrows). The areas of pathology are manifest as low signal areas. **C.** Proton density image reveals the areas of involvement to demonstrate high signal (black and white arrows). **D.** In this patient, subtle irregularities suggesting destruction of the distal fibula are seen (arrows). **E.** Ultrasonogram demonstrates a subperiosteal collection of exudate (arrows). The echogenic line below represents the cortex of the fibula (F). **F.** T1-weighted coronal magnetic resonance study demonstrates extensive edema and exudate (arrows) around the fibula, which itself shows an indistinct cortex. Compare with the normal side. **G.** Low-grade Brodie's abscess in the upper tibia. There is a slight sclerosis of the margins (arrows). **H.** Computed tomography study demonstrates the same lesion (arrows).

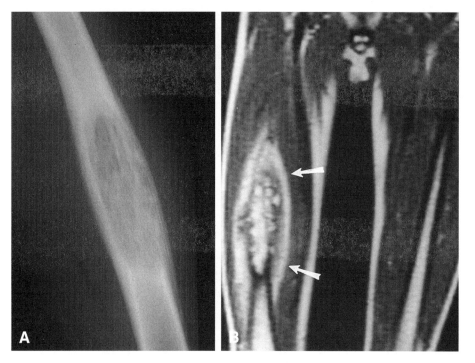

FIGURE 6.115. Chronic diaphyseal osteomyelitis. A. In this patient, a destructive, expanding diaphyseal lesion with periosteal new bone is seen in the midshaft of the femur. At first, Ewing's sarcoma was suspected, but the final diagnosis was chronic osteomyelitis. **B.** Proton density coronal magnetic resonance study demonstrates a halo of edema around the femur (arrows) and numerous pockets of exudate penetrating the cortex.

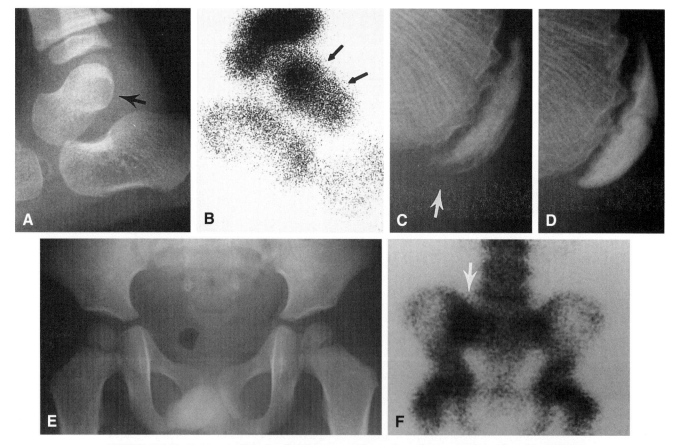

FIGURE 6.116. Osteomyelitis in flat bones: value of nuclear scintigraphy. A. In this patient, the ankle is swollen and a vague area of destruction is seen in the talus (arrow). **B.** Nuclear scintigraphy demonstrates markedly increased activity (arrows) in the talus. **C.** Note the area of destruction in the calcaneal apophysis (arrow). In addition, the calcaneal apophysis has lost its normal sclerosis. **D.** Normal side for comparison. Note the normal density of the calcaneal apophysis. **E.** This patient had pain over the right sacroiliac region, but the pelvic x-rays were normal. **F.** Nuclear scintigraphy demonstrates increased activity around the right sacroiliac joint (arrow). These findings are consistent with sacroiliac osteomyelitis.

by ultrasonography. A means for further successful treatment in pediatric osteomyelitis. Pediatr Radiol 1994;24:336–339.

7. Rosenbaum DM, Blumhagen JD. Acute epiphyseal osteomyelitis in children. Radiology 1985;156:89–92.
8. Hoffman EB, deBeer J, Keys G, et al. Diaphyseal primary subacute osteomyelitis in children. J Pediatr Orthop 1990;10: 250–254.
9. Yousefzadeh DK, Jackson JH. Neonatal and infantile candidal arthritis with or without osteomyelitis: a clinical and radiographical review of 21 cases. Skeletal Radiol 1980;5:77–90.
10. Haliloglu M, Kleinman MB, Siddiqui AR, et al. Osteomyelitis and pyogenic infection of the sacroiliac joint. MRI findings and review. Pediatr Radiol 1994;24:333–335.

Tuberculous and Fungal Osteomyelitis and Arthritis

Tuberculosis of the bones is not particularly common in the United States but is seen with considerable frequency in other parts of the world. Overall, however, tuberculosis is becoming more common on this continent, and more tuberculous osteomyelitis might be expected. Generally, bony destructive changes are indistinguishable from those seen with other causes of osteomyelitis. It should be remembered, however, that tuberculous osteomyelitis, even in older infants, frequently is seen in conjunction with tuberculous arthritis and that both conditions are more indolent than they are with pyogenic infections. For this reason, cystic changes in the bone may develop (1), and in the joints, chronic effusions with scalloped epiphyseal destruction are seen (Fig. 6.117A). In addition, as occurs with any chronic arthritic problem, the epiphyses may overgrow and, together with their osteoporotic appearance, appear large and glassy. Similar bony destructive changes can be seen with fungal infections (Fig. 6.117B). Dactylitis in the hands and lytic lesions in the skull also can be seen (2).

REFERENCES

1. Haygood TM, Wiliamson SL. Radiographic findings of extremity tuberculosis in childhood: back to the future? Radiographics 1994; 14:561–564.
2. Wessels G, Hesseling PB, Beyers N. Skeletal tuberculosis: dactylitis and involvement of the skull. Pediatr Radiol 1998;28:234–236.

Chronic Multifocal Osteomyelitis

Chronic multifocal osteomyelitis represents a distinct entity characterized by multiple sites of indolent, recurrent osteomyelitis (1–4). However, there is some question as to whether the underlying problem truly is one of infection (5–8). The problem here is the same as discitis in the spine: Both are low-grade infections, and in both conditions, it is

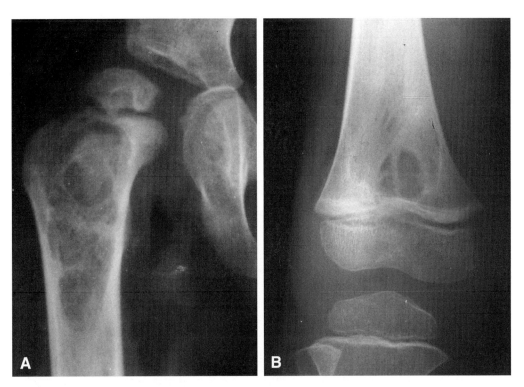

FIGURE 6.117. Tuberculous osteomyelitis. A. Note cystic changes in the upper femur. The epiphysis also is involved, and there is associated arthritis. The joint space is widened and the femoral head is displaced laterally. **B.** Similar cystic-appearing lesions in the distal femur in a patient with **coccidioidomycosis.**

well known that isolation of a pathogen may be difficult. This, however, should not necessarily suggest that the problem is not one of bacterial infection. In my experience, the problem usually is low-grade staphylococcal infection. Characteristically, multiple lesions, often recurrent, produce lytic defects in the involved bones. Considerable sclerosis around the sites of destruction can be seen (Fig. 6.118), and in some cases, periosteal reaction can be exuberant (9). In most cases, as long as the lesions are confined to the metaphyses of the long bones, there usually is little difficulty in determining that osteomyelitis is the most likely problem (Fig. 6.118, B and C). Occasionally, with diaphyseal involvement, Ewing's sarcoma may at first be suggested (Fig. 6.116B). If the flat bones are involved (common), bizarre configurations often result, and again a tumor of some type is first considered (see Fig. 6.118, A, D and E). Epiphyseal involvement also can occur (10) and can be subtle and overlooked.

An interesting association between the Sweet syndrome and chronic multifocal osteomyelitis has been documented (11, 12). In these patients, associated Fanconi's anemia is present, and thus the problem, in terms of genetics, may be more complicated than initially believed. Sweet syndrome is characterized by intracutaneous and extracutaneous neutrophilic infiltrates not unlike those seen with chronic multifocal osteomyelitis (11). An association with ulcerative colitis, Crohn's disease, psoriasis, palmoplantar pustulosis, and acne (SAPHO syndrome) also has been noted to occur (13).

REFERENCES

1. Damharter J, Bohndorf K, Michl W, et al. Chronic recurrent multifocal osteomyelitis: a radiological and clinical investigation of five cases. Skeletal Radiol 1997;26:579–588.
2. Gamble JG, Rinsky LA. Chronic recurrent multifocal osteomyelitis: a distinct clinical entity. J Pediatr Orthop 1986;6:579–584.
3. Chow LT, Griffith JF, Kumta SM, et al. Chronic recurrent multifocal osteomyelitis: a great clinical and radiologic mimic in need of recognition by the pathologist. APMIS 1999;107:369–379.

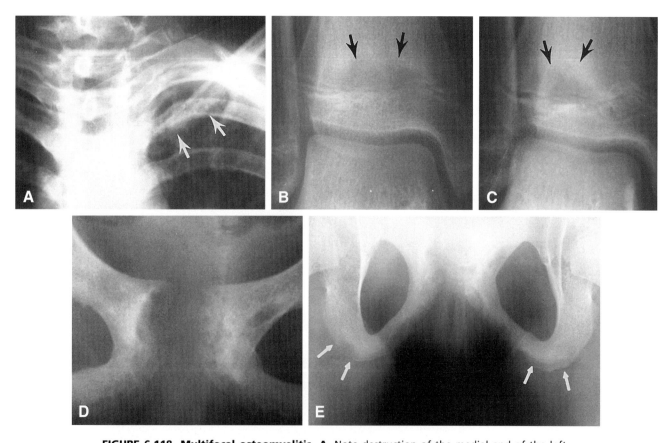

FIGURE 6.118. Multifocal osteomyelitis. A. Note destruction of the medial end of the left clavicle (arrows). **B.** There is an extensive area of bone destruction in the distal right tibia (arrows). The epiphysis and metaphysis are involved. **C.** In the left tibia, a similar lesion but with more surrounding sclerosis is present (arrows). **D.** Another patient with peculiar bony destruction of the pubic bone around the symphysis pubis. **E.** Same patient demonstrating numerous destructive lesions around the ischia (arrows). This patient developed osteomyelitis in the distal tibia approximately 6 months later.

4. Tingley R, Jadavji T, Boag G, et al. Proceeding of the Tumor Board and co-editors' note—chronic recurrent multifocal osteomyelitis: a rare disorder presenting as multifocal bone lesions. Med Pediatr Oncol 2001;37:132–137.
5. Handrick W, Hormann D, Voppmann A, et al. Chronic recurrent multifocal osteomyelitis—report of eight patients. Pediatr Surg Int 1998;14:195–198.
6. King SM, Laxer RM, Manson D, et al. Chronic recurrent multifocal osteomyelitis: a noninfectious inflammatory process. Pediatr Infect Dis J 1987;6:907–911.
7. Meyer zu Reckendorf G, Milton E, Pous JG. Chronic recurrent multifocal osteomyelitis (C.R.M.O.). A case report and review of the literature. Eur J Pediatr Surg 1996;6:312–315.
8. Schultz, C, Holterphus PM, Seidel A, et al. Chronic recurrent multifocal osteomyelitis in children. Pediatr Infect Dis J 1999;18:1008–1013.
9. Starinsky R. Multifocal chronic osteomyelitis with exuberant periosteal formation. Pediatr Radiol 1991;21:455–456.
10. Cuende E, Gutierrez MA, Paniagua G, et al. Chronic recurrent multifocal osteomyelitis: report of a case with epiphyseal and metaphyseal involvement. Clin Exp Rheumatol 1995;13:251–253.
11. Baron F, Sybert VP, Andrews RG. Cutaneous and extracutaneous neutrophilic infiltrates (Sweet syndrome) in three patients with Fanconi's anemia. J Pediatr 1989;115:726–729.
12. Majeed HA, Kalaawi M, Mohanty D, et al. Congenital dyserythropoietic anemia and chronic recurrent multifocal osteomyelitis in three related children and the association with Sweet syndrome in two siblings. J Pediatr 1989;115:730–734.
13. Bazrafshan A, Zanjani KS. Chronic recurrent multifocal osteomyelitis associated with ulcerative colitis: a case report. J Pediatr Surg 2000;35:1520–1522.

Cat-Scratch Disease

Cat-scratch disease can produce lytic lesions in the skeleton (1, 2). In addition, although it has long been known that cat-scratch disease is one of the more common causes of epitrochlear and cervical adenitis (3), it has more recently become evident that granulomas in the liver and spleen also commonly are found in this disease (2). Color flow Doppler is useful in identifying blood flow to the lymph nodes, which in our and others' experience (3) is exuberant.

REFERENCES

1. Carithers HA. Cat-scratch disease associated with an osteolytic lesion. Am J Dis Child 1983;137:968–970.
2. Larsen CE, Patrick LE. Abdominal (liver, spleen) and bone manifestations of cat-scratch disease. Pediatr Radiol 1992;22:353–355.
3. Garcia CJ, Varela C, Abarca K, et al. Regional lymphadenopathy in cat-scratch disease: ultrasonographic findings. Pediatr Radiol 2000;30:640–643.

Septic Arthritis

As noted earlier in the section on osteomyelitis, septic arthritis and osteomyelitis frequently co-exist in infants and young children (1). Generally, pyogenic infections prevail, but candidal infections also can occur (2). In addition, presentation may be that of pseudoparesis of an extremity (3). In infants, most often septic arthritis of the hip and shoulder is first suggested on plain films by demonstration of joint space widening (Fig. 6.119A). This is due to purulent exudate accumulation. Ultrasonography should then be employed to confirm the presence of joint fluid (pus) in the hip (4, 5) and other (6) joints. Ultrasound guidance also is useful for joint aspiration (5). Fluid in the knee is best detected on lateral views of the knee as it accumulates in the suprapatellar bursa.

In the hip, bulging of the joint capsule along the femoral neck (Fig 6.119C) is seen. In the wrist, septic arthritis presents with marked swelling around the wrist and in advanced cases with increased depth of the joint space (Fig. 6.119, D and E). Ultrasound also can be used to demonstrate this finding. In the elbow and ankle, displacement of the anterior and posterior fat pads signifies the presence of joint fluid (see Fig. 6.82). Once again, ultrasound (6) can be used to detect the presence of such fluid.

It is important to diagnose septic arthritis quickly because intraarticular pus accumulation can lead to joint distension and compromise of blood supply, especially in the hip with the femoral head. In addition, articular cartilage destruction occurs early, and thus accurate diagnosis with subsequent drainage is of the essence. For this reason, it has been suggested that even if aspirate cultures are negative, aggressive antibiotic therapy should ensue (7). The causative organism usually is *Staphylococcus aureus*.

REFERENCES

1. Ogden JA, Lister G. The pathology of neonatal osteomyelitis. Pediatrics 1975;55:474–478.
2. Yousefzadeh DK, Jackson JH. Neonatal and infantile candidal arthritis with or without osteomyelitis: a clinical and radiographical review of 21 cases. Skeletal Radiol 1980;5:77–90.
3. Lejman T, Strong M, Michno P. Radial-nerve palsy associated with septic shoulder in neonates. J Pediatr Orthop 1995;15:169–171.
4. Wingstrand H, Egund N, Lidgren L, et al. Sonography in septic arthritis of the hip in the child: report of four cases. J Pediatr Orthop 1987;7:206–209.
5. Fessell DP, Jacobson JA, Craig J, et al. Perspective. Using sonography to reveal and aspirate joint effusions. AJR 2000;174:1353–1362.
6. Lim-Dunham JE, Ben-Ami TE, Yousefzadeh DK. Septic arthritis of the elbow in children: the role of sonography. Pediatr Radiol 1995;25:556–559.
7. Lyon RM, Evanich JD. Culture-negative septic arthritis in children. J Pediatr Orthop 1999;19:655–650.

Transient (Toxic) Synovitis of the Hip (Irritable Hip)

Transient synovitis of the hip commonly afflicts infants under the age of 2 years, in whom there is subacute onset of limp without much discomfort. The infant usually continues to ambulate but definitely favors the affected limb.

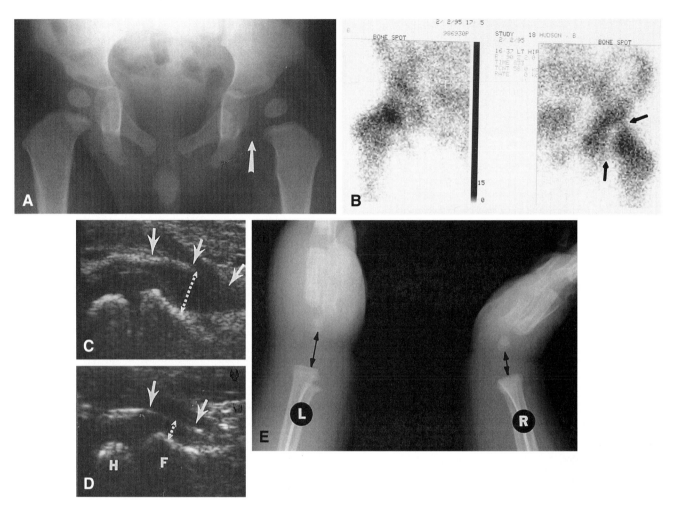

FIGURE 6.119. Septic arthritis. A. Note marked widening of the left hip joint (arrow). **B.** Nuclear scintigraphy demonstrates a photopenic area (arrows) in the left hip. The adjacent acetabulum and femoral neck show increased activity. The photopenic area represents fluid in the joint. **C.** Ultrasonogram clearly demonstrates a bulging joint capsule (solid arrows) with increased distance between the femoral neck and the capsule (dotted arrows). **D.** Normal side demonstrates the normal location of the capsule (solid arrows) and the normal space between the capsule and the femoral neck (dotted arrows). H, femoral head; F, femoral neck. **E. Septic arthritis of wrist.** Note swelling of the distal forearm wrist and hand. In addition, the joint space between the carpal bones and radius is increased (arrows). On the right, the normal space (arrows) is indicated. For examples of joint fluid in other joints, see Fig. 6.62.

Physical examination may be surprisingly benign except that there will be resistance to moving the hip. Systemic response to the problem is mild or nonexistent, and while tapping the joint may yield a turbid aspirate with a few white blood cells, frank pus is not the problem.

Most often, the problem involves the hip, but we have seen an occasional case involve the shoulder or some other large joint. Roentgenograms often are normal but in many cases reveal evidence of fluid in the hip joint manifest by lateral displacement of the femur and widening of the joint space (Fig. 6.120A). Ultrasonography, however, has come to be the most useful imaging tool in detecting fluid in the joints of these patients (1–5). Ultrasonography is sensitive in detecting fluid in the joint, and the findings, although

not diagnostic, are highly suggestive in the proper clinical setting. The reason why they are not diagnostic is that any fluid collection, including that seen with septic arthritis, can produce similar findings. Generally, widening of the joint space as it extends along the femoral neck and bulging of the overlying capsule (Fig. 6.120B) occur. In some cases, echogenic debris can be seen within the joint, and in other cases, synovial thickening is evident. Ultrasound also is useful as guidance for aspiration (5).

Transient synovitis of the hip is, for the most part, a self-limiting condition, but in a few cases, it is eventually determined that the patients have Legg-Perthes disease (6). This probably is because early findings of Legg-Perthes disease mimic those of transient synovitis and not that transient

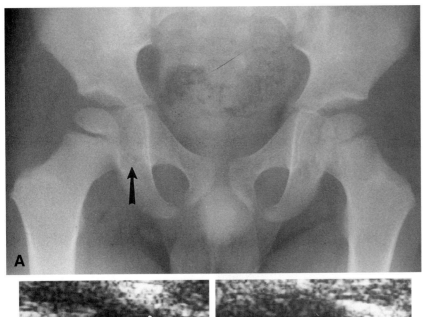

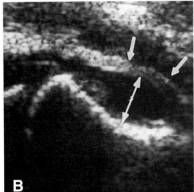

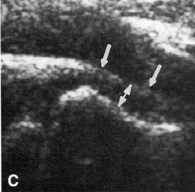

FIGURE 6.120. Transient synovitis: irritable hip. A. Note suggestion of joint space widening on the right (arrow). **B.** Sagittal sonogram of the right hip clearly demonstrates joint capsular bulging (arrows) with increase in joint space (joined arrows). **C.** Normal side for comparison. The capsule (arrows) is not bulging, and the space between the capsule and femoral neck (joined arrows) is normal.

synovitis is the cause of Legg-Perthes disease. In support of this is the fact that the incidence of Legg-Perthes disease in patients with irritable hip usually is quite low, well under 5% (4).

REFERENCES

1. McGoldrick F, Bourke T, Blake N, et al. Accuracy of sonography in transient synovitis. J Pediatr Orthop 1990;10:501–503.
2. Milalles M, Gonzalez G, Pulpeiro JR, et al. Sonography of the painful hip in children: 500 consecutive cases. AJR 1989;152:579–582.
3. Royle SG. Investigation of the irritable hip. J Pediatr Orthop 1992;12:396–397.
4. Terjesen T, Osthus P. Ultrasound in the diagnosis and follow-up of transient synovitis of the hip. J Pediatr Orthop 1991;11:608–613.
5. Zawin JK, Hoffer FA, Rand FF, et al. Joint effusion in children with an irritable hip: US diagnosis and aspiration. Radiology 1993;187:459–463.
6. Haueisen DC, Weiner DS, Weiner SD. The characterization of "transient synovitis of the hip" in children. J Pediatr Orthop 1986;6:11–17.

Rheumatoid Arthritis

Rheumatoid arthritis commonly has onset early in childhood, and usual symptoms consist of transient pain and swelling of various joints. In some cases, however, pain is absent (1). Some patients may have monarticular involvement (2, 3), and in young children, when the polyarthritic syndrome is combined with enlargement of the spleen and lymph nodes and widespread involvement of serous membranes such as the pericardium and pleura, the condition is referred to as "Still's disease." A similar condition has been documented in the neonate (4). If lung involvement occurs, it usually takes the form of interstitial infiltrates or, more rarely, nodules.

Initially, radiographic findings (Fig. 6.121) consist of nothing more than evidence of joint fluid accumulation and demineralization of bones. Eventually, however, because of hyperemia, the individual epiphyses tend to overgrow and become large and radiolucent, and then, as synovial proliferation occurs, the cartilage over the articular surfaces is destroyed. The joint becomes narrowed, the

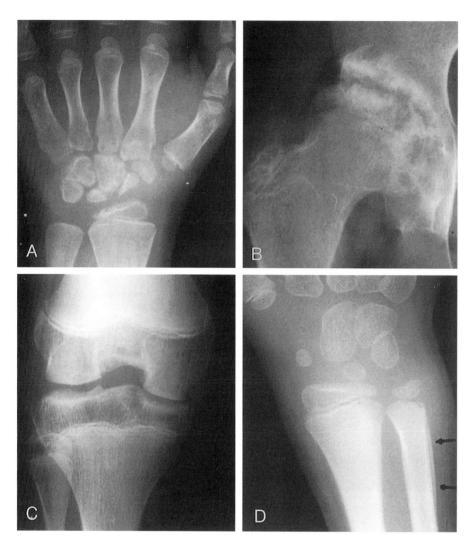

FIGURE 6.121. Rheumatoid arthritis. A. Note extensive changes in the wrist consisting of narrowing of the various joint spaces and smallness and irregularity of the carpal bones. The bones are demineralized. **B.** Advanced changes in the hip consisting of joint space narrowing with associated cystic and sclerotic changes in the femoral head and acetabulum. **C.** Older patient with overgrown epiphyses that are somewhat demineralized and appear glassy. Also note the prominent intercondylar notch. **D.** Still another patient with acute symptoms. Note diffuse swelling around the wrist, demineralization of the bones, and periosteal new bone deposition (arrows).

underlying bone irregular. Juxtaarticular bony erosions are seen, and bony changes in general tend to occur within 2 years of onset (5). In advanced cases, bony ankylosis occurs and intraarticular Rice bodies also have been noted to accumulate in some joints (6). Although these changes tend to predominate in the wrist and small bones of the hands in adults (especially the proximal interphalangeal [IP] joints), children often show more widespread involvement. In addition, periosteal new bone deposition around the involved joints can occur (Fig. 6.121D).

MRI has become useful in demonstrating the presence of synovial thickening and fluid in the joints of patients suffering from rheumatoid arthritis (2, 7). The findings are not pathognomonic (Fig. 6.122) but are especially useful in early cases. Ultrasound also is useful for the detection of fluid and synovial thickening in these patients (8) (Fig. 6.122B).

In longstanding cases, synovial protrusions beyond the joint can develop in the form of diverticula and can extend for long distances in the soft tissues. In other cases, resorp-

tion of the distal ends of the clavicles is seen, and involvement of the spine with apophyseal joint narrowing and eventual fusion also occurs. In the cervical spine, the two areas to show earliest involvement are the C2-3 and C5-7 areas. In advanced cases, extensive fusion of the spine can occur so that a virtual bamboo spine not unlike that seen with ankylosing spondylitis in adults is observed.

REFERENCES

1. Sherry DD, Bohnsack J, Salmonson K, et al. Painless juvenile rheumatoid arthritis. J Pediatr 1990;116:921–923.
2. Herve-Somma GMP, Sebag GH, Prieur AM, et al. Juvenile rheumatoid arthritis of the knee: MR evaluation with Gd-DOTA. Radiology 1992;182:93–98.
3. Jacobsen FS, Crawford AH, Broste S. Hip involvement in juvenile rheumatoid arthritis. J Pediatr Orthop 1992;12:45–53.
4. DeCunto CL, Liberatore DI, San Roman JL, et al. Infantile-onset multisystem inflammatory disease: a differential diagnosis is systemic juvenile rheumatoid arthritis. J Pediatr 1997;130:551–556.
5. Lang BA, Schneider R, Reilly BJ, et al. Radiologic features of sys-

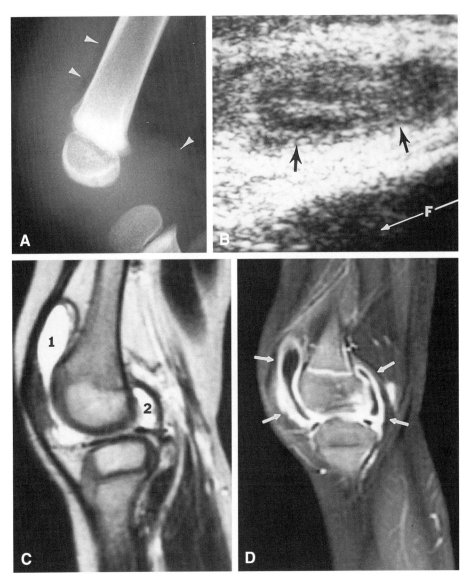

FIGURE 6.122. Rheumatoid arthritis: ultrasound and magnetic resonance findings. A. Note marked bulging of the suprapatellar bursa (arrowheads) and posterior popliteal extension (posterior arrowhead) of the knee joint space. These findings would suggest fluid in the joint. The distended suprapatellar bursa has compressed the prefemoral fat pad against the femur. **B.** Ultrasound, however, demonstrates that the suprapatellar bursa (arrows) contains echogenic debris, and thus the findings probably represent thickened synovium rather than free fluid. The distal femoral metaphysis (F) is located just under the echogenic prefemoral fat, which is located between the femur and the bursa. **C.** Another patient whose sagittal proton density image of the knee demonstrates fluid in the suprapatellar bursa (1) and in the posterior popliteal extension (2). **D.** Fat-suppressed image with gadolinium enhancement demonstrates marked enhancement (arrows) of the synovial membrane of both of the bursae demonstrated in **C.**

temic onset juvenile rheumatoid arthritis. J Rheumatol 1995;22: 168–173.

6. Chung C, Coley BD, Martin LC. Case report. Rice bodies in juvenile rheumatoid arthritis. AJR 1998;170:698–700.

7. Senac MO Jr, Deutsch D, Bernstein BH, et al. Pictorial essay. MR imaging in juvenile rheumatoid arthritis. AJR 1988;150:873–878.

8. Sureda D, Quiroga S, Arnal C, et al. Juvenile rheumatoid arthritis of the knee: evaluation with US. Radiology 1994;190:403–406.

Miscellaneous Arthritides

Lyme disease and its associated arthritis can be seen in children (1, 2), but the radiographic and ultrasonographic findings are nonspecific. Similarly, pigmented villonodular synovitis can be seen in children (3), but it is uncommon. Finally, every so often, one encounters a patient with monarticular arthritis where no cause is determined. It is suspected that many of these cases represent monarticular rheumatoid arthritis, but often the correct diagnosis is never established.

REFERENCES

1. Lawson JP, Rahn DW. Review. Lyme disease and radiologic findings in Lyme arthritis. AJR 1992;158:1065–1069.

2. Rose CD, Fawcett PT, Eppes SC, et al. Pediatric Lyme arthritis: clinical spectrum and outcome. J Pediatr Orthop 1994;14: 238–241.

3. Soifer T, Guirguis S, Vigorita VJ, et al. Pigmented villonodular synovitis in a child. J Pediatr Surg 1993;28:1597–1600.

Infantile Cortical Hyperostosis (Caffey's Disease)

Infantile cortical hyperostosis originally was described in 1945 by Caffey and Silverman (1), but now it is rarely encountered. It still is of unknown etiology, but it is interesting that reports of familial occurrence have been documented (2, 3). However, most cases are sporadic, and there is no predilection for race, sex, or geographic location. Most

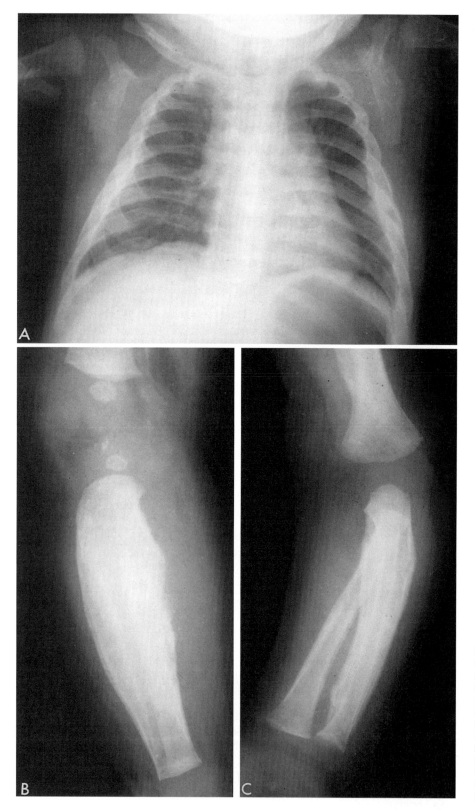

FIGURE 6.123. Caffey's disease. A. Note periosteal new bone deposition along the ribs, both clavicles, and probably the right scapula. **B.** Pronounced periosteal new bone deposition and cortical thickening of the tibia. Also note marked soft tissue swelling and edema. **C.** Same infant as in **B,** demonstrating numerous layers of periosteal new bone along the radius and ulna. Such periosteal new bone deposition is much more exuberant than that seen in normal infants (see Fig. 6.12).

cases usually present in the first few months of life, and onset after the age of 5 months probably does not occur.

In the usual case, there is exuberant and profound periosteal new bone formation (Fig. 6.123). The adjacent soft tissues are markedly edematous and inflamed, and in general, the infant responds as if an infection were present: with irritability, leukocytosis, fever, elevated erythrocyte sedimentation rate, localized swelling, and limited motion of the involved extremity (pseudoparesis). Every bone except the vertebrae and small bones of the hands and feet has been shown to be involved, but most frequently the mandible, clavicles, ribs, and long bones show change. Mandibular involvement is virtually pathognomonic of Caffey's disease (Fig. 6.124) but does not occur in all cases. Involvement estimates range up to 95% but probably generally are in the order of 80% (4). This is important to appreciate because it will cause one less concern when a patient presents without mandibular involvement, especially if the presentation is otherwise atypical. Long bone lytic lesions are rare (5).

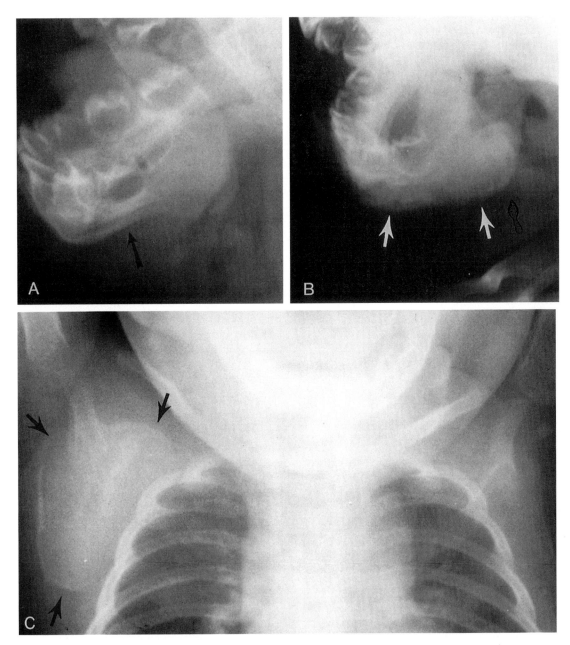

FIGURE 6.124. Caffey's disease: mandibular findings. A. Typical periosteal new bone deposition (arrow). **B.** More exuberant and thick periosteal new bone deposition (arrows). **C. Caffey's disease: scapular involvement.** Note the enlarged right scapula and periosteal new bone deposition (arrows). Also note the increase in soft tissue density representing extensive edema. This infant presented with swelling over the right scapula, pseudoparesis of the right upper extremity, fever, and leukocytosis. No other bones were involved at the time of initial examination, but 5 weeks later, mandibular and clavicular involvement were noted.

Involvement of the flat bones and bones of the face and calvarium is much less common. Calvarial involvement manifests in lytic defects (6), while facial involvement, in some cases isolated (7), presents with swelling over the cheeks. If the disease extends into the orbit, the patient can present with proptosis, ptosis, or glaucoma (8). Scapular involvement (8), also often isolated, is not unusual (Fig. 6.124C) and may present as pseudoparalysis of the extremity. In these patients, the scapula may appear enlarged and swollen and show periosteal new bone deposition to the point that a tumor first is suggested. This misconception can be fortified with the use of CT and MR, which also will erroneously suggest malignant tumor (9). Therefore, the diagnosis should be accomplished on the basis of clinical and plain film findings. In this regard, it should be remembered that Ewing's sarcoma and other sarcomas are rare in this age group and also do not produce so much in the way of inflammatory response.

Late changes or recurrences are uncommon (2) because the natural course of infantile cortical hyperostosis is one of progressive resolution of the periosteal bony reaction. Conversely, in more extensive cases, bony bridging can occur, and persistent bowing deformities with compromised extremity motion can result. Steroid treatment may be of value in controlling the inflammatory response, but more specific treatment is not available. This form of treatment might be considered in the more severe cases where profound periosteal reaction leads to permanent fusion of two adjacent bones (i.e., radius and ulna).

REFERENCES

1. Caffey J, Silverman WA. Infantile cortical hyperostosis: preliminary report on a new syndrome. AJR 1945;54:1–16.
2. Borochowitz Z, Gozal D, Misselevitch I, et al. Familial Caffey's disease and late recurrence in a child. Clin Genet 1991;40: 329–335.
3. Maclachlan AK, Gerrard JW, Houston CS, et al. Familial infantile cortical hyperostosis in a large Canadian family. Can Med Assoc J 1984;130:1172–1174.
4. Gentry RR, Rust RS, Lohr JA, et al. Infantile cortical hyperostosis of the ribs (Caffey's disease) without mandibular involvement. Pediatr Radiol 1983;13:236–238.
5. Leung VC, Lee KE. Infantile cortical hyperostosis with intramedullary lesions. J Pediatr Orthop 1985;5:354–357.
6. Boyd RDH, Shaw DG, Thomas BM. Infantile cortical hyperostosis with lytic lesions in the skull. Arch Dis Child 1972;47: 471–472.
7. Faure C, Beyssac JM, Montagne JP. Predominant or exclusive orbital and facial involvement in infantile cortical hyperostosis (de Toni-Caffey's disease). Report of four cases and a review of the literature. Pediatr Radiol 1977;6:103–106.
8. Katz DS, Eller DJ, Bergman G, et al. Caffey's disease of the scapula: CT and MR findings. AJR 1997;168:286–287.
9. Sanders DGM, Weijers RE. MRI findings in Caffey's disease. Pediatr Radiol 1994;24:325–327.

PERIOSTEAL NEW BONE: OTHER CAUSES AND CONFIGURATIONS

Periosteal New Bone Deposition

Any time the periosteum is irritated, periosteal new bone is deposited, and most often this occurs when intramedullary blood, pus, or tumor extends through the cortex to elevate and irritate the periosteum from its underside. When such periosteal elevation is rapid, single or multiple thin layers of bone result (Fig. 125A), and at the point where the periosteum joins the normal cortex, a triangle often is formed. This is referred to as "Codman's triangle" and almost always is seen with malignant primary or secondary bone tumors (Fig. 6.125B). Occasionally, this same triangle is seen with benign problems such as osteomyelitis, but most often Codman's triangle should be taken as a sign of malignancy. Periosteal new bone associated with vertical spiculations of bone, deposited along stretched Sharpey's fibers, virtually assures a malignant bone tumor, either primary or secondary (Fig. 6.125C). Markedly separated, or "ballooned," periosteal new bone usually indicates marked subperiosteal bleeding as seen with epiphyseal-metaphyseal fractures in scurvy, the battered child syndrome, and neurogenic patients (Fig. 6.125D). It also occurs with subperiosteal bleeding seen with hemophilia and other blood dyscrasias and with neurofibromatosis.

Periosteal new bone deposition also occurs whenever the periosteum is irritated by an adjacent inflammatory process or in association with hypertrophic osteoarthropathy where some centrally mediated or widespread hypoxic or toxic stimulus is present; for example, cyanotic heart disease, chronic inflammatory gastrointestinal disease, a variety of tumors, and chronic pulmonary disease (1–5). It can be seen with vitamin A or D intoxication. Periosteal new bone deposition also is seen in the early stages of infantile gangliosidosis, hereditary pachydermoperiostosis, and primary familial hypertrophic osteoarthropathy (6). It can occur with Engelmann's diaphyseal dysplasia and melorheostosis and is characteristic of Caffey's infantile cortical hyperostosis.

Periosteal new bone formation also can be seen with long-term prostaglandin therapy in infants requiring maintenance of ductal patency (7–9). In some of these latter cases, periosteal new bone deposition can be profound (Fig. 6.126), but it is reversible when such therapy is discontinued. In addition, periosteal new bone deposition on the ribs of newborn infants has been documented with high-frequency jet ventilation therapy (10) and vibrator chest physiotherapy (11).

Finally, it should be recalled that periosteal new bone deposition along the long bones is normal at around 2–3 months in infants, especially in immature infants. It results from exuberant normal bone growth; this is the only time in life when visible periosteal new bone deposition still is normal.

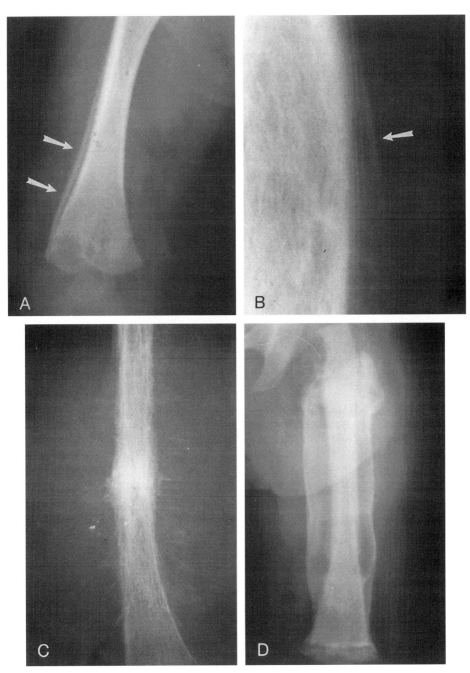

FIGURE 6.125. Periosteal new bone. A. Typical single layer (arrows) associated with osteomyelitis of distal femur. Note the radiolucent area in the distal femoral metaphysis. **B.** Typical multiple layering resulting from a rapidly growing lesion. This patient had an osteosarcoma. The arrow points to a Codman triangle. **C.** Typical spiculated periosteal new bone in Ewing's sarcoma. Linear new bone is seen at the upper extent. **D.** Ballooned periosteal new bone resulting from extensive subperiosteal bleeding in battered child syndrome.

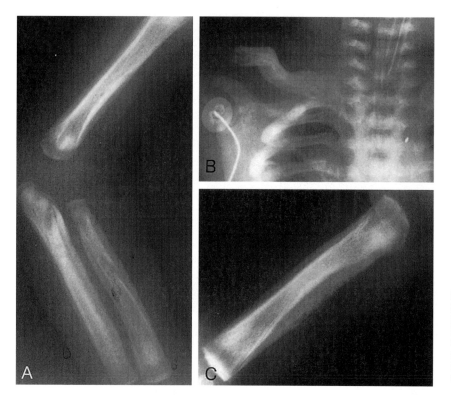

FIGURE 6.126. Prostaglandin E-induced periosteal new bone. A. Note extensive periosteal new bone deposition over the bones of the upper extremity. The bones also are demineralized. **B.** Pronounced periosteal new bone over the clavicles and to a lesser extent over the ribs. **C.** Thick periosteal new bone over the femur.

REFERENCES

1. Erku PE, Ariyurek OM, Altinok D, et al. Colonic hamartomatous polyposis associated with hypertrophic osteoarthropathy. Pediatr Radiol 1994;24:145–146.
2. Hugosson C, Bahabri S, Rifai A, et al. Hypertrophic osteoarthropathy caused by lipoid pneumonia. Pediatr Radiol 1995; 25:482–483.
3. Massicot R, Aubert D, Mboyo A, et al. Localized esophageal leiomyoma and hypertrophic osteoarthropathy. J Pediatr Surg 1997;32:646–647.
4. Varan A, Kutluk T, Demirkazik RB, et al. Hypertrophic osteoarthropathy in a child with nasopharyngeal carcinoma. Pediatr Radiol 2000;30:570–572.
5. Wadhwa N, Balsam D, Ciminera P. Hypertrophic osteoarthropathy in a young child with adult respiratory distress syndrome (ARDS) secondary to burns. Pediatr Radiol 1992;22:539–540.
6. Diren HB, Kutluk MT, Karabent A, et al. Primary hypertrophic osteoarthropathy. Pediatr Radiol 1986;16:231–234.
7. Gardiner JS, Zauk AM, Donchey SS, et al. Prostaglandin-induced cortical hyperostosis: case report and review of the literature. J Bone Joint Surg (Am) 1995;77:932–936.
8. Letts M, Pang E, Simons J. Prostaglandin-induced neonatal periostitis. J Pediatr Orthop 1994;14:809–813.
9. Matzinger MA, Brigs VA, Dunlap HJ, et al. Plain film and CT observations in prostaglandin-induced bone changes. Pediatr Radiol 1992;22:264–266.
10. Hussain M, Wood BP. Periosteal new bone of the ribs with associated extremity fractures after high-frequency jet ventilation. Radiology 1992;183:875.
11. Wood BP. Infant ribs: generalized periosteal reaction resulting from vibrator chest physiotherapy. Radiology 1987;162: 811–812.

BONE INFARCTION

Generally, bone infarction in childhood is seen with sickle cell disease. In older children, it occasionally can be seen with Gaucher's disease. In sickle cell disease, the findings often are difficult to differentiate from osteomyelitis, which, unfortunately, also is a common problem in these patients. Generally speaking, however, osteomyelitis produces greater swelling of the deep soft tissues. With infarction, pain in the absence of significant swelling is more characteristic than pain with the rapidly ensuing swelling of osteomyelitis. Roentgenographically, with infarction, destructive changes usually occur in the metaphyses but in more severe cases can extend into the diaphysis. In any case, differentiation from osteomyelitis often is difficult and requires complete clinical and roentgenographic correlation (Fig. 6.127A). Sclerosis is seen with healing (Fig. 6.127B)

Bone scintigraphy also has been used in the differentiation of infarction from osteomyelitis, and although it has value in the acute case, in those patients with repeated episodes of infarction and osteomyelitis, the findings often are more puzzling than helpful. Generally speaking, in the early "clean" case, bone scintigraphy shows decreased flow to, and uptake of, isotope in the infarcted bone. This, of course, would be expected, but once healing occurs, the bone scan becomes hot and indistinguishable from the hot or positive bone scan of active or healing osteomyelitis. CT and MR (1) also are of questionable value in the majority of

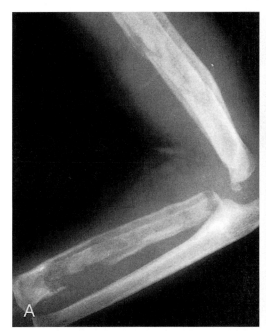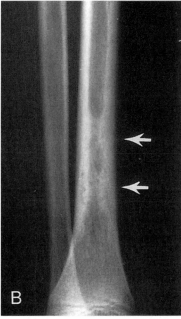

FIGURE 6.127. Bone infarct. A. Extensive and somewhat unusual degree of bone infarction, leading to the long bone shafts becoming sequestra in the newly formed periosteal new bone. **B.** Old infarct demonstrating medullary and endosteal sclerosis (arrows).

cases, and thus diagnosis usually hinges on clinical correlation and plain films.

REFERENCE

1. Munk PL, Helms CA, Holt RG. Immature bone infarcts: findings on plain radiographs and MR scans. AJR 1989;152:547–549.

Meningococcemia and Bone Infarction

Survivors of meningococcemia and disseminated intravascular coagulation can end up with growth-deforming metaphyseal bony lesions resulting from bone infarcts (1, 2). The changes predominantly involve the metaphyses and produce bony destruction. Subsequent growth disturbances are common, including physeal arrest (3). Although most commonly occurring with meningococcemia, any septicemia leading to disseminated intravascular coagulation can produce these findings.

REFERENCES

1. Santos E, Boavida JE, Barroso A, et al. Late osteoarticular lesions following meningococcemia with disseminated intravascular coagulation. Pediatr Radiol 1989;19:199–202.
2. Thompson GH, Morrison SC. Late skeletal deformities following meningococcal sepsis and disseminated intravascular coagulation. J Pediatr Orthop 1985;5:584–588.
3. O'Sullivan ME, Fogarty EE. Distal tibial physeal arrest: a complication of meningococcal septicemia. J Pediatr Orthop 1990;10: 549–550.

Aseptic Necrosis

Aseptic necrosis involves various bones in the body and is largely a problem of older children. Most commonly, the bones involved include the tarsal navicular (Köhler's disease) and the femoral capital epiphysis (Legg-Calvé-Perthes disease). The latter, however, is more common. Aseptic necrosis also can occur after loss of blood supply with trauma. Most commonly, this is seen with the carpal navicular, talar, and displaced femoral head fractures. The femoral head also can undergo necrosis if the blood supply is compromised by marked joint distention such as seen with septic arthritis, and, of course, aseptic necrosis is a common finding throughout the skeleton in sickle cell disease and steroid therapy. Usually, the larger epiphyses are the ones involved in these cases and include the epiphyses of the distal femur, proximal tibia, and proximal humerus.

Köhler's disease of the tarsal navicular usually presents with pain over the forefoot. Fragmentation of the navicular bone is characteristic, and if swelling is seen over the area, the diagnosis is assured (Fig. 6.128). This latter point is important because normal fragmentation of this bone also occurs, and if there is no swelling over the area, one should be cautious about the diagnosis. **Freiberg's disease,** that is, aseptic necrosis of the second metatarsal head, is not commonly seen in children. In the past, **Sever's disease** was considered a form of aseptic necrosis of the calcaneal apophysis. The problem in these cases, however, is an avulsive Achilles tendinitis and not aseptic necrosis of the calcaneus. The calcaneus normally appears sclerotic and fragmented, and in early days, this configuration was

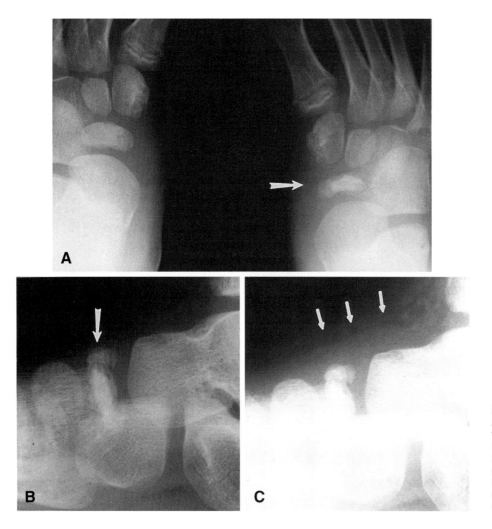

FIGURE 6.128. Köhler's disease.
A. Note irregularity and sclerosis of the tarsal navicular (arrow) on the right. Compare with the normal navicular on the left. **B.** Lateral view demonstrates the same finding (arrow). **C.** Underpenetrated film demonstrates soft tissue swelling over the involved bone (arrows).

misinterpreted for that seen with aseptic necrosis elsewhere in the body.

The most common site of aseptic necrosis in childhood is the femoral capital epiphysis, or so-called. **Legg-Calvé-Perthes disease.** This condition usually occurs in older children and is not a problem of young infants. It has an age range of approximately 4–12 years, with most patients presenting between the ages of 6 and 10 years. Males predominate, and younger children fare better than do older children. In this regard, it has been suggested that children under the age of 4 may require little in the way of treatment (1).

The disease is largely unilateral, and when bilateral, seldom is it completely symmetric; that is, the changes in one hip will be more advanced than in the other. When symmetric fragmentation of the femoral head is seen, one should think of conditions other than Legg-Perthes disease, such as epiphyseal dysplasia, spondyloepiphyseal dysplasia, hypothyroidism with epiphyseal dysgenesis, and infarction seen with sickle cell disease or steroid therapy (2). Aseptic necrosis of the involved or noninvolved hip in congenial

hip dysplasia also can occur during Pavlov harness or casting therapy (3).

The only finding consistently noted to be associated with Legg-Perthes disease is decreased bone maturation as reflected by a decreased bone age (4, 5). Finally, some cases of transient synovitis turn out to be cases of Legg-Perthes disease. The reason for this is that the early clinical and radiographic findings are similar. There is pain around the hip, and fluid may be demonstrated in the joint space. The number of cases of apparent transient synovitis eventually turning out to be Legg-Perthes disease, however, is well under 5–10%. Nonetheless, one should suspect Legg-Perthes disease when symptoms do not disappear within a short time and when there is persistent lateral displacement of the femoral head.

Earliest roentgenographic findings in Legg-Perthes disease (6) consist of smallness of the ossified head (i.e., the head stops growing) and lateral displacement of the femur (Fig. 6.129). This latter finding is a relatively constant feature of Legg-Perthes disease, and a joint effusion also usually is present. However, fluid probably is not the cause of

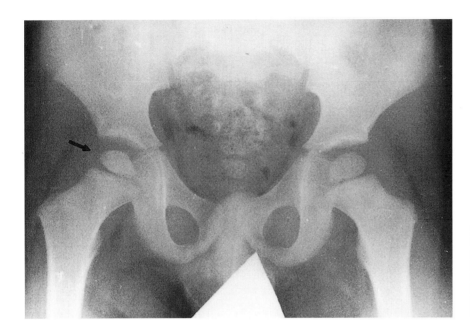

FIGURE 6.129. Legg-Perthes disease: early findings. Note the small, slightly sclerotic femoral head (arrow). In addition, the joint space is slightly widened when compared with that on the left. The teardrop along the medial aspect of the joint space is a little wider than that seen on the left.

the dislocation. Overall, the precise cause of the disease remains unknown. For some reason, blood supply to the femoral head is interrupted, and in this regard, subclinical trauma has been suggested as a possible cause. With long-standing lateral displacement of the head, there is less pressure on the acetabulum, and the so-called "teardrop configuration" of the ischium normally seen in this area becomes wider (7, 8) (Fig. 6.130). This is a useful adjunctive finding but is not seen exclusively with Legg-Perthes disease. Any condition leading to persistent lateral displacement of the femoral head will lead to the same finding.

In terms of the pathogenesis of Legg-Perthes disease, it has been suggested that after initial loss of blood supply,

there is a temporary cessation of growth of the ossified epiphysis and then revascularization of the periphery of the femoral head (9). Subsequently, the entire femoral head revascularizes and reossifies. During this revascularization phase, femoral head subchondral crescent fractures (6) are likely to occur. By no means the earliest radiographic finding, this sign still is relatively common and reflects the presence of a subchondral femoral head fracture (Fig. 6.131, A and B). This fracture frequently is best visualized on frog-leg views because it tends to occur more over the anterior surface of the femoral head. In some cases, a vacuum air phenomenon under the cortical fracture fragment can be seen (Fig. 6.131C). In certain cases, this entire process can

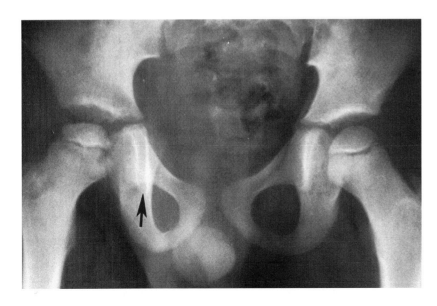

FIGURE 6.130. Legg-Perthes disease: widening of the teardrop. In this patient with a small, slightly sclerotic femoral head and lateral displacement of the femur causing joint space widening, also note widening of the teardrop; the space between the two cortices is increased (arrow). Compare with the other, normal side.

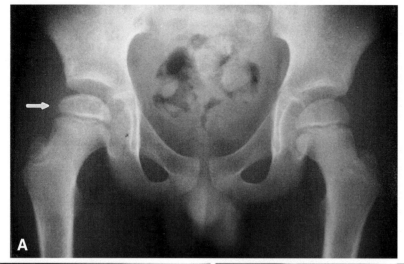

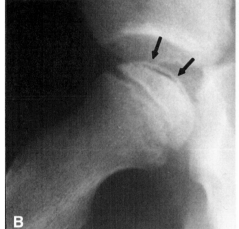

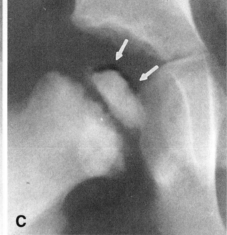

FIGURE 6.131. Legg-Perthes disease: subchondral fracture. A. Note the slightly smaller and more sclerotic femoral head (arrow) on the right. The joint space is widened, and the femur is laterally displaced. **B.** Frog-leg view demonstrates an extensive subchondral fracture (arrows); by Salter's classification, this would forecast a poor result. **C.** Interesting finding of intraepiphyseal gas (arrows), the equivalent of a vacuum joint, in this small, sclerotic, and irregular femoral capital epiphysis.

abort, and in support of this concept, MRI has demonstrated that transient edema of the femoral head only is present in some patients (10).

In terms of correlation of the pathophysiology and imaging of Legg-Perthes disease, as soon as the femoral head loses its blood supply, it stops growing; it becomes smaller, sclerotic, and then flattened (Fig. 6.132). Sclerosis results from lack of washout of calcium because of loss of blood supply and, to some extent, impaction of dead bone. Thereafter, fragmentation of the head occurs because osteoclasts begin to remove dead bone. This is followed by remodeling and reossification of the femoral head (Fig. 6.132), but, at the same time, cystic changes may develop in the metaphysis (11). These areas contain fibrous tissue and probably represent a reparative stage of the disease. They are considered to be somewhat dire in terms of prognosis because once they develop, the head is unlikely to reform properly.

All the foregoing events in Legg-Perthes disease usually take 18–24 months to travel their course, regardless of whether or not therapy is instituted. With early treatment,

however, there is a much better chance that the femoral head will reform in a more normal rounded configuration. If it does not, one ends up with a head that is somewhat flattened (coxa plana) and enlarged (coxa magna) (Fig. 6.133). In addition, the femoral neck becomes fatter, and a coxa vara deformity of the femoral neck develops. All these changes can be modified to some degree if the femoral head is maintained, at an early stage, within the acetabular roof. This is accomplished primarily by using a variety of orthopaedic devices that shift weight bearing to the pelvic bones and off the femoral head. In the past, iliac and subtrochanteric osteotomies were used to move the femoral head medially and under the acetabular roof; currently, surgical treatment of the disease is uncommon. In the end, however, results are poor in older children when there is greater than 50% femoral head involvement and when there is persistent lateral subluxation of the femoral head (2, 12, 13). Chondrolysis is a rare complication in Legg-Perthes disease (14, 15).

In the past, arthrography was used to determine the shape of the cartilaginous femoral head and to determine

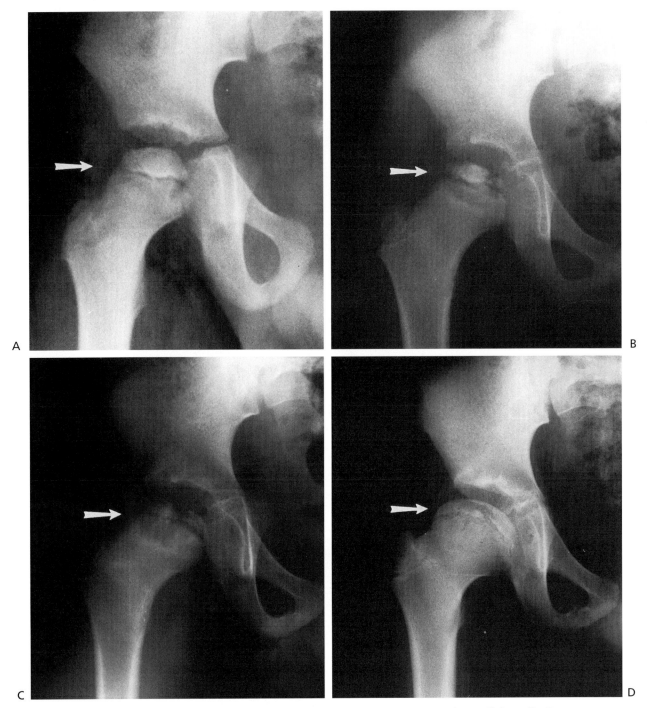

FIGURE 6.132. Legg-Perthes disease: natural progression. A. Note the small, laterally displaced, sclerotic femoral head (arrow). **B.** A few months later, the femoral head is fragmented and the necrotic bone is being resorbed. **C.** Midway through the course of the disease, the femoral capital epiphysis has basically been resorbed and there are radiolucent metaphyseal changes present. **D.** Nearly 2 years later, the femoral head has reconstituted but remains laterally displaced and demonstrates a remaining coxa magna, coxa plana, and coxa vara deformity (arrow).

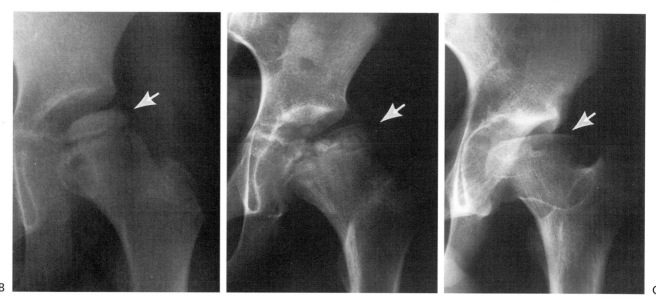

A,B   C

FIGURE 6.133. Legg-Perthes disease: unsuccessful femoral head containment. A. Note the small, laterally displaced femoral head (arrow). **B.** About halfway through the course of Legg-Perthes disease (1 year), the femoral head has become markedly fragmented and partially resorbed (arrow). Lateral displacement of the femur remains, and the femoral head remains well outside the acetabular roof. **C.** Final result. The femoral head (arrow) still remains outside the acetabular roof, and now it is markedly flattened (coxa plana).

whether any of the laterally flattened portion of the cartilage extruded beyond the acetabulum. These changes now can be demonstrated with MRI (Fig. 6.134), and MRI also can be used to demonstrate the early changes in the disease (15–20). **However, if one appreciates the early plain film findings, there is little reason to perform MRI or any other imaging study.** In our institution, we generally do not use MRI but follow the patients with plain films. We relegate nuclear scintigraphy to those cases with no plain film findings and high clinical suspicion. If one uses MRI,

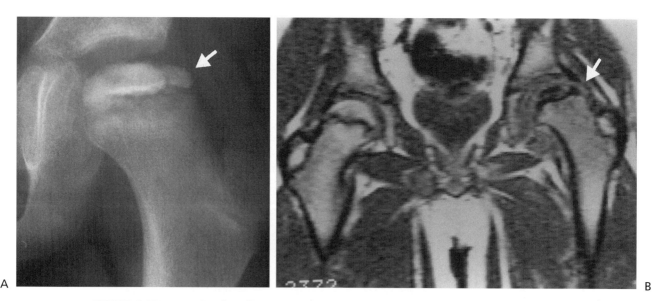

A   B

FIGURE 6.134. Legg-Perthes disease: magnetic resonance findings. A. Note typical plain film findings of a small, sclerotic, and partially fragmented femoral head (arrow). Lateral displacement is present. **B.** T1-weighted magnetic resonance study demonstrates loss of signal in the femoral head (arrow). The femoral head also is laterally displaced and lies outside the edge of the acetabular roof. Fluid in the joint is also present.

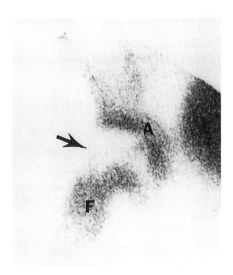

FIGURE 6.135. Aseptic necrosis of the femoral head: scintigraphic findings. Note the photopenic area in the lateral portion of the femoral head (arrow). A, acetabulum; F, femoral neck.

in the early stages of the disease, there will be low signal (edema) in the femoral head on T1-weighted images and variably increased signal on T2-weighted images. With bone scintigraphy, when blood supply is interrupted to the femoral head, a lateral femoral head defect is seen (Fig. 6.135).

Ultrasonography can also be used in the evaluation of Legg-Perthes disease (21, 22), but in the early stages, the findings are no different from those seen with transient synovitis or any other condition in which joint fluid is present. Therefore, ultrasonography plays a minor role in the evaluation of Legg-Perthes disease, but if femoral head cartilage thickening and muscle atrophy are seen, one can suggest the diagnosis (22). Atrophy of the muscles also usually is clearly seen on plain films. Pain in Legg-Perthes disease is due to marrow edema (23).

REFERENCES

1. Mukherjee A, Fabry G. Evaluation of the prognostic indices in Legg-Calvé-Perthes disease: statistical analysis of 116 hips. J Pediatr Orthop 1990;10:153–158.
2. Boechat MI, Winters WD, Hogg RJ, et al. Avascular necrosis of the femoral head in children with chronic renal disease. Radiology 2001;218:411–413.
3. Gore DR. Iatrogenic avascular necrosis of the hip in young children: a long-term follow-up. J Pediatr Orthop 1999;19: 635–640.
4. Loder RT, Farley FA, Herring JA, et al. Bone age determination in children with Legg-Calvé-Perthes disease: a comparison of two methods. J Pediatr Orthop 1995;15:90–94.
5. Keenan W, Clegg J. Perthe's disease after "irritable hip": delayed bone age shows the hip is a "marked man." J Pediatr Orthop 1996;16:20–23.
6. Stansberry SD, Swischuk LE, Barr LL. Legg-Perthes disease: incidence of the subchondral fracture. Appl Radiol 1990;19:30–33.
7. Kahle WK, Coleman SS. The value of acetabular teardrop figure in assessing pediatric hip disorders. J Pediatr Orthop 1992;12: 586–591.
8. Samani DJ, Weinstein SL. The pelvic tear figure: a three-dimensional analysis of the anatomy and effects of rotation. J Pediatr Orthop 1994;14:650–659.
9. Herring JA, Neustadt JB, Williams JJ, et al. The lateral pillar classification of Legg-Calvé-Perthes disease. J Pediatr Orthop 1992; 12:143–150.
10. Pay NT, Singer WS, Bartal E. Hip pain in children accompanied by transient abnormal findings on MR images. Radiology 1989; 171:147–149.
11. Hoffinger SA, Rab GT, Salamon PB. Metaphyseal cysts in Legg-Calvé-Perthes disease. J Pediatr Orthop 1991;11:301–307.
12. Herring JA, Williams JJ, Neustadt JN, et al. Evolution of femoral head deformity during the healing phase of Legg-Calvé-Perthes disease. J Pediatr Orthop 1993;13:41–45.
13. Kamegaya M, Shinada Y, Moriya H, et al. Acetabular remodelling in Perthes disease after primary healing. J Pediatr Orthop 1992;12:308–314.
14. Joseph B, Pydisetty RV. Chondrolysis and the stiff hip in Perthes' disease: an immunological study. J Pediatr Orthop 1996;16: 15–19.
15. Jaramillo D, Kasser JR, Villegas-Medina OL, et al. Cartilaginous abnormalities and growth disturbances in Legg-Calvé-Perthes disease: evaluation with MR imaging. Radiology 1995;197: 767–773.
16. Jaramillo D, Galen TA, Winalski CS, et al. Legg-Calvé-Perthes disease: MR imaging evaluation during manual positioning of the hip—comparison with conventional arthrography. Radiology 1999;212:519–525.
17. Lahdes-Vasama T, Lamminen A, Merikanto J, et al. The value of MRI in early Perthes disease: an MRI study with a 2-year follow-up. Pediatr Radiol 1997;27:517–522.
18. Sebag G, Ducou Le Pointe H, Klein I, et al. Dynamic gadolinium-enhanced subtraction MR imaging—a simple technique for the early diagnosis of Legg-Calvé-Perthes disease: preliminary results. Pediatr Radiol 1997;27:216–220.
19. Uno A, Hattori T, Noritake K, et al. Legg-Calvé-Perthes disease in the evolutionary period: comparison of magnetic resonance imaging with bone scintigraphy. J Pediatr Orthop 1995;15: 362–367.
20. Weishaupt D, Exner GU, Hilfiker PR, et al. Technical innovation. Dyamic MR imaging of the hip in Legg-Calvé-Perthes disease—comparison with arthrography. AJR 2000;174: 1635–1637.
21. Kaniklides C, Lonnerholm T, Moberg A, et al. Legg-Calvé disease: comparison of conventional radiography, MR imaging, bone scintigraphy and arthrography. Acta Radiol 1995;36: 434–439.
22. Robben SG, Meradji M., Diepstraten AM, et al. US of the painful hip in childhood: diagnostic value of cartilage thickening and muscle atrophy in the detection of Perthes disease. Radiology 1998;208:35–42.
23. Wirth T, LeQuesne GW, Paterson DC. Ultrasonography in Legg-Calvé-Perthes disease. Pediatr Radiol 1992;22:498–504.

Meyer Dysplasia

Meyer dysplasia is a benign disorder that results in fragmentation of the femoral heads. The radiographic findings resemble those of Legg-Perthes disease, but there is no pain associated. No positive ultrasound findings are seen, and the entire condition is self-limiting (1).

REFERENCE

1. Harel L, Kornreich L, Ashkenazi S, et al. Meyer dysplasia in the differential diagnosis of hip disease in young children. Arch Pediatr Adolesc Med 1999;153:942–945.

METABOLIC AND ENDOCRINOLOGIC DISEASE

Juvenile Osteoporosis

Juvenile osteoporosis is of unknown etiology and presents in adolescence with profound osteoporosis. Skeletal pain is common, especially in the spine, where universal collapse of the vertebral bodies is common (Fig. 6.136). The condition is largely self-limiting, but it is interesting that similar bony changes have been identified in lysinuric protein intolerance (1).

REFERENCE

1. Svedstrom E, Parto K, Marttinen M, et al. Skeletal manifestations of lysinuric protein intolerance: a followup study of 29 patients. Skeletal Radiol 1993;22:11–16.

Hypothyroidism

The most common cause of hypothyroidism in the neonate is congenital absence or underdevelopment of the thyroid gland, the so-called "athyrotic" or "hypothyrotic cretinism." Hypothyroidism also can be seen in the infants of mothers who ingest excessive iodide or antithyroid medication during pregnancy and in a few infants who are unable to convert inorganic iodine into active hormone. Endemic hypothyroidism, resulting from dietary deficiency of iodine, is uncommon in this day and age.

Athyrotic infants tend to present with more florid findings in the neonatal period than do hypothyrotic infants. The findings include prolonged gestation, large size at birth, prominent fontanelles, respiratory distress, hypothermia, hypoactivity, poor feeding, delayed stooling, abdominal distension, peripheral cyanosis, and edema. In other infants, there may be enough circulating maternal thyroid hormone to delay and mask the development of classic findings until 2 or 3 months of age.

Roentgenographically, abnormal bony changes can be present in the neonate but are easily missed. Basically, they stem from a general immaturity of the skeleton, and in this regard, the vertebral bodies may be unduly rounded or oval (immature configuration), with prominent central vein grooves (Fig. 6.137A). Later on, because these infants are hypotonic, increased thoracolumbar kyphosis and vertebral notching can occur (Fig 6.137B). Such notching probably is not caused by underdevelopment of the vertebral bodies but by anterior compression because of hypotonia and increased kyphosis (1). While inspecting the spine in lateral projection, it also is helpful to note the configuration of the anterior aspect of the ribs because often they lose their normal cupping and become more flat and square.

Delayed bone age is typical in hypothyroidism and can be seen in the neonate. Irregularity of epiphyseal ossification (i.e., fragmentation caused by epiphyseal dysgenesis) is not usually seen until the patient becomes much older (Fig. 6.138A), but dislocation of the hips can be a feature in the neonatal period. In addition, the bones of these infants may be more dense than usual. This is of unexplained etiology, but hypercalcemia can be seen in some of these patients.

The skull shows evidence of delayed ossification with unduly wide sutures, overly dense bones, and large fontanelles. In addition, excessive wormian bone formation is common, and there is delay in development of the mastoid and paranasal sinus air cavities. In older infants and children, the sella turcica can become enlarged in a symmetrical rounded fashion (2–5). This is caused by rebound hypertrophy of the anterior portion of the pituitary gland that, with treatment, can regress (3). This rounded sella often is referred to as a "cherry" sella and, in combination with other calvarial findings, can be highly suggestive of hypothyroidism (Fig. 6.138B). In some cases, an actual adenoma can develop, and currently the enlarged pituitary gland can best be demonstrated with MRI (3–5). The gland enhances uniformly with gadolinium (5).

Some infants with hypothyroidism may show enlargement and goitrous transformation of the thyroid gland (2, 6). In such cases, the enlarged gland may extend into the retropharyngeal space and lead to airway compromise and obstruction (7). Airway obstruction, however, also can be the result of myxedematous retropharyngeal thickening of the soft tissues. The thyroid gland in infants is readily evaluated with ultrasound, and in congenital hypothyroidism, the findings are variable, ranging from no gland at all (Fig. 6.139A) to a small gland or, later on, a multinodular goiter. Occasionally, cardiomegaly with congestive heart failure or pericardial effusion can be encountered and can develop. When thyroid tissue is found to be absent in the newborn, it is important to look for sublingual tissue, either with ultrasound or with nuclear scintigraphy (Fig. 6.139B). Hypothyroidism also can be seen with cystinosis (8).

REFERENCES

1. Swischuk LE. The beaked, notched, or hooked vertebra: its significance in infants and young children. Radiology 1970;95: 661–664.

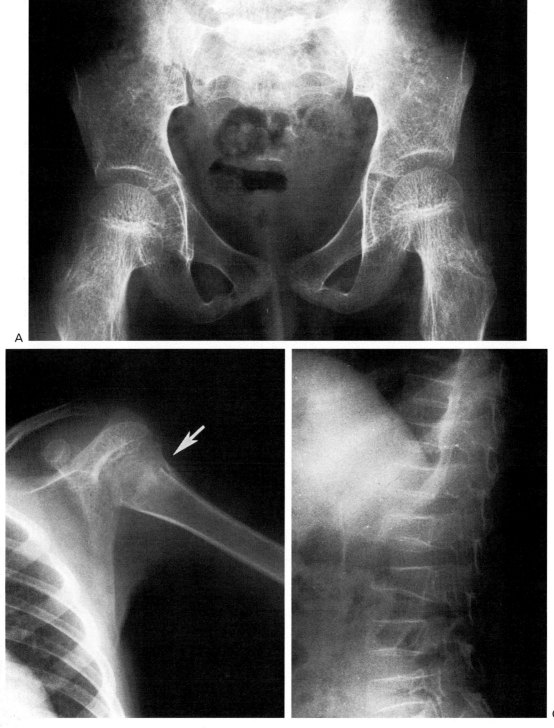

A

B

C

FIGURE 6.136. Juvenile osteoporosis. A. Note marked osteoporosis of the pelvis and upper femurs. **B.** Demineralized humerus demonstrating a pathologic fracture (arrow). **C.** Severe osteoporosis of the spine is present, and virtually every vertebral body has suffered a compression fracture.

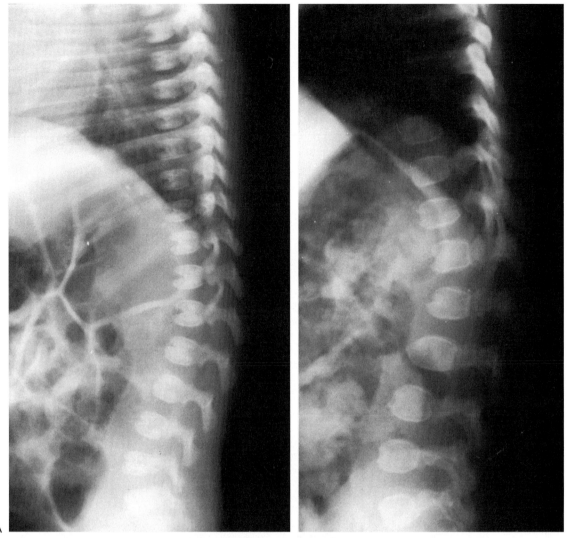

A   B

FIGURE 6.137. Hypothyroidism: spine changes. A. This 3-month-old infant demonstrates an immature spine wherein the vertebral bodies are rounded, the disc spaces in between are deeper than usual, and the central vein grooves are prominent. **B.** Older infant demonstrating increased kyphosis at the thoracolumbar junction, vertebral notching, and immature, oval vertebrae.

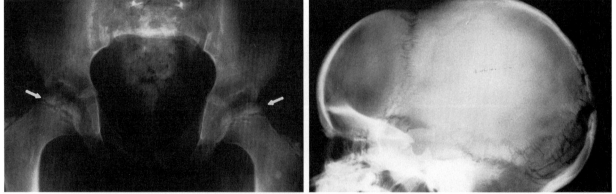

A   B

FIGURE 6.138. Hypothyroidism. A. Epiphyseal dysgenesis. Note that both femoral heads are somewhat small and irregularly ossified (arrows). At first, Legg-Perthes disease might be suggested. **B. Calvarial changes.** First, note the increased density of the calvarium. Then, note the numerous wormian bones and prominent sutures. The sella is slightly larger than normal and well rounded. This is an early "cherry" sella. The findings become more pronounced in older children.

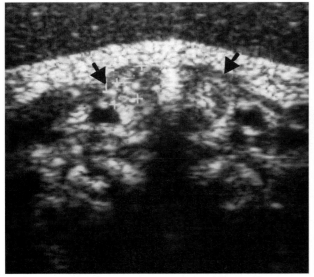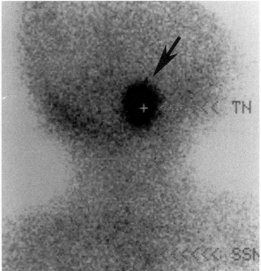

FIGURE 6.139. Absent thyroid tissue in neonate: ultrasound findings. A. Note absence of normal thymic tissue (arrows). **B.** Nuclear scintigraphy demonstrates a focus of lingual thyroid tissue (arrow).

2. Swischuk LE, Sarwar M. The sella in childhood hypothyroidism. Pediatr Radiol 1977;6:1–3.
3. Hutchins WW, Crues JV III, Miya P, et al. MR demonstration of pituitary hyperplasia and regression after therapy for hypothyroidism. AJNR 1990;11:410.
4. Desai MP, Mehta RU, Choksi CS, et al. Pituitary enlargement on magnetic resonance imaging in congenital hypothyroidism. Arch Pediatr Adolesc Med 1996;150:623–628.
5. Kuroiwa T, Okabe Y, Hasuo K, et al. MR imaging of pituitary hypertrophy due to juvenile primary hypothyroidism: a case report. Clin Imag 1991;15:202–205.
6. Optican RJ, White KS, Effmann EL. Case report. Goiterous cretinism manifesting as newborn stridor: CT evaluation. AJR 1991;157:557–558.
7. Ueda D, Mitamura R, Suzuki N, et al. Sonographic imaging of the thyroid gland in congenital hypothyroidism. Pediatr Radiol 1992;22:102–105.
8. Rezvani I, DiGeorge AM, Cote ML. Primary hypothyroidism in cystinosis. J Pediatr 1977;91:340–341.

Hyperthyroidism

Hyperthyroidism can be seen in the neonate, and in such cases, the mother usually is suffering from hyperthyroidism at the time of delivery or has undergone surgical or medical thyroidectomy for the disease during gestation. In the latter instance, even though the mother may be euthyroid during the remainder of the pregnancy, the infant may be born hyperthyroid.

Patients with hyperthyroidism demonstrate hyperactivity, restlessness, increased hunger, weight loss, increased pulse rate, cardiac failure, and other features of typical hyperthyroidism such as myopathy and exophthalmos. In those patients whose thyroid gland is enlarged, airway obstruction may result.

Roentgenographically, the findings consist of accelerated bone maturation and premature closure of the cranial sutures (1). In addition, premature epiphyseal fusion can occur in the hands, leading to brachydactyly. Thyrotoxic myopathy and cardiomyopathy can occur in older children, but it is not a recognized problem in neonates. Thyroid acropachy is rare in children.

REFERENCE

1. Riggs W Jr, Wilroy RS Jr, Etteldorf JN. Neonatal hyperthyroidism with accelerated skeletal maturation, craniosynostosis, and brachydactyly. Radiology 1972;105:621—625.

Hypopituitarism and Growth Hormone Deficiency

Hypopituitarism and growth hormone deficiency produce somewhat similar findings. Congenital hypopituitarism is uncommon and often unrecognized until postmortem studies are obtained. These infants have aplasia or hypoplasia of the pituitary gland and also show underdevelopment or absence of the adrenal glands, thyroid gland, and gonads. They are prone to severe hypoglycemia and often die before the condition is recognized. If recognized, however, it can be treated and the infant saved. Roentgenographically, the only finding in the skull is a small pituitary fossa, but since most of these infants are not subject to calvarial roentgenograms, there is seldom a chance to note this finding. MRI is the most expedient way with which to image the pituitary gland in these patients. The findings range from

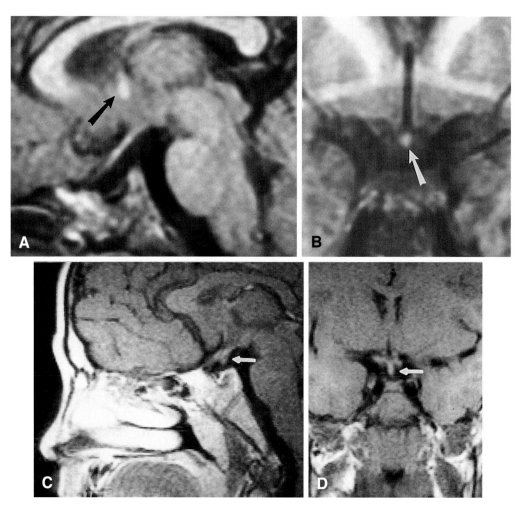

FIGURE 6.140. Pituitary abnormalities in hypopituitarism and growth hormone deficiency. A. In this patient, the posterior pituitary lobe (arrow) is ectopically located. The sella itself is empty. **B.** Coronal view demonstrates the ectopic bright posterior pituitary (arrow). **C.** Another patient with a thick, truncated pituitary stock (arrow). The sella is empty. **D.** Frontal view demonstrates the thick pituitary stock (arrow).

virtually no change to severe underdevelopment or absence of the anterior pituitary lobe and pituitary stock (1).

With idiopathic growth hormone deficiency, bone age and growth are delayed. On MRI, absence of the posterior pituitary bright spot, a small pituitary stock, and very often ectopic posterior pituitary tissue in the hypothalamic region (2–5) (Fig. 6.140) can be seen. In addition to these findings, midline central nervous system anomalies are common in both growth hormone deficiency and hypopituitarism (4, 6). It is interesting, however, that the pituitary gland is normal in cases of hereditary isolated growth hormone deficiency (7).

REFERENCES

1. Rofanova O, Takamura N, Kimoshita E-I, et al. MR imaging of the pituitary gland in children and young adults with congenital combined pituitary hormone deficiency associated with PROP1 mutations. AJR 2000;174:555–559.
2. Abrahams JJ, Trefelner E, Boulware SD. Idiopathic growth hormone deficiency: MR findings in 35 patients. AJR 1991;156:599–604.
3. Argyropoulou M, Perignon F, Brauner R, et al. Magnetic resonance imaging in the diagnosis of growth hormone deficiency. J Pediatr 1992;120:886–891.
4. Hamilton J, Blaser S, Daneman D. MR imaging in idiopathic growth hormone deficiency. AJNR 1998;19:1609–1615.
5. Chen S, Leger J, Garel C, et al. Growth hormone deficiency with ectopic neurohypophysis: anatomical variations and relationship between the visibility of the pituitary stalk asserted by magnetic resonance imaging and anterior pituitary function. J Clin Endocrinol Metab 1999;84:2408–2413.
6. Triulzi F, Scotti G, deNatale B, et al. Evidence of a congenital midline brain anomaly in pituitary dwarfs: a magnetic resonance imaging study in 101 patients. Pediatrics 1994;93:409–416.
7. Kornreich L, Horev G, Lazr L, et al. MR findings in hereditary isolated growth hormone deficiency. AJNR 1997;18:1743–1747.

Acromegaly and Gigantism

In acromegaly and gigantism, a pituitary adenoma is present and accelerates body growth. In childhood, the problem usually is gigantism and not acromegaly.

Cushing's Syndrome

Cushing's syndrome can occur in infancy. Clinical findings in any patient consist of obesity, moon facies, hypertension, hirsutism, and glycosuria. Many of these infants also demonstrate marked atrophy of the thymus, resulting from excessive cortisol production. The disease is usually caused by functioning tumors or hyperplasia of the adrenal glands (1, 2), although pituitary adenomas have also been described (3, 4). Roentgenographic findings consist of widespread osteoporosis, pathologic bone fractures, vertebral compressions, and retarded bone maturation (1) (Fig. 6.141). Ultrasound (2), CT, and MRI can demonstrate the adrenal adenomas, but MRI (3) is best for the demonstration of pituitary adenomas. Neither of these tumors shows any specific features except that they are solid tumors that enhance.

REFERENCES

1. Neville AM, Symington T. Bilateral adrenocortical hyperplasia in children with Cushing's syndrome. J Pathol 1972;107:95–106.
2. Zia-ul-Miraj M, Usmani GN, Yaqub MM, et al. Cushing's syndrome caused by an adrenal adenoma. J Pediatr Surg 1998;33:644–646.
3. Maeer P, Gudinchet F, Rillet B, et al. Cushing's disease due to a giant pituitary adenoma in early infancy: CT and MRI features. Pediatr Radiol 1996;26:48–50.
4. Summer TE, Volberg FM. Cushing's syndrome in infancy due to pituitary adenoma. Pediatr Radiol 1982;12:81–83.

Hypophosphatasia

Hypophosphatasia is inherited as an autosomal recessive condition, and depending on the severity of the disease, a wide gamut of clinical and roentgenographic change is seen (1). The severe form is manifest in the neonate, and many of these infants are stillborn. Others develop severe respiratory distress due to chest cage weakness and hypoplastic lungs and die soon after birth.

The basic defect is believed to lie in an inability of osteoblasts to produce alkaline phosphatase, and as a consequence, normal mineralization of bones does not occur. Serum alkaline phosphatase levels are low, and there is excessive urinary phosphoethanolamine excretion. The roentgenographic changes resemble rickets or metaphyseal dysostosis, and in the more severe cases, the bones are extremely poorly ossified (Fig. 6.142). Pathologic fractures are common, and in this regard, osteogenesis imperfecta is mimicked. The teeth are also involved and show defective mineralization. There also is premature loss of the deciduous teeth. Bowed bones without metaphyseal abnormalities and bony spurs over the convex surfaces of the bent bones also have been seen (2).

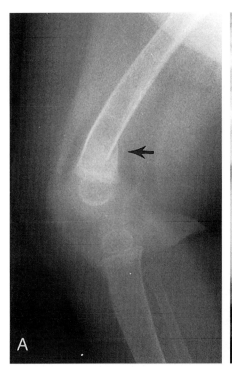
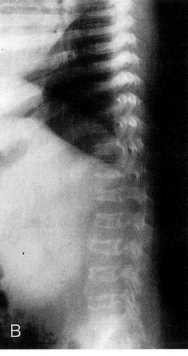

FIGURE 6.141. Cushing's syndrome. A. Note marked demineralization of the bones and associated pathologic fracture through the femur (arrow). Also note that the extremities are fat, but that muscle bulk is diminished. **B.** Another patient with numerous compression fractures of demineralized vertebral bodies.

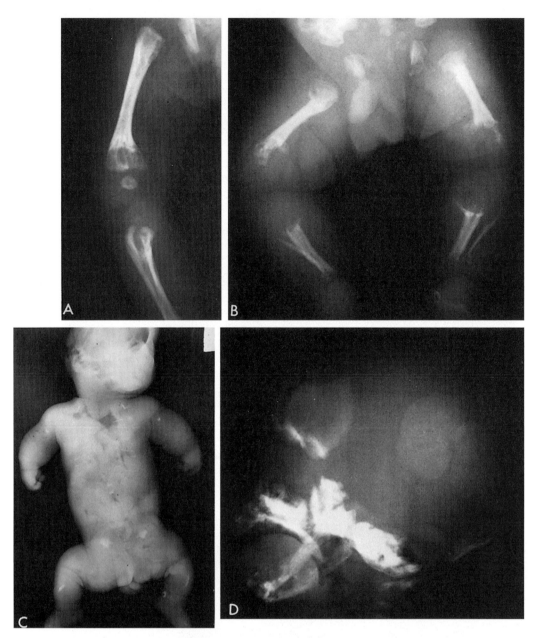

FIGURE 6.142. Hypophosphatasia. A. Classic, "celery stalk-like" metaphyseal radiolucencies in the long bones. **B.** Another infant with more profound changes in the metaphyses. In both cases, the findings might be confused with metaphyseal dysostosis or congenital lues. **C.** Postmortem examination showing severe bony underossification in hypophosphatasia. These findings might be confused with achondrogenesis. **D.** Skull in an infant with severe hypophosphatasia showing marked underossification of the membranous calvarial bones and pseudowidening of the sutures and fontanelles. Tooth formation is also impaired. Sclerosis of the base of the skull is partially the result of an artifact in reproduction. (**A, B,** and **D** reproduced with permission from Macpherson RI, Kroeker M, Houston CS. Hypophosphatasia. J Can Assoc Radiol 1972;23:16–26; **C** reproduced with permission from Houston CS, Awen CF, Kent HP. Fatal neonatal dwarfism. J Can Assoc Radiol 1972;23:45–61).

Calvarial changes consist of gross underossification, pseudowidening of the sutures, and excessive wormian bone formation (Fig. 6.142D). It is interesting, however, that even though the calvarium is grossly underossified, many of these infants eventually develop secondary premature closure of the sutures. Recently, treatment with alkaline phosphatase-rich plasma from patients with Paget's bone disease has been successful as a form of treatment (3).

REFERENCES

1. Kozlowski K, Sutcliffe J, Barylak A, et al. Hypophosphatasia. Review of 25 cases. Pediatr Radiol 1976;5:102–117.
2. Oestreich AE, Bofinger MK. Prominent transverse (Bowdler) bone spurs as a diagnostic clue in a case of neonatal hypophosphatasia without metaphyseal irregularity. Pediatr Radiol 1996;19:341–342.
3. White MP, Values R Jr, Ryan LM, et al. Infantile hypophosphatasia: enzyme replacement therapy by intravenous infusion of alkaline phosphatase-rich plasma from patients with Paget's bone disease. J Pediatr 1982;101:379–386.

Pseudohypophosphatasia

Pseudohypophosphatasia is a recently described condition with changes similar to classic hypophosphatasia except that serum alkaline phosphatase activity is normal. It is therefore termed "pseudohypophosphatasia." The case reported by Scriver and Cameron (1) had onset at 3 months of age. Whether this is a separate entity or a variation of hypophosphatasia is yet to be determined.

REFERENCE

1. Scriver CR, Cameron D. Pseudohypophosphatasia. N Engl J Med 1969;281:604–606.

Familial Hyperphosphatasemia (Hyperphosphatasia)

This rare abnormality now generally is termed "familial hyperphosphatasemia," and an autosomal recessive pattern of inheritance is likely (1). The basic problem is an overproduction of bone and collagen by osteocytes. Normal maturation into compact lamellar bone does not occur, and thus there is resultant diaphyseal widening and ballooning of the long bones. Corticomedullary differentiation is poor, and the bones generally are quite demineralized. In addition, periosteal cloaking around the widened bones is a common occurrence in infancy (Fig. 6.143). Except for demineralization, the skull at this stage may appear normal. Later on, the bones of the calvarium become thickened, and the long bones become bowed and even more ballooned. Tumoral calcinosis also has been noted with hyperphosphatemia (2, 3).

Generally, the condition is not manifest at birth, but more severe cases tend to present earlier. The bony changes are progressive, and biochemically, both serum alkaline and acid phosphatases are elevated. Recently, treatment with human thyrocalcitonin has been shown to be successful (4).

REFERENCES

1. Mikati MA, Melhem RE, Najjar S. The syndrome of hyperostosis and hyperphosphatemia. J Pediatr 1981;99:900–904.
2. Narchi H. Hyperostosis with hyperphosphatemia: evidence of familial occurrence and association with tumoral calcinosis. Pediatrics 1997;99:745–748.
3. Wilson MP, Lindsley CB, Warady BA, et al. Hyperphosphatemia associated with cortical hyperostosis and tumoral calcinosis. J Pediatr 1989;114:1010–1013.
4. Tuysuz B, Mercinmek S, Ungur S, et al. Calcitonin treatment in osteoectasia with hyperphosphatasia (juvenile Paget's disease): radiographic changes after treatment. Pediatr Radiol 1999;29:838–841.

Idiopathic Hypercalcemia

There are two types of idiopathic hypercalcemia of infancy. The first is a transient variety with a benign clinical course and relatively prompt return to normal. There are no roentgenographic changes in this type. In the other, more severe form, a number of clinical and roentgenographic findings have been described. Most infants with this form of hypercalcemia show a specific facial appearance consisting of broad maxillae, a full prominent upper lip, an upturned nose, hypertelorism, a relatively small mandible, and prominent ears (elfin facies). They are usually mentally retarded and show progressive muscular weakness. The etiology of idiopathic hypercalcemia is unknown, but a deficiency in thyrocalcitonin production by the C cells of the thyroid gland is likely. Familial occurrence also has been documented (1).

Supravalvular aortic stenosis is part of the syndrome, but probably less than half of patients demonstrate this abnormality. In addition, hypercalcemia may not be present in all patients. Peripheral pulmonary artery stenoses are common, and systemic and intracranial arterial stenoses frequently are encountered (2–5). Multiple bladder diverticula can be associated. An additional skeletal finding is a variable increase in sclerosis of the entire skeleton (Fig. 6.144).

REFERENCES

1. White RA, Preus M, Watters GV, et al. Familial occurrence of the Williams syndrome. J Pediatr 1977;91:614–616.
2. Ingelfinger JR, Newburger JW. Spectrum of renal anomalies in patients with Williams syndrome. J Pediatr 1991;119:771–773.
3. Kaplan P, Levinson M, Kaplan BA. Cerebral artery stenoses in Williams syndrome cause strokes in childhood. J Pediatr 1995;126:943–945.

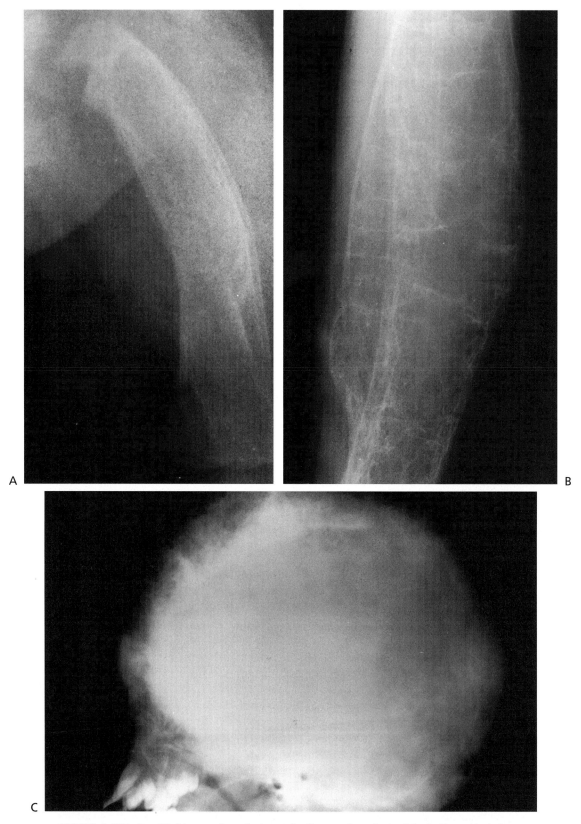

FIGURE 6.143. Familial hyperphosphatasemia (hyperphosphatasia). A. Femur in infancy demonstrates widening of the diaphysis, periosteal new bone formation, and early ballooning of the femur. **B.** Older child demonstrating more extensive ballooning. **C.** Same patient demonstrating marked thickening of the calvarium.

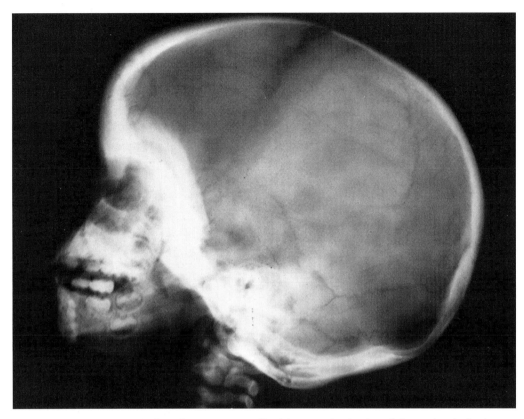

FIGURE 6.144. Hypercalcemia. Note generalized increase in density of the entire skull. The entire skeleton in this older infant was more sclerotic than normal.

4. Putman CM, Chaloupka JC, Eklund JE, et al. Multifocal intracranial occlusive vasculopathy resulting in stroke: an unusual manifestation of Williams syndrome. AJNR 1995;16:1536–1538.
5. Soper R, Chaloupka JC, Fayad PB, et al. Ischemic stroke and intracranial multifocal cerebral arteriopathy in Williams syndrome. J Pediatr 1995;126:945–948.

Hyperparathyroidism

Primary hyperparathyroidism is rare in childhood and extremely rare in the newborn infant (1, 2), and some cases are familial (2). In other instances, hyperparathyroidism develops as a secondary phenomenon in infants delivered of hypoparathyroid mothers and also of mothers with renal insufficiency (3). This probably represents secondary hyperparathyroidism, which is much more common in older infants and in children with renal disease leading to renal rickets or renal osteodystrophy. In such infants, a glomerular deficiency in addition to tubular abnormality is present. Infants with primary hyperparathyroidism usually are very ill, and the condition is often fatal. Clinically, such infants present with failure to thrive, poor feeding, hypotonicity, irritability, and constipation.

Roentgenographic findings (4) consist of profound demineralization of the skeleton, marked subperiosteal bone resorption (Fig. 6.145), and, in infants surviving the neonatal period, metastatic soft tissue calcification. Bone demineralization often is so profound that the findings might be confused with hypophosphatasia or the Jansen type of metaphyseal dysostosis.

In secondary hyperparathyroidism, changes of rickets are intermingled with those of hyperparathyroidism. Often, however, flaring of the metaphyses is not as pronounced. On the other hand, the epiphyseal line is wide, there is extreme indistinctness of the metaphyseal edge, and there is characteristic sub- and endosteal bone resorption along the middle phalanges of the hand, upper inner metaphyseal edges of the tibiae, the distal radius and ulna, and both the inner and the outer aspects of the femoral neck (Fig. 6.146). In addition, there also is bone resorption at other sites such as the flat bones, ribs, and lateral ends of the clavicles. Brown tumors are uncommon (5, 6). Secondary hyperparathyroidism also can be seen in infants on long-term furosemide therapy, where hypercalcemia also leads to gallbladder and renal calculi.

REFERENCES

1. Blair JW, Carachi R. Neonatal primary hyperparathyroidism—a case report and review of the literature. Eur J Pediatr Surg 1991;1:110—114.

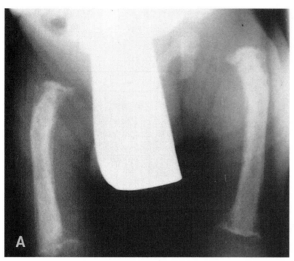
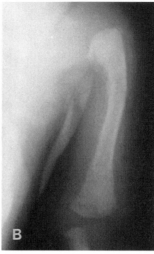

FIGURE 6.145. Hyperparathyroidism. A. Lower extremities. Note extensive demineralization, subperiosteal bone resorption, and fragmentation of the metaphyses. The bones are coarsely trabeculated. **B.** Upper extremity demonstrating similar changes in the humerus and, in addition, some bowing of the upper humerus. The upper femurs also are slightly bowed. Films taken approximately 2 months later showed complete healing of all these lesions.

2. Powell BR, Blank E, Benda G. Neonatal hyperparathyroidism and skeletal demineralization in an infant with familial hypocalciuric hypercalcemia. Pediatrics 1993;91:144–145.

3. Levin TL, States L, Greig A, et al. Maternal renal insufficiency: a cause of hyperparathyroidism. Pediatr Radiol 1992;22:315–316.

4. Eftekhari F, Yusefzadeh DK. Primary infantile hyperparathyroidism: clinical, laboratory, and radiographic features in 21 cases. Skeletal Radiol 1982;8:201–208.

5. Fasanelli S, Graziani M, Boldrini R, et al. "Brown tumor" of the maxilla. Pediatr Radiol 1992;22:142–144.

6. Gurumurthy K, Solomon M, Butt KMH, et al. Maxillary brown tumor caused by secondary hyperparathyroidism in an infant. J Pediatr 1982;100:245–247.

Hypoparathyroidism and Pseudohypoparathyroidism

Neonatal hypoparathyroidism is uncommon and often familial (1). Roentgenographic skeletal findings usually are normal, and clinically these infants often present with tetany or some other manifestation of hypocalcemia (1).

Pseudohypoparathyroidism also is rare in infancy, and, as with hypoparathyroidism, the presenting problem usually is that of tetany. Congenital absence of the parathyroid gland often is seen with absence of the thymus gland and associ-

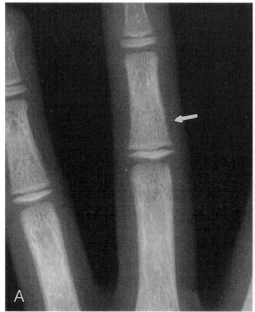
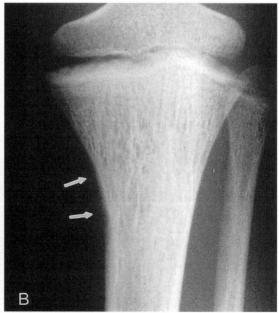

FIGURE 6.146. Renal osteodystrophy: secondary hyperparathyroidism. A. Typical subperiosteal bone deposition of the fingers (arrow). **B.** Subperiosteal bone resorption along the upper medial tibia (arrows).

ated immunologic deficiencies. Roentgenographically, radiographic findings in the majority of these patients are absent in infancy and early childhood. With pseudohypoparathyroidism, however, shortening of the fourth and fifth or even third metacarpals is commonly encountered and becomes more pronounced as the patient grows older (Fig. 6.147). In addition, calcifications in the basal ganglia can be seen in these patients.

REFERENCE

1. Whyte MP, Weldon VV. Idiopathic hypoparathyroidism presenting with seizures during infancy: X-linked recessive inheritance in a large Missouri kindred. J Pediatr 1981;99:608–611.

Phenylketonuria

Although phenylketonuria is manifest at birth, the described bony changes usually develop in older children. When seen, they consist of exaggerated cupping of the ends of the long bones, bony spicules in the metaphyseal regions, and demineralization of the bones (1). With proper treatment, however, these changes usually now are not seen. On MRI of the brain, there is increased signal in the basal ganglia on T1-weighted images (2, 3). These changes have been noted to reverse with treatment (2). If untreated, brain damage will result with subcortical white matter changes and calcification of the basal ganglia (4, 5). In addition, hypoplasia of the corpus callosum has been noted (3). When a baby is born of a phenylketonuric mother, if maternal phenylalanine levels are not under control, the infant's brain may not grow properly. It has been suggested that this might be prevented with proper treatment of the mother from the twentieth week of gestation (2).

REFERENCES

1. Carson DJ, Greeves LG, Sweeney LE, et al. Osteopenia and phenylketonuria. Pediatr Radiol 1990;20:598–599.
2. Cleary MA, Walter JH, Wraith JE, et al. Magnetic resonance imaging in phenylketonuria: reversal of cerebral white matter change. J Pediatr 1995;127:251–255.
3. Pearsen KD, Gean-Marton AD, Levy HL, et al. Phenylketonuria: MR imaging of the brain with clinical correlation. Radiology 1990;177:437–440.
4. Gudinchet F, Maeder PH, Meuli RA, et al. Cranial CT and MRI in malignant phenylketonuria. Pediatr Radiol 1992;22:223–224.
5. Levy HL, Lobbregt D, Barnes PD, et al. Maternal phenylketonuria: magnetic resonance imaging of the brain in offspring. J Pediatr 1996;128:770–775.

Diabetes Mellitus

The changes in diabetes mellitus in children are much the same as those in adulthood. These patients have chronic problems with infections and vascular insufficiency involving almost all the organs of the body. Diabetes is uncommonly seen in the newborn infant but has been documented secondary to congenital absence of the islets of Langerhans. In addition, a transient form of neonatal diabetes mellitus exists and is presumed to be caused by delayed maturation of the pancreatic β-cells.

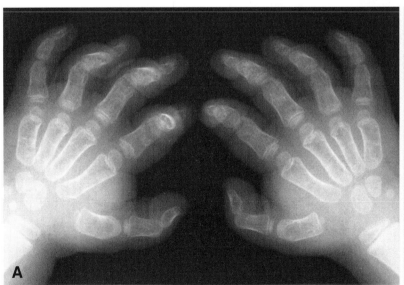
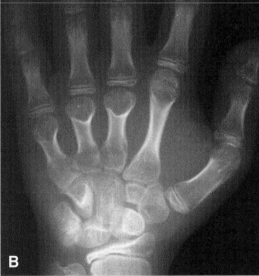

FIGURE 6.147. Pseudohypoparathyroidism. A. Young child with slightly ballooned bones in the hands. **B.** Another older patient demonstrates characteristic shortening of the third, fourth, and fifth metacarpals. The findings are variable in this condition; in some patients, only one of the metacarpals is short, while in others, all the metacarpals are short.

Infants of Diabetic Mothers

Infants of diabetic mothers are notoriously large for their gestational age and show generalized visceromegaly, cardiomegaly, and hypoglycemia. Cardiomegaly and other visceromegaly are believed to be caused by cellular hypertrophy and hyperplasia. Such hypertrophy of the left ventricle and interventricular septum can lead to transient hypertrophic subvalvular aortic stenosis. Structural congenital heart disease also is somewhat more common than it is in the general infant population (1, 2), and there is an increase in subcutaneous fat. These are big, fat babies, but still immature.

Respiratory distress can occur secondary to hypoglycemia, but it also should be noted that these infants are prone to develop hyaline membrane disease because they are immature. The lungs also are hypoplastic, secondary to compressive cardiomegaly and visceromegaly. Vascular problems such as vascular thrombosis are more common in these infants, as is the meconium plug or small left colon syndrome (3). Congenital deformities involving other systems also have an increased incidence (1, 2). One of the more serious of these anomalies is the so-called "caudal regression syndrome" or "mermaid deformity." Hypoplastic femurs and micrognathia also have been described (4). Roentgenographically, the findings are nonspecific but in conjunction with one another can suggest the diagnosis, that is, hepatosplenomegaly, cardiomegaly, and hypoplastic lungs (Fig. 6.148).

REFERENCES

1. Day RE, Insley J. Maternal diabetes mellitus and congenital malformation: survey of 205 cases. Arch Dis Child 1976;51:935–938.
2. Ziereisen F, Courtens W, Clercx A, et al. Maternal diabetes and fetal malformations: a case associating cardiovascular, facial and skeletal malformations. Pediatr Radiol 1997;27:945–947.
3. Dunn V, Nixon GW, Jaffe RB, et al. Review: infants of diabetic mothers: radiographic manifestations. AJR 1981;137:123–128.
4. Johnson JP, Carey JS, Gooch M III, et al. Femoral hypoplasia—unusual facies syndrome in infants of diabetic mothers. J Pediatr 1983;102:866–872.

Trace Element Abnormalities

In terms of trace element deficiencies, hypomagnesemia in the neonatal period can lead to convulsions, and hypermagnesemia to extreme lethargy, flaccidity, and cyanosis. Hypermagnesemia can also lead to metaphyseal sclerosis (1). No bony changes have been documented with hypomagnesemia. Zinc deficiency can cause failure of normal growth and is important in certain enzyme systems. Copper deficiency commonly occurs in premature infants and in those on total parenteral nutrition, and skeletal changes resembling those of rickets have been documented. It is likely, however, that copper deficiency is intertwined with other deficiencies, including vitamin D, and probably is best discussed with metabolic bone disease of the premature infant (see next section). Failure to absorb copper from the intestinal tract also recently has been incriminated as the basic defect in the kinky hair syndrome.

Excessive aluminum intake most often occurs in patients requiring excessive amounts of aluminum hydroxide therapy. Such patients show profound osteoporosis with irregularities and fraying of the metaphysis and widening of the physis (2). To a minor degree, the changes resemble those of certain types of rickets. Once the aluminum hydroxide is removed from the diet, the bones repair.

REFERENCES

1. Cumming WA, Thomas VJ. Case report: hypermagnesemia: a cause of abnormal metaphyses in the neonate. AJR 1989;152:1071–1072.
2. Andreoli SP, Smith JA, Bergstein JM. Aluminum bone disease in

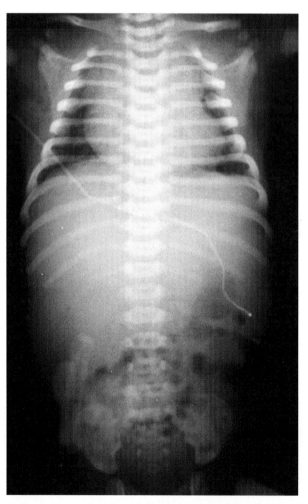

FIGURE 6.148. Infant of diabetic mother. Note hepatosplenomegaly along with cardiomegaly. The lungs are clear but small (hypoplastic).

children: radiographic features from diagnosis to resolution. Radiology 1985;156:663–668.

Metabolic Bone Disease of the Premature (Copper Deficiency, Rickets of Prematurity)

Metabolic bone disease in the premature infant is a common problem in infants on total parenteral nutrition. Although in the past, the problem was considered to be caused by copper deficiency, it is now generally believed to be a problem of multiple mineral, trace element, and vitamin deficiencies. Overall, however, the resulting osteomalacic bones most resemble those of rickets (1, 2). For this reason, the term **metabolic bone disease of the premature** often is preferred.

Roentgenographically, the changes in these infants consist of osteomalacia, subperiosteal bone resorption, and fraying of the metaphyses (Figs. 6.149). Corner fractures are common. In the healing phases, periosteal new bone deposition is seen, and pathologic fractures are common (1, 3). These fractures often are detected incidentally and are especially prone to occur in the ribs. For this reason, the condition frequently is misinterpreted for the battered child syndrome (4). However, this should not occur because the bones in the battered child syndrome show no metabolic

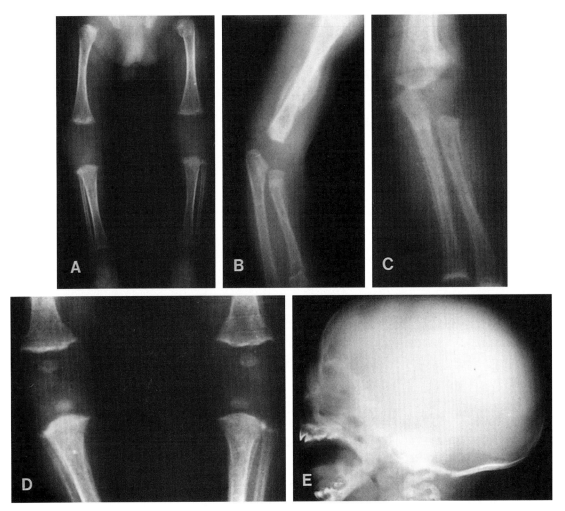

FIGURE 6.149. Metabolic bone disease of the premature (copper deficiency, rickets of prematurity). A. Early findings consisting of extensive demineralization and fragmentation and irregularity of the metaphyses. A healing pathologic fracture of the upper left femur also is present. **B.** Another infant demonstrating a pathologic fracture of the distal radius, slight cupping of the distal ulna, demineralization of the bones, and periosteal new bone deposition around the humeral shaft. This probably is caused by subperiosteal bleeding. Overall, the findings are a mixture of those seen with rickets and scurvy. **C.** Another infant demonstrating healing changes with more pronounced cupping of the bones and early periosteal new bone deposition. **D.** Another infant showing typical metaphyseal changes. **E.** Another infant demonstrating extensive demineralization of the calvarium and facial structures.

disturbances. Generally, all these changes slowly clear, and eventually the bones become normal. Even when they fracture, conservative therapy is advised.

REFERENCES

1. Koo K, Sherman R, Succop P, et al. Fractures and rickets in very low birth weight infants: conservative management and outcome. J Pediatr Orthop 1989;9:326–330.
2. Lyon AJ, McIntosh N, Wheeler K, et al. Radiological rickets in extremely low birth weight infants. Pediatr Radiol 1987;17: 56–58.
3. Amir J, Katz K, Grunebaum M, et al. Fractures in premature infants. J Pediatr Orthop 1988;8:41–44.
4. Swischuk LE. Not everything is child abuse. Emerg Radiol 2000; 7:218–224.

Oxalosis

Oxalosis is known primarily for the nephrocalcinosis and renal failure it produces. However, metaphyseal changes not unlike those seen with rickets also can be seen in these patients, however (1–3). In addition, in the early stages, radiolucent transverse bands in the long bones can be seen along with marked bony resorption (1). When the kidneys fail, changes of renal osteodystrophy predominate (1). The bony changes result from oxalate crystals being deposited in the bone marrow and the resultant chronic inflammatory response.

REFERENCES

1. Fisher D, Hiller N, Drukker A. Oxalosis of bone: report of four cases and a new radiological staging. Pediatr Radiol 1995;254: 293–295.
2. Schnitzler CM, Kok JA, Jacobs DWC, et al. Skeletal manifestations of primary oxalosis. Pediatr Nephrol 1991;5:193–199.
3. Vichi GF, Bongini U, Seracini D, et al. Progression of bone lesions

in a child with primary hyperoxaluria type 1: evaluation by roentgenology and MRI. Pediatr Radiol 1995;25:S102–S104.

Lead and Heavy Metal Intoxication

Any heavy metal intoxication can lead to bony changes, but lead intoxication is the most common. Lead can cross the placenta, and intrauterine or neonatal poisoning can occur (1, 2). This generally results in neurologic disturbances, and the typical white lines of lead poisoning do not develop. These lines take time to develop and usually are seen in older infants and in children with chronic lead poisoning. They usually are quite dense, 3–4 mm in thickness, and discretely delineated from the adjacent normal bone (Fig. 6.150A) (3). They result from abnormally thick trabeculae being formed in the metaphyseal growth zone. In addition, however, actual lead deposition occurs in these areas. However, it might be noted that the most common cause of a rather dense white line in the metaphysis, mimicking the lead line, is a normal line seen in response to abundant sunlight and vitamin D production (Fig. 6.150B). Rarely, in longstanding intoxication, abnormal growth of the metaphyses can result, causing undue widening of this portion of the bone. White lines similar to those seen with lead poisoning also have been documented with bisphosphonate therapy (4). Rarely, lead intoxication can occur from chronic lead pellet entrapment in the appendix (5).

REFERENCES

1. Singh N, Donovan CM, Hanshaw JB. Neonatal lead intoxication in a prenatally exposed infant. J Pediatr 1978;93:1019–1021.
2. Timpo AE, Amin JS, Casalino MB, et al. Congenital lead intoxication. J Pediatr 1979;94:765–767.
3. Pearl M, Boxt LM. Radiographic findings in congenital lead poisoning. Radiology 1980;136:83–84.
4. Van Persijn van Meerten EL, Kroon HM, Papapoulos SE. Epi- and metaphyseal changes in children caused by administration of bisphosphonates. Radiology 1992;184:249–254.

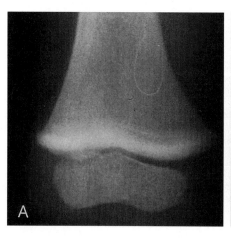 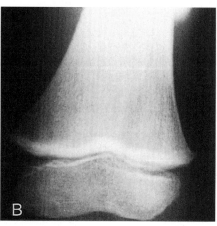

FIGURE 6.150. Lead lines. A. Note typical dense lead line. **B.** Normal physiologic white line mimicking lead line.

5. Lyons JD, Filston HC. Lead intoxication from a pellet entrapped in the appendix of a child: treatment considerations. J Pediatr Surg 1994;29:1618–1620.

VITAMIN DEFICIENCIES AND EXCESSES

Excessive Vitamin Intake

Excessive vitamin intake is not a problem of the neonate, but as the infant grows older, excess intake of vitamins A and D can result in toxicity. With hypervitaminosis D, roentgenographic findings usually consist of increased density of the bones, very dense zones of provisional calcification, and calcification of structures such as the falx, kidneys, and various soft tissues. In some cases, excessive periosteal new bone deposition may be seen, but periosteal new bone deposition is more the hallmark of chronic vitamin A intoxication. Other manifestations of vitamin A intoxication include increased intracranial pressure and itchiness of the skin. These patients also develop yellow pigmentation and, sooner or later, bone pain. This pain largely is restricted to the extremities, and roentgenographically there is evidence of periosteal new bone deposition (Fig. 6.151A). In addition, we have seen one other patient with evidence of tendinitis (Fig. 6.151B). For some reason, the most commonly involved bones demonstrating periosteal new bone deposition are the tibiae, ulnae, and fourth and fifth metatarsals.

Bone scintigraphy also has been employed in the investigation of hypervitaminosis A and results in increased nuclear activity along the shafts of the involved bones (1, 2). This is not to suggest that such scanning be performed in every case, but in puzzling cases, it may be useful. In addition, some of these patients can develop metaphyseal growth disturbances, which lead to shortening of the extremities.

REFERENCES

1. James MB, Leonard JC, Fraser JJ Jr, et al. Hypervitaminosis A: a case report. Pediatrics 1982;69:112–115.
2. Miller JH, Hayon II. Bone scintigraphy in hypervitaminosis. AJR 1985;144:767–768.

Rickets (Vitamin D Deficiency)

Congenital rickets is uncommon but occurs if there is decreased vitamin D intake or synthesis in the mother. This

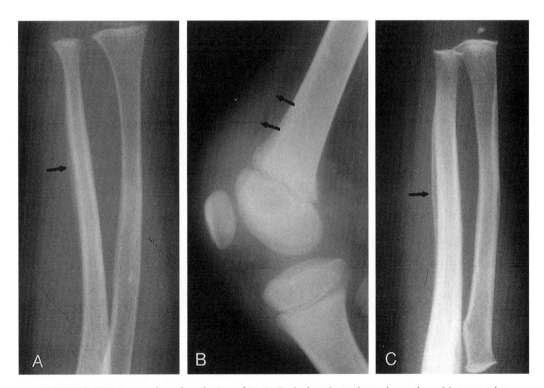

FIGURE 6.151. Hypervitaminosis A and D. A. Typical periosteal new bone deposition over the ulna (arrow) in hypervitaminosis A. **B.** Another patient with tendinitis manifest in thickening of the quadriceps tendon (arrows) secondary to vitamin A intoxication. Swelling extends down to the patella. **C.** Combined vitamin A and D intoxication. Note periosteal new bone deposition (arrow), and then note the prominent, albeit thin, white zones of provisional calcification in the ends of the long bones. The latter finding is the result of hypervitaminosis D.

latter situation is likely to occur in those ethnic groups where, because of certain cultural and clothing practices, exposure to sunlight during pregnancy is diminished. In the postnatal period, dietary deficiency rickets can occur as a result of inadequate vitamin D intake for many reasons (1). Usually, however, rickets does not develop for 3 months or so after birth because enough vitamin D is transferred from the mother to the infant to protect the infant from this condition. Rickets in low birth weight infants was discussed earlier, in Metabolic Bone Disease of the Premature.

The two most common forms of rickets to present in infants are those secondary to nutritional disturbances and so-called "vitamin D-dependent rickets." Familial hypophosphatemic rickets usually does not present in early infancy, and it is uncommon for patients with renal osteodystrophy to present under 6 months of age. Rickets secondary to proximal renal tubular acidosis, however, can present in the first 3–6 months of life. Rickets secondary to cystinosis and anticonvulsive drug therapy appears in older children.

The roentgenographic changes in rickets are well known (Fig. 6.152). In the active stage, coarse demineralization of the bones (osteomalacia), loss of cortical distinction, cupping, fraying and irregularity of the metaphyseal regions, loss of definition of the epiphyses, widening of the epiphyseal-metaphyseal junctions (physes), and, in severe cases, pathologic epiphyseal-metaphyseal fractures (Figs. 6.152D) occur. With healing, periosteal new bone is deposited around the diaphyses, cupping of the metaphyses becomes more clearly apparent, and the zones of provisional calcifi-

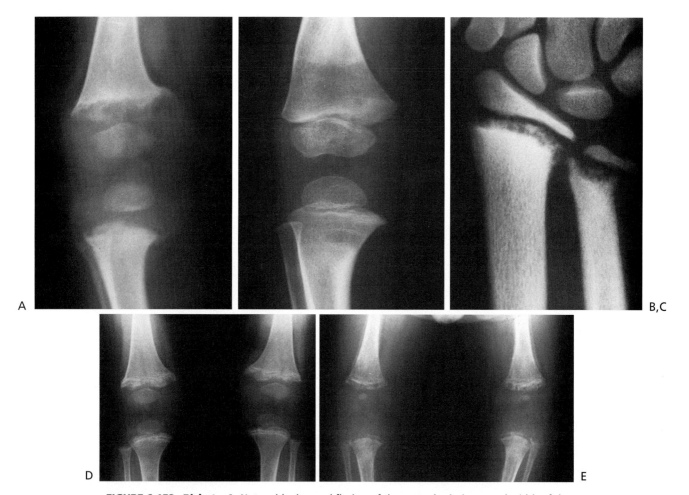

FIGURE 6.152. Rickets. A. Note widening and flaring of the metaphysis, increased width of the epiphyseal line, and absence of the zone of provisional calcification. **B.** Healing demonstrates a near-normal bone configuration. This patient had vitamin D-dependent rickets. **C. Fanconi's rickets.** Note irregularity and widening of the metaphysis. Irregular sclerosis is evidence of partial healing. The changes are not as pronounced as with nutritional and vitamin D-dependent rickets. **D. Renal osteodystrophy.** Note widening of the epiphyseal line and irregularity of the metaphysis. Also note that the epiphyses are indistinct. Coarse, fuzzy trabeculation is typical of osteomalacia. **E.** Brush border in healing rickets secondary to renal tubular acidosis.

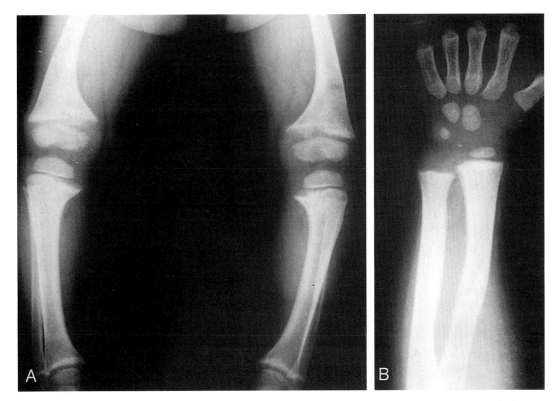

FIGURE 6.153. Hypophosphatemic vitamin D-resistant rickets, type A. A. Note typical bowing, near-normal mineralization of the bones, but pronounced widening of the epiphyseal plates medially at the knees. **B.** Wrist in the same patient shows virtually no abnormal changes. The ulna may be slightly broadened and cupped.

cation become more definite and white. With renal tubular acidosis, a peculiar brush border along the metaphysis can be seen in the healing phase (Fig. 6.152E).

Familial hypophosphatemic vitamin D-resistant rickets is caused by a tubular defect of the kidneys, not because of vitamin D deficiency. The condition is familial and has variable penetrance, and roentgenographically, classic findings consist of bowing of the legs, medial widening of the epiphyseal plates of the femur and to some extent the distal tibia, and a paucity of findings in the wrist (Fig. 6.153). A few of these patients may demonstrate more generalized epiphyseal-metaphyseal changes more typical of rickets and short, squat bones somewhat suggestive of the bones seen in the storage diseases (Fig. 6.154). These latter patients are less resistant to vitamin D and phosphorus therapy, even though their initial roentgenographic changes are more striking. For these reasons, we have designated this type of rickets as type B hypophosphatemic rickets and the other as type A (2).

The various types of rickets one can encounter can be classified on the basis of their roentgenographic appearance (2). The classification depends on the degree and type of metabolic change reflected in the bones and on the presence or absence of bowlegs or knock-knees. Bowing usually is seen in ambulatory patients; knock-knees are seen in

patients who are hypotonic, and hypotonia usually is part of the underlying disease process in patients with Fanconi's rickets, cystinosis, etc. Our proposed classification and categorization of the various types of rickets based on these parameters are presented in Fig. 6.155. The classification also includes renal osteodystrophy, in which the findings are those of rickets with superimposed secondary hyperparathyroidism. Indeed, the latter changes often predominate.

Finally, in terms of clinical presentation, some infants present with tetany or seizures (3, 4) secondary to marked hypocalcemia. Clinically, a neurologic disturbance often first is suspected. Hormonally mediated rachitic changes in the bones also can be seen with a variety of bony or other tumors (5–7). A relatively new form of rickets is that associated with ifosfamide therapy (8).

REFERENCES

1. Bhowmick SK, Johnson KR, Rettig KR. Rickets caused by vitamin D deficiency in breast-fed infants in the southern United States. Am J Dis Child 1991;145:127–130.
2. Swischuk LE, Hayden CK Jr. Rickets: a roentgenographic scheme for diagnosis. Pediatr Radiol 1979;8:203–208.
3. Jagdeo DG, Rambihar VS, Liu PC. Rickets presenting as seizures in the emergency department: medico-cultural implications. Pediatr Emerg Care 1998;14:215–216.

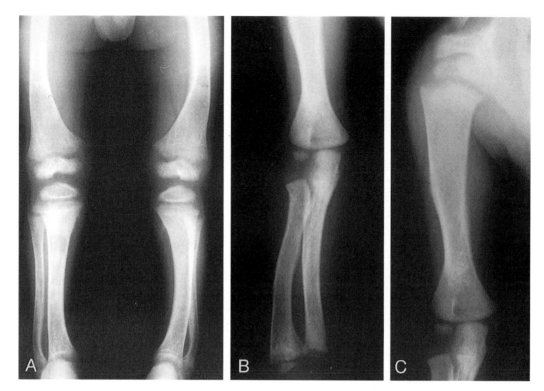

FIGURE 6.154. Hypophosphatemic vitamin D-resistant rickets, type B. A. Note broad-appearing bones, marked demineralization as a result of osteomalacia, and typical rachitic changes in all the metaphyseal regions. **B and C.** Upper extremity. Note similar findings but especially that the humerus is short and squat and somewhat similar to the humerus seen in the storage diseases.

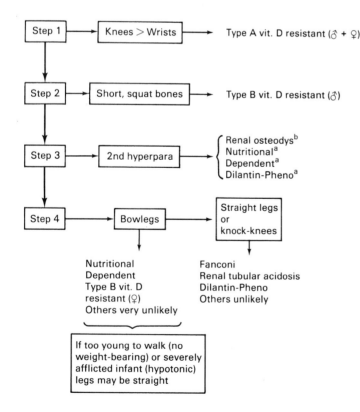

FIGURE 6.155. Rickets: roentgenographic classification. Step 1 identifies patients with type A hypophosphatemic vitamin D-resistant rickets. **Step 2** identifies type B hypophosphatemic vitamin D-resistant rickets in males. Females with this form of rickets are not identified in this step and with all other patients pass on to the next step. **Step 3** identifies patients with renal osteodystrophy and the occasional case of severe nutritional, dependent, or dilantin-phenobarbital rickets. **Step 4** deals with the remaining patients and allows one to offer a practical, short differential diagnosis in each instance. [a]A few severe cases only; [b]accounts for most cases.

4. Swischuk LE, Hayden CK Jr. Seizures and demineralization of the skull. A diagnostic presentation of rickets. Pediatr Radiol 1977; 6:65–67.

5. Amir G, Boneh A, Tochner Z, et al. Widespread hemangiomatosis of bone associated with rickets: recovery after irradiation. J Pediatr 1993;123:269–272.

6. Lee DY, Chooi IH, Lee CK, et al. Acquired vitamin D-resistant rickets caused by aggressive osteoblastoma in the pelvis: a case report with ten years' follow-up and review of the literature. J Pediatr Orthop 1994;14:793–798.

7. Nuovo MA, Dorfman HD, Sun C-CJ, et al. Tumor-induced osteomalacia and rickets. Am J Surg Pathol 1989;13:588–599.

8. Silberzweig JE, Haller JO, Miller S. Case report. Ifosfamide: a new cause of rickets. AJR 1992;158:823–824.

Scurvy

Scurvy is an uncommon condition in any age group, at least on this continent. It is caused by vitamin C deficiency. Roentgenographically, the bony changes are typical and consist of osteoporotic demineralization of the bones with preservation of the zones of provisional calcification, resulting in the so-called "white lines of Frankel." Beneath this

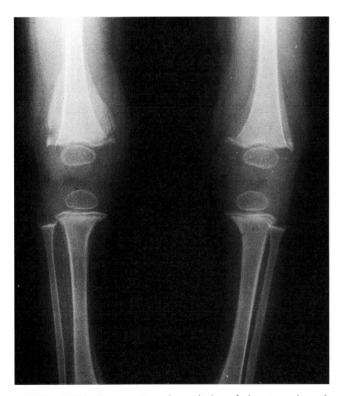

FIGURE 6.156. Scurvy. Note irregularity of the metaphyseal regions. The dense white lines are the lines of Frankel, the radiolucent zones beneath are the scurvy zones, and the beaks or fragments at the corner of the metaphyses, when healed, produce the Pelkan spurs. The changes in this patient represent those seen with partial healing; thus, there is evidence of periosteal new bone calcification around the diaphyses. The periosteal new bone is displaced far from the diaphyses because of extensive subperiosteal bleeding. Pathologic fractures have occurred through the scurvy zones.

white line is a radiolucent line, or the scurvy zone. Pathologic fractures occur through this area, and corner metaphyseal fractures are common. In their healing phase, these are termed "Pelkan spurs." The epiphyses are ringed by a fine white line, Wimberger's ring, and, all in all, the findings are typical (Fig. 6.156). Subperiosteal bleeding and bleeding elsewhere in the body are extensive, and when the subperiosteal bleeds heal, large cloaks of ballooned periosteal new bone form around the bones.

HEMATOLOGIC DISEASE

Anemias

Although congenital anemias such as congenital spherocytosis, Fanconi's anemia, sickle cell anemia, and thalassemia can manifest themselves at birth, it is uncommon for them to produce secondary skeletal changes at this early stage. In infancy, however, with sickle cell disease, the hand-foot syndrome is a common problem. This syndrome results from infarction of the various small bones of the hands and feet, and osteolysis along with periosteal new bone deposition usually is pronounced (Fig. 6.157). When multiple bones are involved, the diagnosis is relatively easy, but if only one bone is involved, the differential diagnosis includes osteomyelitis, tuberculous dactylitis, and metastatic disease from neuroblastoma. Later, as the child grows older, sickle cell disease leads to numerous skeletal infarcts and, in some cases, aseptic necrosis of the femoral or humeral heads. Other epiphyses may undergo necrosis, but the most common are the femoral heads (Fig. 6.158A). In the long bones, infarction may occasionally be massive but more often is focal. In the acute stages, the findings mimic those of osteomyelitis (Fig. 6.158B), and with healing, patchy medullary sclerosis results (Fig. 6.158C). In addition to these findings, biconcave deformities of the vertebral bodies, caused by endplate infarction, are characteristic (Fig. 6.159A). In the long bones, differentiation from osteomyelitis often is difficult, no matter which imaging modality one uses.

In the skull, changes associated with any of the anemias, including sickle cell anemia, consist of thickening of the diploë with vertical striations (Fig. 6.159B). In sickle cell disease and iron deficiency anemia, the thickenings tend to be somewhat focal, while with Cooley's thalassemia, widespread thickening of the calvarium and facial bones is more likely to occur. Indeed, the calvarial and bony findings are startling, with massive thickening and spiculation of the calvarium and ballooning of the long bones with very coarse trabeculations (Fig. 6.160). All these findings result from massive proliferation of hemopoietic tissue in the bone marrow.

Sludging of blood in sickle cell disease leads to thrombosis and variable end-organ insult, namely acute chest syndrome, infarcts of the spleen, cerebrovascular accidents, bone

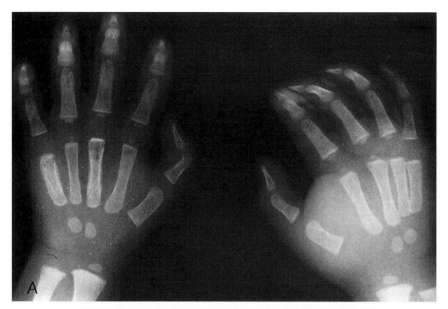

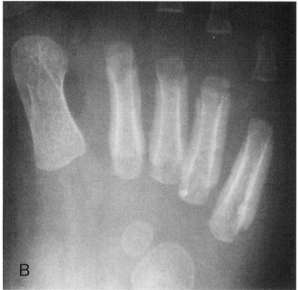

FIGURE 6.157. Hand-foot syndrome. A. Note extensive swelling of the soft tissues around the thumb and metacarpals of the left hand. On the right, note destructive changes in the third and fifth metatarsals. Also note periosteal new bone deposition. The changes on the right are older than those on the left. **B.** Another infant with extensive periosteal new bone deposition on four of the metatarsals.

infarcts, orbital infarcts (1), and mesenteric vessel involvement leading to acute abdominal problems. In addition, microthrombi also lead to eventual renal involvement. As a result, it is not uncommon to encounter hyperechoic kidneys in sickle cell disease. With cerebrovascular accidents, although transcranial Doppler has been utilized to evaluate the vessels, it is probably best to evaluate these vessels with MR angiography (2–4).

Patients with sickle cell disease frequently present with symptoms of an acute abdomen (sickle crisis), and almost invariably the plain films and other studies are normal. These patients also are prone to gallstone formation and cholecystitis; although in sickle cell disease, the spleen becomes infarcted and small, in sickle cell SC disease, the spleen tends to remain normal. Overall, symptoms are less pronounced in sickle SC disease. The so-called **acute chest syndrome** also is a common feature of sickle cell disease.

Many times, it is difficult to determine whether the problem is pneumonia or infarction, but there is growing evidence that the problem is more the result of infarction from microthrombi (5–7) and that pneumonia may be a secondary phenomenon. Nonetheless, the pulmonary findings are about the same because these patients present with what appear to be consolidations.

Osteomyelitis is a significant problem in sickle cell disease because the chronic hypoxia of sickle cell disease predisposes to infection by less-than-common organisms. In this regard, salmonella osteomyelitis is common, but the imaging findings generally are not different from those of osteomyelitis due to other organisms and seen in other children. Finally, because of repeated transfusions, iron deposition in the liver and other organs occurs (8, 9). On CT, the involved organs show increased density; on MRI, there is decreased signal (i.e., black liver) on T1-weighted images.

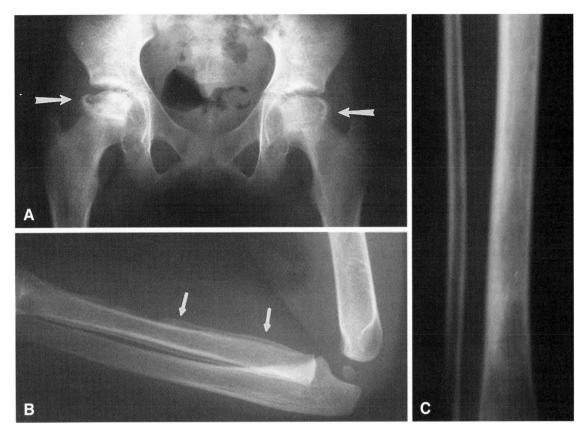

FIGURE 6.158. Bone infarcts. A. Note bilateral aseptic necrosis of the femoral heads (arrows), worse on the right. **B.** Healing total infarction of the radius. Note periosteal new bone (arrows) and lytic lesions in the distal radius. **C.** Another patient demonstrating patchy sclerotic areas throughout both tibiae, indicating the presence of old healed infarcts.

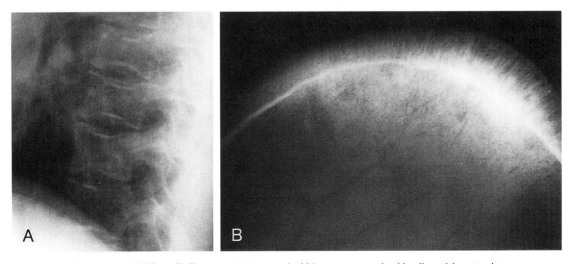

FIGURE 6.159. Sickle cell disease. A. Note typical biconcave vertebral bodies with central step-off. **B.** Typical localized thickening of the calvarium with vertical striations.

With iron deficiency anemia, about the only bony change seen with any consistency is focal thickening of the calvarium, while hypoplasia or absence of the radius and thumb often occurs in Fanconi's anemia (Fig. 161A) and in the related condition thrombocytopenia with absent radius (TAR syndrome). The thumb, however, usually is present in these latter patients (Fig. 6.161B). There are no specifically abnormal findings with congenital spherocytosis, but mild changes secondary to hemopoietic hypertrophy in the bone marrow, similar to those of Cooley's anemia, can be encountered.

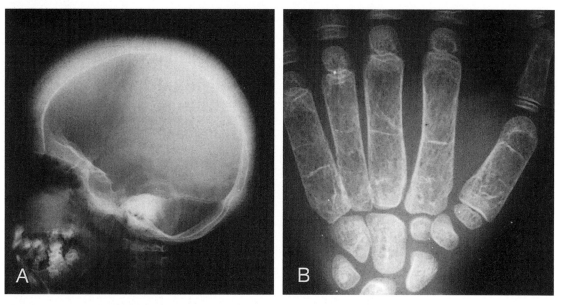

FIGURE 6.160. Cooley's anemia. A. Note the markedly thickened calvarium and facial bones. **B.** Hand demonstrating coarse trabecular pattern and somewhat ballooned bones.

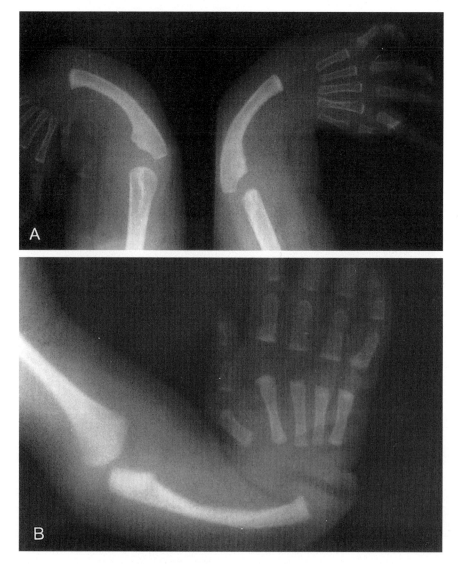

FIGURE 6.161. A. Fanconi's anemia. Severe case showing bilateral absent radii and hypoplastic thumbs. **B. Thrombocytopenia absent radius syndrome.** Note absence of the radius but presence of the thumb.

Finally, extramedullary hematopoiesis can be a complication of any chronic anemia. These sites of extramedullary hematopoiesis can be located anywhere in the body, and if they are located next to a critical organ or structure, symptoms related to that organ or structure may be the presenting problem (10). In addition to these considerations, a bony dysplasia has been documented with deferoxamine treatment for thalassemia major (11, 12). Although the precise etiology is not known, the problem probably lies in hypertransfusion and celation, in which the end result is flattening of the vertebra into an irregular vertebra plana configuration along with metaphyseal changes suggesting metaphyseal dysostosis.

REFERENCES

1. Naran AD, Fontana L. Sickle cell disease with orbital infarction and epidural hematoma. Pediatr Radiol 2001;31:257–259.
2. Verlhac S, Bernaudin F, Tortrat D, et al. Detection of cerebrovascular disease in patients with sickle cell disease using transcranial Doppler sonography: correlation with MRI, MRA and conventional angiography. Pediatr Radiol 1995;25:S14–S19.
3. Kogutt MS, Goldwag SS, Gupta KL, et al. Correlation of transcranial Doppler ultrasonography with MRI and MRA in the evaluation of sickle cell disease patients with prior stroke. Pediatr Radiol 1994;24:204–206.
4. Seibert JJ, Miller SF, Kirby RS, et al. Cerebrovascular disease in symptomatic and asymptomatic patients with sickle cell anemia: screening with duplex transcranial Doppler US—correlation with MR imaging and MR angiography. Radiology 1993;189:447–466.
5. Aquino SL, Gamsu G, Fahy JV, et al. Chronic pulmonary disorders in sickle cell disease: findings at thin-section CT. Radiology 1994;193:807–811.
6. Bhalla M, Abboud MR, McLoud TC, et al. Acute chest syndrome in sickle cell disease: CT evidence of microvascular occlusion. Radiology 1993;187:45–49.
7. Castro O, Brambilla DJ, Thorington B, et al. The acute chest syndrome in sickle cell disease: incidence and risk factors. Blood 1994;84:643–649.
8. Flyer MA, Haller JO, Sundaram R. Transfusional hemosiderosis in sickle cell anemia: another cause of an echogenic pancreas. Pediatr Radiol 1993;23:140–142.
9. Levin TL, Sheth SS, Hurlet A, et al. MR marrow signs of iron overload in transfusion-dependent patients with sickle cell disease. Pediatr Radiol 1995;25:614–619.
10. Khandelwal N, Malik N, Khosla VK, et al. Spinal cord compression due to epidural extramedullary hematopoiesis in thalassemia. Pediatr Radiol 1992;22:70–71.
11. Brill PW, Winchester P, Giardina PJ, et al. Deferoxamine-induced bone dysplasia in patients with thalassemia major. AJR 1991;156:561–565.
12. Miller TT, Caldwell G, Kaye JJ, et al. MR imaging of deferoxamine-induced bone dysplasia in an 8-year-old female with thalassemia major. Pediatr Radiol 1993;23:523–524.

Myelofibrosis and Congenital Neutropenia

Myelofibrosis can be primary or secondary, and profound anemia and decreased production of other elements of the blood are common. About the only radiographic finding that can be encountered is increased sclerosis of the bones. In addition, as with any chronic anemia, extramedullary hematopoiesis can produce masses anywhere in the body (1).

REFERENCE

1. Fernbach SK, Feinstein KA. Extramedullary hematopoiesis in the kidneys in infant siblings with myelofibrosis. Pediatr Radiol 1992;22:211–212.

Erythroblastosis Fetalis

Erythroblastosis fetalis results when an Rh-negative mother becomes sensitized to Rh-positive blood (from previous pregnancies or transfusions). Other blood type incompatibilities can also occur, but in any case, the problem is circulating antibodies crossing the placenta and entering the fetal circulation. They subsequently act on the fetal red blood cells, causing hemolysis and anemia. In mild cases, few or no roentgenographic changes are noted, but in the more severe cases (hydrops fetalis), changes that may be seen include generalized edema of the soft tissues, ascites, hydrothorax, pericardial effusion, and cardiomegaly (Fig. 6.162). Pulmonary vascular congestion is common in

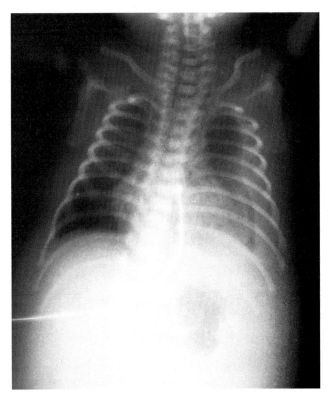

FIGURE 6.162. Erythroblastosis fetalis. Extremely edematous infant (note thickness of soft tissues) who also shows a good deal of peritoneal fluid and a large pleural effusion on the left.

patients with profound anemia and high output failure. In addition to hydrops fetalis developing in patients with erythroblastosis fetalis, many nonimmune cases also occur. These include twin or twin transfusion, fetomaternal transfusion, severe fetal cardiac failure, large arteriovenous malformations, and cardiac or pericardial tumors.

Leukemia

In the neonate, leukemia is relatively uncommon and is most apt to present with cutaneous infiltrates (leukemia cutis), pallor, fever, jaundice, hepatosplenomegaly, and hemorrhagic manifestations. The disease also is more common in infants with trisomy 21 and other chromosomal abnormalities. Bony changes in the neonatal period are uncommon; when they do occur, they consist of bony demineralization and transverse radiolucent lines through the metaphyses (Fig. 6.163A).

Later in childhood, destructive changes primarily in the metaphyses may develop (Fig. 6.163B), and these can be accompanied by periosteal new bone deposition, spiculated periosteal new bone, and pathologic fractures. Destructive

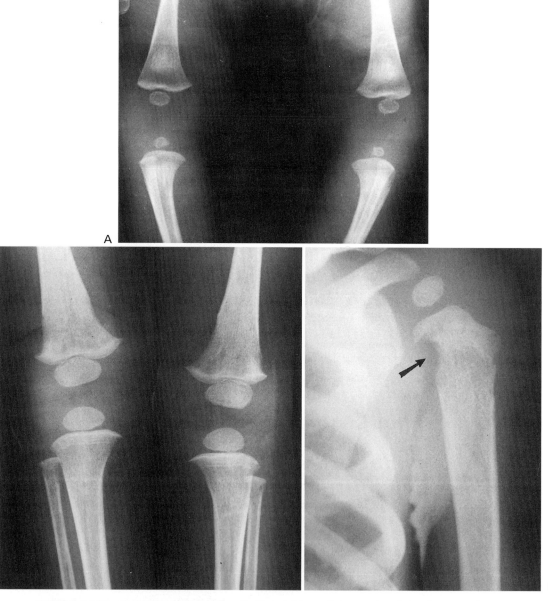

FIGURE 6.163. Congenital leukemia. A. Note wide radiolucent bands in the metaphyses (arrows) in this infant with Down's syndrome. **B** and **C.** Older infant. Notice destructive changes in the various metaphyses and notching of the proximal humerus (arrow).

lesions also can occur in the skull and spine, and overall, the changes are not unlike those seen with metastatic neuroblastoma. In some cases, destruction in the metaphysis produces notching of long bones such as the tibia, femur, and humerus (1) (Fig. 6.163C). Transverse radiolucent bands in the metaphyses of the long bones are a common early finding in acute leukemia. In the early stages, these lines are nonspecific and probably trophic in nature. In more advanced cases, however, pressure erosion of the bony trabeculae also probably occurs as the bone marrow becomes packed with leukemic cells. This probably further weakens the bone, and pathologic fractures are common. These lines can be seen in any of the long bones but are especially well visualized in the distal femur, proximal tibia, proximal femur, and proximal humerus (Fig. 6.164). These lines are of more than passing interest because they may be the first clue to the presence of leukemia in patients with nonspecific bone pain, limps, etc. This is important because bone pain may be the first presenting problem in these patients.

Another finding not uncommonly seen with leukemia, and even as the initial roentgenographic manifestation, is reactive periosteal new bone deposition along the clavicles and ribs. In addition, elevation of the pleura by tumor extending beyond the cortex of the ribs also can occur. Acute lymphocytic leukemia in infants may present with massive thymic enlargement because the thymus gland itself can become completely infiltrated by leukemic cells. Finally, a tumor of the periorbital region, known as a chloroma (2), can be encountered, but chloromas can arise at other sites.

REFERENCES

1. Melhem RE, Saber TJ. Erosion of the medial cortex of the proximal humerus. A sign of leukemia on the chest radiograph. Radiology 1980;137:77–79.
2. Bulas RB, Laine FJ, das Narla L. Bilateral orbital granulocytic sarcoma (chloroma) preceding the blast phase of acute myelogenous leukemia: CT findings. Pediatr Radiol 1995;25:488–489.

Hemophilia

In young infants, the findings associated with hemophilia deal primarily with acute bleeding at various sites. If such bleeding occurs next to a vital structure such as the spinal cord (1), symptoms related to compression rather than to

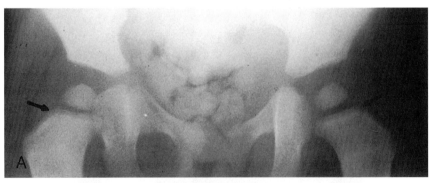

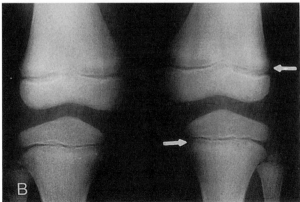

FIGURE 6.164. Leukemia lines. A. Note typical radiolucent lines in the upper femurs of this infant (arrow). **B.** Older patient with radiolucent lines in the distal femur and proximal tibia (arrows).

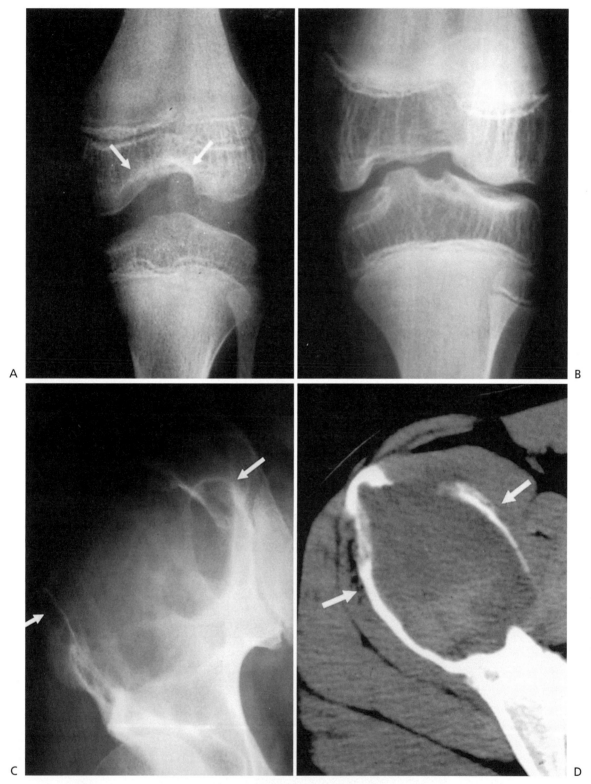

FIGURE 6.165. Hemophilic arthritis and other bony changes. A. The bones are demineralized, and the intracondylar notch (arrows) is large and smooth. **B.** In this patient, the epiphyses of the distal femur and proximal tibia have overgrown, are irregular, and demonstrate a "glassy" appearance. **C.** Bone cyst (hemorrhagic) in the iliac bone (arrows). **D.** Computed tomography study demonstrates the same bone cyst (arrows).

the bleed itself can be the presenting problem. Bony changes such as hemophiliac pseudotumor (bleeding into the bone) and arthritic changes usually do not develop until later childhood. In such cases, the epiphyses become overgrown, demineralized, and even scalloped (Fig. 6.165, A and B). Hyperemia leads to overgrowth and synovial hypertrophy to scalloping. In the knee, a deep intercondylar notch caused by such erosion is characteristic but not pathognomonic. The finding can be seen with other chronic arthritides. When bleeding occurs into a bone, a pseudotumor or cyst-like lesion eventually develops (Fig 6.165, C and D).

REFERENCE

1. Irwin SL, Attia MW. A traumatic spinal epidural hematoma in an infant with hemophilia A. Pediatr Emerg Cardiol 2001;17:40–41.

THE RETICULOENDOTHELIOSES (HISTIOCYTOSIS X-LANGERHANS' CELL HISTIOCYTOSIS)

The diseases in this group include Hand-Schüller-Christian disease, eosinophilic granuloma, and Letterer-Siwe disease. All have similar roentgenographic abnormalities, but none are a particular problem in the neonate. In those rare cases with neonatal presentation, one almost exclusively is dealing with acute disseminated Letterer-Siwe disease. The diagnosis usually is suspected on the basis of skin lesions, anemia, lymphadenopathy, and hepatosplenomegaly. Bone changes are not a usual feature in the neonate, but pulmonary cystic lesions can be seen (1). Familial hemophagocytic or erythrophagocytic reticulosis (2) is a peculiar form of reticulosis that also has clinical features similar to those of the more acute forms of histiocytosis X or Langerhans' cell histiocytosis.

Roentgenographically, the bony changes in the reticuloendothelioses are well known and consist of discrete, punched-out destructive lesions scattered throughout the skeleton. The edges of the lesions usually show little sclerosis in the initial stages, but as healing occurs, peripheral sclerosis can develop. Any bone can be involved, and new lesions may appear after old lesions regress. Vertebral body collapse is common, and the classic vertebral plana should be considered the result of histiocytosis X until proven otherwise (Fig. 6.166A). More rarely, destruction of the posterior elements can occur (3).

Not all patients demonstrate classic bone changes, and overall, a variety of presentations are common. In this regard, one should be aware of the patient presenting with proptosis secondary to orbital disease, diabetes insipidus secondary to pituitary gland involvement, pseudoparesis as a result of involvement of the scapula, and middle ear disease as a result of destruction of the petrous bone. In addition, the so-called **floating teeth sign,** secondary to massive destruction of the mandible, should be recalled. Finally, pulmonary infiltrates, cystic changes, and nonspecific reticulonodular pulmonary infiltrates and hilar adenopathy can be seen in some patients (Fig. 6.166B). All of these changes now are vividly demonstrable with high-resolution CT.

Hepatic, splenic, and pancreatic lesions also can be documented with ultrasound and CT. With ultrasound, the

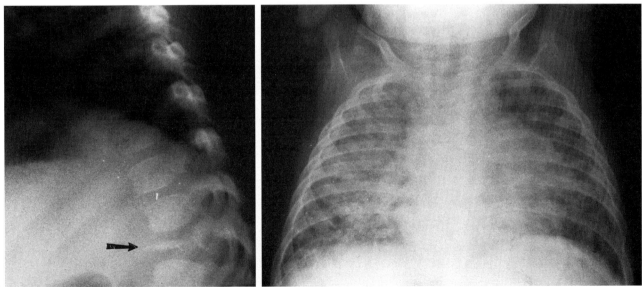

A   B

FIGURE 6.166. Histiocytosis X: vertebral plana. A. Note typical collapse of the vertebra (arrow). The disc spaces above and below are preserved. **B.** Same patient with diffuse reticulonodular infiltrates in the chest.

lesions appear somewhat hypoechoic (4), while on CT, they present with low attenuation. In addition, primary meningeal and brain involvement can occur and is best demonstrated with MRI where the lesions show decreased signal on both T1- and T2-weighted images (5). However, MR findings generally are variable (Fig. 6.167), and the study is not necessary in most cases of Langerhans' cell histiocytosis.

A variety of radiographically demonstrable lesions can be encountered in histiocytosis X or Langerhans' cell histiocytosis, and both solitary and multiple bone involvement occurs. The flat bones are as susceptible as the long bones, and overall a variety of lesions can be encountered (Fig. 6.168). Also note that periosteal new bone is not uncommon and is especially likely with lesions in the femur and humerus (Fig. 6.168F). In such cases, it is most important not to misinterpret the lesion for a malignant bone tumor. In this regard, even though CT and MRI (6) may be helpful, it is the plain films that steer one in the proper direction from the beginning (5). Nonetheless, CT is of considerable value when petrous bone involvement is being evaluated (Fig. 6.169), and MRI is of value in demonstrating infiltrative involvement of the hypothalamus and pituitary stock (7).

In terms of imaging of the bony lesions of histiocytosis X, there has been considerable debate as to whether the total body bone scintigram or radiographic bone survey is more worthwhile. In this regard, it is well known that lesions visible on plain radiographs may not be positive on regular bone scintigraphy. The reason for this is that there is low bony reactive activity with most of these lesions, and therefore, they do not manifest their presence on the nuclear scintigram. For this reason, it has been suggested that both first and follow-up examinations be performed with regular radiography but that bone scintigraphy should be included with the first examination (8).

Finally, one might note a few other peculiarities about histiocytosis X. First, the disease can involve the epiphyses of bones (9), and second, it has been demonstrated that the rate of resolution of the bony lesions depends little on the form of therapy or whether therapy is administered (10). In this regard, it has been demonstrated that if the lesions are confined to the bones and no organ dysfunction exists, the prognosis is relatively good (11). Last, thymic involvement can occur in the form of cystic transformation and tissue calcification (12–15). In addition, the disease process can manifest in unusual places such as the nose (16). This underscores the fact that in the pediatric age group, **the diagnosis of histiocytosis X (Langerhans' cell histiocytosis) should always be considered, even if the possibility of its existence seems remote.**

REFERENCES

1. Vade A, Hayani A, Pierce KL. Congenital histiocytosis X. Pediatr Radiol 1993;23:181–182.
2. Imashuku S, Hibi S, Todo S. Hemophagocytic lymphohistiocytosis in infancy and childhood. J Pediatr 1997;130:352–357.
3. Damry N, Hottat N, Azzi N, et al. Unusual findings in two cases of Langerhans' cell histiocytosis. Pediatr Radiol 2000;30: 196–199.
4. Muwakkit S, Gharagozloo A, Souid AK, et al. The sonographic appearance of lesions of the spleen and pancreas in an infant with Langerhans' cell histiocytosis. Pediatr Radiol 1994;14:222–223.
5. Poe LB, Dubowy RL, Hochhauser L, et al. Demyelinating and

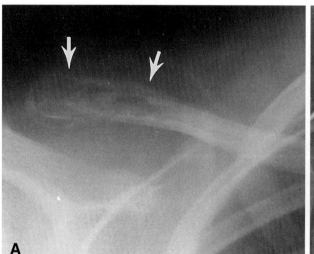
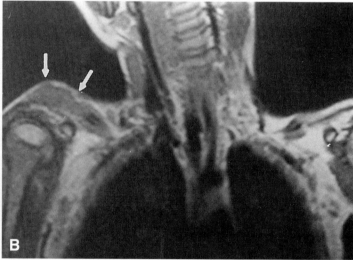

FIGURE 6.167. Histiocytosis X: magnetic resonance findings. A. Note the destructive expanding lesion of the distal clavicle (arrows). **B.** T1-weighted magnetic resonance study demonstrates a nonspecific mass (arrows) around the clavicle.

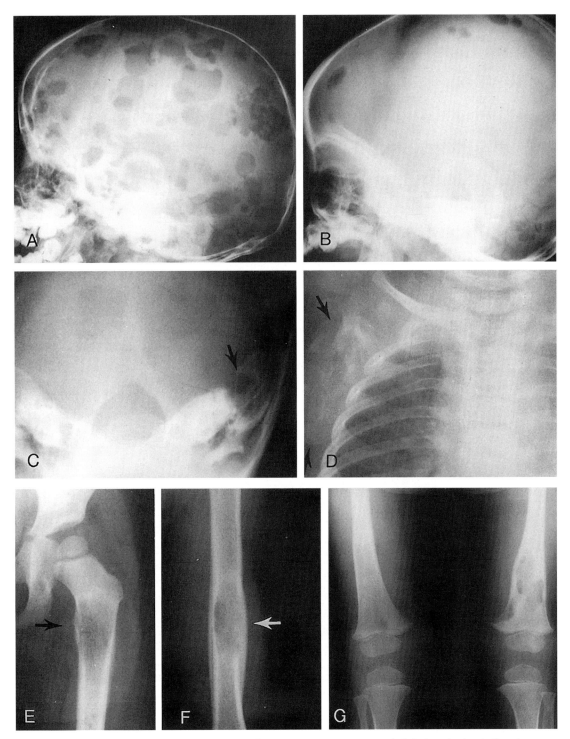

FIGURE 6.168. Histiocytosis X: various lesions. A. Note numerous lytic lesions in the skull and the absence of peripheral sclerosis. In some cases, however, some sclerosis may occur, especially with eosinophilic granuloma. **B.** Another patient with fewer lesions. **C.** Destructive lesion of the left petrous bone (arrow). **D.** Solitary expanding lesion of the right scapula (arrow). **E.** Destructive lesion of the upper right femur (arrow). Note that the edges of the lesion are not as discrete as are those of lesions in the skull. **F.** Another infant with a destructive lesion in the humerus. Note associated periosteal new bone deposition (arrow). This can occur with histiocytosis X, especially in the humerus and femur. **G.** Older patient with typical scalloped-out lesions in both distal femurs and proximal left tibia.

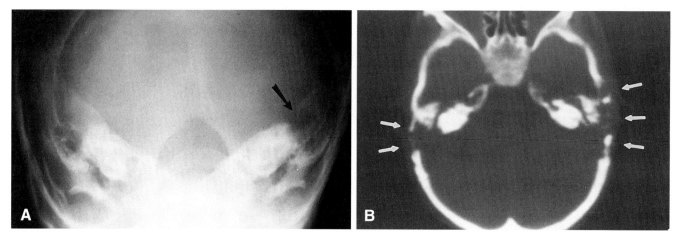

FIGURE 6.169. Histiocytosis X: petrous bone involvement. A. In this patient, note destruction of the left petrous bone (arrows). **B.** Another patient showing extensive bilateral petrous and temporal bone destruction (arrows).

gliotic cerebellar lesions in Langerhans' cell histiocytosis. AJNR 1994;15:1921–1928.

6. George JC, Buckwalter KA, Cohen MD, et al. Langerhans' cell histiocytosis of bone: MR imaging. Pediatr Radiol 1994;24: 29–32.

7. Maghnie M, Arico M, Villa A, et al. MR of the hypothalamic-pituitary axis in Langerhans' cell histiocytosis. AJNR 1992;13: 1365–1371.

8. Van Nieuwenhuyse J-P, Clapuyt P, Malghem J, et al. Radiographic skeletal survey and radionuclide bone scan in Langerhans' cell histiocytosis of bone. Pediatr Radiol 1996;26:734–738.

9. Leeson MC, Smith A, Carter JR, et al. Eosinophilic granuloma of bone in the growing epiphysis. J Pediatr Orthop 1985;5: 147–150.

10. Sartoris DJ, Parker BR. Histiocytosis X: rate and pattern of resolution of osseous lesions. Radiology 1984;152:679–684.

11. Meyer JS, Harty MP, Mahboubi S, et al. Langerhans' cell histiocytosis: presentation and evolution of radiologic findings with clinical correlation. Radiographics 1995;15:1135–1146.

12. Heller GD, Haller JO, Berdon WE, et al. Punctate thymic calcification in infants with untreated Langerhans' cell histiocytosis: report of four new cases. Pediatr Radiol 1999;29:813–815.

13. Odagiri K, Hishihira K, Hatekeyama S, et al. Anterior mediastinal masses with calcifications on CT in children with histiocytosis X (Langerhans' cell histiocytosis). Pediatr Radiol 1991;21: 550–551.

14. Junewick JJ, Fitzgerald NE. The thymus in Langerhans' cell histiocytosis. Pediatr Radiol 1999;29:904–907.

15. Sumner TE, Auringer ST, Preston AA. Thymic calcifications in histiocytosis X. Pediatr Radiol 1993;23:204–205.

16. Kulkarni A, Lakheeram D, Haller JO, et al. Histiocytosis presenting as a nasal mass. Pediatr Radiol 2000;30:87–89.

Juvenile Xanthogranuloma

Juvenile xanthogranuloma is a nonhistiocytic X granulomatous condition that presents with clinical and imaging findings similar to those of histiocytosis X or Langerhans' histiocytosis (1, 2). Both systemic and bony involvement occur.

REFERENCES

1. Eggli KD, Caro P, Quioque T, et al. Juvenile xanthogranuloma: non-X histiocytosis with systemic involvement. Pediatr Radiol 1992;22:374–376.

2. Garcia-Pena P, Mariscal A, Abellan C, et al. Juvenile xanthogranuloma with extracutaneous lesions. Pediatr Radiol 1992;22: 377–378.

CHROMOSOMAL ABNORMALITIES

Down's Syndrome (Trisomy 21)

In Down's syndrome, formerly known as mongolism and now referred to as trisomy 21, there is an extra chromosome at the 21 location. Initial diagnosis in the newborn is primarily clinical, as these infants show hypotonia, hyperextensibility of the joints, a simian crease, and a typical facial appearance with slanted palpebral fissures. The fifth finger may also be in-curved. Definitive diagnosis, however, is now usually made with a study of the chromosomes. Although in the past, much emphasis was placed on skeletal changes, these have now become of lesser importance. Nonetheless, it is of some value to be familiar with a few of them.

Pelvic changes consist of flattening of the acetabular angles, outward flaring of the iliac wings, and hypoplasia of the ischial rami (Fig. 6.170A). Normal acetabular angles in the neonate average approximately 20–30°, whereas those in trisomy 21 are substantially less, averaging somewhere between 10 and 15°. Other skeletal changes include an increase in the number of ossification centers in the sternum (1) (Fig. 6.170B), the presence of only 11 ribs in approximately one-quarter of cases (1), and, as previously mentioned, a short in-curved fifth finger with a hypoplastic middle phalanx.

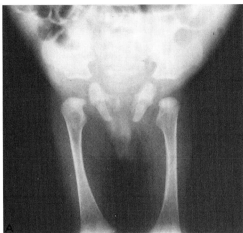

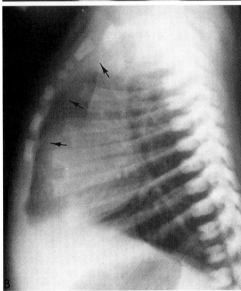

FIGURE 6.170. Trisomy 21. A. Note that the iliac wings are flared outwardly and that the acetabular roofs are horizontal, resulting in an acetabular angle near 0°. **B.** Sternum. Note hypersegmentation of sternum. At least six, and possibly seven, ossification centers are seen (arrows). This patient also had only 11 ribs and congenital heart disease (atrioventricular communis).

Calvarial changes are less specific than once believed, and the skull, although usually small and round, can be of variable shape. However, an increase of the basal angle beyond 140° in a calvarium that also is small and round should be looked on as highly suspicious for Down's syndrome. In the spine, hypotonia often leads to exaggerated kyphosis of the dorsolumbar region and development of hooking or notching of the vertebra. In addition, and probably more commonly, hypotonia leads to lessened vertical axial stresses on the vertebra and tall vertebra.

Atlantoaxial and atlantooccipital instability also are a problem in patients with trisomy 21 (2–7). In this regard, it has been known for some time that these patients are subject to hypoplasia of the dens and C1 and, in some cases, increased mobility of the upper cervical spine. In those cases

where C1 is hypoplastic (8), the findings are profound and symptoms are present early in infancy (Fig. 6.171). In other patients (the majority), the findings are not associated with symptoms and are a problem only when contact sports are being considered. In these patients, the imaging workup consists of obtaining plain films with flexion and extension (Fig. 6.172) and then MRI as required (7). **However, all of this is not a great clinical problem in my experience. The only time I have seen serious problems arise is when the posterior arch of C1 is hypoplastic or absent.**

Numerous other abnormalities involving many systems also occur in Down's syndrome. Some of the more serious ones include cardiac anomalies such as atrioventricular canal, ventricular septal defect, patent ductus arteriosus (9), and gastrointestinal abnormalities such as duodenal atresia, duodenal bands, malrotation of the small bowel, esophageal atresia, tracheoesophageal fistula, and anorectal anomalies (10). There also is a higher than usual incidence of leukemia in infants with Down's syndrome. Usually, it is lymphoblastic leukemia and may be related to a thymic cell abnormality that may be the cause of immune deficiency in some of these patients.

Other findings seen in trisomy 21 include a prominent coronoid process of the clavicle (11) (Fig. 6.173), a rheumatoid-like arthropathy (12), and an increased incidence of celiac disease (13, 14).

REFERENCES

1. Edwards DK III, Berry CC, Hilton SvW. Trisomy 21 in newborn infants: chest radiographic diagnosis. Radiology 1988;167: 317–318.
2. Davidson RG. Atlantoaxial instability in individuals with Down syndrome: a fresh look at the evidence. Pediatrics 1988;81: 857–865.
3. El-Khoury CY, Clark CR, Dietz FR, et al. Posterior atlanto-occipital subluxation in Down syndrome. Radiology 1986;159: 507–509.
4. Parfenchuck TA, Bertrans SL, Powers MJ, et al. Posterior occipitoatlantal hypermobility in Down syndrome: an analysis of 199 patients. J Pediatr Orthop 1994;14:304–308.
5. Peuschel SM, Scola FH. Atlantoaxial instability in individuals with Down syndrome. Epidemiologic, radiographic, and clinical studies. Pediatrics 1987;80:555–560.
6. Stein SM, Kirchner SG, Horey G, et al. Atlanto-occipital subluxation in Down syndrome. Pediatr Radiol 1991;21:121–124.
7. White KS, Ball WS, Prenger EC, et al. Evaluation of the craniocervical junction in Down syndrome: correlation of measurements obtained with radiography and MR imaging. Radiology 1993;186:377–382.
8. Martich V, Ben-ami T, Yousefzadeh DK, et al. Hypoplastic posterior arch of C-1 in children with Down syndrome: a double jeopardy. Radiology 1992;183:125–128.
9. Wells GL, Barker SE, Finley SC, et al. Congenital heart disease in infants with Down's syndrome. South Med J 1994;87: 724–727.
10. Torres R, Levitt MA, Tovilla JM, et al. Anorectal malformations and Down's syndrome. J Pediatr Surg 1998;33:194–197.
11. Weinberg B, Maldjian C, Kass EG, et al. Case report. The promi-

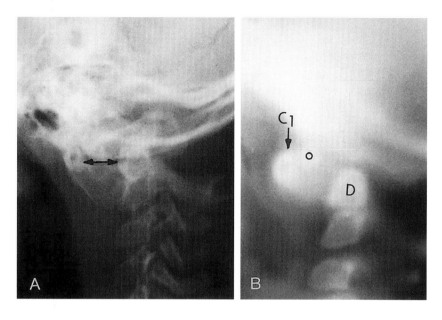

FIGURE 6.171. Trisomy 21: C1-2 dislocation. A. Note anterior dislocation of C1 on C2. This causes the C1-dens distance to be increased (arrow). **B.** Tomogram demonstrating the marked degree of anterior displacement of the anterior arch of C1 (arrow). The dens (D) is hypoplastic. A displaced os terminale (o) also is present.

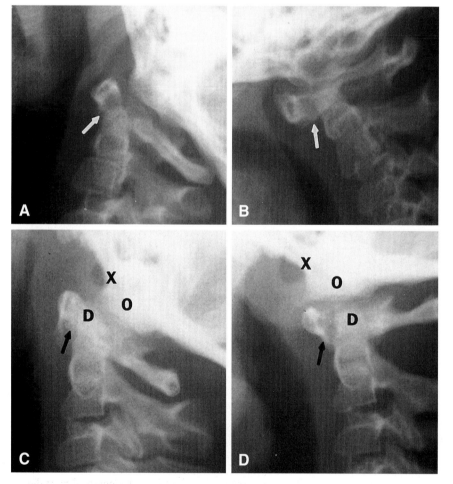

FIGURE 6.172. Trisomy 21: upper cervical spine instability. A. Atlantoaxial instability. In extension, the C1-dens distance (arrow) is normal. **B.** With flexion, the C1-dens distance widens (arrow), consistent with mild atlantoaxial instability. **C. Atlantooccipital instability.** On extension, note the position of the dens (D), anterior rim of the foramen magnum (X), and the occipital condyles (O). Also note the C1-dens distance (arrow). **D.** With flexion, note how movement has occurred between the dens (D), anterior margin of the foramen magnum (X), and the occipital condyles (O). In addition, the C1-dens distance has increased (arrow), suggesting mild associated atlantoaxial instability.

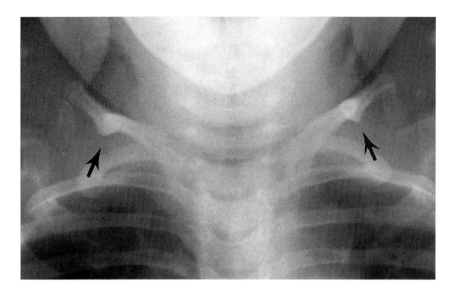

FIGURE 6.173. Trisomy 21: prominent coronoid process of the clavicle. Note bilateral prominent coronoid processes (arrows) of the clavicles in this patient with trisomy 21.

nent coronoid process of the clavicle: a new radiographic sign in Down's syndrome. AJR 1993;160:591–592.

12. Olson JC, Bender JC, Levinson JE, et al. Arthropathy of Down syndrome. Pediatrics 1990;86:931–936.
13. Cizmadia CG, Mearin ML, Oren A, et al. Accuracy and cost-effectiveness of a new strategy to screen for celiac disease in children with Down syndrome. J Pediatr 2000;137:756–761.
14. Walker-Smith JA. Celiac disease and Down syndrome. J Pediatr 2000;137:743–744.

Trisomy 18 Syndrome

Trisomy 18 syndrome is associated with an extra chromosome in the 16—18 group (Group E), and many of these infants die in the neonatal period. Clinical features consist of low birth weight, growth and mental retardation, muscular hypotonicity, characteristic facial appearance (micrognathia, a small mouth, and a high palate), and a typical grasp of the hand consisting of flexion of all the digits, hypoplasia of the first digit, and overlapping of the third digit by the second (Fig. 6.174A).

Other typical roentgenographic findings consist of thin ribs (often only 11 ribs are present), thin clavicles (especially laterally), a short, undersegmented sternum, and an increase in the anteroposterior diameter of the chest (Fig. 6.175). A rocker-bottom (pes calcaneovalgus) deformity is characteristic of the feet (Fig. 6.174B), while the pelvis usually shows an increase in the acetabular angles and an in-turning of the iliac wings (see Fig. 6.175C). Dislocated hips are common, and the entire pelvic configuration is opposite that of mongolism: the so-called "antimongoloid pelvis." The skull is often reported as being dolichocephalic, but this is not a consistent finding. The mandible is usually small, and other commonly occurring abnormalities include ventricular septal defect, eventration of the diaphragm, and genitourinary anomalies (rotational abnormalities of the kidneys, hydronephrosis).

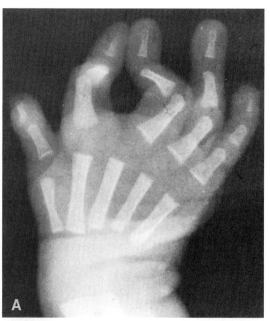

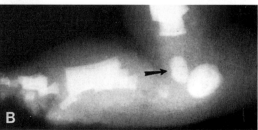

FIGURE 6.174. Trisomy 18. A. Hand. The thumb, especially the first metacarpal, is hypoplastic. Overlapping of the third digit over the second digit has been partially obliterated by positioning of the hand. **B. Foot.** Note the extreme flatfoot deformity with a vertical talus (arrow). Actually, a mild rocker-bottom deformity is present.

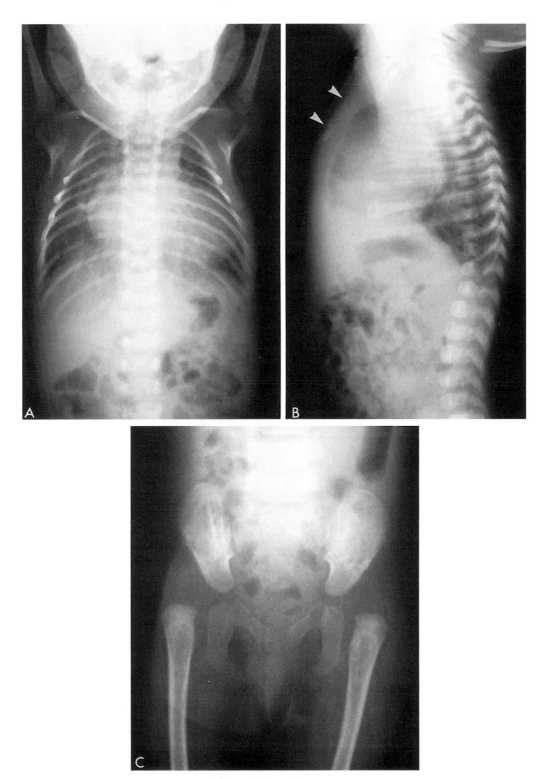

FIGURE 6.175. Trisomy 18. A. Typical chest configuration showing thin ribs and clavicles. A large ventricular septal defect is producing cardiomegaly and pulmonary vascular congestion. **B.** Lateral view showing deepened anteroposterior diameter of the chest and a markedly shortened sternum (arrowheads). Only two sternal segments are visualized. **C.** Inward turning of the iliac wings produces an antimongoloid slant of the acetabula. In this patient, bilateral hip dislocations also are present.

Trisomy 13—15

Trisomy 13–15 is a chromosomal abnormality associated with an extra chromosome in the 13—15 group (Group D). These infants are usually grossly malformed and severely retarded, and most die at birth or shortly thereafter. Alobar holoprosencephaly, profound hypotelorism, and severe midline cleft deformities involving the lip, nose, and palate are usually present. Ocular hypoplasia and cataracts also usually occur, and congenital heart disease in the form of ventricular septal defect and dextroposition of the heart is common. Other abnormalities include umbilical hernia, abdominal wall deficiencies, anomalies of the genitourinary system, coronal cleft vertebrae, and, occasionally, micrognathia. Lenticulostriate vessel prominence on ultrasonography has been demonstrated in trisomy 13—15, probably representing a vasculopathy (1).

REFERENCE

1. Kriss VM, Kriss TC. Doppler sonographic confirmation of thalamic and basal ganglia vasculopathy in three infants with trisomy 13. J Ultrasound Med 1996;15:523–526.

4p Syndrome (Wolf Syndrome)

The 4p syndrome is a rare chromosomal abnormality consisting of partial deletion of the short arm of the number 4 chromosome. Numerous congenital anomalies have been documented, including microcephaly, midline facial defects, hypertelorism, a small sella, scoliosis, square vertebrae, 13 thoracic vertebrae, thin fibulae, radioulnar synostosis, coxa valga of the hips, steep iliac wings, flat acetabular angles, underdeveloped pelvic bones, sternal anomalies, medial tipping of the tibial epiphysis, polydactyly, and synostoses of various long bones (1).

REFERENCE

1. Katz DS, Smith TH. Wolf syndrome. Pediatr Radiol 1991;21: 369–372.

The Cri-du-Chat Syndrome (Trisomy 5p)

The cri-du-chat or cat-cry syndrome is a chromosomal abnormality of the B group (partial deletion of the short arm of the number 5 chromosome). The cry these infants have resembles that of a cat meowing, hence the name "cat-cry syndrome." Marked growth and mental retardation, microcephaly, micrognathia, and oblique palpebral fissures with an antimongoloid slant are observed. Hypertelorism, as opposed to hypotelorism as seen in the trisomy 13–15 syndrome, is present. Congenital heart lesions and a simian crease can also be seen in this abnormality.

Miscellaneous Trisomies

With the advent of chromosomal studies, numerous other trisomies have been identified. Generally, **the roentgenographic findings in these entities are noted in retrospect, and when enough patients are reported, a grouping of abnormalities is possible.** On a practical basis, however, what usually occurs is that first it is noted that these patients look peculiar, and then someone will decide to investigate the possibility that a chromosome abnormality exists. If an abnormality is detected, the radiologist is asked to assist in confirming the diagnosis, and, at this point, familiarity with the various anomalies present in these trisomies is useful. **However, to remember them all is difficult, and for this reason, one usually consults the available literature.**

Turner's Syndrome (Bonnevie-Ullrich Syndrome): Gonadal Dysgenesis

In the neonate, Turner's syndrome is often referred to as the "Bonnevie-Ullrich syndrome" and is usually characterized by redundancy of the skin along the neck and shoulders and edema of the extremities (Fig. 6.176, A and B). In addition, one is usually able to clinically demonstrate the typical shield-shaped chest and widespread nipples. As the infant grows older, the characteristic cubitus valgus deformity, retarded growth, and sexual infantilism with amenorrhea become apparent.

Other anomalies (not always present) seen in patients with Turner's syndrome include drumstick terminal phalanges, a decreased (more acute) carpal angle, and short fourth and fifth metacarpals (Fig. 6.176C) (1). In addition, there is an increased incidence of coarctation of the aorta and bicuspid aortic valve. Rotational abnormalities of the kidneys also are common, especially horseshoe kidney, and cystic hygromas and hemangiomas can be encountered in the extremities. Simple renal cysts also have been documented (1), and the gonads have been demonstrated to be "streak" to normal (2).

REFERENCES

1. Herman TE, Siegel MJ. Renal cysts associated with Turner's syndrome. Pediatr Radiol 1994;24:139–140.
2. Massarano AA, Adams JA, Preece MA, et al. Ovarian ultrasound appearances in Turner's syndrome. J Pediatr 1989;114:568–573.

Noonan's Syndrome (Ullrich-Noonan Syndrome, Pseudo-Turner's Syndrome)

Many of the clinical and roentgenographic features of Noonan's syndrome are similar to those of Turner's syndrome, hence the name "pseudo-Turner's syndrome." These patients, however, have normal chromosomes, and the condition can also occur in males. The most common

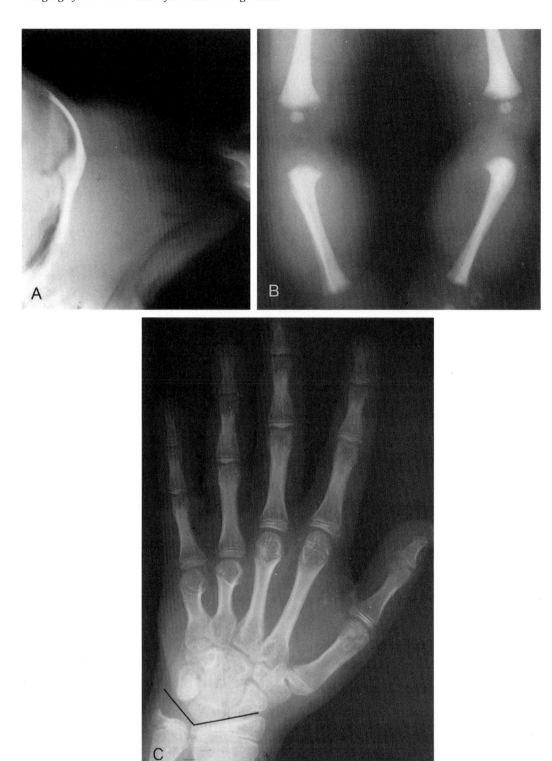

FIGURE 6.176. Neonatal Turner's syndrome. A. Characteristic soft tissue web of the cervicooccipital region. The web is being stretched out posteriorly. Intracranial air noted in this infant is from a pneumogram performed for another reason. **B.** Note extensive edema of both lower extremities. Edema of the upper extremities was also present in this infant. **C.** Older child. Note short fourth and fifth metacarpals, increased angle of the proximal row of carpal bones (lines), and fat (drumstick) terminal phalangeal ends.

congenital heart lesions are pulmonary stenosis and atrial septal defect. Lymphatic vessel dysplasia throughout the body also occurs, and thus spontaneous chylothorax can be a problem (1).

REFERENCE

1. Goens MB, Campbell D, Wiggins JW. Spontaneous chylothorax in Noonan's syndrome: treatment with prednisone. Am J Dis Child 1992;146:1453–1456.

Klinefelter's Syndrome

The findings of Klinefelter's syndrome are only rarely documented in the neonate. One must usually wait until puberty or later, when gynecomastia and eunuchoidism appear. The testes are small in these patients, and the chromosome pattern is XXY. Recently, abdominal, probably prostate-centered germ cell and other tumors have been documented in these patients (1–3).

REFERENCES

1. Czauaderna P, Stoba C, Wysocka B, et al. Association of Klinefelter syndrome and abdominal teratoma: a case report. J Pediatr Surg 1998;33:774–775.
2. Gohji K, Goto A, Takenaka A, et al. Extragonadal germ cell tumor in the retrovesical region associated with Klinefelter's syndrome: a case report and the review of the literature. J Urol 1989; 141:133–135.
3. Tay HP, Bidair M, Shabaik A, et al. Primary yolk sac tumor of the prostate in a patient with Klinefelter's syndrome. J Urol 1995;153: 1066–1069.

THE STORAGE DISEASES

The Mucopolysaccharidoses

Generally, the mucopolysaccharidoses include Hurler's disease (type I), Hunter's disease (type II), Maroteaux-Lamy syndrome (type VI), Sanfilippo's syndrome (type III), Scheie's syndrome (type V), and Morquio's disease (type IV). The most striking roentgenographic findings usually are seen in infants with Hurler's disease (type I), Maroteaux-Lamy syndrome (type VI), and Morquio's disease (type IV). The other types show either lesser degrees of roentgenographic abnormality or no abnormality at all, but none usually show roentgenographic manifestations in the neonatal period.

In older children (usually age 2 and older) with the mucopolysaccharidoses, typical calvarial enlargement with frontal bossing and bone thickening, paddle-shaped ribs, notched vertebra in the thoracolumbar region, narrowing and underdevelopment of the neck of the iliac wings, broad small bones of the hands with proximal tapering of the metacarpals (bullet shape), and squat long bones are characteristic (Figs. 6.177–6.179). In addition, these patients also demonstrate shallow glenoid fossae, hypoplasia of the scapulae, and broad, short clavicles. In those storage diseases in which lesser degrees of change are present, **it is useful to examine the pelvic bones and scapulae.** The reason for this is that it seems that underdevelopment of the iliac wing and acetabular roof, along with the glenoid fossa, seems to penetrate more than do the other bony changes in these conditions.

Other problems that can occur in the storage diseases include hypoplasia of the odontoid with atlantoaxial subluxation (1) and infiltration with thickening of the

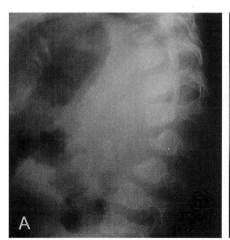
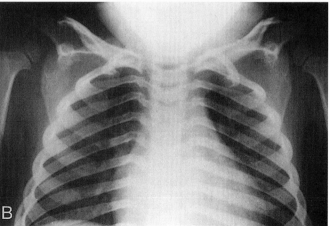

FIGURE 6.177. Hurler's disease. A. Note typical kyphosis with beaking of the upper lumbar vertebral bodies. In general, the vertebral bodies are somewhat cuboid. **B.** Note the short and dysplastic-appearing clavicles. The ribs also are somewhat broadened, and the glenoid fossae are shallow.

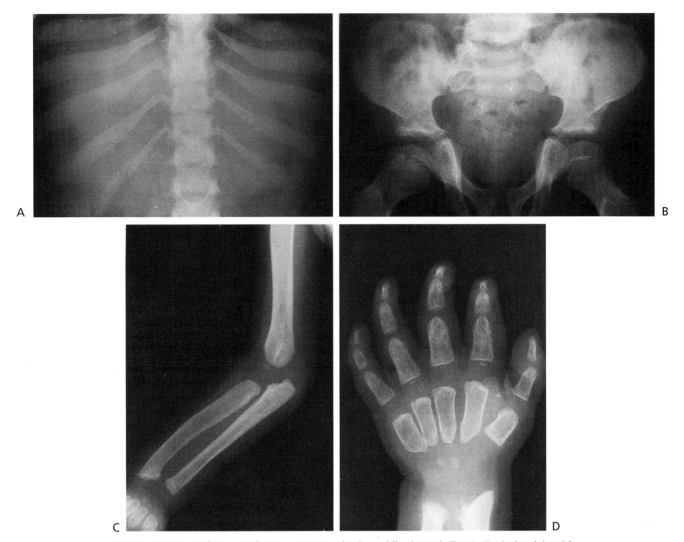

FIGURE 6.178. Hurler's syndrome. A. Note classic paddle-shaped ribs. **B.** Typical pelvis with narrowed (constricted) lower iliac wings. **C.** Upper extremity. Note the short, squat long bones. **D.** Hand. All of the bones are short and squat, and the proximal phalanges along with the metacarpals are somewhat "bullet" shaped. The radiocarpal angle is increased.

meninges (2). In addition, narrowing of the trachea as a result of infiltration with the mucopolysaccharide has been noted (3), and we have seen this in two patients ourselves. Similar infiltration can occur in the vocal cords.

Mucopolysaccharidosis (type IV), or **Morquio's disease,** presents with roentgenographic changes quite different from those of Hurler's syndrome. The condition strongly resembles spondyloepiphyseal dysplasia congenita. These patients usually do not present with problems until the end of the first year of life. Older infants with Morquio's disease present with muscular atrophy and hypotonia, deep barrel chests, and knock-knee deformity. In most cases, by the time clinical findings are appreciated, roentgenographic changes are present. Characteristically, these consist of universal platyspondylia (with or without pear-shaped verte-

brae), widespread epiphyseal dysplasia, and a pelvic appearance consisting of square iliac bones and flat acetabular roofs (Fig. 6.180). Shortening and varus deformity of the femoral necks and undertubulated, bullet-shaped small bones of the hands also are present. The skull is normal, but the dens often is absent or hypoplastic.

REFERENCES

1. Pizzutillo PD, Osterkamp JA, Scott CI Jr, et al. Atlantoaxial instability in mucopolysaccharidosis. J Pediatr Orthop 1989;9:76–78.
2. Taccone A, Donati PT, Marzoli A, et al. Mucopolysaccharidosis: thickening of dura mater at the craniocervical junction and other CT/MRI findings. Pediatr Radiol 1993;23:349–352.
3. Peters ME, Arya S, Langer LO, et al. Narrow trachea in mucopolysaccharidoses. Pediatr Radiol 1985;15:225–228.

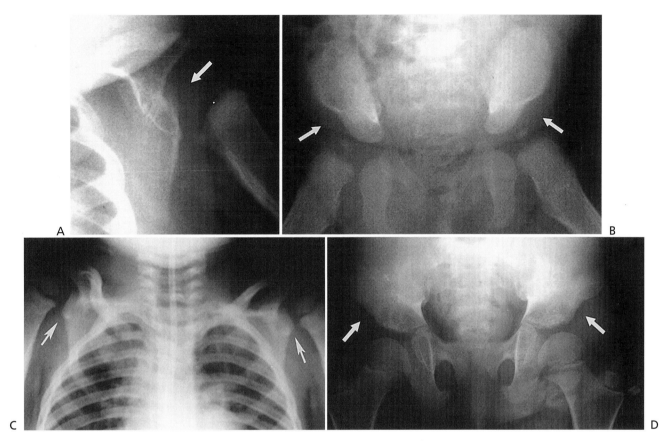

FIGURE 6.179. Storage diseases: less classic findings. A. Sanfilippo type. Note that the glenoid fossa (arrow) is markedly underdeveloped. **B.** Pelvis demonstrating underdeveloped (constricted) lower iliac wings with a false (pseudoacetabular) formation (arrows). **C.** This older patient demonstrates underdevelopment of the glenoid fossa (arrows). The clavicle is slightly shortened. **D.** Subtle changes in the pelvis consist of underdevelopment of the lower portions of the iliac wings.

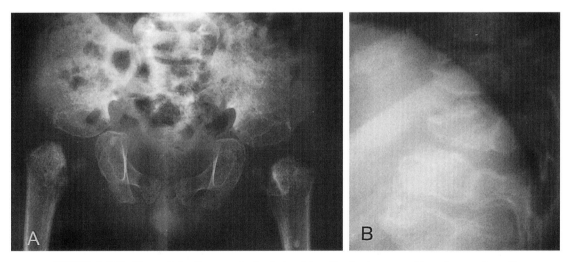

FIGURE 6.180. Morquio's disease. A. Typical pelvis with short, square iliac wings and small, irregular femoral capital epiphyses. The metaphyseal regions also are underdeveloped, and a coxa vara deformity is present. **B.** Flat vertebra with slight kyphosis and notching.

Generalized Gangliosidosis

Generalized gangliosidosis is one of the few storage diseases that presents with changes in the newborn period. These infants present with skeletal changes consisting of poor mineralization of the bones, extreme cupping, irregularity and fragmentation of the metaphyses, and periosteal new bone formation around the shaft of the long bones (Fig. 6.181). These changes slowly resolve and are replaced by changes strongly resembling those of Hurler's syndrome (Fig. 6.182).

Winchester Syndrome

Winchester syndrome is an unusual storage disease (1). The skeletal changes strongly resemble those of advanced rheumatoid arthritis with juxtaarticular demineralization and joint space narrowing (Fig. 6.183).

REFERENCE

1. Winchester P, Grossman H, Lim WN, et al. A new acid mucopolysaccharidosis with skeletal deformities simulating rheumatoid arthritis. AJR 1969;106:128.

Mucolipidoses (I-Cell Disease)

Infants with these storage diseases often resemble those with Hurler's disease and thus often are referred to as cases of pseudo-Hurler's disease. The problem, however, lies in the abnormal accumulation of various mucolipids and not mucopolysaccharidoses. Subdivision into three types has been suggested, but types II and III show the more pronounced bony changes. The type II abnormality also often is referred to as I (inclusion)-cell or Leroy's disease.

In the neonatal period, the coarse facial features, moderate joint limitation, and Hurler-like appearance call attention to the underlying problem. Radiographically, periosteal cloaking of the long bones much as in generalized gangliosidosis, especially the humeri and femurs, is seen. In older children, the changes are not unlike those of classic Hurler's disease or generalized gangliosidosis.

Mannosidosis and Fucosidosis Type II

These are less common storage diseases that present with a Hurler-like appearance in later childhood. Fucosidosis has been classified by some as a mucolipidosis. Generally speaking, both conditions present in the older child.

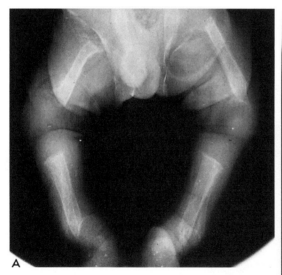
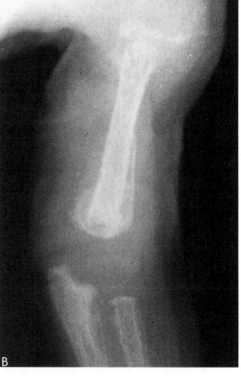

FIGURE 6.181. Generalized gangliosidosis. A. Bones of the lower extremity show coarse trabeculation, undertubulation of the long bones (they appear wide and swollen), and extreme metaphyseal irregularity with pathologic fracture. **B.** Similar changes in the upper extremity, but, in addition, periosteal new bone formation (cloaking) around the humerus is noted. (Reproduced with permission from Scott CR, Lagunoff D, Trump BF. Familial neurovisceral lipidosis. J Pediatr 1967;71:357–366).

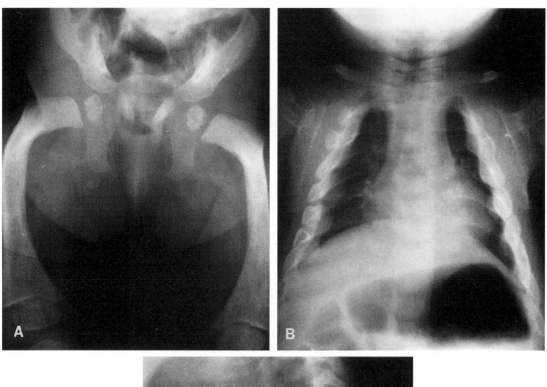

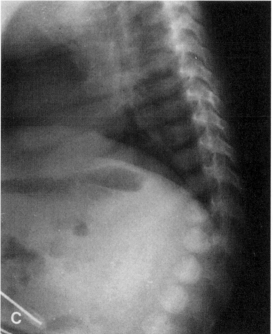

FIGURE 6.182. Generalized gangliosidosis: pseudo-Hurler's syndrome. A. Note the typical appearance of the femurs with a pronounced coxa vara deformity. The iliac wings are thin and narrow through their inferior aspects. The findings are not unlike those seen in Hurler's disease. **B.** Chest film demonstrating short, thick ribs and short clavicles. **C.** Lateral view of the spine demonstrates increased kyphosis at the thoracolumbar junction, rounded vertebral bodies, but no notching. Eventually, notching develops and the spine is indistinguishable from that seen with Hurler's disease. This patient also had hypoplasia of the dens.

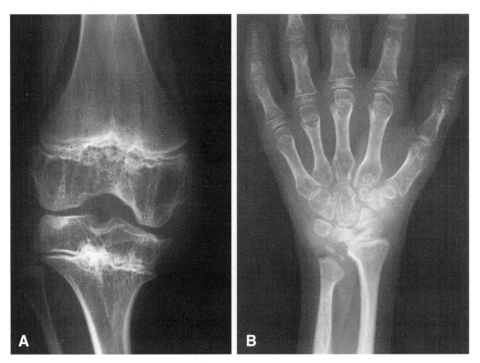

FIGURE 6.183. Winchester's syndrome. A. Knee demonstrating demineralization, glassy-appearing irregular epiphyses, with overall changes resembling those of rheumatoid arthritis. **B.** Similar changes in the hands and wrists. (Courtesy of Derek Harwood-Nash, M.D.).

Gaucher's Disease and Niemann-Pick Disease

The infantile form of Gaucher's disease usually is acute and fulminating. It often appears shortly after birth, but bony change is absent. The earliest I have seen widening of the metaphyses is in an 8-month-old infant. Changes occur predominantly in the viscera and leptomeninges, and thus the presentation most often, but not always, is that of an acute neuropathic problem. In this regard, pronounced meningeal

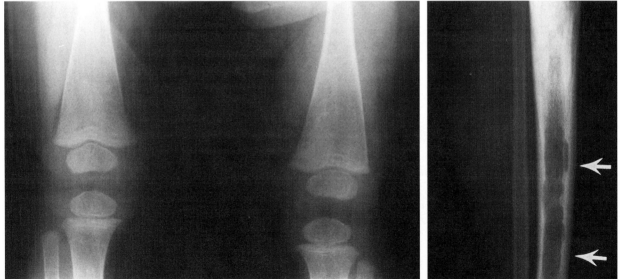

FIGURE 6.184. Gaucher's disease. A. Note widening (Erlenmeyer flask deformity) of the distal femurs in this young infant with Gaucher's disease. **B.** Older patient with scalloped-out areas in the diaphysis of the tibia and sclerosis in the proximal portion of the tibia. These findings often mimic those of chronic osteomyelitis.

irritation can lead to opisthotonos, and cranial nerve involvement to difficulties with swallowing. Similar manifestations can be seen with the more severe forms of Niemann-Pick disease, but, as with Gaucher's disease, these patients also demonstrate bony changes later on. The changes consist of widening of the metaphysis and complicating aseptic necrosis of the femoral heads or infarcts of the long bones, resulting in changes similar to those seen with osteomyelitis (Fig. 6.184). Interstitial pulmonary infiltrates, now best demonstrated with CT (1), can be seen in both conditions, and enlargement of the liver and spleen is common. Finally, one can encounter a proximal humeral notch in some of these patients (2), a finding that disappears with appropriate therapy (3).

REFERENCES

1. Tunaci A, Berkmen YM, Gokmen E. Pulmonary Gaucher's disease: high-resolution computed features. Pediatr Radiol 1995;25: 237–238.
2. Li JKW, Birch PD, Davies AM. Proximal humeral defects in Gaucher's disease. Br J Radiol 1988;61:579–583.
3. Pastores GM, Hermann G, Norton K, et al. Resolution of a proximal humeral defect in type-1 Gaucher disease by enzyme replacement therapy. Pediatr Radiol 1995;25:486–487.

Glycogen Storage Disease

Glycogen storage disease in the neonate manifests primarily with muscular abnormalities, cardiomegaly, and visceromegaly. Bone changes do not become apparent until the infant becomes older. The form in which muscular and cardiac hypertrophy occur is referred to as "type II glycogen storage disease" (Pompe's disease).

In later childhood, bony changes consist primarily of widening of the metaphyses (undertubulation) of the long bones. In addition, a smooth colon, devoid of haustral markings, and medullary renal nephrocalcinosis can occur in type I hepatorenal glycogen storage disease (1).

REFERENCE

1. Fick JJ, Beek FJ. Echogenic kidneys and medullary calcium deposition in a young child with glycogen storage disease type 1A. Pediatr Radiol 1992;22:72–73.

THE BONY "DYSPLASIAS"

Osteogenesis Imperfecta

Mild and severe forms of osteogenesis imperfecta exist, and although heterogenicity of the condition extends beyond these two basic groups (1), for simplicity's sake, it still is best to consider the condition under the congenita or tarda forms. The tarda form (type I) may or may not present with problems in the neonate, but the congenita form (type II)

often is a lethal neonatal problem (Fig. 6.185). Inheritance in the type II form is autosomal recessive; in the type I form, it is autosomal dominant.

The abnormality in osteogenesis imperfecta is believed to lie in a basic deficiency of collagen formation (2). Even though the basic mechanism of subsequent bony mineralization is intact, overall bone development is impaired. Although the bones often receive primary consideration, the collagen disturbance present in this condition also afflicts the skin, sclera (blue sclera), and other connective tissue structures.

Roentgenographically, in type I osteogenesis imperfecta, changes may be mild to moderate (Fig. 6.185A) and, as noted earlier, may or may not present in the neonatal period. The changes largely consist of thinning of all the long bones, ribs, and clavicles. Fractures are variable but usually occur through the shafts of the long bones. Epiphyseal-metaphyseal fractures also can be seen but are uncommon. As these fractures heal, callus formation is exuberant and residual curvature deformities of the bones are usual. Nontraumatic bowing of the various long bones also is commonly seen, and the bones remain thin and fragile throughout life (Fig. 6.186). The ribs also show increased flaring at the costochondral junctions.

In type II osteogenesis imperfecta (i.e., osteogenesis imperfecta congenita), the changes usually are profound and can be seen in utero. Almost every long bone, rib, and clavicle shows numerous fractures, and the long bones are very ballooned, short, and squat (Fig. 6.185). These patients often are stillborn or die shortly after birth. Severe respiratory compromise caused by a restricted thorax and hypoplastic lungs is a significant factor in their early demise. In type III osteogenesis imperfecta, the bones are short and accordion-like (Fig. 6.185C).

The skull in osteogenesis imperfecta usually is underossified, and pseudospreading of the calvarial sutures (i.e., pseudowidening) results from underossification of the calvarial bones. There also is exaggerated parietal bone fissuring, fragmentation, or actual wormian or mosaic bone formation (Fig. 6.187). In severe cases, ossification of the calvarium virtually is absent, and the skull consists of a membranous primordium. The skull in general is round, and in the tarda form, platybasia with basilar invagination and cord compression can occur.

In the spine, the characteristic finding is multiple compression fractures. In some cases, the vertebrae assume a biconcave appearance as the disc expands into the soft bone, but more often the compression fractures are more ordinary appearing (Fig. 6.187C). Most of these patients also demonstrate disuse atrophy of the muscles because they are less ambulant than normal. Their tooth bud precursors also show underdevelopment and underdemineralization, resulting in so-called "odontogenesis imperfecta."

Malignant degeneration in patients with the tarda form occurs in a small number of patients. Enlargement of the

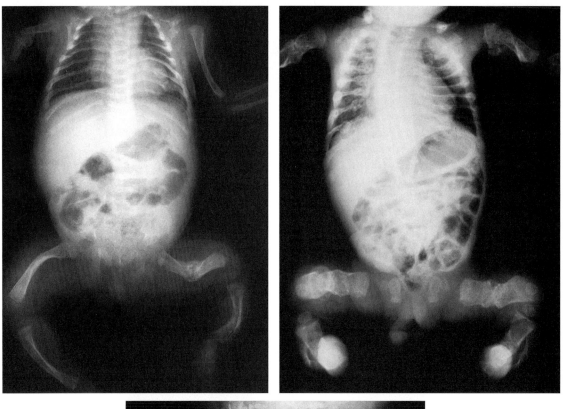

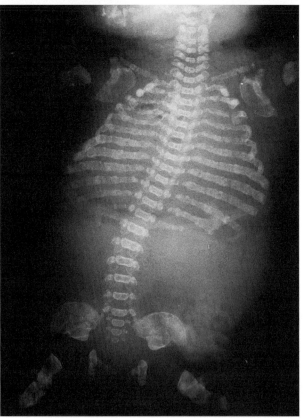

FIGURE 6.185. Osteogenesis imperfecta, Type II. A. In this infant, note the fragile-appearing ribs and long bones. Most of the long bones show the aftermath of intrauterine bending and fracturing. The bones in the right upper extremity and left lower extremity have lost their thin, delicate appearance and have become markedly short and squat. **B.** Another infant with the more severe form. Note numerous fractures with hypercallosis involving almost all the ribs and bones of the extremities. The bones are markedly shortened, squat, and bent. **C. Type III.** Note marked shortening of the bones and an accordion-like appearance to the multiple fractures of the ribs and long bones.

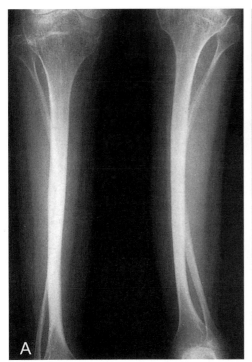
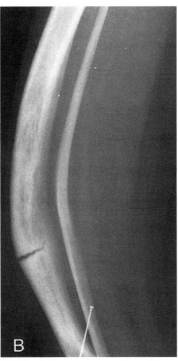

FIGURE 6.186. Osteogenesis imperfecta tarda, Type I. A. Typical thin extremities with thin, curving long bones and atrophy of the muscles. **B.** Another patient with typical bony changes and a classic fracture.

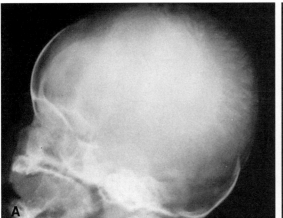
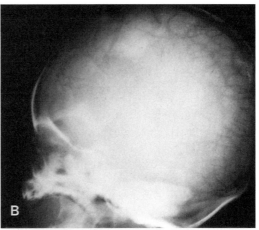
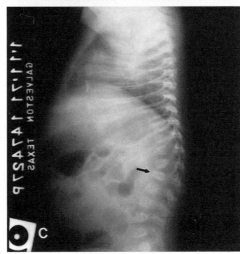

FIGURE 6.187. Osteogenesis imperfecta: calvarial and spinal findings. A. Skull in an infant with osteogenesis imperfecta shows pseudowidening of the coronal suture (secondary to underossification of the skull) and characteristic fissuring (wormian bone formation) of the parietal bones. **B.** Another pattern of abnormal ossification of the calvarial bones (mosaic bones) in an infant with osteogenesis imperfecta. **C.** Lateral view of a chest showing thin, anteriorly cupped ribs, generalized osteoporosis of the skeleton, and a number of vertebral compression fractures, best visualized at L1 (arrow).

metaphyseal regions with irregular calcification, however, is more common and at first may erroneously suggest malignant degeneration. The "popcorn" calcifications commonly seen in these areas probably result from an abnormality of bone formation at the epiphyseal plate (3).

REFERENCES

1. Spranger J, Cremin B, Beighton P. Osteogenesis imperfecta congenita. Features and prognosis of a heterogeneous condition. Pediatr Radiol 1982;12:21–27.
2. Cole WG, Campbell PE, Rogers JG, et al. The clinical features of osteogenesis imperfecta resulting from a nonfunctional carboxy terminal Pro 1(1) propeptide of type I procollagen and a severe deficiency of normal type I collagen in tissues. J Med Genet 1990;27:545–551.
3. Goldman AB, Davidson D, Pavlov H, et al. "Popcorn" calcifications: a prognostic sign in osteogenesis imperfecta. Radiology 1980;136:351–358.

Osteopetrosis (Marble Bones, Albers-Schönberg Disease)

Osteopetrosis is believed to result from a failure to resorb primary spongiosa, and abnormal osteocytes have been implicated in this role (1). Osteoid formation and bone mineralization are normal, but the primary spongiosa is not resorbed, and consequently the bones become extremely dense. In the neonate, the disease often presents in the so-called "malignant" form and is characterized by rapid deterioration of the infant. Typical roentgenographic findings are always present in such cases, but attention is usually first called to the problem because of hepatosplenomegaly, profound anemia, jaundice, and, in some cases, calvarial enlargement. In somewhat milder cases, the course may be more protracted, and in the very mild tarda form, survival into late adulthood can occur. It is believed that the malignant form is transmitted as an autosomal recessive trait, while the benign form is transmitted as an autosomal dominant trait.

The anemia of osteopetrosis generally is believed to be the result of obliteration of the bony medullary cavities. In addition, marked, bony thickening of the calvarium can lead to encroachment on the optic foramina and other foramina for the cranial nerves. In some cases, even the foramen magnum is involved, and hydrocephalus may result. Imaging of the face, calvarium, and upper cervical spine now is best accomplished with CT and MR (2, 3). Serum calcium, phosphorus, and alkaline phosphatase values are usually normal or near normal.

The roentgenographic findings in infancy consist of a marked increase in density of all bones, and in most cases, involvement of the diaphysis, metaphysis, and epiphysis is equal (Fig. 6.188). The marrow cavities are all but obliterated, and alternating areas of increased and decreased density may be seen in the metaphyses (i.e., fluctuating activity in the disease). This often leads to the well-known bone-within-bone appearance. Fractures are not uncommon because the bones are unduly brittle, even though they appear dense.

In the tarda form, the skull and long bones are more dense (Fig. 6.189, A and B) and the vertebral bodies are usually square and dense. They almost always demonstrate the so-called "sandwich vertebra" configuration (Fig. 6.189C). Another interesting finding is that of squaring off of the anterior rib margins where normal cupping is lost (Fig. 6.188B). In all cases, the skull is usually dense and thick, over both the base and the calvarium, and premature closure of the sutures is a frequent complication. In the newborn, care should be taken not to misdiagnose idiopathic, transient osteosclerosis of the newborn for osteopetrosis.

REFERENCES

1. Krook LM, Whalen JP, Dorfman HD, et al. Osteopetrosis: an interpretation of its pathogenesis. Skeletal Radiol 1981;7:185–189.
2. Elster AD, Theros EG, Key LL, et al. Cranial imaging in autosomal recessive osteopetrosis. 1. Facial bones and calvarium. Radiology 1992;183:129–135.
3. Elster AD, Theros EG, Key LL, et al. Cranial imaging in autosomal recessive osteopetrosis. II. Skull base and brain. Radiology 1992;183:137–144.

Lethal Neonatal Dwarfism

Many of the conditions to be discussed in subsequent sections result in stillbirths or infants who die shortly after birth. In many cases, this results from severe thoracic dysplasia and hypoplastic lungs. Most of these dwarfs have discriminating roentgenographic features, and thus the radiologist plays an important role in their identification and further genetic counseling.

Achondroplasia

The bony disorder of achondroplasia can be inherited as an autosomal dominant condition but most often is a fresh mutation. It is readily recognizable at birth, both clinically and roentgenographically, and the diagnosis can even be made in utero. The basic defect appears to lie in faulty growth of the normal zone of proliferating cartilage in enchondral bone. Consequently, the long bones and ribs are shortened, the vertebral bodies lack their normal height, and the cartilaginous portion (base) of the skull is underdeveloped. Flat bones such as the pelvis and the scapula are also smaller than normal. In the extremities, shortening is characteristically most pronounced in the proximal segment (humerus-femur), resulting in the so-called "rhizomelic" type of dwarfism.

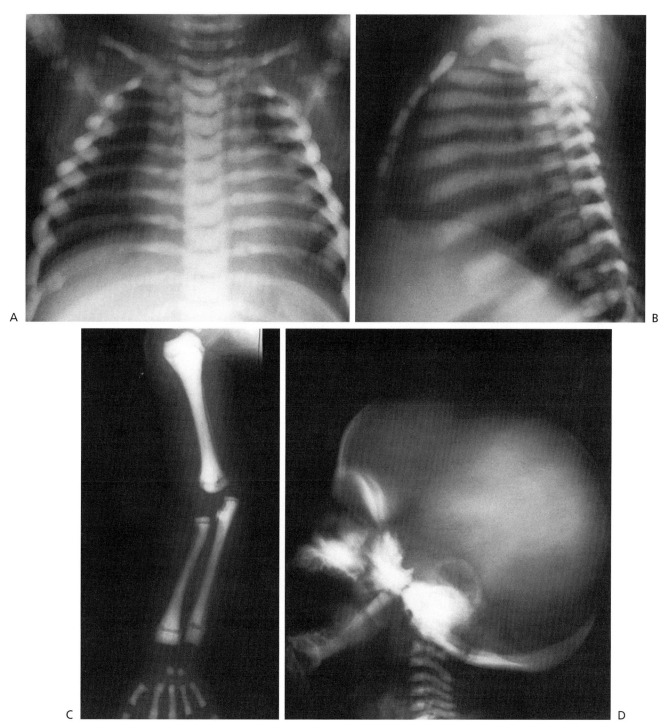

FIGURE 6.188. Osteopetrosis. A. Chest. Note increased density of all of the bones. **B.** Lateral view demonstrating similar density and loss of normal cupping of the anterior ribs. **C.** Long bone demonstrating typical increased density and bone-within-bone appearance. **D.** Calvarium demonstrating sclerosis, especially over the face and basal regions.

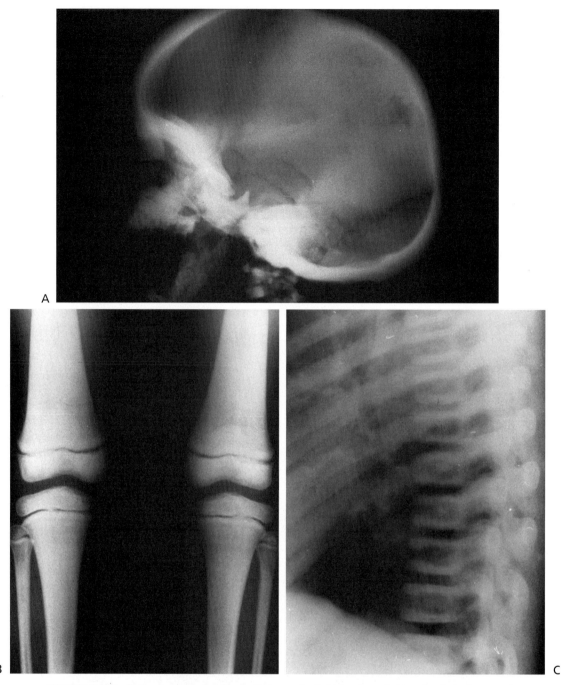

FIGURE 6.189. Osteopetrosis tarda. A. Note marked thickening of the calvarium, face, and base of the skull. **B.** Sclerosis of the femurs and tibiae with slight widening of the metaphyses. **C.** Typical spine with deep transverse bands resulting in the so-called "sandwich" vertebra configuration.

Roentgenographically, the characteristically short extremities and marked flaring of the metaphyses strongly suggest the diagnosis. The epiphyses are relatively spared, although some secondary irregularity and fragmentation may be seen in the more severe cases. The narrowed spinal canal, short, squared-off iliac wings due to flat acetabular roofs, and bulky proximal femurs make the diagnosis (Fig.

6.190). In later life, the narrowed spinal canal with associated intervertebral disc protrusion can lead to symptoms of cord and nerve root compression.

As the patient becomes older, these changes persist, but the long bones become more squat in appearance. The epiphyses become deep-set in the metaphyses, leading to the so-called "ball-and-socket" appearance (Fig. 6.191A). The

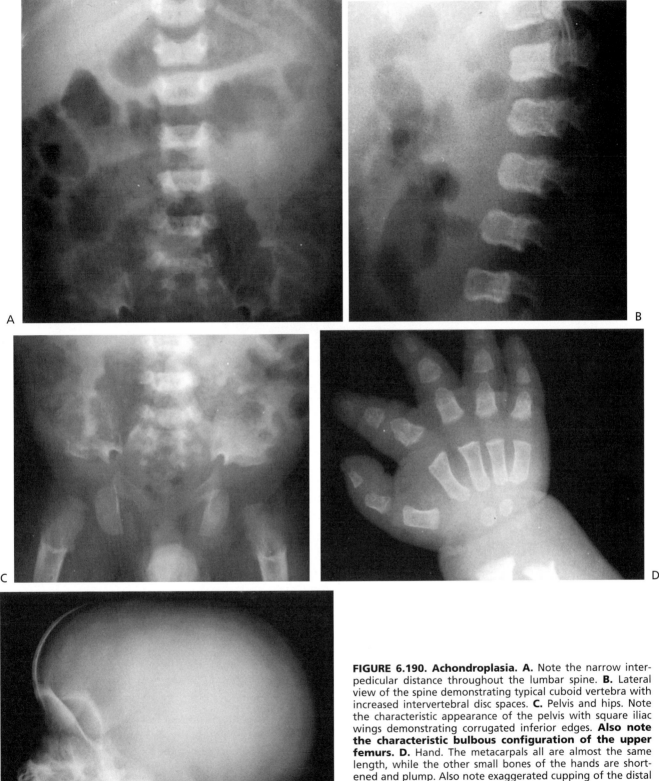

FIGURE 6.190. Achondroplasia. A. Note the narrow interpedicular distance throughout the lumbar spine. **B.** Lateral view of the spine demonstrating typical cuboid vertebra with increased intervertebral disc spaces. **C.** Pelvis and hips. Note the characteristic appearance of the pelvis with square iliac wings demonstrating corrugated inferior edges. **Also note the characteristic bulbous configuration of the upper femurs. D.** Hand. The metacarpals all are almost the same length, while the other small bones of the hands are shortened and plump. Also note exaggerated cupping of the distal ulna and that the ulna is shorter than the radius. **E.** Lateral skull. Typical configuration showing enlarged membranous calvarium and a relatively underdeveloped (enchondral) base. The face is also relatively small and underdeveloped, especially the maxilla. Frontal bossing is moderately prominent.

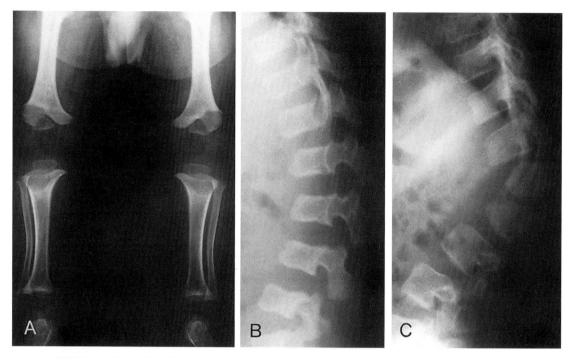

FIGURE 6.191. Achondroplasia. A. Note typical shortening of the long bones. Also note flaring and widening of the metaphyses and a ball-and-socket appearance of the epiphyseal-metaphyseal junctions. **B.** Typical cuboid vertebra with thick disc spaces, slight suggestion of notching of one or two of the vertebral bodies, pronounced posterior scalloping, and a narrow spinal canal. **C.** An older patient with similar changes in the spine, but this time there is marked kyphosis with severe wedging or notching of the vertebral bodies.

fibula also tends to be longer than the tibia, and the vertebral bodies continue to be somewhat cuboid. Kyphosis at the thoracolumbar junction can become pronounced (1) and be associated with anterior notching of the vertebrae (Fig. 6.191, B and C).

In severe neonatal cases (homozygous form), the findings may resemble those of thanatophoric dwarfism, and these infants usually have severe respiratory distress and may, in fact, be stillborn or die shortly after birth. Hypoplastic lungs, secondary to the small thorax, are the rule, and the changes are much more pronounced than in the ordinary case (Fig. 6.192).

The skull is enlarged and shows relative underdevelopment and constriction of the base (Fig. 6.190). Frontal and biparietal bossing of the membranous calvarium is pronounced. Initial enlargement of the calvarium is not the result of hydrocephalus but eventually can be exaggerated since constriction of the base of the skull results in obstructive hydrocephalus. This aggravates the problem. In keeping with this, the foramen magnum is small (Fig. 6.193), and some patients may require shunting for the hydrocephalus. Evaluation of this area now most often is relegated to MRI in which dynamic flexion studies can elicit brainstem and cord compression (Fig. 6.194). In patients with acute or chronic compression of the medulla

by the narrowed foramen magnum, recurrent apnea can result (2, 3).

REFERENCES

1. Herring JA, Winter RB. Kyphosis in an achondroplastic dwarf. J Pediatr Orthop 1983;3:250–252.
2. Fremion AS, Garg BP, Kalsbeck J. Apnea as the sole manifestation of cord compression achondroplasia. J Pediatr 1984;104:398–400.
3. Pauli RM, Scott CI, Wassman ER, et al. Apnea and sudden unexpected death in infants with achondroplasia. J Pediatr 1984;104:342–348.

Hypochondroplasia

Hypochondroplasia does not usually present in infancy. It differs from true achondroplasia in that the skull usually is normal and shortening of the long bones and changes in the spine are less pronounced than in true achondroplasia. Many times, the diagnosis is suggested on the basis of spinal changes and shortening of the extremities (1).

REFERENCE

1. Prinster C, Del Maschio M, Beluffi G, et al. Italian Study Groups

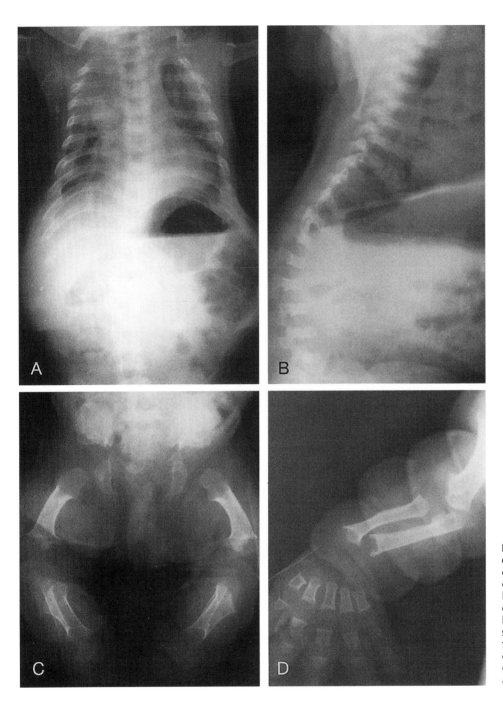

FIGURE 6.192. Severe achondroplasia. A. Note marked shortening of the ribs and underdevelopment of the thorax. Hypoplastic lungs were present. **B.** Lateral view demonstrating small vertebral bodies, pronounced kyphosis, and short ribs. **C.** Marked shortening of the long bones with exaggerated cupping of their ends. **D.** Upper extremity with typical long bone and hand changes.

for Hypochondroplasia: diagnosis of hypochondroplasia: the role of radiological interpretation. Pediatr Radiol 2001;31:203–208.

Pseudoachondroplasia

The term "pseudoachondroplasia" stems from the fact that a clinically achondroplasia-like appearance can be seen in other patients. These largely include those with multiple epiphyseal dysplasia or spondyloepiphyseal dysplasia. In the spondyloepiphyseal type of pseudoachondroplasia, the ver-

tebrae are flat and severely underdeveloped, but the spinal canal is not narrowed. Scoliosis and kyphosis also become a problem, but generally only those infants with the severe congenita form of spondyloepiphyseal dysplasia present in the neonatal period.

In differentiating these patients from those with achondroplasia, it should be noted that the skull is relatively normal and that the epiphyses are markedly underdeveloped, irregular, and delayed in ossification. Changes in the metaphyses causing confusion with achondroplasia are believed

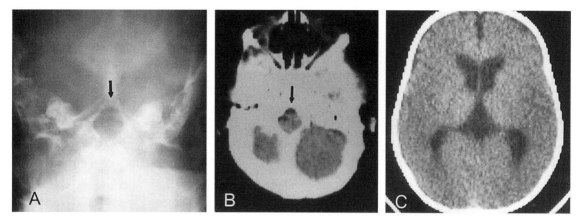

FIGURE 6.193. Achondroplasia: small foramen magnum and hydrocephalus. A. Note small foramen magnum (arrow) on this Towne's view of the skull. **B.** Computed tomography study in another patient demonstrates a small foramen magnum (arrow). **C.** Same patient demonstrating mild hydrocephalus.

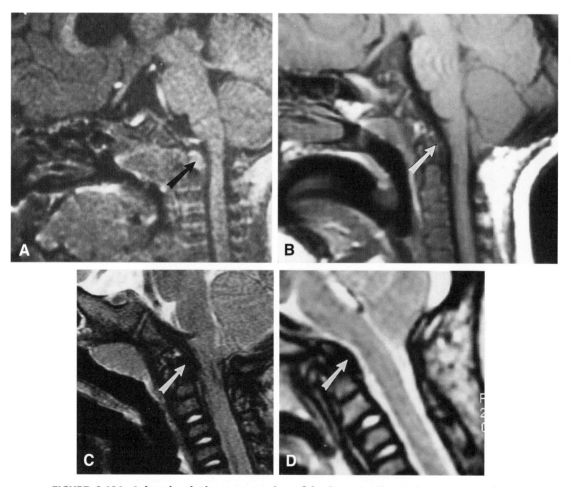

FIGURE 6.194. Achondroplasia: compromise of brainstem. Magnetic resonance findings. A. Sagittal T1-weighted image demonstrates compression of the cervicomedullary junction (arrow). **B.** After occipital craniectomy, the foramen magnum was enlarged and the cervical cord now is not compressed (arrow). **C.** Preoperative T2-weighted study demonstrates absence of high-signal cerebrospinal fluid around the cervical cord in the involved area (arrow). **D.** Postoperative T2-weighted image with slight flexion demonstrates the presence of high-signal cerebrospinal fluid both anterior (arrow) and posterior to the upper cervical cord. All of this indicates that decompression has been accomplished.

secondary to the epiphyseal changes. In this regard, since the epiphyses develop poorly, they do not afford proper protection to the metaphysis, and over a period of time, metaphyseal growth disturbances occur.

Thanatophoric Dwarfism

Thanatophoric dwarfism is a congenital skeletal dysplasia characterized by marked underdevelopment of the skeleton, short-limbed dwarfism, and early death. Most of these infants are either stillborn or die shortly after birth. If they live, severe respiratory distress is present because the thoracic cage is small and extremely restricted in its motion. Hypoplastic lungs are the eventual cause of demise.

Two forms of thanatophoric dwarfism have been defined, but the most common form is referred to as "thanatophoric dwarfism type I." These infants demonstrate marked underdevelopment of the entire skeleton, extremely short, bent, or curved long bones, and considerable flaring of the metaphyses (Fig. 6.195). The pelvic bones are markedly underdeveloped, and the acetabular roof is flat. The skull, spinal curvature, and spinal canal narrowing are somewhat similar in configuration to those seen in achondroplasia, but in thanatophoric dwarfism, the vertebral bodies are very flat and underdeveloped (Fig. 6.195, C and D). In the usual form of achondroplasia, the vertebral bodies are generally more squat and cuboid. Cloverleaf skull is also seen in type I thanatophoric dwarfism (1). In type II thanatophoric dwarfism, the long bones are not as short, and they are not bent or bowed. Their metaphyses, however, still are flared and cupped. The vertebral bodies are underdeveloped but not as flat and thin as those of type I thanatophoric dwarfism.

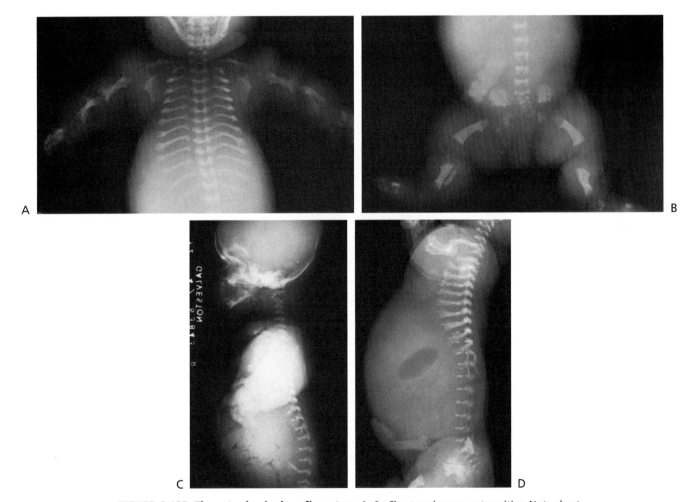

FIGURE 6.195. Thanatophoric dwarfism, type I. A. Chest and upper extremities. Note shortening of the ribs and of the long bones of the extremities. **B.** Pelvis and lower extremities. Again, note shortening of the long bones and the typical appearance of the pelvis with square iliac wings and corrugated inferior edges. The findings are similar to those of achondroplasia. **C.** Lateral view demonstrating short ribs and generalized platyspondyly. **D.** Another patient demonstrating severe platyspondyly.

REFERENCE

1. Isaacson G, Blakemore KJ, Chervenak FA. Thanatophoric dysplasia with cloverleaf skull. Am J Dis Child 1983;137:896–898.

Achondrogenesis

There can be some confusion between achondrogenesis and thanatophoric dwarfism, both clinically and roentgenographically. Clinically, however, most of these infants are much more deformed than are thanatophoric dwarfs, and roentgenographically, distinction is possible. Many are stillborn, and those born alive show severe respiratory distress and early demise. Once again, restricted thoracic motion and underlying pulmonary hypoplasia are contributing factors.

Although a certain degree of heterogenicity exists (1), basically two types of achondrogenesis exist: types I and II.

In the past, the type I form was the one usually described. Roentgenographically, both are examples of severe short-limbed dwarfism, but most importantly, the identifying feature in both is the absence of vertebral body ossification. Almost all other lethal neonatal dwarfs show vertebral body ossification. The only exception is the severe form of hypophosphatasia congenita. In achondrogenesis, depending on the severity of involvement, the entire spine or just the lower regions will show lack of ossification.

In type I achondrogenesis, the long bones are extremely short and cuboid as are the iliac bones. At the same time, they have peculiar metaphyseal scallopings and diaphyseal bendings (Fig. 6.196A). The ribs are thin and fractured and show pronounced anterior cupping, most commonly seen in type IA. However, there is heterogenicity within the type I grouping, and in this regard, in type IB achondrogenesis, the changes are more severe. These patients virtually show no bony ossification of the skeleton (1). In the type II form,

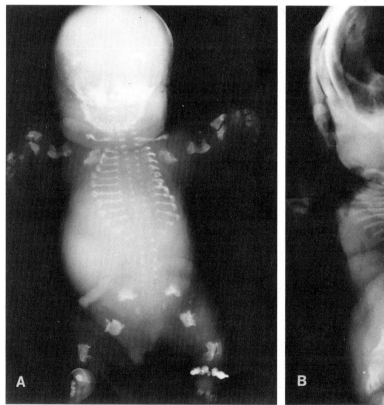
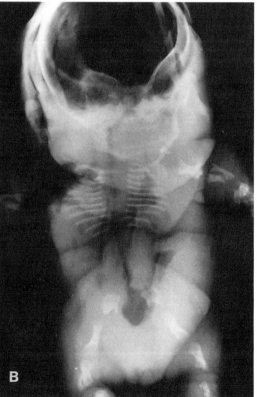

FIGURE 6.196. Achondrogenesis. A. Type I. Note biparietal prominence of the skull, severely underdeveloped and shortened extremities, thin and short ribs with pronounced anterior cupping, and virtually absent vertebral bodies. The long bones are cuboid and peculiarly scalloped. **B. Type II.** Note the overall similarity of bony maldevelopment, but also note that the long bones are not as cuboid or shortened. The pubic bone underdevelopment is more pronounced. (**A** reproduced with permission from Houston CS, Awen CF, Kent HP. Fatal neonatal dwarfism. J Can Assoc Radiol 1972;23:45–61; **B** reproduced with permission from Yang SS, Brough AJ, Garewal GS, et al. Two types of heritable lethal achondrogenesis. J Pediatr 1974;85:796–801).

the long bones are longer and less bowed or bent, the ribs are not as thin, and the pubic bones are generally unossified (2). The pubic bones also are unossified in the type I form, but underossification of the pubic bones is more pronounced in the type II form (Fig. 6.196B). A distinguishing feature of both types is that the width of the spinal canal usually is normal. In thanatophoric dwarfism and achondroplasia, the spinal canal is narrowed.

REFERENCES

1. Jaeger HJ, Schmitz-Stolbrink A, Hulde J, et al. The boneless neonate: a severe form of achondrogenesis type I. Pediatr Radiol 1994;24:319–321.
2. Dilmen U, Kaya IS, Ceyhan M, et al. Achondrogenesis type II. Pediatr Radiol 1988;19:53.

Asphyxiating Thoracic Dystrophy (Jeune's Syndrome)

Asphyxiating thoracic dystrophy is probably inherited on an autosomal recessive basis and is characterized by short-limbed dwarfism, restrictive thoracic cage deformity, and subsequent severe respiratory distress (due to hypoplastic lung) at birth. Many, but not all, infants die either immediately after birth or shortly thereafter. These infants are the most severely afflicted and die from underlying pulmonary hypoplasia. There is, however, a considerable spectrum of abnormality in this condition, and many patients can survive into childhood. In such patients, the skeletal changes may, with time, become less pronounced, but renal failure and death resulting from associated nephritis may ensue (1). In terms of the renal lesion in these patients, it has been demonstrated in one study that the problem is juvenile nephrophthisis (2).

The long bones in asphyxiating thoracic dystrophy are short, but not nearly as short or as abnormal appearing as in achondroplasia, thanatophoric dwarfism, and achondrogenesis. In more severe cases, however, there may still be some confusion with these entities. This is especially true when one examines only the pelvis because the square iliac wings and underdeveloped pelvic bones are similar (Figs. 6.197 and 6.198). In asphyxiating thoracic dystrophy, however, the upper ends of the femurs do not have the same

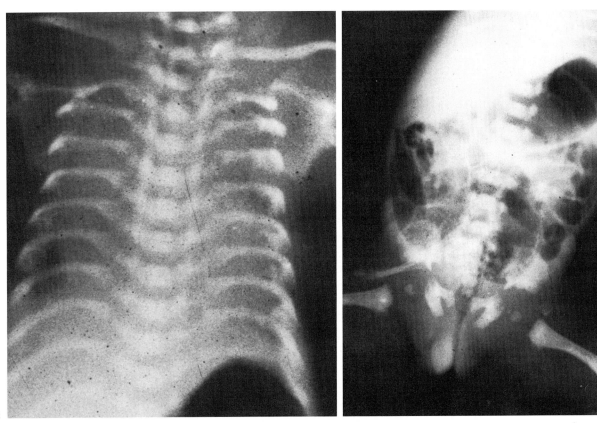

FIGURE 6.197. Asphyxiating thoracic dystrophy. A. Chest. Note the elongated thorax and short ribs. There is anterior cupping of the ribs. **B.** Pelvis and lower extremities. Note the square iliac wings and flat acetabular angles. Also note premature ossification of the proximal femoral epiphysis. (Reproduced with permission from Houston CS, Awen CF, Kent HP. Fatal neonatal dwarfism. J Can Assoc Radiol 1972;23:45–61).

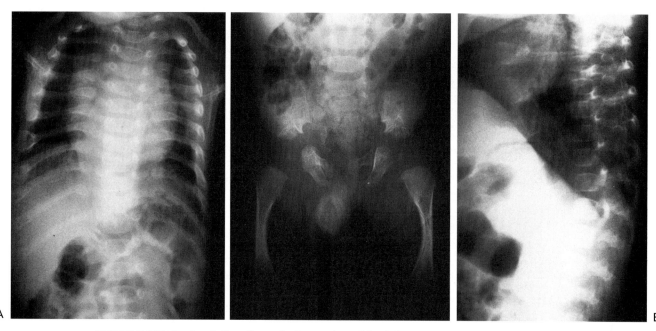

A

B,C

FIGURE 6.198. **Asphyxiating thoracic dystrophy: older infant. A.** Chest. Note narrow chest with short ribs. **B.** Pelvis. Note the squared-off iliac wings. **C.** Spine. Note normal configuration of the vertebral bodies.

bulbous appearance as they do in achondroplasia. Furthermore, the proximal femoral epiphyses are prematurely visible in asphyxiating thoracic dystrophy, and this in itself constitutes an abnormal and highly suggestive finding for the entity.

Another major diagnostic point used in differentiating achondroplasia and/or thanatophoric dwarfism from asphyxiating thoracic dystrophy lies in the configuration of the spine. In asphyxiating thoracic dystrophy, there is neither significant underdevelopment of the vertebral bodies nor narrowing of the spinal canal (Fig. 6.198C). Curvatures in lateral projection are near normal, and the skull also is normal. There is no foramen magnum constriction. All these features handsomely serve to differentiate asphyxiating thoracic dystrophy from achondroplasia, thanatophoric dwarfism, and achondrogenesis. There is, however, difficulty in differentiating asphyxiating thoracic dystrophy from the Ellis-van Creveld syndrome because the skeletal abnormalities, including polydactyly, are similar. Differentiating points are covered in the next section.

REFERENCES

1. Herdman RC, Langer LO. The thoracic asphyxiant dystrophy and renal disease. Am J Dis Child 1968;116:192–201.
2. Shah KJ. Renal lesion in Jeune's syndrome. Br J Radiol 1980;53:432–436.

Ellis-van Creveld Syndrome

Ellis-van Creveld syndrome presenting in the neonatal period has skeletal changes similar to those of asphyxiating thoracic dystrophy. However, they represent different conditions. The two can be differentiated as follows: (a) Polydactyly in asphyxiating thoracic dystrophy is less common and involves the lateral side of the hand, whereas in Ellis-van Creveld syndrome, it usually involves the medial side; (b) congenital heart disease is almost always present in Ellis-van Creveld syndrome but is not a particularly common feature of asphyxiating thoracic dystrophy; (c) consanguinity is more common in the Ellis-van Creveld syndrome; and (d) the thoracic cage deformity is usually not as pronounced in the Ellis-van Creveld syndrome. As far as the roentgenographic changes are concerned, the long bones usually are shorter and more bowed in the Ellis-van Creveld syndrome than in asphyxiating thoracic dystrophy (Fig. 6.199).

One of the roentgenographic hallmarks of Ellis-van Creveld syndrome is carpal fusion (Fig. 6.200). In addition, it has been demonstrated that some of these patients may also demonstrate polycarpaly, with a ninth carpal bone appearing in the distal row (1).

REFERENCE

1. Taylor GA, Jordan CE, Dorst SK, et al. Polycarpaly and other

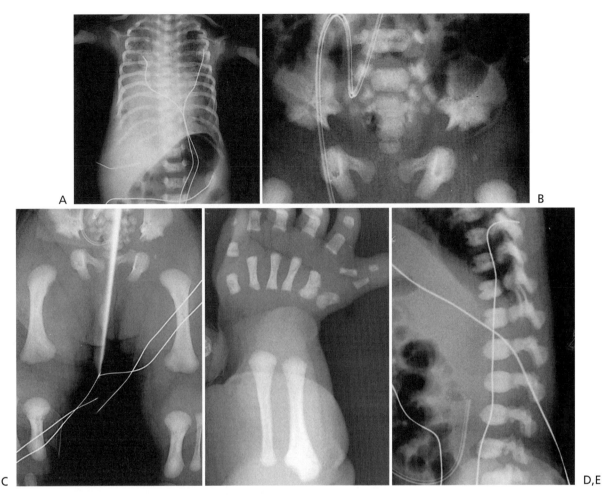

FIGURE 6.199. Ellis-van Creveld syndrome: infancy. A. Thorax. The thorax is elongated and the ribs are shortened. **B.** Pelvis. Note typical square iliac wings with corrugated inferior edges. The findings are similar to those of thanatophoric dwarfism and achondroplasia. **C.** Lower extremities. Note the short, slightly dumbbell-shaped long bones. **D.** Upper extremity. Similar dumbbell configuration of the radius and ulna, which are markedly shortened. All of the small bones of the hands are shortened, but note polydactyly. **E.** Spine. The vertebral bodies are normal.

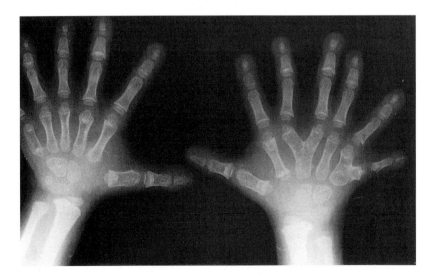

FIGURE 6.200. Ellis-van Creveld syndrome. Note bilateral polydactyly and also that the distance between the ossified carpal bones is narrower than normal and heralds future fusion.

abnormalities of the wrist in chondroectodermal dysplasia: the Ellis-van Creveld syndrome. Radiology 1984;151:393–396.

Short Rib-Polydactyly Syndrome (Majewski and Saldino-Noonan Types)

The short rib-polydactyly syndrome is a syndrome consisting of severe micromeric dwarfism, marked thoracic dystrophy, and polydactyly. Two forms have been defined—the Majewski and Saldino-Noonan types (1)—but intrinsic variability does exist (2). The Saldino-Noonan type is more common and is characterized by severe shortening of the ribs, anterior cupping of the ribs, and marked shortening of the extremities. In addition, the ends of the long bones are cupped and ragged or scooped out (Fig. 6.201, A–C). The appearance of the pelvis is not unlike that seen in asphyxiating thoracic dystrophy or the Ellis-van Creveld syndrome. Vertebral body underdevelopment is variable in both types, and in the Majewski type, the very short tibia and fibula without cupping is characteristic (Fig. 6.201, D-F).

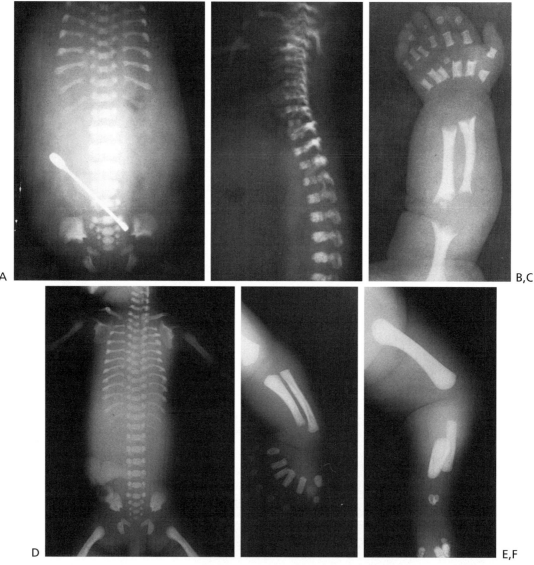

FIGURE 6.201. Short rib-polydactyly syndrome: Saldino-Noonan type. A. Note the elongated thorax and markedly shortened ribs. Also note the square appearance of the iliac wings. **B.** Lateral view demonstrating the extremely short ribs and the markedly underdeveloped vertebrae. **C.** Upper extremity demonstrating polydactyly and typical appearance of the scooped-out metaphyseal regions of the shortened long bones. **D. Majewski type.** Note somewhat similar changes, but the iliac wings are not as hypoplastic. **E.** Upper extremity shows short bones but no metaphyseal cupping. Note polydactyly. **F.** Lower extremity showing short tibia and fibula. (**C** courtesy of David Rogers, M.D.).

REFERENCES

1. Saldino RM, Noonan CD. Severe thoracic dystrophy with striking micromelia, abnormal osseous development, including the spine, and multiple visceral anomalies. AJR 1972;114:257–263.
2. Sillence D, Kozlowski K, Bar-Ziv J, et al. Perinatally lethal short rib-polydactyly syndrome. 1. Variability in known syndromes. Pediatr Radiol 1987;17:474–480.

Metatropic Dwarfism

Metatropic dwarfism can be confused with achondroplasia and thanatophoric dwarfism because there are marked shortening of the extremities and a resemblance in their pelvic configuration. The calvarium usually is normal, however, and there is no foramen magnum constriction. A few infants may be so severely afflicted that they present with hypoplastic lungs and respiratory distress at birth, but this is rare (1). Roentgenographically (2), the key findings consist of a dumbbell-like appearance to the shortened bones of the extremities and severe generalized platyspondyly (Fig. 6.202). The more severely afflicted the infant, the more pronounced these changes, and overall the changes resemble those seen in the Kniest syndrome (see next section).

In addition to the foregoing findings, the ribs are short and the spinal canal variably narrowed, being more evident in the more severe cases (1). In addition, as with many chondrodystrophies, hypoplasia of C1 and the dens can lead to upper cervical spine instability (3). Recently, a new subtype with advanced skeletal age and radial head dislocation has been described (4).

REFERENCES

1. Perri G. A severe form of metatropic dwarfism. Pediatr Radiol 1978;7:183–185.
2. Kozlowski K, Morris L, Reinwein H, et al. Metatropic dwarfism and its variants. Australas Radiol 1976;20:367–385.
3. Shohat M, Lachman R, Rimoin L. Odontoid hypoplasia with vertebral cervical subluxation and ventriculomegaly in metatropic dysplasia. J Pediatr 1989;114:239–243.
4. Nishimura G, Satoh M, Aihara T, et al. A distinct subtype of "metatrophic dysplasia variant" characterized by advanced carpal skeletal age and subluxation of the radial heads. Pediatr Radiol 1998;28:120–125.

Kniest Syndrome

Kniest syndrome is characterized by retinal detachment, deafness, and bony dysplasia (1). Myopia also occurs, along with limited joint motion and large painful joints. The long bones are short and have a dumbbell appearance as a result of marked splaying of the metaphysis and enlargement of the epiphyses (Fig. 6.203). Punctate epiphyseal calcifications can occur, and the bony changes are progressive from infancy. In addition, coxa vara deformity is marked, and

there is generalized platyspondyly with irregular vertebral endplates. Upper cervical spine underdevelopment with instability also can be seen (2). These skeletal changes can be seen from birth, and overall they most closely resemble those of metatropic dwarfism and Dyggve-Melchior-Clausen syndrome.

REFERENCES

1. Kozlowski K, Barylak A, Kobielowa Z. Kniest syndrome. Australas Radiol 1977;21:60–67.
2. Merrill KD, Schmidt TL. Occipitoatlantal instability in a child with Kniest syndrome. J Pediatr Orthop 1989;9:338–340.

Cleidocranial Dysostosis

Cleidocranial dysostosis is transmitted as an autosomal dominant trait and has a strong familial incidence. Sporadic cases, however, also occur. The roentgenographic diagnosis of cleidocranial dysostosis can be made at birth because many of the typical skeletal features are readily apparent at this stage. Clinically, the diagnosis is often suspected by the presence of slight frontal and biparietal bossing of the calvarium and palpably absent clavicles (1). In addition, extreme thinness and underossification of the membranous bones of the calvarium are seen. As a consequence, the fontanelles are unduly large and the sutures excessively "wide" (Fig. 6.204B). In other infants, these findings may be less striking.

The clavicles may be totally absent, absent only in part, or merely mildly hypoplastic. In some cases, the clavicles may be almost normal in appearance, but most patients show some clavicular underdevelopment. Changes in the pelvis include underossification and underdevelopment of the pelvic bones (Fig. 6.204A). In the hands and feet, one may note hypoplasia and underossification of the terminal phalanges.

Most of the skeletal changes just described persist into later childhood, and in the skull, wormian bone formation often becomes exuberant (Fig. 6.205). The calvarial sutures remain unusually prominent, and the base of the skull along with the petrous bone becomes sclerotic. Clavicular and pelvic changes also persist into adulthood, and late long bone changes consist of abnormalities in tubulation and curvature. Associated hearing loss also has been reported (2).

REFERENCES

1. Tan KL, Tan LKA. Cleidocranial dysostosis in infancy. Pediatr Radiol 1981;11:114–116.
2. Hawkins HB, Shapiro R, Petrillo CJ. The association of cleidocranial dysostosis with hearing loss. AJR 1975;125:944–947.

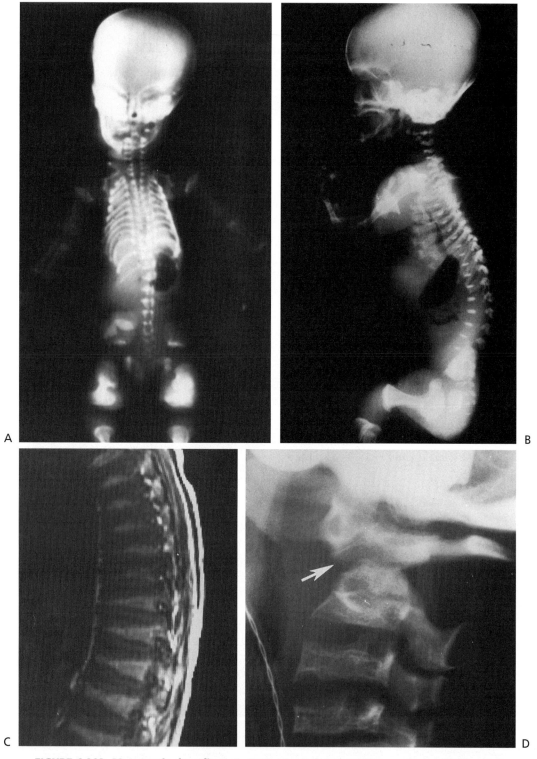

FIGURE 6.202. Metatropic dwarfism. A. Note extremely narrow thorax, shortened ribs, and typical dumbbell configuration of the long bones. This is the result of exceptional widening of the metaphyses. Also note the squared iliac wings and what would appear to be a narrowed spinal canal. **B.** Lateral view showing shortening of the ribs and marked flattening and underdevelopment of the vertebral bodies. **C.** Sagittal T2-weighted magnetic resonance study of the spine demonstrates universal platyspondyly and thick discs. **D.** Same patient demonstrating a hypoplastic dens and an anomalous upper cervical spine. (**A** and **B** reproduced with permission from Houston CS, Awen CF, Kent HP. Fatal neonatal dwarfism. J Can Assoc Radiol 1972;23:45–61).

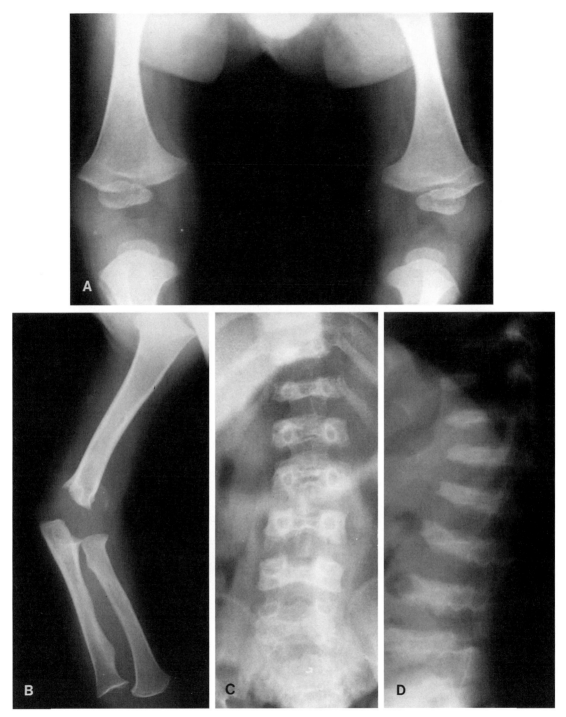

FIGURE 6.203. Kniest syndrome. A. Lower extremities. Note the markedly shortened long bones and dumbbell appearance resulting from enlargement and flaring of the metaphyses. **B.** Upper extremity demonstrating similar changes. **C.** Spine demonstrating universal platyspondyly and narrowing of the spinal canal. **D.** Lateral view of the spine demonstrating pronounced platyspondyly.

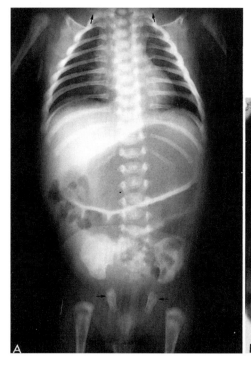

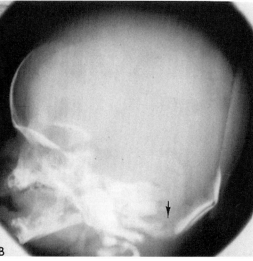

Figure 6.204. Cleidocranial dysostosis. A. Note the extremely hypoplastic clavicles (upper arrows) and partial absence of the pubic bones (lower arrows). In normal newborn infants, the transverse portions of the pubic bones are always well visualized. In cleidocranial dysostosis, these bones remain unossified, and only the ischia are seen. Frequently, they appear somewhat more oval than normal. **B.** Marked under-ossification of the membranous portion of the calvarium with no visualization of the parietal bone. Note the large anterior fontanelle and the unusually wide innominate or posterior occipital synchondrosis (arrow).

Pyknodysostosis

Pyknodysostosis is usually diagnosed after the neonatal period, whereupon the infants closely resemble those with cleidocranial dysostosis (1). Calvarial and clavicular changes are similar (including wide sutures), except that generalized skeletal osteosclerosis is present (Fig. 6.206). Such osteosclerosis does not occur in typical cleidocranial dysostosis. Infants with pyknodysostosis can also show acro-osteolysis of the dis-tal phalanges, increased bone fragility with pathologic fracture, dental abnormalities, and hypoplasia of the mandible.

REFERENCE

1. Srivastava KK, Bhattacharya AK, Galatius-Jensen F, et al. Pycnodysostosis (report of four cases). Australas Radiol 1978;22: 70–78.

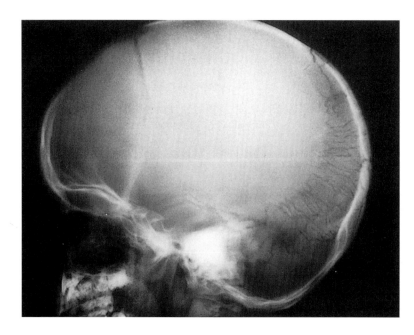

FIGURE 6.205. Cleidocranial dysostosis: marked wormian bone formation. Note exaggerated wormian bone formation in this patient with a large, round calvarium and flattened base of the skull.

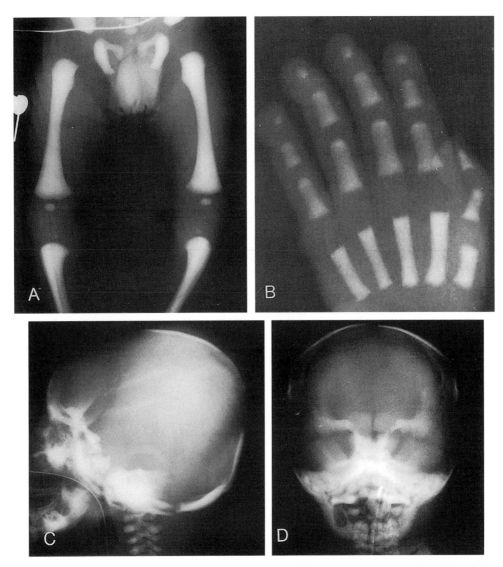

FIGURE 6.206. Pyknodysostosis. A. Typical sclerosis of the long bones. Note that the pubic bones are intact. **B.** Hands demonstrating sclerosis of the bones and hypoplasia of the terminal phalanges. **C and D.** Calvarium demonstrating sclerosis of the facial bones and base of the skull. Note that the sutures are unusually prominent.

Progeria (Hutchinson-Gilford Syndrome)

Progeria may have onset at birth, but changes usually develop later. Typically, features include thinning of the skin, alopecia, hypoplasia of the nails, and progressive loss of subcutaneous fat. Periarticular fibrosis also is usually present, and limitation of movement of the extremities occurs early. The life span of these infants is markedly shortened by the development of premature senility, arteriosclerosis, vascular calcification, and myocardial infarction.

Roentgenographic findings consist of generalized skeletal osteoporosis and hypoplasia, thin calvarial bones, persistently open fontanelles, thin long bones, ribs, and clavicles (Fig. 6.207), a small thoracic cage, and hypoplasia of the facial bones and mandible. Progressive bony resorption occurs at various sites, but it is especially pronounced in the clavicles and long bones. Some of these infants may also demonstrate early scleroderma-like changes, and coronary heart disease eventually becomes a problem.

Metaphyseal Dysostosis (Dysplasia)

The terms "metaphyseal dysostosis" and "metaphyseal dysplasia" are nonspecific but generally are used to refer to those cases demonstrating dysplastic bone changes confined primarily to the metaphyseal regions. In this regard, there are at least three known types: the Jansen (1, 2), Schmid (3, 4), and McKusick (5) forms. The Schmid type of metaphyseal dysostosis usually is not a problem in the neonate, but

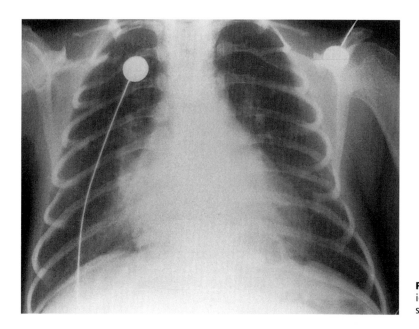

FIGURE 6.207. Progeria. Older child with thin clavicles and ribs. The heart is enlarged, and there is passive congestion secondary to myocardial disease.

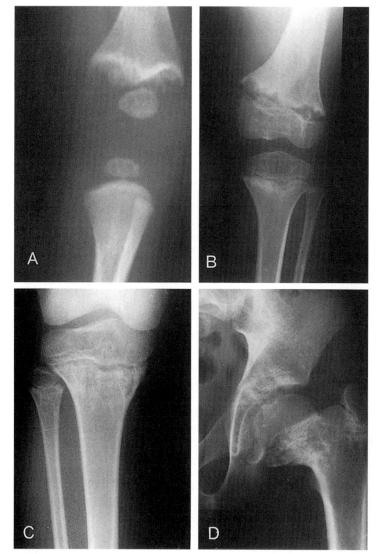

FIGURE 6.208. Metaphyseal dysostosis: Schmid type.
A. Infant with typical flaring and scalloping of the metaphysis. Note the sclerotic zone of provisional calcification. **B.** An older child with typical changes of metaphyseal dysostosis. **C.** Less typical changes of metaphyseal dysostosis in the upper tibia and fibula. **D.** Same patient demonstrating similar changes in the femoral neck.

the Jansen type tends to appear in the neonate and young infant, manifesting with radiographic changes mimicking those of hyperparathyroidism.

Roentgenographically, the metaphyseal findings of metaphyseal dysostosis, especially in the Schmid type, can be confused with those of rickets, hypophosphatasia, or even the battered child syndrome. The reason for this is that there are excessive cupping and fraying of the metaphyses. Usually, however, the zone of provisional calcification is still quite dense, and thus both rickets and hypophosphatasia become less likely possibilities (Fig. 6.208). Later, as the patient matures, the metaphyseal changes become less pronounced and merely consist of somewhat poorly formed metaphyses and irregular epiphyseal-metaphyseal junctions (Fig. 6.208). Eventually, even though there is persistent shortening of the bones, metaphyseal changes disappear (3). In the Jansen type, cortical erosions just proximal to the frayed and poorly mineralized metaphyses of these young infants more closely resemble the changes of hyperparathyroidism (Fig. 6.209). Those infants who survive demonstrate more grotesque deformities and severe growth and joint function impairment. The metaphyses and adjoining epiphyses become large and bulbous (2, 3). Eventually, the skull in these patients becomes thickened along the base, and the zygomatic bones become overly prominent.

The cartilage-hair hypoplasia syndrome of McKusick usually presents because of problems with malabsorption or failure to thrive. The reason for this is that pancreatic insufficiency and neutropenia are part of the syndrome. Skeletal changes consist of metaphyseal abnormalities similar to those of the Schmid type of metaphyseal dysostosis, shortening of the ribs with anterior cupping, vertebral body flattening, and dwarfism. The hair in these individuals is fine and sparse, and generalized hypotonicity of the muscles is common. Related conditions include the Shwachman-Diamond syndrome and the metaphyseal dysostosis-thymolymphopenia syndrome.

REFERENCES

1. Nazara Z, Hernandez A, Corona-Rivera E, et al. Further clinical and radiological features in metaphyseal chondrodysplasia—Jansen type. Radiology 1981;140:697–700.
2. Silverthorn KG, Houston CS, Duncan BP. Murk Jansen's metaphyseal chondrodysplasia with long-term follow-up. Pediatr Radiol 1987;17:119–123.
3. Beluffi G, Fiori P, Notarangelo CD, et al. Metaphyseal dysplasia type Schmid—early x-ray detection and evolution with time. Ann Radiol 1983;26:237–243.
4. Lachman RS, Rimoin DL, Spranger J. Metaphyseal chondrodysplasia, Schmid type clinical and radiographic delineation with a review of the literature. Pediatr Radiol 1988;18:93–102.
5. Stanley P, Sutcliffe J. Metaphyseal chondrodysplasia with dwarfism, pancreatic insufficiency, and neutropenia. Pediatr Radiol 1973;1:119–126.

Diastrophic Dwarfism

On clinical grounds, the rare diastrophic dwarfism can be confused with achondroplasia, but the roentgenographic features usually clearly differentiate the two conditions. The most striking findings are in the spine, feet, and hands. In the spine, scoliosis (not a feature of achondroplasia), although not usually present in early infancy, becomes pronounced as the child grows older. The spinal canal is narrowed in some cases.

Severe clubfoot deformity is usually present at birth, as are the typical abnormalities in the upper extremity. More specifically, these consist of short bones in general, an especially short thumb, and an almost oval first metacarpal (Fig. 6.210A). Similar changes occur in the feet (Fig. 6.10B). The thumb is often markedly abducted and has been termed a "hitchhiker's thumb." The long bones are somewhat flared at their ends, and dislocation of the radial heads and hips can occur. Cervical spine defects also may be seen and can lead to such pronounced kyphosis that neurologic deficit results (1). This, however, is usually more of a problem in older children. Limitation of motion of the joints can cause some confusion with arthrogryposis, but in diastrophic dwarfism, muscle atrophy is not as prominent a feature. Some of these infants also have cysts behind the ears.

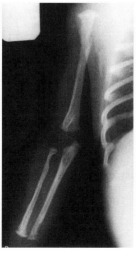

A,B

FIGURE 6.209. Metaphyseal dysostosis: Jansen type. A and B. Seven-week-old infant showing coarse trabecular pattern and numerous metaphyseal cortical erosions. These, at least in roentgenographic appearance, are not unlike the subperiosteal cortical bony absorptive lesions of hyperparathyroidism. Also note a pathologic fracture in the proximal humerus. (Reproduced with permission from Ozonoff MB. Metaphyseal dysostosis of Jansen. Radiology 1969;93:1047–1050).

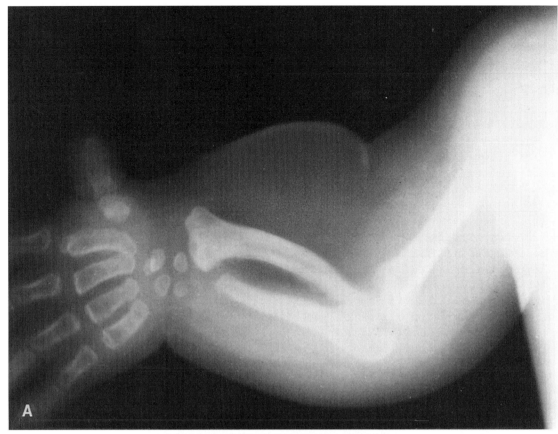

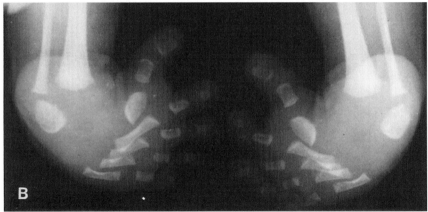

FIGURE 6.210. Diastrophic dwarfism. A. Note the shortened bones of the forearm, underdevelopment of the ulna, bowing of the radius, shortening of the metacarpals and small bones of the hands, and the characteristic extended "hitchhiker's thumb." Also note that the first metacarpal is extremely small and almost oval and that the ends of the long bones are flared. The radial head is also partially dislocated. **B.** Note severe bilateral clubfoot deformity. The small bones of the feet are shortened, and especially note the small oval first metatarsal. (Reproduced with permission from Stover CN, Hayes JT, Holt JF. Diastrophic dwarfism. AJR 1963;89:914–922).

Chondrodystrophia Calcificans Congenita (Conradi's Disease, Stippled Epiphyses)

The relatively uncommon chondrodystrophia calcificans congenita is characterized by stippling of the epiphyses and bones such as the carpal bones, tarsal bones, patella, pelvic bones, and pedicles of the vertebrae. The biochemical abnormality in this condition has been determined to be a lack of phytanic acid oxidation (1, 2). Stippling of the epiphysis is the hallmark of this condition, but stippling need not be uniformly distributed throughout all the bones. In addition, stippling is not exclusive to this condition because it is seen in many other conditions (3) such as Zellweger syndrome and warfarin embryopathy.

Generally speaking, two forms are identified: dominant and recessive varieties. The recessive variety is the one in which the infant is more severely afflicted and frequently dies shortly after birth or in the first year of life. These infants usually show one or more of the following clinical manifestations: shortening and flexion contractures of the extremities, saddle nose deformity, frontal bossing, hypertelorism, cataracts, optic atrophy, renal cysts, and, in some cases, cardiac abnormalities and hypoplastic lungs. It is often one of these associated abnormalities that leads to the early death of these infants. Consanguinity is common in the recessive form. In the more mildly afflicted patients, that is, those with a dominant form of the disease, their problems may pass unnoticed until stippling of the epiphyses is discovered when radiographs are obtained for some other reason.

Typical roentgenographic findings center around punctate calcifications in the epiphyses of the long bones, the tarsal and carpal bones, the patellae, some flat bones, the vertebrae, and cartilaginous structures such as the larynx, trachea, and bronchi. The calcifications are typical and should strongly suggest the diagnosis (Fig. 6.211), but, as

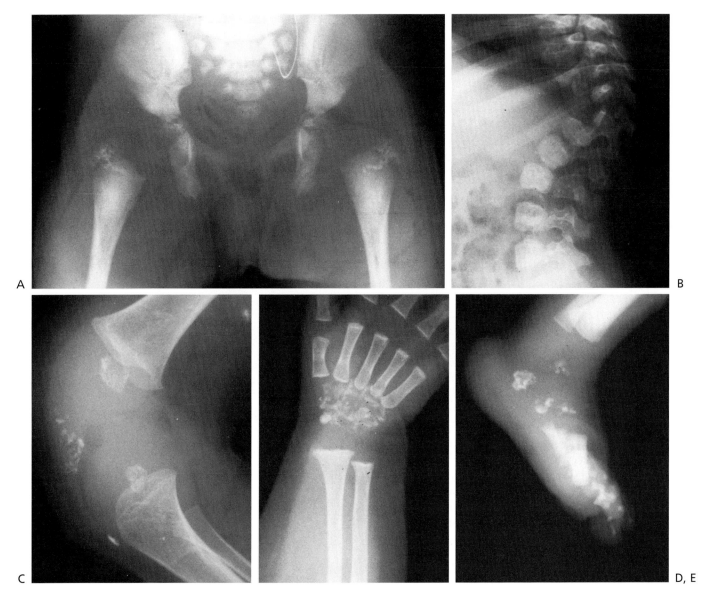

FIGURE 6.211. Chondrodystrophia calcificans congenita: stippled epiphyses. A. Note typical punctate calcifications in the upper femurs and pubic bones. **B.** Note marked kyphosis of the lower thoracic spine caused by severe vertebral underdevelopment. Also note multiple stippled calcifications scattered throughout the spine and along the anterior aspects of the ribs. **C.** Typical calcifications in the patella. **D.** Note multiple calcifications of the carpal bones. **E.** Similar calcifications in the tarsal bones of another infant.

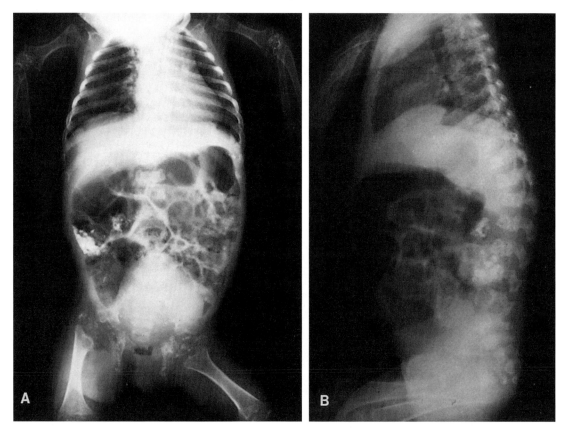

FIGURE 6.212. Chondrodystrophia calcificans congenita: recessive or rhizomelic type. A.
First, note extensive stippling of the various epiphyses. Then, note marked shortening of the
humeri and femurs. The other long bones also are shortened, but predominant shortening occurs
in the proximal segment. **B.** Lateral view demonstrating multiple coronal clefts in the vertebral
bodies. Also note stippling along the spine. (Courtesy of William Culp, M.D.).

mentioned earlier, their distribution can be erratic. This latter phenomenon occurs in the dominant form primarily; in
the recessive form, symmetric distribution is the rule, and
the long bones are shorter. This is especially true of the
proximal segment of the extremities (i.e., humerus, femur),
hence the term "rhizomelic type of punctate epiphyseal dysplasia" (Fig. 6.212). In those infants who survive, calcifications gradually disappear so that virtually all are gone by 6
months to 1 year of age. In more severe cases, residual
deformities of the extremities persist.

The spine characteristically is involved in both types. In
the recessive or rhizomelic type, multiple coronal clefts are
seen on lateral view (Fig. 6.212); in the dominant form,
focal hypoplasia of the vertebrae occurs and can result in
severe kyphoscoliosis (Fig. 6.211) or atlantoaxial dislocation.

REFERENCES

1. Hoefler G, Hoefler S, Watkins PA, et al. Biochemical abnormalities in rhizomelic chondrodysplasia punctata. J Pediatr 1988;112:
726–733.

2. Poulos A, Sheffield L, Sharp P, et al. Rhizomelic chondrodysplasia
punctata: clinical, pathologic, and biochemical findings in two
patients. J Pediatr 1988;113:685–690.

3. Poznanski AK. Punctate epiphyses: a radiological sign, not a disease. Pediatr Radiol 1994;24:418–424.

Multiple Epiphyseal Dysplasia and Spondyloepiphyseal Dysplasia

Chondrodystrophia calcificans congenita (preceding section) is considered a form of multiple epiphyseal dysplasia,
but apart from this, multiple epiphyseal dysplasia is difficult
to diagnose in the neonate. Indeed, often it is an incidental
diagnosis, even in older children. All epiphyses are not normally ossified in infancy, and it is only when the child
becomes older that the characteristic smallness and delayed
development of epiphyses become apparent.

Spondyloepiphyseal dysplasia, on the other hand, has a
congenital form that can present in the neonate and occasionally is lethal (1). Development of the epiphysis is
delayed, and in addition, tarsal bones such as the talus and
calcaneus will not be ossified (Fig. 6.213). Spinal abnormalities consist of universal platyspondylia with small,

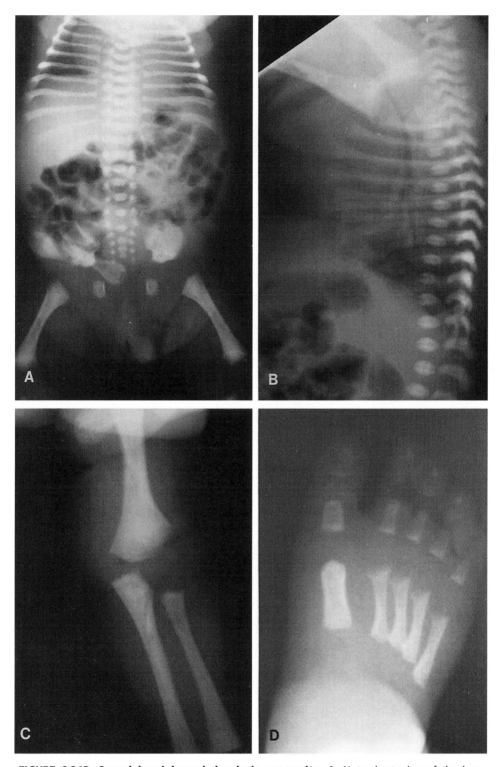

FIGURE 6.213. Spondyloepiphyseal dysplasia congenita. A. Note shortening of the long bones of the lower extremities. There is some metaphyseal flaring present, and the distal femoral and proximal tibial epiphysis are not ossified in this 1-month-old infant (i.e., delay in epiphyseal development). Also note delayed ossification of the pubic bones and that the iliac wings are somewhat square and outwardly flared. The width of the spinal canal is normal. **B.** Lateral view demonstrating typical underdevelopment of the vertebral bodies, which have an oval configuration and demonstrate universal platyspondylia. The bodies in the cervical spine are absent, and the ribs are short. **C.** Upper extremity demonstrating shortening of the long bones and slight flaring of the metaphyses. **D.** Foot demonstrating lack of ossification of the talus and calcaneus. Normally, both of these bones are well ossified at birth. (Courtesy of R. Bombet, M.D., and J. Sims, M.D.).

oval vertebral bodies, abnormal spinal curvatures, and absent vertebral bodies (Fig. 6.213). In older patients, the changes persist and, in fact, become more dramatic. In addition, there is shortening of the long bones, and often this is what causes these patients to first come to the attention of the physician. When the roentgenograms are obtained, cupping and flaring of the metaphyses may at first suggest achondroplasia; thus, this condition often is erroneously considered as the diagnosis. For this reason, these patients often are said to have pseudoachondroplasia. The epiphyseal abnormalities in these patients result in secondary metaphyseal growth impairment and short bones (Fig. 6.214). The vertebrae demonstrate generalized platyspondylia and irregularities of the vertebral bodies (Fig. 6.215A). In some cases, a pear-shaped vertebra results (Fig. 6.215B). In any form of epiphyseal dysplasia, as the patient grows older, the epiphyses remain small and most often have smooth edges. The tarsal and carpal bones also characteristically show underdevelopment, irregularity, and scalloping (Fig. 6.214, B and D). These latter findings are valuable in subtle cases where the smallness of the epiphysis may elude the observer.

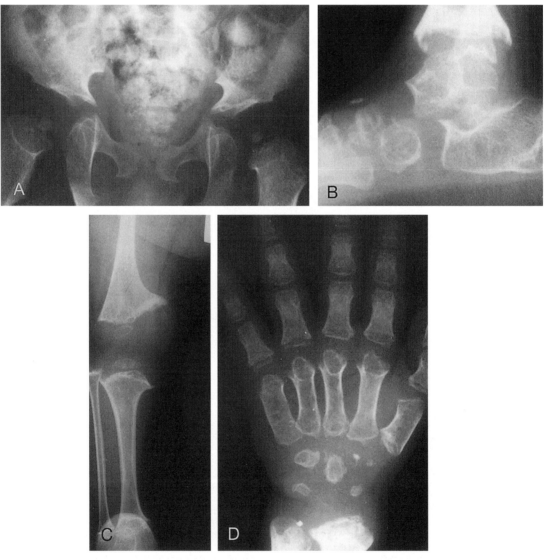

FIGURE 6.214. Spondyloepiphyseal dysplasia: older child. A. Note the small femoral head epiphyses and characteristic appearance of the iliac wings and pelvis. **B.** Scalloped-appearing tarsal bones characteristic of an epiphyseal dysplasia. **C.** Cupping and flaring of the metaphyses and shortening of the bones produce a pseudoachondroplastic appearance. As opposed to achondroplasia, however, the epiphyses are fragmented and underdeveloped. **D.** Hand with short, small bones, small, irregular carpals, and cupping of the distal radius and ulna.

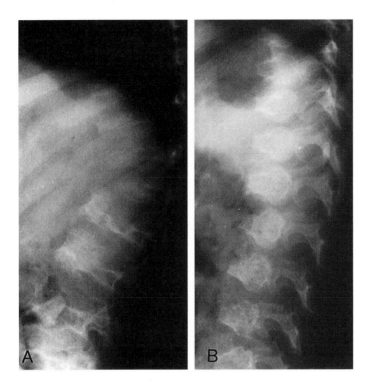

FIGURE 6.215. Spondyloepiphyseal dysplasia: older child. A. Flat vertebral bodies with wide disc spaces and associated kyphosis. **B.** Another patient with pear-shaped vertebrae seen in some patients with spondyloepiphyseal dysplasia.

REFERENCE

1. Macpherson RI, Wood BP. Spondyloepiphyseal dysplasia congenita. A cause of lethal neonatal dwarfism. Pediatr Radiol 1980; 9:217–224.

Spondylometaphyseal Dysplasia

Spondylometaphyseal dysplasia often is familial and is inherited as an autosomal dominant trait (1). Findings are not usually present at birth but develop early in infancy. Findings consist of shortness of stature, generalized platyspondylia (1, 2), coxa vara deformity of the femoral necks (2, 3), irregularity of the acetabula, and dysplastic changes in the metaphyses of the long bones. Changes are often most marked in the metaphyses of the lower extremities and resemble those of metaphyseal dysostosis. Spinal changes are not unlike those of Morquio's disease or spondyloepiphyseal dysplasia. The epiphyses remain relatively normal (Fig. 6.216).

REFERENCES

1. Diren HB, Buyukgebiz B, Buyukgebiz A, et al. Spondylometaphyseal dysplasia, type VII. Pediatr Radiol 1992;22:87–89.
2. Maroteaux P, Spranger J. The spondylometaphyseal dysplasias. A tentative classification. Pediatr Radiol 1991;21:293–297.
3. Langer LO Jr, Brill PW, Ozonoff MB, et al. Spondylometaphyseal dysplasia, corner fracture type: a heritable condition associated with coxa vara. Radiology 1990;175:761–766.

Dysplasia Epiphysealis Hemimelia

In dysplasia epiphysealis hemimelia, unilateral deformity and overgrowth of an epiphysis and adjacent metaphysis (1) occur. The condition may or may not be symptomatic and is more common in the lower extremities, especially in the knee and ankle (Fig. 6.217). MRI is very effective in demonstrating the bony, cartilaginous, and soft tissue changes in these patients (2, 3).

REFERENCES

1. Keret D, Spatz DK, Caro PA, et al. Dysplasia epiphysealis hemimelia: diagnosis and treatment. J Pediatr Orthop 1992;12: 365–372.
2. Peduto AJ, Frawley KJ, Bellemore MC, et al. Original report. MR imaging of dysplasia epiphysealis hemimelica: bony and soft-tissue abnormalities. AJR 1999;172:819–823.
3. Kuo RS, Bellemore MC, Monsell FP, et al. Dysplasia epiphysealis hemimelica: clinical features and management. J Pediatr Orthop 1998;18:543–548.

Progressive Diaphyseal Dysplasia (Engelmann-Camurati Disease)

Progressive diaphyseal dysplasia, frequently referred to as "Engelmann-Camurati disease," is rarely detected before an infant begins to walk. Characteristically, marked muscular weakness (1, 2) and pain and progressive cortical thickening of the diaphyses of the long bones (Fig. 6.218) are

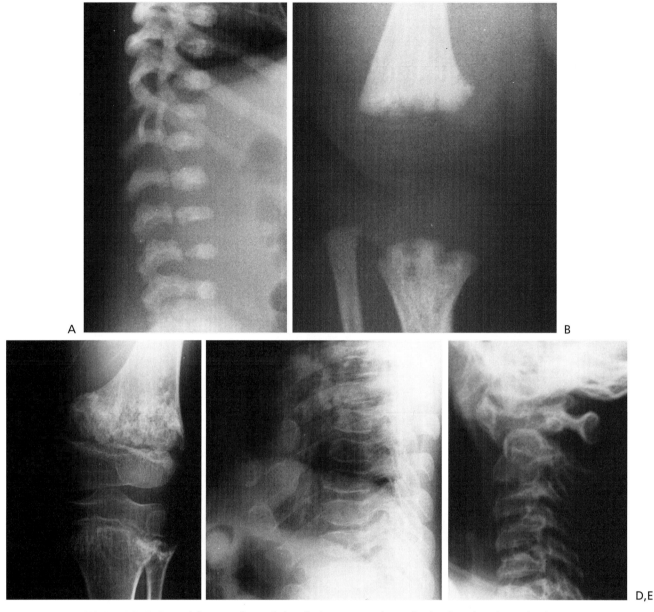

FIGURE 6.216. Spondylometaphyseal dysplasia. A. Note the underdeveloped oval vertebral bodies similar to those seen with spondyloepiphyseal dysplasia. **B.** The metaphyses, however, demonstrate metaphyseal irregularity and lucencies. Slight widening is present. **C.** Older child. Note marked irregularity and flaring of the metaphyses. **D.** Lateral view of the spine demonstrates flat vertebral bodies and marked shortening of the ribs with excessive anterior cupping. **E.** Note hypoplasia of the dens and anomalous development of the upper cervical spine.

present. All the long bones are usually involved, and marked sclerosis of the skull can also be seen. In some of these patients, steroids can be helpful. Similar changes can be seen in Ribbing's disease, another condition manifesting in diaphyseal sclerosis (3).

REFERENCES

1. Naveh Y, Ludatscher R, Alon U, et al. Muscle involvement in progressive diaphyseal dysplasia. Pediatrics 1985;76:944–949.
2. Kaftori JK, Kleinhaus U, Naveh Y. Progressive diaphyseal dysplasia (Camurati-Englemann): radiographic follow-up and CT findings. Radiology 1987;164:777–782.
3. Seeger LL, Hewel KC, Yao L, et al. Ribbing disease (multiple diaphyseal sclerosis): imaging and differential diagnosis. AJR 1996;167:639–694.

Pyle's Disease and Craniometaphyseal Dysplasia

Pyle's disease and craniometaphyseal dysplasia may be interrelated, for both conditions demonstrate marked widening

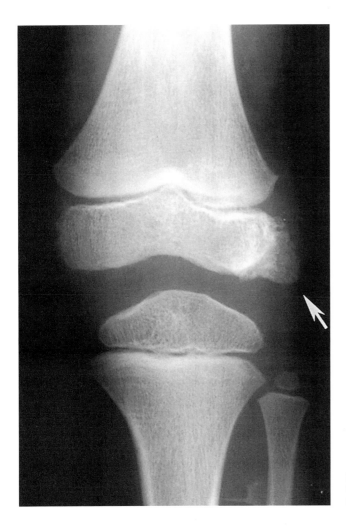

FIGURE 6.217. Epiphyseal dysplasia hemimelica. Note hypertrophy and a unilateral exostotic appearance of the distal femoral epiphysis (arrow).

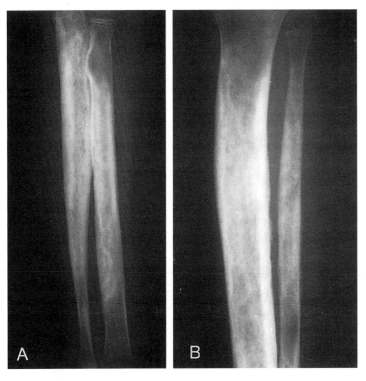

A

B

FIGURE 6.218. Englemann's disease (diaphyseal dysplasia). A and B. Note characteristic periosteal thickening with widening of the shafts of the long bones.

of the metaphyses of the long bones and the findings can be seen in infancy but are exaggerated in older children (Fig. 6.219). In the craniometaphyseal dysplasia type, hyperostosis of the skull may be so profound that visual impairment and facial nerve paralysis result. The widened metaphyseal deformities often are referred to as "Erlenmeyer flask deformities" and are more pronounced in older patients. A similar configuration, along with expansion of other bones such as the clavicles, ribs, and bones of the hands, can be seen in the otopalatodigital syndrome (see next section). Recently, platyspondylia has also been noted to occur in Pyle's disease

(1). Craniometaphyseal dysostosis can be treated with calcitonin (2, 3).

REFERENCES

1. Turra S, Gigante C, Pavanini G, et al. Spinal involvement in Pyle's disease. Pediatr Radiol 2000;30:25–27.
2. Fanconi S, Fischer JA, Wieland P, et al. Craniometaphyseal dysplasia with increased bone turnover and secondary hyperparathyroidism: therapeutic effect of calcitonin. J Pediatr 1988;112: 587–591.

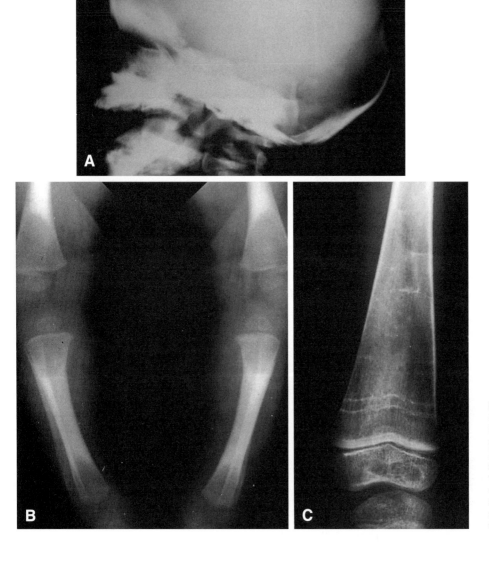

FIGURE 6.219. Pyle's disease (metaphyseal dysplasia). A. Note hyperostosis of the base of the skull and facial bones. The skull itself is a little large, and the patient demonstrated biparietal widening on frontal view. **B.** Lower extremities demonstrate metaphyseal flaring and lucency as compared with the sclerotic diaphyses. **C.** Older patient with metaphyseal widening.

3. Key LL Jr, Volberg F, Baron R, et al. Treatment of craniometaphyseal dysplasia with calcitriol. J Pediatr 1988;112:583–587.

Otopalatodigital Syndrome

In the otopalatodigital syndrome, the overall bony findings are similar to those seen in Pyle's disease (Fig. 6.220). These consist of widening of the metaphyses, eventually some curvature to the long bones, and characteristic-appearing hands. The individual bones show shortening of the first digit and slight ballooning and metaphyseal widening of the individual small bones. The terminal phalanges also are broad. Other findings include frontal bossing, facial hypoplasia, cleft palate, and conductive deafness. These features are seen in type I otopalatodigital syndrome. In type II otopalatodigital syndrome (1–4), which usually presents in the neonate, the mandible is small, the midface hypoplastic, and the long bones may be bowed, hypoplastic, or absent (fibula). Metacarpals and metatarsals are hypoplastic, as are the phalanges. Type II dwarfism often is lethal at birth (1).

REFERENCES

1. Gendall PW, Kozlowski K. Oto-palato-digital syndrome type II. Report of two related cases. Pediatr Radiol 1992;22:267–269.
2. Kozlowski K, Turner G, Scougall J, et al. Oto-palato-digital syn-

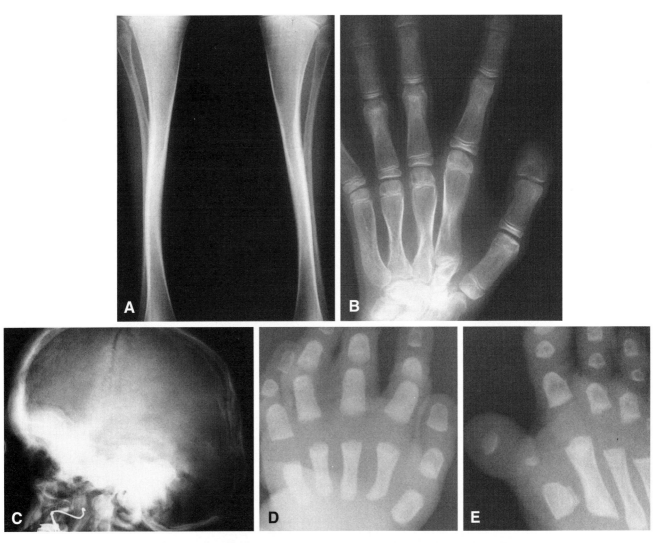

FIGURE 6.220. Otopalatodigital syndrome. A. Tibia and fibula demonstrating characteristic curvature and metaphyseal widening. **B.** Typical appearance of the hands, showing ballooning of the bones. **C.** Note facial hypoplasia and marked thickening of the calvarium involving both the membranous and the basal portions. **D.** Hand in an infant. The bones are short and broad. Exaggerated shortening of the thumb and clinodactyly of the fifth digit are seen. **E.** Foot in the same infant demonstrating similar findings but more pronounced hypoplasia of the first digit.

drome with severe x-ray changes in two half-brothers. Pediatr Radiol 1977;6:97–102.

3. Langer LO. The roentgenographic features of the otopalatodigital (OPD) syndrome. AJR 1967;100:63.
4. Taybi H. Generalized skeletal dysplasia with multiple anomalies. AJR 1962;88:450.

Frontometaphyseal Dysplasia

Frontometaphyseal dysplasia is rare in the neonate and infant (1). In older infants and children, widening of the metaphyses is not as pronounced as in Pyle's disease, and as opposed to craniometaphyseal dysplasia, it is the frontal bone that becomes hyperostotic in these patients. Similar changes in association with craniosynostosis have been documented in the Shprintzen-Goldberg syndrome (2).

REFERENCES

1. Nishimura G, Takano H, Aihara T, et al. Radiological changes of frontometaphyseal dysplasia in the neonate. Pediatr Radiol 1995; 25:S143–S146.

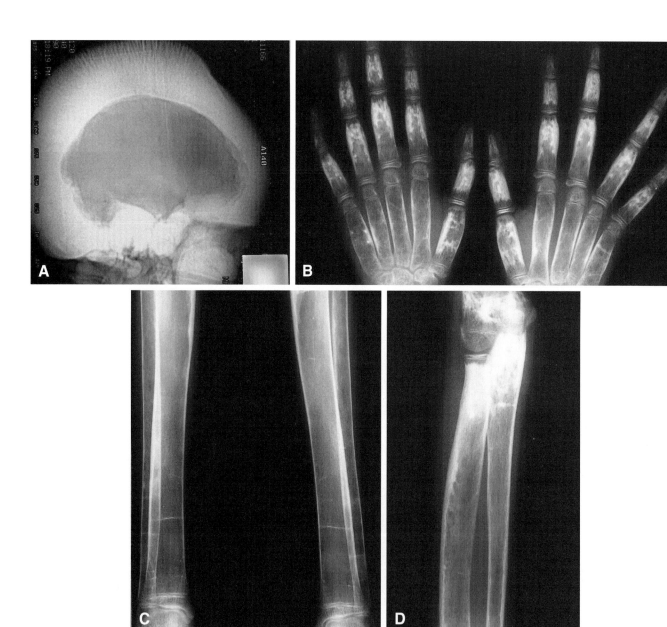

FIGURE 6.221. Craniodiaphyseal dysostosis. A. Note profound thickening of the calvarium and facial bones. **B.** Small bones of the hands show diaphyseal widening and ballooning of the bones along with patchy sclerosis. **C.** Lower extremities demonstrate widening of the diaphyses. **D.** Similar changes in the bones of the forearm.

2. Nishimura G, Nagai T. Radiographic findings in Shprintzen-Goldberg syndrome. Pediatr Radiol 1996;26:775–778.

Craniodiaphyseal Dysplasia

Craniodiaphyseal dysplasia can present in infancy and consists of dilation of the diaphyses of the bones, relatively normal metaphyses, and hyperostosis of the long bones, face, and skull. Widening of the ribs and clavicles also can occur, and the disease is progressive (Fig. 6.221).

Dyschondrosteosis

Dyschondrosteosis is characterized by shortening of the middle segment of the extremities. In the upper extremity, Madelung's deformity is characteristic (Fig. 6.222), and Madelung's deformity is believed to represent the simplest form of this syndrome.

Spondylothoracic Dysplasia

Spondylothoracic dysplasia consists of a grotesque and bizarre deformity of the ribs and almost the entire spine (1, 2). Marked vertebral column shortening, widening of the spinal canal, and numerous vertebral anomalies consisting of hemivertebra, absent vertebra, cleft vertebra, and open neutral arches are present. Marked deepening of the anteroposterior diameter of the chest cage and severe deformity of the spinal column lead to posterior crowding and a fan-like appearance of the ribs on frontal roentgenograms (Fig. 6.223).

REFERENCES

1. Fogarty EE, Beatty T, Dowling F. Spondylo-costal dysplasia in identical twins. J Pediatr Orthop 1985;5:720–721.
2. Kozlowski K. Spondylo-costal dysplasia: severe and moderate types (report of 8 cases). Australas Radiol 1981;25:81–90.

Mesomelic Dwarfism

Mesomelic dwarfism presents at birth and is characterized by marked shortening of the middle segment of the extremities (i.e., radius and humerus, tibia, and fibula). In the Nievergelt type, shortening of these bones is extreme, and synostoses between the radius and ulna are common. In the Langer type, shortening is a little less pronounced (Fig. 6.224), and in the lower extremities, the fibula often is more involved than is the tibia (1). To a lesser degree, the same is true of the ulna. In addition, there is hypoplasia of the mandible.

Pelvis-Shoulder Dysplasia

Pelvis-shoulder dysplasia is a rare condition that can present in infancy and is characterized by symmetrical hypoplasia of the iliac wings and scapulae. The iliac wings are square, and the acetabular roof is flat. Unstable hips can be associated, and lumbar lordosis, along with a waddling gait, can accompany the syndrome. Minor bony changes occur in the femurs, lumbar spine, and ribs. Pelvic dysplasia without shoulder involvement has recently been documented (1), and scapular (glenoid) dysplasia also can occur alone (2).

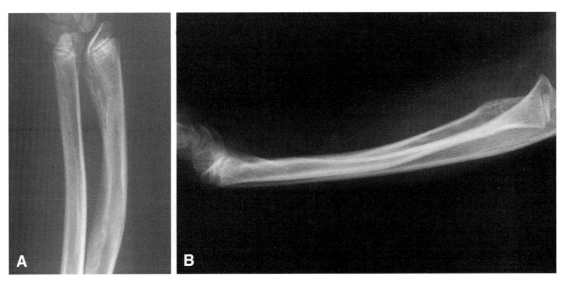

FIGURE 6.222. Madelung's deformity: dysosteochondrosis. A. Note typical bowing of the bones of the forearm, hypoplasia of their distal ends, and characteristic slant of the distal radius. **B.** Lateral view demonstrates the typical deformity of the wrist.

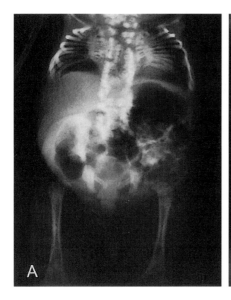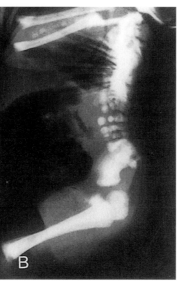

FIGURE 6.223. Spondylothoracic dysplasia. A. Note typical fan-like radiation of ribs resulting from posterior crowding secondary to numerous vertebral and neural arch anomalies. **B.** Lateral view showing pronounced shortening of the spine and prominent dorsolumbar lordosis. Once again, the numerous vertebral anomalies are visible. (Reproduced with permission from Moseley JE, Bonforte RJ. Spondylothoracic dysplasia—a syndrome of congenital anomalies. AJR 1969;106: 166–169).

REFERENCES

1. Hauser SE, Chemke JM, Bankier A. Pelvis shoulder dysplasia. Pediatr Radiol 1998;28:681–682.
2. Currarino G, Sheffield E, Twickler D. Congenital glenoid dysplasia. Pediatr Radiol 1998;28:30–37.

Dyssegmental Dwarfism

Dyssegmental dwarfism is a rare lethal anisospondylic camptomicromelic form of dwarfism. Most likely, it is inherited on an autosomal recessive basis and is characterized by a short neck, short, bent long bones, a narrow chest, cleft

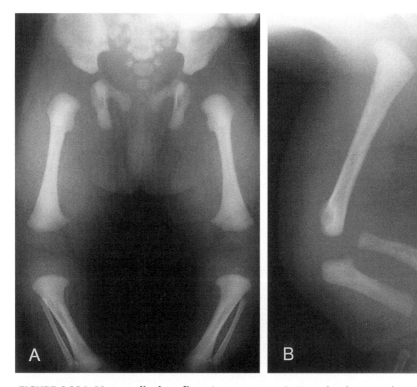

FIGURE 6.224. Mesomelic dwarfism: Langer type. A. Note the short, stocky extremities with some degree of metaphyseal flaring. Note, however, that the tibiae and the fibulae show more shortening than the femur. The fibula is the shortest bone of all. **B.** Upper extremity demonstrating marked shortening and deformity of the radius and ulna.

palate, and reduced joint mobility. Roentgenographically, the short, bent long bones show metaphyseal flaring and to some extent resemble other dysplasias with such flaring. Most commonly, the condition is confused with Kniest syndrome, but the fact that the vertebral bodies are of variable size and of bizarre round to oval shape should distinguish the two conditions. Indeed, the variable-sized vertebral bodies distinguish this form of dwarfism from all other forms.

DRUG-INDUCED SYNDROMES

Aminopterin-Induced Syndrome

If aminopterin, a folic acid antagonist, is ingested by the mother during the first trimester of pregnancy, abnormalities in the fetus can occur (aminopterin fetopathy). The primary problem is one of skeletal dysplasia, with a variety of calvarial and skeletal changes present. In the skull, changes consist of sutural synostosis, hypoplasia of various calvarial bones, and maxillary hypoplasia. Clubfoot deformity, hypoplasia of the bones of the extremities, and narrowing of the medullary space of the long bones occur.

Fetal Alcohol Syndrome

Clinically, infants suffering from the fetal alcohol syndrome are smaller than normal and fail to thrive. Microcephaly is common (1), along with short, flat palpebral fissures and limitation of joint motion. In addition, congenital abnormalities of almost every system can occur. There also is an increased incidence of neuroblastoma and ganglioneuroma and other adrenal tumors in these infants. Abnormal external genitalia also can occur.

The DiGeorge syndrome (2) and punctate epiphyseal dysplasia (3) also have been documented in this syndrome,

and from a radiographic standpoint, fusion of the carpal bones along with radioulnar synostosis (4) and tibial exostoses (5) also have been noted. In addition, we have encountered two infants demonstrating peripheral phalangeal abnormalities consisting of hypoplasia of the terminal phalanges in one patient and overgrown terminal phalanges with shortened fingers in another (Fig. 6.225). In another infant, dumbbell-shaped long bones and thick ribs with overall dwarfism suggesting a chondrodystrophy were seen (Fig. 6.226).

REFERENCES

1. Swayze WW II, Johnson VP, Hanson JW, et al. Magnetic resonance imaging of brain anomalies of fetal alcohol syndrome. Pediatrics 1997;99:232–240.
2. Ammann AJ, Wara DW, Cowan MJ, et al. The DiGeorge syndrome and the fetal alcohol syndrome. Am J Dis Child 1982; 136:906–908.
3. Leicher-Duber A, Schumacher R, Spranger J. Stippled epiphyses in fetal alcohol syndrome. Pediatr Radiol 1990;20:369–370.
4. Cremin BJ, Jaffer A. Radiological aspects of the fetal alcohol syndrome. Pediatr Radiol 1981;11:151–153.
5. Azouz EM, Kavianian G, Der Kaloustian VM. Fetal alcohol syndrome and bilateral tibial exostoses. A case report. Pediatr Radiol 1993;23:615–616.

Cocaine-Induced Syndrome

In cocaine-induced syndrome, believed to result from cocaine-induced vasospasm in the fetus (1, 2), many anomalies have been documented, including central nervous system abnormalities (3), genitourinary malformations, prune belly syndrome, terminal limb reduction defects, and ileal atresia. In addition, basal ganglia infarcts and intracranial vascular hemorrhage can occur (1, 4).

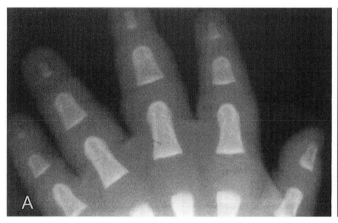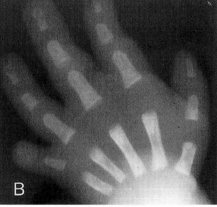

FIGURE 6.225. Fetal alcohol syndrome. A. Note peripheral phalangeal hypoplasia. **B.** Another patient with hypoplasia of the fifth digit and peculiar, somewhat overgrown terminal phalanges of the second, third, and fourth digits.

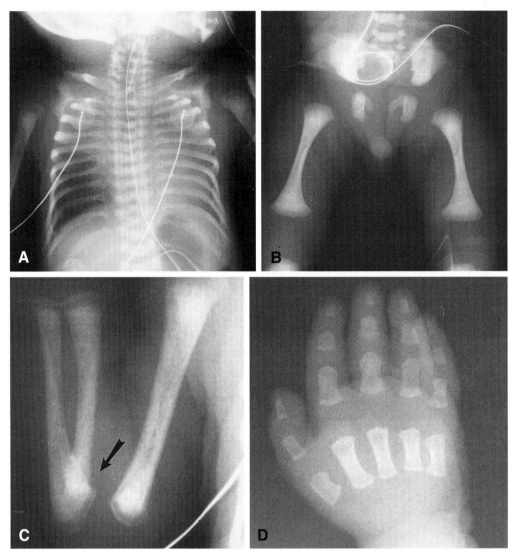

FIGURE 6.226. Fetal alcohol syndrome. A. Chest demonstrating broad medial clavicles. **B.** Long bones show slight dumbbell configuration. **C.** Radioulnar synostosis (arrow) is present in the elbow. **D.** The long bones of the hands are short and squat, and the terminal phalanges are underdeveloped. The thumb is relatively hypoplastic.

REFERENCES

1. Heier LA, Carpanzano CR, Mast J, et al. Maternal cocaine abuse: the spectrum of radiologic abnormalities in the neonatal CNS. AJR 1991;157:1105–1110.
2. Hoyme HE, Jones KL, Dixon SD, et al. Prenatal cocaine exposure and fetal vascular disruption. Pediatrics 1990;85:743–747.
3. Dogra VS, Shyken JM, Menon PA, et al. Neurosonographic abnormalities associated with maternal history of cocaine use in neonates of appropriate size for their gestational age. AJNR 1994; 15:697–702.
4. Singer LT, Yamashita TS, Hawkins S, et al. Increased incidence of intraventricular hemorrhage and developmental delay in cocaine-exposed, very low birth weight infants. J Pediatr 1994;124: 765–771.

Anticonvulsant Drug Syndrome

Infants with the anticonvulsant drug syndrome often are small and show poor growth after birth. Frontal bossing, large fontanelles, a broad nasal bridge, hypertelorism, and low-set ears constitute the calvarial abnormalities. Although some infants demonstrate visceral anomalies, the radiographic hallmark of the syndrome is hypoplasia or absence of the terminal phalanges of the hands and feet (Fig. 6.227A). In older children, these phalanges may develop in two parts, giving rise to pseudohyperphalangism (Fig. 6.227B). Abnormal external genitalia and cardiac anomalies also have been described, and there is an increased incidence of neuroblastoma in these infants (1).

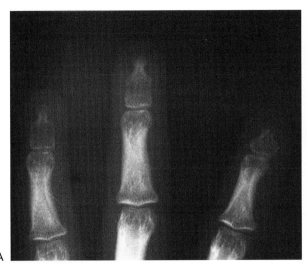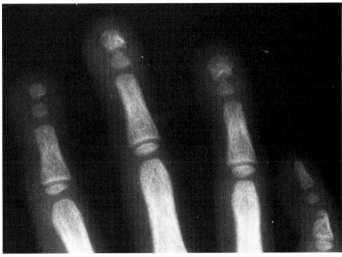

FIGURE 6.227. Dilantin embryopathy. A. Older patient demonstrating typical terminal phalangeal hypoplasia. **B.** Another patient demonstrating pseudohyperphalangism of the terminal phalanges.

REFERENCE

1. Allen RW Jr, Ogden B, Bently FL, et al. Fetal hydantoin syndrome, neuroblastoma, and hemorrhagic disease in a neonate. JAMA 1980;244:1464–1465.

Warfarin Embryopathy

In warfarin embryopathy, frontal bossing and terminal phalangeal hypoplasia in the hands and feet are seen and are somewhat similar to those seen with anticonvulsant drug-induced malformation. The finding of most interest, however, is chondrodysplasia punctate or stippled epiphyses, remarkably similar to that seen in congenital stippled epiphyses (1). The changes are postulated to be caused by bleeding into the cartilage primordia of the fetal bones.

REFERENCE

1. Tamburrini O, Bartolomeo-De Iuri A, Di-Guglielmo GL. Chondrodysplasia punctata after warfarin. Pediatr Radiol 1987;17:323–324.

MISCELLANEOUS SYNDROMES WITH SKELETAL CHANGES

Marfan's Syndrome and Marfan's Contractural Arachnodactyly

Marfan's syndrome usually is diagnosed in older children. The long fingers, toes, and long bones along with acetabulae protrusio are typical. In addition, lens dislocation and cardiac disease such as dissecting aneurysm of the ascending aorta (cystic medial necrosis), mitral insufficiency, and, occasionally, aortic insufficiency caused by connective tissue disease of these valves are seen. Occasionally, the problem can be detected in the neonate, in which dislocated hips, dissecting aneurysms of the ductus arteriosus (1, 2), and pulmonary emphysema (3) have been reported. These manifestations undoubtedly are the result of the connective and elastic tissue disorder present in these patients.

Marfan's contractural arachnodactyly (4, 5) probably is a related condition, but in addition to long thin bones, these patients also show changes in the muscles not unlike those of arthrogryposis. Severe contractural abnormalities of the extremities exist, and scoliosis of the spine is seen (Fig. 6.228). Both of these conditions have been linked to abnormalities of chromosomes 5 and 15 (6).

REFERENCES

1. Gillan JE, Costigan DC, Keeley FW, et al. Spontaneous dissecting aneurysm of the ductus arteriosus in an infant with Marfan's syndrome. J Pediatr 1984;105:952–954.
2. Muller NL, Mayo J, Culham JAG, et al. Ductus arteriosus aneurysm in Marfan's syndrome. J Can Assoc Radiol 1986;37:195–197.
3. Dominguez R, Weisgrau RA, Santamaria M. Pulmonary hyperinflation and emphysema in infants with the Marfan syndrome. Pediatr Radiol 1987;17:365–369.
4. Bass HN, Sparkes RS, Crandall BF, et al. Congenital contractural arachnodactyly, keratoconus, and probably Marfan's syndrome in the same pedigree. J Pediatr 1981;98:591–593.
5. Travis RC, Shaw DG. Congenital contractural arachnodactyly. Br J Radiol 1985;58:1115–1117.
6. Tsipouras P. International Marfan Syndrome Collaborative Study: genetic linkage of the Marfan syndrome, ectopia lentis, and congenital contractural arachnodactyly to the fibrillin genes on chromosomes 15 and 5. N Engl J Med 1992;326:905–909.

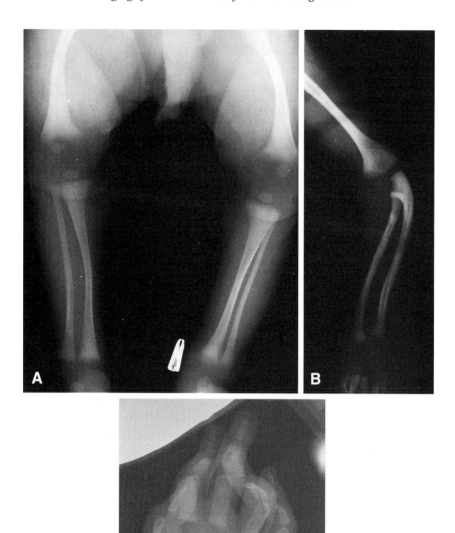

FIGURE 6.228. Marfan's contractural arachnodactyly. A. Note the long, thin long bones with variable bending. **B.** Upper extremity show similar findings. **C.** Hands demonstrate long fingers and camptodactyly.

Homocystinuria

Patients with homocystinuria tend to resemble those with Marfan's syndrome but in distinction show flattening of the vertebral bodies with a biconcave configuration and both epiphyseal and metaphyseal dysplastic changes. Often, the epiphyses are overgrown. The condition, however, seldom presents in early infancy and has not been documented in the neonate. Megaepiphyseal dwarfism may be a related condition. In adult life, calcification of the intervertebral discs can occur. Recently, vascular thrombotic disease resulting in a hyperlucent lung has been documented (1) in this condition.

REFERENCE

1. Herman J, Miller JH, Wang F. Hyperlucent lung secondary to homocystinuria. Pediatr Radiol 1996;26:672–674.

Lenz-Majewski Hyperostotic Dwarf

In Lenz-Majewski hyperostotic dwarfism, there is hyperostosis of the calvarium, especially along the base (Fig. 6.229), but the anterior fontanelle is widely patent. Progressive sclerosis of the diaphyses of the long bones along with the ribs is seen. The vertebral bodies also show increased sclerosis. In some ways, the findings resemble those of Engelmann-Camurati disease.

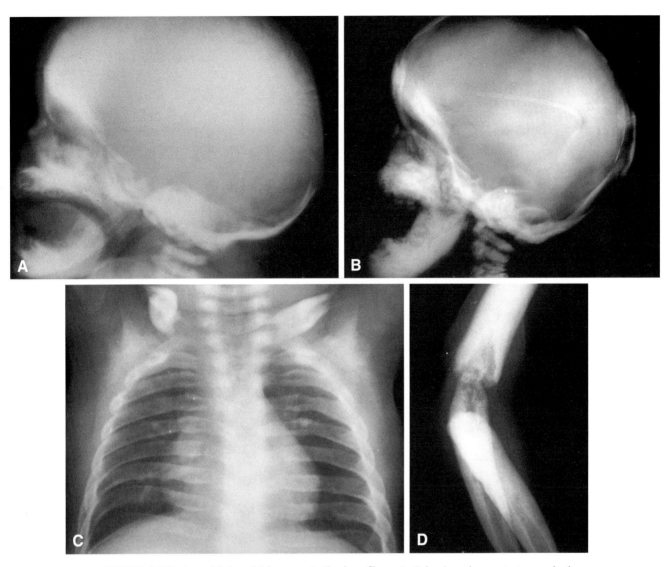

FIGURE 6.229. Lenz-Majewski hyperostotic dwarfism. A. Calvarium demonstrates marked hyperostosis of the base of the skull and the facial bones. **B.** More pronounced changes later in life. **C.** Note thickening and sclerosis of the clavicles and thickening of the ribs. The vertebrae also are sclerotic and thicker than normal. **D.** Long bones show marked hyperostosis and virtual obliteration of the medullary canals.

Kinky Hair (Menkes') Syndrome

The sex-linked kinky hair syndrome consists of failure to thrive, mental and motor retardation, seizures, and abnormal hair. Roentgenographic findings consist of metaphyseal spurring or beaking of the long bones similar to those seen with intrauterine infections, flaring of the ribs, periosteal reaction along the clavicles and long bones, bladder diverticula, and widespread dysplastic-stenotic arterial changes (Fig. 6.230). These now can be demonstrated with MRI (1). The bony changes tend to resolve as the infants grow older.

REFERENCE

1. Kim OH, Suh JH. Intracranial and extracranial MR angiography in Menkes disease. Pediatr Radiol 1997;27:782–784.

Cerebrohepatorenal Syndrome (Zellweger Syndrome)

Cerebrohepatorenal syndrome is a rare condition manifest by abnormal facies, marked hypotonia, flexion contractures of the extremities, cataracts, congenital iron overload, multiple renal cortical cysts (1), liver disease,

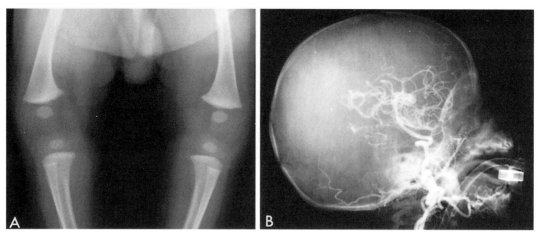

FIGURE 6.230. Kinky hair syndrome. A. Note metaphyseal beaking in the lower femurs. **B.** Note the disorganized, extremely tortuous course of the intracerebral vessels. They are also somewhat dilated. Extensive vascular changes including tortuosity, focal dilation, and focal narrowing also can be seen in other arteries of the body. (Reproduced with permission from Wesenberg RL, Gwinn JL, Barnes GR. Radiologic findings in the kinky hair syndrome. Radiology 1969;92:500–506).

extramedullary hematopoiesis, and failure to thrive. Liver biopsy frequently shows fibrosis and increased hemosiderin deposits. Cerebral abnormalities include lissencephaly and sudanophilic leukodystrophy. In terms of imaging, the significant finding consists of chondral calcification and is most frequently seen in the patella (Fig. 6.231A). Renal dysplasia with cortical cysts also is seen (Fig. 6.231B). Subependymal germinal matrix cysts also have been reported in these infants (1). The irregular pattern of calcification of the patellae can be confused with chondrodystrophia calcificans congenita.

REFERENCE

1. Russel IMB, van Sonderen L, van Straaten HLM, et al. Subependymal germinolytic cysts in Zellweger syndrome. Pediatr Radiol 1995;25:254–255.

Hand-Foot-Uterus Syndrome

Clinically, patients with hand-foot-uterus syndrome have small feet, short great toes with hallux deformity (1), and abnormal thumbs. Females also show duplication anomalies of the genital tract. The syndrome is transmitted as an

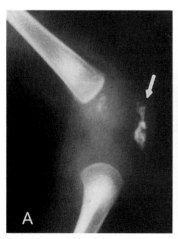
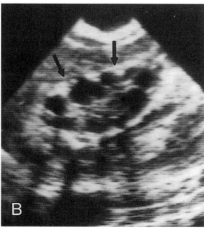

FIGURE 6.231. Cerebrohepatorenal syndrome (Zellweger syndrome). A. Note typical, extensive, irregular calcification of the patella (arrow). The findings are not unlike those seen in chondrodystrophia calcificans congenita, except that in the latter condition, irregular cartilaginous calcification involves other structures besides the patellae. **B.** Another patient whose ultrasonogram demonstrates typically small, echogenic kidneys with numerous cysts (arrows). [**A** reproduced with permission from Poznanski AK, Nosanchuk J, Baublis J, et al. The cerebrohepatorenal syndrome (CHRS): Zellweger syndrome. AJR 1970;109:313–322].

autosomal dominant trait, and in some patients, minor abnormalities of the chromosomes in the D and E groups have been noted.

REFERENCE

1. Cleveland RH, Holmes LB. Hand-foot-genital syndrome: the importance of hallux varus. Pediatr Radiol 1990;20:339–343.

Holt-Oram Syndrome

Basically, Holt-Oram syndrome consists of congenital heart disease and upper limb abnormalities. Most frequently, the underlying heart lesion is a left-to-right shunt, either an atrial or a ventricular septal defect. The most common skeletal abnormality is hypoplasia or complete absence of the radius and thumb, but handlebar clavicles also are common (Fig. 6.232). Other upper limb anomalies of the carpal and small bones of the hands also occur.

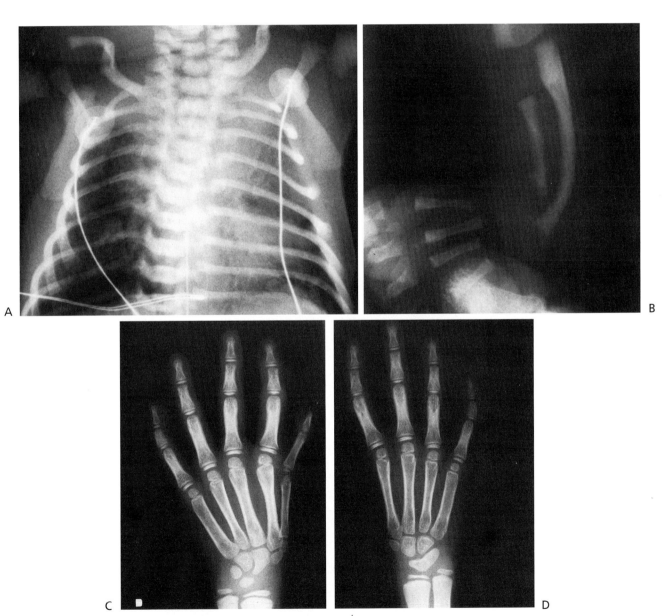

FIGURE 6.232. Holt-Oram syndrome. A. Infant demonstrating "handlebar" clavicles. **B.** Arm in the same infant demonstrates severe radial ray underdevelopment and severe deformity through the wrist. **C** and **D.** Note typical hypoplasia of the thumb on one side and absence on the other in this older patient.

Poland's Syndrome

Poland's syndrome is a congenital malformation consisting of partial or complete absence of the pectoralis major muscle and abnormalities of the upper extremity (hypoplasia and syndactylism) on the same side. Roentgenographically, unilateral absence of the pectoralis muscle leads to relative hyperlucency of the involved hemithorax and, in some cases, underlying rib hypoplasia (Fig. 6.233). The finding must be differentiated from hyperlucency caused by obstructive emphysema, congenital hypoplasia of the lung, and the hyperlucent lung of the Swyer-James syndrome.

Familial Idiopathic Osteoarthropathy (Pachydermoperiostosis)

Neonates with familial idiopathic osteoarthropathy usually are normal but shortly thereafter develop periosteal proliferation along the shafts of the long bones, clubbing of the terminal phalanges, and broadening of the terminal phalangeal tufts. In the skull, the sutures (often most pronounced in the lambdoid suture) appear unusually wide (underossified), and wormian bone formation is often exuberant. The calvarial defects usually disappear after a year or two, but the long bone periosteal new bone deposition persists.

Cornelia de Lange Syndrome (Brachmann-de Lange Syndrome)

Cornelia de Lange syndrome is characterized by severe motor and mental retardation, retarded growth, and multi-ple skeletal anomalies (1). Most often, these occur in the upper extremities and range from extreme phocomelia to mild hypoplasia. Frequently, this consists of hypoplasia of the radius and first digit and dorsal dislocation of the radial head along with radioulnar synostosis.

Clinically, dwarfism is present, and typical facies comprises a small nose, flat nasal bridge, anteverted nostrils, downward-curving mouth, bushy eyebrows that fuse in the center, and long, curly eyelashes. Hirsutism is present, the feet are usually small, and syndactyly of the second and third toes is common. The mandible often also is small, and mandibular and supracondylar spurs of the humerus occur. In addition, a nuchal web similar to that seen in Turner's syndrome along with a cleft palate and hypopituitarism can occur (1).

REFERENCE

1. Kousseff BG, Newkirk P, Root AW. Brachmann-de Lange syndrome: 1994 update. Arch Pediatr Adolesc Med 1994;148: 749–755.

Seckel Syndrome (Bird-Headed Dwarf)

Infants with Seckel syndrome are of low birth weight (prenatal growth deficiency), mentally retarded, and microcephalic. The face is small, but the nose is prominent, thus leading to the term "bird-headed dwarf." The radius may be hypoplastic and the fifth finger in-curved. Hypoplasia of the proximal fibula and dislocation of the hip also can occur.

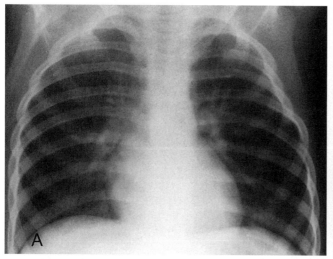 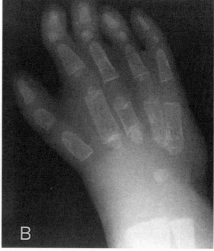

FIGURE 6.233. Poland's syndrome. A. Note radiolucency of the left hemithorax and hypoplasia of the upper ribs. **B.** Deformed left hand with hypoplasia of the various small bones, including the thumb.

Nail-Patella Syndrome (Hereditary Osteo-onychodysplasia)

Nail-patella syndrome usually manifests beyond the neonatal period and consists of hypoplastic nails that split easily, hypoplasia or absence of the patella, hypoplasia of the head of the fibula and radius, radial head dislocation (1), and a peculiar bony spur, or Fong's lesion (2), in the midposterior iliac wings (Fig. 6.234). A similar exostosis has been demonstrated on the superior distal aspect of the clavicle (3). Absence of the ischium and inferior pubic ramus also has been documented (4, 5). Renal disease, consisting of interstitial fibrosis with resultant proteinuria, hematuria, and eventually renal insufficiency, also occurs.

REFERENCES

1. Guidera KJ, Scatterwhite Y, Ogden JA, et al. Nail-patella syndrome: a review of 44 orthopaedic patients. J Pediatr Orthop 1991;11:737–742.
2. Fong EE."Iliac horns" (symmetrical bilateral central posterior iliac processes): case report. Radiology 1946;47:517–518.
3. Yarali HN, Erden GA, Karaarslan F, et al. Clavicular horn: another bony projection in nail-patella syndrome. Pediatr Radiol 1995; 25:549–550.
4. Azouz EM, Kozlowski K. Small patella syndrome: a bone dyspla-

sia to recognize and differentiate from the nail-patella syndrome. Pediatr Radiol 1997;27:432–435.

5. Habboub HK, Thneibat WA. Ischio-pubic-patellar hypoplasia: is it a new syndrome? Pediatr Radiol 1997;27:430–431.

Cockayne's Syndrome

In the neonate, roentgenographic changes of Cockayne's syndrome consist only of a small head (secondary to cerebral underdevelopment). In the older child, calcifications may be seen in the region of the basal ganglia and other parts of the brain (Fig. 6.235). The vertebral bodies are typically flat, and the long bones are thin (1). Enophthalmia, impaired vision, and impaired hearing also are common.

REFERENCE

1. Silengo MC, Franceschini P, Bianco R, et al. Distinctive skeletal dysplasia in Cockayne's syndrome. Pediatr Radiol 1986;16:264–266.

Acrocephalosyndactyly

Temtamy and McKusick (1) divided arachnocephalosyndactyly into five types: type I (Apert's syndrome), type II (Vogt cephalosyndactyly), type III (acrocephalosyn-

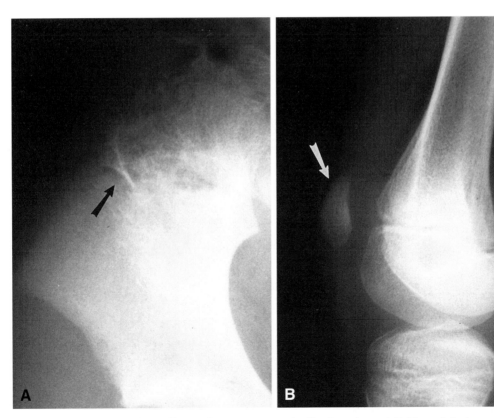

FIGURE 6.234. Nail-patella syndrome. A. Note the iliac horn (arrow). **B.** The patella (arrow) is hypoplastic.

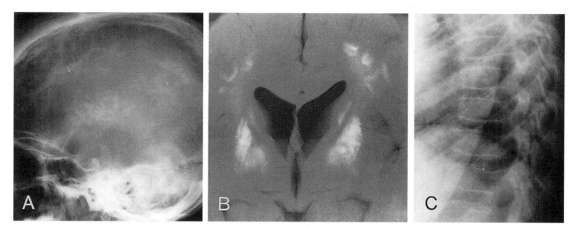

FIGURE 6.235. Cockayne's syndrome. A. Note thickening of the calvarium and intracranial calcifications. **B.** Postmortem coronal slice through the brain demonstrates calcifications in the basal ganglia and in white matter. This patient also had calcifications in the cerebellum. **C.** Note flat vertebral bodies.

dactyly with asymmetry of the skull and mild syndactyly), type IV (Wardenburg type), and type V (Pfeiffer type). All types show some degree of syndactyly and cranial malformation secondary to a variety of patterns of premature closure of the cranial sutures. When polydactyly is also present, the condition is referred to as "acrocephalopolysyndactyly."

REFERENCE

1. Temtamy S, McKusick VA. Synopsis of hand malformations with particular emphasis on genetic factors. Natl Found March Dimes Birth Defects 1969;5:125–184.

Rubinstein-Taybi Syndrome

Rubinstein-Taybi syndrome consists of mental retardation, abnormal facial appearance, short stature, and broad thumbs and toes. Other skeletal anomalies include syndactyly, polydactyly, and in-curving of the fifth finger. Roentgenographically, the bones and soft tissues of the thumb and great toes are markedly broadened and enlarged (Fig. 6.236A). In addition, a duplicated proximal phalanx

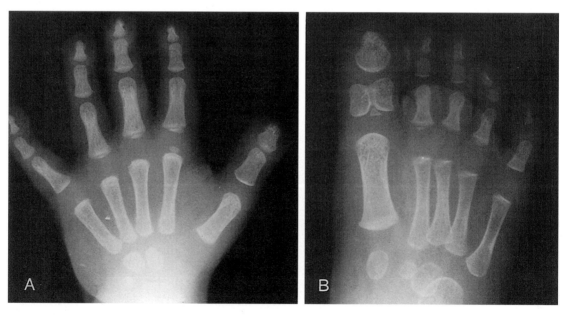

FIGURE 6.236. Rubinstein-Taybi syndrome. A and B. Note the typical broad thumb and great toe.

of the thumb or great toe, the so-called "kissing delta phalanx," also has been described (1) (Fig. 6.236B).

REFERENCE

1. Wood VE, Rubinstein J. Duplication longitudinal bracketed epiphysis "kissing delta phalanx" in Rubinstein-Taybi. J Pediatr Orthop 1999;19:603–606.

Oral-Facial-Digital Syndrome

In the oral-facial-digital syndrome, webbing between the lip and alveolar ridge, partial clefts in the mid-upper lip, variable degrees of cleft palate, shortening of the digits, in-curving of the fifth digit, and, in some cases, syndactyly occur (1–3). Mental retardation and hydrocephalus are common; in addition, agenesis of the corpus callosum, cerebral cortical cysts, and other cerebral abnormalities are seen. Multiple clefts in the tongue usually also are present.

Goldenhar's Syndrome (Oculoauriculovertebral Dysplasia)

Goldenhar's syndrome is characterized by ocular, aural, and vertebral anomalies. In addition, congenital heart lesions, lipoma of the corpus callosum, and intracranial dermoids occur. Roentgenographic findings consist of a variety of vertebral anomalies and hypoplasia of the zygomatic arches, malar bones, and mandible. On occasion, mandibular hypoplasia and subsequent retropositioning of the tongue can produce hypopharyngeal compromise and respiratory distress. In this regard, the problem is similar to that of the Pierre-Robin syndrome and the mandibulofacial dysostosis of Treacher Collins.

REFERENCES

1. Beltinger C, Saule H. Imaging of lipoma of the corpus callosum and intracranial dermoids in the Goldenhar syndrome. Pediatr Radiol 1988;18:72–73.
2. Greenwood RD, Rosenthal A, Wolff G, et al. Cardiovascular malformations in oculoauriculovertebral dysplasia (Goldenhar's syndrome). J Pediatr 1974;85:816–818.
3. Friedman S, Saraclar M. The high frequency of congenital heart disease in oculoauriculovertebral dysplasia (Goldenhar's syndrome). J Pediatr 1974;85:873–874.

Möbius' Syndrome

Möbius' syndrome produces an extraordinary immobility of the face that is recognizable at birth. It is secondary to facial nerve palsy. Other cranial nerves can be involved, and associated abnormalities of the skeletal system include micrognathia, syndactylism, Klippel-Feil deformity, and clubfeet. The condition is also referred to as "nuclear agen-

esis," and with ultrasound, brainstem calcifications suggesting prenatal insult (schemia, infections) to the brainstem have been documented (1).

REFERENCE

1. Yoon KH, Yoo SJ, Suh DC, et al. Mobius syndrome with brain stem calcification: prenatal and neonatal sonographic findings. Pediatr Radiol 1997;27:150–152.

Mastocytosis

Mastocytosis is a relatively uncommon disease that, because of mast cell proliferation, causes histamine release and clinical manifestations such as urticaria, flushing, diarrhea, and vomiting. In the bones, fibroblasts and granulomatous tissue proliferate to replace the bone marrow and cause pressure erosion of the bony trabeculae. With healing, however, osteosclerosis occurs, and often a mixed picture of bone destruction and repair is present. In infancy, the initial roentgenographic changes frequently consist of marked expansion of the long bones, thin cortices, and irregularly thickened residual trabeculae (Fig. 6.237). Diffuse and local forms of the disease exist, and the differential diagnosis includes the storage diseases such as Gaucher's disease and Niemann-Pick disease.

Russell-Silver Dwarfism

Infants with Russell-Silver dwarfism are usually small for their gestational age, and craniofacial disproportion produces relative calvarial enlargement. This often leads to an appearance suggesting hydrocephalus. However, the ventricles are not particularly dilated. There is asymmetry of the body, often more pronounced over the lower half (Fig. 2.238), and at times, the condition is referred to as "hemiatrophy." General stature is smaller than normal, and sexual development may be abnormal (i.e., sexual precocity, ambiguous genitalia, early appearance of gonadotropin, and premature onset of estrogen effects). Café-au-lait spots may be present, the fifth finger is frequently inwardly curved, and renal anomalies such as ureteropelvic junction obstruction and posterior urethral valves (1) can occur. In addition, growth hormone deficiency and hypopituitarism can be associated.

REFERENCE

1. Ortiz C, Cleveland RH, Jaramillo D, et al. Urethral valves in Russell-Silver syndrome. J Pediatr 1991;119:776–778.

Prader-Willi Syndrome (Fanconi III)

The only manifestation of Prader-Willi syndrome in the neonate is extreme hypotonia. By 2 or 3 years of age, the

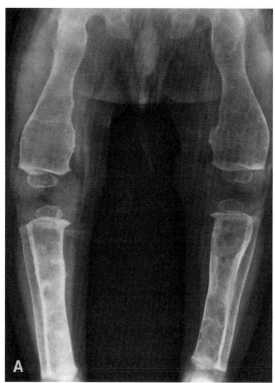
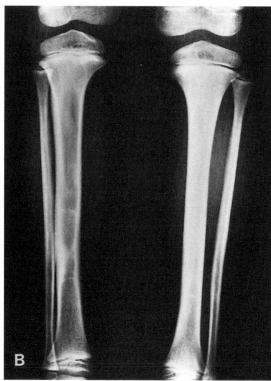

FIGURE 6.237. Mastocytosis. A. Note marked osteoporosis and extensive ballooning of the bones. The cortices are thin, and the trabeculae are irregularly thickened. **B.** Five years later, note that remodeling of the bone has occurred but that patchy sclerosis is present on the right and generalized sclerosis on the left. (Reproduced with permission from Wooten WB, de Santos LA, Finkelstein JB. Case report 61, diagnosis: systemic mastocytosis. Skeletal Radiol 1978;3:53–55).

more classic findings of sexual infancy, marked obesity, and mental retardation become apparent. Changes secondary to hypotonia also become more pronounced, and, as a result, one may note such bony abnormalities as coxa valga deformity of the hips, dislocation of the hips, scoliosis of the spine, and thinning of the long bones. Recently, MRI of the pituitary gland has demonstrated absence of the posterior bright spot, in keeping with frequently present lack of growth hormone (1).

REFERENCE

1. Miller L, Angulo M, Price D, et al. MR of the pituitary in patients with Prader-Willi syndrome: size determination and imaging findings. Pediatr Radiol 1996;26:43–47.

Diencephalic Syndrome in Infancy

Onset of diencephalic syndrome is usually beyond the neonatal period. It consists of a "silent" hypothalamic brain tumor inferior to the third ventricle, growth failure, and loss of subcutaneous fat (1). The key roentgenographic findings consist of a striking loss of subcutaneous fat (Fig. 6.239A) and the presence of a tumor encroaching on the

anterior third ventricle (Fig. 6.239B). The brain tumor may be of a variety of cell types but is usually a low-grade astrocytoma.

REFERENCE

1. Poussaint TY, Barnes PD, Nichols K, et al. Diencephalic syndrome: clinical features and imaging findings. AJNR 1997;18: 1499–1505.

Generalized Lipodystrophy

Generalized lipodystrophy produces soft tissue changes similar to those seen in the diencephalic syndrome. Its etiology is unknown, but pituitary-hypothalamic dysfunction is suspected.

Cerebral Gigantism (Sotos Syndrome)

Cerebral gigantism is characterized by advanced height and weight from birth. Skeletal maturation is accelerated, and the physical findings suggest gigantism. Nonprogressive mental retardation is usually present, and the ventricles usually are slightly dilated. It is not known just what the stim-

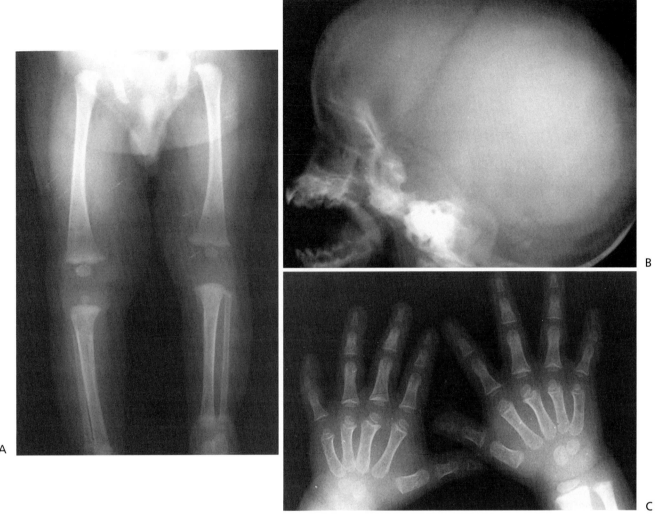

FIGURE 6.238. Russell-Silver dwarfism. A. Note that the left lower extremity is smaller than the right. **B.** Lateral view of the skull demonstrates a large calvarium. **C.** Older infant demonstrating a smaller right hand (hemiatrophy).

ulus to growth is, but it is believed to arise in the hypothalamus.

Laurence-Moon-Biedl Syndrome

Laurence-Moon-Biedl syndrome is characterized by mental retardation, obesity, genital underdevelopment, retinitis pigmentosa, and, on occasion, polydactyly. It does not usually become manifest in the neonate except for the obesity. As the infant grows older, a more typical clinical picture develops, and, at times, confusion with the Prader-Willi syndrome arises. Renal structural and parenchymal abnormalities also can occur.

Hallermann-Streiff Syndrome

Hallermann-Streiff syndrome is recognizable at birth and consists of brachycephaly, frontal bossing, malar and mandibular hypoplasia, microphthalmia, congenital cataracts, congenital heart defects, and a small, thin nose. The mouth is small, and dentition is abnormal. The skin is usually atrophic, and the hair is thin and light. Roentgenographically, craniofacial disproportion is present, and the calvarial bones often are thin and poorly ossified. Because of this, the sutures may appear unusually wide. Small orbits reflect the microphthalmia.

Oculodentodigital Syndrome

Oculodentodigital syndrome has findings similar to the Hallermann-Streiff syndrome. Generally, the findings consist of small orbits, small eyes, a thin nose, small teeth, syndactyly, camptodactyly of the fourth and fifth fingers, hypoplasia of the middle phalanx of some of the fingers and toes, and undertubulation of the long bones.

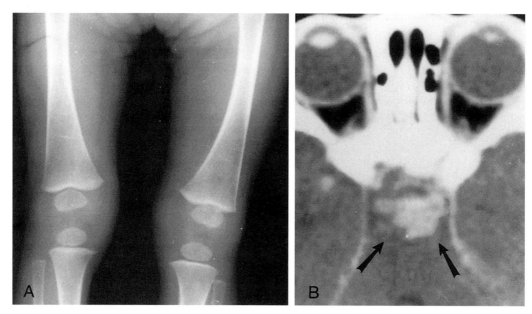

FIGURE 6.239. Diencephalic syndrome. A. Note the uniform density of the soft tissues of the lower extremities. This results from lack of subcutaneous and intermuscular fat tissue. **B.** Typical suprasellar location of brain tumor (arrows) in these patients.

Oculocerebrorenal Syndrome of Lowe

Oculocerebrorenal syndrome is characterized by failure to thrive, hypotonia, mental deficiency, and renal tubular dysfunction (limited ammonia production with resultant renal tubular acidosis). Other findings include hyperphosphaturia, hypophosphatemia, amino aciduria, and hyperchloremic acidosis with white matter disease. Eventually, the bones become osteoporotic, and changes of rickets develop.

Smith-Lemli-Opitz Syndrome

Smith-Lemli-Opitz syndrome is characterized by low birth weight, failure to thrive, moderate to severe mental deficiency, micrognathia, microcephaly, polydactyly, syndactyly, brachydactyly, and other bony anomalies such as hypoplasia of the thumb, stippled epiphyses, and equinovarus deformity of the foot (1).

REFERENCE

1. Herman TE, Siegel MJ, Lee BCP, et al. Smith-Lemli-Opitz syndrome type II: report of a case with additional radiographic findings. Pediatr Radiol 1993;23:37–40.

Ectodermal Dysplasia

In ectodermal dysplasia, absence of the sebaceous and sweat glands of the skin, generalized hypotrichosis, and partial or

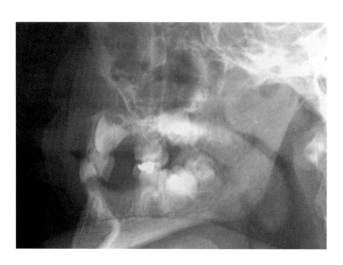

FIGURE 6.240. Ectodermal dysplasia. Note the pointed mandible and absence of teeth in the mandible and maxilla.

complete absence of teeth are observed. Absence of the sweat glands leads to heat intolerance, and because mucous glands of the bronchial tree are absent, respiratory tract infections are common. Roentgenographically, no specifically abnormal features are present except for the lack of normal tooth buds (Fig. 6.240). The deciduous teeth are normally calcified at birth, but in ectodermal dysplasia, the individual teeth are either absent or severely underdeveloped.

Larsen's Syndrome

The manifestations of Larsen's syndrome, probably a connective tissue disorder, are heterogeneous and consist of multiple joint dislocations (1), flat facies, and bony abnor-malities consisting of anterior dislocation of the knee (genu recurvatum), dislocations of the hip and elbows, and equinovarus or valgus deformity of the feet (Fig. 6.241). Hypoplasia and shortening of the various long bones, vertebral anomalies (2), and short, squat metacarpals and small bones of the hands and feet also occur.

REFERENCES

1. Laville JM, Lakermance P, Limouzy F. Larsen's syndrome: review of the literature and analysis of thirty-eight cases. J Pediatr Orthop 1994;14:63–73.
2. Weisenbach J, Melegh B. Vertebral anomalies in Larsen's syndrome. Pediatr Radiol 1996;26:682–683.

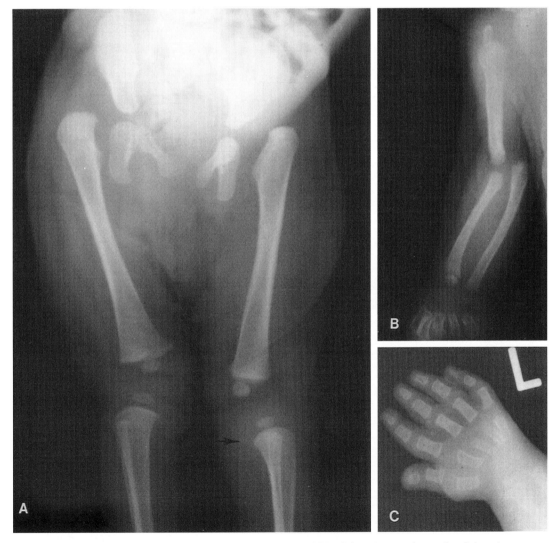

FIGURE 6.241. Larsen's syndrome. A. Note bilateral hip dislocations and anterior dislocation of the tibia on the left (arrow), where extreme hypermobility of the joint allows the tibia and fibula to be projected in an almost lateral position. **B.** Another infant demonstrating dislocation through the elbow and shortening of the humerus whose distal end is markedly underdeveloped and somewhat tapered. **C.** Same infant as in **B.** Note shortening of all the small bones of the hand.

Desbuquois Syndrome

Desbuquois syndrome is an uncommon condition presenting with coxa vara deformity of the hips, hypoplastic femoral necks, ligament laxity leading to multiple joint dislocations, short limbs, increased bone age, and metaphyseal spurs (1–3). Early demise in the neonatal period is common in the more severe forms (2, 3).

REFERENCES

1. Jequier S, Perreault G, Maroteaux P. Desbuquois syndrome presenting with severe neonatal dwarfism, spondyloepiphyseal dysplasia, and advanced carpal bone age. Pediatr Radiol 1992;22:440–442.
2. de-Orey MC, Mateus M, Guimaraes H, et al. Dyssegmental dysplasia: a case report of a Rolland-Desbuquois type. Pediatr Radiol 1997;27:948–950.
3. Hall BD. Lethality in Desbuquois dysplasia: three new cases. Pediatr Radiol 2001;31:43–47.

Camptomelic Dwarfism

Camptomelic dwarfism is associated with respiratory distress, hypotonia, peculiar facies, multiple bowing abnormalities of the long bones, and scoliosis. In addition, cartilaginous deformities exist, and dislocation of various joints can be seen. There is some suggestion that the condition is inherited as an autosomal recessive trait, but familial cases also can occur. Roentgenographically, prenatal bowing of the various long bones is seen, and the bones are variably shortened and undertubulated (Fig. 6.242). In some cases, the bones are of near-normal length; in others, they are markedly shortened and fatter than usual. Clubfoot deformity, dislocation of the hips and other joints, a bell-shaped thorax, widening of the interpedicular space in the upper lumbar region, and hypoplasia of the lower cervical spine also occur. In addition, underdevelopment of the radius and first digits can be seen, and tracheobronchial tree cartilage underdevelopment can lead to respiratory distress.

Pena-Shokeir Syndrome

Infants with Pena-Shokeir syndrome often are misdiagnosed as having some type of arthrogryposis multiplex congenita problem because they show severe joint contractures and marked loss of muscle bulk. They also demonstrate severe camptodactyly, clubfeet, facial anomalies, and pulmonary hypoplasia. The kidneys in these patients are nor-

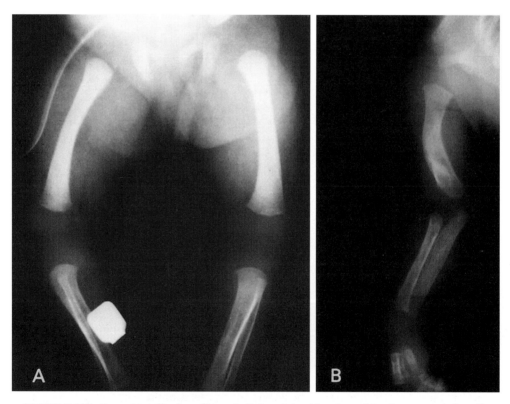

FIGURE 6.242. Camptomelic dwarfism. A. Note minimal bowing of the femurs and virtually no bowing of the tibiae. **B.** Same patient as in **A.** The humerus is markedly bowed, and there is a severe modeling disturbance. The bone is wider and shorter than normal. Similar changes are seen in the radius and ulna.

mal, and pulmonary hypoplasia seems to be primary in nature. It may be related to restricted thoracic cage movement in utero.

Cephaloskeletal Dysplasia (Taybi-Linder Syndrome)

Cephaloskeletal dysplasia is a form of familial dwarfism with severe microcephaly, mental retardation, low birth weight, and bony abnormalities. These latter abnormalities consist of shortening of all the long bones, but especially those of the hands and feet, splaying of the metaphyses of the long bones, and cup-shaped ends of the short tubular bones of the hands and feet.

Beckwith-Wiedemann Syndrome

Beckwith-Wiedemann syndrome is characterized by fetal gigantism, pronounced visceromegaly, macroglossia, microcephaly, nevus flammeus, diaphragmatic hernia, hemihypertrophy, increased bone age, pancreatic and adrenal hyperplasia, polycythemia, hyperglycemia, and an omphalocele or umbilical hernia (1). In addition, hemorrhagic cysts (2) and subsequent calcifications of the adrenal gland of these infants can be seen. Of more importance, however, is the increased incidence of intraabdominal tumors such as Wilms' tumor of the kidney, neuroblastoma and other tumors (3) of the adrenal gland, and nesidioblastomatosis of the pancreas (1–6).

REFERENCES

1. Andrews MW, Amparo EG. Case report. Wilms' tumor in a patient with Beckwith-Wiedemann syndrome: onset detected with 3-month serial sonography. AJR 1993;160:139–140.
2. McCauley RGK, Beckwith JB, Elias ER, et al. Benign hemorrhagic adrenocortical macrocysts in Beckwith-Wiedemann syndrome. AJR 1991;157:549–552.
3. Sbragia-Neto L, Melo-Filho AA, Guerra-Junior G, et al. Beckwith-Wiedemann syndrome and virilizing cortical adrenal tumor in a child. J Pediatr Surg 2000;35:1269–1271.
4. Sirinelli D, Silberman B, Baudon JJ, et al. Beckwith-Wiedemann syndrome and neural crest tumors. A report of two cases. Pediatr Radiol 1989;19:242–245.
5. Tank ES, Kay R. Neoplasms associated with hemihypertrophy, Beckwith-Wiedemann syndrome, and aniridia. J Urol 1980;124: 266–268.
6. Yamaguchi T, Fukuda T, Uetani M, et al. Renal cell carcinoma in a patient with Beckwith-Wiedmann syndrome. Pediatr Radiol 1996;26:312–314.

Pierre-Robin Syndrome

In the Pierre-Robin syndrome, the main problem is underdevelopment of the mandible and retropositioning of the tongue, causing severe respiratory distress. These aspects of the syndrome are discussed in Chapter 2 with

micrognathia. However, patients with the Pierre-Robin syndrome can show other abnormalities including palatal defects, hypophalangism, and clinodactyly. Rib defects also have been documented, and the condition is then termed the "cerebrocostomandibular syndrome" (see next section).

Cerebrocostomandibular Syndrome

Cerebrocostomandibular syndrome is characterized by posterior rib defects (fibrous) and micrognathia (1–4). The micrognathia portion of the syndrome often is referred to as the "Pierre-Robin anomaly," and some consider the cerebrocostomandibular syndrome to be a variation of the Pierre-Robin syndrome. These patients also have vertebral anomalies, subluxation of the elbows, stippled epiphyses (1), tracheal cartilage abnormalities, and brain defects. Their main clinical problem is a flail chest, which leads to severe respiratory distress. This is caused by the numerous rib defects (Fig. 6.243) and can be aggravated by the associated presence of abnormal costovertebral articulations.

REFERENCES

1. Burton EM, Oestreich AE. Cerebro-costo-mandibular syndrome with stippled epiphysis and cystic fibrosis. Pediatr Radiol 1988;18: 365–367.
2. Flodmark P, Wattsgard C. Cerebro-costo-mandibular syndrome. Pediatr Radiol 2001;31:36–37.
3. Leroy JG, Devos EA, Bulcke LJV, et al. Cerebro-costo-mandibular syndrome with autosomal dominant inheritance. J Pediatr 1981; 99:441–443.
4. Silverman FN, Strefling AM, Stevenson DK, et al. Cerebro-costo-mandibular syndrome. J Pediatr 1980;97:406–416.

VATER Syndrome

Although any of the abnormalities occurring in VATER syndrome can occur alone, when all are associated, the term "VATER syndrome" is applied (1). Originally, the condition included vertebral abnormalities, vascular abnormalities, anorectal malformations, tracheoesophageal fistula, esophageal atresia, and radial limb hypoplasia (Fig. 6.244). **It now has been so expanded that it no longer really means anything except that one should look for a lot of other anomalies when one encounters one of the basic anomalies of VATER syndrome.** In this regard, tracheal agenesis, horseshoe lung (2), cardiac anomalies, and renal abnormalities can occur. In addition, in keeping with the imperforate anus problem, spinal cord abnormalities, primarily in the form of a tethered cord (3), are common and are best detected with ultrasound or MRI. Finally, note that VACTERAL syndrome is just an expanded VATER syndrome.

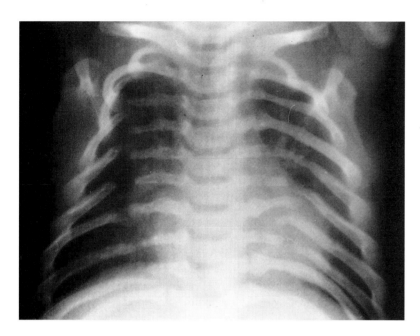

FIGURE 6.243. Cerebrocostomandibular syndrome. Note numerous bilateral rib defects in this 11-day-old infant with respiratory distress. (Reproduced with permission from Williams HJ, Sane SM. Cerebrocostovertebral syndrome. AJR 1976;126: 1223–1228).

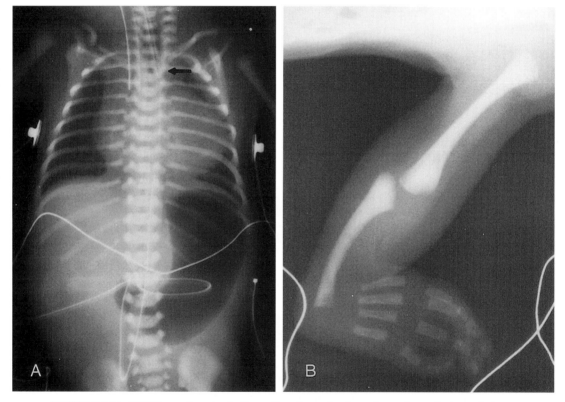

FIGURE 6.244. VATER syndrome. A. Note dilated pouch of esophageal atresia (arrow), large heart resulting from underlying congenital heart disease, congenital pseudoarthrosis of the right clavicle, and gas in the stomach and duodenal bulb constituting the double-bubble sign of duodenal atresia. Also note fusion of two vertebrae of the lower lumbar spine. **B.** Same patient demonstrating absence of the radius and thumb.

REFERENCES

1. Fernbach SK, Glass RBJ. The expanded spectrum of limb anomalies in the VATER association. Pediatr Radiol 1988;18:215–220.
2. Obregon MG, Giannotti A, Digillio MC, et al. Horseshoe lung: an additional component of the VATER association. Pediatr Radiol 1992;22:158.
3. James HE, Chestnut R, Krous H, et al. Distal spinal cord pathology in the VATER association. J Pediatr Surg 1995;29:1501–1503.

CHARGE Syndrome

The CHARGE syndrome consists of colobomas, heart disease, choanal atresia, growth and mental retardation, genital hypoplasia, and ear anomalies with deafness (1, 2). Esophageal atresia also has been documented (3).

REFERENCES

1. August GP, Rosenbaum KN, Friendly D, et al. Hypopituitarism and the CHARGE association. J Pediatr 1983;103:424–425.
2. Russell-Eggitt IM, Blake KD, Taylor DSI, et al. The eye in the CHARGE association. Br J Ophthalmol 1990;74:421–426.
3. Kutyanawala M, Wyse RKH, Brereton RJ, et al. CHARGE and esophageal atresia. J Pediatr Surg 1992;27:558–560.

Marshall Syndrome (Marshall-Smith Syndrome)

Marshall syndrome is characterized by accelerated prenatal maturation and the premature appearance of ossification centers at birth (1). In addition, these patients demonstrate hypoplastic mandibular rami, prominence of the forehead, and thinning of the long bones. The bones of the hand, however, show broadening of the middle and proximal phalanges and tapering or thinning of the distal phalanges.

REFERENCE

1. Eich GF, Silver MM, Weksberg R, et al. Marshall-Smith syndrome: new radiographic, clinical, and pathologic observations. Radiology 1991;181:183–188.

Weaver Syndrome

Weaver syndrome is rare and in some ways resembles the Marshall-Smith syndrome. It is characterized by overgrowth of the infant, accelerated skeletal maturation, macrocephaly, and camptodactyly. There may be mild mental and motor retardation (1).

REFERENCE

1. Ramos-Arroyo MA, Weaver DD, Banks ER. Weaver syndrome: a

case without early overgrowth and review of the literature. Pediatrics 1991;88:1106–1111.

Mccune-Albright Syndrome

McCune-Albright syndrome usually presents in the older child but can be seen in infancy. It is characterized by fibrous dysplasia of the bones, café-au-lait spots, and precocious puberty. Although it most commonly occurs in girls, it can occur in boys. Pituitary enlargement with adenomas can be seen in some patients.

Whistling Face Syndrome (Craniocarpotarsal Dystrophy)

Whistling face syndrome is characterized by microstomia and lip protrusion that mimics the configuration seen when whistling (1). In addition, these patients show hypertelorism, ulnar deviation of the hands, finger contractures, nonopposable thumbs, and camptodactyly. Clubfoot deformity also can be seen.

REFERENCE

1. Kousseff BG, McConnachie P, Hadro TA. Autosomal recessive type of whistling face syndrome in twins. Pediatrics 1982;69: 328–331.

Weissenbacher-Zweymuller Syndrome

Weissenbacher-Zweymuller syndrome can present in infancy and is a form of chondrodysplasia that at birth is characterized by a small retropositioned mandible and rhizomelic shortening of the extremities. The metaphyses of the long bones are widened and flared, and the bones themselves are shortened.

Aarskog Syndrome (Facial-Digital-Genital Syndrome)

In Aarskog syndrome, patients have short stature and shortening of the fingers and toes. The shortening is the result primarily of hypoplasia of the terminal phalanges. In addition, one can see clinodactyly of the fifth finger, mild syndactyly, and camptodactyly (1). Other findings include the presence of 13 ribs, hypertelorism, and a decreased bone age (1).

REFERENCE

1. Porteous MEM, Gudie DR. Aarskog syndrome. J Med Genet 1991;28:44–47.

Melnick-Needles Syndrome (Osteodysplasia)

Patients with Melnick-Needles syndrome usually do not present in early infancy. As they grow older, however, they develop extensive changes of almost all the bones of the skeleton (Fig. 6.245). The ribs, clavicles, and long bones show ribbon-like waviness and cortical irregularity. S-shaped bowing of the radius and tibia also commonly occurs, and the flat bones also are involved in the dysplastic process (1). The vertebral bodies are tall, and the mandible is underdeveloped. Older children may demonstrate wide metaphyses (Erlenmeyer flask configuration), persistent wavy bones, and clubfoot deformities (Fig. 6.246).

REFERENCE

1. Eggli K, Giudici M, Ramer J, et al. Melnick-Needles syndrome. Four new cases. Pediatr Radiol 1992;22:257–261.

Dyggve-Melchior-Clausen Syndrome

Dyggve-Melchior-Clausen syndrome is characterized by short trunk dwarfism, mental retardation, and bony changes not unlike those seen in Morquio's disease or spondyloepiphyseal dysplasia. However, it is not believed to be a mucopolysaccharidosis. The skull in these patients often is small, the vertebra markedly flattened and associated with deep anterior corner notches, the iliac wings squared, and the epiphyses dysplastic. The metaphyses may eventually become wide, mimicking those of the Kniest and metatrophic dwarf syndromes. The metaphyses become wide on a secondary basis, however, much as do the metaphyses of the pseudoachondroplastic forms of spondyloepiphyseal and epiphyseal dysplasia.

Ehlers-Danlos Syndrome (Cutis Laxa)

Ehlers-Danlos syndrome is inherited on an autosomal dominant basis and is characterized by hypermobility of the joints, hyperelasticity of the skin, and fragility of the skin and blood vessels (1). As these patients grow older, bony changes related to hypermobility of the joints arise, but in infancy, bony changes are minimal. These patients can demonstrate abnormalities of other systems, including diaphragmatic eventrations, a variety of hernias, urinary tract and gastrointestinal diverticula (2–4), aortic rupture (1), severe progressive pulmonary emphysema, and lung cysts (5). The latter problems are believed to be caused by a widespread defect in the development of the elastic tissue of the respiratory tree.

REFERENCES

1. Blickman JG, Griscom NT. Aortic rupture in a previously undiagnosed case of the Ehlers-Danlos syndrome. Pediatr Radiol 1982;12:86–88.
2. Janik JS, Shandling B, Mancer K. Cutis laxa and hollow viscus diverticula. J Pediatr Surg 1982;17:318–320.

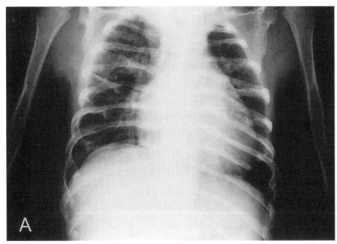

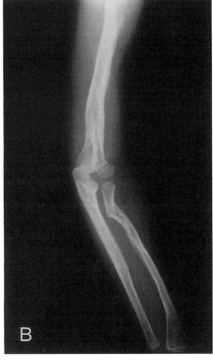

FIGURE 6.245. Melnick-Needles syndrome. A. Typical twisted, thin ribs and clavicles. **B.** Note the twisted, thin long bones.

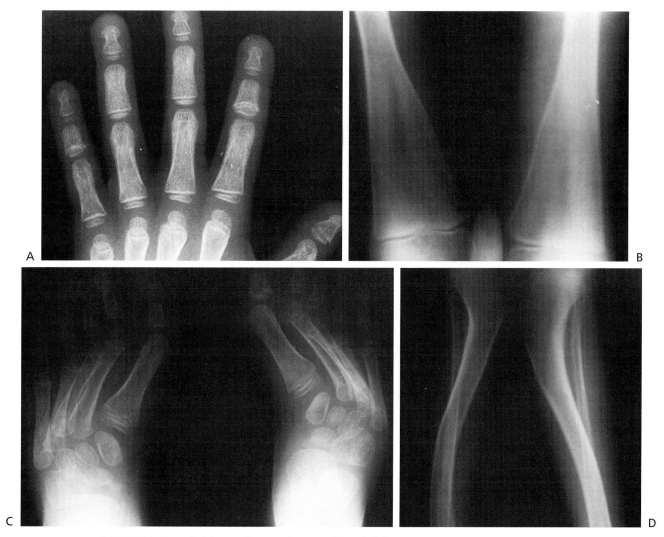

FIGURE 6.246. Melnick-Needles syndrome: older child. A. Hand demonstrating small bones but especially underdevelopment of the terminal phalanges. **B.** Distal femurs demonstrate widening of the metaphyses, constituting the so-called "Erlenmeyer flask" configuration. **C.** Marked metatarsus varus and alteration of midtarsal bone alignment are present. **D.** Note the persistent tortuosity and waviness of the long bones of the lower extremities.

3. Schippers E, Dittler HJ. Multiple hollow organ dysplasia in Ehlers-Danlos syndrome. J Pediatr Surg 1989;24:1181–1183.
4. Toyohara T, Kaneko T, Araki H, et al. Giant epiphrenic diverticulum in a boy with Ehlers-Danlos syndrome. Pediatr Radiol 1989; 19:437.
5. Herman TE, Mcalister WH. Cavitary pulmonary lesions in type IV Ehlers-Danlos syndrome. Pediatr Radiol 1994;24:263–265.

Robinow Syndrome

Robinow syndrome is characterized by mesomelic (middle segment) shortening of the limbs, hypoplastic external genitalia, a characteristic facial appearance, growth delay, and hemivertebrae (1, 2).

REFERENCES

1. Kelly TE, Benson R, Temtamy S, et al. The Robinow syndrome. Am J Dis Child 1975;129:383–386.
2. Wadlington WB, Tucker VL, Schimke RN. Mesomelic dwarfism with hemivertebrae and small genitalia (the Robinow syndrome). Am J Dis Child 1973;126:202–205.

Metaphyseal Dysostosis-Thymolymphopenia Syndrome

Patients with metaphyseal dysostosis-thymolymphopenia syndrome have a combined immunologic deficiency and adenosine deaminase deficiency of the red blood cells (1).

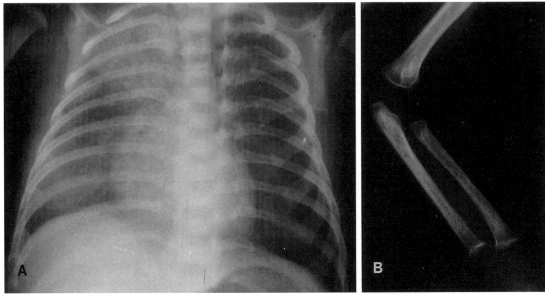

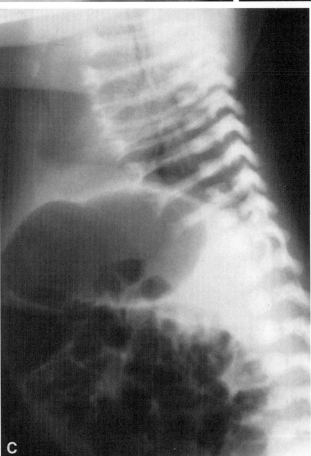

FIGURE 6.247. Metaphyseal dysostosis-thymolymphopenia syndrome. A. Note cupping of the anterior aspect of the ribs. Also note diffuse interstitial infiltrates secondary to *Pneumocystis carinii* pneumonia. **B.** Upper extremity demonstrating typical cupping of the metaphyses and nonspecific trophic bands. **C. Shwachman-Diamond syndrome.** Note marked shortening and cupping of the ribs. Minimal metaphyseal cupping of the upper femurs was present in this patient. Otherwise, the long bones appeared relatively normal.

Roentgenographically, they are identified by the presence of rachitic or chondrodystrophic bony changes resulting from metaphyseal dysostosis. The changes consist of cupping and widening of the anterior ends of the ribs and the metaphyses of the long bones (Fig. 6.247, A and B). The condition is related to the McKusick form of metaphyseal dysostosis and the Shwachman-Diamond syndrome (see next section).

REFERENCE

1. Chakravarti VS, Borns P, Lobell J, et al. Chondro-osseous dysplasia in severe combined immunodeficiency due to adenosine deaminase deficiency (chondro-osseous dysplasia in ADA deficiency SCID). Pediatr Radiol 1992;21:447–448.

Shwachman-Diamond Syndrome

Shwachman-Diamond syndrome is characterized by metaphyseal dysostosis, neutropenia, and pancreatic insufficiency. It is also termed the "MMN syndrome" (1) and is related to the McKusick form of metaphyseal dysostosis and the metaphyseal dysostosis-thymolymphopenia syndrome. These patients show variable shortening of the extremities, metaphyseal cupping and widening (also variable), and short ribs with pronounced cupping, usually visible at birth (Fig. 6.247C). Repeated pulmonary infections and malabsorption are major problems in all these syndromes.

REFERENCE

1. Berrocal T, Simon MJ, Al-Assir I, et al. Shwachman-Diamond syndrome: clinical, radiological, and sonographic findings. Pediatr Radiol 1995;25:356–359.

Aglossia-Adactylia Syndrome

Aglossia-adactylia syndrome is characterized by the absence or severe underdevelopment of the tongue, micrognathia, and hypoplasia of the extremities with absence of the distal digits. Dental anomalies also exist.

Laron Dwarfism

In Laron dwarfism, a large head and a small face are present. The posterior fossa is large, but the membranous calvarium is thickened. The long bones are slender, and wormian bones are present in the skull (1).

REFERENCE

1. Vasil M, Baxova A, Kozlowski K. Radiographic abnormalities in Laron dwarfism. Pediatr Radiol 1994;24:260–262.

Aplasia Cutis Congenita

In aplasia cutis congenita, scalp defect, often an associated skull defect, and terminal phocomelia of the limbs are seen.

Coffin-Siris Syndrome

Coffin-Siris syndrome is characterized radiographically by terminal phalangeal hypoplasia and clinically by deformed and absent fingernails, especially of the fifth finger and toe. In addition, these patients are hypotonic and show joint hypermobility.

REFERENCES

1. Franceschini P, Silengo MC, Bianco R, et al. The Coffin-Siris syndrome in two siblings. Pediatr Radiol 1986;16:330–333.
2. Lucaya J, Garcia-Conesa JA, Bosch-Banyeras JM, et al. The Coffin-Siris syndrome. A report of four cases and review of the literature. Pediatr Radiol 1981;11:35–38.

Septo-optic Dysplasia (de Morsier's Syndrome)

Septo-optic dysplasia is characterized by agenesis of the septum pellucidum, hypoplasia of the anterior optic tracts, a variety of ocular findings, and hypopituitarism or deficient growth hormone production (1–3). The absent septum pellucidum along with the heart-shaped single ventricle on coronal section are characteristic (Fig. 6.248A). The hypoplastic optic nerves are best demonstrated with MRI (Fig. 6.248 B).

REFERENCES

1. O'Dwyer JA. Radiologic features of septo-optic dysplasia. AJNR 1980;1:443.
2. Stewart C, Castro-Magana M, Sherman J, et al. Septo-optic dysplasia and median cleft face syndrome in a patient with isolated growth hormone deficiency and hyperprolactinemia. Am J Dis Child 1983;137:484–487.
3. Williams JL, Faerber EN. Septo-optic dysplasia (de Morsier's syndrome). J Ultrasound Med 1985;4:265–266.

Trichorhinophalangeal Syndrome (Giedion Syndrome)

Features of trichorhinophalangeal syndrome consist of sparse scalp hair, thin fingernails, short small bones of the hands, midfacial hypoplasia, and tooth abnormalities. The radiographic finding (1) considered to be the hallmark of the condition, however, is the cone-shaped epiphysis of the hand, usually of the middle phalanges (Fig. 6.249).

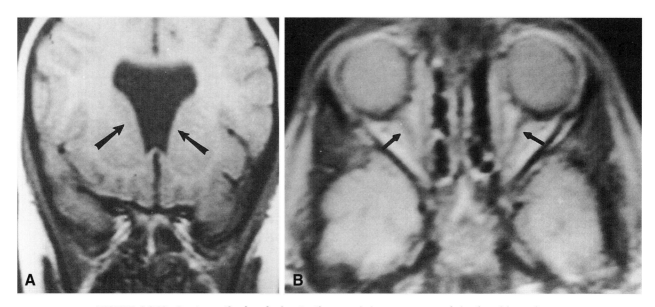

FIGURE 6.248. Septo-optic dysplasia. A. Characteristic appearance of the fused lateral ventricles (arrows) because of the absence of the septum pellucidum. **B.** Note the atrophic optic nerves (arrows).

REFERENCE

1. Cope R, Beals RK, Bennett RM. The trichorhinophalangeal dysplasia syndrome: report of eight kindreds, with emphasis on hip complications, late presentations, and premature osteoarthrosis. J Pediatr Orthop 1986;6:133–138.

McKusick-Kaufman Syndrome

McKusick-Kaufman syndrome consists of vaginal atresia with hydrometrocolpos and postaxial polydactyly (1).

REFERENCE

1. Chitayat D, Hahm SYW, Marion RW, et al. Further delineation of the McKusick-Kaufman hydrometrocolpos-polydactyly syndrome. Am J Dis Child 1987;141:1133–1136.

Blue Rubber Bleb Nevus Syndrome

Blue rubber bleb nevus syndrome, which can be autosomal dominant, presents with rubbery, raised, bluish, subcutaneous hemangiomas (nevi). Gastrointestinal bleeding (1, 2)

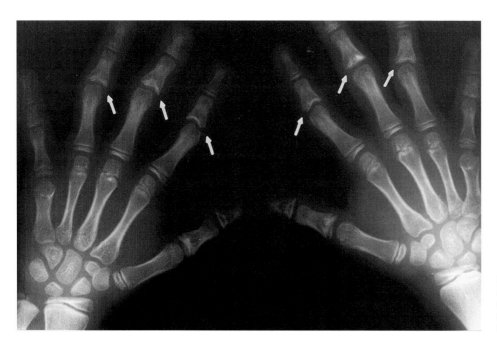

FIGURE 6.249. Trichorhinophalangeal syndrome. Note the characteristic cone-shaped epiphyses (arrows) of the shortened middle phalanges.

secondary to mucosal hemangiomatosis is seen, and hemangiomas can occur in other parts of the body and in almost any organ. There are no bony abnormalities.

REFERENCES

1. Moodley M, Ramdial P. Blue rubber bleb nevus syndrome: case report and review of the literature. Pediatrics 1993;92:160–162.
2. Wong Y-C, Li Y-W, Chang M-H. Gastrointestinal bleeding and paraparesis in blue rubber bleb nevus syndrome. Pediatr Radiol 1994;24:600–601.

Kenny-Caffey Syndrome

Kenny-Caffey syndrome is characterized by low birth weight, dwarfism, and transient hypocalcemia with convulsions. There may be delayed closure of the anterior fontanelle, but the single most striking radiographic finding is thickening of the cortex of the long bones with narrowing of the medullary cavity. The bones, therefore, appear thin, but their cortices are thick. There also is lack of differentiation of the calvarium into the inner and outer tables and diploic space.

Acrodysostosis

Acrodysostosis is characterized by short stature, psychomotor retardation, and shortening of the extremities, more marked in the upper limbs. Hypogonadism also is present, and radiographically the most impressive finding is marked shortening of the small bones of the hand (Fig. 6.250A). In addition, cone-shaped epiphyses are seen in the proximal phalanges, but the long bones, although somewhat shortened and thickened, are not nearly as dramatic in their change. Irregularity of the vertebral endplates also can be seen along with a dorsal kyphosis.

Juberg-Hayward Syndrome

Juberg-Hayward syndrome is composed of oral, cranial, and digital abnormalities consisting of microcephaly, cleft lip, and cleft palate. Radiographically, the most striking findings are a short thumb and great toe, with a short first metacarpal or metatarsal and hypoplasia of the small bones of the hands and feet (Fig. 6.250, B and C).

Acromesomelic Dysplasia

The hand in acromesomelic dysplasia resembles that of acrodysostosis except that the individual bones may be shorter and fatter. In addition, coned epiphyses are not present, and the long bones show much greater changes in modeling and are shortened. In some regards, they resemble those of achondroplasia, although metaphyseal cupping with the ball-and-socket epiphysis phenomenon is more pronounced. These patients also have large great toes and thoracic kyphosis but normal intelligence. Shortening of the long bones is most manifest in the forearms and the hands (1, 2).

REFERENCES

1. Borelli P, Fasanelli S, Marini R. Acromesomelic dwarfism in a child with an interesting family history. Pediatr Radiol 1983;13:165–168.
2. Langer LO. Acromesomelic dysplasia. Radiology 1980;137:349.

Klippel-Trenaunay Syndrome

Klippel-Trenaunay syndrome is characterized by port wine telangiectatic nevi throughout the body and soft tissue and bone hypertrophy. If the intestines are involved, protein-losing enteropathy occurs, and disfiguring deformities of the various involved portions of the body are often rather grotesque.

Macrodystrophia Lipomatosa Syndrome

In macrodystrophia lipomatosa syndrome, gigantism of the extremities occurs (1) and is secondary to a mesenchymal defect, resulting in a disproportionate increase in the deposition of fibroadipose tissue at different sites of the body (Fig. 6.251A). In addition to excessive subcutaneous fat, enlarged extremity bones may show marginal erosions and even secondary periosteal reaction. In some ways, the findings resemble those of the Proteus syndrome (see next section).

REFERENCE

1. Moran V, Butler F, Colzille J. X-ray diagnosis of macrodystrophia lipomatosa. Br J Radiol 1984;57:523–525.

Proteus Syndrome

In Proteus syndrome, numerous skeletal and mesodermal malformations exist. Foremost are hemihypertrophy and fatty or lymphangiomatous tumors throughout various parts of the body (1–3). In the extremities, associated gigantism causes confusion with macrodystrophia lipomatosa (Fig. 6.251, B and C). Macrocephaly may be profound and focal thickening of the calvarium pronounced. The fatty and lymphangiomatous tumors are readily imaged with ultrasound and MR (4). Other tumors encountered include fibroma, osteoma, osteochondroma, and enchondroma. Cystic lung disease also has been seen in this condition (5).

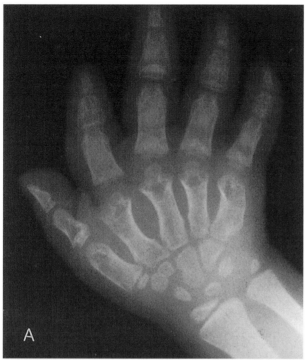

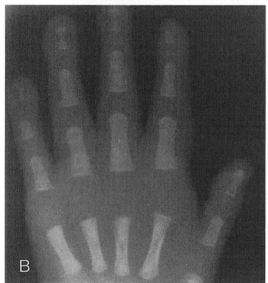

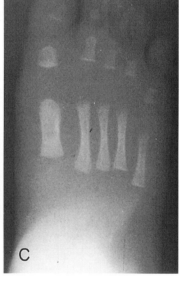

FIGURE 6.250. A. Acrodysostosis. Note typical short, squat small bones of the hands. Also note suggestion of coned epiphyses in the proximal phalanges. **B. Juberg-Haywood syndrome.** Note the recessed thumb with hypoplastic metacarpal. The peripheral phalanges also are underdeveloped, especially that of the index finger. All the small bones are somewhat underdeveloped, however. **C.** Toes demonstrating a short first metatarsal and general underdevelopment of the small bones.

REFERENCES

1. Azouz EM, Costa T, Fitch N. Radiologic findings in the Proteus syndrome. Pediatr Radiol 1987;17:481–485.
2. Demetriades D, Hager J, Nikolaides N, et al. Proteus syndrome: musculoskeletal manifestations and management: a report of two cases. J Pediatr Orthop 1992;12:106–113.
3. Strickler S. Musculoskeletal manifestations of Proteus syndrome: report of two cases with literature review. J Pediatr Orthop 1992; 12:667–674.
4. Cremin BJ, Biljoen DL, Wynchank S, et al. The Proteus syndrome: the magnetic resonance and radiological features. Pediatr Radiol 1987;17:486–488.
5. Newman B, Urbach AH, Orenstein D, et al. Proteus syndrome: emphasis on the pulmonary manifestations. Pediatr Radiol 1994; 24:189–193.

Acro-osteolysis

In acro-osteolysis, there is progressive lysis of various portions of the skeleton. Eventually, virtual dissolution of the

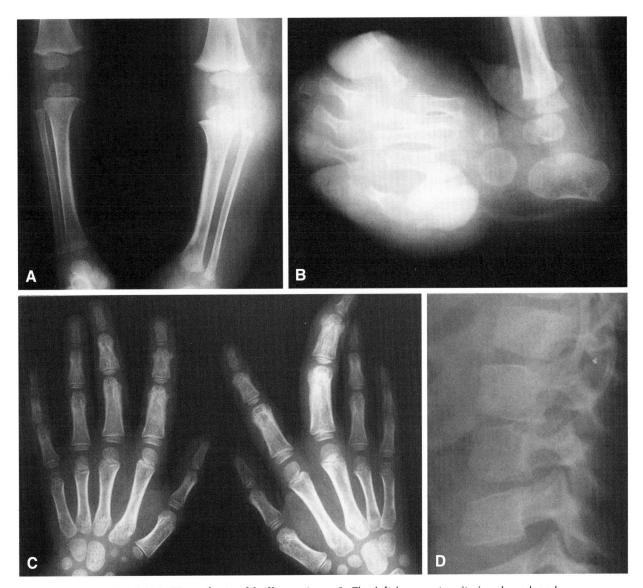

FIGURE 6.251. Macrodystrophia lipomatosa. A. The left lower extremity is enlarged, and there is increased fat in the soft tissues. **B.** Foot on the same side shows marked enlargement, deformity of the bones, and abundant fatty tissue. **C. Proteus syndrome.** Note the enlarged digits on both sides. There is less adipose tissue deposited than in macrodystrophia lipomatosa. **D.** Lateral view demonstrates dysplastic vertebra in the lumbar region.

bones occurs, and the findings are characteristic, especially in the familial carpal-tarsal osteolysis (Fig. 6.252). In addition to lysis of the carpal, tarsal, and other bones, a nephropathy exists in familial cases.

Hajdu-Cheney Syndrome

In the rare Hajdu-Cheney syndrome, terminal phalangeal osteolysis occurs along with persistence of the calvarial sutures, basilar invagination, radial head dislocation, and dislocation of the hips (1, 2).

REFERENCES

1. Diren HB, Kovanlikaya I, Suller A, et al. The Hajdu-Cheney syndrome: a case report and review of the literature. Pediatr Radiol 1990;20:568–569.
2. Pellegrini V, Widdowson DJ. CT findings in the Hajdu-Cheney syndrome. Pediatr Radiol 1991;21:304.

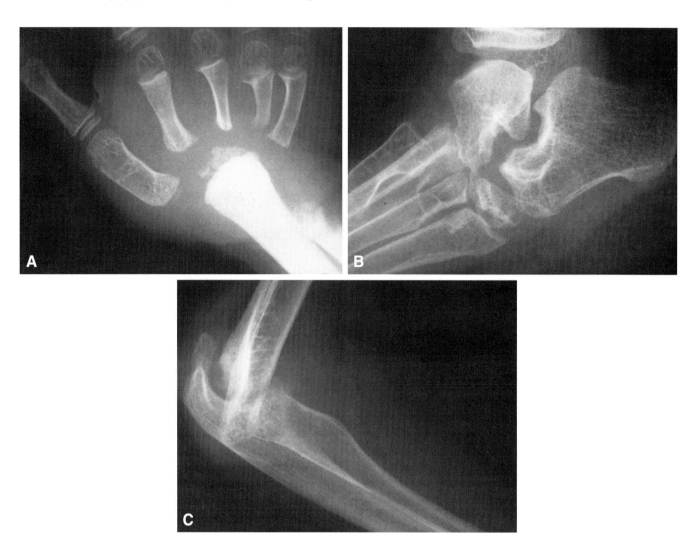

FIGURE 6.252. Carpal-tarsal osteolysis. A. The carpal bones are basically absent and totally resorbed. There also is resorption of the proximal metacarpals and of the radius and ulna, especially the ulna. **B.** The tarsal bones appear irregular because of resorption. **C.** Elbow demonstrates dissolution of the humerus and proximal ulna.

Gorlin's Syndrome (Basal Cell Nevus Syndrome)

In Gorlin's syndrome, basal cell nevi are found in the skin, but, in addition, dentigerous cysts (Fig. 6.253, A and B) are characteristically found in the mandible (1). In addition, scoliosis and wavy rib deformities are characteristic, as is calcification of the falx (Fig. 6.253, C and D).

REFERENCE

1. Lovin JD, Talarico CL, Wegert SL, et al. Gorlin's syndrome with associated odontogenic cysts. Pediatr Radiol 1991;21:584–587.

Stickler Syndrome

The key radiographic features of Stickler syndrome, a connective tissue disease, include rhizomelic limb shortening, under tubulation of the diaphyses, coxa valga, wide femoral neck, and wide iliac wing bases (1) (Fig. 6.254). Scheuermann-like changes occur in the spine, and clinically retinal detachments, glaucoma, and other ocular problems are present.

REFERENCE

1. Vintiner GM. Genetic and clinical heterogenicity of Stickler. Am J Med Genet 1991;41:44–48.

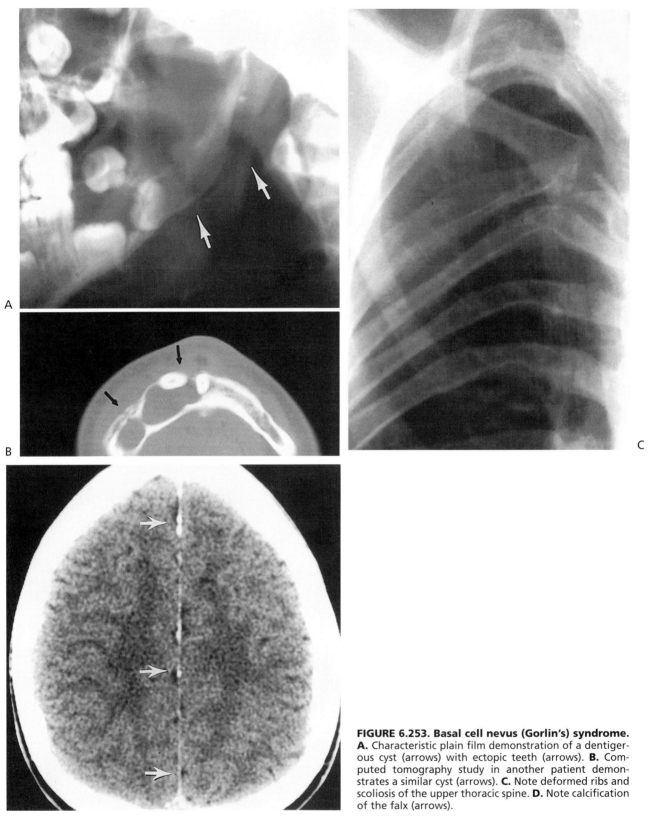

FIGURE 6.253. Basal cell nevus (Gorlin's) syndrome.
A. Characteristic plain film demonstration of a dentiger-ous cyst (arrows) with ectopic teeth (arrows). **B.** Computed tomography study in another patient demonstrates a similar cyst (arrows). **C.** Note deformed ribs and scoliosis of the upper thoracic spine. **D.** Note calcification of the falx (arrows).

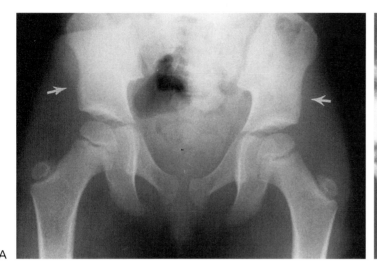

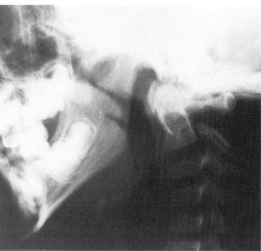

A

B

FIGURE 6.254. Stickler syndrome. A. Note that the necks of the iliac wings (arrows) are wider than normal. **B.** Lateral view of the skull demonstrates a hypoplastic mandible with a pointed anterior configuration. Also note anomalies of the upper cervical spine.

Nager's Syndrome

Nager's syndrome, or Nager acrofacial dysostosis, consists of mandibular and malar bone hypoplasia, macrostomia, cleft palate, thumb hypoplasia, absence of the radius (radial ray syndrome), and radioulnar synostosis (1).

REFERENCE

1. Halal F, Herrmann J, Pallister PD, et al. Differential diagnosis of Nager acrofacial dysostosis syndrome: report of four patients with Nager syndrome and discussion of other related syndromes. Am J Med Genet 1983;14:209–224.

Melorheostosis

Melorheostosis of Leri is a rare condition consisting of hyperostotic, flowing, periosteal new bone deposition (Fig. 6.255) along the diaphysis of the long bones. Its etiology is unknown, but the radiographic findings are characteristic. In addition, dense spotted areas may occur in the epiphysis and other bones, reminiscent of osteopoikilosis.

Osteopathia Striata and Osteopoikilosis

In osteopathia striata, vertical dense linear striations are seen in the ends of the long bones. They generally are of little clinical significance, but the condition can be seen in association with sclerosis of the base of the skull. It also can be seen with osteopoikilosis, which consists of numerous dense cortical bone islands scattered throughout the skeleton but especially prolific in the metaphyses of the long bones, tarsals, and carpals (Fig. 6.256). Generally speaking, neither of these conditions is considered pathologic (1).

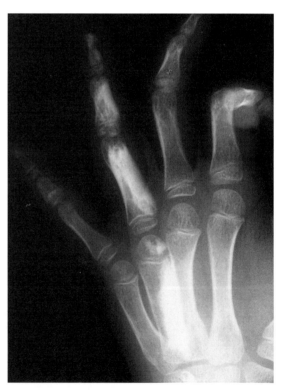

FIGURE 6.255. Melorheostosis. Note thick periosteal new bone deposition or cortical thickening of the bones of the fourth digit.

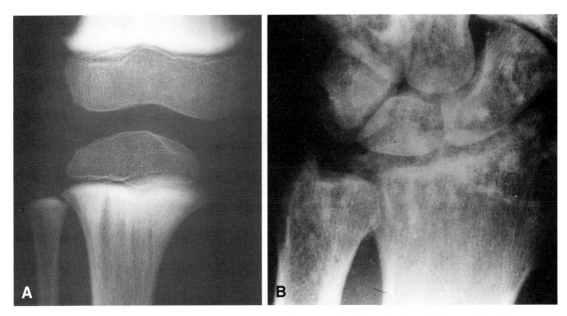

FIGURE 6.256. A. Osteopathia striata. Note dense vertical lines in the tibial metaphysis. **B. Osteopoikilosis.** Numerous small islands of compact bone are seen scattered throughout the carpal bones and distal radius and ulna.

REFERENCE

1. Gay BB Jr, Elsas LJ, Wyly JB, et al. Osteopathia striata with cranial sclerosis. Pediatr Radiol 1994;24:56–60.

SOFT TISSUE ABNORMALITIES

Soft Tissue Edema

Edema of the soft tissues, whether widespread as in the nephrotic syndrome or localized as with infection or trauma, is easily demonstrable roentgenographically. The characteristic appearance is that of coarse reticulation of the soft tissues and loss of the normally distinct planes between the skin, subcutaneous fat, and muscle (Fig. 6.257). In other instances, probably where fluid accumulation is greater, the soft tissues assume a more uniform opaque appearance.

Soft tissue edema also can be seen in conditions such as neonatal Turner's syndrome (Bonnevie-Ullrich syndrome), congenital absence of the lymphatics, or primary lymphedema and in extremities where venous return is compromised. It can also be seen in association with generalized lymphangiectasis and distal to an amniotic constricting ring.

Soft Tissue Calcification

In the neonate, soft tissue calcification can occasionally be seen with **fat necrosis** (1). In these cases, it is believed that

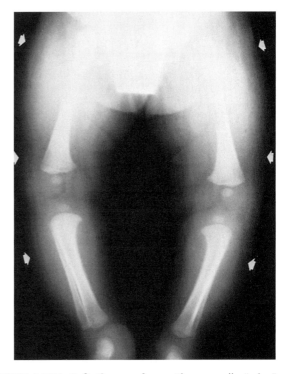

FIGURE 6.257. Soft tissue edema. The normally "crisp" and distinct tissue planes between the subcutaneous fat and muscle bundles are replaced by an extremely reticular appearance of the soft tissues (arrows). This is characteristic of edema in the soft tissues and, in this case, was the result of extensive cellulitis of both lower extremities.

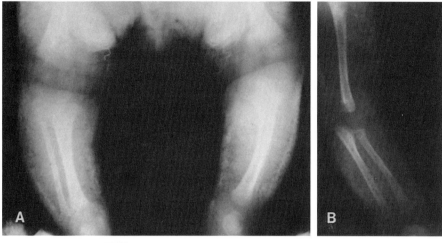

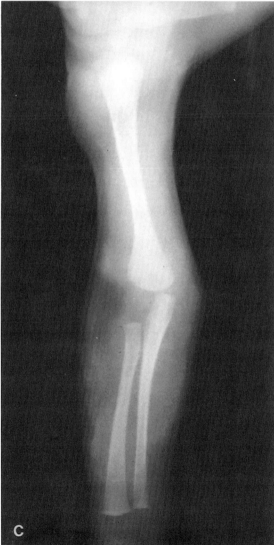

FIGURE 6.258. A and B. Fat necrosis. Widespread, irregular subcutaneous soft tissue calcification in both the upper and the lower extremities of this infant with fat necrosis secondary to hypothermia. These calcifications gradually disappeared. **C. Calcium injection.** Inadvertent leaking of calcium chloride solution into soft tissues of forearm produces a configuration suggesting soft tissue calcification. (**A** and **B** reproduced with permission from Duhn R, Schoen EJ, Siu M. Subcutaneous fat necrosis with extensive calcifications after hypothermia in two newborn infants. Pediatrics 1968;41:661–664).

obstetrical trauma leads to local schemia and subsequent calcification of necrotic fat tissue. Fat necrosis, with subsequent calcification, can also be seen after prolonged hypothermia (2, 3) and soft tissue trauma (4). Roentgenographically, the findings often are striking but should not be cause for undue alarm (Fig. 6.258, A and B). The prognosis is good, and both the calcifications and the associated soft tissue masses eventually disappear. Calcification in the soft tissues has also been described with generalized infantile fibromatosis and can be encountered with organizing intramuscular hematomas (5) or myositis ossificans (Fig. 6.259A).

Calcification in hemangiomas, other soft tissue tumors, dermatomyositis, calcinosis universalis, Ehlers-Danlos syndrome, tumoral calcinosis, and progressive myositis ossificans usually is seen in older children and not in neonates. Hemangiomas produce punctate calcifications (Fig. 6.259B), while dermatomyositis (Fig. 6.260B) and most of the other conditions produce sheath-like calcifications, and with tumoral calcinosis, the calcifications are bulky, lumpy, and juxtaarticular (Fig. 6.260A). With progressive myositis ossificans, the calcifications are linear and tend to follow tendons, and, in addition, the condition is associated with a short first digit (Fig. 6.261). Calcification secondary to hyperparathyroidism and vascular calcifications with progeria and arteriosclerosis are also occasionally encountered in young infants.

Calcium salts inadvertently injected into the soft tissues can produce changes that at first might suggest pathologic calcification (Fig. 6.258C). They disappear quickly, however. Calcification after subcutaneous emphysema in the neonate also has been described.

REFERENCES

1. Norton KI, Som PM, Shugar JM, et al. Subcutaneous fat necrosis of the newborn: CT findings of head and neck involvement. AJNR 1997;18:547–550.
2. Craig JE, Scholz TA, Vanderhooft SL, et al. Fat necrosis after ice application for supraventricular tachycardia termination. J Pediatr 1998;133:727.
3. Lee SK, Lee JH, Han CH, et al. Calcified subcutaneous fat necrosis induced by prolonged exposure to cold weather: a case report. Pediatr Radiol 2001;31:294–295.
4. Tsai TS, Evans HA, Donnelly LF, et al. Fat necrosis after trauma: a benign cause of palpable lumps in children. AJR 1997;169:1623–1626.
5. Gindel A, Schwamborn D, Tsironie K, et al. Myositis ossificans traumatica in young children: report of three cases and review of the literature. Pediatr Radiol 2000;30:451–459.

Congenital Soft Tissue Rings (Amniotic Band Syndrome)

Some infants are born with tight, constricting soft tissue amniotic rings, and in some cases, underlying bone underdevelopment is present. Some rings are so tight that they induce autoamputation (1–3). Edema of the extremity distal to the ring is often present, and the findings are clearly visible both clinically and roentgenographically (Fig. 6.262A). The etiology is uncertain, but the pathogenesis

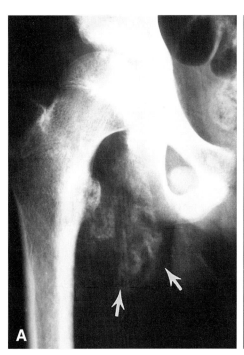

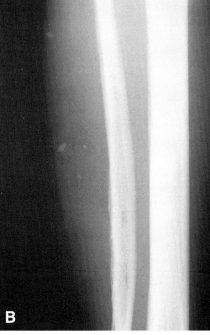

FIGURE 6.259. A. Posttraumatic myositis ossificans. Note irregular calcification along the medial aspect of the right femur (arrows) caused by a healing hematoma of the iliopsoas muscle. **B. Hemangioma with punctate calcifications.** Note numerous punctate calcifications (phleboliths) in the soft tissues of this patient with a longstanding hemangioma. Also note secondary changes in the fibula consisting of bending and some reactive periosteal new bone deposition.

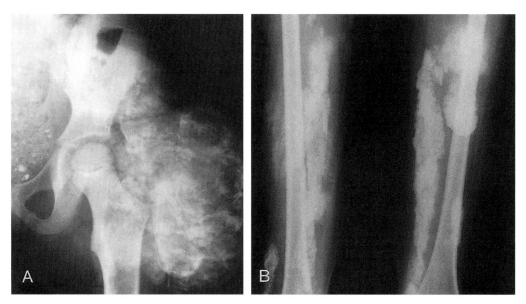

FIGURE 6.260. A. Tumoral calcinosis. Note flocculent, bulky paraarticular calcification around the hip. **B. Dermatomyositis.** Note sheet-like calcifications with some areas that are more lumpy.

probably lies with premature rupture of the amniotic membrane and its subsequent encirclement of the fetal extremities. If these bands involve the head (4), grotesque deformities can result (Fig. 6.262B). Such deformities are likely to occur if amniotic membrane rupture occurs early in pregnancy. Rupture later in pregnancy is likely to result in extremity bands.

REFERENCES

1. Askins G, Ger E. Congenital constriction band syndrome. J Pediatr Orthop 1988;8:461–466.
2. Bourne MH, Klassen RA. Congenital annular constricting bands: review of the literature and a case report. J Pediatr Orthop 1987;7:218–221.
3. Tada K, Yonenobu K, Swanson AB. Congenital constriction band syndrome. J Pediatr Orthop 1984;4:726–730.
4. McCarthy S, Sarwar M, Birapongse C, et al. Craniofacial anomalies in the amniotic band disruption complex. Pediatr Radiol 1984;14:44–46.

Arthrogryposis Multiplex Congenita

The striated muscle in arthrogryposis multiplex congenita, a very heterogeneous syndrome (1), is extremely atrophic, and widespread fatty replacement is seen. These findings are clearly evident on roentgenograms of the extremities (Fig. 6.263). Flexion contractures of the extremities are part of the syndrome and usually are pronounced and progressive. The bones become osteoporotic, thin, and gracile and show a distinct tendency to pathologic fracture. Many different types exist, and, overall, the syndrome is heterogeneous.

REFERENCE

1. Houston CS, Chudley AE. Separating monostomy-21 from the "arthrogryposis basket." J Can Assoc Radiol 1981;32:220–223.

Soft Tissues and Bones in Neurogenic and Neuromuscular Disease

Many conditions including meningomyelocele, sacral agenesis, diastematomyelia, spinal cord tumors, intracranial lesions, and muscular abnormalities such as arthrogryposis, amyotonia congenita, and myotonic dystrophy can lead to atrophy of the muscles of the extremities. This is clearly visualized roentgenographically and is a valuable clue to the detection of such underlying abnormalities. Typically, muscle bulk is decreased, subcutaneous fat is increased, and the fatty stripes between the muscle bundles become more prominent. The findings are the same as those seen in Fig. 6.263. Joint dislocations (especially the hip) are also commonly seen, and the bones become osteoporotic and thin. Pathologic fractures are common.

MRI can detect muscle atrophy and its associated increased fat replacement in these conditions (1, 2). With ultrasound, there is increased echogenicity of the muscle as it is replaced with fat (3).

REFERENCES

1. Liu G-C, Jong Y-J, Chiang C-H, et al. Spinal muscular atrophy MR evaluation. Pediatr Radiol 1992;22:584–586.
2. Schreiber A, Smith WL, Ionasescu V, et al. Magnetic resonance

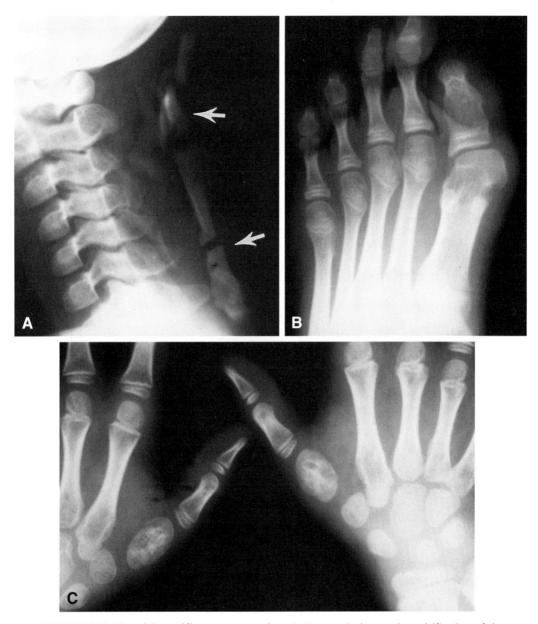

FIGURE 6.261. Myositis ossificans progressiva. A. Note typical extensive calcification of the posterior cervical (nuchal) ligament (arrows). **B.** Typical short first digit of the foot. **C.** Same patient demonstrating short and oval first metacarpals.

imaging of children with Duchenne's muscular dystrophy. Pediatr Radiol 1987;17:495–497.

3. Reimers K, Reimers CD, Wagner S, et al. Skeletal muscle sonography: a correlative study of echogenicity and morphology. J Ultrasound Med 1993;12:73–77.

Hemihypertrophy

If pronounced, hemihypertrophy may be evident at birth. It can involve all the structures on one side of the body or be more marked in the lower extremities. There is an increase in both soft tissue bulk and bone length and size. Hemihypertrophy is of unknown etiology, but such factors as unilateral

vascular and lymphatic tumors, incomplete twinning, and central nervous system abnormalities have been invoked. None of these explains the abnormality in all cases.

It is important to know that there is a more than coincidental association of certain intraabdominal tumors and hemihypertrophy. Although this can occur with almost any intraabdominal tumor, most commonly it is seen with Wilms' tumor of the kidney or adrenal tumors. In addition, hypertrophy can occur after the tumor appears, and the abnormality can persist after the tumor is removed. Hemihypertrophy also occurs in the Beckwith-Wiedemann syndrome and conditions such as renal polycystic disease.

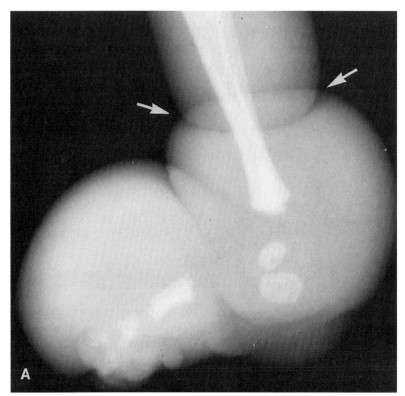

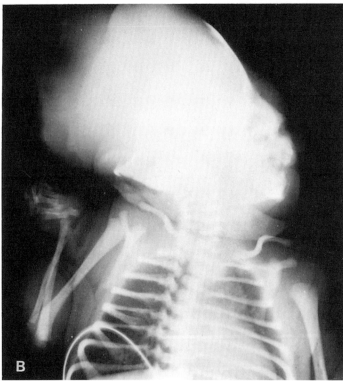

FIGURE 6.262. Congenital soft tissue amniotic bands. A. Note the constricting soft tissue band (arrows) producing extensive edema of the ankle and foot below it. **B.** Another infant with involvement of the head. Note the grotesque deformity of the head.

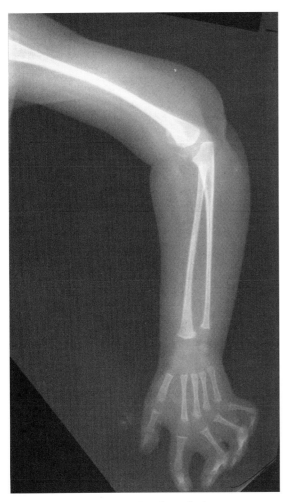

FIGURE 6.263. Arthrogryposis. The soft tissues are extremely radiolucent as a result of pronounced muscular atrophy and replacement with fatty tissue. Only a few thin muscular strands are seen in the upper extremity. Also note that the bones are extremely thin, gracile, and underdeveloped.

Soft Tissue Infections

Soft tissue infections can take the form of cellulitis, abscess, myositis, or adenopathy. In terms of cellulitis, radiographic changes consist of superficial soft tissue edema with reticulation of the soft tissues (Fig. 6.264A). When infection involves the muscles, the term "pyomyositis" often is used (1–4). The findings are often most vividly demonstrable with ultrasound or MR (Fig. 6.264, B and C). When pyomyositis involves the deep pelvic soft tissues, a hip problem can be mimicked (5). In some cases, an actual abscess develops, and these abscesses are readily detected with ultrasound (Fig. 6.264D). With necrotizing fasciitis, ultrasound demonstrates echogenic thickened soft tissues with small interspersed fluid collections (6).

With inflammatory adenopathy, no matter where it occurs, it once again is most readily detected with ultrasonography. The inflamed lymph nodes are variably enlarged and may be clustered in groups. The nodes are variably hypoechoic to the adjacent fat, and in addition, exuberant blood flow can be seen (7) (Fig. 6.265, A and B). When lymph nodes suppurate, they become liquid in the center and much more echoic. A residual rim of tissue usually is present. In some cases, the enlarged, edematous lymph nodes are very hypoechoic and may at first suggest liquefaction or suppuration (Fig. 6.265C). However, with color flow Doppler, it becomes evident that only an inflamed lymph node is present (Fig. 6.265D).

Lymph nodes occurring in the epitrochlear region produce epitrochlear lymphadenitis (1, 2) and again are readily identified with ultrasound as well as plain film (Fig. 6.266). Many times, epitrochlear adenitis results from cat-scratch disease.

REFERENCES

1. Bibbo X, Patel DV, Mackessy RP, et al. Pyomyositis of the left with early neurologic compromise. Pediatr Emerg Care 2000;16: 352–354.
2. Spiegel DA, Meyer DA, Dormans JP, et al. Pyomyositis in children and adolescents: report of 12 cases and review of the literature. J Pediatr Orthop 1999;19:143–150.
3. Viani RM, Bromberg K, Bradley JS. Obturator internus muscle abscess in children: report of seven cases and review. Clin Infect Dis 1999;28:117–122.
4. Wheeler DS, Vasquez WD, Vaux KK, et al. Streptococcal pyomyositis: case report and review. Pediatr Emer Care 1998;14: 412.
5. Hernandez RJ, Strouse PJ, Craig CL, et al. Original report: focal pyomyositis of the perisciatic muscles in children. AJR 2002;179: 1267.
6. Chao H, Kong MS, Ling TY. Diagnosis of necrotizing fasciitis in children. J Ultrasound Med 1999;18:277–281.
7. Swischuk LE, Desai PB, John SD. Exuberant blood flow in enlarged lymph nodes: findings on color-flow Doppler. Pediatr Radiol 1992;22:419–421.

Tendinitis

Tendinitis can be inflammatory or traumatic; in regard to the latter, it most commonly is associated with avulsion injuries such as Osgood-Schlatter disease, Sinding-Larsen-Johansson disease, and Sever's disease. Sever's disease, often believed to be aseptic necrosis of the calcaneal apophysis, actually is an Achilles tendinitis. Sinding-Larsen-Johansson disease represents a tendon-avulsion injury of the inferior pole of the patella. The most common problem of all, that is, Osgood-Schlatter disease, constitutes a tendinous avulsion of the tibial tubercle by the infrapatellar tendon. When tendon inflammation is associated with tendon avulsion injuries, the underlying bone often becomes demineralized

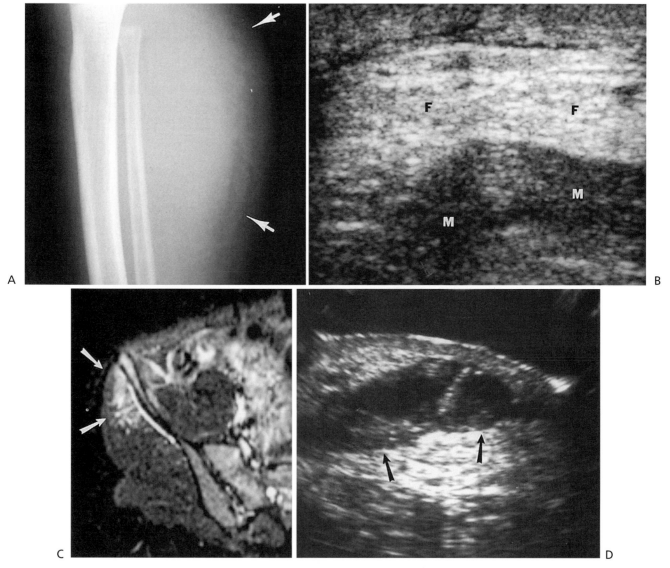

FIGURE 6.264. Soft tissue infection. A. Note the enlarged muscle mass and reticulated, edematous superficial tissues of the calf (arrows). **B.** Ultrasonogram demonstrates thickening and edema of the muscle (M) and increased echogenicity and thickness of the overlying subcutaneous fat (F). **C.** Another patient whose magnetic resonance study demonstrates increased irregular signal in the gluteus muscle (arrow). **D.** Abscess formation. Note the hypoechoic abscess (arrows) within the echogenic muscle mass.

and fragmented. This is what classically is seen with active Osgood-Schlatter disease (Fig. 6.267). Similar fragmentation occurs along the inferior pole of the patella in Sinding-Larsen-Johansson disease. These conditions are generally self-limiting, but a rare complication of tibia recurvatum has been documented with Osgood-Schlatter disease (1).

Finally, a subclinical avulsion injury commonly occurs along the distal medial supracondylar ridge of the femur in adolescence. Irregularity of the bone in this area should not be misinterpreted for a more dire problem such as infection or tumor. The location and configuration of the lesion are characteristic (Fig. 2.267A). This particular lesion has been variably referred to as a benign cortical defect or desmoid tumor, but most likely it represents a healing subclinical avulsion injury.

When tendinitis results from inflammation, the findings merely consist of thickening of the involved tendon with surrounding edema (Fig. 6.268). All these tendon problems usually are clearly apparent on plain films but also can be imaged with CT and MRI (2–5).

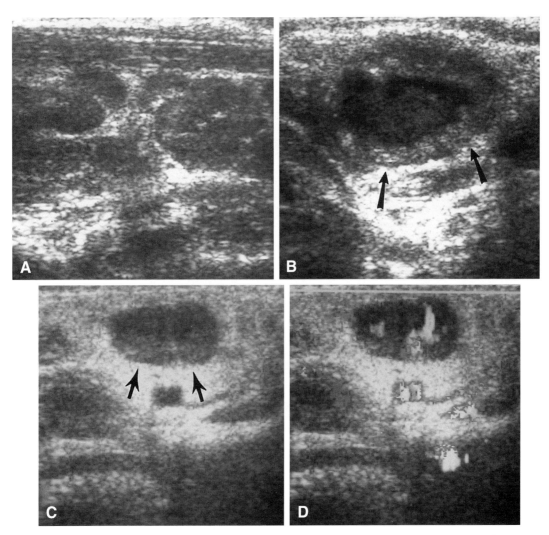

FIGURE 6.265. Inflammatory adenopathy. A. Note numerous enlarged hypoechoic, oval to round lymph nodes. **B.** In another area, one of the nodes has enlarged and liquefied (suppurated), leaving a residual rim of tissue (arrows). **C.** Another patient with a single inflamed lymph node (arrows). The surrounding fat is echogenic secondary to superimposed edema. **D.** Color flow Doppler demonstrates exuberant blood flow to the lymph node (white streaks inside the lymph node).

REFERENCES

1. Lynch MC, Walsh HPJ. Tibia recurvatum as a complication of Osgood-Schlatter disease: a report of two cases. J Pediatr Orthop 1991;11:543–544.
2. Davies SG, Baudouin CJ, King JB, et al. Ultrasound, computed tomography, and magnetic resonance imaging in patellar tendinitis. Clin Radiol 1991;43:52–56.
3. El-Khoury GY, Wira RL, Berbaum KS, et al. MR imaging of the patellar tendinitis. Radiology 1992;184:849–854.
4. Lanning P, Heikkinen E. Ultrasonic features of the Osgood-Schlatter lesions. J Pediatr Orthop 1991;11:538–540.
5. Rosenberg ZS, Kawelblum M, Cheung YY, et al. Osgood-Schlatter lesion: fracture or tendinitis? Scintigraphic, CT, and MR imaging features. Radiology 1992;185:188.

Soft Tissue Hematomas

Soft tissue hematomas are common after trauma and can be seen with bleeding disorders. They are most readily detected with ultrasound, where, in their early stages, they are echogenic. In their later stages, they undergo liquefaction and become hypoechoic. The hematomas also can be demonstrated with CT and MRI, but plain films and ultra-

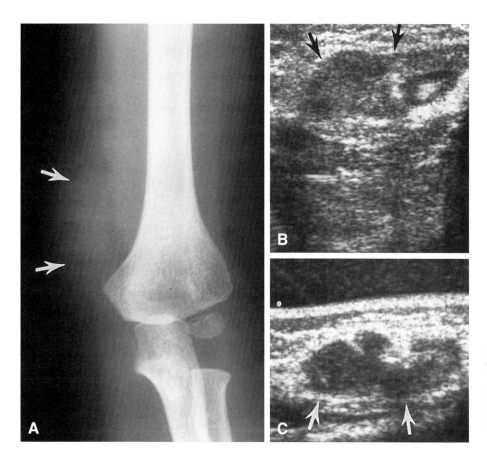

FIGURE 6.266. Epitrochlear adenitis. A. Anteroposterior view of the forearm demonstrates enlarged nodes (arrows) in the epitrochlear region. **B.** Ultrasound demonstrates an echogenic enlarged lymph node (arrows). **C.** In another area, another lymph node has liquefied (arrows).

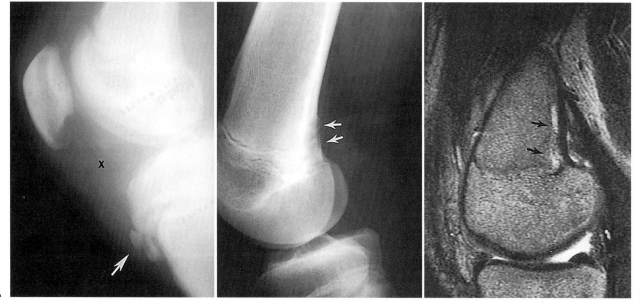

FIGURE 6.267. Traumatic tendinitis: avulsion injuries. A. Osgood-Schlatter disease. There is edema involving the infrapatellar fat pad (X), which has caused it to become partially obliterated. Edema and swelling extend over the tibial tubercle, which itself is fragmented (arrow). **B. Normal distal femoral irregularity.** Note irregularity of the cortex (arrows) over the medial supracondylar ridge. This configuration often erroneously is interpreted for a tumor. **C.** Another patient who had a similar lesion in the femur and whose magnetic resonance study demonstrates inflammatory changes in both the cortex and the surrounding soft tissues (arrows).

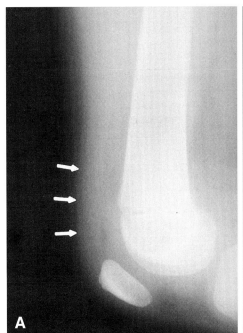
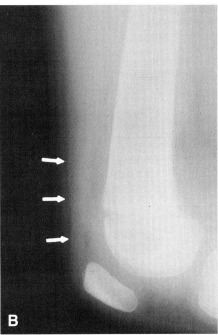

FIGURE 6.268. Nonspecific tendinitis. A. The quadriceps tendon in this patient (arrows) is thickened and fuzzy both anteriorly and posteriorly, attesting to edema in and around the tendon. **B.** Compare with the normal appearance of the tendon (arrows) on the other side.

sound usually suffice. Hematomas can calcify in their later stages, leading to posttraumatic myositis ossificans.

Soft Tissue Foreign Bodies

Soft tissue foreign bodies may be opaque or nonopaque. If they are opaque, they are readily identified and localized on plain films. If nonopaque, however, they can be a greater problem, and in this regard, ultrasonography has become extremely useful in their detection (Fig. 6.269). Ultrasonography also can be used as guidance for removing these

foreign bodies (1). Fish and chicken bones, if they are large, usually are detectable with plain films, but smaller bones may require ultrasonography for detection. Most glass is visible with plain films.

REFERENCE

1. Leung A, Patton A, Navoy J, et al. Intraoperative sonography-guided removal of radiolucent foreign bodies. J Pediatr Orthop 1998;18:259–261.

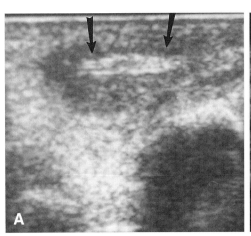
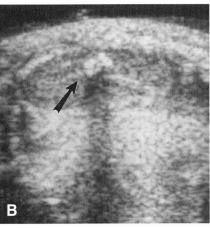

FIGURE 6.269. Soft tissue foreign body: ultrasonographic demonstration. A. Sagittal view demonstrates the echogenic elongated foreign body (arrows) surrounded by a ring of edema. **B.** Cross-section demonstrates the echogenic foreign body (arrow) with distal shadowing.

TUMORS OF THE SKELETON AND SOFT TISSUES

Soft Tissue Tumors

Soft tissue tumors in the neonate and young infant usually are lymphangiomatous, hemangiomatous, lipomatous, or fibromatous in origin. The latter are dealt with later in the section on fibromatous soft tissue and bony tumors in the infant. Lymphangiomas tend to be solitary, but hemangiomas and fibromas often are multiple and involve the viscera. As far as soft tissue tumors in general are concerned, ultrasound and MR are one's best imaging modalities for their delineation (1–3).

Ultrasonographically, cystic hygromas are multiloculated with variable-sized hypoechoic collections of fluid separated by thin echogenic septa (Fig. 6.270A). With MRI, the fluid

shows medium signal on T1-weighted images (Fig. 6.270, B and C), but it increases in signal on T2-weighted images (Fig 6.270D). This does not occur to the same degree that it does with hemangiomas. When bleeding occurs, echogenic debris can be seen within the various cysts, and on MR, signal increases (Fig. 6.271). MR and CT may show greater extent of the lesion than originally anticipated (4–6) and in this way also aid in directing possible biopsy intervention.

Hemangiomas are solid and echogenic on ultrasound. The pattern of echogenicity is coarse, and sinusoids along with vascular feeders and drainers can be identified (Fig. 6.272). Color flow Doppler is excellent in demonstrating blood flow to these tumors (7) and in many cases also identifies the feeders and drainers. It should be noted, however, that with capillary hemangiomas, because blood flow is

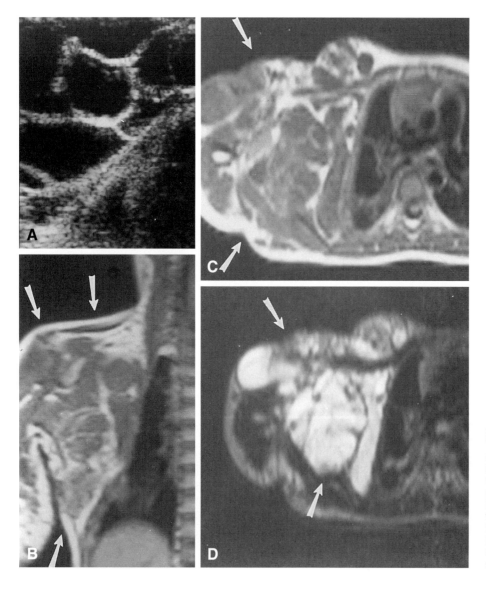

FIGURE 6.270. Cystic hygroma. A. Typical ultrasonographic appearance of multiple anechoic cystic structures separated by echogenic septa. **B.** T1-weighted magnetic resonance image demonstrates an extensive multiloculated lesion (arrows). It is deforming the rib cage. **C.** Axial T1-weighted image demonstrates similar findings (arrows). Fluid in the cyst is of low signal. **D.** T2-weighted image demonstrates high signal in the cyst (arrows).

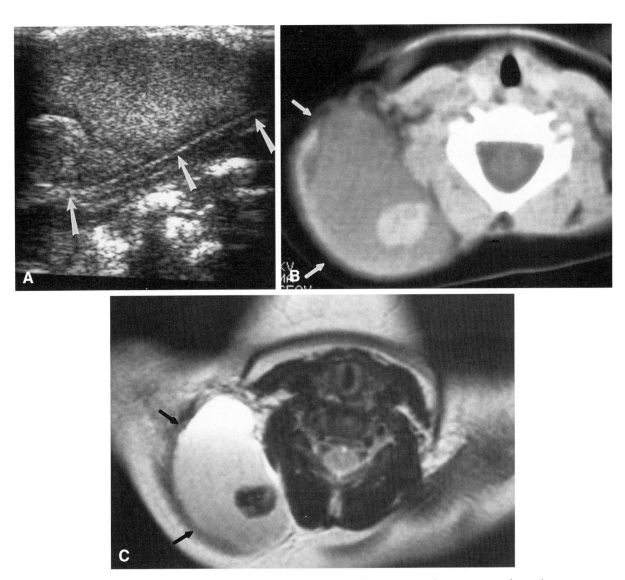

FIGURE 6.271. Cystic hygroma with bleeding. A. Ultrasonogram demonstrates echogenic debris within the cystic hygroma (arrows). On the far left, an echogenic ball is suggested. This is a blood clot. **B.** Computed tomography study demonstrates the cystic hygroma (arrows) with the high signal blood clot. **C.** Proton density magnetic resonance imaging demonstrates increased signal in the fluid (arrows). The blood clot is of low signal.

sluggish, it might not be detected with color flow Doppler. With MRI, hemangiomas tend to be high in signal on T2-weighted images and remain high on second-echo T2-weighted images (Fig. 6.273). In addition, feeders and drainers can be identified. Finally, cerebrovasculopathy with large craniofacial angiomas has been noted (8). Customarily, systemic steroids are used for treated hemangiomas, but intralesional corticosteroid therapy also has been suggested (9).

Lipomas also are echogenic and solid on ultrasound, but as opposed to hemangiomas, the pattern of echogenicity is delicate and finely granular (Fig. 6.274). On plain films and CT, lipomas are radiolucent; on MRI, they show increased

signal on T1-weighted images (Fig. 6.274D). An interesting syndrome called the Bannayan-Zonana syndrome manifests in the presence of multiple soft tissue tumors, primarily lipomas, hemangiomas, and lymphangiomas (10).

Although not a true tumor in the sense that it is not a neoplasm, a common problem in infancy is that of torticollis with shortening of the sternocleidomastoid muscle secondary to a fibroma in the belly of the muscle (11–13). The mass produced is readily identified with ultrasound (Fig. 6.275), where it will be echogenic and oval shaped and seen to blend into normal muscle.

Malignant soft tissue tumors are much less common than benign tumors and consist primarily of rhab-

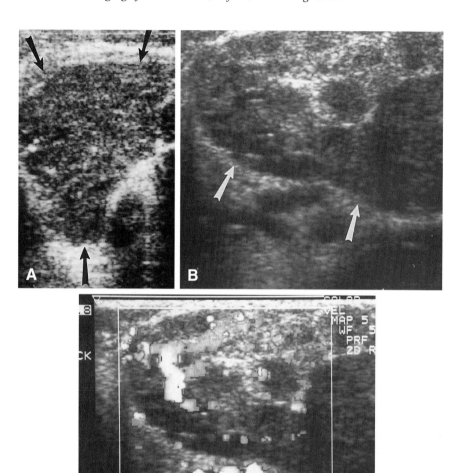

FIGURE 6.272. Hemangioma: ultrasonographic features. A. Typical coarse echogenic pattern of a hemangioma (arrows). **B.** Another patient with a similar coarse echogenic pattern and anechoic areas representing sinusoids. **C.** Color flow Doppler demonstrates increased flow throughout the lesion.

domyosarcoma and fibrosarcoma. These tumors are generally echogenic on ultrasound and show increased signal with MRI (Fig. 6.276). The findings are nonspecific, and it is difficult to differentiate one tumor from another. Because of this, almost invariably with malignant tumors (which clinically are firm and hard), one will obtain both ultrasound and MRI. With soft benign tumors (i.e., hemangiomas, lymphangiomas, and lipomas), because the ultrasonographic features are so characteristic, MRI is required only if surgical or other therapy is contemplated.

REFERENCES

1. Abiezzi SS, Miller LS. The use of ultrasound for the diagnosis of soft-tissue masses in children. J Pediatr Orthop 1995;15:566–573.
2. Glasier CM, Seibert JJ, Williamson SL, et al. High-resolution ultrasound characterization of soft tissue masses in children. Pediatr Radiol 1987;17:233–237.
3. Jabra AA, Taylor GA. MRI evaluation of superficial soft tissue lesions in children. Pediatr Radiol 1993;23:425–428.
4. Fung K, Poenaru D, Soboleski DA, et al. Impact of magnetic resonance imaging on the surgical management of cystic hygromas. J Pediatr Surg 1998;33:839–841.
5. Konez O, Vyas PK, Goyal M. Disseminated lymphangiomatosis presenting with massive chylothorax. Pediatr Radiol 2000;30:35–37.
6. Wunderbaldinger P, Paya K, Partik B, et al. Original report. CT and MR imaging of generalized cystic lymphangiomatosis in pediatric patients. AJR 2000;174:827–832.
7. Latifi HR, Siegel MJ. Color-flow Doppler imaging of pediatric soft tissue masses. J Ultrasound Med 1994;13:165–169.
8. Burrows PE, Robertson RL, Mullilken JB, et al. Cerebral vasculopathy and neurologic sequelae in infants with cervicofacial hemangioma: report of eight patients. Radiology 1998;207:601–607.
9. Chen MT, Yeong EK, Horng SY. Intralesional corticosteroid therapy in proliferating head and neck hemangiomas: a review of 155 cases. J Pediatr Surg 2000;35:420–423.
10. Hayashi Y, Ohi R, Tomita T, et al. Bannayan-Zonana syndrome associated with lipomas, hemangiomas, and lymphangiomas. J Pediatr Surg 1992;27:722–723.

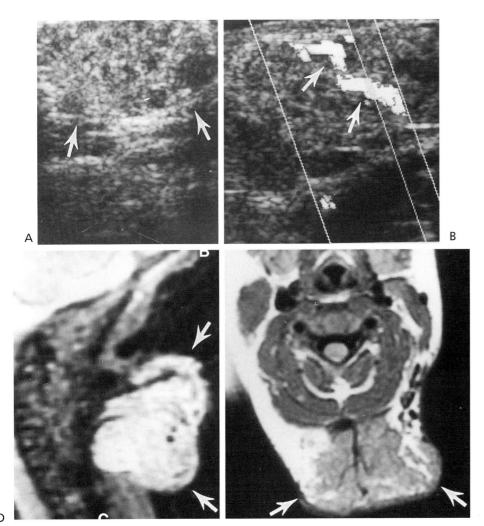

FIGURE 6.273. Hemangioma: ultrasonographic and magnetic resonance findings. A. Typical echogenic pattern with small sinusoids (arrows). **B.** Color flow Doppler demonstrates a large feeding vessel (arrows). **C.** Proton density magnetic resonance imaging demonstrates the high signal in the hemangioma (arrows) located over the posterior neck. Note linear and circular dark areas demonstrating the feeding vessels. **D.** T1-weighted image demonstrates the low signal hemangioma (arrows) and the branching feeding vessel (black branching structure).

11. Chan YL, Cheng JCY, Metreweli C. Ultrasonography of congenital muscular torticollis. Pediatr Radiol 1992;22:356–360.
12. Ablin DS, Jain K, Howell L, et al. Ultrasound and MR imaging of fibromatosis colli (sternomastoid tumor of infancy). Pediatr Radiol 1998;28:230–233.
13. Lin J-N, Chou M-L. Ultrasonographic study of the sternocleidomastoid muscle in the management of congenital muscular torticollis. J Pediatr Surg 1997;32:1648–1651.

Bone Cysts and Other Cyst-Like Lesions

These lesions consist of simple bone cysts, aneurysmal bone cysts, giant cell tumor, osteofibrous dysplasia, benign cortical defects, and their intimately related lesion, the nonossifying fibroma. In addition, it should be remembered that low-grade infections such as tuberculosis can result in cystic-appearing lesions of the bone and that cystic bony lesions also can be seen with histiocytosis X (Langerhans' histiocytosis) (Fig. 6.277).

Bone cysts most commonly occur in the proximal humerus but can be seen in other long bones. They also are not uncommonly seen in flat bones such as the iliac wing and calcaneus (1). In the long bones, these cysts are prone to pathologic fracture (Fig. 6.278A), and most present after such fractures occur. Otherwise, they are innocuous and benign lesions, producing no symptoms. Bone cysts contain fluid, and because of this, if a piece of cortex falls into the cyst, it will be seem to be suspended in the cyst, constituting the so-called "fallen fragment sign" (Fig. 2.278A). Repeated fracturing may cause healing of the bone cyst, but most often, some form of intervention is required. Over the years, bone chips, steroids (2), demineralized bone matrix (3), and autogenic bone marrow (4) have been used. The bottom line here appears to be that, somehow or other, you have to irritate the cyst and then it will heal. MRI has been employed in the evaluation of benign bone cysts (5), but its results are confusing, and it is recommended that one utilize plain films for the diagnosis. They are usually definitive.

Aneurysmal bone cysts are, by definition, aneurysmally expanded bone cystic lesions (Fig. 6.278D). They have been shown to occur most commonly in the tibia (6), and

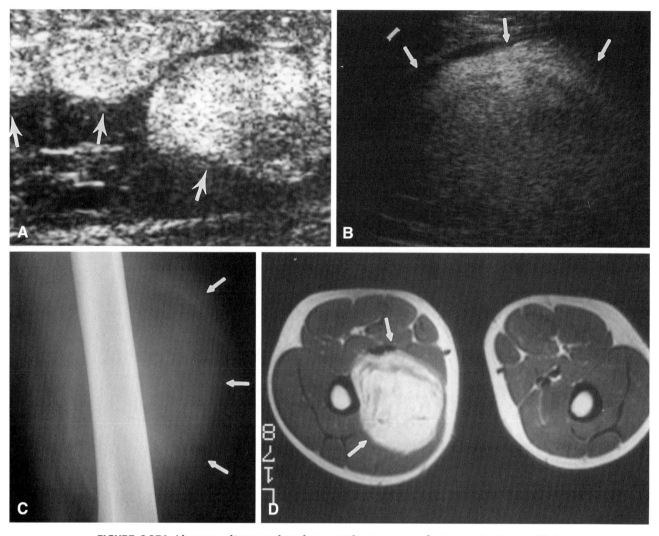

FIGURE 6.274. Lipoma: ultrasound and magnetic resonance features. A. Note multiple highly echogenic lipomas (arrows) in this patient with Bannayan-Zonana syndrome. **B.** Another large lipoma demonstrating a delicate echogenic pattern (arrows). **C.** Same patient whose plain films demonstrate the radiolucent lipoma (arrows). **D.** T1-weighted magnetic resonance image demonstrates the characteristic high signal of a lipoma (arrows). (Courtesy of C. Keith Hayden, Jr., M.D.).

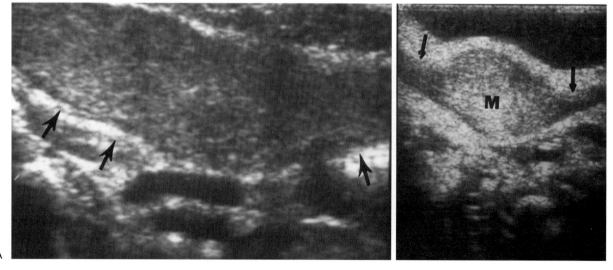

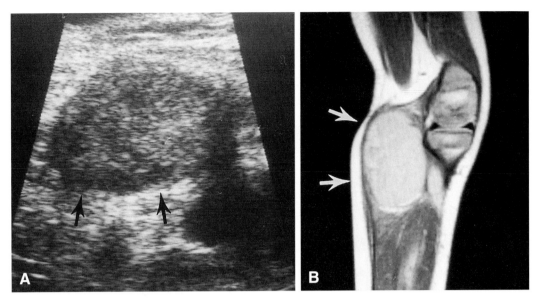

FIGURE 6.276. Rhabdomyosarcoma. A. Ultrasonogram demonstrates nonspecific echogenicity in the round mass (arrows). **B.** Sagittal T1-weighted magnetic resonance image demonstrates the reasonably well-defined tumor (arrows), which shows moderately high signal. (Courtesy of C. Keith Hayden, Jr., M.D.).

also they tend to recur (7). The current theory for the development of aneurysmal bone cysts is bleeding into a preexisting bony lesion, often a previous benign cyst or tumor (7). Because of the bleeding, a blood-fluid level (Fig. 6.278E) frequently is seen within the substance of these cysts, with both ultrasound and MRI (8, 9). Aneurysmal bone cysts most commonly are located in the medullary cavity but also can be cortical (Fig. 6.279). Aneurysmal bone cysts can be treated by embolization (10–12). Giant cell tumors of the bone can resemble aneurysmal bone cysts but generally are rare in children (13).

Benign cortical defects are common in children and adolescents. They most commonly are seen in the distal femur and proximal tibia (Fig. 6.278B) and are characteristically cortical in location. They usually have sclerotic margins, although in some of the lesions, this finding is minimal. There is an increased incidence of benign cortical defects in neurofibromatosis, but otherwise they are benign and innocuous lesions. A closely related lesion is the nonossifying fibroma (Fig. 6.278C). Again, this lesion is eccentric, occurs in the long bones (primarily in the lower extremities), and shows a sclerotic, often scalloped border. Gener-

ally, these lesions also are innocuous and self-limiting. They usually heal by sclerosis (Fig. 6.280), and with benign cortical defects, avulsion of the overlying cortex can occur (13) (Fig. 6.280C). MRI imaging can be confusing (14), and thus, once again, the diagnosis is accomplished with plain films.

A peculiar cystic, somewhat dysplastic lesion of the long bones in infants is the so-called "osteofibrous dysplasia of bone" (15–18). This lesion has been described in the neonate (19) and has a nonspecific and yet highly suggestive cystic-dysplastic appearance (Fig. 6.281A). In some patients, the lesion may appear more cystic and with pathologic fracturing can appear almost malignant (Fig. 6.281B).

REFERENCES

1. Moreau G, Letts M. Unicameral bone cyst of the calcaneus in children. J Pediatr Orthop 1994;14:101–104.
2. Rosenborg M, Mortensson W, Hirsch G, et al. Considerations in the corticosteroid treatment of bone cysts. J Pediatr Orthop 1989;9:240–243.
3. Killian JT, Wilkinson L, White S, et al. Treatment of unicameral

---

FIGURE 6.275. Fibroma: sternocleidomastoid muscle. A. Note the typical oval configuration of the echogenic fibromatous mass. **B.** In this patient, the muscle mass (M) is more echogenic, and the two ends of the normal sternocleidomastoid muscle are seen (arrows).

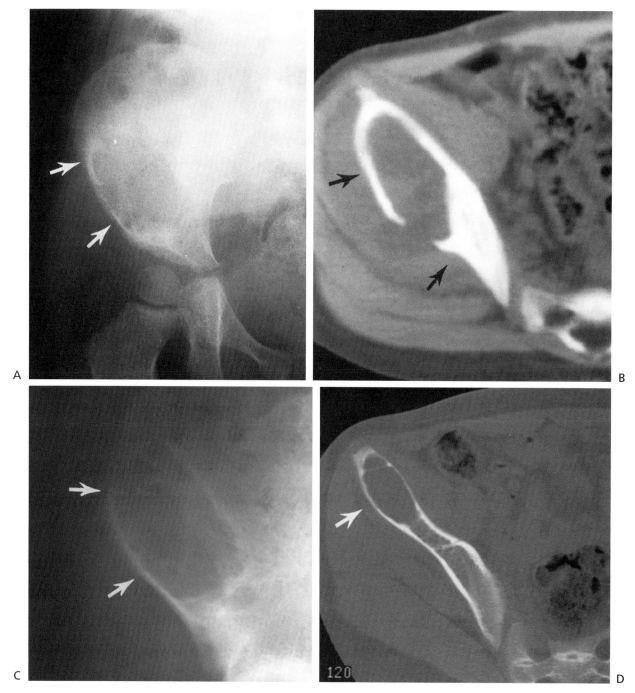

FIGURE 6.277. Pelvic cystic lesions. A. Note the cystic lesion of the right iliac wing (arrows). Its margin is slightly indistinct. **B.** Computed tomography study demonstrates the same cystic mass. In one area, the cortex has been eroded and there is a significant surrounding soft tissue mass (arrows). This patient had histiocytosis X. **C.** Benign bone cyst in the right iliac wing shows a lytic center and a sclerotic margin (arrows). **D.** Computed tomography study demonstrates the same features of the cyst (arrow). Note, however, that there is no associated soft tissue mass.

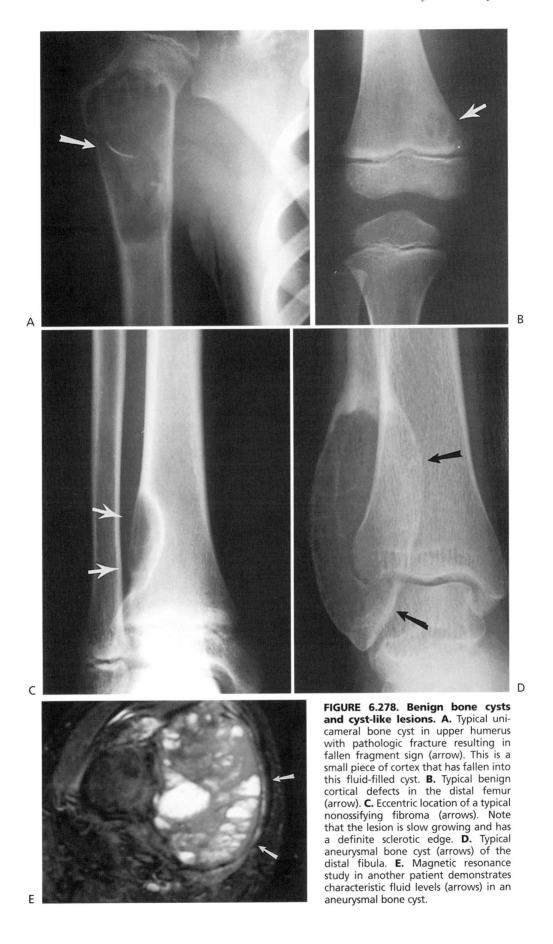

FIGURE 6.278. Benign bone cysts and cyst-like lesions. A. Typical unicameral bone cyst in upper humerus with pathologic fracture resulting in fallen fragment sign (arrow). This is a small piece of cortex that has fallen into this fluid-filled cyst. **B.** Typical benign cortical defects in the distal femur (arrow). **C.** Eccentric location of a typical nonossifying fibroma (arrows). Note that the lesion is slow growing and has a definite sclerotic edge. **D.** Typical aneurysmal bone cyst (arrows) of the distal fibula. **E.** Magnetic resonance study in another patient demonstrates characteristic fluid levels (arrows) in an aneurysmal bone cyst.

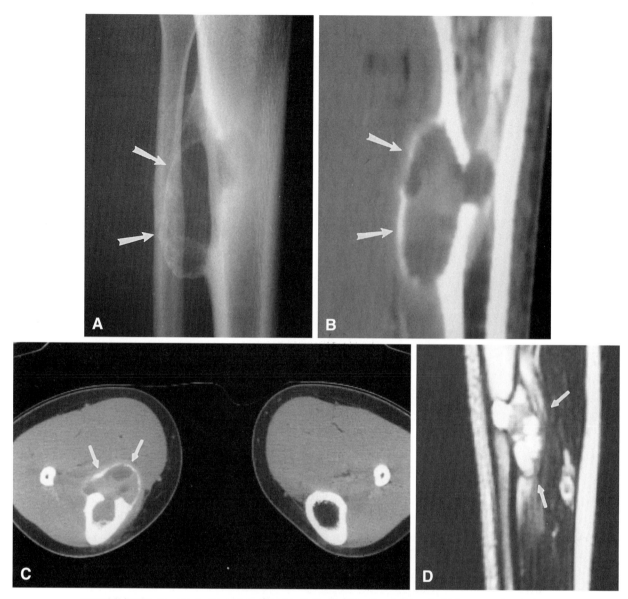

FIGURE 6.279. Cortical aneurysmal bone cyst. A. Note the delicate bubbly-appearing lesion (arrows). **B.** Sagittal reconstructed computed tomogram demonstrates similar findings (arrows). **C.** Axial computed tomography study demonstrates a markedly thinned, bulging cortex (arrows). The internal content of the cyst is heterogeneous. **D.** T1-weighted magnetic resonance image demonstrates high signal in the multiple lobules consistent with bleeding (arrows).

bone cyst with demineralized bone matrix. J Pediatr Orthop 1998;18:621–624.

4. Yandow SM, Lundeen GA, Scott SM, et al. Autogenic bone marrow injections as a treatment for simple bone cyst. J Pediatr Orthop 1998;18:616–620.

5. Margau R, Babyn P, Cole W, et al. MR imaging of simple bone cysts in children: not so simple. Pediatr Radiol 2000;30:551–557.

6. Rodriguez-Ramirez A, Stanton RP. Aneurysmal bone cyst in 29 children. J Pediatr Orthop 2002;22:533–539.

7. Balci P, Obuz F, Gore O, et al. Aneurysmal bone cyst secondary to infantile cartilaginous hamartoma of rib. Pediatr Radiol 1997; 27:767–769.

8. Freiberg AA, Loder RT, Heidelberger KP, et al. Aneurysmal bone cysts in young children. J Pediatr Orthop 1994;14:86–91.

9. Haber HP, Drews K, Scheel-Walter H, et al. Aneurysmal bone cysts in early childhood. Ultrasound findings. Pediatr Radiol 1993;23:405–406.

10. Krajca-Radcliffe JB, Thomas JR, Nicholas RW. Giant-cell tumor of bone: a rare entity in the hands of children. J Pediatr Orthop 1994;14:776–780.

11. Guibaud L, Herbreteau D, Dubois J, et al. Aneurysmal bone cysts: percutaneous embolization with an alcoholic solution of Zein—series of 18 cases. Radiology 1998;208:369–373.

12. Green JA, Bellemore MC, Marsden FW. Embolization in the

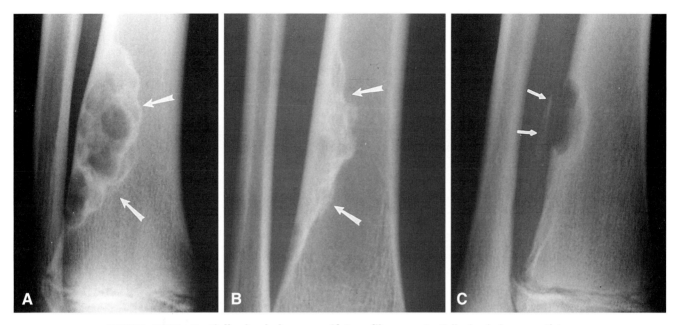

FIGURE 6.280. Partially healed, nonossifying fibroma. Partially healed, nonossifying fibroma (arrows) is shown. The eccentric location is characteristic. **B.** Another almost completely healed, nonossifying fibroma (arrows). **C. Benign cortical defect.** An associated avulsion fracture (arrows) is demonstrated.

treatment of aneurysmal bone cysts. J Pediatr Orthop 1997;17:440–443.

13. Hemmadi SS, Cole WG. Treatment of aneurysmal bone cysts with saucerization and bone marrow injection in children. J Pediatr Orthop 1999;19:540–542.

14. Kumar R, Swischuk LE, Madewell JE. Benign cortical defect: site for an avulsion fracture. Skeletal Radiol 1986;15:553–555.

15. Jee WH, Choe BY, Kang HS, et al. Nonossifying fibroma; char-

acteristics at MR imaging with pathologic correlation. Radiology 1998;209:197–202.

16. Komiya S, Inoue A. Aggressive bone tumorous lesion in infancy: osteofibrous dysplasia of the tibia and fibula. J Pediatr Orthop 1993;13:577–581.

17. Smith NM, Byard RW, Foster B, et al. Congenital ossifying fibroma (osteofibrous dysplasia) of the tibia—a case report. Pediatr Radiol 1991;21:449–451.

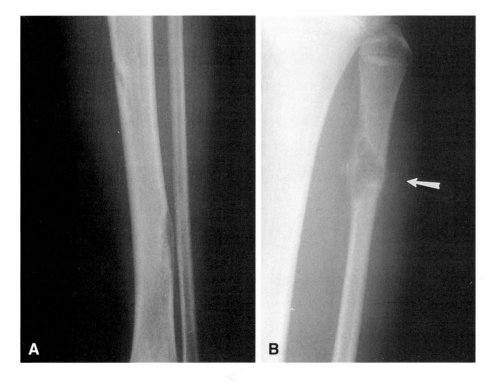

FIGURE 6.281. Osteofibrous dysplasia. A. Note the typically dysplastic appearance of the tibial and scattered cortical cystic lesions. **B.** Another patient with a pathologic fracture through one of the lesions (arrow).

18. Sweet DE, Vinh TN, Devaney K. Cortical osteofibrous dysplasia of long bone and its relationship to adamantinoma. Am J Surg Pathol 1992;16:282–290.

19. Hindman BW, Bell S, Russo T, et al. Neonatal osteofibrous dysplasia: report of two cases. Pediatr Radiol 1996;26: 303–306.

Osteoid Osteoma

Although not a cystic lesion, the osteoid osteoma characteristically presents with a central radiolucent nidus and considerable surrounding sclerosis (Fig. 6.282). The central nidus is

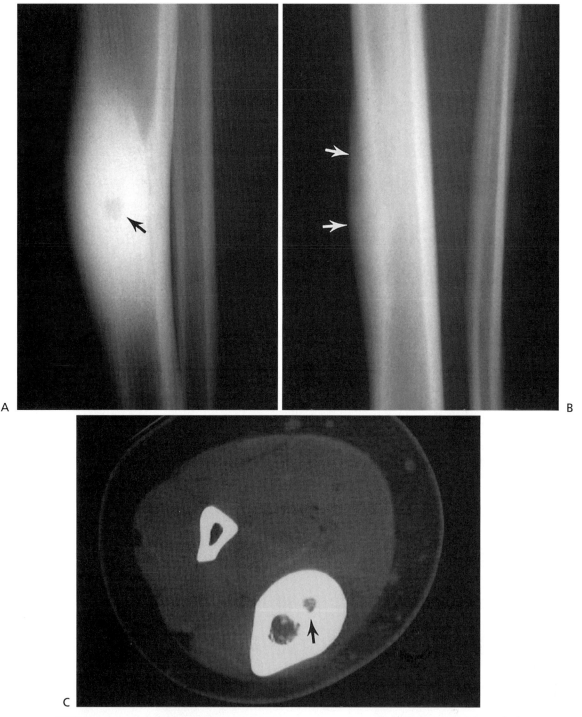

FIGURE 6.282. Osteoid osteoma. A. Classic appearance of an osteoid osteoma with marked sclerosis and thickening of the cortex along with a typical nidus (arrow). **B.** In this patient, only focal sclerosis (arrows) is seen. **C.** On computed tomography, however, a definite nidus (arrow) is seen within the thickened cortex.

vascular and evokes considerable irritation of the surrounding bone (1). Characteristically, there is pain in the extremity or involved portion of the skeleton that worsens at night and is relieved with aspirin. Not all patients have such a classic clinical presentation, however. Currently, these lesions can be resected percutaneously under CT guidance. Occasionally, osteoid osteomas are subperiosteal or epiphyseal (2, 3).

REFERENCES

1. Kransdorf MJ, Stull MA, Gilkey FW, et al. Osteoid osteoma. Radiographics 1991;11:671–696.
2. Shankman S, Desai P, Beltran J. Subperiosteal osteoid osteoma: radiographic and pathologic manifestations. Skeletal Radiol 1997; 26:457–462.
3. Kayser F, Resnick D, Haghighi P, et al. Evidence of the subperiosteal origin of osteoid osteomas in tubular bones: analysis by CT and MR imaging. AJR 1998;170:609–614.

Fibromatous Tumors of Infancy

There is a wide spectrum of fibromatous tumors seen in infancy (1–4). These can involve the soft tissues or the bony skeleton and may be solitary or multiple. Furthermore, they may be benign or aggressive (5). The benign variety, when it involves the bone, often occurs in the tibia (Fig. 6.283).

Congenital fibromatosis usually is widespread (6–8), and multiple areas of involvement are seen (Fig. 6.284). The lesions are typically destructive and, in the long bones, affect the metaphyses. There may be pathologic fractures, periosteal proliferation, and even calcification of the adjacent soft tissues. Because of the metaphyseal distribution and periosteal proliferation, the roentgenographic findings may at first suggest conditions such as congenital lues, osteomyelitis, hypophosphatasia, rubella, metaphyseal dysostosis, or even metastatic neuroblastoma.

There are two forms of congenital generalized fibromatosis: The first is limited to the skeleton (Fig. 6.284), whereas the second shows widespread visceral involvement (Fig. 6.285). Prognosis in the form limited to the skeleton is usually good, and regression of the lesions occurs over a period of years. In the other form, widespread visceral involvement, including the brain (8), usually leads to early death. Histopathologically, the lesions are not always purely fibromatous, and smooth muscle was demonstrated in the case illustrated in Fig. 6.284. Consequently, the term "hamartomatosis" is used (9).

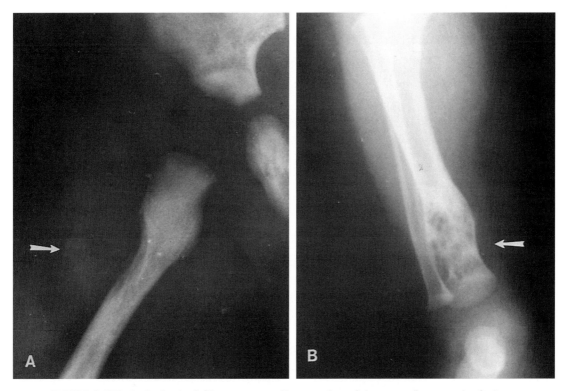

FIGURE 6.283. A. Periosteal fibrosarcoma. Note erosion of the upper femur and soft tissue calcification (arrow) produced by this periosteal fibrosarcoma in a newborn infant. **B. Benign fibrous bone tumor.** Note the cystic, expanding, multiloculated bone tumor of the distal tibia in this young infant (arrow). Histologically, this was a benign lesion comprising fibrous tissue that, as the infant grew older, became smaller. (**A** courtesy of Stuart Houston, M.D.).

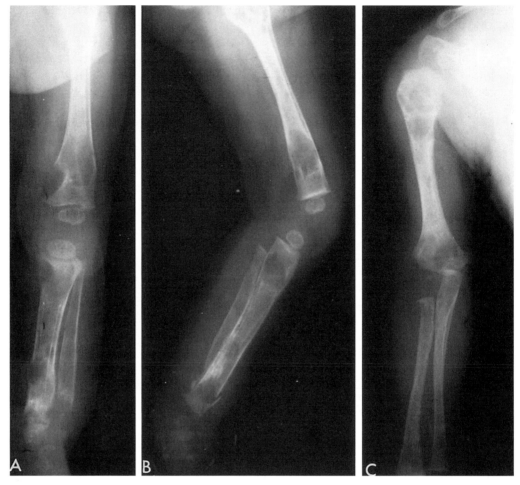

FIGURE 6.284. Generalized fibromatosis. A–C. There are extensive destructive lesions in the metaphyses of all the long bones. In the lower extremities, the findings closely resemble those of congenital lues, including Wimberger's sign in the upper tibiae. Also note periosteal new bone formation along the shafts of the long bones. Pathologic fracture is seen at various sites. [Reproduced with permission from Morettin LB, Mueller E, Schreiber M. Generalized hamartosis (congenital generalized fibromatosis). AJR 1972;114:722–734].

REFERENCES

1. Eich GF, Hoeffel JC, Tschappeler H, et al. Fibrous tumours in children: imaging features of a heterogeneous group of disorders. Pediatr Radiol 1998;28:500–509.
2. Patrick LE, O'Shea P, Simoneaux SF, et al. Pictorial essay. Fibromatoses of childhood: the spectrum of radiographic findings. AJR 1996;166:163–169.
3. Schrodt B, Callen JP. A case of congenital multiple myofibromatosis developing in an infant. Pediatrics 1999;104:113–115.
4. Humar A, Chou S, Carpenter B. Fibromatosis in infancy and childhood: the spectrum. J Pediatr Surg 1993;28:1446–1450.
5. Herring JA, Watts HG, Enneking WF. Aggressive fibromatosis. J Pediatr Orthop 1987;7:107–108.
6. Brill PW, Yandow DR, Langer LO, et al. Congenital generalized fibromatosis. Pediatr Radiol 1982;12:269–278.
7. Capusten BM, Azouz EM, Rosman MA. Fibromatosis of bone in children. Radiology 1984;152:693–694.
8. Spadola L, Anooshiravani M, Sayegh Y, et al. Generalized infantile myofibromatosis with intracranial involvement: imaging findings in a newborn. Pediatr Radiol 2002;32:872.
9. Soper JR, DeLisva M. Infantile myofibromatosis: a radiological review. Pediatr Radiol 1993;23:189–194.

Benign Bone Tumors

The osteoid osteoma, although not a true tumor, has been discussed previously. Other benign bone tumors include osteochondroma, enchondroma, chondromyxoid fibroma, chondroblastoma, lymphangioma, and hemangioma. Chondromyxoid fibromas are rare and produce lytic lesions with variably sclerotic margins. They may be multiloculated. Chondroblastomas characteristically occur in the proximal humerus, femur, or tibia and involve both the metaphysis and the epiphysis. Calcifications in the center of the lesion are common (Fig. 6.286). Osteochondromas are

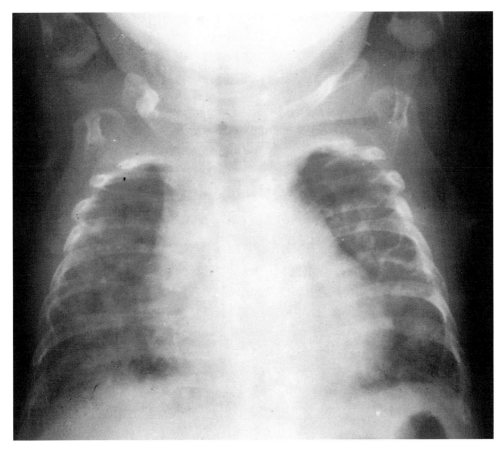

FIGURE 6.285. Generalized fibromatosis: lung involvement. There are extensive infiltrates throughout both lungs, with some suggestion of cystic or honeycombing changes. This infant is the same infant as in Fig. 6.284 and had generalized visceral fibromatosis. [Reproduced with permission from Morretin LB, Mueller E, Schreiber M. Generalized hamartosis (congenital generalized fibromatosis). AJR 1972;114:722–734].

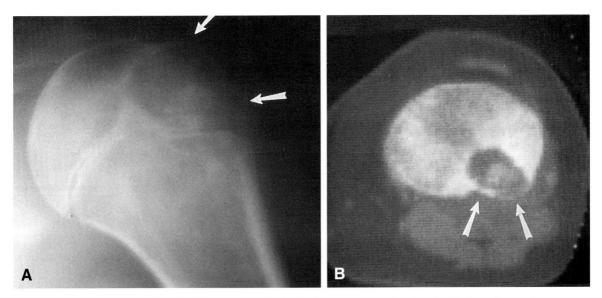

FIGURE 6.286. Chondroblastoma. A. Typical lytic appearance of a chondroblastoma (arrows) with some central calcification. Note that the lesion involves both the epiphysis and the metaphysis. **B.** Cross-sectional computed tomography study through the upper tibia in another patient demonstrates a similar appearance to this chondroblastoma (arrows).

bony outgrowths of the skeleton and can be seen in almost any long or flat bone in the body. In the long bones, they are attached to tendons and therefore when elongated point away from the joint. Basically, there are two morphologic forms: sessile and pedunculated (Fig. 6.287, A and B). Osteochondromas may be singular or multiple; when multiple, they are familial and often referred to as "Fairbanks' disease." There is an increased incidence of malignant degeneration in these latter patients, but this does not occur in childhood and probably does not occur in more than

5–10% of cases. However, mechanical and asymptomatic problems associated with osteochondromas, such as tendinitis and vascular compromise by pressure (1, 2), are common. In addition, large osteochondromas are prone to injury and even can be fractured. Because osteochondromas have a cartilaginous cap, they behave much as do epiphyses and thus will continue to grow until epiphyses close. When osteochondromas occur close to the growth plate, they may cause progressive deformity of the involved bone and interfere with joint function (3). This is most likely to occur in

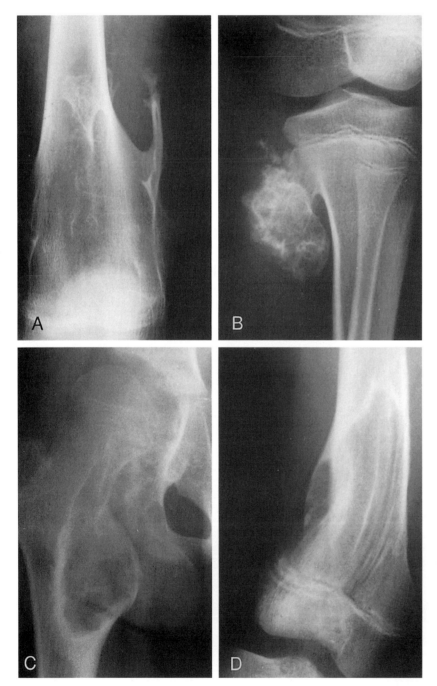

FIGURE 6.287. Benign bone tumors. A. Typical sessile osteochondroma of the distal femur. **B.** Another osteochondroma, peduculated, of the upper tibia. The irregular calcification may cause concern, but the finding is normal and not an indication of malignant degeneration. **C.** Typical enchondroma in the upper femur with sclerotic margins. **D.** Same patient with typical longitudinal striations in the distal femur as a result of an enchondroma. This patient had Ollier's disease.

the multiple form of the condition. In this regard, it has been suggested that the problem may not be so much that of a tumor but rather one of defective remodeling of the bone because of a localized defect in transition of cartilage to bone (4).

Enchondromas can be single or multiple and are much less common than osteochondromas. They produce lytic lesions with moderate sclerosis around them (Fig. 6.287C). When they are multiple, they occur in the condition known as Ollier's disease, where the lesions are predominantly unilateral, are usually discovered incidentally, and tend to have a somewhat multilinear (parallel lucent lines) configuration (Fig. 6.287D). When enchondromas are associated with soft tissue hemangiomas, the term "Maffucci's syndrome" is used. In the neonate, Ollier's disease presents with cupped and widened metaphyses (3).

Lymphangiomas and hemangiomas of bone, on a solitary basis, are uncommon. On a multiple basis, however, they are a little more common, especially hemangiomas. Multiple lytic-cystic lesions of the long bones and skeleton in general are seen (3, 5), and the findings may mimic those of congenital fibromatosis (Fig. 6.288). Visceral involvement is not uncommon and usually carries a worse progno-

sis. As with hemangiomas elsewhere, high signal is present on T2-weighted images (6). With lymphangiomatosis, cystic lesions of the long bones again are seen, and the bones can appear dysplastic (Fig. 6.289). They are prone to pathologic fracture (Fig. 6.289A), and when chylous pleural effusions are associated, the prognosis is dire (7, 8). The condition is also referred to as "vanishing bone disease" or "Gorham's disease" (8–10).

REFERENCES

1. Karasick D, Schweitzer ME, Eschelman J, et al. Pictorial essay. Symptomatic osteochondromas: imaging features. AJR 1997; 168:1507–1512.
2. Shore RM, Poznanski AK, Anandappa EC, et al. Arterial and venous compromise by an osteochondroma. Pediatr Radiol 1994;24:39–40.
3. Raupp P, Kemperdick H. Neonatal radiological aspect of enchondromatosis (Ollier's disease). Pediatr Radiol 1990;20:337–338.
4. Pazzaglia UE, Pedrotti L, Beluffi G, et al. Radiographic findings in hereditary multiple exostoses and a new theory of the pathogenesis of exostoses. Pediatr Radiol 1990;20:594–597.
5. Winterberger AR. Radiographic diagnosis of lymphangiomatosis of bone. Radiology 1972;102:321–324.

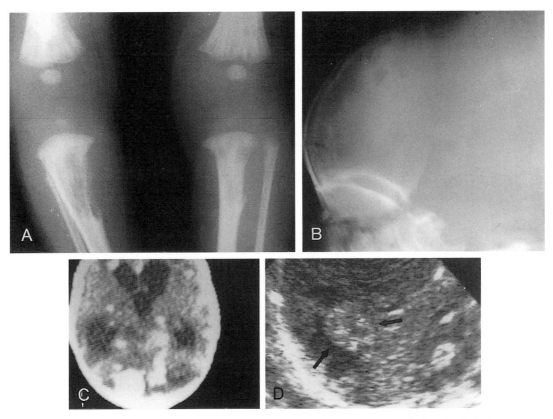

FIGURE 6.288. Multiple bone hemangiomas. A. Note typical destructive lesions in all the long bones. **B.** Lytic destructive lesions in the calvarium. **C.** Contrast-enhanced computed tomography study demonstrates numerous hemangiomas in the brain. **D.** Ultrasonogram demonstrating a hemangioma in the liver (arrows).

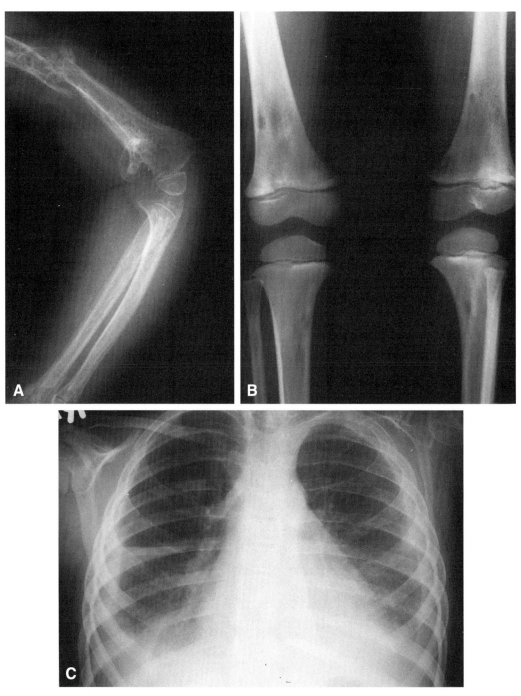

FIGURE 6.289. Multiple lymphangiomas of bone. A. Note the reticular and dysplastic bones of the forearm. A pathologic fracture is present through the humerus. **B.** Lower extremity demonstrating multiple lytic lesions that appear less aggressive. **C.** Bilateral pleural effusions secondary to chylothorax in the same patient.

6. Cohen MD, Rougraff B, Faught P. Cystic angiomatosis of bone: MR findings. Pediatr Radiol 1994;24:256–257.

7. Meller JL, Curet-Scott M, Dawson P, et al. Massive osteolysis of the chest in children: an unusual cause of respiratory distress. J Pediatr Surg 1994;28:1539–1542.

8. Mitchell CS, Parisi MT, Osborn RE. Gorham's disease involving the thoracic skeleton. Plain films and CT in two cases. Pediatr Radiol 1993;23:543–544.

9. Dominguez R, Washowich TL. Gorham's disease or vanishing bone disease: plain film, CT, and MRI findings of two cases. Pediatr Radiol 1994;24:316–318.

10. Kozlowski K, Bacha L, Brachimi L, et al. Multicentric/massive idiopathic osteolysis in a 17-year-old girl. Pediatr Radiol 1990; 21:48–51.

Malignant Bone Tumors

Malignant bone tumors can be either primary or secondary, with the latter being much more common. Secondary metastatic disease can occur from any number of primaries, but in the pediatric age group, most commonly it occurs from metastatic neuroblastoma. Characteristically, lytic, permeative changes are seen in the long and flat bones (Fig. 6.290A), and in the skull, similar destructive changes along with spreading of the sutures secondary to meningeal involvement are characteristic (Fig. 6.290B).

In terms of primary malignant bone tumors, the two most common are osteosarcoma and Ewing's sarcoma. Most often, these lesions are solitary, but multiple bone involvement can occur, it being more common with Ewing's sarcoma (1). Osteogenic sarcoma may be primarily lytic, or it may evoke considerable irregular intramedullary new bone formation and be "osteogenic." There usually is considerable permeative bony destruction, layered periosteal new bone deposition, and formation of a Codman's triangle (Fig. 6.291). The presence of a significant soft tissue mass is common. Both CT and MRI can be used for determining extent of tumor, but MRI is preferred (Fig. 2.291, D and E).

With Ewing's sarcoma, bone destruction often is extensive and lytic. Bone sequestra can be seen. Although the lesion is supposedly characteristically located in the diaphysis, metaphyseal involvement is common (Fig. 6.292). Once again, MRI amply demonstrates the extent of the lesion (Fig. 2.292), where T1 sequence images may be better than T2 sequence images (2). Fibrosarcoma is much rarer in the pediatric age group, and the changes resemble those of Ewing's sarcoma (Fig. 6.293). Ewing's sarcoma frequently involves the small bones of the hand and feet. In such cases, the findings may resemble those of low-grade osteomyelitis (3) or metastatic disease from neuroblastoma. Ewing's sarcoma in general has a great propensity to mimic low-grade osteomyelitis and vice versa. In addition, the so-called "malignant fibrous histiocytoma" can have a similar appearance, although in other cases, it may appear more benign, with more marginated edges and a more cystic appearance.

Finally, it should be recalled that in infancy, histiocytosis X can produce lesions in the skeleton that strongly resemble malignant tumors. Destruction, expansion of bone, and periosteal new bone deposition occur. Periosteal new bone deposition, however, usually is layered and not spiculated. With malignant bone tumors, spiculated periosteal new bone formation is seen and is characteristic.

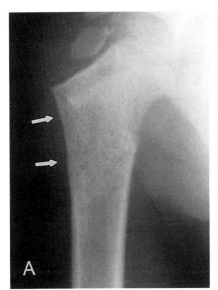 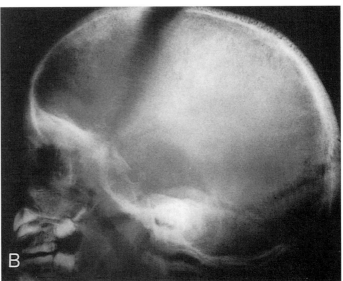

FIGURE 6.290. A. Metastatic bone disease. A. Note typical destructive changes in the long bones secondary to metastatic neuroblastoma (arrows). **B.** Typical calvarial changes demonstrating spread sutures and early moth-eaten destruction of the calvarial bones in the frontoparietal regions.

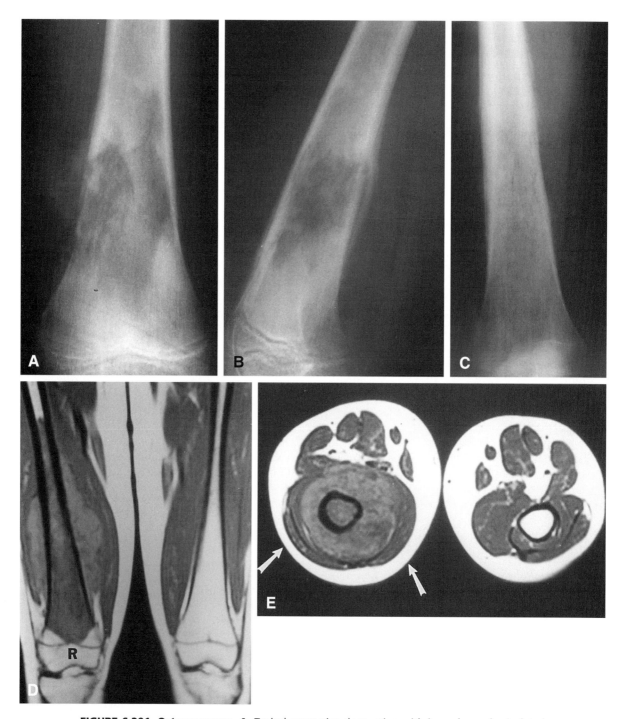

FIGURE 6.291. Osteosarcoma. A. Typical aggressive destruction with irregular and spiculated periosteal new bone medially. **B.** Lateral view demonstrates similar destruction and periosteal new bone posteriorly. **C.** Another patient with less destruction and more sclerosis of the femoral shaft. **D.** T1-weighted magnetic resonance imaging demonstrates the tumor in the right femur (R) to involve the marrow cavity from the epiphyseal plate upward into the femur. The involved marrow shows low signal, while normal marrow is of high signal. Compare with the normal femur on the left. Also note the bulky tumor mass extending into the adjacent soft tissues. **E.** Axial T1-weighted image demonstrates expansion of the thigh (arrows) as a result of the underlying tumor that has produced a mass around the femur and caused the normally high bone marrow to be of low signal. Compare with the normal left side.

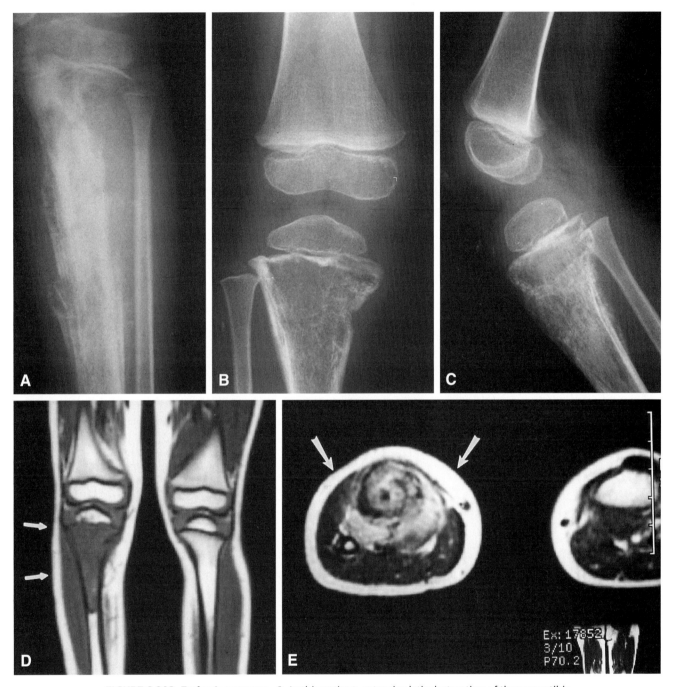

FIGURE 6.292. Ewing's sarcoma. A. In this patient, extensive lytic destruction of the upper tibia is present. Periosteal new bone along with a Codman triangle is present. The dense bone in the center has been sequestrated. **B.** Another patient with a delicate, lacy pattern of destruction of the upper tibia. A pathologic fracture is present medially. **C.** Lateral view demonstrates similar destruction and periosteal new bone deposition with early spiculation posteriorly. **D.** T1-weighted magnetic resonance image demonstrates the area of the tumor (arrows). The tumor causes the bone marrow to be of low signal. Note that some low signal is present in the tibial epiphysis, indicating that the tumor has crossed the epiphyseal line. **E.** T1-weighted magnetic resonance image in the axial plane demonstrates the soft tissue component of the tumor surrounding the upper tibia (arrows). The tibial cortex is almost completely destroyed.

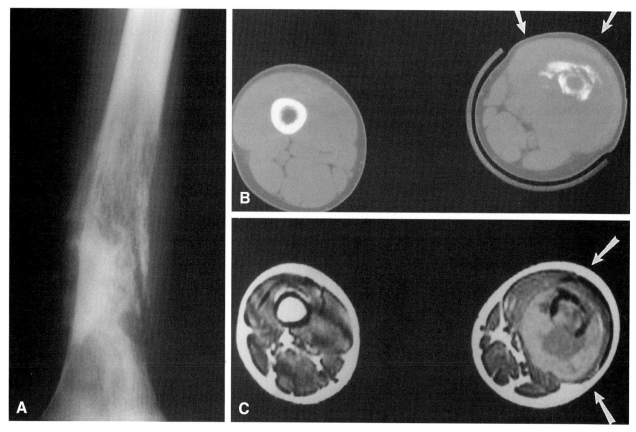

FIGURE 6.293. Fibrosarcoma. A. Note extensive permeated destruction of the femur. A pathologic fracture is present. Periosteal new bone deposition also is present. The findings are not unlike those of Ewing's sarcoma and osteolytic osteosarcoma. **B.** Computed tomography demonstrates the expanded thigh (arrows) with a soft tissue mass surrounding the destroyed femur. Compare with normal side. **C.** T1-weighted magnetic resonance image demonstrates the extent of the soft tissue mass (arrows) and again demonstrates destruction of the cortex and alteration in the signal of the bone marrow. Compare with the normal high signal on the normal side.

Malignant bone tumors seldom involve the epiphysis, but in some cases, they can cross the epiphyseal line (Fig. 6.292D) (4). In addition, response to therapy both with osteosarcoma and with Ewing's sarcoma can be accomplished with multiple imaging modalities, but MRI is especially useful. With contrast enhancement, residual areas of tumor tend to retain the contrast and are bright on T1-weighted images. White trophic lines in the metaphyses of the long bones can be seen after methotrexate therapy for malignant tumor such Ewing's tumor (5, 6). Finally, a rare tumor is the lipoblastoma (7).

Before we leave the topic of malignant bone tumors, it should be appreciated that in their early stages, the plain film findings may be very subtle (Fig. 6.294A). For this reason, even with the slightest suspicion that such a tumor is present, one should proceed to further imaging, either CT or MR (Fig. 6.294).

REFERENCES

1. Beluffi G, Kozlowski K, Arico M. Simultaneous (synchronous) occurrence of Ewing's sarcoma. Pediatr Radiol 1991;21: 452–454.
2. OnikulE, Fletcher BD, Parham DM, et al. Accuracy of MR imaging for estimating intraosseous extent of osteosarcoma. AJR 1996; 167:1211–1215.
3. Baraga J, Amrami KK, Swee RG. Radiographic features of Ewing's sarcoma of the bones of the hands and feet. Skeletal Radiol 2001; 30:121–126.
4. Norton KI, Hermann G, Abdelwahab IF, et al. Epiphyseal involvement in osteosarcoma. Radiology 1991;180:813–816.
5. Ecklund K, Laor T, Goorin AM, et al. Methotrexate osteopathy in patients with osteosarcoma. Radiology 1997;202:543–547.
6. Roebuck DJ. Skeletal complications in pediatric oncology patients. Radiographics 1999;19:873–885.
7. Reiseter T, Nordshus T, Borthne A, et al. Lipoblastoma: MRI appearances of a rare pediatric soft tissue tumour. Pediatr Radiol 1999;29:542–545.

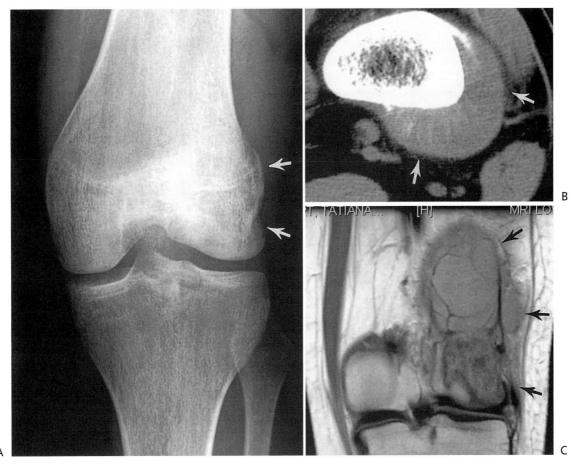

A

B

C

FIGURE. 6.294. Ewing's sarcoma: early findings. A. Note vague suggestion of bony destruction (arrows) in the distal femur. **B.** Computed tomography study demonstrates a large muscle mass with typical spiculated bone through the destroyed cortex. **C.** Coronal magnetic resonance study demonstrates the extent of the tumor (arrows), not suspected as being this large on plain films. The large soft tissue component was not appreciated.

HEAD, BRAIN, AND MENINGES

Unlike the skull of the older child and adult, the newborn and young infant's skull is a dynamic structure. Not only can it reflect changes in intracranial pressure, but it frequently offers valuable clues to the presence of underlying bone dysplasias, metabolic disease, hematologic disease, chromosomal abnormalities, and intracranial pathology. However, there is probably as much trouble in interpreting normal findings, variations, and artifacts as there is in pathologic change. **Therefore, it becomes important that one acquire a firm foundation in the recognition of these normal variations and common artifacts, especially because skull films are obtained less frequently than in the past and one's database for these findings becomes eroded.**

NORMAL SKULL AND VARIATIONS

The newborn infant's skull is variable in size and shape, because not only is one dealing with hereditary factors, but the specific fetal presentation and degree of molding can produce configurations that, on first inspection, suggest abnormality (Fig. 7.1). As a consequence, one must allow a considerable degree of latitude when assessing the shape of the newborn infant's skull. In the newborn and young infant, the facial structures definitely are diminutive as compared with the calvarium. In this regard, normal face-to-skull ratios are about 3:1; a general rule of some help in making a gross assessment of calvarial size.

Degree of ossification and thickness of the calvarial bones is also variable. The frontal and occipital bones usually show more advanced ossification than do the parietal bones; the parietal bone is often so thin that it is barely visible (Fig. 7.2). This is not abnormal and is seen in exaggerated form in the premature infant. Inner table convolutional markings, generally speaking, are absent or scant in the newborn infant. Therefore, when encountered in this age group, one should consider the possibility of primary or secondary premature closure of the sutures. In normal infants and children, they later become more prominent and can be striking in some cases. They are a direct reflection of normal brain growth, which at this stage of life is exuberant.

Sutures, Synchondroses, and Fontanelles

One should become familiar with the numerous normal sutures, synchondroses, and fontanelles that are present in the newborn infant. To be sure, they are often misinterpreted as fractures, calvarial defects, or the like. The major sutures consist of the coronal, sagittal, lambdoid, squamosal, metopic, and mendosal, and the major synchondroses (1) are the intersphenoid, spheno-occipital, frontosphenoidal, and posterior occipital (innominate) (Figs. 7.3 and 7.4). The major fontanelles are the anterior, posterior, and lateral fontanelles. Occasionally, small accessory fontanelles are seen along the suture lines, especially along the sagittal suture. The one occurring in the posterior parietal region often is called the third fontanelle. A fontanelle occasionally occurs in the metopic bone, the so-called metopic fontanelle. The normal metopic suture extends anteriorly from the anterior fontanelle and divides the frontal bone in half (Fig. 7.5). It may persist into childhood. Accessory sutures are most common in the parietal bone and are very frequently confused with fractures (Fig. 7.6). These sutures are called "intraparietal" sutures and generally are relatively horizontal in position. They have a tendency to be symmetric and in exaggerated cases may present with a picture resembling that of an eggshell fracture of the calvarium.

The intersphenoid, posterior occipital, and frontosphenoid synchondroses usually are obliterated by 2 years of age, but the spheno-occipital synchondrosis does not become obliterated until the late teens. The anterior fontanelle closes by 2 years of age, and the posterior and lateral fontanelles usually close by 9 months to 1 year. However, these latter fontanelles may close earlier; in a few infants they are nearly closed at birth. Most of the regularly seen cranial sutures remain open well into late childhood, but the mendosal is often difficult to identify after 6 months. **In some infants, the anterior fontanelle can be small but normal.**

The infantile sella, although bearing a general resemblance to the sella in older children, does possess certain differences (Fig. 7.1). Primarily these consist of lack of ossification of the planum sphenoidale, prominence of the

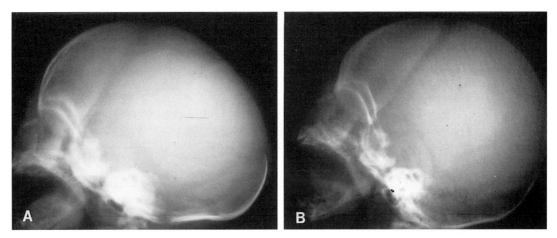

FIGURE 7.1. A and B. Normal skull shape variations. Striking variation in shape of two normal neonatal skulls. Also note the difference in size and shape of the anterior and posterior fossae. Such variations often result from intrauterine molding or lack thereof. The parietal bone is least well ossified. The long skull demonstrated in **A** commonly is seen in breech deliveries and results from the head being molded by the fundus of the uterus. (From Swischuk LE. The normal pediatric skull: variants and artefacts. Radiol Clin North Am 1972;10:277–290, with permission.)

various sphenoidal synchondroses, and smallness and underossification of the bony structures in general. Consequently, the dorsum sella and the anterior and posterior clinoid processes appear small and underdeveloped. The auditory canal produces an oval area of radiolucency surrounded by a thin bony margin in the base of the skull in the petrous bone (Fig. 7.1B).

Vascular markings are absent or scant in the newborn infant, and the only ones seen in this early age period are those produced by the supraorbital artery in the frontal bone. Otherwise, vascular markings in older children result from diploic veins and the middle meningeal artery. All of these vascular channels can be confused with fractures, both on plain films and computed tomography (CT).

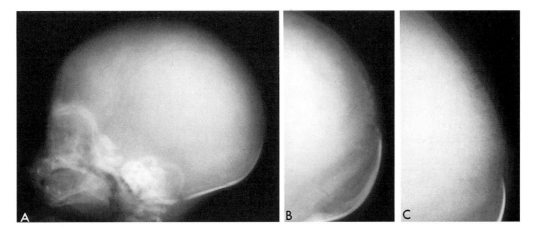

FIGURE 7.2. Normal underossification. A. Extreme underossification of the calvarium frequently seen in the premature infant. Also note that the calvarium is proportionately larger than in the full-term newborn. **B.** Normal irregular ossification and fragmentation of the parietal bone in a newborn infant. **C.** Normal underossification and fissuring of the parietal bone in another newborn infant. (From Swischuk LE. The normal pediatric skull: variants and artefacts. Radiol Clin North Am 1972;10:277–290, with permission.)

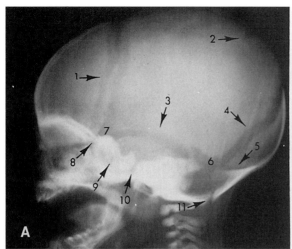

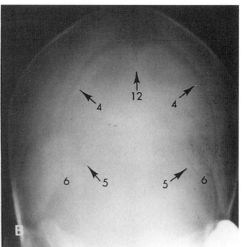

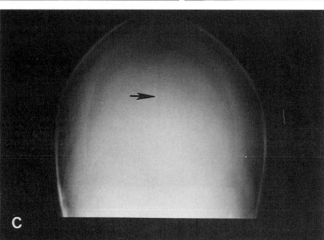

FIGURE 7.3. Normal sutures, fissures, and synchondroses. Normal lateral (**A**) and Towne's (**B**) projections of the neonatal skull. Note that the sutures appear unduly wide and prominent. 1, coronal suture; 2, posterior parietal fissure; 3, squamosal suture; 4, lambdoid suture; 5, mendosal suture; 6, posterior lateral fontanelle; 7, anterior lateral fontanelle; 8, frontosphenoid synchondrosis; 9, intersphenoid synchondrosis; 10, spheno-occipital synchondrosis; 11, innominate or posterior occipital synchondrosis; 12, median occipital fissure. **C.** Exceptionally long median occipital fissure (arrow). A fissure of this length occurs only occasionally but should not be confused with a fracture. (**A** and **B** from Swischuk LE. The normal pediatric skull: variants and artefacts. Radiol Clin North Am 1972;10:277–290, with permission.)

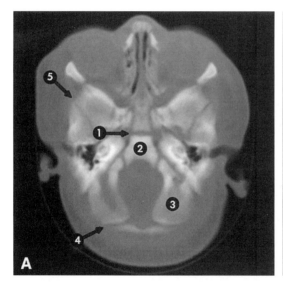

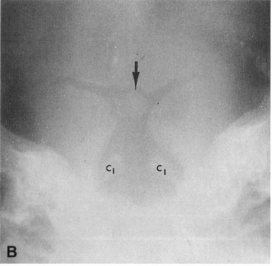

FIGURE 7.4. Base of skull: sutures and synchondroses. A. CT study demonstrates the spheno-occipital synchondrosis (1), basioccipital bone (2), exoccipital bone (3), innominate synchondrosis (4), and coronal suture (5). **B.** Towne's projection demonstrates an occipital ossicle (arrow) located along the posterior edge of the foramen magnum. To either side extend the innominate synchondroses. Posterior arch of C1 (C₁).

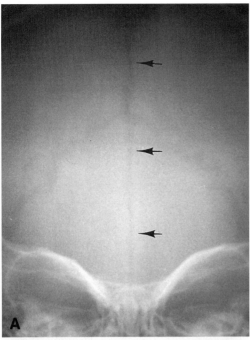

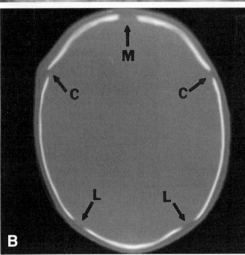

FIGURE 7.5. Metopic and other sutures. A. Note the metopic suture (arrows) extending downward from the anterior fontanelle. **B.** CT study demonstrates the metopic suture (M), coronal sutures (C), and lambdoid sutures (L).

Bathrocephaly and the Interparietal (Inca) Bone

Bathrocephaly is a peculiar deformity of the occipital portion of the skull (Fig. 7.7A). It consists of posterior occipital bulging and, although it can be striking, it is of no particular significance. It probably results from intrauterine molding, and spontaneous remodeling is the rule. The bulge slowly becomes less prominent and eventually disappears. It is frequently seen in association with the interpari-

etal (inca) bone. This bone is located just at or above the posterior fontanelle (Fig. 7.7B). It is often triangular in shape and on lateral view appears as a thin sclerotic fragment of bone. It should not be misinterpreted as representing a depressed fracture fragment. At times, it can be bipartite or even tripartite.

Anterior Fontanelle Bones

An accessory anterior fontanelle bone occasionally is encountered in normal infants (Fig. 7.8, A and B). For the most part, it is a normal variation and does not alter calvarial growth. Rarely, multiple anterior fontanelle bones can be seen, and rarely, they can be very large (Fig. 7.8C).

Wormian Bones

Although wormian bone formation is a normal phenomenon, when excessive, one should consider conditions such as cleidocranial dysostosis, osteogenesis imperfecta, congenital hypophosphatasia, cretinism, pyknodysostosis, pachydermoperiostosis, and a variety of trisomies (Fig. 7.9). Wormian bones are intrasutural bones occurring most frequently along the lambdoid and posterior sagittal sutures. Eventually, they become incorporated into the adjacent calvarial bones.

Occipital Ossicles

These small round bones, located just above the foramen magnum, can present a problem in diagnosis. They are usually round or oval and can be single or multiple (Fig. 7.10). They represent separate areas of ossification of the occipital bone, just at the level of the posterior occipital synchondrosis. They are of no particular significance except that they are recognized as normal variations. In some cases, a midline bony process just above the foramen magnum can also be seen, the so-called Kerckring's process.

Posterior Parietal Fissures, Irregularities, and Parietal Foramina

The parietal bone is the most poorly ossified bone of the normal neonatal skull. Its posterosuperior aspect can show extensive fissuring and irregularity (Fig. 7.2). Similar fissuring is also usually present in the adjacent occipital bone, and often, one or two fissures so predominate that a fracture is suggested (Fig. 7.2). However, they represent entirely normal findings, and with future growth the parietal bones become more uniformly ossified and the fissures disappear. It is of some interest that the fissure occurs in the same area as do congenital parietal foramina, and it may be that the two findings are associated (Fig. 7.11A). If the defect is large it is often referred to as the "third fontanelle" (Fig. 7.11B).

(Text continues on page 985)

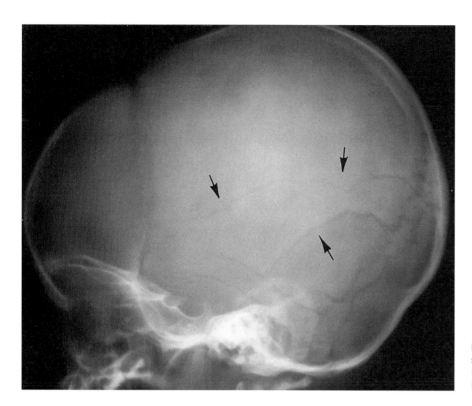

FIGURE 7.6. Intraparietal (accessory) sutures. Note the bilateral, somewhat undulating but basically symmetric, intraparietal sutures (arrows).

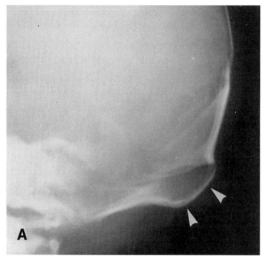

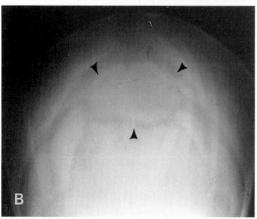

FIGURE 7.7. A. Bathrocephaly and interparietal bone. Peculiar bulging of occipital bone is called bathrocephaly (arrows). The dense, triangular bony fragment above the bathrocephalic deformity is an interparietal bone. This latter structure can be seen with bathrocephaly, but it is more often seen as an isolated finding. **B. Interparietal bone.** Towne's projection demonstrates a typical interparietal (inca) bone in another infant (arrows). Also note the normal skin folds. (From Swischuk LE. The normal pediatric skull: variants and artefacts. Radiol Clin North Am 1972;10:277–290, with permission.)

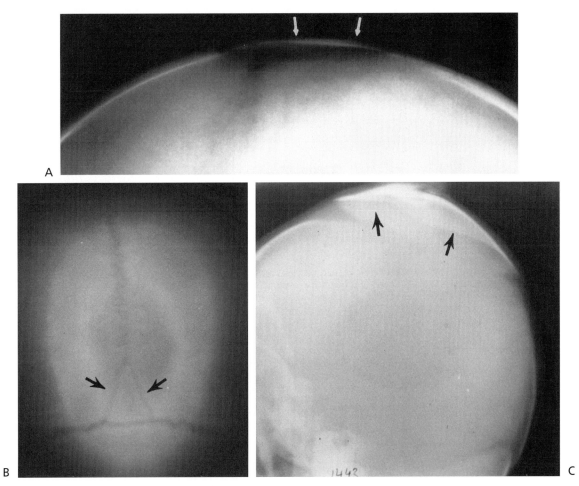

FIGURE 7.8. Anterior fontanelle bone. A. Typical appearance of an anterior fontanelle bone (arrows) seen on lateral view. **B.** CT demonstrates the triangular appearance of the anterior fontanelle bone (arrows). **C.** Note the large anterior fontanelle bone (arrows) with a peculiar bony spicule. This patient was otherwise normal, and it is presumed that this represents a large anterior fontanelle bone. (**A** from Swischuk LE. The normal pediatric skull: variants and artefacts. Radiol Clin North Am 1972;10:277–290, with permission; **C** courtesy of F. Eftekharin, M.D.)

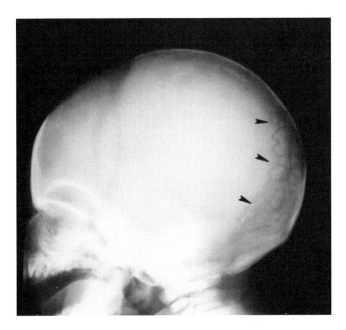

FIGURE 7.9. Wormian bones. Note the numerous wormian bones (arrows) in this infant with an F chromosome translocation.

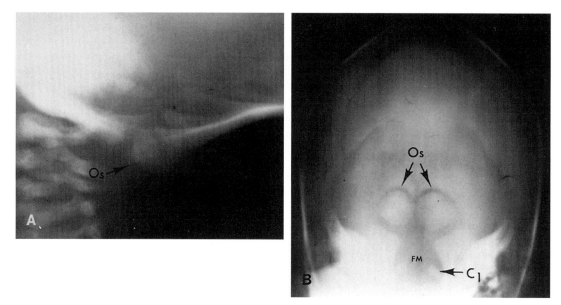

FIGURE 7.10. Occipital ossicles. A. Lateral view showing typical location and configuration of occipital ossicles (Os). **B.** Towne's projection showing two occipital ossicles (Os), an incompletely ossified arch of the first cervical vertebra (C1), and the foramen magnum (FM). (From Swischuk LE. The normal pediatric skull: variants and artefacts. Radiol Clin North Am 1972;10:277–290, with permission.)

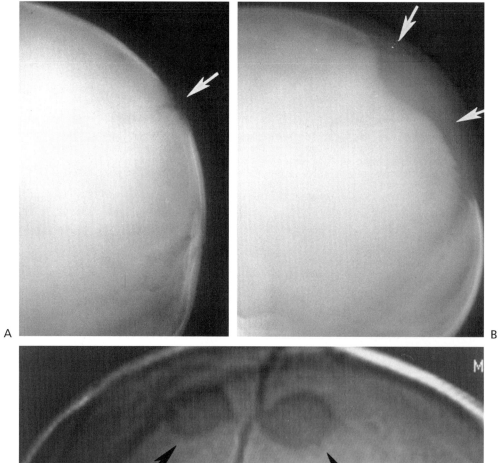

FIGURE 7.11. Posterior parietal fissure and foramen. A. Note the posterior parietal foramen (arrow) with a small fissure associated. **B.** In this infant, the confluent posterior parietal bony defects result in a so-called third fontanelle (arrows). **C.** Persistent biparietal foramen (arrows). (**A** and **B** from Swischuk LE. The normal pediatric skull: variants and artefacts. Radiol Clin North Am 1972;10:277–290, with permission.)

Normal Brain

The brain can be studied with CT, magnetic resonance imaging (MRI), and in the neonate and young infant, with ultrasound. Color flow sonography is useful in evaluating blood flow in the various intercerebral vessels. Normally, in premature infants the ventricles are slightly dilated and easier to visualize than in newborns where they are generally slit-like (Fig. 7.12). The normal ventricles also often are asymmetric, with the left usually being a little larger than the right (1).

Ultrasonography is best suited for the premature infant and neonate where the anterior fontanelle is open and serves as a window for imaging of the brain. It is used most for evaluating midline structures, and hence it has become the primary imaging modality for the evaluation of germinal matrix bleeds in premature infants. This study generally is performed in multiple coronal and mid-sagittal-parasagittal planes, and the important anatomy is readily visualized (Figs. 7.13 and 7.14). The posterolateral fontanelle also can be used as a window for posterior fossa abnormalities (2).

In terms of identifying germinal matrix bleeds, it is important not to misinterpret the caudothalamic groove, which often is echogenic and separates the head of the caudate nucleus from the thalamus. It also marks the site of the foramen of Monroe and is most often seen on parasagittal

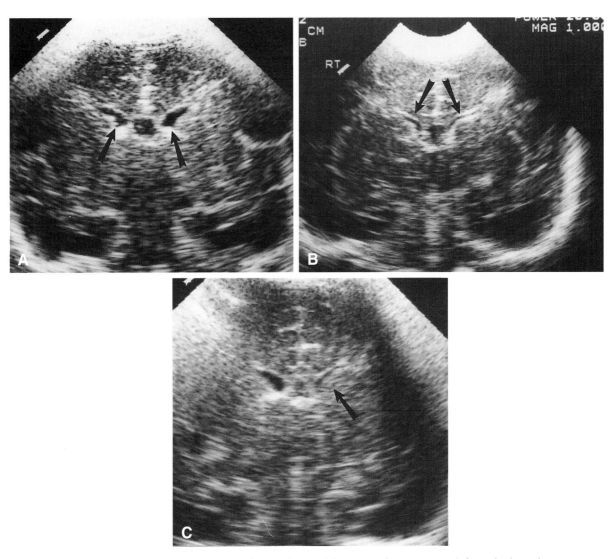

FIGURE 7.12. Normal variation of lateral ventricles. A. In this premature infant, the lateral ventricles (arrows) are slightly dilated but normal. In the center is the septum cavum pellucidum. **B.** In this infant the ventricles are more slit-like (arrows), a configuration more characteristic of a full-term infant. **C.** Asymmetry of the lateral ventricles (arrow) is normal.

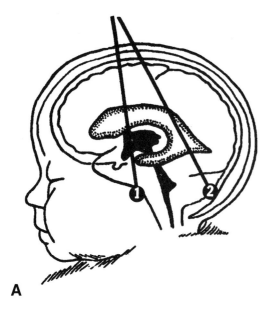

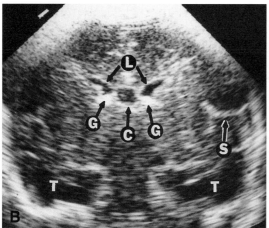

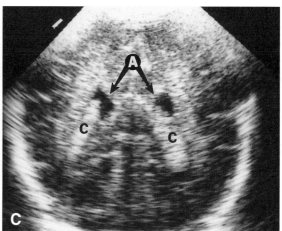

FIGURE 7.13. Normal cranial ultrasound: coronal views. A. Imaging in the two planes numbered 1 and 2 is most informative. **B.** Image obtained through plane 1. Lateral ventricles (L), cavum septum pellucidum (C), germinal matrix (G), sylvian fissure (S), and temporal lobe (T). **C.** Image obtained through plane 2. Atria of the lateral ventricles (A) and choroid plexus (C) extending into the temporal horns.

images (Fig. 7.15). Overall, however, in evaluating the pediatric brain, CT is the workhorse imaging study. It is the best overall study for imaging the bony and intracranial structures (Fig. 7.16). MRI is more useful when parenchymal disease is suspected. Drawbacks of MRI include poor visualization of calcifications, prolonged studies, and inability to identify acute bleeding. Nonetheless, it provides exquisite detail of the brain (Fig. 7.17).

In the premature infant cerebral gray-white matter differentiation is not as well defined as in older infants, because myelinization has not progressed to this level of the brain. Myelinization in infants occurs in a set pattern (3–6). First it is seen below the brainstem; then it progresses into the brainstem and internal capsule; and finally, the peripheral white matter of the corona radiata. A detailed summary of normal myelinization is presented in Figure 7.18, while imaging studies of the immature brain are seen in Figure

7.19. A near-adult appearance of the brain is seen by 2 years and the corpus callosum appears adult-like by 8 months (3). On T1-weighted MR images, cerebral spinal fluid has a low signal intensity (gray), but on T2-weighted images, the signal reverses and becomes high and bright or white. With CT, the immature brain is hypodense because the white matter is nonmyelinated (Fig. 7.19A). On T1-weighted MR images, it is of low signal intensity, whereas on T2-weighted images, it has high signal intensity (Fig. 7.19, B and C). This is the opposite of its behavior in older infants and children, and therefore myelinization is best evaluated on T1-weighted images until 6–9 months (Fig. 7.20), and then it is more readily evaluated on T2-weighted images. On FLAIR imaging, normal CSF is gray, but at the same time FLAIR images are excellent in detecting demyelinization in older infants (Fig. 7.21). It also has been demonstrated that sulcal and gyral development in immature

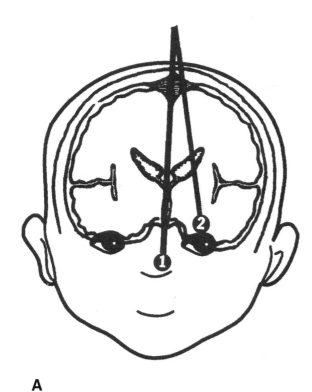

FIGURE 7.14. Normal cranial ultrasound: sagittal planes. A. The midsagittal (1) and parasagittal (2) planes illustrated are most informative. **B.** Midsagittal view (plane 1) demonstrates the corpus callosum (1), choroid plexus of third ventricle (2), third ventricle (3), fourth ventricle (4), cerebellum (5), cisterna magna (6), aqueduct of Sylvius (7), cavum septum pellucidum (8), and cavum vergae (9). **C.** Parasagittal view (plane 2) through area of the trigone. Lateral ventricle (L), temporal horn (T), choroid plexus (C), and atrium (A) of the lateral ventricle are seen.

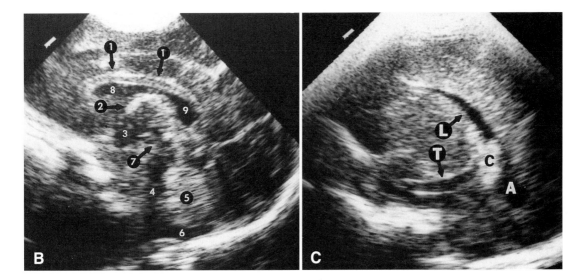

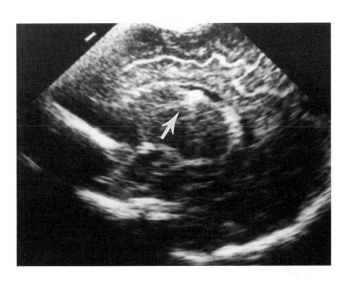

FIGURE 7.15. Normal caudothalamic groove. Note the echogenic caudothalamic groove (arrow), which should not be misinterpreted for a germinal matrix bleed. It is usually seen on parasagittal views.

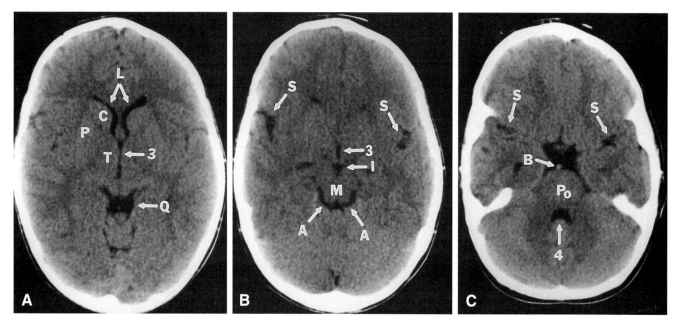

FIGURE 7.16. Normal brain: CT imaging. A. Upper axial slice. **B.** Lower axial slice. **C.** Infratentorial axial slice. Lateral ventricles (L), caudate nucleus (C), putamen (P), thalamus (T), third ventricle (3), ambient cistern (A), quadrigeminal plate cistern (Q), medulla (M), aqueduct of Sylvius (A), sylvian fissures (S), fourth ventricle (4), basilar artery (B), and pons (Po) are illustrated. Also note the normal white and gray matter distribution on all slices. In **C,** the cerebellum surrounds the fourth ventricle.

infants follows a predicted pathway which can be documented with MRI (7). In patients who are anesthetized, the increased oxygen content of the blood leads to hyperintensity of the CSF over the brain surface (8).

Arteriography is seldom used for the investigation of intracranial problems in infants and children. The reason for this is that magnetic resonance arteriography and venography are readily available and easily performed. They provide exquisite imaging of the vascular tree with little, if any, trouble to the patient (Fig. 7.22).

REFERENCES

1. Winchester P, Brill PW, Cooper R, et al. Prevalence of "compressed" and asymmetric lateral ventricles in healthy full-term neonates: sonographic study. AJR 1986;146:471–475.
2. Luna JA, Goldstein RB. Sonographic visualization of neonatal posterior fossa abnormalities through the posterolateral fontanelle. AJR 2000;174:561–567.
3. Ballesteros MC, Hansen PE, Soila K. MR imaging of the developing human brain. Part 2. Postnatal development. Radiographics 1993;13:611–622.
4. Barkovich AJ, Kjos BO, Jackson DE Jr, et al. Normal maturation of the neonatal and infant brain: MR imaging at 1.5 T. Radiology 1988;166:173–180.
5. Holland BA, Haas DK, Norman D, et al. MRI of normal brain maturation. AJNR 1986;7:201–208.
6. Staudt M, Schropp C, Staudt F, et al. Myelination of the brain in MRI: a staging system. Pediatr Radiol 1993;23:169–176.
7. van der Knapp MS, van Wezel-Meijler G, et al. Normal gyration and sulcation in preterm and term neonates: appearance on MR images. Radiology 1996;200:389–396.
8. Frigon C, Jardine DS, Weinberger E, et al. Fraction of inspired oxygen in relation to cerebrospinal fluid hyperintensity on FLAIR MR imaging of the brain in children and young adults undergoing anesthesia. AJR 2002;179:791.

Normal Pituitary Gland

The pituitary gland is readily imaged with MRI, and it has been demonstrated that in the newborn infant the gland is somewhat plump and shows increased signal intensity in both its anterior and posterior portions (1–4). After about 2 months of age, the anterior portion of the gland begins to loose its signal, but the posterior lobe retains high signal intensity, the so-called "bright" posterior pituitary (1–4). As the infant grows older, the pituitary gland becomes flatter (1, 2, 4) and the pituitary stock is readily visualized. All of these features are demonstrated in (Fig. 7.23).

(Text continues on page 993)

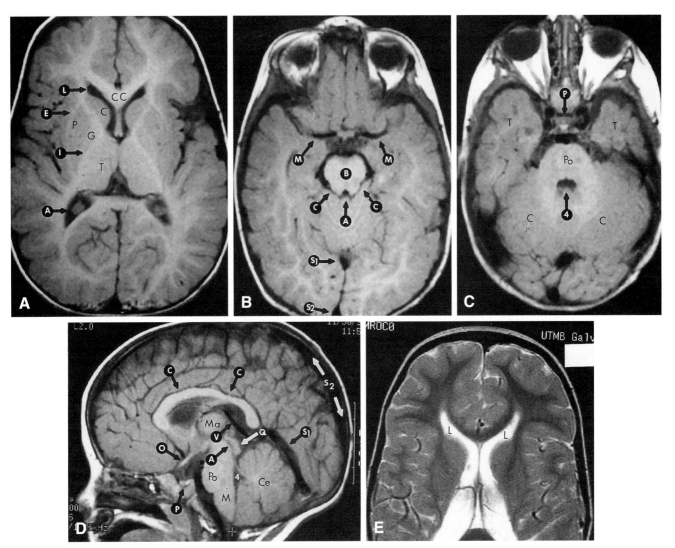

FIGURE 7.17. Normal brain: T1-weighted MRI. A. Upper axial slice demonstrates the corpus callosum (CC), lateral ventricle (L), caudate nucleus (C), putamen (P), globus pallidus (G), external capsule (E), internal capsule (I), thalamus (T), and atrium of the lateral ventricle (A) within which lies the choroid plexus. **B.** Lower slice shows the middle cerebral arteries (M), brainstem (B), ambient cistern (C), aqueduct of Sylvius (A), superior sagittal sinus (S2), and straight sinus (S1). **C.** Slice through the base of the brain shows the fourth ventricle (4), cerebellum (C), pons (Po), pituitary gland and sella (P), and temporal lobes (T). **D.** Midsagittal view demonstrates the corpus callosum (C), massa intermedia (Ma), internal cerebral vein (V), aqueduct of Sylvius (A), pons (Po), medulla (M), fourth ventricle (4), cerebellum (Ce), pituitary gland and sella (P), optic nerve (O), quadrigeminal plate (Q), superior sagittal sinus (S2), and straight sinus (S1). **E.** T2-weighted image demonstrating that fluid in the lateral ventricles (L) is of high signal intensity and normal. On T1-weighted images, cerebral spinal fluid shows low signal intensity (**A**).

AREAS	FETAL MONTHS		BIRTH	POST-NATAL MONTHS			
	3	6		3	6	9	12
MEDULLA		▪▪▪▪▪▪ ➞➞➞➞					→
CEREBELLUM		▪▪▪ ➞➞➞					→
PONS MESENCEPHALON		▪▪▪ ➞➞➞					→
POSTERIOR LIMB INTERNAL CAPSULE		▪▪▪ ➞➞➞					→
BASAL NUCLEI			▪▪▪ ➞➞				→
CENTRUM SEMIOVALE			▪▪ ➞➞				→
OPTIC RADIATIONS				▪▪▪ ➞➞			→
SPLENIUM CORPUS CALLOSUM				▪▪▪ ➞➞			→
ANTERIOR LIMB INTERNAL CAPSULE				▪▪▪▪▪▪ ➞			→
GENU CORPUS CALLOSUM					▪▪▪ ➞		→
PERIPHERAL OCCIPITAL WHITE MATTER					▪▪▪ ➞		→
PERIPHERAL PARIETAL WHITE MATTER						▪▪▪ ➞	→
PERIPHERAL FRONTAL WHITE MATTER						▪▪▪ ➞	→
PERIPHERAL TEMPORAL WHITE MATTER							▪▪▪ ➞

FIGURE 7.18. **Ages when changes of myelinization appear.** Arrows indicate time frame for myelinization of each structure. (From Ballesteros MC, Hansen PE, Soila K. MR imaging of the developing human brain. Radiographics 1993;13:611–622, with permission.)

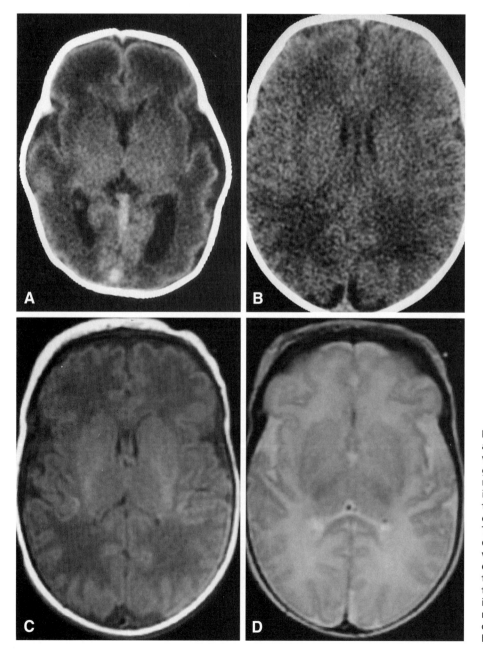

FIGURE 7.19. **Immature brain: CT and MR appearance. A.** Thirty-week-old infant. Note the absence of gyri and an overall appearance that resembles that of lissencephaly. There is poor gray-white matter differentiation. **B.** Another infant, showing typical hypodense white matter on CT. **C.** T1-weighted image in the same infant demonstrates low-signal-intensity white matter. **D.** T2-weighted image demonstrates high signal intensity in the white matter. The MR signals are the reverse of those seen in older infants and children where the white matter has become myelinated (i.e., compare with white matter signal in Fig. 7.20).

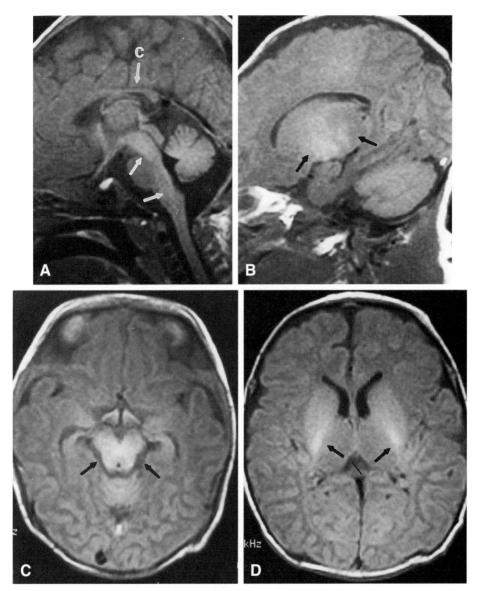

FIGURE 7.20. Early myelinization pattern: T1-weighted images. A. Sagittal view demonstrates slightly increased signal intensity in the brainstem (arrows) and cerebellum. This is consistent with early myelinization. The corpus callosum (C) shows low signal intensity because it is not myelinated. **B.** Parasagittal view demonstrates early myelinization in the internal capsule (arrows). **C.** Axial view through brainstem demonstrates increased signal intensity in the brainstem (arrows). **D.** Slightly higher view demonstrates increased signal intensity resulting from early myelinization in the internal capsule (arrows). The anterior and posterior white matter (corona radiata) show low signal intensity because of lack of myelinization.

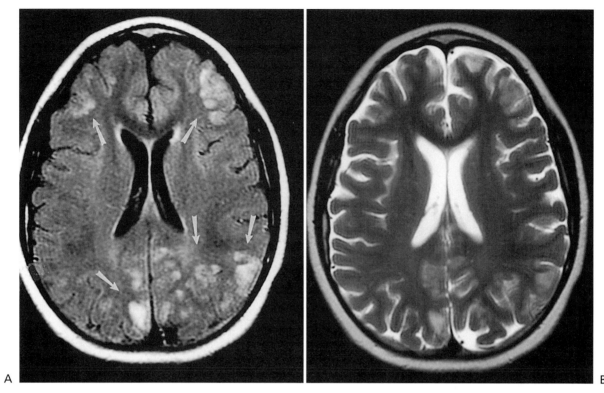

FIGURE 7.21. Value of FLAIR imaging. A. On this FLAIR image, note the easily recognizable high-signal-intensity abnormal white matter (arrows). **B.** On the T2-weighted study, the findings are much less pronounced for a patient with drug-induced white matter disease.

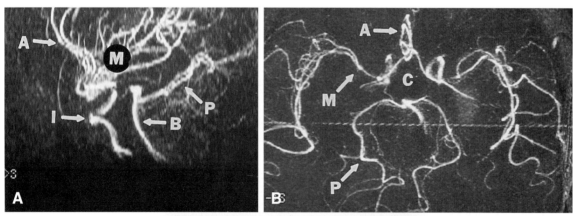

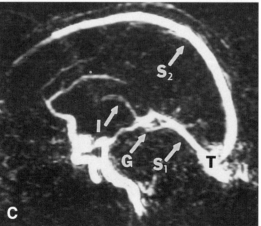

FIGURE 7.22. Normal intracranial vessels: magnetic resonance angiography and venography. A. MRA, midsagittal view, demonstrates the basilar artery (B), posterior cerebral artery (P), internal cerebral artery (I), anterior cerebral artery and its branches (A), and the middle cerebral artery (M) and its branches. **B.** Axial view demonstrates the circle of Willis (C) and the anterior cerebral arteries (A), middle cerebral artery (M), and posterior cerebral artery (P). **C.** MRV, midsagittal plane. Note the superior sagittal sinus (S₂), straight sinus (S₁), vein of Galen (G), internal cerebral vein (I), and the torcular herophili (T). The basilar artery and anterior cerebral artery along with the pericallosal and callosal marginal branches also are visualized.

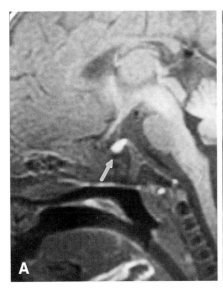 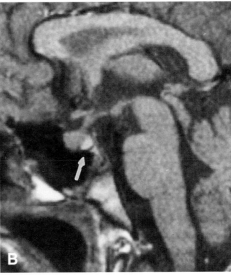

FIGURE 7.23. Normal pituitary gland. A. Neonate. In the neonate, the anterior lobe of the pituitary gland (arrow) normally shows increased signal. The slightly brighter posterior pituitary lobe also is visualized. Note the thin pituitary stalk above the gland. **B. Older child,** demonstrating that the anterior lobe now has lost its high signal intensity. The posterior lobe (arrow) remains bright. Again note the pituitary stalk above the pituitary gland.

REFERENCES

1. Argyropoulou M, Perignon F, Brunelle F, et al. Height of normal pituitary gland as a function of age evaluated by magnetic resonance imaging in children. Pediatr Radiol 1991;21:247–249.
2. Cox TD, Elster AD. Normal pituitary gland: changes in shape, size and signal intensity during the 1st year of life at MR imaging. Radiology 1991;179:721–724.
3. Dietrich RB, Lis LE, Greensite FS, et al. Normal MR appearance of the pituitary gland in the first 2 years of life. AJNR 1995;16: 1413–1419.
4. Tien RD, Kucharczyk J, Bessette J, et al. MR imaging of the pituitary gland in infants and children: changes in size, shape, and MR signal with growth and development. AJR 1992;158:1151–1154.

Prominent Arachnoid Spaces

It has been known for some time that the subarachnoid spaces in infants are more prominent than those in older children (1,2). In the past, this space was considered subdural but more recently it has been determined that the space is subarachnoid. This has been vividly substantiated by the so-called cortical vein sign (3, 4). Cortical veins traverse the subarachnoid space, but not the subdural space. Therefore, with ultrasound, or any other imaging modality if traversing vessels are seen within a fluid-filled space the diagnosis should be subarachnoid fluid accumulation (Fig. 7.24, A–C).

Subarachnoid fluid collections lead to calvarial enlargement, often familial. In this regard, upper normal measurements for the width of these fluid collections over the convexities are 4 mm, and 6 mm at the widest point along the interhemispheric fissure (Fig. 7.24). The range of measurements at these two sites is 0.3–6.3 and 0.5–8.2 mm respectively (2). However, I still consider 1 cm for the latter measurement to be normal if no other abnormal clinical

findings, other than a large head, are present. This condition is benign and as noted earlier, often familial. However similar subarachnoid fluid collections have been seen in premature infants (5). The fluid collection in all of these cases is anterior, over the frontoparietal regions of the brain and not posterior. Vessels can be seen traversing the fluid (Fig. 7.24, B and C), and this solidifies the fact that the fluid is subarachnoid fluid. Generally, the problem resolves by 2 years of age and generally is believed to be due to inefficient clearing of cerebral spinal fluid by the pacchionian granulations.

REFERENCES

1. Kleinman PK, Zito JL, Davidson RI, et al. The subarachnoid spaces in children: normal variations in size. Radiology 1983;147: 455–457.
2. Libicher M, Troger J. US measurement of the subarachnoid space in infants: normal values. Radiology 1992;184:749–751.
3. McCluney KW, Yeakley JW, Fenstermacher MJ, et al. Subdural hygroma versus atrophy on MR brain scans: "the cortical vein sign." Amer J Neuroradiol 1992;13:1335–1339.
4. Chen CY, Chou TY, Zimmerman RA, et al. Pericerebral fluid collections: differentiation of enlarged subarachnoid spaces from subdural collections with color Doppler US Radiol 1996;201: 389–392.
5. Al-Saedi SA, Lemke RP, Debooy VD, et al. Subarachnoid fluid collections: a cause of macrocrania in preterm infants. J Pediatr 1996;128:234–236.

Normal Spectroscopy

Spectroscopy plays a complimentary role in the evaluation of a number of brain abnormalities. It probably has not provided as much specific information as was expected but nonetheless it is in common use. A normal spectroscopy

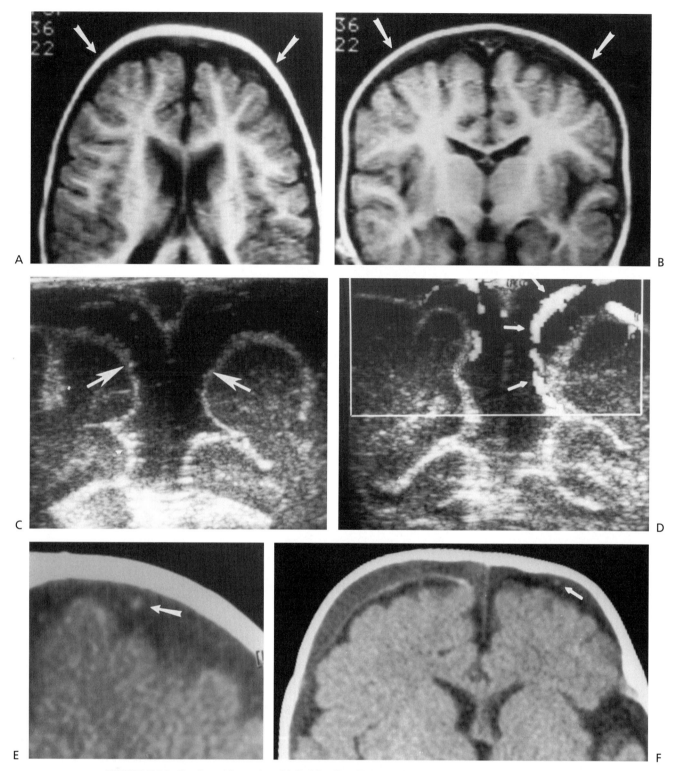

FIGURE 7.24. Benign subarachnoid fluid collections. A. Typical location and appearance of normal subarachnoid fluid over the frontal region (arrows). Note that the underlying gyri and sulci appear normal. They are not compressed. **B.** Coronal view demonstrates similar findings (arrows). **C.** Ultrasound study demonstrates typical fluid over the convexities and in the inter-hemispheric fissure (arrows). **D.** Color flow Doppler demonstrates the presence of blood vessels (arrows) in the fluid. **E.** CT study demonstrates a blood vessel (arrow) in the subarachnoid fluid. **F.** In this patient, normal subarachnoid fluid and a blood vessel (arrow) are present on the left. On the right the fluid is "dirty," and the brain is compressed by a subdural empyema.

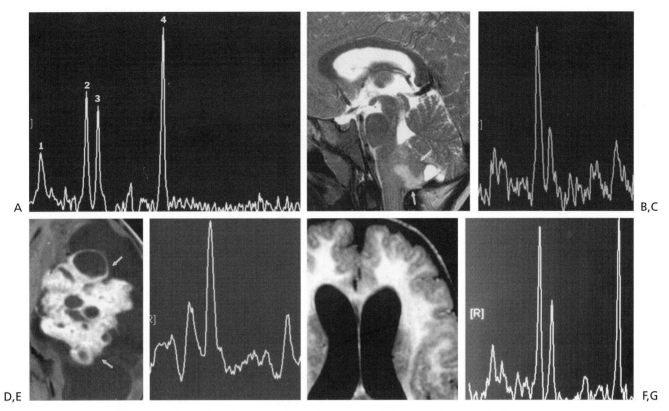

FIGURE 7.25. Normal and abnormal spectroscopy. A. Normal spectroscopy. Peak 1 measures myo-inositol (sugar), peak 2 measures choline (cell wall) metabolism, peak 3 measures creatine (cell energy), and peak 4 measures *N*-acetyl aspartate. Often, with tumors, peaks 2 and 4 are reversed. **B and C. Medulloblastoma. D and E. Cystic glioma. F and G. Alexander's disease.**

tracing is presented in Figure 7.25A, and a few abnormalities for comparison also are included.

CRANIOSYNOSTOSIS

Craniosynostosis occurs in primary or secondary forms. The secondary form is usually seen with conditions such as healing rickets and hypophosphatasia, idiopathic hypercalcemia, anemias with diploë involvement, and hyperthyroidism. All of these conditions represent hypermetabolic states that accelerate suture closure. Sutures also close prematurely (secondary synostosis) with decreased intracranial pressure as seen with brain atrophy or after successful shunting for hydrocephalus. It is most important to differentiate these latter forms of craniosynostosis from the primary type. The etiology of **primary premature synostosis of the calvarial sutures is unknown, but the problem may well lie in faulty dural development in utero.**

When premature closure of a suture occurs, normal bone growth perpendicular to the edges of the suture is impaired. Growth in other directions, however, continues normally and, in most cases, is compensatorily excessive. It is the combination of retarded growth in one direction and exu-

berant compensatory overgrowth in other directions that leads to the specific calvarial deformities encountered. For each suture that closes prematurely, a specific deformity occurs, and the deformity is usually apparent at birth. Characteristic changes along the involved suture also occur. These consist of sutural narrowing, sharpening of the edges (the suture appears as though it were cut with a knife), sclerosis and ridging along the margins of the suture, and bony bridging across the suture line. In newborns, the sutures often have the sharp sclerotic edge appearance.

A suture may be totally or partially obliterated, and in cases of partial fusion only a small bony bridge may be seen. However, even in such cases, characteristic deformity is readily apparent, and even though the suture still appears roentgenographically open, functionally the whole suture is involved and eventually will close. This is most likely to occur with the coronal suture (Fig. 7.26), where CT is very helpful. CT in general is helpful with prematurely closed sutures and is even more helpful as a three-dimensional study (1). The three-dimensional study is considered gold standard. Ultrasound also can be used as a preliminary study (2, 3).

As the infant grows older, calvarial deformity, if uncorrected, becomes more profound, and inner table convolu-

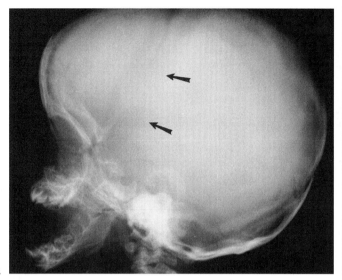

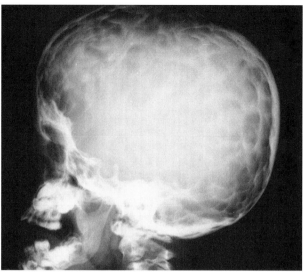

A   B

FIGURE 7.26. Early synostosis. A. In this patient with developing Crouzon's disease, note the facial hypoplasia and a large skull. The coronal sutures, however, merely appear indistinct over their lower portions (arrows). **B.** Years later, classic findings of premature closure of all the sutures are seen.

tions (due to increased intracranial pressure) often become more pronounced. For the same reason sellar erosion and enlargement also occur and all of these late changes result from chronically increased intracranial pressure. They usually are more pronounced when more than one suture is involved and are most striking when all sutures are prematurely closed. In such cases, corrective craniotomy is mandatory, otherwise brain growth is not accommodated. This is less of a problem when only one suture is involved, especially if it is the sagittal suture. Nonetheless, almost all of these patients undergo surgical correction, both for cosmetic reasons and to avert potential damage to the brain.

Sagittal Craniosynostosis

Sagittal suture craniosynostosis is the most common form of synostosis, and when it is the only suture involved, the head becomes extremely long from front to back. It is narrow from side to side, and the deformity produced has been called scaphocephaly or dolichocephaly. The characteristic long head is easily detected both clinically and roentgenographically, and the typical sharpening of the sagittal suture margins, along with sclerosis, ridging, and bridging are readily discernible (Fig. 7.27). As the infant grows older, if untreated, convolutional markings increase in prominence. Currently, three-dimensional CT exquisitely demonstrates these findings (Fig. 7.28).

Coronal Craniosynostosis

The coronal suture is the second most common suture to be involved in primary premature synostosis. The resulting

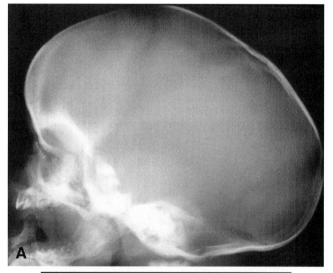

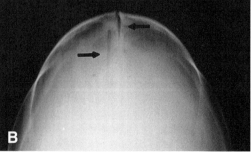

FIGURE 7.27. Sagittal craniosynostosis. A. Lateral view showing characteristically elongated (dolichocephalic or scaphocephalic) skull. In normal newborns, the parietal bone is least well ossified (see Fig. 7.1), but in premature closure of the sagittal suture, the parietal bone is usually thickened and sclerotic. **B.** Frontal view showing thin, sharp-edged sagittal suture (arrows). Also note slight ridging and partial bony bridging.

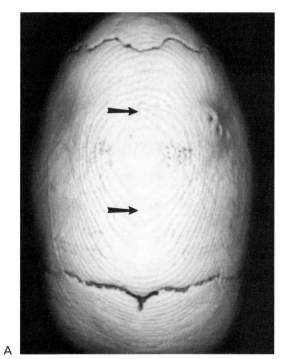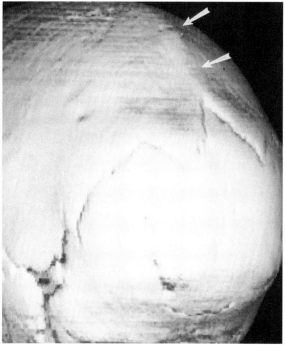

FIGURE 7.28. Sagittal craniosynostosis: three-dimensional CT. A. View from the top demonstrates open coronal (anterior), and lambdoid (posterior) sutures. The sagittal suture, however, is obliterated (arrows). **B.** Tangential view in another patient demonstrates characteristic ridging (arrows).

deformity produces a calvarium that is short from front to back and wide from side to side (Fig. 7.29). This particular configuration has been called bradycephaly or brachycephaly, in which the bregma is somewhat high in position, and on frontal projection the calvarium is wide. There is marked uptilting of the sphenoid wings and a characteristic oval obliquity to the orbital margins. This results in a "harlequin" appearance to the orbits (Fig. 7.29). Hypertelorism is also present, and in addition to the coronal suture, the frontosphenoid synchondrosis is also probably involved. Consequently, there is marked shortening of the anterior fossa, and proptosis often is pronounced. As with sagittal craniosynostosis, if the deformity is uncorrected, convolutional markings become more pronounced, and the sella may show signs of enlargement and erosion.

Coronal synostosis is often the primary deformity in such conditions as Crouzon's disease and Apert's syndrome. Crouzon's disease is a craniofacial dysostosis in which the facial structures are underdeveloped and the calvarium is involved in premature closure of the sutures. It is usually familial, and the sagittal suture also may be involved. In Apert's syndrome, calvarial changes are similar to those of Crouzon's disease, but abnormalities of the hands and feet are also present. These consist primarily of fusion-segmentation anomalies and symphalangism.

Unilateral Coronal Synostosis

The changes of unilateral coronal synostosis are similar to those of bilateral coronal suture synostosis, except that they are one-sided. Primarily, they consist of flattening of the ipsilateral frontoparietal region, elevation of the ipsilateral sphenoid wing, and a unilateral harlequin appearance to the involved orbit (Fig. 7.30). The coronal suture on the involved side shows the usual changes of premature closure: narrowness of the suture line, sharpening of the sutural edges, and sclerosis along the bony margins. The anterior fontanelle may show unilateral smallness, and the nasal septum is usually obliquely tilted, giving rise to the **"skewed nasal septal"** sign. Other findings such as unilateral exophthalmos (secondary to smallness of the anterior fossa) and compensatory enlargement of the ipsilateral middle and posterior fossae are occasionally seen.

Lambdoid Craniosynostosis

Isolated synostosis of the lambdoid sutures is less common than both sagittal and coronal synostosis. When present, there is marked flattening and underdevelopment of the lower portion of the posterior fossa. There may be severe

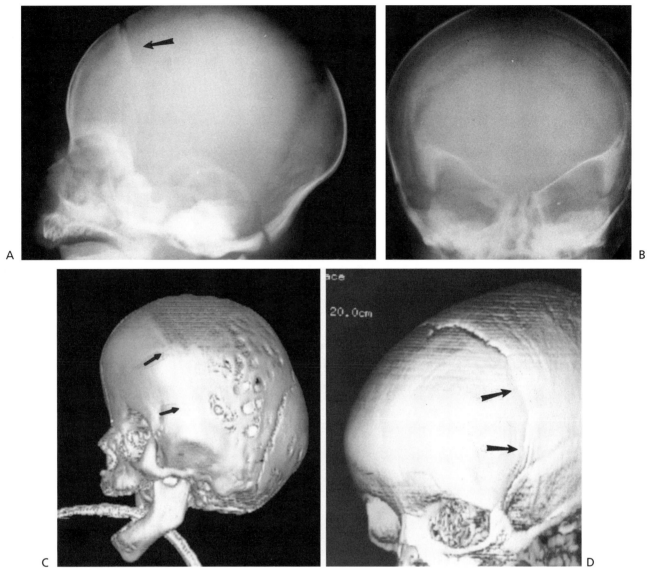

FIGURE 7.29. Bilateral coronal synostosis. A. Lateral view showing typical brachycephalic skull, shallow anterior fossa, highly arched orbital roofs, and characteristic appearance of the coronal sutures (arrow). They are thin, sharply demarcated, and show sclerosis along their edges. The lower two thirds of the suture already have fused. **B.** Frontal view showing biparietal widening, moderate hypertelorism, and upward sloping orbital margins and sphenoid wings resulting in a typical harlequin appearance. **C.** Three-dimensional CT in another patient demonstrates the fused coronal suture (arrows). Note the brachycephaly and underdevelopment of the anterior skull and face. **D.** Partial closure (arrows) of coronal suture in another patient.

overgrowth of the bregma, giving rise to an oxycephalic or turricephalic skull. Unilateral lambdoid suture premature closure produces similar posterior fossa findings, but on one side only (Figs. 7.31 and 7.32). Pseudolambdoid synostosis is more common and is due to chronic posterior positioning, which is now commonplace. This subject is discussed later.

Metopic Craniosynostosis

When there is isolated metopic suture synostosis, the forehead becomes pointed. On tangential view the typical pointed configuration is easily demonstrable. It is called trigonocephaly and is associated with various degrees of hypotelorism (Figs. 7.33 and 7.34).

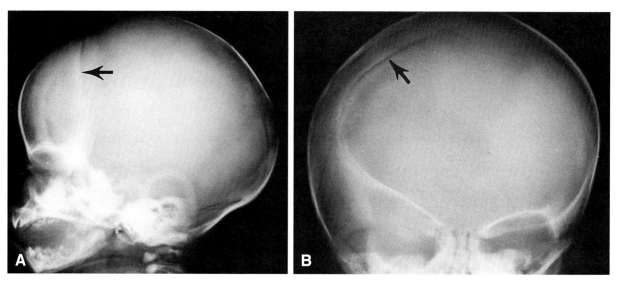

FIGURE 7.30. Unilateral coronal synostosis. A. Lateral view showing complete obliteration of the right coronal suture (arrow). The left coronal suture, just barely visible, is wide open. **B.** Frontal view showing flattening of the right parietal region and the prematurely closed, sharp-appearing coronal suture (arrow). A unilateral harlequin appearance is present.

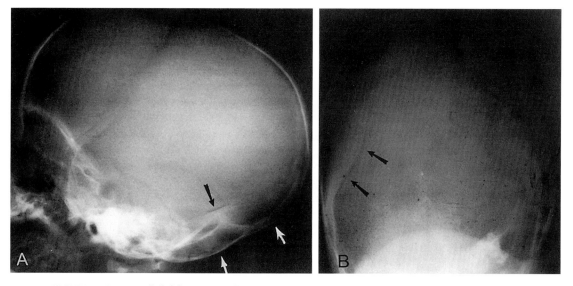

FIGURE 7.31. Lambdoid synostosis. A. Lateral view showing characteristic flattening and deformity of the occipital region (white arrows). Also note the sclerotic, thin, sharp-edged lambdoid suture (black arrow). **B.** Town's projection showing unilateral lambdoid synostosis with a thin, sclerotic, sharp-edged suture (arrows). Also note pronounced and characteristic asymmetry of the posterior fossa.

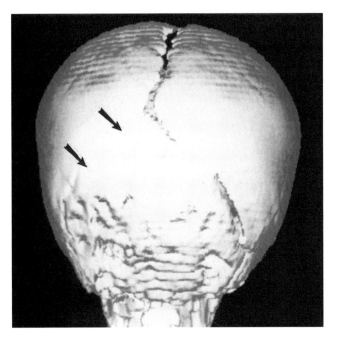

FIGURE 7.32. Lambdoid synostosis: three-dimensional findings. Note the fused and obliterated right lambdoid suture (arrows). The left suture is basically open although closed in its midportion.

Mixed Craniosynostoses

When mixed sutural synostoses occur, bizarre combinations can result (Fig. 7.35). The **cloverleaf skull** is a most grotesque deformity in which prominent bulging of the temporal regions is seen (Fig. 7.36). Other skeletal abnormalities can occur with cloverleaf skull, including synostosis and hypoplasia of the bones around the elbows (4), hips, and shoulders and changes not unlike those of thanatophoric dwarfism.

Universal Craniosynostosis

Occasionally, all sutures can close prematurely and, as a result, severe microcephaly is seen. If untreated, mental retardation occurs, and it is most important that this form of microcephaly be differentiated from that resulting from brain atrophy. The main differential point is that infants with primary universal premature closure of the sutures show markedly increased inner table convolutions and other signs of chronically increased intracranial pressure (Fig. 7.37), while those with brain atrophy show a paucity of convolutional markings and other evidence of decreased intracranial pressure (Fig. 7.38). Hydrocephalus is more common when primary craniosynostosis occurs as part of a syndrome (5, 6). These include Crouzon's and Apert's syndromes.

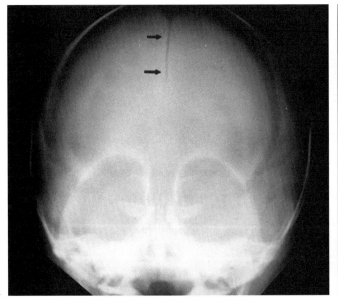

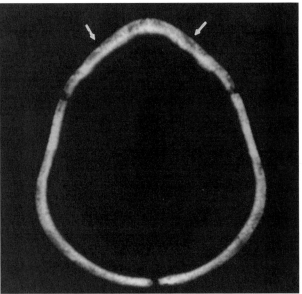

A   B

FIGURE 7.33. Metopic synostosis. A. On this frontal view, note the prematurely closed metopic suture (arrow) which appears thin and sclerotic. There also is associated hypotelorism. The configuration results in a "worried look" appearance. **B.** CT findings. Note the keel-shaped forehead (arrows), consistent with trigonocephaly. The coronal and sagittal sutures are open.

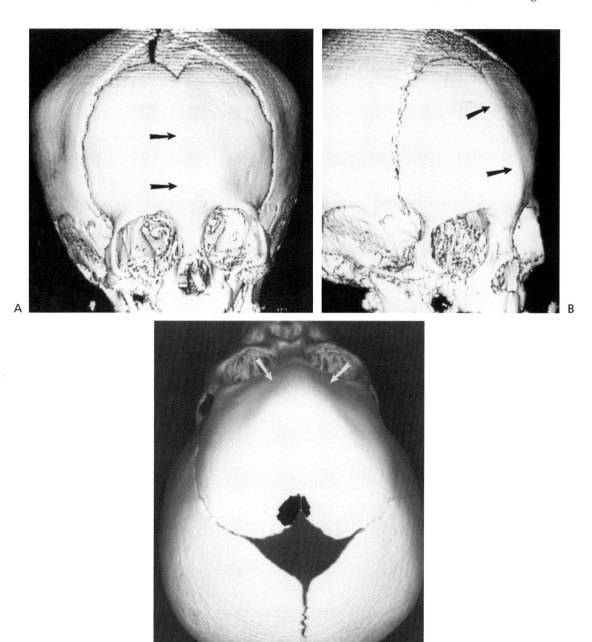

FIGURE 7.34. Metopic synostosis: three-dimensional CT findings. A. Frontal projection demonstrates fusion of the metopic suture (arrows). It is obliterated. Also note the hypotelorism and the "worried look." **B.** Oblique view demonstrates typical prominence and ridging (arrows) along the fused metopic suture. **C.** Overhead view demonstrates the typical keel-shaped "trigonocephaly" configuration of the frontal bones (arrows).

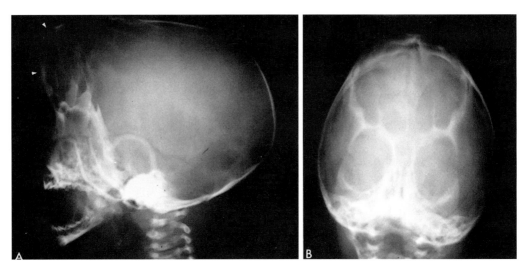

FIGURE 7.35. Mixed craniosynostosis. A. Mixed coronal and metopic craniosynostosis produces extremely shallow anterior fossa, high-arched orbital roofs, and an extremely prominent bregma (arrows). Also note increased convolutions in the frontal region. **B.** Frontal view demonstrates the increased frontal inner table convolutions and vividly shows hypotelorism secondary to metopic suture synostosis. The orbital roofs are high, and the orbits are elongated. (From Jabbour JT, Taybi H. Craniotelencephalic dysplasia, an unusual example of dysplasia of the frontal bone. Am J Dis Child 1964;108:627–632, with permission.)

REFERENCES

1. Vannier MW, Pilgram JL, Marsh JL, et al. Craniosynostosis: diagnostic imaging with three-dimensional CT presentation. AJNR 1994;15:1861–1869.
2. Sobeleski D, McCloskey D, Mussari B, et al. Sonography of normal cranial sutures. AJR 1997;168:819–821.
3. Sobeleski D, Mussari B, McCloskey D, et al. High-resolution sonography of the abnormal cranial suture. Pediatr Radiol 1998:28:79–82.
4. Kitoh H, Nogami H, Oki T, et al. Antley-Bixler syndrome: a disorder characterized by congenital synostosis of the elbow joint and the cranial suture. J Pediatr Orthop 1996;16:243–246.
5. Noetzel MJ, Marsh JL, Palkes H. Hydrocephalus and mental retardation in craniosynostosis. J Pediatr 1985;107:885–892.
6. Cinalli G, Sainte-Rose C, Kollar EM, et al. Hydrocephalus and craniosynostosis. J Neurosurg 1998;88:209–214.

Secondary Synostosis

Secondary craniosynostosis as noted earlier, can be seen with a number of metabolic disturbances either in their active or reparative stages. These include such conditions as rickets, hypophosphatasia, hypercalcemia, and hyperthyroidism. Secondary craniosynostosis can also be seen in association with calvarial thickening secondary to underlying anemia. More importantly, however, is that secondary craniosynostosis is frequently seen when the brain fails to grow normally. Insult to the brain may result from infection, trauma, or hemorrhage, and when the brain ceases to grow, the calvarium ceases to expand. There is no stimulus to keep the cranial sutures open, and they become increasingly narrow and finally close.

Roentgenographically, the changes in patients with impaired brain growth consist of a small skull, occipital flattening (postural from prolonged lying on the back), narrowing and eventual closing of the sutures, small fontanelles, absence of inner table convolutions, and thickening of the calvarium (Figs. 7.38). All of these changes result from absent normal brain growth and hence a lack of normal intracranial pressure. It is most important to differentiate these findings from those seen in patients with primary universal craniosynostosis, because surgical intervention is not indicated in these infants. There is no problem of compromised room for brain growth in these patients and, as opposed to primary synostosis, bridging, ridging, and sclerosis of the sutural edges are absent. At times, ridging may be suggested clinically, but the roentgenographic study will show that such ridging is the result of persistently overlapped bones. Other less consistent calvarial changes associated with microcephaly include excessive roundness of the orbits, elevation of the superior orbital margins, and a variable degree of hypotelorism.

Secondary premature closure of the sutures also occurs in infants in whom hydrocephalus has been successfully treated by a shunting procedure. In these infants, if the shunt is functioning, intracranial pressures decrease, and even though the brain continues to grow it grows inwardly, encroaching upon the ventricles. Outward growth is less than normal, and the stimulus for calvarial expansion is lost. As with atrophy, the skull shows persistence of its original size and shape, progressive thickening, and eventually, premature closure of the sutures. However, it must be

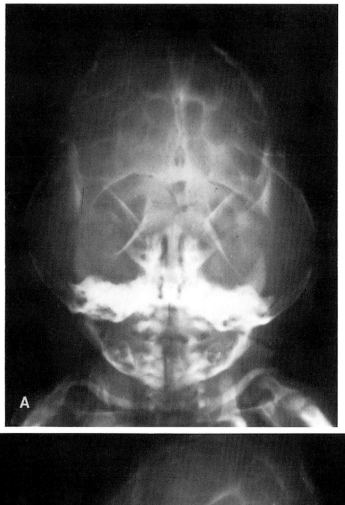

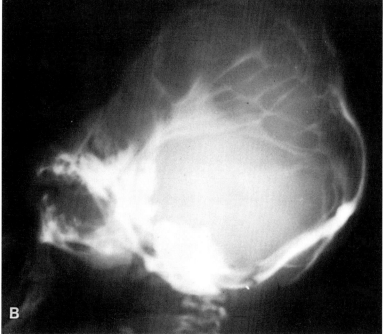

FIGURE 7.36. Cloverleaf skull. A. Frontal view showing typical cloverleaf configuration with bitemporal and bregmatic bulging. **B.** Lateral view showing typical deformities and pronounced lacunar skull. (Courtesy of S. E. Garrison, M.D.)

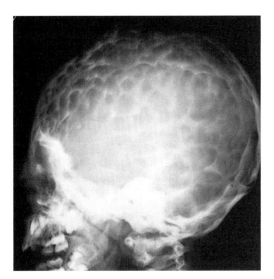

FIGURE 7.37. Universal craniosynostosis. Older child showing end result of universal craniosynostosis. The skull is microcephalic and the inner table convolutions markedly increased. This is not lacunar skull but rather represents prominent inner table convolutions resulting from longstanding increased intracranial pressure. Although not clearly visualized in this reproduction, the sella was markedly demineralized and even enlarged. Universal craniosynostosis requires early operative intervention.

emphasized that for this given situation this picture is "normal" and expected.

Factitious Lambdoid Synostosis

Persistent posturing (turning) to one side or the other over the occiput, infants can cause the calvarial bones to overlap along the lambdoid suture and the suture to appear prematurely closed. The reason for this is that the suture will appear sclerotic along its edge, but it has been determined that this is the result of overlapping of the sutures (1). This is important, because it has been suggested in the past that sclerosis along the suture is an indication that it will close prematurely. However, sclerosis must occur on both sides of the suture, and in cases of factitious suture closure, sclerosis is present on one side only (Fig. 7.39, A and B). The problem simply is one due to overlapping of the sutures, but it may become more common now that infants are being made to sleep in the supine position (2–7). If other positions are used, other deformities occur (7). In most cases CT with three-dimensional reconstruction solve the problem (Fig. 7.39, C and D).

REFERENCES

1. Rollins N, Sklar F. Factitious lambdoid perisutural sclerosis: does the "sticky suture" exist? Pediatr Radiol 1996;26:356–358.
2. Hunt CE, Puczynski MS. Does supine sleeping cause asymmetric heads? Pediatrics 1996;98:127–129.
3. Kane AA, Mitchell LE, Craven KP, et al. Observations on a recent increase in plagiocephaly without synostosis. Pediatrics 1996;97:877–885.
4. McAlister WH. Invited commentary: posterior deformational plagiocephaly. Pediatr Radiol 1998;28:727–728.
5. Fernbach SK. Craniosynostosis 1998: concepts and controversies. Pediatr Radiol 1998;28:722–727.
6. Pollack IF, Losken WH, Fasick P. Diagnosis and management of posterior plagiocephaly. Pediatrics 1997;99:180–185.
7. Huang C-S, Cheng H-C, Lin W-Y, et al. Skull morphology affected by different sleep positions in infancy. Cleft Palate Craniofac J 1995;32:413–419.

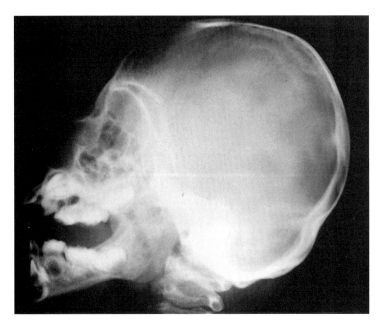

FIGURE 7.38. Brain atrophy with secondary craniosynostosis. Note that the sutures all have been obliterated and are closed. Note also that the calvarium is very thick. These findings are characteristic of secondary craniosynostosis due to decreased intracranial pressures.

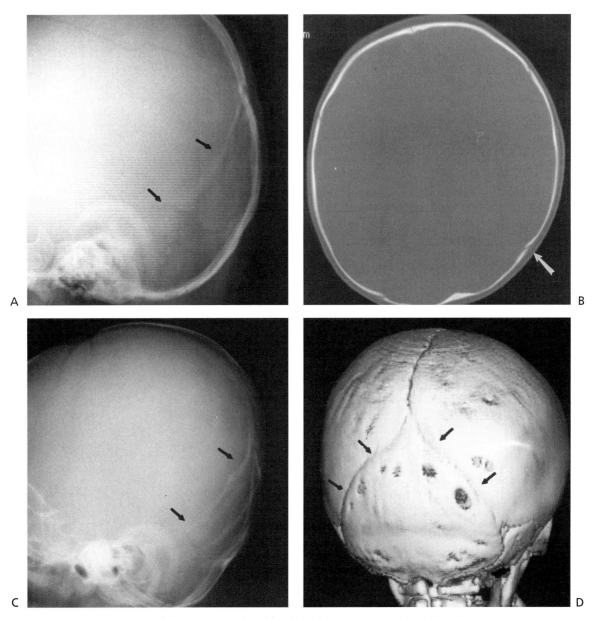

FIGURE 7.39. Factitious synostosis of lambdoid suture. A. In this patient, there is suggestion of lambdoid suture synostosis (arrows). **B.** CT scan, however, demonstrates that the problem is mere overlapping of the open suture (arrow). Note the ipsilateral flattening of the calvarium. **C.** Another patient demonstrating what would appear to be bilateral lambdoid synostosis (arrows) with associated flattening of the occiput. **D.** Three-dimensional reconstructed tomography demonstrates that both lambdoid sutures (arrows) are open. In both patients, the problem was postural-induced deformity of the head.

SPREAD SUTURES: INCREASED INTRACRANIAL PRESSURE

Before the advent of CT, ultrasonography, and MRI, considerable attention was placed on evaluating the infantile skull for evidence of spread sutures. The finding translated into increased intracranial pressure, but today it is of minor significance. However, it still is useful to briefly review the problem, and in this regard the coronal suture is the first to show spread secondary to increased intracranial pressure. It is assessed on the lateral view of the skull where in the neonate and young infant it assumes an exaggerated V-shaped configuration (Fig. 7.40A). After the coronal, the sagittal suture is next to spread, and finally the lambdoid and squamosal sutures spread. Spread sutures in older children present with increased lucency and sharpness of the

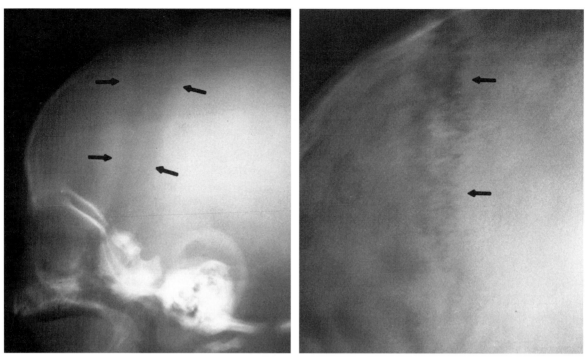

FIGURE 7.40. Increased intracranial pressure: spread sutures. A. Neonate with increased intracranial pressure demonstrating a markedly spread, V-shaped coronal suture (arrows). **B.** Older child with spreading of the coronal suture manifesting in a stretched appearance of the suture interdigitations (arrows).

sutures and with subacute spread elongation of the sutural interdigitations (Fig. 7.40B). Spread sutures in infants also can be detected with ultrasound (1).

The sutures also can spread when there is ***rebound normal brain growth*** after a period of growth suppression. This commonly occurs in chronically ill newborns and almost all premature infants, as well as in recovering deprivational dwarfism. Deprivational dwarfs are physically and emotionally deprived, but once removed from their negative environment, they rapidly begin to thrive, gain weight, and grow. As the brain partakes in this resurgence of normal growth, cranial sutures often spread. I have seen a similar phenomenon occur in one older child with treated hypothyroidism.

If the calvarium is underossified, the sutures are brought into exaggerated prominence and erroneously suggest spread. Conditions in which this phenomenon occurs consist of osteogenesis imperfecta, cleidocranial dysostosis, hypophosphatasia, active rickets, hyperparathyroidism, progeria, the trisomies, Jansen-type metaphyseal dysostosis, hypothyroidism, prostaglandin E therapy (2, 3), and prematurity. Pseudospreading (i.e., underossification) and prominence of the lambdoid and other sutures, excessive wormian bone formation, and other cranial defects are frequently seen in idiopathic osteoarthropathy (i.e., pachydermoperiostosis) of childhood. This is an uncommon abnor-

mality that tends to be familial and is of unknown etiology. As these infants grow older, the calvarial defects and suture prominence disappear.

REFERENCES

1. Sobeleski D, Mussari B, McCloskey D, et al. High resolution sonography of the abnormal cranial suture. Pediatr Radiol 1998; 28:79–82.
2. Beitzke A, Stein J. Pseudo-widening of cranial sutures as a feature of long-term prostaglandin E1 therapy. Pediatr Radiol 1986;16: 57–58.
3. Hoevels-Guerich H, Haferkorn L, Persigehl M, et al. Widening of cranial sutures after long-term prostaglandin E2 therapy in two newborn infants. J Pediatr 1984;105:72–74.

CRANIOTABES

This term refers to palpable soft spots in the neonatal infant's calvarium. The finding can be seen with conditions such as osteogenesis imperfecta, prematurity, rickets of prematurity, cleidocranial dysostosis, and any number of conditions with poor membranous bone ossification. It also can be seen in normal infants, but whatever, it is benign and self-correcting with time.

THE LARGE HEAD

A large calvarium can result from megalencephaly, chronic subdural hematoma or hygroma, brain tumor, hydrocephalus, and with benign subarachnoid effusions of infancy. Disproportionately large calvaria also are seen with bone dysplasias such as cleidocranial dysostosis, achondroplasia, Hurler's disease, or Russel-Silver dwarfism. The premature infant has a disproportionately large head, and this finding is normal. Many premature infants, once they begin to grow more rapidly, show rapid increase in head size. In terms of investigation of a large head, if the anterior fontanelle is open, one can use ultrasound as the initial screening procedure. Thereafter, CT or MRI is required.

Hereditary Megalencephaly

This is a rare hereditary condition that results in enlargement of the brain and head. The etiology is unknown, but a genetic or metabolic defect is speculated. Infants with this condition are usually severely retarded, and their brains are extremely large. Imaging reveals normal or small ventricles and readily differentiates megalencephaly from hydrocephalus. Unilateral megalencephaly also occurs (1). In these infants refractory seizures are a problem, and there is overgrowth of half the brain with abnormally thick gray matter. The problem is now considered a of gray matter migrational abnormality.

REFERENCES

1. Kalifa GL, Chiron C, Sellier PD, et al. Hemimegalencephaly: MR imaging in five infants. Radiology 1987;165:29–33.

Subdural Hematoma, Hygroma, and Hydroma

Subdural hematoma, hygroma, and hydroma all refer to collections of fluid in the subdural space. If the fluid is bloody, it is referred to as a subdural hematoma; if xanthochromic, it is often referred to as a hygroma; and if clear, it is called a hydroma. Subdural hematomas can occur anywhere, but are most common over the frontoparietal region. Frequently they can extend along the temporal horns into the middle fossae. Posterior fossa subdural hematomas are uncommon. In newborns, subdural hematoma usually is related to difficult deliveries and fractures are uncommon. In older infants and children, subdural hematomas usually are the result of trauma, including the battered child syndrome.

Subdural hematomas are best identified with CT or MRI (Fig. 7.41). With CT, the subdural hematoma appears different at different stages of its evolution. Early on, the blood is radio-opaque, but after 10 days or so it becomes isodense and invisible on regular scanning. Rapid high-dose contrast CT scanning can obviate this problem, but in other cases, one should suspect the presence of such a

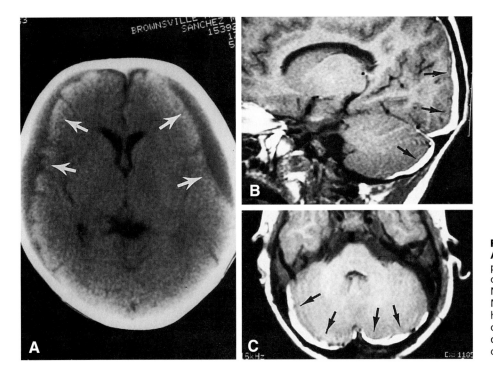

FIGURE 7.41. Subdural hematoma. A. Bilateral fluid collections causing partial compression and effacement of the underlying brain (arrows). **B.** Newborn infant with a T1-weighted MR image demonstrating subdural hematomas over the occipital and cerebellar regions. **C.** Axial view demonstrates the bleeds over the cerebellum (arrows).

hematoma by the presence of other findings, such as a shift of the midline structures and compression of the ipsilateral ventricle. With MRI, blood in the early stages of a bleed produces low signal intensity and may be missed. However, within a day or two, hemoglobin changes to methemoglobin, and high signal intensity is seen on both T1- and T2-weighted images (Fig. 7.41C). Subdural hygromas or hydromas also produce high signal intensity on T2-weighted images and calcifications of subdural hematomas also can occur.

Hydrocephalus

Hydrocephalus usually results from obstruction to the normal flow of cerebrospinal fluid. As a consequence, fluid accumulates in excessive quantities and the ventricular system dilates. Faulty absorption of cerebrospinal fluid has also been considered and, occasionally, excessive fluid production, as seen with choroid plexus papilloma, is the cause.

In terms of classification of hydrocephalus, if obstruction occurs within the ventricles, it is usually referred to as noncommunicating hydrocephalus, while if it occurs outside the ventricles, the term "communicating" hydrocephalus is applied. Communication, in the latter cases, indicates only that cerebral spinal fluid can leave the fourth ventricle and enter the subarachnoid space and not that cerebral spinal fluid flow is entirely normal. In the usual case of communicating hydrocephalus, secondary to obliterative arachnoiditis resulting either from inflammation or

hemorrhage, circulation through the subarachnoid space is impaired.

Conditions producing noncommunicating hydrocephalus include stenosis of the aqueduct of Sylvius, Arnold-Chiari syndrome, Dandy-Walker cyst, and the relatively rare congenital obstruction of the foramina of Monro. Intraventricular or paraventricular tumors or vascular abnormalities also can produce obstructive hydrocephalus, but this section deals only with nontumoral causes. Communicating hydrocephalus, as noted earlier, usually is produced by posthemorrhagic or inflammatory arachnoiditis. In the latter, depending on the site of the adhesions, obstruction can occur in the posterior fossa, basal cisterns, or over the convexity of the brain. Most frequently, it occurs in the posterior fossa or along the basal cisterns. A similar pattern of obstruction can be seen in infants with meningeal infiltrates secondary to leukemia, lymphoma, carcinomatosis, or histiocytosis X, but these are not usually a problem in the neonatal period.

In the **imaging of hydrocephalus**, plain films are of limited value. Definitive imaging is accomplished with ultrasound, CT, or MR. With ultrasound, the study is useful only if the anterior fontanelle is open, because this is the usual window for the study. CT and MRI basically provide identical information and on both studies, in patients with marked degrees of hydrocephalus, periventricular transudation of cerebral spinal fluid into the brain substance can be seen (Fig. 7.42). The finding is reversible and disappears when the ventricles are decompressed. Resistive indices, as

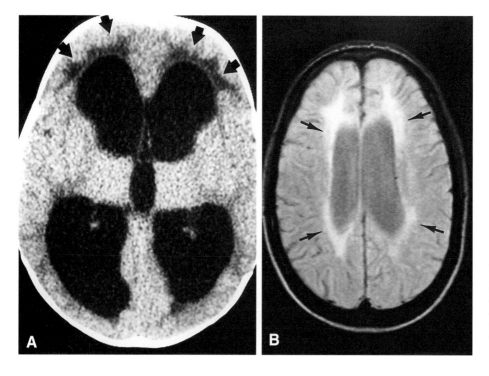

FIGURE 7.42. Hydrocephalus with transudation of fluid. A. CT study demonstrates marked hydrocephalus with dilation of the lateral and third ventricle. Note the transudation of fluid (arrows) over the frontal horns. **B.** Circumferential transudation of fluid (arrows) demonstrated on this proton density MR image.

detected with color flow Doppler also can be used to monitor intracranial pressure in hydrocephalus (1).

Once a patient has been shunted for hydrocephalus, shunt patency must be maintained. Breaks and discontinuity of the shunt tubing along with spread sutures can be assessed with regular radiography (Fig. 7.43, A–C). However, in some cases, contrast radiography is required (2). Contrast material is injected into the shunt tubing, and then under fluoroscopic control it is determined whether it flows retrograde into the ventricles or antegrade into the peritoneal cavity or other receiving compartment. Nuclear

scintigraphy also can be employed in the same manner, but contrast shuntography is more expedient. After shunting has been accomplished, if pressures decrease too rapidly, the brain may fall away from the dura and cause the dural veins to tear and result in subdural hematomas (2) (Fig. 7.43D). Calvarial findings after successful shunting, because of chronically decreased intracranial pressure include thickening of the skull, premature closure of the sutures, and diminution in size of the sella.

The phenomenon of the isolated fourth ventricle after shunting also should be considered. In these cases, the

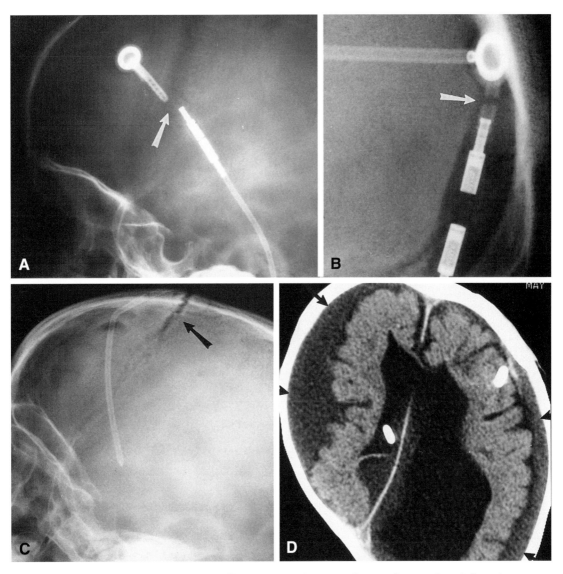

FIGURE 7.43. Postshunting complications. A. The coronal suture is spread, and there is a frank break (arrow) in the shunt tubing. **B.** More subtle break (arrow) through shunt tubing. **C.** Acutely spread coronal suture (arrow) resulting from shunt malfunction. Because the sutures are closing prematurely in these patients, when they spread, they have a sharp, black appearance. **D.** Postshunting subdural hematoma. The ventricles are dilated, and the atrophic brain is surrounded by subdural hematomas (arrows).

fourth ventricle is obstructed at the aqueduct (e.g., stenosis, kinking) or the foramina of Luschka and Magendie (e.g., congenital, adhesions). Most often, this occurs after supratentorial shunting for Dandy-Walker cyst, but it also can be seen with other causes of hydrocephalus (3–5). Whatever the underlying problem, after supratentorial shunting there is progressive enlargement of the "trapped" or "isolated" fourth ventricle (Fig. 7.44). In some cases, there may be transtentorial herniation of the trapped fourth ventricle (3, 4).

Congenital obstruction of the aqueduct of Sylvius, or aqueductal stenosis is a common cause of hydrocephalus in the newborn and young infant and often produces the largest ventricles seen. Although some cases are secondary to inflammatory structure or stenosis, most cases are probably the result of developmental abnormality where the problem can be; the presence of a membrane in the aqueduct, actual ductal stenosis, or, more commonly, forking of the aqueduct. The latter abnormality consists of the formation of multiple small aqueductal channels, many of which are blind ending. All imaging modalities vividly demonstrate the characteristic dilation of the lateral (occipital horn often most dilated) and third ventricles, and no dilation of the fourth ventricle (Fig. 7.45). The third ventricle also may show cystic dilation of the suprapineal recess, and in some cases, posteroinferior transtentorial herniation of the posterior portion of the third ventricle can occur. Similarly, a diverticulum of the atrium of the lateral ventricles can herniate below the tentorium and produce an apparent pseudocyst (Fig. 7.46).

An uncommon cause of supratentorial obstructive hydrocephalus is **unilateral obstruction of the foramen of Monro.** One or the other of the foramina of Monro is obstructed and unilateral hydrocephalus results. In pronounced cases there may be unilateral enlargement of the calvarium, but otherwise diagnosis depends on demonstrating the unilaterally enlarged lateral ventricle with some imaging modality (Fig. 7.47).

In the abnormality known as **Dandy Walker cyst** there is congenital obstruction of the fourth ventricular foramina of Magendie and Luschka and subsequent cystic dilation of the fourth ventricle. Obliteration of these foramina is occasionally secondary to inflammatory disease, but most cases represent congenital atresia. In addition to cystic enlargement of the fourth ventricle, the cerebellum is usually underdeveloped, dysplastic, and displaced anterosuperiorly

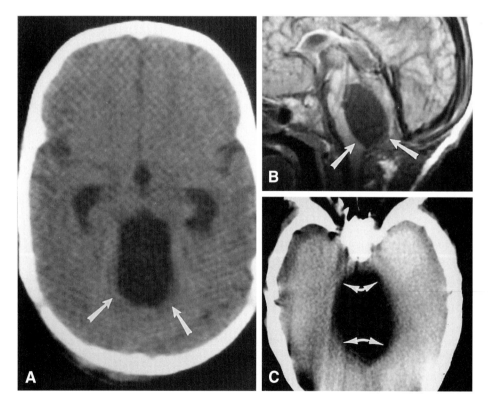

FIGURE 7.44. Isolated fourth ventricle. A. Note the isolated, dilated fourth ventricle (arrows). **B.** MR study in another patient demonstrates similar findings (arrows). **C.** In this patient, the isolated fourth ventricle is black (arrows). The dilated lateral ventricles surrounding the fourth ventricle are white because of the introduction of contrast material into the lateral ventricles. The contrast material did not pass into the isolated fourth ventricle, and it therefore remains unopacified (i.e., black).

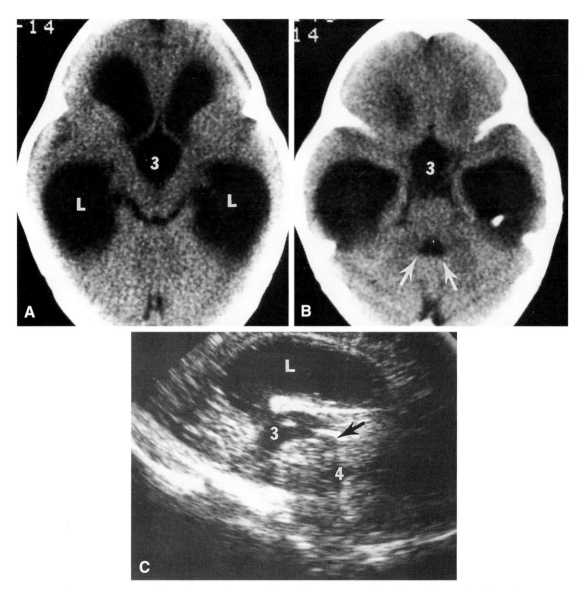

Figure 7.45. Aqueductal stenosis. A. Axial CT demonstrates dilated lateral ventricles (L) and a dilated third ventricle (3). **B.** Slightly lower slice demonstrates the dilated lateral and third (3) ventricles. Because the fourth ventricle (arrows) is normal, obstruction at the aqueductal level is presumed. **C.** Sagittal ultrasound study demonstrates a dilated lateral ventricle (L), a dilated third ventricle (3), but a normal fourth ventricle (4). Obstruction is at the level of the aqueduct (arrow).

by the enlarging fourth ventricle. In milder cases, fourth ventricular dilation is less striking; and the associated cerebellar changes, less dramatic.

All of the findings are vividly demonstrable with any of the available imaging modalities (6). The findings consist of a large central, posterior fossa cystic structure (the abnormal fourth ventricle) and a hypoplastic cerebellum with an absent or dysplastic inferior vermis (Fig. 7.48). The cystic fourth ventricle may be so large so as to push the tentorium and supratentorial structures far forward. In other cases, the enlarged fourth ventricle may herniate upward through the dysplastic tentorium, but in others, it may extend into the cervical spine through the foramen magnum. The foramen magnum in these latter cases is enlarged. In those cases with lesser abnormality, or the so-called Dandy-Walker variant, the cerebellum shows less underdevelopment, but the inferior vermis, although present, is usually markedly underdeveloped. The size of the resulting cyst may not be as large as in the classic case (Fig. 7.49, A and B). Other abnormalities commonly seen with Dandy-Walker cyst include agenesis of the corpus callosum and interhemispheric arachnoid cysts. There is some trend towards a unifying concept of

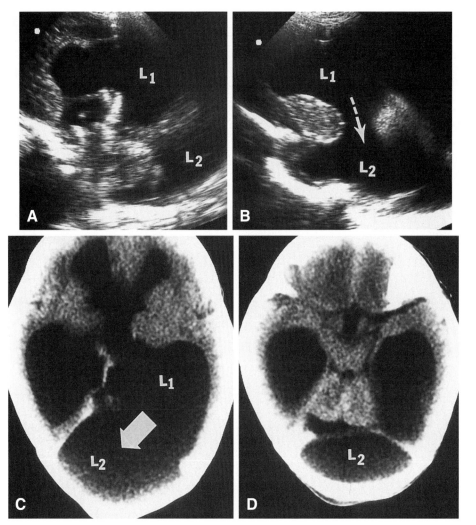

FIGURE 7.46. Aqueductal stenosis with transtentorial herniation of lateral ventricle. A. Sagittal ultrasound demonstrates the dilated lateral ventricle (L1) with a portion having herniated into the posterior fossa (L2). Note the dilated third ventricle and normal fourth ventricle. **B.** Parasagittal view demonstrates the dilated lateral ventricle (L1) herniating (arrow) into the posterior fossa (L2). **C.** Axial CT study demonstrates marked ventricular dilation with the left lateral ventricle (L1) herniating (arrow) into the posterior fossa (L2). **D.** Slice through the posterior fossa demonstrates the herniated portion of the lateral ventricle (L2) located in the posterior fossa.

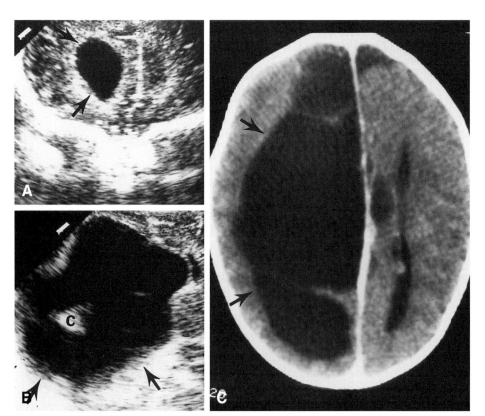

FIGURE 7.47. Unilateral foramen of Monro obstruction. A. Coronal sonogram through the frontal horns demonstrates a dilated right lateral ventricle (arrows). **B.** A posterior cut through the trigone demonstrates massive dilation of the right lateral ventricle (arrows). The choroid plexus (C) is floating in the ventricle. **C.** CT study in another patient demonstrates unilateral dilation of the right ventricle (arrows). The midline structures and the other ventricle are contralaterally displaced and compressed.

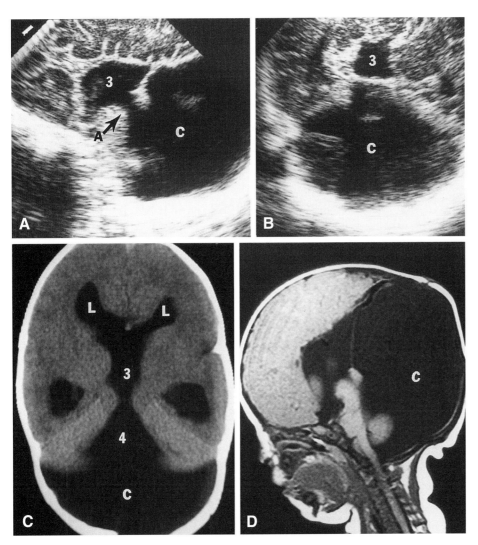

FIGURE 7.48. Dandy-Walker cyst. A. Sagittal ultrasonogram demonstrates a dilated third ventricle (3) communicating via the aqueduct (A) with the large Dandy-Walker cyst (C). A fourth ventricle as such is not identified. **B.** Coronal view demonstrates the dilated third ventricle (3) and Dandy-Walker cyst (C). There is no vermis present. **C.** Another patient with a large Dandy-Walker cyst (C) communicating with the dilated fourth ventricle (4), which communicates with a dilated third ventricle (3) by way of a dilated aqueduct. The lateral ventricles (L) are dilated and assume the characteristic appearance when associated agenesis of the corpus callosum is present. **D.** Sagittal MR study in another infant demonstrates an extremely large Dandy-Walker cyst (C) displacing the tentorium and supratentorial structures far anteriorly.

Dandy-Walker cyst, including Dandy-Walker cyst, Dandy-Walker variant, and large cisterna magna (6) (Fig. 7.49, C and D). A Dandy-Walker cyst also needs to be differentiated from an extraaxial posterior fossa cyst. With extraaxial posterior fossa cysts, the off midline location of the cyst, causing associated distortion and displacement of the cerebellum and fourth ventricle, secures the diagnosis (Fig. 7.50). There is no underdevelopment of the vermis and cerebellum.

In the **Arnold-Chiari malformation**, there is downward displacement of the cerebellum and fourth ventricle, through the foramen magnum and into the cervical spinal canal. Three types exist: types I through III. In the type I deformity, there is only slight downward displacement of the cerebellar tonsils. No cerebellar hypoplasia exists, but syringomyelia is seen in some cases. The type II abnormality consists of pronounced downward displacement of the

cerebellum, medulla, lower pons, and fourth ventricle into the cervical spinal canal. It is invariably associated with a spinal or cranial meningocele or meningomyelocele and in many cases syringomyelia and tethering of the cord. In the rare type III abnormality, there is abnormal displacement of the entire cerebellum into a large cervical spina bifida (7). In the type II anomaly, the most common in the newborn, associated hydrocephalus is believed to result from secondary aqueductal stenosis resulting from stretching and compression of the aqueduct as the fourth ventricle is displacement into the foramen magnum. The intracranial abnormalities in the Chiari II malformation are readily demonstrated with any imaging modality, but especially well with MRI. The findings include; (a) a V-shaped configuration of the quadrigeminal cistern resulting in so-called "tectal" beaking; (b) downward displacement of the cerebellum; (c) absence of the septum pellucidum; (d) enlarge-

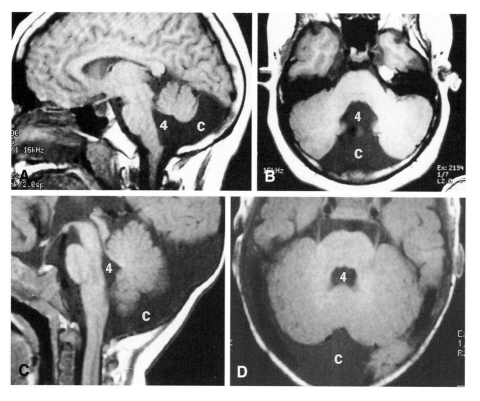

FIGURE 7.49. Dandy-Walker cyst variant and large cisterna magna. A. Dandy-Walker cyst variant. Note that the cyst (C) freely communicates with the slightly dilated fourth ventricle (4). There is no hydrocephalus. **B.** Axial view demonstrates the cyst (C) freely communicating with the fourth ventricle (4). The vermis is severely hypoplastic and actually absent. **C. Large cisterna magna.** Note the large cisterna magna (C) and normal fourth ventricle (4). The distal foramina of the fourth ventricle also are normal. There is no hydrocephalus. **D.** Axial view demonstrates the large cisterna magna (C) and the normal fourth ventricle (4). There is no communication between the two structures.

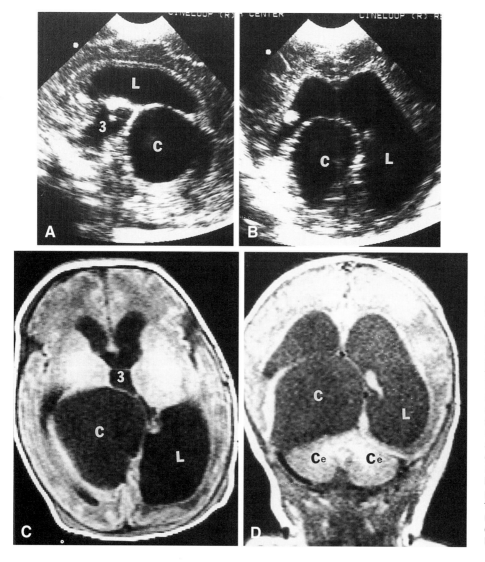

FIGURE 7.50. Extraaxial posterior fossa cyst. A. Ultrasonogram demonstrates a dilated lateral ventricle (L), a dilated third ventricle (3), and a large cyst (C). **B.** Coronal sonogram demonstrates the large cyst (C) to lie in the posterior fossa. The left lateral ventricle (L) is markedly dilated resulting from compressive aqueductal obstruction. **C.** Axial MR study demonstrates the large posterior fossa extraaxial cyst (C) causing aqueductal obstruction and hydrocephalus. The left occipital horn (L) is markedly dilated. Third ventricle (3). **D.** Coronal view demonstrates the posterior fossa cyst (C), dilation of the lateral ventricles (L), and a normal cerebellum (Ce). The findings are completely different from those of a Dandy-Walker cyst.

ment of the massa intermedia; and (e) a heart-shaped, common ventricle on coronal view with pointed inferior recesses (Figs. 7.51 and 7.52). In the Arnold-Chiari type I malformation, symptoms usually are absent unless an associated syrinx is present (8, 9). Symptoms may include one of more of the following: neck or occipital pain, scoliosis, torticollis, apnea, and motor disturbances. The syrinx is believed to develop because of the piston-like action of the low tonsils on the CSF fluid of the spinal canal, causing pressure waves and subsequent dilatation (10). A case of spontaneous resolution has been documented (11).

With **communicating hydrocephalus,** the findings are readily demonstrable with any imaging modality and consist of dilation of the lateral, third, and fourth ventricles (Fig. 7.53). The aqueduct and cisterna magna often are large and dilated.

REFERENCES

1. Goh D, Minns RA, Hendry GMA. Cerebrovascular resistive index assessed by duplex Doppler sonography and its relationship

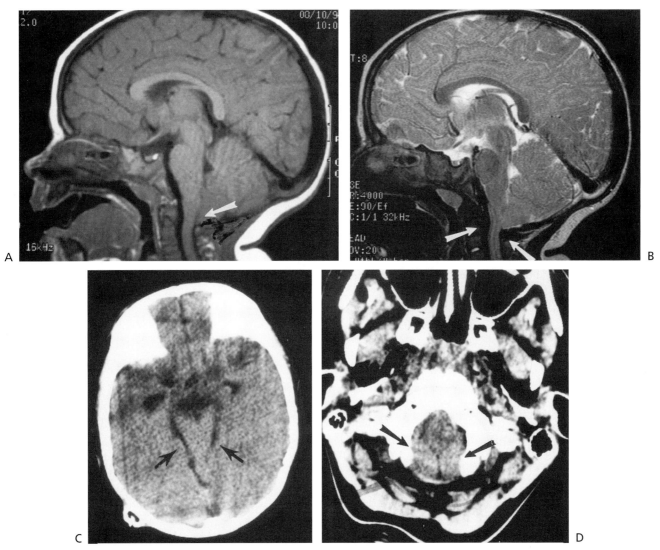

FIGURE 7.51. Arnold-Chiari malformation: type I. A. Note the downwardly displaced cerebral tonsils (arrow). **B.** T2-weighted image demonstrates the same findings (arrow). Note that there is very little if any cerebral spinal fluid (high signal intensity) around the tonsillar herniation. **C.** CT study demonstrating typical V-shaped configuration (arrows) of the perimesencephalic cisterns. **D.** On this CT study, note the herniation of the cerebral tonsils (arrows) into the foramen magnum.

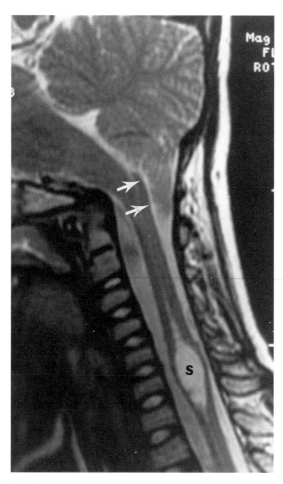

FIGURE 7.52. Arnold-Chiari malformation: type II. Note the marked downward displacement of the cerebral tonsils (arrows). They extend far into the upper cervical spine. Also note the presence of a syrinx (S) in the cervical spinal cord.

to intracranial pressure in infantile hydrocephalus. Pediatr Radiol 1992;22;246–250.

2. Sweeney LE, Thomas PS. Contrast examination of cerebrospinal fluid shunt malfunction in infancy and childhood. Pediatr Radiol 1987;17:177–183.

2. Kirkpatrick PJ, Knibb AA, Downing HA. Rapid decompression of chronic hydrocephalus resulting in bilateral extradural hematomas; a general surgical complication. J Pediatr Surg 1993; 28:744–745.

3. Hall TR, Choi A, Schellinger D, et al. Isolation of the fourth ventricle causing transtentorial herniation: neurosonographic findings in premature infants. AJR 1992;159;811–815.

4. Castillo M, Wilson JD. Spontaneous resolution of a Chiari I malformation: MR demonstration. AJNR 1995;16:1158–1160.

4. Rosenfeld DL, Lis E, DeMarco K. Transtentorial herniation of the fourth ventricle. Pediatr Radiol 1995;25:436–439.

5. Scotti G, Musgrave MA, Fitz CR, et al. The isolated fourth ventricle in children: CT and clinical review of 16 cases. AJR 1980; 135:1233–1238.

6. Strand RD, Barnes PD, Poussaint TY, et al. Cystic retrocerebellar malformations: unification of the Dandy-Walker complex and the Blake's pouch cyst. Pediatr Radiol 1993;23:258–260.

7. Castillo M, Quencer RM, Dominguez R. Chiari III malformation: imaging features. AJNR 1992;13:107–113.

8. Elster AD, Chen MYM. Chiari I malformations: clinical and radiological reappraisal. Radiology 1992;183:347–353.

9. Listernick R, Tomita T. Persistent crying in infancy as a presentation of Chiari type I malformation. J Pediatr 1991;118: 567–569.

10. Heiss JD, Patronas N, DeBroom HL. Elucidating the pathophysiology of syringomyelia. J Neurosurg 1999;91:553–562.

11. Sun PP, Harrop J, Sutton LN. Complete spontaneous resolution of childhood Chiari I malformation and associated syringomyelia. Pediatrics 2001;107:182–185.

Hydranencephaly

Hydranencephaly is a relatively uncommon condition believed to represent a severe form of intrauterine cere-

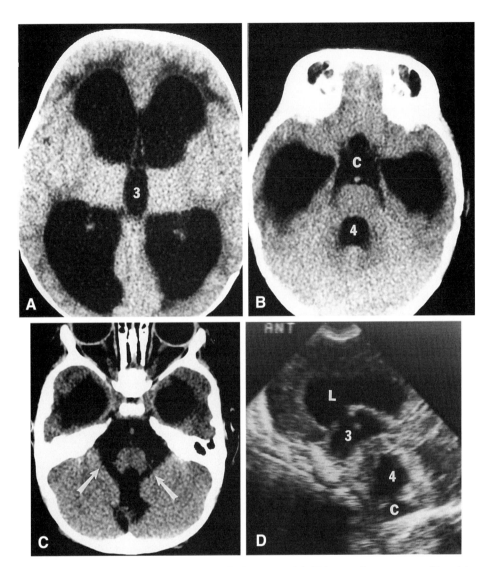

FIGURE 7.53. Communicating hydrocephalus. A. Axial CT image demonstrates dilated lateral ventricles and a dilated third (3) ventricle. **B.** Lower slice demonstrates dilation of the fourth ventricle (4) and the cisterna magna (C). **C.** Axial slice through the base of the skull demonstrates a prominent cisterna magna (arrows). **D.** Sagittal ultrasonogram demonstrates the dilated lateral ventricle (L) communicating through a dilated foramen of Monro with the dilated third ventricle (3). The fourth ventricle (4) also is dilated, and the cisterna magna (C) is clearly visible.

bral degeneration secondary to a vascular insult. These infants show markedly dilated fluid-filled ventricles with virtually no remaining cortex. All that is left is a thin glial and meningeal sac. On frontal view, the falx often is very clearly visualized, and residual thalamic structures may be seen as lumps of tissue along the base of the skull (Fig. 7.54). The posterior fossa structures remain relatively normal, and one also can determine with ultrasound whether the common carotid artery is smaller than normal, because it usually is underdeveloped with hydranencephaly (Fig. 7.54).

Colpocephaly

This is a descriptive term reflecting predominant dilation of the occipital horns of the lateral ventricles. This is seen in association with hydrocephalus, as is present in aqueductal stenosis and the Arnold-Chiari malformation, but is more properly called "colpocephaly" when it occurs alone. Its etiology is not known, but it is suspected that it represents "central" atrophy secondary to loss of surrounding white matter. The findings are readily demonstrable with any imaging modality (Fig. 7.55).

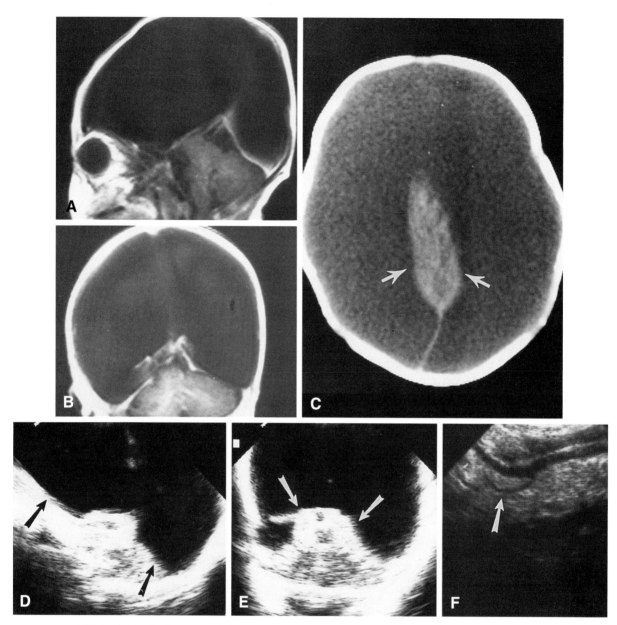

FIGURE 7.54. Hydranencephaly. A. MR study demonstrates a completely fluid-filled supratentorial compartment. Only the brainstem remains. **B.** Coronal view shows similar findings. **C.** CT study in another patient demonstrates a fluid-filled calvarium, and only the brainstem (arrows) is visible. **D.** Sagittal ultrasonogram demonstrates a totally fluid-filled supratentorial compartment. **E.** Coronal view demonstrates similar findings. Only the brainstem is seen. **F.** Carotid vessel ultrasonogram demonstrates a small internal cerebral artery (arrow).

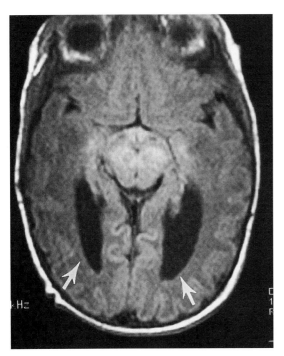

FIGURE 7.55. Colpocephaly. Note the preferential dilation of the occipital horns (arrows) of the lateral ventricles.

THE SMALL HEAD

A small head usually is the result of anencephaly and cerebral atrophy. These patients usually are mentally retarded to a marked degree. In all of these cases, lack of normal brain growth fails to provide a stimulus for the skull to expand.

As a consequence the sutures are narrower than normal and eventually close prematurely. Just when this occurs, and the rate at which it does, depends on when the insult is sustained. If it occurs in utero, the infant is born with a very small head and persistently narrow sutures (Fig. 7.56). Molding may be excessive and often never disappears (Fig. 7.57). **In such cases, the overlapped bones fuse and the ridge they produce often is misinterpreted for the one seen with primary synostosis.** Clinically, both feel about the same, but radiographically, they appear different.

Brain atrophy is readily demonstrable with any imaging modality and the findings consist of large ventricles, prominent sulci, and dilation of the various basal cisterns (Fig. 7.58). In cases of unilateral cerebral atrophy, the plain film findings consist of ipsilateral flattening of the calvarium and elevation of the ipsilateral petrous pyramid and sphenoid wing, and brain imaging delineates the underlying atrophy (Fig. 7.59). This findings are now exquisitely delineated with CT or MRI (Fig. 7.59). The phenomenon of unilateral atrophy often is referred to as the **Davidoff–Mason–van Dyke syndrome.**

CRANIOLACUNIA

Craniolacunia (lacunar skull, Lückenshadel) is almost exclusively associated with meningomyelocele, meningocele, and encephalocele. Occasionally, it can be seen in the absence of any of these or other neurologic abnormalities but this is rare. Lacunar skull disappears by 4–6 months of age, a phenomenon that occurs regardless of whether intracranial pressure is normal, increased, or decreased. This is most important to appreciate, because lacunar skull was

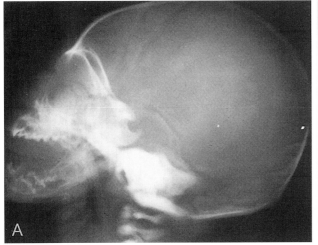
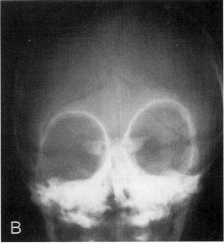

FIGURE 7.56. Microcephaly. A. Note the small, round calvarium; relatively narrow sutures; and persistent overlapping of the bones in this infant almost 1 week old. The calvarium is definitely small when compared with the face. **B.** Frontal view shows extremely round orbits and hypotelorism. This is common with severe microcephaly.

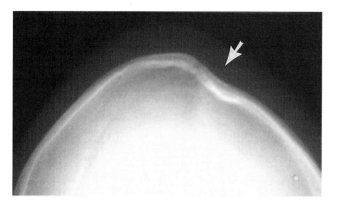

FIGURE 7.57. Persistent molding with closed sutures. Note the wavy configuration (arrow) of the calvarium along the sagittal suture resulting from persistent molding.

once considered a manifestation of increased intracranial pressure (hydrocephalus). Lacunar skull, in itself, is probably of little consequence to the infant. It is the associated meningomyeloceles and Arnold-Chiari malformations seen in these infants that are a problem. Because of this, hydrocephalus has always been associated with lacunar skull, but it does not result in lacunar skull.

The calvarial defects (lacunae) in lacunar skull probably represent areas of defective membranous bone formation, but the precise etiology is unknown. Thinning in the region of the lacunae can involve the inner table, diploë, or even the outer table. Most frequently, however, only the inner table and diploë are involved. The dura is thinned over the lacunae, but is of normal thickness over the intervening bony struts. Roentgenographically, lacunar skull has a very characteristic and absolutely diagnos-

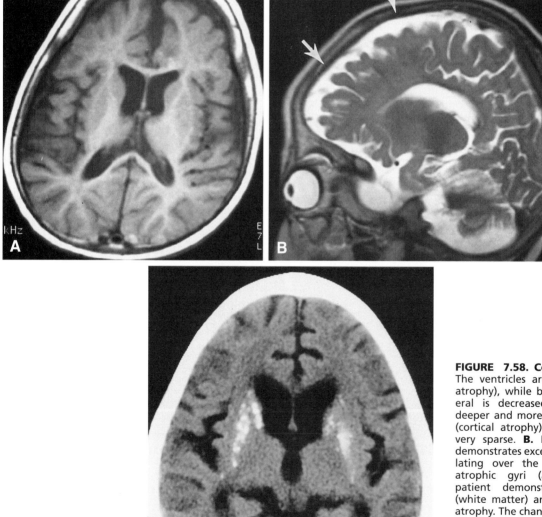

FIGURE 7.58. Cerebral atrophy. A. The ventricles are dilated (i.e., central atrophy), while brain substance in general is decreased, and the sulci are deeper and more prominent than usual (cortical atrophy). The white matter is very sparse. **B.** Parasagittal MR study demonstrates excessive CSF fluid accumulating over the prominent sulci and atrophic gyri (arrows). **C.** Another patient demonstrating both central (white matter) and peripheral (cortical) atrophy. The changes are similar to those seen in **A** and **B**. Note the calcification of the basal ganglia. All of these changes resulted from severe hypoxia.

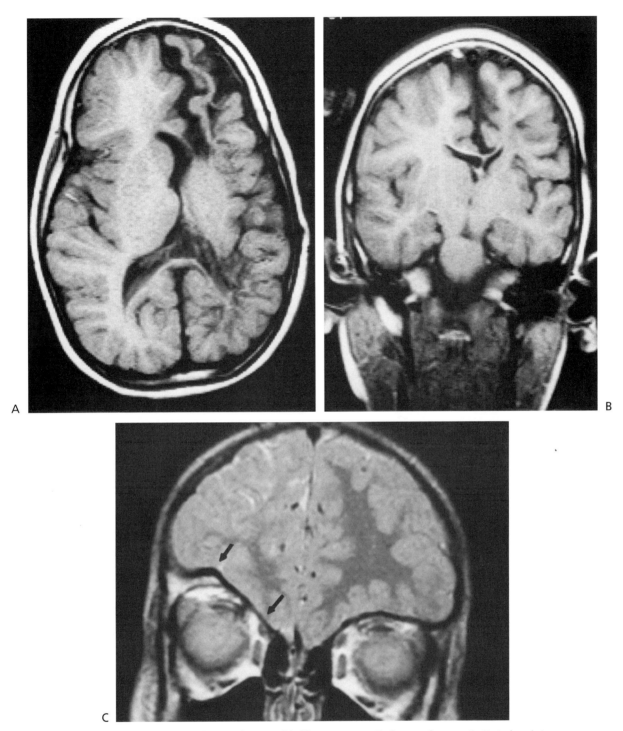

FIGURE 7.59. Unilateral atrophy: Davidoff Mason-van Dyke syndrome. A. Note hemiatrophy of the left cerebral hemisphere. The ipsilateral calvarium also is small, and there is some midline shift toward the atrophic left side. **B.** Similar findings on the coronal view. **C.** Another patient with a small right brain. Also note smallness of the calvarium and elevation (arrows) of the anterior fossa floor.

tic appearance (Fig. 7.60A). The fenestrations or lacunae produce a very striking and roentgenographically aesthetic picture. Generally, the lacunae are most pronounced in, and in some cases limited to, the parietal bone. In other cases, the frontal and upper occipital bones are also involved, but the base of the skull and lower half of the occipital bone (enchondral portions of the skull) do not show these abnormal inner table defects. The abnormality is one of faulty membranous bone formation. It is important to differentiate lacunar skull from

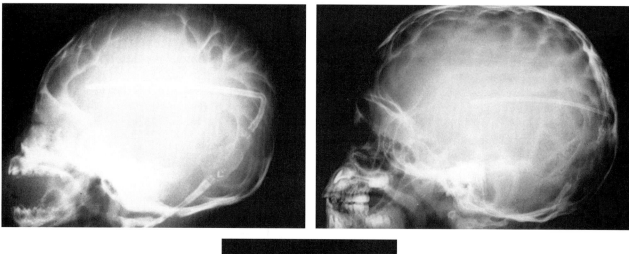

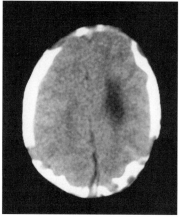

FIGURE 7.60. Lacunar skull. A. Lateral view showing typical lacunae. These calvarial defects are not the result of increased intracranial pressure but rather the result of inner table bony defects. A shunt tube is in place. **B.** Years after premature closure of the sutures secondary to successful shunting, shunt failure results in chronically increased intracranial pressure with typical findings of so-called "silver beaten skull." Compare the convolutions at this time with those seen with lacunar skull in **A. C.** Lacunar skull. CT study demonstrates the characteristic scalloped irregularity of the calvarial bones seen with lacunar skull.

"silver beaten" or "copper beaten" skull. The latter results when chronically increased intracranial pressure is present and, although appearing somewhat similar, on closer inspection will be determined to appear different from lacunar skull (Fig. 7.60B). A frontal cranium bifidum defect along the upper metopic suture is also frequently present with lacunar skull. Soft tissue bulging through the defect is palpable and readily visualized roentgenographically. The frontal bone is defective, but it is probably not a true encephalocele, because as the infant grows older, the defect fills in and the soft tissue bulge disappears.

ENCEPHALOCELE AND CRANIUM BIFIDUM

Encephaloceles of the skull are the counterpart of meningoceles or myelomeningoceles of the spine. They are most commonly located in the midline, and by far, most arise in the occipital region. Next most common are those in the

nasofrontal area. Occipital encephaloceles usually are more serious, because they frequently contain portions of the occipital lobes and cerebellum. Frontal encephaloceles are more of a cosmetic problem; even if brain tissue is present in the outpouching, it is that of the frontal lobes, and its removal does not produce as much neurologic defect.

Although midline occipital and frontal encephaloceles are most common, one can occasionally encounter lateral encephaloceles, anterior fontanelle encephaloceles, or even ones in the base of the skull. The latter lesions extend inferiorly (1, 2) and often present as masses in the nasopharynx or neck. In rare instances, one may encounter orbital encephaloceles; in such cases, the sphenoid bone is defective and brain tissue protrudes into the orbit. Such patients can present with pulsating exophthalmos and often have neurofibromatosis as their basic underlying problem.

Encephaloceles usually are readily apparent clinically and radiographically. The bulging soft tissue and underlying calvarial defect are characteristic (Figs. 7.61 and 7.62).

MRI is best for demonstrating brain in the encephalocele (Fig. 7.61C). In the frontal region, it is of some importance to determine whether the encephalocele is nasofrontal or nasoethmoidal, because the information facilitates proper neurosurgical correction. The nasofrontal encephalocele occurs above the nasal bone, while the nasoethmoidal encephalocele occurs below the nasal bone. Consequently, in the latter the nasal bones are elevated, while in the former they are depressed. The crib-riform plate also is depressed in nasofrontal encephaloceles, and a large V-shaped defect is present in the frontal bone (Fig. 7.61). This causes a slanting lateral displacement or bowing of the superior aspect of the medial orbital walls, but no true hypertelorism. With nasoethmoidal encephaloceles, a circular defect is present between the orbits and below the nasal bone, and definite hypertelorism is present. With basal encephaloceles, a mass may be seen in the nasopharynx (Fig. 7.62B), and any imaging

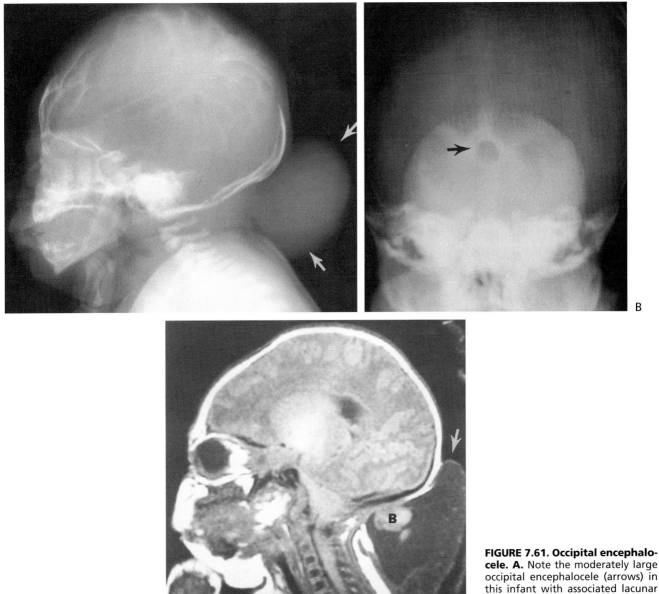

FIGURE 7.61. Occipital encephalocele. A. Note the moderately large occipital encephalocele (arrows) in this infant with associated lacunar skull and microcephaly. **B.** Town's projection shows the bony defect (arrow). **C.** MR scan in another patient, demonstrates a large encephalocele (arrows) extending through a large occipital defect. Brain tissue (B) is contained within the encephalocele.

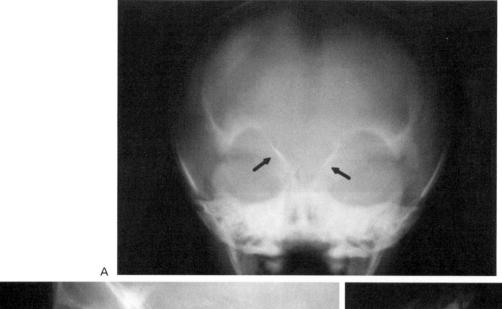

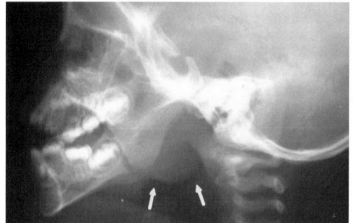

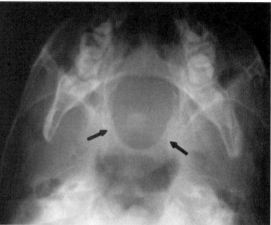

FIGURE 7.62. Other encephaloceles. A. Frontonasal encephalocele. Note the V-shaped frontal bone defect (arrows), above the nasal bone area. **B. Basal encephalocele.** Note the nasopharyngeal mass (arrows). **C.** Basal view demonstrates the defect in the base of the skull (arrows).

modality can vividly demonstrate this form of encephalocele.

REFERENCES

1. Larsen CE, Hudgins PA, Hunter SB. Skull-base meningoencephalocele presenting as a unilateral neck mass in a neonate. AJNR 1995;16:1161–1163.
2. Yokota A, Matsukado Y, Fuwa I, et al. Anterior basal encephalocele of the neonatal and infantile period. Neurosurgery 1986;19: 468–478.

CONGENITAL DERMAL SINUS

In congenital dermal sinus there is a persistent midline sinus connection from the surface of the skin to the brain or meninges. Most commonly these sinuses occur in the occiput, but frontal and lateral sinus tracts can also be encountered. A mass or dimpling of the skin over the sinus

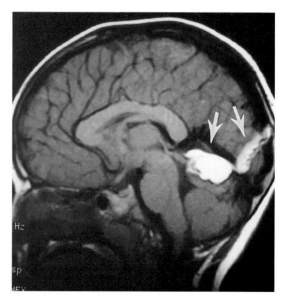

FIGURE 7.63. Congenital dermal sinus. Note the fatty tissue (arrows) in this congenital dermal sinus extending to the occiput.

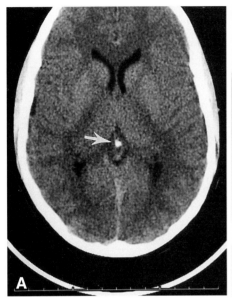 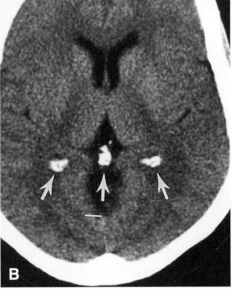

FIGURE 7.64. Physiologic calcifications. A. Note the calcification of the pineal gland (arrow) in this 15-year-old boy. **B.** Calcifications in the pineal gland (central arrow) and the choroid plexuses (outer arrows) of the lateral ventricles.

is usually present, and the tract itself may extend just under the inner table or deep into the meninges or brain. Because of such intracranial extension, congenital dermal sinus tracts provide a ready route for infection and predispose to meningitis or intracranial abscess. A small dermoid cyst is often associated and can be located just below the skin, in the diploic space , or intracranially. Intracranial cystic dermoids can present with symptoms of an intracranial tumor. Lipomatous tissue is not an uncommon component of these cysts. The intracranial and extracranial components of this lesion are perhaps best demonstrated with MRI or CT imaging (Fig. 7.63).

INTRACRANIAL CALCIFICATIONS

Physiologic calcifications such as those seen in the pineal gland (Fig. 7.64, A and B), choroid plexus of the lateral ventricles (Fig. 7.64B), habenular commissure, petroclinoid ligaments, and falx are not seen in the newborn infant. For that matter, they are uncommon below the age of 6 years. Consequently, if one sees intracranial calcification in infants and young children, some pathologic basis for the development probably exists. An exception is seen with the so-called pituitary stone, a rare calcification occasionally encountered in otherwise healthy patients (Fig. 7.65).

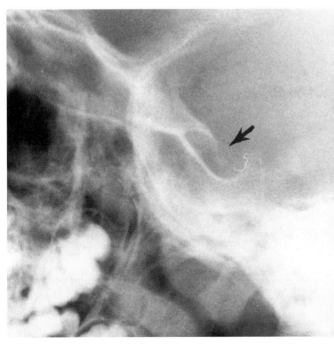 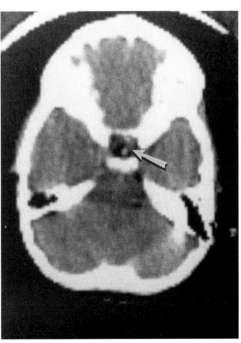

FIGURE 7.65. Pituitary stone. A. Note the calcification in the middle of the pituitary fossa (arrow). **B.** CT scan demonstrates the same calcification (arrow).

Pathologic calcifications are much more common and can be seen in association with vascular disease, brain infarcts, tumors, metabolic conditions, infections, and the neurophakomatoses. All of these conditions are discussed at later points but generally, pathologic calcifications tend to be irregular, clumpy, linear, or curvilinear. All of them are more exquisitely defined with CT than with plain films. Irregular calcifications usually are seen with old infarcts, old inflammatory processes, and tumors. Large,

clumpy calcifications tend to be seen with old infarcts and some tumors, while curvilinear calcifications are seen within vessel walls, cyst walls, and cystic tumors. Linear calcifications are seen along the tentorium and falx and can be seen with certain metabolic diseases, hypervitaminosis D, the basal cell nevus syndrome, and occasionally after meningitis. Similar calcifications can occur over the convexities of the brain and result from calcified subdural hematomas.

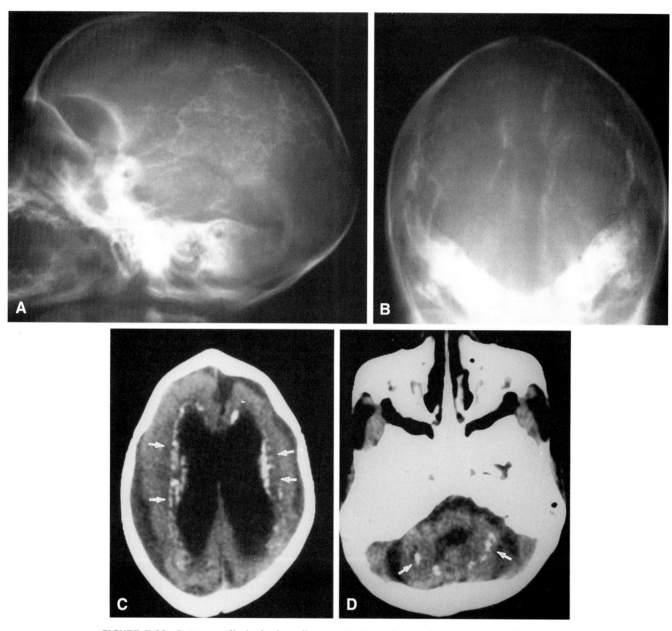

FIGURE 7.66. Cytomegalic inclusion disease. A. Lateral view shows extreme microcephaly and typical irregular periventricular calcifications. **B.** Town's projection in the same infant more clearly demonstrates the periventricular distribution of the calcifications. The ventricles are dilated, but the brain and calvarium are small (brain atrophy). **C.** CT study in another patient demonstrates classic periventricular calcifications (arrows). The head is small, the brain atrophic, and the ventricles dilated. **D.** Same patient, demonstrating punctate calcifications in the cerebellum (arrows).

Serpentine calcifications are characteristic of Sturge-Weber disease, but similar calcifications can occur after intrathecal methotrexate therapy for leukemia and with folic acid deficiency. Finally, basal ganglia calcifications also are common and usually are the result of infarction, hypoxia, or vasculopathy of the basal ganglia. For the most part, they tend to be irregular and frequently are bilateral. They also can be seen with metabolic problems such as hypoparathyroidism and pseudohyperparathyroidism.

Perinatal Central Nervous System Infection: TORCH Syndromes

Conditions generally included in the TORCH infections include cytomegalic inclusion disease (cytomegalovirus (CMV)), herpes, rubella, and toxoplasmosis. In the past, considerable effort was directed at separating these condi-

tions on the basis of the appearance of their intracranial calcifications, even though overall there was some lack of specificity. This latter point has become even more evident when CT arrived on the scene, where more calcifications are seen in more places. Nonetheless, with cytomegalic inclusion disease (cytomegalic virus disease) one still can depend on the fact that a small skull with a small atrophic brain showing dilated ventricles with periventricular calcifications is most suggestive of this infection (Fig. 7.66). Less commonly, similar calcifications have been noted with rubella (1). Acute changes often are best demonstrated with MR, and in this regard in the postnatal period periventricular edema leading to a pseudomass has been documented (3). Calcifications in the basal ganglia also occur and both these and the periventricular calcifications can be identified with ultrasound (Fig. 7.67). They are, however, more clearly seen with CT.

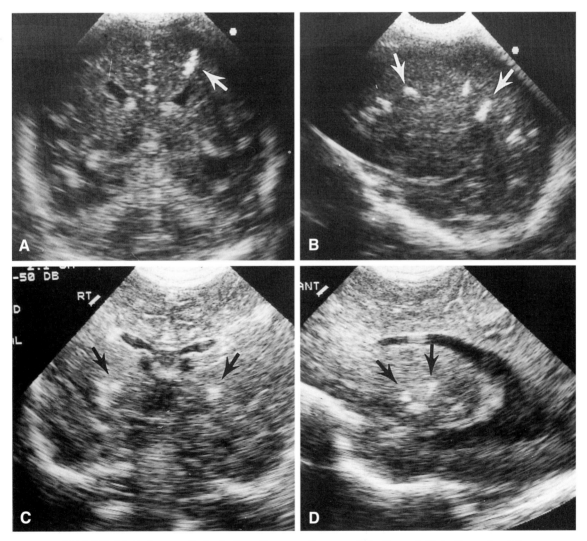

FIGURE 7.67. Cytomegalic inclusion disease: ultrasound findings. A. Note the periventricular calcification (arrow). **B.** Parasagittal scan demonstrates numerous punctate periventricular calcifications (arrows). **C.** Bilateral calcifications (arrows) in the basal ganglia. **D.** Lateral view demonstrates calcifications (arrows) in the basal ganglia.

Calcifications resulting from herpes simplex type II intrauterine infections are less common than those seen with cytomegalic inclusion viral infection. However, the infection is serious and usually involves the whole brain (4) with massive necrosis and subsequent atrophy (Fig. 7.68). The final result may be massive calcification of the brain (Fig. 7.68). Toxoplasmosis, a protozoal infection caused by the organism **Toxoplasma gondii** often has more insidious onset than the other intrauterine infections. Complicating hydrocephalus frequently is present, and therefore these patients may present with a large, rather than a small calvarium. Calcifications are nonspecific and can occur almost anywhere in the brain or meninges (Fig. 7.69). These calcifications have been showed to regress with therapy (5).

Other manifestations of all these intrauterine infections include white matter degeneration (2, 6), subependymal or paraventricular degenerative cysts, and a peculiar lenticulostriate vasculopathy of the basal ganglia (7–9). Although the latter is a nonspecific finding (see next section), it is perhaps most commonly seen with intrauterine infections. Color flow Doppler has documented increased flow in these vessels (7), basically substantiating that a vasculopathy is present (Fig. 7.70).

Although the central nervous system manifestations of these infections often take the spotlight, these infections are generalized infections with rashes and hemorrhages, hepatosplenomegaly, chorioretinitis, and in some cases, pneumonitis. It should be recalled that both rubella and

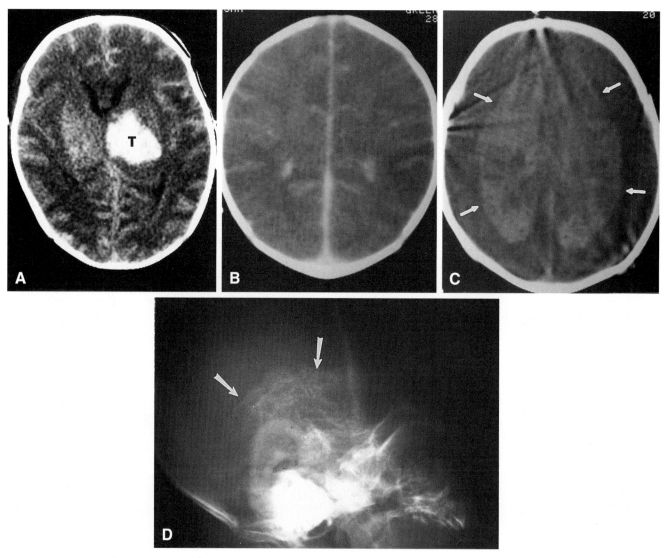

FIGURE 7.68. A. Herpes simplex encephalitis. Note the marked edema of the entire brain and a large thalamic (T) bleed. **B.** Another patient with extensive edema of the brain resulting from widespread necrosis. **C.** One month later, the brain has become markedly atrophic (arrows). **D.** Massive calcification in an atrophic brain (arrows) after herpes simplex encephalitis.

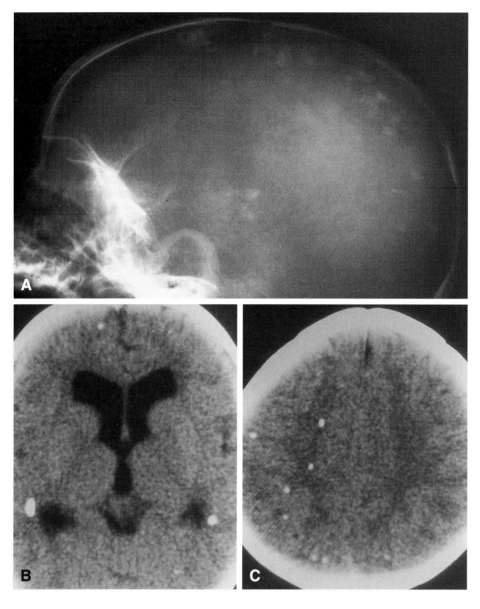

FIGURE 7.69. Toxoplasmosis. A. Note the flaky calcifications over the convexities and central calcifications in the basal ganglia. **B and C.** Another patient demonstrating moderate hydrocephalus and numerous calcifications scattered throughout the brain. (**B** and **C** courtesy of Bill Anderson, M.D.)

cytomegalic inclusion disease produce characteristic metaphyseal long bone changes consisting of irregularity of the metaphysis and the so-called celery stalk appearance.

REFERENCES

1. Parisot S, Droulle P, Feldmann M, et al. Unusual encephaloclastic lesions with paraventricular calcification in congenital rubella. Pediatr Radiol 1991;21:229–230.
2. Sugita K, Ando M, Makino M, et al. Magnetic resonance imaging of the brain in congenital rubella virus and cytomegalovirus infections. Neuroradiology 1991;33:239–242.
3. Alonso A, Alvarez A, Seara MJ, et al. Unusual manifestations of postnatally acquired cytomegalovirus infection: findings on CT and MR. Pediatr Radiol 1996;26:772–774.
4. O'Reilly MAR, O'Reilly PMR, de Bruyn R. Neonatal herpes simplex type 2 encephalitis: its appearances on ultrasound and CT. Pediatr Radiol 1995;25:68–69.
5. Patel DV, Holfels EM, Vogel NP, et al. Resolution of intracranial calcifications in infants with treated congenital toxoplasmosis. Radiology 1996;199:433–440.
6. Barkovich AJ, Lindan CE. Congenital cytomegalovirus infection of the brain: imaging analysis and embryologic considerations. AJNR 1994;15:703–715.
7. Ben-Ami T, Yousefzadeh D, Backus M, et al. Lenticulostriate vasculopathy in infants with infections of the central nervous system sonographic and Doppler findings. Pediatr Radiol 1990;20:575–579.

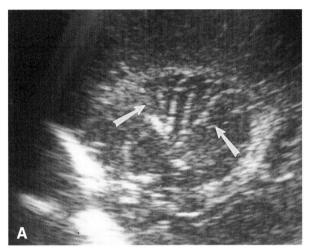

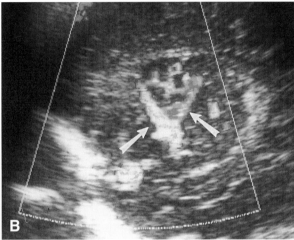

FIGURE 7.70. Basal ganglia vasculitis. A. Note the prominent striations (arrows) in the basal ganglia. **B.** Color flow Doppler demonstrates hypervascularity along the striations (arrows). These findings represent those of lenticulostriate vasculopathy of the basal ganglia.

8. Estroff JA, Parad RB, Teele RL, et al. Echogenic vessels in the fetal thalami and basal ganglia associated with cytomegalovirus infection. J Ultrasound Med 1992;11:686–688.
9. Ogino MT, Hahn JS, Skew SB, et al. Linear echodensities in the basal ganglia in newborn infants: an indicator of congenital infection and/or in utero drug exposure. J Ultrasound Med 1991;10(Suppl):S20.

Basal Ganglia Vasculopathy

Basal ganglia vasculopathy is a common finding with the intrauterine TORCH infections. However, it also can be seen as an incidental finding, with trisomies such as trisomy 13 and the storage diseases (1–4), and it has been seen with twin-to-twin transfusion (5). The findings are readily detectable with ultrasound and enhanced with color flow Doppler imaging (Fig. 7.70). Almost surely some of these patients eventually develop calcifications of the basal gan-

glia. Similar changes have been demonstrated with human immunodeficiency virus (HIV) infection (see next section).

REFERENCES

1. Hughes P, Weinberger E, Shaw DWW. Linear areas of echogenicity in the thalami and basal ganglia of neonates: an expanded association. Work in progress. Radiology 1991;179:103–105.
2. Kriss VM, Kriss TC. Doppler sonographic confirmation of thalamic and basal ganglia vasculopathy in three infants with trisomy 13. J Ultrasound Med 1996;15:523–526.
3. Ries M, Deeg K-H, Wolfel D, et al. Colour Doppler imaging of intracranial vasculopathy in severe infantile sialidosis. Pediatr Radiol 1992;22:179–181.
4. Weber K, Riebel Th, Nasir R. Hyperechoic lesions in the basal ganglia: an incidental sonographic finding in neonates and infants. Pediatr Radiol 1992;22:182–186.
5. de Vries LS, Beek FJ, Stoutenbeek P. Lenticulostriate vasculopathy in twin-to-twin transfusion syndrome: sonographic and CT findings. Pediatr Radiol 1995;25:S41–S42.

HIV Infection and Acquired Immunodeficiency Syndrome (AIDS)

HIV infection produces a progressive encephalopathy with progressive white matter degeneration (1). Vasculopathy of the basal ganglia, similar to that seen with intrauterine infections, has been documented (2) and can lead to calcification of the basal ganglia (2). Cerebral artery aneurysms also have been documented (3) and primary lymphoma is not uncommon (4, 5). There is nothing particularly specific about any of these manifestations.

REFERENCES

1. Lobato MN, Caldwell B, Ng P, et al. Pediatric spectrum of disease clinical consortium: encephalopathy in children with perinatally acquired human immunodeficiency virus infection. J Pediatr 1995;126:710–715.
2. Bode H, Rudin C. Calcifying arteriopathy in the basal ganglia in human immunodeficiency virus infection. Pediatr Radiol 1995; 25:72–73.
3. Husson RN, Saini R, Lewis LL, et al. Cerebral artery aneurysms in children infected with human immunodeficiency virus. J Pediatr 1992;121;927–930.
4. Bouek P, Bertrand Y, Tran Minh VA, et al. Case report: primary lymphoma of the CNS in an infant with AIDS: imaging findings. AJR 1991;156:1037–1038.
5. Cordoliani Y-S, Derosier C, Pharaboz C, et al. Primary cerebral lymphoma in patients with AIDS: MR findings in 17 cases. AJR 1992;159:841–847.

Neurophakomatoses

Conditions generally included in this group of diseases are tuberous sclerosis, neurofibromatosis, von Hippel-Lindau disease, and Sturge-Weber disease. All of these conditions are characterized by dysplasia or neoplasia of organs derived from the embryonic ectoderm (i.e., skin, central and peripheral nervous system, and eyes). In some cases, structures derived from the mesoderm and endoderm also are involved. These conditions now are generally most expediently imaged with CT or MR, but CT is preferred when one is searching for the commonly occurring calcifications.

In the newborn infant, the diagnosis of **tuberous sclerosis** usually depends on the recognition of characteristic cutaneous lesions consisting of a yellowish white maculopapular rash (1, 2) and the presence of cardiac tumors such as rhabdomyomas (1, 2). These patients can present with cysts and hamartomas of the kidney and later in life with angiomyolipomas of the kidney and the characteristic adenoma sebaceum (angiofibroma of the face). However, it is the intracranial tubers that are the focal imaging findings in the diagnosis of tuberous sclerosis.

The tubers consist of dysplastic tissue, composed mainly of abnormal, giant astrocytes. They can be found in the ventricles (subependymal) or in the peripheral cortex and even in the subcortical white matter (2). When calcified, they are readily demonstrable with CT (Fig. 7.71) and even can be seen on plain films. Noncalcified tubers also can be seen with CT but are more vividly demonstrable with MR, especially if they are limited to the cortical regions (Fig. 7.71). Some of these tubers can undergo transformation to gliomas, and it has been suggested that, if tubers enhance with gadolinium on MRI, they should be considered premalignant (3, 4). When tumors develop, they have an appearance similar to that seen with patients without underlying tuberous sclerosis (Fig. 7.72). Patients with tuberous sclerosis also may demonstrate other central nervous system abnormalities such as heterotropic gray matter, white matter cystic lesions (6), gliosis, and neuronal migrational abnormalities such as pachygyria (7) and schizencephaly. An interesting association with aortic aneurysm also has been documented (8–10), but overall, the cause of the condition remains unknown.

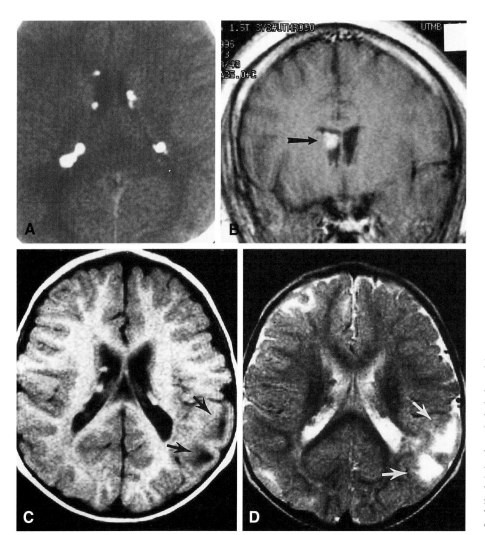

FIGURE 7.71. Tuberous sclerosis. A. Typical subependymal calcified tumors seen on CT. **B.** Enhancing tuber (arrow) after gadolinium administration. Such enhancement generally is taken as a sign of early or potential transformation to a glial tumor. **C.** T1-weighted MR study demonstrates the presence of numerous subependymal tubers projecting into the ventricles. Also note the hypodense areas in the occipital region (arrows) consistent with cortical tubers. **D.** T2-weighted study demonstrates the subependymal tubers and high signal intensity in the cortical tubers (arrows).

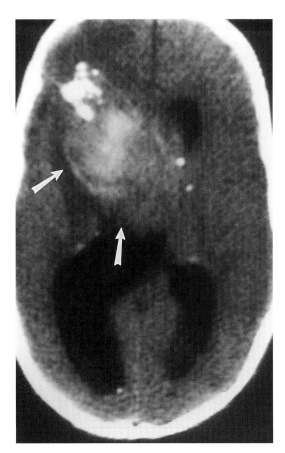

FIGURE 7.72. Tuberous sclerosis with complicating tumor. Note the large glioma (arrows) causing obstruction of the foramina of Monro and hydrocephalus. Also note numerous typical and atypical calcifications.

In **Sturge-Weber disease**, also known as encephalotrigeminal angiomatosis or meningofacial angiomatosis, a facial hemangioma leading to a port wine stain along with a similar lesion of the leptomeninges is characteristic. Meningeal angiomatosis consists of multiple small venous channels that are matted together on the surface of the brain. The angiomatosis is not visualized as such on any imaging study, but its sequelae, cortical calcification and brain atrophy, usually are readily identified both with CT and MR. The calcifications characteristically occur in the cerebral cortex underlying the angiomatosis and typically are gyriform or serpentine (Fig. 7.73). Although the gyriform-serpentine calcifications are characteristic of the condition, they generally are not seen in young infants, but in infancy, calvarial involvement can occur. The disease usually is unilateral, but bilateral

involvement can be seen and involvement of the cerebellum also has been noted (11). The Sturge-Weber syndrome also can be associated with large intracranial arteriovenous malformations (12).

The **von Hippel-Lindau syndrome** consists of angiomas of the cerebellum, with associated cystic change, and hemangiomas of the retina. Polycystic kidney disease and cysts in other organs also occur, and any of the hemangiomas can calcify.

REFERENCES

1. Allison JW, Stephenson CA, Angtuaco TL, et al. Radiological case of the month—tuberous sclerosis with myocardial and central nervous system involvement at birth. Am J Dis Child 1991; 145:470–471.
2. Christopher C, Bartholome J, Blum D, et al. Neonatal tuberous sclerosis: US, CT and MR diagnosis of brain and cardiac lesions. Pediatr Radiol 1998;19:446–448.
3. Martin N, Debussche C, DeBroucker T, et al. Gadolinium-DTPA enhanced MR imaging in tuberous sclerosis. Neuroradiology 1990;31:492–497.
4. Menor F, Marti-Bonmati L, Mulas F, et al. Neuroimaging in tuberous sclerosis: a clinicoradiological evaluation in pediatric patients. Pediatr Radiol 1992;22:485–489.
6. Van Tassel P, Cure JK, Holden KR. Cyst-like white matter lesions in tuberous sclerosis. AJNR 1997;18:1367–1373.
7. Sener RN. Tuberous sclerosis associated with pachygyria. CT findings. Pediatr Radiol 1993;23:489–490.
8. Baker PC, Furnival RA. Tuberous sclerosis presenting with bowel obstruction and an aortic aneurysm. Pediatr Emerg Care 2000; 16:255–257.
9. Jost CJ, Gloviczki P, Edwards WD. Aortic aneurysms in children and young adults with tuberous sclerosis: report of two cases and review of the literature. J Vasc Surg 2001;33:639–642.
10. Tsukui A, Noguchi R, Honda T, et al. Aortic aneurysm in a four-year-old child with tuberous sclerosis. Pediatr Anesth 1995;5: 67–70.
11. Decker T, Jones K, Barnes P. Sturge-Weber syndrome with posterior fossa involvement. AJNR 1994;15:389–392.
12. Laufer L, Cohen A. Sturge-Weber syndrome associated with a large left hemispheric arteriovenous malformation. Pediatr Radiol 1994;24:272–273.

HEAD TRAUMA

Neonatal Trauma

In the neonate, trauma to the calvarium and brain is almost always related to delivery. Bleeding in these infants can be subarachnoid, subdural, and occasionally intraventricular (1–4). However, not all newborn infants who demonstrate bleeding have a history of trauma during delivery, and

FIGURE 7.74. Skull fracture. A. Typical linear skull fracture with slight diastases (arrow). **B.** Occipital synchondrotic diastatic fracture (arrow).

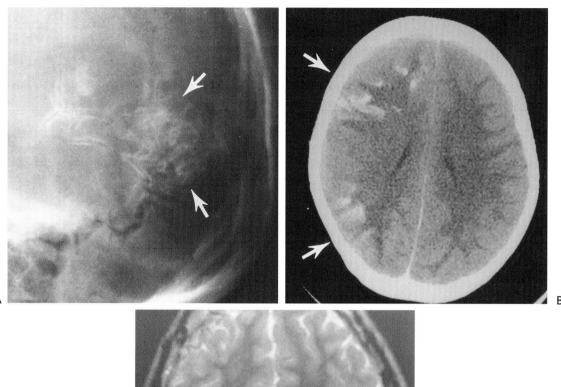

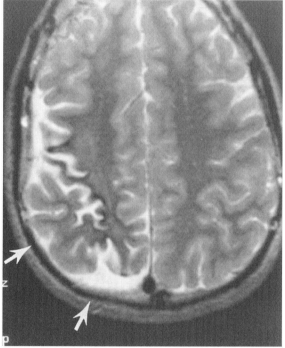

FIGURE 7.73. Sturge-Weber disease. A. Typical calcifications in an older child (arrows). B. CT in another patient demonstrates typical cortical calcification (arrows). C. T2-weighted MR study demonstrates atrophy over the right occipital lobe and increased subarachnoid fluid (arrows). On this T2-weighted image, fluid appears white, and the adjacent black serpentine lines represent the arachnoid calcifications.

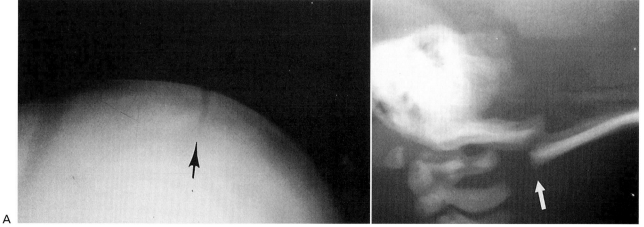

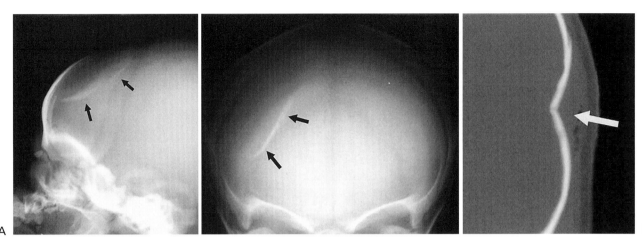

FIGURE 7.75. Depressed fracture. A. Lateral view demonstrates the depressed fracture (arrow). **B.** Frontal view demonstrates the same depressed fracture (arrows). **C.** CT in another patient shows a depressed fracture (arrow).

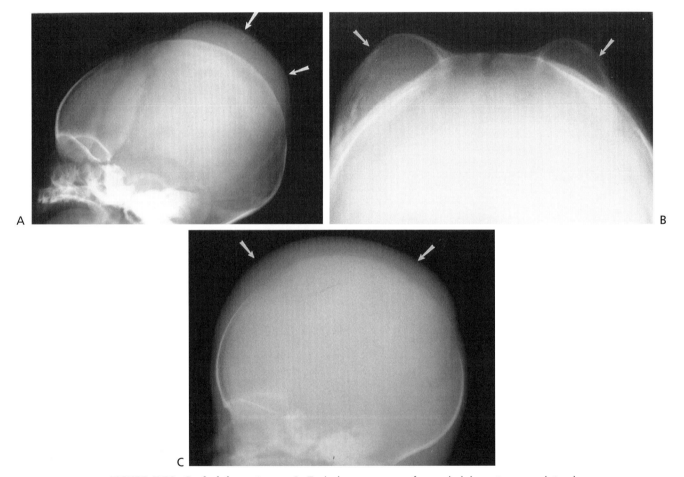

FIGURE 7.76. Cephalohematoma. A. Typical appearance of a cephalohematoma on lateral view (arrows). **B.** Healing phase demonstrates peripheral calcification of bilateral cephalohematomas (arrows) and slight inward depression of the underlying bone. **C.** Caput succedaneum. Note the extensive swelling of the scalp (arrows) that crosses multiple sutures.

upwards of 14% of asymptomatic newborn infants have been estimated to have grossly bloody, or at least xanthochromic, fluid. This would suggest that these infants have hemorrhages that are clinically occult. Although most hemorrhages in the neonate are supratentorial, posterior fossa hemorrhages also can occur. Hemorrhages near midline can be detected with ultrasound, but CT is the best imaging modality with which to demonstrate bleeds in general. MRI can be used later to detect injuries that might not have been apparent on initial CT examination.

Skull fractures in the neonate can be linear, buckle, or depressed (Figs. 7.74 and 7.75). Depressions can occur anywhere without actual fracturing and usually result from chronic pressure by one of the infant's extremities. Depressed fractures, as in any age group, may require elevation, and although seen on plain films, are best seen on CT studies (Fig. 7.75C). One also may encounter occipital osteodiastatic fractures (5).

REFERENCES

1. Castillo M, Smith JK. Imaging features of acute head and spine injuries secondary to difficult deliveries. Emerg Radiol 1995;2:7–12.
2. Hanigan WC, Morgan AM, Stahlberg LK. Tentorial hemorrhage associated with vacuum extraction. Pediatrics 1990;85:534–539.
3. Lam A, Cruz GB, Johnson I. Extradural hematoma in neonates. J Ultrasound Med 1991;10:205–209, Apr.
4. Roland EH, Flodmark O, Hill A. Thalamic hemorrhage with intraventricular hemorrhage in the full-term neonate. Pediatrics 1990;85:737–742.
5. Currarino G. Occipital osteodiastasis: presentation of four cases and review of the literature. Pediatr Radiol 2000;30:823–829.

Cephalohematoma

Cephalohematoma is a very common manifestation of calvarial injury in the newborn infant. It is always secondary to birth trauma and typically presents as a soft fluctuant mass or swelling of the scalp. It most commonly occurs over the middle and posterior parietal regions and can be bilateral (Fig. 7.76). The next most common site is over the occiput (Fig. 7.77). Cephalohematoma must be differentiated from caput succedaneum, the rare epicranial hydroma (leak of cerebrospinal fluid through a fracture into the subcutaneous space), and the more serious massive subgaleal or subaponeurotic bleed. Bleeding, in these latter cases, may be secondary to birth trauma or part of a bleeding disorder such as hemophilia or hemorrhagic disease of the newborn. It is potentially lethal, because exsanguination can occur. Radiographically, **subgaleal bleeding and caput succedaneum** produce uniform thickening of the scalp that crosses the calvarial sutures (Fig. 7.76B). In cephalohematoma, bleeding is subperiosteal, and the accumulation of blood is limited to the suture edges by the firm attachment of the periosteum (7.76A). Ultrasound, CT, and MR scanning all

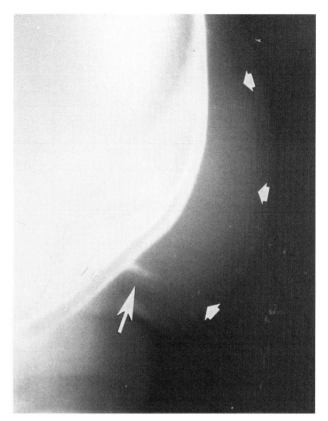

FIGURE 7.77. Occipital cephalohematoma. Note the characteristic soft tissue bulge (short arrows) and early peripheral calcification (long arrow).

can identify cephalohematomas (Fig. 7.78), but these studies seldom are required, because plain films are much simpler to obtain and just as informative. Underlying fracture in cephalohematoma generally is uncommon and probably is most common when forceps deliveries are involved.

In a few cases, bleeding also occurs intracranially, and small extradural collections of blood may be present. These are often referred to as internal cephalohematomas.

Healing of cephalohematomas consists of progressive resorption and decrease in size of the hematoma. In most cases, peripheral curvilinear calcification develops within 10–14 days (Fig. 7.77). Eventually, the calcification outlines the entire hematoma, and the finding is readily demonstrable with both plain films and CT scanning. As the calcification becomes thicker, a pseudocystic lesion of the calvarium can be encountered.

Postnatal Head Trauma in Infants and Children

Head trauma in older infants and children usually is accidental, but it also frequently is seen in the battered child syndrome. The latter is more common under 2 years of age. Nonetheless, the manifestations of head trauma are about the same no matter how the injury is sustained. Skull frac-

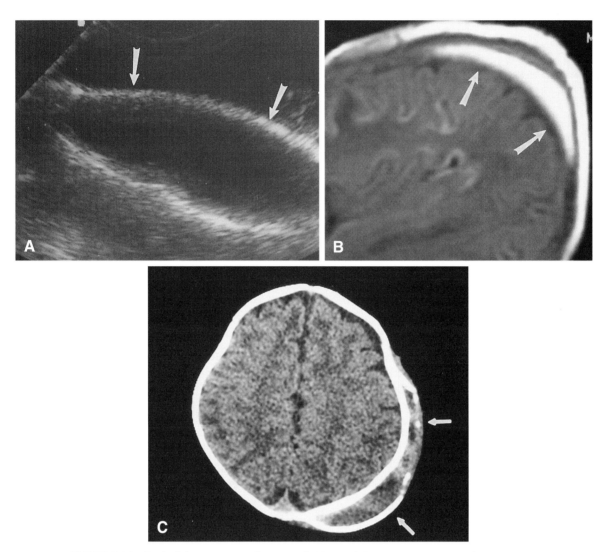

FIGURE 7.78. Cephalohematoma: ultrasound, MR, and CT appearances. A. Ultrasonogram demonstrates a typical elliptical, hypoechoic, fluid-filled structure (arrows). In other cases, echogenic debris may be present. **B.** T1-weighted MR image demonstrates a high-signal cephalohematoma (arrows) over the occiput. **C.** CT study demonstrates a calcifying cephalohematoma (arrows).

tures are common and assume a variety of configurations, but generally, skull films are no longer obtained for head trauma. However, there still is a role for plain film radiography when depressed fractures or the battered child syndrome are suspected. The reason for this is that some fractures, primarily those that are horizontal in the parietal bone often are not seen on axial CT studies.

In terms of facial injuries, the Waters' view still is useful, but CT is much more rewarding in terms of evaluating facial and orbital fractures (Fig. 7.79). A detailed dissertation of facial fractures and calvarial fractures is beyond the scope of this book, but **suffice it to say that it is the intracranial injury that is much more important than the calvarial fracture and this is best assessed with CT and MR.**

In terms of intracranial injury, one can encounter epidural hematomas (arterial bleeds), subdural hematomas (venous bleed), intraparenchymal hematoma-contusion, intraventricular bleeding, and subarachnoid bleeding. Almost invariably one's first line of imaging, when one suspects these injuries, is CT. MRI is not effective at detecting very early bleeds (i.e., less than 24 hours old), and ultrasonography is used only in the neonate. In the average case, one should proceed directly to CT.

Acute arterial bleeding results in epidural hematomas, while subdural hematomas are caused by tearing of dural vessels. Subdural bleeds tend to parallel the calvarium, while epidural bleeds tend to be elliptical (Fig. 7.80). On CT studies, subdural hematomas can appear isodense in the

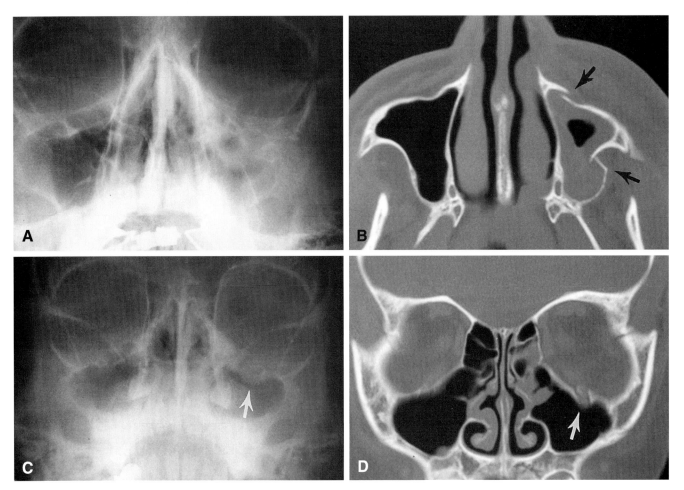

FIGURE 7.79. Facial fractures. A. On this Waters' view, the left maxillary sinus area is indistinct, but overall bony detail is obscured. **B.** Axial CT clearly demonstrates a comminuted fracture of the maxillary sinus (arrows). Blood also is present in the maxillary sinus. **C.** Another patient with blunt trauma to the left orbit demonstrating a slight soft tissue bulge (arrow) in the roof of the left maxillary sinus. **D.** CT more clearly demonstrates the bulge resulting from a blowout fracture of the orbital floor (arrow).

middle of their healing phase. As such, they can be missed unless one looks for evidence of ventricular compression or midline shift. When subdural hematomas break down and become more fluid-like, they can be referred to as subdural hygromas. After the acute phase, subdural hematomas are readily demonstrable on MR, where they have increased signal intensity on T1-weighted, T2-weighted, and FLAIR images.

Subarachnoid bleeding, when it occurs along the falx and tentorium, is difficult to detect with certainty. The reason for this is that the falx normally appears white on nonenhanced CT scans. When subarachnoid blood is seen over the convexities, one can be more confident of the diagnosis (Fig. 7.81, A and B) Subarachnoid blood can accumulate in the basal cisterns. Intraparenchymal bleeds and

contusions are readily identified with CT and MR, as is intraventricular blood (Figs. 7.82 and 7.83). However, it should be remembered that MRI does not detect early bleeds and that the signal of blood differs on T1- and T2-weighted sequences, depending on the age of the bleed (1). It is important to appreciate these variations, which are summarized in Figure 7.84.

In terms of calvarial trauma, it should be remembered that contrecoup injuries are common. In these cases, while the point of impact may be on one side of the head, the parenchymal injury occurs on the other side as the brain is compressed against the calvarium (Fig. 7.85). Shearing injuries of the brain commonly occur with more severe head trauma. They often are difficult to detect on initial CT studies but, when seen, manifest as small, almost pinpoint

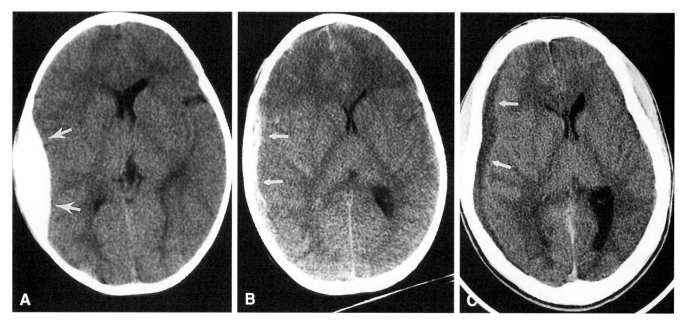

FIGURE 7.80. Epidural and subdural bleeding. A. Epidural hematoma producing an elliptical collection of fluid (arrows). **B.** Deceptively small subdural hematoma is layered along the right calvarium (arrows). Note that there is contralateral mediastinal shift and some compression of the ipsilateral ventricle. **C.** Older, hypodense subdural hematoma (arrows) producing shift of the midline structures to the left and compression of the ipsilateral ventricle.

areas of hemorrhage in the white matter and at the white-gray matter interfaces (Fig. 7.86). They are also common in the corpus callosum and brainstem. MRI 2 or 3 days after the injury usually detects these lesions with greater clarity (2) (Fig. 7.86B). This is especially true of FLAIR images (4). It is important that this type of injury be appreciated, because it is associated with considerable morbidity and is

considered a serious injury. The underlying mechanism of injury is the result of acceleration-deceleration and rotation, and with these forces at work, the white matter tracks can shear and separation can occur along the white-gray matter interfaces. Another important feature of brain injury is the development of cerebral edema. When such edema develops, the basal cisterns become obliterated and there is

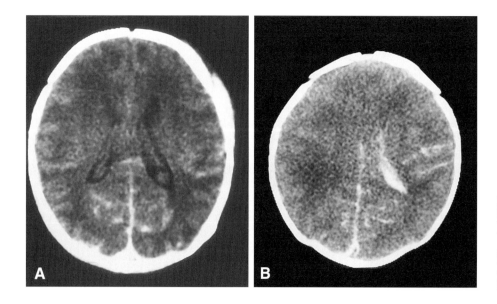

FIGURE 7.81. Subarachnoid bleeding. A. Note the bleeding along the falx and over the sulci of the brain. This infant had a traumatic delivery. **B.** Another patient with evidence of bleeding along the falx and over the various sulci. Some intraventricular blood also is present.

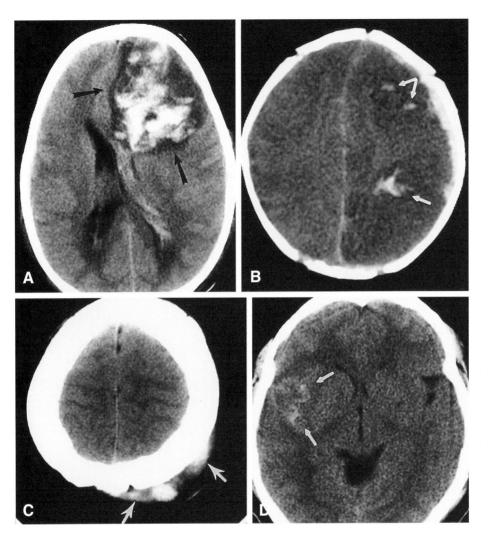

FIGURE 7.82. Parenchymal bleeding. A. Large intraparenchymal bleed (arrows). There is a mass effect with displacement of the midline structures and compression of the ipsilateral ventricle. **B.** Multiple focal parenchymal bleeds (arrows) in a patient with severe brain injury (i.e., battered child). **C. Contrecoup injury.** This patient sustained a blow over the left occipital region. Note the blood (arrows) in the scalp. **D.** However, a contrecoup contusion hemorrhage also has occurred in the right frontoparietal region (arrows).

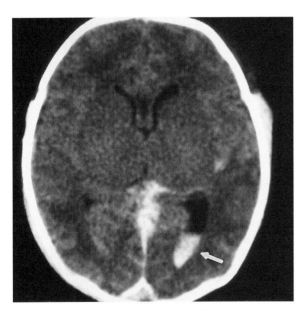

FIGURE 7.83. Intraventricular bleeding. Intraventricular blood (arrow) in an infant after traumatic delivery. Blood also is seen along the falx and over the sulci, consistent with associated subarachnoid hemorrhage.

downward herniation of the brainstem into the foramen magnum (Fig. 7.87). Death will ensue unless immediate decompression is accomplished.

A late manifestation of calvarial fractures, although not very common, is the so-called leptomeningeal cyst, or growing fracture. Most often, the initial fracture is linear and diastatic, and rather than healing, the fracture becomes progressively wider, because the meninges herniate through it. In such cases, there is an associated tear in the dura, which allows the arachnoid membrane to herniate into the fracture. This produces a pulsating mass that slowly increases in size and widens the fracture line. Clinically the mass is soft, fluctuant, and pulsatile and roentgenographically it appears as a scalloped, smooth-edged calvarial defect (Fig. 7.88). Herniation of cerebral tissue into such cysts also can occur, and CT or MRI are useful in its evaluation (4). Leptomeningeal cysts also have been described after vacuum extraction in newborns (5).

In the past, plain films were obtained for skull trauma but these have become more or less archaic except for depressed skull fractures and in the battered child syn-

Evolution of Parenchymal Hematomas as Seen at MR Imaging

				Intensity Compared to Brain	
Stage	**Age**	**Compartment**	**Hemoglobin**	**T1-weighted Image**	**T2-weighted Image**
Hyperacute	< 24 h	Intracellular	Oxyhemoglobin	Isointense	Slightly hyperintense
Acute	1-3 d	Intracellular	Deoxyhemoglobin	Slightly hypointense	Very hypointense
Subacute					
Early	> 3 d	Intracellular	Methemoglobin	Very hyperintense	Very hypointense
Late	> 7 d	Extracellular	Methemoglobin	Very hyperintense	Very hyperintense
Chronic	> 14 d	Extracellular	Hemichromes	Isointense	Slightly hyperintense
Center					
Rim		Intracellular	Hemosiderin	Slightly hypointense	Very hypointense

FIGURE 7.84. MR appearance of blood. The signal of blood on MR images depends both on whether they are T1- or T2-weighted and their age. A summary is provided in the illustration. (From Bradley WG Jr. MR appearance of hemorrhage in the brain. Radiology 1993;189:15–26, with permission.)

drome. Examination of the brain, after trauma, largely has been supplanted with CT and to some extent MR. However many CT studies are obtained because of medical legal issues and not because of clinical problems (6). The role of CT is being examined more closely, and in one communication, it was determined that, with head trauma and normal neurologic examination results in the emergency room setting, intracranial injury occurs in less than 5% of cases (7). At the same time, it has been suggested that "children with head injuries who are otherwise stable can be safely discharged from the ER if they have a normal CT scan" (8). Undoubtedly, there will be

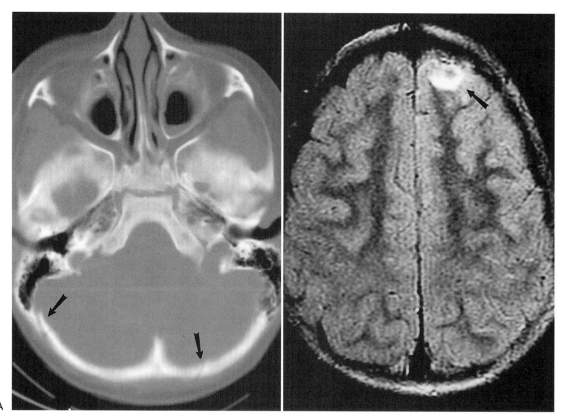

FIGURE 7.85. Contra coup injury. A. Note the bilateral occipital fractures (arrows). **B.** A contusion (arrow), however is located in the anterior portion of the left frontal lobe.

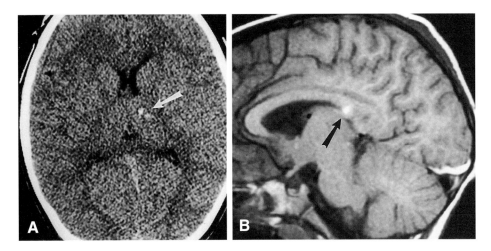

FIGURE 7.86. Shearing injuries. A. Note the punctate hemorrhages (arrow) in the thalamus. **B.** Focal bleed in the corpus callosum (arrow). Also note blood over the occipital lobe.

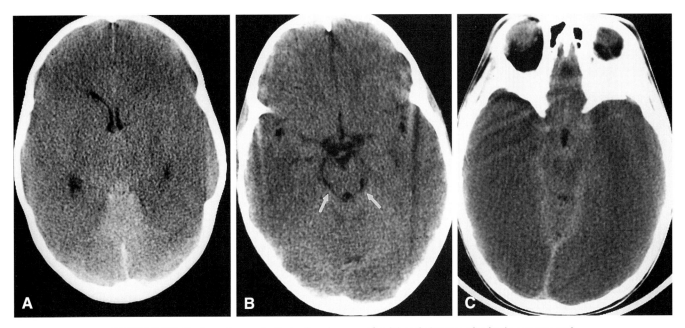

FIGURE 7.87. Brain edema. A. Note the absence of sulci and cisterns. The brain appears uniformly gray and the ventricles are slit-like. The posterior fossa contents, however, are white, constituting the so-called "bright" posterior fossa sign. **B.** Another patient with early edema, causing the sylvian fissures and ventricles to be small. The ambient cistern (arrows) is still visible but appears a little small. **C.** Three days later, profound edema has caused the brain to become darker gray and the ambient cistern to virtually become obliterated.

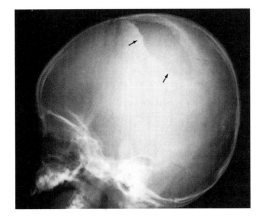

FIGURE 7.88. Leptomeningeal cyst. Typical configuration of a leptomeningeal cyst consisting of a scalloped radiolucent defect (arrows). The edges are usually smooth and moderately sclerotic.

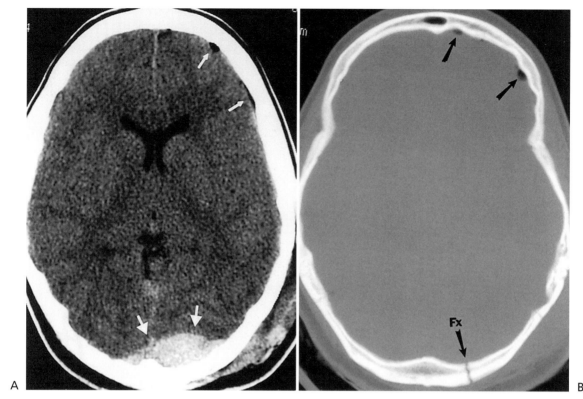

FIGURE 7.89. Skull fracture with pneumocephalus. A. CT study demonstrates an occipital epidural hematoma (lower arrows). Also note air under the calvarium on the left (upper arrows). **B.** CT study with bone windows demonstrates one of the fractures (FX) and air bubbles (arrows) under the left frontal bone.

continued examination of the exact role that CT is to play in head trauma.

Pneumocephalus is a significant finding when seen in association with head trauma. It generally indicates that an air containing structure (e.g., paranasal sinus, mastoid air cells) has been violated. Infection in the form of meningitis then becomes a potential complication, and pneumocephalus is important to detect (Fig. 7.89). Almost invariably, it is secondary to traumatic violation of the air spaces but it also has been demonstrated on a nontrauma basis from a forceful Valsalva maneuver (9).

REFERENCES

1. Bradley WG Jr. MR appearance of hemorrhage in the brain. Radiology 1993;189:15–26.
2. Mittl RL Jr, Grossman RI, Hiehle JF Jr, et al. Prevalence of MR evidence of diffuse axonal injury in patients with mild head injury and normal head CT findings. AJNR 1994;15:1583–1589.
3. Ashikaga R, Araki Y, Ishida O. MRI of head injury using FLAIR. Neuroradiology 1997;39:239–242.
4. Husson B, Pariente D, Tammam S, et al. The value of MRI in the early diagnosis of growing skull fracture. Pediatr Radiol 1996; 26:744–747.
5. de Dijientcheu V, Rilliet B, Delavelle J, et al. Leptomeningeal cyst in newborns due to vacuum extraction: report of two cases. Childs Nerv Syst 1996;12:399–403.
6. Carty H, Lloyd D. Commentary: head injury in children. Who needs a skull x-ray? Pediatr Radiol 1998;28:815–816.
7. Schunk JE, Rodgerson JD, Woodward GA. The utility of head computed tomographic scanning in pediatric patients with normal neurologic examination in the emergency department. Pediatr Emergency Care 1996;12:160–165.
8. Davis RL, Hughes M., Gubler KD, Waller PL, Rivera FP. The use of cranial CT scans in the triage of pediatric patients with mild head injury. Pediatrics 1995;95:345–349.
9. Babl FE, Arnett AM, Barnett E, et al. A traumatic pneumocephalus: a case report and review of the literature. Pediatr Emerg Care 1999;15:106–109.

INTRACRANIAL HEMORRHAGE IN PREMATURE INFANTS

Intracranial hemorrhage in low-birth-weight, premature infants is very common, and especially vulnerable is the infant under 35 weeks' gestation weighing less than 1500 g. It is generally accepted that hypoxia and prematurity are the two most significant predisposing factors to bleeding in these infants, and such bleeding originates in the subependymal germinal matrix of the choroid plexus of the lateral ventricles. The choroid plexus is extremely vascular and, although present in all the ventricles, is most abundant in the lateral ventricles. For this reason, bleeds arise here most often, but can occur elsewhere, including the posterior fossa.

The choroid plexus reaches maximum size by 32 weeks' gestation and then subsides in size towards term. Because of its rich vascularity, it is susceptible to rupture with increases in pressure and rate of blood flow. In this regard, hypoxia leads to vascular dilation, distention, and congestion of the blood vessels in the germinal matrix and so that is why hemorrhages occur here. This can result from any number of causes, but in all cases the end result is vessel rupture and bleeding. Potential predisposing factors include transient increases in systemic blood pressure and back pressure from venous drainage impairment as seen with heart failure, neck vein kinking due to faulty head positioning, and increased intrathoracic pressures secondary to problems such as pneumothorax and positive pressure ventilation.

In preterm infants, it has been demonstrated that the resistive index in the middle cerebral artery, anterior cerebral artery, and basilar artery are decreased in comparison to that in full-term infants (1). This means that velocities would be less, but mean blood flow would be greater. This being the case, volume overload of dilated capillaries in the germinal matrix could occur. This can be aggravated by the presence of a patent ductus arteriosus (common in preterm infants). In these cases, there is an exaggerated diastolic run off through the patent ductus and the resulting jolt in the delivery of blood to the dilated capillaries can add to the propensity to their rupture and hemorrhage. To this end it has been demonstrated that the administration of indomethacin to close a patent ductus arteriosus reduces the incidence of intracranial hemorrhage (2). Phenobarbital also has been demonstrated to decrease the incidence of bleeding in preterm infants (3). Clearly then, the problem is multifactorial but almost all of the secondary factors probably would go by the wayside if it were not for the facts that the germinal matrix is very vascular and that hypoxia causes its vessels to dilate and become more vulnerable to rupture. Grade IV bleeds probably are hemorrhagic infarcts and may have PVL as their precursor (4).

The original bleed in the germinal matrix may remain confined to this area or become larger and extend further into the ventricle. Accordingly, these bleeds are graded from grade I through IV (Fig. 7.90) and are defined as follows: grade I, the hemorrhage is confined to the germinal matrix and does not extend past the caudothalamic groove; grade II, the bleed protrudes into the ventricle but only reaches the choroid plexus in the trigone; grade III, the bleed fills the ventricle and causes it to enlarge (dilate), and it may extend into the temporal horn; grade IV, there is extension or associated bleeding in the adjacent parenchyma (Figs. 7.91). Although ventricular dilation has been used in grad-

GRADE I.	BLEEDING CONFINED TO THE GERMINAL MATRIX AND DOES NOT EXTEND BEYOND THE CAUDOTHALAMIC GROOVE.
GRADE II.	BLEEDING EXTENDS TO BUT DOES NOT INVOLVE THE CHOROID PLEXUS OF THE TRIGONE.
GRADE III.	BLEEDING EXTENDS INTO THE CHOROID PLEXUS AND/OR TEMPORAL HORN.
GRADE IV.	BLEEDING OCCURS IN THE ADJACENT PARENCHYMA.

FIGURE 7.90. Grades of intracranial hemorrhage. Generally, with grade I and II bleeds, the prognosis is good, but with grade III and IV bleeds, the prognosis is poor, and complications such as atrophy, porencephalic cysts, hydrocephalus, and gliosis are much more common.

ing bleeds, **I believe that differentiation needs to be made as to whether the ventricles dilate because of the size of the bleed (grade III) or because of complicating hydrocephalus.** The latter should not be used for grading purposes. Hydrocephalus is a complication of bleeding.

Even though grade II and III bleeds are considered intraventricular, they probably are not free intraventricular bleeds. Their appearance would suggest that they are confined by the ependyma for they tend to have a discrete margin and are surrounded by clear cerebral spinal fluid (Fig. 7.91, A–D). There is no question that some leakage of blood also must occur into the ventricle itself, but the bulk of the bleed remains confined and subependymal, and merely protrudes into the ventricle. In terms of prognosis, almost all agree that patients with grade I or II bleeds do relatively well, while those with grade III or IV bleeds tend to develop complications such as progressive hydrocephalus, porencephalic cysts, areas of brain gliosis and atrophy, and subsequent cerebral palsy. With hydrocephalus, the obstruction may occur at the level of the aqueduct or over the meninges resulting in communicating hydrocephalus. In infants with more severe bleeds, clinical findings in the form of apnea, lethargy, seizures, and a dropping hematocrit bring attention to the problem, but many infants with the smaller bleeds are relatively asymptomatic. For this reason, high-risk infants (i.e., premature infants weighing less than 1500 g) are routinely examined with ultrasound.

When intraventricular bleeds resorb, they get smaller and often totally disappear. This is especially true of grade I bleeds. On the other hand, some may undergo cystic degeneration in the interim, and the cysts are especially well visualized if associated ventricular dilation also is present (Fig. 7.92, A and B). Cystic degeneration of grades III and IV bleeds also occurs (Fig. 7.92, C and D) and with grade IV bleeds the cystic degeneration may result in porencephaly (Fig. 7.93). In terms of the cysts resulting from degeneration of grades I and II bleeds, it should be noted that these cysts also have been found in totally asymptomatic infants,

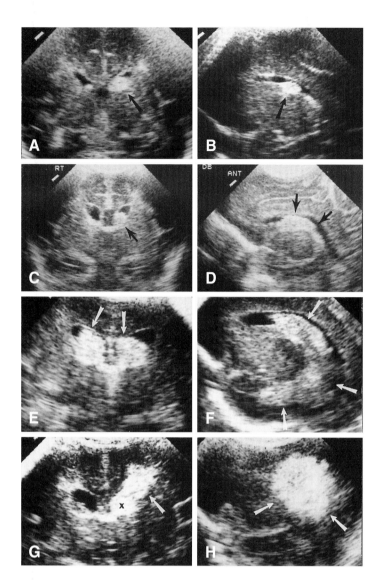

FIGURE 7.91. Intraventricular bleeds: various grades.
A. Grade I bleed on the left (arrow). **B.** Parasagittal view demonstrates the typical oval or round appearance of a grade I bleed (arrow). It is confined to the germinal matrix. **C.** Grade II bleed. Note that the appearance of the bleed (arrow) on a coronal view is not much different from that of a grade I bleed. **D.** On sagittal view, however, note that the bleed is much larger and that it extends posteriorly toward the trigone (arrows). **E.** Bilateral grade III bleeds (arrows) filling and dilating the lateral ventricles. Note the caps of clear cerebral spinal fluid over the convex surface of the bleeds, suggesting that they are confined and not free intraventricular bleeds. **F.** Parasagittal view demonstrates that the bleed (arrows) virtually completely fills the dilated lateral ventricle. **G. Grade IV bleed.** The intraventricular bleed has extended into the brain parenchyma (arrow). This patient also had a grade II intraventricular bleed (X). **H.** Parasagittal view demonstrates the echogenic parenchymal portion of the bleed (arrows).

before and after birth, and in the absence of documented germinal matrix bleeding (see next section). It is not known whether these cysts represent degenerative phenomenon after undocumented prenatal bleeds or normal developmental abnormalities, but whatever their etiology, they generally are considered of little importance. After any type of bleed, the lining of the ventricles often becomes thickened and echogenic. This is a relatively benign finding and results from deposition of degenerating blood products and proliferation of subependymal glial cells (5, 6) (Fig. 7.94).

REFERENCES

1. Nishimaki S, Shima Y, Yoda H, et al. Blood flow velocities in the cerebral arteries and descending aorta in small-for-dates infants. Pediatr Radiol 1993;23:575–577.
2. Van Bel F, Van Zwietan PHT, Den Ouden LL. Contribution of color Doppler flow imaging to the evaluation of the effect of indomethacin on neonatal cerebral hemodynamics. J Ultrasound Med 1990;9:107–109.
3. Kaemof JW, Porreco R, Molina R, et al. Antenatal phenobarbital for the prevention of periventricular and intraventricular hemorrhage: a double-blind, randomized, placebo-controlled, multihospital trial. J Pediatr 1990;117:933–938.
4. Schellinger D, Grant EG, Manz HJ, et al. Intraparenchymal hemorrhage in preterm neonates: a broadening spectrum. AJR 1988; 150:1109–1115.
5. Gaisie G, Roberts MS, Bouldin TW, et al. The echogenic ependymal wall in intraventricular hemorrhage: sonographic-pathologic correlation. Pediatr Radiol 1990;20:297–300.
6. Rypens F, Avni EF, Dussaussois L, et al. Hyperechoic thickened ependyma: sonographic demonstration and significance in neonates. Pediatr Radiol 1994;24:550–553.

Subependymal Germinal Matrix Cysts

Degenerating grade I and II bleeds often develop cysts in the germinal matrix region. These cysts first came to atten-

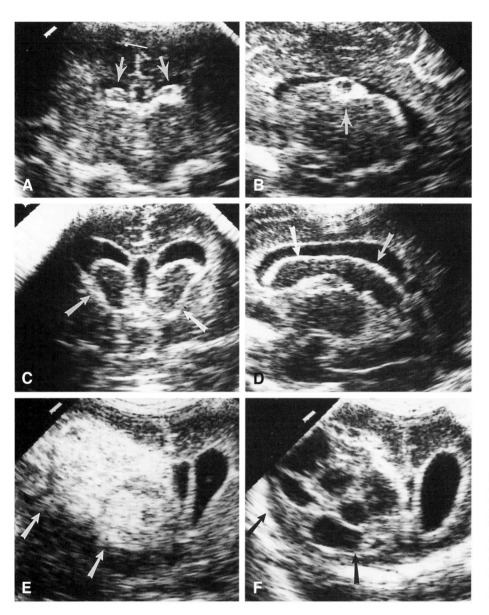

FIGURE 7.92. Cystic degeneration of bleeds. A. Cystic degeneration (arrows) of bilateral grade I bleeds. **B.** Parasagittal view demonstrates the same cystic change (arrow). **C.** Note the bilateral grade III bleeds (arrows). **D.** Later, cystic degeneration of the bleeds occurs (arrows). **E.** Large, grade IV bleed (arrows). **F.** At a later date, cystic degeneration of the bleed occurs (arrows).

tion because of the extensive use of ultrasonography, which demonstrated that they also could exist in normal infants before and after birth. Unfortunately, it has at the same time become apparent that these cysts frequently are seen with trisomies 18 and 21. However, even then, they are generally of no particular consequence although, if large, can obstruct the foramina of Monro and produce hydrocephalus. Their appearance on ultrasonography is typical and no different from that seen with cysts resulting from grades I bleeds.

Periventricular Leukomalacia in Preterm Infants

Periventricular leukomalacia is another manifestation of hypoxia in low-birth-weight infants (1–4). Prematurity and hypoxia lead to hypotension and underprofusion of the periventricular watershed zone, the critical zone between ventriculofugal and ventriculopedal circulations of the brain. When blood supply to this zone is diminished, tissue schemia occurs, and leukomalacia develops. This has been noted pathologically on postmortem specimens for some time, but only with modern imaging has its real prevalence come to the forefront. In addition to the initial hypoxic-ischemic insult to this portion of the brain, secondary hemorrhages are common, and one may have hemorrhagic and nonhemorrhagic periventricular leukomalacia. The former is more devastating, as the latter may regress. Nonetheless, periventricular leukomalacia is a serious problem and remains a common cause of cerebral palsy later in life (3).

In the past, periventricular leukomalacia was overdiagnosed on CT studies. It was not known at that time that,

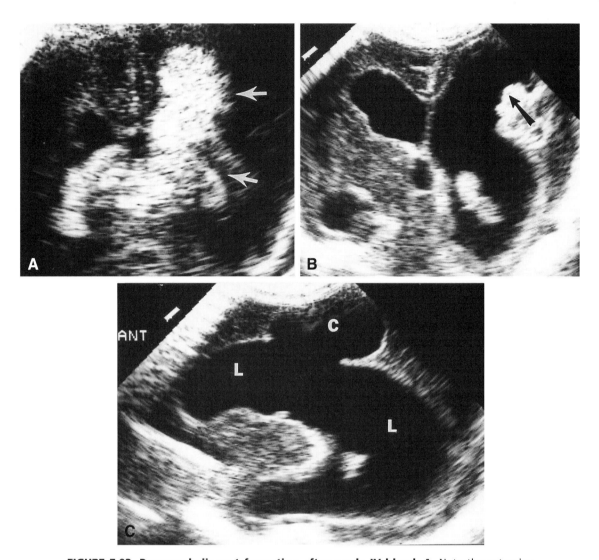

FIGURE 7.93. Porencephalic cyst formation after grade IV bleed. A. Note the extensive grade IV bleed (arrows). **B.** Later, with the bleed resolving, a porencephalic cyst (arrow) adjacent to the dilated ventricle is seen. **C.** Parasagittal view demonstrates the dilated lateral ventricle (L) and the porencephalic cyst (C).

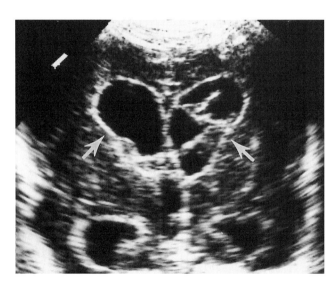

FIGURE 7.94. Ventriculitis. Note the dilated ventricles (arrows) with an echogenic lining and some internal echogenic debris.

because of lack of normal myelinization, the periventricular white matter was radiolucent and normal. In the meantime, ultrasound has become the primary imaging modality for detecting periventricular leukomalacia. Characteristically, increased echogenicity is seen immediately adjacent to the lateral ventricles both anteriorly and posteriorly (Fig. 7.95). The posterior location is most common, but must be differentiated from normal echogenicity seen in this area in full-term infants (Fig. 7.96). As the lesion heals, echogenicity may decrease, and in mild cases findings may disappear completely. In such cases, one probably is dealing with non-hemorrhagic periventricular leukomalacia. In more severe cases echogenicity persists, and cystic degeneration (breakdown of brain tissue) develops and may be very extensive (Fig. 7.97).

MRI of infants with periventricular leukomalacia is not usually performed in the initial stages of the disease, but later has been shown to demonstrate the presence of edema, hemorrhage, and gliosis (4). In the early stages on T1-weighted images, areas of white matter abnormality are seen as linear, high-signal periventricular stripes (Fig. 7.98C). Both CT and MRI also can demonstrate bleeding into these areas, substantiating the concept that most often the problem is hemorrhagic periventricular leukomalacia, at least in the more pronounced cases.

REFERENCES

1. Carson SC, Hertzberg BS, Bowie JD, et al. Value of sonography in the diagnosis of intracranial hemorrhage and periventricular

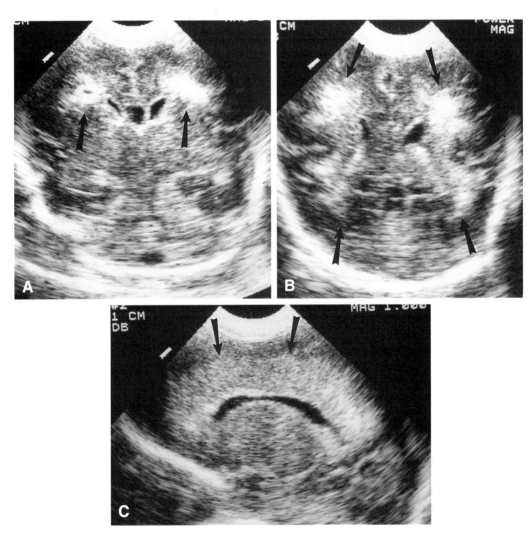

FIGURE 7.95 Periventricular leukomalacia, ultrasonographic features. A. Note the characteristic periventricular echogenicity (arrows). **B.** Similar but more extensive echogenicity (arrows) is seen posteriorly. **C.** Parasagittal view demonstrates extensive periventricular echogenicity (arrows) all along the lateral ventricle.

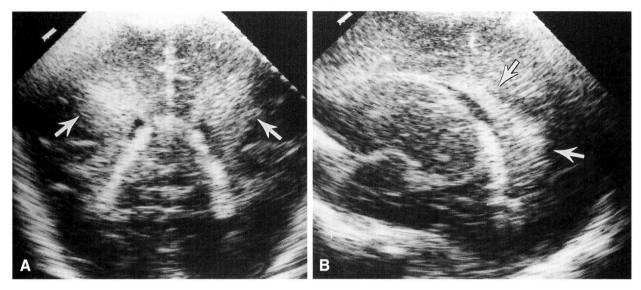

FIGURE 7.96. Normal occipital periventricular echogenicity. A. Note the bilateral echogenicity over the posterior occipital regions (arrows). **B.** Lateral view similarly demonstrates the same area of echogenicity (arrows).

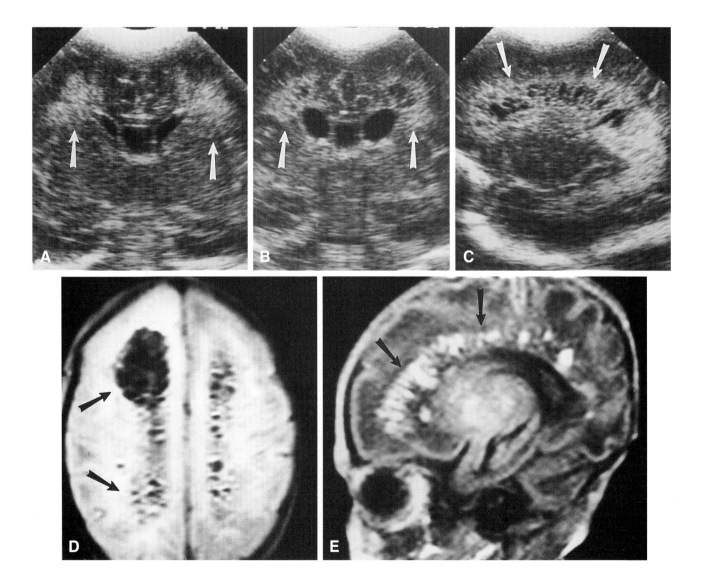

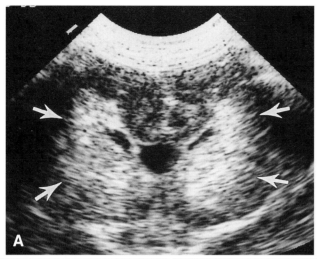

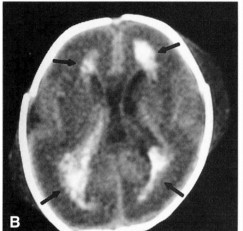

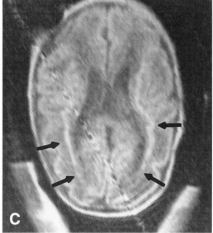

FIGURE 7.98. Periventricular leukomalacia: CT and MR findings. A. Ultrasound demonstrates typical periventricular echogenicity (arrows). **B.** CT study demonstrates that the areas demonstrated on the ultrasound scan are hemorrhagic (arrows). **C.** MR study in another patient demonstrates typical high signal intensity in the periventricular white matter (arrows) on T1-weighted images.

leukomalacia. A postmortem study of 35 cases. AJNR 1990;11: 677–683.

2. Paneth N, Rudelli R, Monte W, et al. White matter necrosis in very low birth weight infants: neuropathologic and ultrasonographic findings in infants surviving six days or longer. J Pediatr 1990;116:975–984.

3. Pidcock FS, Graziani LJ, Stanley C, et al. Neurosonographic features of periventricular echodensities associated with cerebral palsy in preterm infants. J Pediatr 1990;116:417–422.

4. Schouman-Claeys E, Henry-Feugeas M-C, Roset F, et al. Periventricular leukomalacia: correlation between MR imaging and autopsy findings during the first 2 months of life. Radiology 1993;189:59–64.

5. DiPietro MA, Brody BA, Teele RL. Peritrigonal echogenic "blush" on cranial sonography: pathologic correlates. AJNR 1986;7: 305–309.

Central Nervous System Findings with Extracorporeal Oxygenation Therapy

Ultrasonography plays a key role in evaluation of the brain in patients being placed and/or maintained on extracorporeal oxygenation therapy (EMCO). Because these patients are to be anticoagulated, they are examined for the presence of germinal matrix bleeds before being placed on such therapy. Any bleeds after ECMO therapy is initiated need to be detected promptly, and ultrasonography is excellent for their detection. These bleeds often are large and hypoechoic or sonolucent because the blood does not clot. However, some still are echogenic, and there is a propensity for these bleeds to occur in the posterior fossa (1). Originally, when

FIGURE 7.97. Periventricular leukomalacia: cystic degeneration. A. Typical periventricular echogenicity (arrows) in the early stages. **B.** Early cystic degeneration is occurring (arrows). **C.** Parasagittal view demonstrates extensive cystic degeneration (arrows). **D.** Cystic degeneration (arrows) on MRI. On this T2-weighted image, the cysts exhibit low signal intensity, suggesting the presence of blood. **E.** On the T1-weighted image, the cystic areas with high signal intensity (arrows) suggest the presence of blood.

venous (jugular) and arterial (carotid) cannulas were used, the right carotid artery often was sacrificed, and it was believed that considerable neurologic deficit would result. However, this has not proved to be the case, and it is remarkable how little damage to the central nervous system occurs after the carotid artery is ligated. This has been substantiated with MRI (2). The problem is circumvented if a single venous cannula is used.

A question often arises as to how often should cranial ultrasound be performed in this patients. More and more it is being generally accepted that bleeding usually occurs within five days (3). It also has been suggested that if a second ultrasound study, within a twenty-three hour period is normal subsequent bleeding is unlikely to occur (4). In our institution we perform the study for five consecutive days.

REFERENCES

1. Bulas DI, Taylor GA, Fitz C, et al. Posterior fossa intracranial hemorrhage in infants treated with extracorporeal membrane oxygenation: sonographic findings. AJR 1991;156:571–575.
2. Wiznitzer M, Masaryk TJ, Lewin J, et al. Parenchymal and vascular magnetic resonance imaging of the brain after extracorporeal membrane oxygenation. Am J Dis Child 1990;144:1323–1326.
3. Khan AM, Shabarek FM, Zwischenberger JB, et al. Utility of daily head ultrasonography for infants on extracorporeal membrane oxygenation. J Pediatr Surg 1998;33:1229–1232.
4. Heard ML, Clark RH, Pettignano P, et al. Daily cranial ultrasound during ECMO: a quality review cost analysis project. J Pediatr Surg 1997;32:1260–1261.

ANOXIC BRAIN INJURY

Prolonged periods of anoxia result in severe damage to the brain and no matter what age group one is dealing with, and the findings are generally the same. One can encounter focal infarcts or severe global hypoxia of the entire brain. On CT, global hypoxia produces a progressively hypodense brain, obliteration of the basal cisterns, sulci and ventricles, and the so-called white cerebellar sign due to sparing of the cerebellum (Fig. 7.99, A and C). On ultrasound, the early findings are those of loss of normal parenchymal architecture secondary to edema (Fig. 7.99D). Other configurations include decreased density of the white matter due to edema extending up to the cortex (Fig. 7.100A), complete loss of architecture of the brain with the falx standing out as a white line (Fig. 7.100C), infarction of the basal ganglia (Fig. 7.100D). Later changes often are better demonstrated with MRI (Fig. 7.100B).

In severe cases the brain undergoes necrosis and subsequent cystic degeneration (Fig. 7.101). MRI has demonstrated that initial changes occur in the cortex, subcortical white matter, and the deep white matter itself (1–3). It also has been demonstrated that there is hyperperfusion of the brain after the initial hypoxic insult (4). Hypoxia in the preterm infant leads to periventricular leukomalacia and germinal matrix bleeding, and both conditions have been covered in previous sections. In some patients, the brunt of the hypoxic episode may be reflected in infarction of the basal ganglia and thalamus (5) (see Fig. 7.100D). Currently diffusion weighted imaging is being used more and more to evaluate cerebral infarction (6–9). It is more sensitive than CT (6), but this method of imaging may not detect all infarcts in the hyperacute phase (8, 9).

REFERENCES

1. Barkovich AJ, Westmark K, Partridge C, et al. Perinatal asphyxia: MR findings in the first 10 days. AJNR 1995;16:427–438.
2. Christophe C, Clercx A, Blum D, et al. Early NMR detection of cortical and subcortical hypoxia; ischemic encephalopathy in full term infants. Pediatr Radiol 1994;24:581–584.
3. Moorcraft J, Bolas NM, Ives NK, et al. Spatially localized magnetic resonance spectroscopy of the brains of normal and asphyxiated newborns. Pediatrics 1991;87:273–282.
4. van Bel F, Dorrepaal CA, Benders MJNL, et al. Changes in cerebral hemodynamics and oxygenation in the first 24 hours after birth asphyxia. Pediatrics 1993;92:365–372.
5. Connolly B, Kelehan P, O'Brien N, et al. The echogenic thalamus in hypoxic ischaemic encephalopathy. Pediatr Radiol 1994;24:268–271.
6. Barber PA, Darby DG, Desmond PM, et al. Identification of major ischemic change: diffusion-weighted imaging versus computed tomography. Stroke 1999;30:2059–2065.
7. Inder T, Huppi PS, Zientara GP, et al. Early detection of periventricular leukomalacia by diffusion-weighted magnetic resonance imaging techniques. J Pediatr 1999;134:631–634.
8. Lefkowitz D, LaBena M, Nudo ST, et al. Hyperacute ischemic stroke missed by diffusion-weighted imaging. AJNR 1999;20:1871–1875.
9. Schaefer PW, Grant PE, Gonzalez RG. Diffusion-weighted MR imaging of the brain. Radoil 2000;217:331–345.

CYSTIC ENCEPHALOMALACIA

Cystic encephalomalacia results from massive brain destruction. Most often, this is the result of severe hypoxia, but infections such as herpes encephalitis also can produce similar changes (1). In any of these cases, the initial findings are those of widespread edema or necrosis of the brain, eventually cystic degeneration develops, calcifications may be seen, and imaging of the brain can be accomplished with any imaging modality (Fig. 7.101).

REFERENCE

1. Gray PH, Tudehope DI, Masel J. Cystic encephalomalacia and intrauterine herpes simplex virus infection. Pediatr Radiol 1992;22:529–532.

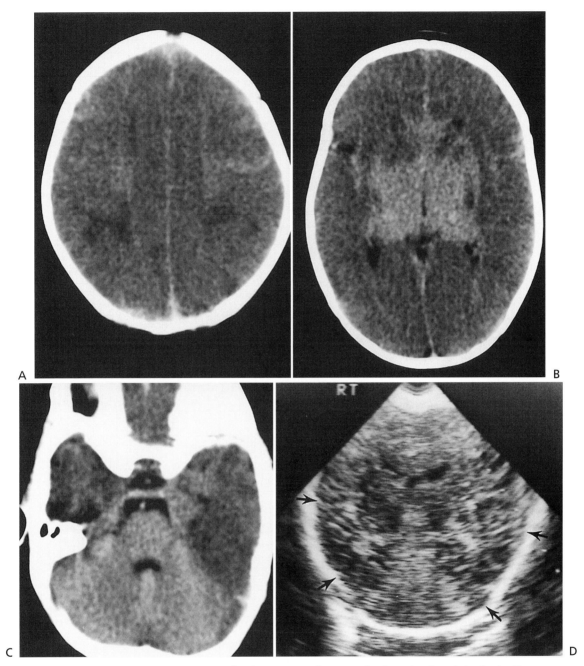

FIGURE 7.99. Hypoxic injury to brain. A. Note the extensive hypodensity of the brain. **B.** Another slice demonstrates preservation of the central basal ganglia. **C.** Axial view through the posterior fossa demonstrates a preserved cerebellum (i.e., white cerebellar sign). **D.** Ultrasonogram in another patient demonstrates loss of gray-white matter differentiation and a coarsely echogenic pattern of the brain (arrows).

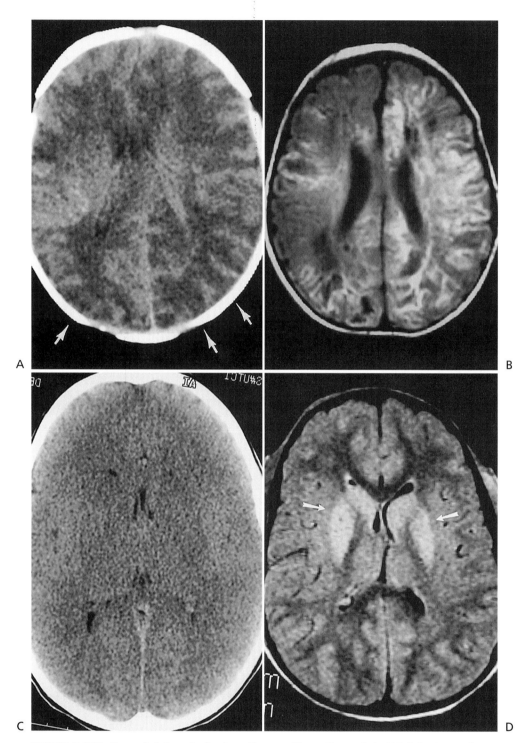

FIGURE 7.100. Hypoxic injury to brain: other configurations. A. In this infant, note hypodensity of the white matter extending to the surface of the brain (arrows). Also note that the sutures are spread and the ventricles are compressed. **B.** MR study at a later date demonstrates early, widespread cystic degeneration. **C.** In this patient, gray-white matter differentiation has been lost, the brain has a uniform "no personality" appearance, and the ventricles are compressed. The falx stands out as a white line posteriorly. **D.** In this patient, increased signal intensity in the basal ganglia (arrows) signifies basal ganglia infarction.

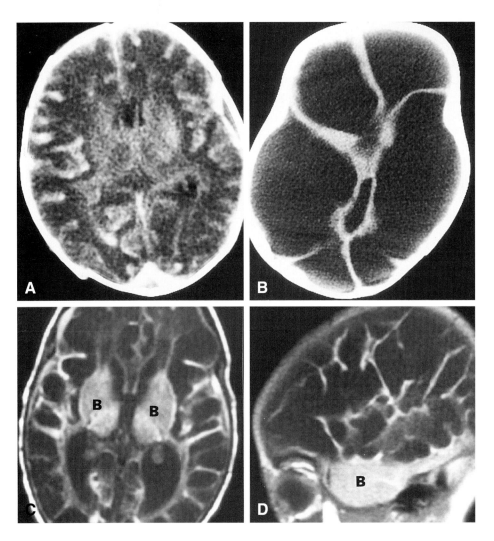

FIGURE 7.101. Cystic encephalo-malacia. A. Note the extensive edema of the brain, producing wide-spread hypodensity. The brain is necrotic. **B.** End-stage disease demonstrates multiple cystic areas but no remaining brain tissue. **C.** T1-weighted MR study demonstrates cystic encephalomalacia of the brain with only the basal ganglia (B) remaining visible. **D.** Sagittal view demonstrates the same findings.

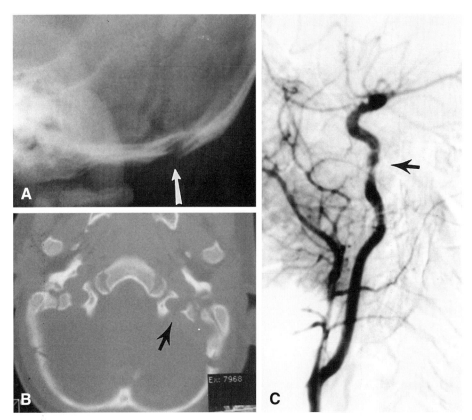

FIGURE 7.102. Traumatic carotid dissection. A. Note the occipital skull fracture (arrow). **B.** Note the fracture through the base of the skull (arrow) involving the jugular foramen (arrow). **C.** Digital subtraction arteriogram demonstrates irregularity of the internal cerebral artery (arrow).

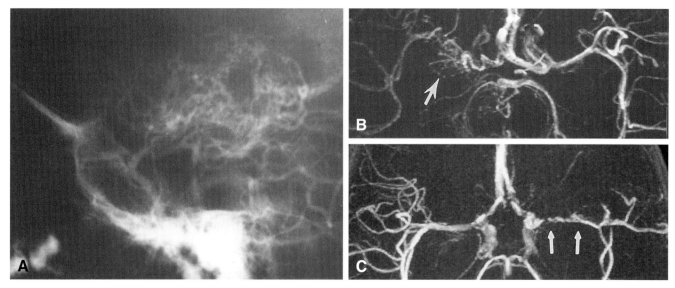

FIGURE 7.103. Moyamoya. A. Note the leash of telangiectatic collaterals characteristic of this condition. **B.** MRA study demonstrates underperfusion of the right middle cerebral artery region and a similar leash (arrow) of telangiectatic vessels. **C.** In this patient, the left middle cerebral artery is irregular (arrows), and the area of brain it supplies is underperfused.

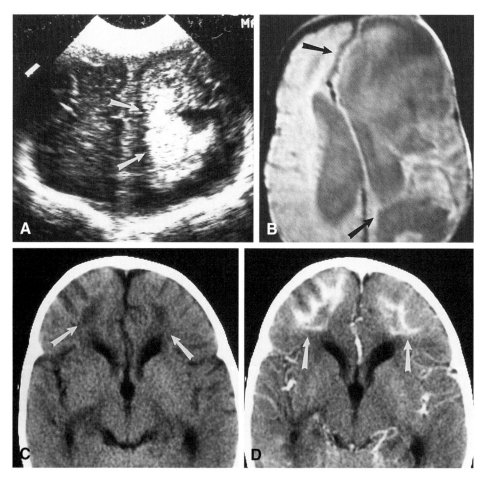

FIGURE 7.104. Cerebral infarction with early and late findings. A. Ultrasonogram demonstrates a large area of echogenicity in the left cerebral hemisphere (arrows). **B.** T1-weighted MR study demonstrates the low signal intensity in the area of infarction (arrows). There is midline shift. **C.** On CT, bilateral hypodense areas (arrows) are seen in the frontal lobes of this patient. **D.** CT study with contrast obtained a few days later demonstrates hyperperfusion of the previously noted areas of infarction (arrows).

VASCULAR ABNORMALITIES

Cerebral Infarction

Cerebral infarction can occur from intraluminal arterial or venous occlusion (i.e., thrombosis) or vasospasm induced by hypoxia or infection. Although more commonly a problem in older children, arterial occlusions can occur in infants. Such occlusions usually results from thrombosis precipitated by trauma to arteries with dissection (1, 2) (Fig. 7.102), infection, hypoxia, or dehydration. Vascular occlusions also can be seen with sickle cell disease due to vascular sludging (3, 4), the collagen vascular diseases, HIV infection (5), and embolism from the systemic venous circulation in infants with congenital heart defects such as tetralogy of Fallot.

In infancy, primary, progressive arterial occlusion, often called **infantile hemiplegia**, is a common problem. The cause of the condition is unknown, and stenotic lesions are seen in the large vessels. However, the most characteristic finding is the presence of telangiectatic collaterals distal to the site of arterial occlusion. These produce a fine mesh-like conglomeration of vessels, and the condition also is known as **moyamoya disease** (Fig. 7.103). On T1-weighted, gadolinium-enhanced MR images, a similar phenomena in which the leptomeninges show marked linear tortuous areas of enhancement has been noted and referred to as the "Ivy sign" (6). Cerebral infarction or stroke also has been documented with

migraine headaches (7, 8). Vasculopathy with microthrombi can be seen with cervicofacial hemangiomas (9, 10). Cerebral infarction has been documented in patients with L-carnitine deficiency (11).

With ultrasound, cerebral infarction presents as an echogenic lesion (Fig. 7.104A), while on CT, the area of infarction initially is hypodense (Fig. 7.104C). However, within a few days contrast-enhanced hypervascularity of the infarct is demonstrable (Fig. 7.104D). One T1-weighted MR images, areas of infarction show decreased signal intensity (Fig. 7.104B), but on T2-weighted images, they show increased signal intensity (Fig. 7.105B). For the most part, infarcts follow the distribution of larger arteries, but one also can see global infarction and infarction of the basal ganglia (Fig. 7.105).

Most of the comments thus far have dealt with single vessel occlusion, and in these cases the infarcted portion of the brain can be massive (Fig. 7.106A). However, it should be remembered that multiple small vessel (peripheral) infarcts also occur and are characteristic of septic emboli. Many of these infarcts are hemorrhagic (Fig. 7.106B), and in general, hemorrhage superimposed on infarction is not uncommon.

MRI with spectroscopy and proton-density profusion and diffusion scans can be employed for further delineation of infarcts (Fig. 7.107). Screening with color and power Doppler can be used to detect possible vascular occlusions in sickle cell disease (4, 12, 13).

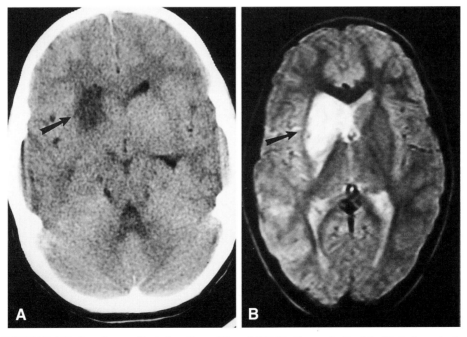

FIGURE 7.105. Basal ganglia infarction: CT and MR findings. A. On this CT study, note the hypodense area (arrow) reflecting an infarct in the basal ganglia. **B.** T2-weighted MR image demonstrates high signal intensity in the area of infarction (arrow). On T1-weighted images, nonhemorrhagic infarctions have low signal intensity (see Fig. 7.104B).

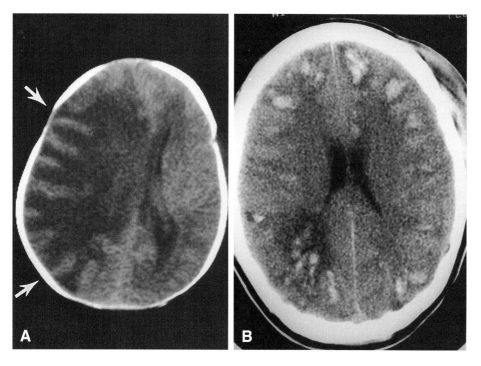

FIGURE 7.106. Cerebral infarction, other findings. A. Massive infarction of the right cerebral hemisphere (arrows) in a patient with meningitis. Note the extensive hypodensity and enlargement of the right hemisphere. There is associated midline shift. **B.** Multiple hemorrhagic cortical infarcts scattered throughout the periphery of both cerebral hemispheres in this patient with a streptococcal empyema and septic emboli.

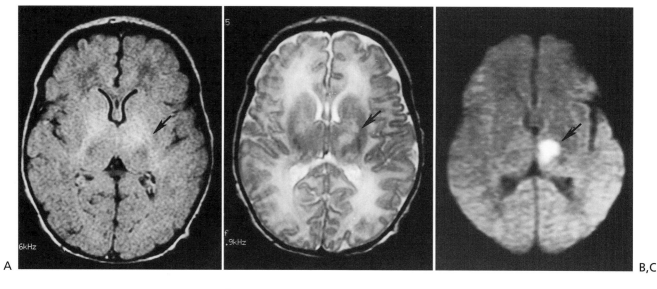

FIGURE 7.107. Cerebral infarction: MR diffusion study. A. FLAIR image of this patient shows very little in the way of abnormality in the left thalamic region (arrow). **B.** A T2-weighted study demonstrates an area of increased signal intensity in the left thalamic region (arrow). **C.** Diffusion image more clearly demonstrates the area of infarction (arrow).

REFERENCES

1. Cheon J-E, Kim I-O, Kim WS, et al. MR diagnosis of cerebellar infarction due to vertebral artery dissection in children. Pediatr Radiol 2001;31:163–166.
2. Velkey I, Lombay B, Harkanyi Z. Ischemic stroke due to traumatic carotid artery dissection. Pediatr Radiol 1999;29:223.
3. Powars DR, Conti PS, Wong W-Y, et al: Cerebral vasculopathy in sickle cell anemia: diagnostic contribution of positron emission tomography. Blood 1999;93:71–79.
4. Seibert JJ, Glasier CM, Kirby RS, et al. Transcranial Doppler, MRA, and MRI as a screening examination for cerebrovascular disease in patients with sickle cell anemia: an 8-year study. Pediatr Radiol 1998;28:138–142.
5. Shah SS, Zimmerman RA, Rorke LB, et al. Cerebrovascular complications for HIV in children. AJNR 1996;17:1913–1917.
6. Yoon H-K, Shin H-J, Chang YW. "Ivy Sign" in childhood Moyamoya disease: depiction and FLAIR and contrast-enhanced T1-weighted MR images. Radiology 2002;223:384–389.
7. Ebinger F, Boor R, Gawehn J, et al. Ischemic stroke and migraine in childhood: coincidence or causal relation? J Child Neurology 1999;14:451–455.

8. Hoekstra-van Dalen RA, Cillessen JP, Kappelle LJ, et al. Cerebral infarcts associated with migraine: clinical features, risk factors and follow-up. J Neurology 1999;243:511–515.
9. Burrows PE, Robertson RL, Mulliken JB, et al. Cerebral vasculopathy and neurologic sequelae in infants with cervicofacial hemangioma: report of eight patients. Radiology 1998;207:601–607.
10. Pascual-Castroviejo I, Viano J, Moreno F, et al. Hemangiomas of the head, neck and chest with associated vascular and brain anomalies: a complex neurocutaneous syndrome. AJNR 1996;17:461–471.
11. Thompson JE, Smith M, Castillo M, et al. MR in children with L-carnitine deficiency. AJNR 1996;17:1585–1588.
12. Bulas DI, Jones A, Seibert JJ, et al. Transcranial Doppler (TCD) screening for stroke prevention in sickle cell anemia: pitfalls in technique variation. Pediatr Radiol 2000;30:733–738.
13. Malouf AJ Jr, Hamrick-Turner JE, Doherty MC, et al. Implementation of the STOP protocol for stroke prevention in the sickle cell anemia by using duplex poster and Doppler imaging. Radiology 2001;219:359–365.

Hypernatremic Brain Abnormalities

With severe hypernatremia, it has been documented that the brain can be damaged and demonstrate multifocal areas of hemorrhage, hemorrhagic infarction, and generalized edema (1, 2).

REFERENCES

1. Han BK, Lee M, Yoon HD. Cranial ultrasound and CT findings in infants with hypernatremic dehydration. Pediatr Radiol 1997;27:739–742.
2. Mocharla R, Schexnayder SM, Glsier CM. Fatal cerebral edema and intracranial hemorrhage associated with hypernatremic dehydration. Pediatr Radiol 1997;27:785–787.

Arterial Aneurysms

In the neonate and young infant, arterial aneurysms are relatively uncommon and rupture is rare. Occult intracranial aneurysms can be seen with polycystic kidney disease (1) and are commonly associated with coarctation of the aorta. Posttraumatic aneurysms are uncommon (Fig. 7.108), as are mycotic aneurysms. In any of these cases, secondary changes associated with bleeding and infarction are demonstrable with CT and MR, and the vascular anatomy is demonstrable with MRA, CT angiography (2), and arteriography.

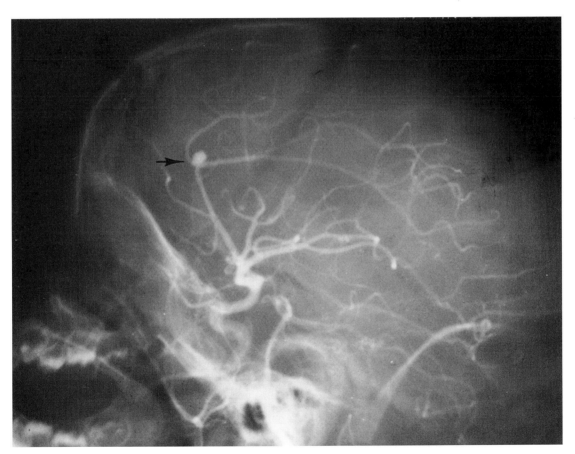

FIGURE 7.108. Traumatic aneurysm. Note the traumatic aneurysm of anterior cerebral artery (arrow). The proximal portion of the anterior cerebral artery is somewhat straightened, probably secondary to bleeding and surrounding hematoma. Also note frontal and parietal skull fractures of the 7-week-old infant who was in an automobile accident.

REFERENCES

1. Ruggieri PM, Poulos N, Masaryk TJ, et al. Occult intracranial aneurysms in polycystic kidney disease: screening with MR angiography. Radiology 1994;191:33–39.
2. White PM, Teasdale EM, Wardlaw JM, et al. Intracranial aneurysms: CT angiography and MR angiography for detection-prospective blinded comparison in a large patient cohort. Radiology 2001;219–739–749.

Vein of Galen Aneurysm

This aneurysm, actually an arteriovenous malformation, is the most common intracranial aneurysm of the neonate. They range in size from relatively small to enormous and, with the larger aneurysms, obstruction in the region of the posterior third ventricle and aqueduct of Sylvius is not uncommon. Consequently, hydrocephalus may be the presenting problem. Feeders and drainers are variable (1), and many of these infants also have a cranial bruit. Others may present with hyperkinetic congestive heart failure secondary to massive arteriovenous shunting through the aneurysm (2). This usually occurs in the immediate neonatal period or in early infancy. In such cases, chest roentgenography often reveals a diffusely enlarged heart and congested lungs. However, in other cases there may be slightly diminished pulmonary vascularity (Fig. 7.109A). This is accounted for by a combination of increased pulmonary vascular resistance (normal in the neonate) and a large right-to-left shunt through a patent ductus arteriosus (2). The first factor promotes increased right-side pressures and, with the ductus open, facilitates right-to-left ductal shunting. The end result is that blood flow to the lungs is diminished, and this phenomenon may be further enhanced by the presence of lower than usual aortic pressures seen with this lesion. This occurs because of the "stealing" effect present when the arteriovenous fistulous component of this anomaly is marked.

Cardiomegaly is an important finding in this condition and should aid one in suspecting the correct diagnosis in an infant with a cranial bruit, possibly an enlarging head, and evidence of congestive heart failure. However, the cardiac findings may so predominate that primary cardiac disease is at first suspected; even with cardiac ultrasonography, catheterization, and angiocardiography, the condition can elude early diagnosis. During angiocardiography a clue to the diagnosis lies in the fact that the carotid and vertebral arteries often appear exceptionally large and dilated and that most of the contrast material flows into the head (Fig. 7.109, B and C). Decreased intracranial circulation time is also noted, and not infrequently, large dilated jugular veins are seen in the drainage phase. If hydrocephalus is present, the calvarium is enlarged. Occasionally, calcification in a vein of Galen, probably secondary to thrombosis (3, 4), can

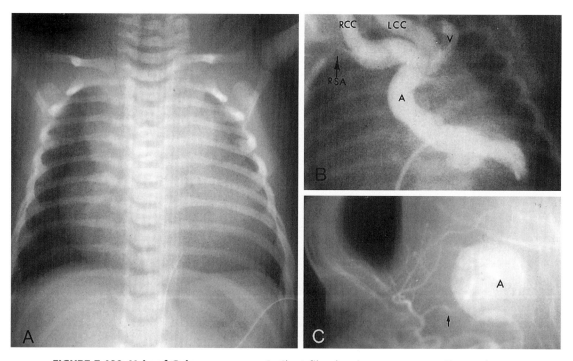

FIGURE 7.109. Vein of Galen aneurysm. A. Chest film showing enormous cardiomegaly, predominant right atrial and right ventricular enlargement, and in this case, slightly decreased pulmonary vascularity. In other instances, the vascularity is increased. In the neonate and young infant, massive cardiomegaly is a common feature of systemic arteriovenous malformations and is secondary to high-output failure. **B.** Cineangiogram in the same infant showing predominant flow into large right (RCC) and left (LCC) carotid arteries. The left vertebral artery (V) also is large. The right subclavian artery (RSA) is thin and just barely visible, and the left subclavian artery is not visible. A, aorta. **C.** Cerebral arteriogram in the same infant shows the large aneurysm (A) being supplied by the posterior cerebral artery (arrow). Air is present in the ventricles.

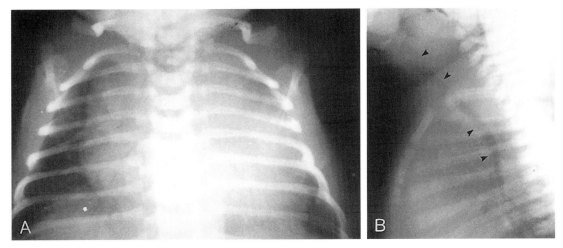

FIGURE 7.110. Vein of Galen aneurysm: chest and neck findings. A. Note the cardiomegaly with right atrial and right ventricular enlargement and widening of the superior mediastinum. Although this widening could be from the thymus gland, in these patients, it is the result of enlargement of the brachiocephalic vessels (see Fig. 7.118). **B.** Lateral view of the chest demonstrates posterior displacement of the intrathoracic portion of the trachea (lower arrows) and forward displacement of the upper airway (upper arrows). These changes also are the result of the large brachiocephalic vessels. In the neck the large jugular veins and cranial arteries act as a retropharyngeal mass. However, since the mass is not solid, stridor is not a problem. (From Swischuk LE, Crowe JE, Mewborne EB Jr. Large vein of Galen aneurysms in the neonate. A constellation of diagnostic chest and neck radiologic findings. Pediatr Radiol 1977;6:4–9, with permission.).

be seen, but this is a rare occurrence. Spontaneous regression also has been documented (5).

Many times, these infants demonstrate a **constellation of plain film findings that can suggest the correct diagnosis (2).** These include cardiomegaly with right atrial and right ventricular enlargement (increased venous return from the head), widening of the superior mediastinum, retropo-

sitioning of the intrathoracic portion of the trachea, and forward displacement of the upper airway and pharynx. All of these latter changes result from the large brachiocephalic vessels pushing the intrathoracic portion of the trachea backward and the upper airway and pharynx forward (Fig. 7.110). Appreciating these findings is most helpful in those cases that elude early clinical diagnosis.

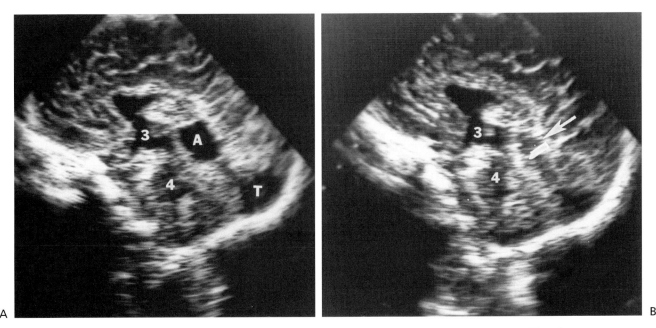

FIGURE 7.111. Vein of Galen aneurysm. A. Sagittal ultrasound demonstrates the third (3) and fourth (4) ventricles. Behind the third ventricle is the vein of Galen aneurysm (A), and more inferiorly is the enlarged torcular herophili (T). **B.** After embolization the aneurysm has markedly decreased in size (arrow).

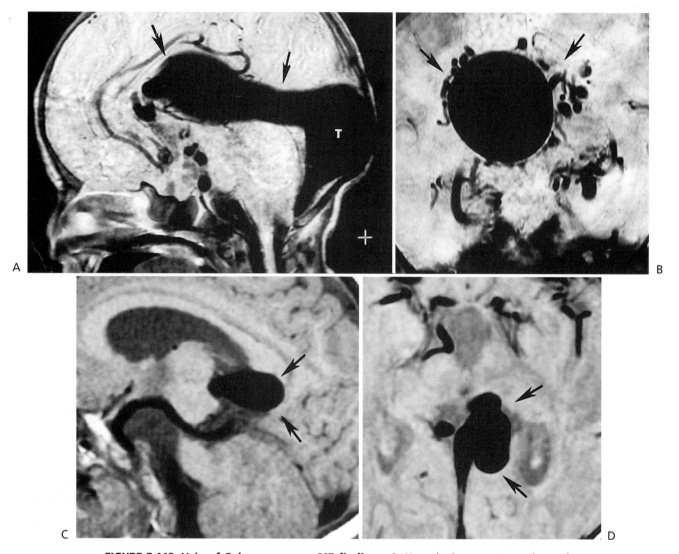

FIGURE 7.112. Vein of Galen aneurysm: MR findings. A. Note the large aneurysm (arrows) draining through the straight sinus into the large torcular herophili (T). Also note numerous collaterals. **B.** Cross-sectional view demonstrates the same large aneurysm (arrows) and the numerous collaterals. **C.** A smaller aneurysm is present in this patient (arrows). No collateral circulation is seen. **D.** Cross-sectional view of the aneurysm (arrows). Note that no collaterals are seen and that there is only slight dilatation of the straight sinus as it drains into the torcular herophili.

These aneurysms now are most commonly first diagnosed with cranial ultrasound or MRI (1, 6). With ultrasound, the findings are typical and consist of a round or oval sonolucent area posterior to the third ventricle (Fig. 7.111). The highly mobile speckles seen within the lesion result from turbulence. The feeding and draining vessels also may be delineated with ultrasound, but this aspect of the lesion usually is relegated to MRI (Fig. 7.112) or angiography. Angiography is necessary before treatment to precisely identify the feeding vessels before currently favored embolization (7). For the most part, these lesions are inoperable, and embolization therefore becomes an important mode of treatment. Nonetheless, there is variable success with such therapy, and there is always the problem of inducing permanent brain damage. These lesions have a tendency to recur, because they are not aneurysms but arteriove-nous malformations, and as old channels are obliterated, new ones open. On MRI, the findings are comparable to those on angiography.

REFERENCES

1. Desprechins B, Debaere C, Machies F, et al. A vein of Galen aneurysm with an abnormal drain system: MRI findings. Pediatr Radiol 1995;25:442–443.
2. Swischuk LE, Crowe JE, Mewborne EB Jr. Large vein of Galen aneurysms in the neonate. A constellation of diagnostic chest and neck radiologic findings. Pediatr Radiol 1977;6:4–9.
3. Chapman S, Hockley AD. Calcification of an aneurysm of the vein of Galen. Pediatr Radiol 1989;19:541–542.
4. Schulman H, Laufer L, Hertzanu Y. Complete calcification of an aneurysm of the vein of Galen. Pediatr Radiol 1998;28:233.

5. Hurst RW, Kagetsu NJ, Berenstein A. Angiographic findings in two cases of aneurysmal malformation of vein of Galen prior to spontaneous thrombosis: therapeutic implications. AJNR 1992; 13:1446–1450.
6. Taccone A, Oddone M, Cariati M, et al. Vein of Galen aneurysm: MRI with a fast gradient refocusing pulse sequence. Pediatr Radiol 1993;23:202–203.
7. Friedman DM, Verma R, Madrid M, et al. Recent improvement in outcome using transcatheter embolization techniques for neonatal aneurysmal malformations of the vein of Galen. Pediatrics 1993;91:583–586.

Arteriovenous Malformations

Arteriovenous malformations are not particularly common in infancy or childhood except for the vein of Galen aneurysm just discussed. Smaller arteriovenous malformations may bleed and cause meningeal irritation or focal cerebral signs. They also may be associated with seizures and can be demonstrated with CT, MR, or angiography (Fig. 7.113 and 7.114). Treatment can be surgical with stereotactic radiosurgery (1) or nonsurgical with embolization. In neonates and young infants, as long as the anterior fontanelle is open, the abnormalities can be imaged with ultrasound (2). Venous angiomas occupy one end of the spectrum of arteriovenous malformations and now that MRI is being performed so commonly, these small lesions often are discovered incidentally (Fig. 7.115A). For the most part, they are innocuous, and conservative management is suggested (3). However, some may bleed (Fig. 7.115B).

REFERENCES

1. Lunsford LD, Kondziolka D, Flickinger JC, et al. Stereotactic radiosurgery for arteriovenous malformations of the brain. J Neurosurg 1991;75:512–524.
2. Westra SJ, Curran JG, Duckwiler GR, et al. Pediatric intracranial vascular malformations: evaluation of treatment results with color Doppler ultrasound. Work in progress. Radiology 1993;186: 775–783.
3. Kondziolka D, Dempsey PK, Lunsford LD. The case for conservative management of venous angiomas. Can J Neurol Sci 1991;18: 295–299.

Deep Venous Thrombosis

Deep venous thrombosis is not uncommon in infancy and childhood, and dehydration and infection are the most common predisposing factors (1–3). However, it has also been seen with leukemia, the nephrotic syndrome (4), and systemic lupus. Hydrocephalus also may be a complication, and thrombosis is best demonstrated with CT or MRI (5–7). On nonenhanced CT studies, increased density in the region of the superior sagittal sinus may be seen, but this also commonly is seen as a normal finding. Therefore, it is with contrast enhancement that a characteristic triangular defect, called the "delta sign" ensures the diagnosis (Fig. 7.116A). With MRI, the thrombus shows high signal intensity on T1-weighted images (Fig. 7.116, B and C). With MRV, no flow is seen in the thrombosed sinus, and with gadolinium enhancement, although the wall of the sinus may enhance, the lumen does not.

There also is an association between deep venous thrombosis and infarction and hemorrhage of the thalamus associated with intraventricular bleeding in full-term neonates (1, 3). When one sees the latter combination of findings, one should suspect underlying deep vein thrombosis, and finally polycythemia has been noted to mimic the findings of deep vein thrombosis on CT (8).

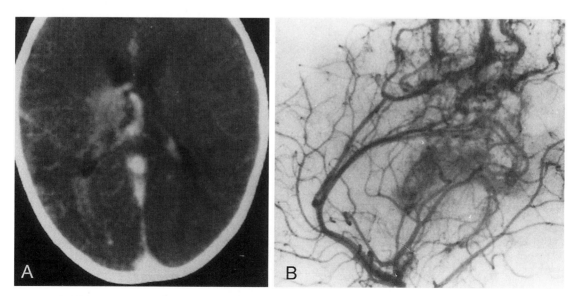

FIGURE 7.113. Arteriovenous malformation. A. Note the spidery vessels in the left cerebral hemisphere in this contrast-enhanced CT study. There is no mass effect, no deformity of the ventricles, and no shift of the midline structures. **B.** Cerebral arteriogram demonstrating the blotchy spidery vessels of this arteriovenous malformation.

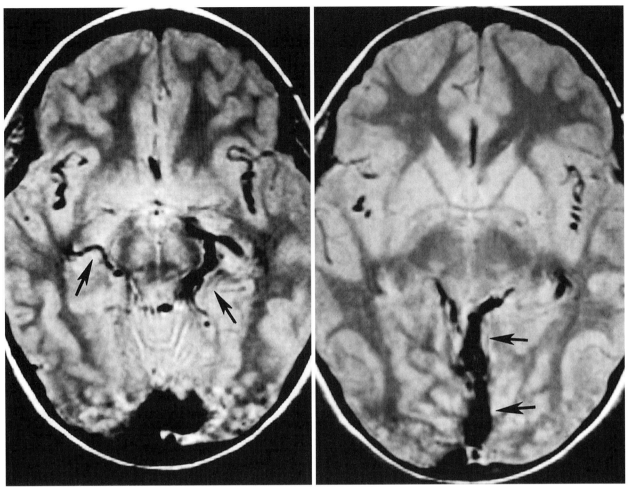

A   B

FIGURE 7.114. Arteriovenous malformation: MRI findings. A. Note the feeding vessels (arrows) around the brainstem. **B.** Draining vessels (arrows) drain to the torcular herophili.

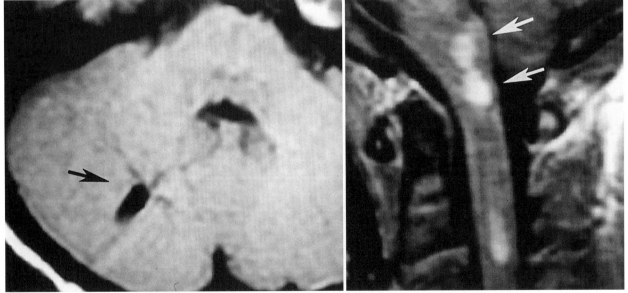

A   B

FIGURE 7.115. Venous angiomas. A. Note the small cerebellar venous angioma (arrow). **B.** Bleeding (arrows) has occurred into this small venous angioma present in the upper cervical cord and brainstem.

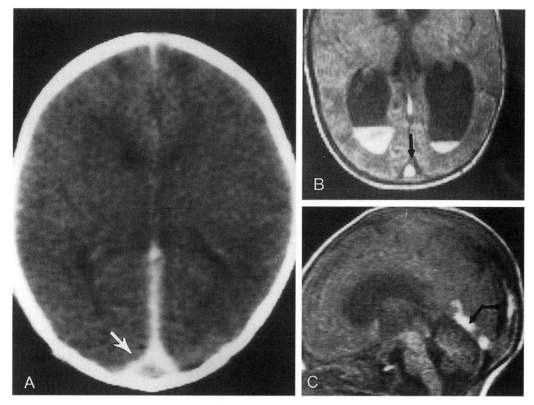

FIGURE 7.116. Deep venous thrombosis. A. Enhanced CT scan demonstrates typical triangular hypodensity in the sagittal sinus (arrow). This constitutes the "empty triangle" or "delta" signs. **B.** T1-weighted MR study demonstrates high signal intensity in the superior sagittal sinus (arrow) in a premature infant. The ventricles are dilated, and there is blood (high signal intensity) in their dependent portions. **C.** Midsagittal, T1-weighted study demonstrates high signal intensity in the straight and superior sagittal sinuses (arrows). Although these findings in isolated form may be seen with stasis, their extensive and persistent distribution in this patient should suggest deep vein thrombosis.

REFERENCES

1. Govaert P, Achten E, Vanhaesebrouck F, et al. Deep cerebral venous thrombosis in thalamo-ventricular hemorrhage of the term newborn. Pediatr Radiol 1992;22:123–127.
2. Garcia RDJ, Baker AS, Cunningham MJ, et al. Lateral sinus thrombosis associated with otitis media and mastoiditis in children. Pediatr Infect Dis J 1995;14:617–623.
3. Roland EH, Flodmark O, Hill A. Thalamic hemorrhage with intraventricular hemorrhage in the full-term newborn. Pediatrics 1990;85:737–742.
4. Pirogovsky A, Aki M, Dagan A, et al. Superior sagittal sinus thrombosis: a rare complication in a child with nephrotic syndrome. Pediatr Radiol 2001;31:709–711.
5. Medlock MD, Olivero WC, Hanigan WC, et al. Children with cerebral venous thrombosis diagnosed with magnetic resonance imaging and magnetic resonance angiography. Neurosurgery 1992;31:870–876.
6. Tsuruda JS, Shimakawa A, Pelc NJ, et al. Dural sinus occlusion: evaluation with phase-sensitive gradient-echo MR imaging. AJR 1991;157:139–146.
7. Yuh WTC, Simonson TM, Wang A-M, et al. Venous sinus occlusive disease: MR findings. AJNR 1994;15:309–316.
8. Healy JF, Nichols C. Polycythemia mimicking venous sinus thrombosis. AJNR 2002;23:1402–1403.

INFLAMMATORY DISEASE OF THE BRAIN AND MENINGES

Inflammatory lesions of the brain and meninges include brain abscess, epidural abscess, subdural empyema, meningitis, and diffuse or focal cerebritis. On CT examination, brain abscesses usually are well circumscribed and demonstrate a hyperemic margin resulting from inflammatory neovascularity (Fig. 7.117A). A similar appearance is seen with gadolinium-enhanced MRI (Fig. 7.117D), but on T2-weighted images the abscess may be lost in the surrounding edema (Fig. 7.117E). On T1-weighted images, an area of focal decreased signal intensity is seen (Fig. 7.117A). Abscesses also can result from tuberculosis (tuberculomas) (1) and fungal disease, and appear the same as do bacterial abscesses (Fig. 7.117, C and D). With AIDS, fungal infections may be more diffuse and *Cryptococcus* is a particularly common offender (2). The latter also can produce large gelatinous pseudocysts (3).

With subdural empyema, the findings are not unlike those of subdural hematoma except that contrast-enhanced CT scanning can demonstrate hyperemia over the underly-

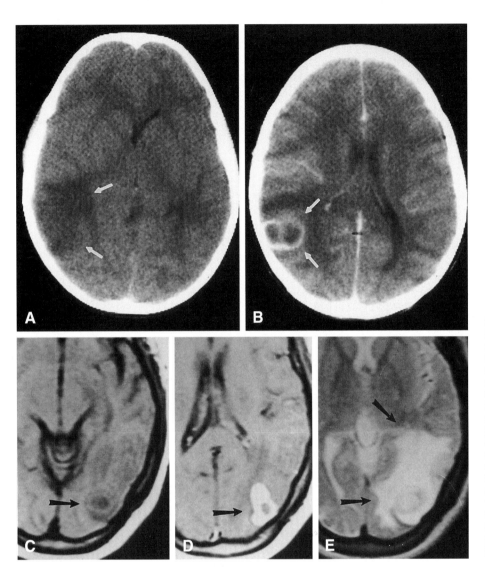

FIGURE 7.117. Brain abscess. A. Nonenhanced CT scan. Note the area of edema (arrows) in the right posterior parietal region. **B.** With contrast enhancement, a typical enhancing ring develops (arrows). The ring is typical, but not pathognomonic. Similar findings can be found on T1-weighted MR images with gadolinium enhancement. **C. Tuberculoma.** Note the hypodense center with a ring-like structure (arrow) in the left occipital region. Some edema is seen anteriorly. **D.** With gadolinium enhancement, a typical ring-like configuration (arrow) results. **E.** T2-weighted image, however, demonstrates extensive edema (arrows) around the abscess, and the abscess itself is more difficult to visualize.

ing brain (i.e., cerebritis) (Fig. 7.118B). If there is high protein content, the fluid may show increased density on CT (Fig. 7.118D), increased signal intensity on gadolinium-enhanced MRI (Fig. 7.118C), and stranding with ultrasound (4). Epidural abscesses behave the same as do subdural empyemas, and both can show enhancement with gadolinium on MRI.

Meningitis most often is bacterial in origin, although viral meningitis also commonly occurs. With bacterial meningitis CT findings usually are normal (5). In some cases, brain edema can be seen, and with contrast enhancement, some increased uptake of contrast material in the inflamed meninges occurs. This is most pronounced with tuberculous (6) (Fig. 7.118A) and other forms of granulomatous (fungal) meningitis. With MRI, the inflamed meninges also demonstrate increased signal intensity with gadolinium enhancement, but MRI of the brain for meningitis, like CT, usually is not required. Most often, one uses these imaging modalities for the detection of complications of meningitis such as subdural empyema and cerebral infarction. Steroids are of use in treating tuberculous meningitis with improved outcome (7).

Encephalitis, as opposed to meningitis, usually is of viral origin (8, 12) but occasionally can be encountered with mycoplasma infections (12). Focal areas of inflammation on CT produce blotchy or focal areas of decreased density (Fig. 7.119). These can be seen scattered throughout the brain and enhance on contrast studies. Complicating necrosis may result in lesions similar to those seen with brain abscess. With MRI, areas of focal encephalitis produce areas of decreased signal intensity on T1-weighted images and areas of increased signal intensity on T2-weighted images (Fig. 7.119, B and C). Enhancement occurs with gadolinium, and in some cases, an abscess-like configuration can result (Fig. 7.119D).

Herpes encephalitis in childhood deserves some special attention. In type II infections, the most common infection in the perinatal period, involvement of the brain is diffuse and massive, often resulting in total destruction of the brain and subsequent cystic encephalomalacia. All of this has been covered earlier in the section on TORCH infections. Herpes 1 infection, on the other hand, is the type of herpes infection contracted after birth. The findings in these cases

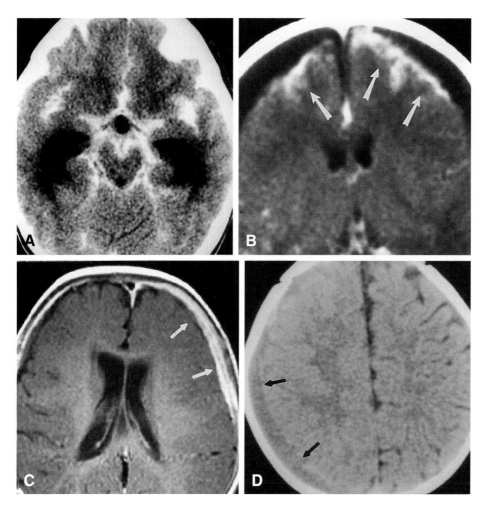

FIGURE 7.118. Meningitis. A. Note the marked enhancement of the meninges after administration of contrast in this patient with tuberculous meningitis. Such enhancement does not usually occur with ordinary meningitis. **B.** Subdural empyemas are seen on both sides. There is some enhancement of the underlying cerebral cortex (arrows), indicating associated cerebritis. **C.** Another patient with MR demonstration of a gadolinium-enhancing subdural empyema (arrows). **D.** In this patient, the subdural empyema (arrows), because of high protein content, shows increased density. Also note that the ipsilateral hemisphere is compressed and edematous. There are no remaining sulci and gyri.

resemble those seen in adults. The infection actually is a reactivation of the virus in the trigeminal ganglion (6). Thereafter, there is involvement of the temporal lobe, but eventually more, if not all, of the brain becomes involved. It is the initial temporal lobe involvement, however, that strongly signals the fact that herpes 1 infection is the problem (Fig. 7.120). Herpes encephalitis also can diffusely involve the cortex and subcortical white matter (9).

An interesting type of encephalitis, although not particularly common, is brainstem encephalitis (13–17). Also referred to as mesenrhombencephalitis (18), it usually is caused by a viral infection, including herpes. Clinical findings center around the brainstem, and with CT and MRI, swelling and edema of the brainstem becomes apparent. Another interesting feature of viral encephalitis deals with varicella encephalitis, which generally produces very little in the way of imaging findings during the course of the disease. However, infarction of the basal ganglia can occur after the infection (12, 19). Gyral calcifications after purulent meningitis have been documented (20), and gyriform and punctate calcifications have been seen after viral encephalitis (21).

REFERENCES

1. Jamieson DH. Imaging intracranial tuberculosis in childhood. Pediatr Radiol 1995;25:165–170.
2. Tien RD, Chu PK, Hesselink JR, et al. Intracranial cryptococcosis in immunocompromised patients: CT and MR findings in 29 cases. AJR 1991;156:1245–1251.
3. Caldemeyer KS, Mathews VP, Edwards-Brown MK, et al. Central nervous system cryptococcosis: parenchymal calcification and large gelatinous pseudocysts. AJNR 1997;18:107–109.
4. Chen C-Y, Huang C-C, Chang Y-C. Subdural empyema in 10 infants: US characteristics and clinical correlates. Radiology 1998;207:609–617.
5. Friedland IR, Paris MM, Rinderknecht S, et al. Cranial computed tomographic scans have little impact on management of bacterial meningitis. Am J Dis Child 1992;146:1484–1487.
6. Hooijboer A, van der Vliet AM, Sinnige LF. Tuberculous meningitis in native Dutch children: a report of four cases. Pediatr Radiol 1996;26:542–546.
7. Schoeman JF, Van Zyl LE, Laubscher JA, et al. Effect of corticosteroids on intracranial pressure, computed tomographic findings, and clinical outcome in young children with tuberculosis meningitis. Pediatrics 1997;99:226–231.
8. Khong P-L, Ho H-K, Cheng P-W, et al. Childhood acute disseminated encephalomyelitis: the role of brain and spinal cord MRI. Pediatr Radiol 2002;32:59–66.

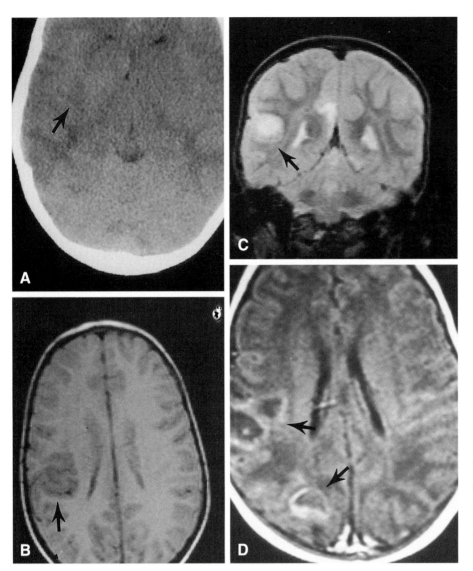

FIGURE 7.119. Viral encephalitis. A. On this CT scan, there is very little abnormality to be seen. There may be a vague hypodense area in the right parietal region (arrow). **B.** T1-weighted MR image demonstrates an area of low signal intensity (arrow) consistent with edema. **C.** T2-weighted coronal image demonstrates increased signal intensity in the area of inflammation (arrow). **D.** Another patient with herpes encephalitis, whose T1-weighted MR image with gadolinium enhancement demonstrates numerous areas of inflammation with enhancing rings (arrows).

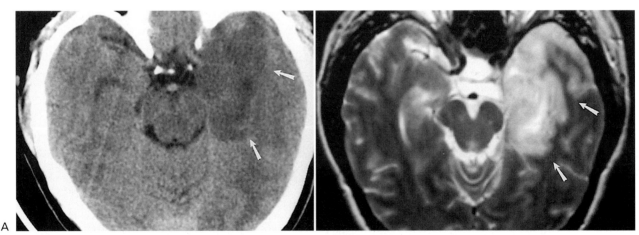

FIGURE 7.120. Herpes encephalitis: temporal lobe involvement. A. On the CT study, note the hypodense left temporal lobe (arrows). **B.** The T2-weighted MR study demonstrates increased signal intensity in the same area (arrows).

9. Leonard JR, Moran CJ, Cross D III. MR imaging of Herpes simplex type I encephalitis in infants and young children: a separate pattern of findings. AJR 2000;174:1651–1655.

10. Noah DL, Bresee JS, Gorensek MJ. Cluster of five children with acute encephalopathy associated with cat-scratch disease in south Florida. Pediatr Infect Dis J 1995;14:866–869.

11. Ono J, Shimizu K, Harada K, et al. Characteristic MR features of encephalitis caused by Epstein-Barr virus: a case report. Pediatr Radiol 1998;28:569–570.

12. Kumada S, Kusaka H, Koaniwa M. Encephalomyelitis subsequent to mycoplasma infection with elevated serum anti-Gal antibody. Pediatr Neurol 1997;16:241–244.

13. Darling CF, Larsen MB, Byrd SE, et al. MR and CT imaging patterns in post-varicella encephalitis. Pediatr Radiol 1995;25:241–244.

14. Gregorio L, Sutton CL, Lee DA. Central pontine myelinolysis in a previously healthy 4-year-old child with acute rotavirus gastroenteritis. Pediatrics 1997;99:738–743.

15. Shian WJ, Chi CS. Fatal brainstem encephalitis caused by Epstein-Barr virus. Pediatr Radiol 1994;24:596–597.

16. Unsal E, Olgun N, Sarialioglu F, et al. Posterior fossa pseudotumour due to vital encephalitis in a child. Pediatr Radiol 1997;27:788–789.

17. Tarhan NC, Firat A, Otken A, et al. Central pontine myelinolysis secondary to cytomegalovirus hepatitis in a 10-month-old child. Pediatr Radiol 2003;33:44.

18. Soo MS, Tien RD, Gray L, et al. Mesenrhombencephalitis: MR findings in nine patients. AJR 1993;160:1089–1093.

19. Silverstein FS, Brunberg JA. Postvaricella basal ganglia infarction in children. AJNR 1995;16:449–452.

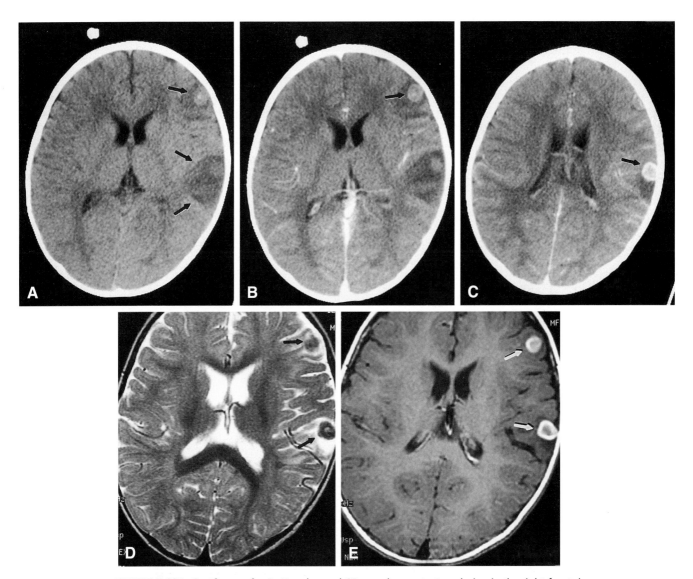

FIGURE 7.121. Cysticercosis. A. Unenhanced CT scan demonstrates a lesion in the right frontal area (upper arrow) with a central calcification and surrounding edema. Another lesion (lower arrows) has a central density with surrounding edema. **B.** After contrast administration, the anterior lesion (arrow) shows minimal peripheral enhancement. **C.** The lower lesion, however, demonstrates more pronounced peripheral enhancement (arrow). **D.** T2-weighted MR image demonstrates both of the lesions (arrows), but the posterior lesion shows more surrounding high-signal-intensity edema. This is the more active lesion. **E.** Gadolinium-enhanced, T1-weighted image demonstrates ring-like enhancement of both lesions (arrows).

20. Sener RN. Gyriform calcifications following purulent meningitis. Pediatr Radiol 1993;23:491.
21. Somekh E, Glode MP, Reiley TT, et al. Multiple intracranial calcifications after western equine encephalitis. Pediatr Infect Dis J 1991;10:408–409.

Neurocysticercosis

Neurocysticercosis is a parasitic infection caused by the encysted form of *Taenia solium*. Humans are the intermediate hosts, and the organism usually is acquired by accidental ingestion of the tapeworm eggs. The eggs subsequently hatch in the small intestine, burrow into the mucosa, and penetrate venules to enter the circulation. Thereafter, when they lodge in the brain, there is variable expression of the disease, but seizures are almost invariably present (1). When the larvae die, antigen stimulus results in local inflammation, breakdown of the blood-brain barrier, and surrounding edema. With contrast administration, ring-like enhancement of the periphery of the lesion is seen with both CT and MRI (Fig. 7.121). Later, the dead larvae undergo calcification, and a small punctate calcification in the center of the lesion is seen, best with CT (Fig. 7.121A).

REFERENCE

1. Chang KH, Lee JH, Han MH, et al. The role of contrast-enhanced MR imaging in the diagnosis of neurocysticercosis. AJNR 1991;12:509–512.

BRAIN TUMOR

A detailed discussion of brain tumors is beyond the scope of this book, and only a summary of their findings and investigation is provided. In most cases, with modern imaging, it is relatively easy to detect the presence of a tumor. Assigning histologic type is more difficult and of questionable importance, as almost all of these lesions will be biopsied before treatment. **Therefore, it is more important that the imager locate the lesion and identify critical surrounding structures than try to assign a histologic diagnosis in every case.**

Brain tumors in the neonatal period are relatively rare, a little more common in young infants, but quite common in older infants and children. In newborn infants both supratentorial and infratentorial lesions occur with almost the same frequency (1, 2), but in the older child posterior fossa tumors predominate. In the neonate, the most common presenting finding of a brain tumor is a markedly enlarged, or rapidly enlarging, head. One often believes that hydrocephalus resulting from a nontumoral cause is the problem, because the tumors, no matter what type, tend to be large when the patients present (Fig. 7.122). The more common of these include germ cell tumors or teratomas (3), gliomas, and neuroepithelial tumors (2). One also may encounter choroid plexus papillomas (4, 5), hamartomas (6), hemangiomas (7), rhabdoid tumor (8), and even craniopharyngiomas. Choroid plexus papillomas are more common in infancy than in childhood and produce large, lobulated masses in the ventricle (Fig. 7.123) along with excessive accumulation of cerebral spinal fluid and hydrocephalus (5). Some of these tumors are malignant and are recognized by their invasion of the brain parenchyma. Most often, the choroid plexus papillomas are unilateral, but bilateral occurrence can occur (5). Primary neuroblastoma is rare and may be solid or cystic. Most likely, what has been called primary neuroblastoma in the past is really a primitive neuroectodermal tumor. Neuroblastoma from the neck also can extend into the cranial vault (9).

In older infants and children, posterior fossa tumors, primarily involving the cerebellum or pons, include medulloblastoma, glioma, ependymoma, and hemangioblastoma. Medulloblastomas and gliomas are most common, and tumors in the pons are almost always gliomas. The most

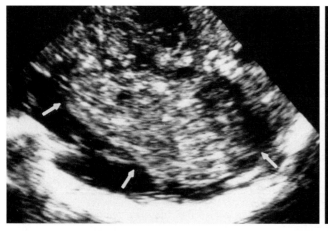
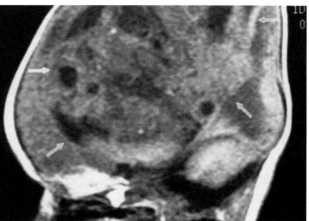

FIGURE 7.122. Neonatal teratoma. A. Sagittal sonogram demonstrates a large, echogenic heterogenous and lobulated mass (arrows). **B.** Sagittal, T1-weighted MR image demonstrates the marked heterogenicity of the tumor.

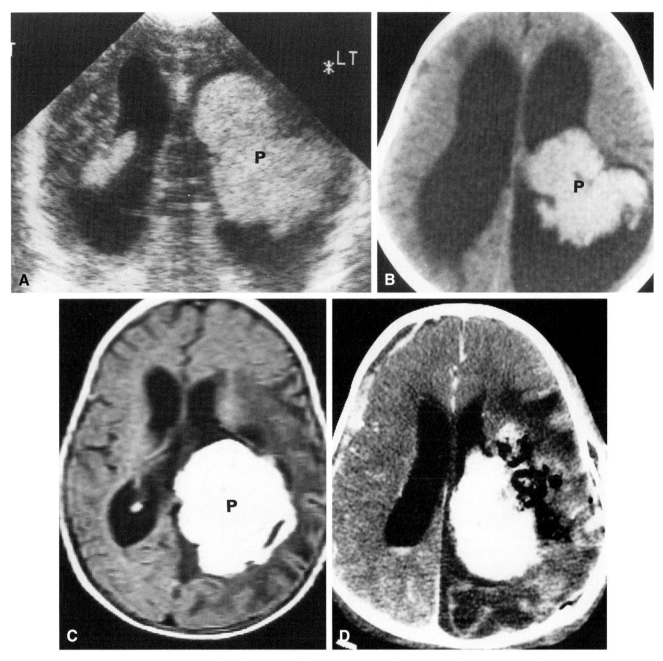

FIGURE 7.123. Choroid plexus papilloma. A. Coronal sonogram demonstrates a large, echogenic, lobulated choroid plexus papilloma (P) in the dilated left ventricle. The right ventricle also is dilated. The large echogenic area in the right ventricle is the normal choroid plexus. **B.** Axial CT study demonstrates a dilated lateral ventricle and the large papilloma (P). **C.** T1-weighted MR study of another patient demonstrates a large choroid plexus papilloma (P). It shows high signal intensity, indicating the presence of fluid with high protein content. There is edema in the adjacent brain tissue (low-density area). The ventricles are dilated. **D.** Another slice demonstrates invasion of the parenchyma by this malignant choroid plexus papilloma. Extensive surrounding brain edema is present.

common supratentorial tumor is some type of glioma, or a craniopharyngioma. Other tumors encountered include ependymomas, meningiomas (1, 10, 11), choroid plexus papillomas, hamartomas, and atypical teratomas or dysgerminomas. Primary lymphoma is relatively rare (12, 13).

Pinealomas are now generally considered to be atypical teratomas (dysgerminomas), and often these tumors occur at two sites, anteriorly just in front of the third ventricle and posteriorly around the pineal gland (14). The anterior tumors often produce endocrinologic problems such as diabetes insipidus, while the posterior tumors result in Parinaud's phenomenon. These tumors often calcify and can be detected on plain films but are more vividly demonstrated with CT or MRI (Fig. 7.124). Hamartomas of the tuber

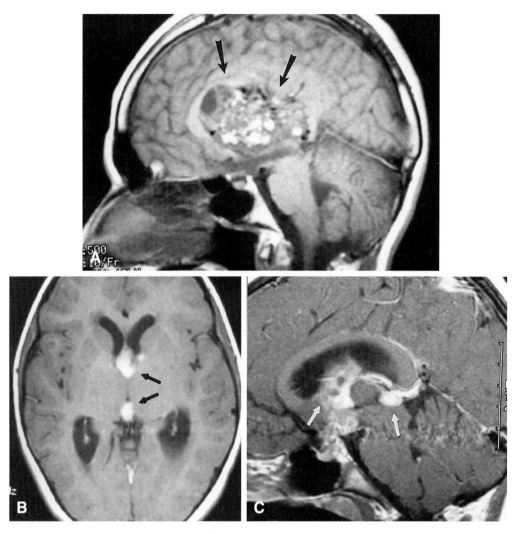

FIGURE 7.124. Atypical teratoma (dysgerminoma). A. Large, atypical teratoma (arrows) with characteristic heterogeneous signal pattern. **B. Double teratomas (dysgerminomas).** On this T1-weighted, gadolinium-enhanced MR image, note the double tumors (arrows) in their characteristic location. **C.** Sagittal view demonstrates the typical location of the tumors (arrows).

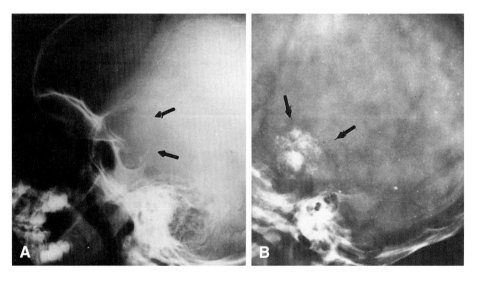

FIGURE 7.125. Craniopharyngioma: calcifications. A. Note the typical curvilinear calcifications (arrows) in this suprasellar craniopharyngioma extending into the pituitary fossa and causing it to enlarge. The coronal suture also is spread, indicating increased intracranial pressure. **B.** Heavily calcified craniopharyngioma in a 1-day-old infant (arrows). (From Milhorat TH. Hydrocephalus and the cerebrospinal fluid. Baltimore: Williams & Wilkins, 1972, with permission.)

cinereum are not uncommon in children and are associated with endocrinologic abnormality (15). They can be large and their location just inferior to the third ventricle serves as a clue to diagnosis. Optic gliomas can occur in isolated form or in association with neurofibromatosis. They produce enlargement of the optic canal, deformities of the optic chiasm, and in some cases may extend along the optic tracts to the occipital lobes of the brain (16).

Craniopharyngioma characteristically are mixed cystic and solid tumors and produce calcifications in the suprasellar region (17). These may be curvilinear or irregular, and when the tumor extends into the sella, the sella can be enlarged (Fig. 7.125). Visual disturbances often are the first presentation, as the lesion can become extremely large before it produces increased intracranial pressure. CT and MRI readily demonstrate the extent of the tumor (Fig. 7.126). Other intrasellar tumors are less common in chil-

dren than in adults, but still one can encounter a variety of adenomas, including the microadenoma. If adenomas are large enough, they produce enlargement of the sella, which can be seen on plain films (Fig. 7.127A). However, most often CT or MRI is required for their delineation. Bleeding into adenomas can occur and constitutes the syndrome of pituitary apoplexy (18, 19) (Fig. 7.127B). Gadolinium-enhanced MRI can identify pituitary adenomas most readily (Fig. 7.127, C and D). Rarely, one can encounter a suprasellar retinoblastoma, usually an extension of a ocular retinoblastoma but some times occurring before the primary lesion (20).

Gangliogliomas are a benign form of astrocytoma which can be identified by their occurrence in; (1) patients under two years, and (2) the frontoparietal region. They have a peripheral dura-based solid component along with a central cystic component (20, 21) (Fig. 7.128). The tumors often

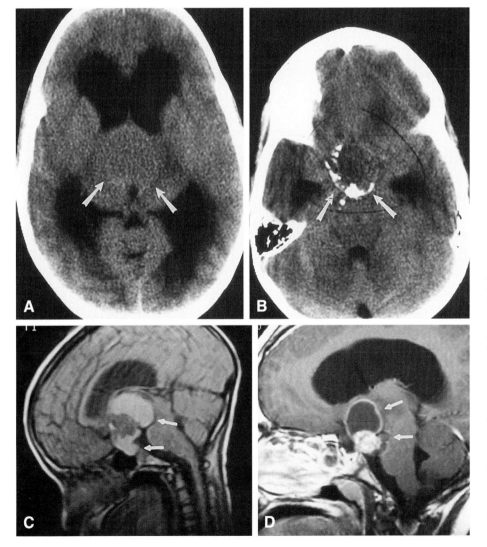

FIGURE 7.126. Craniopharyngioma: CT and MR findings. A. Note the large suprasellar mass (arrows) with faint calcification around its rim. Marked hydrocephalus is present. **B.** Lower cut demonstrates typical calcifications (arrows) within the walls of the tumor. **C.** T1-weighted, sagittal MR study demonstrates the heterogeneous nature of this tumor. There is a large suprasellar cystic component (upper arrow) with high signal intensity because of increased protein content. There also is extension of the cystic component (lower arrow) into the sella. Between lies solid tumor. **D.** Another patient whose T1-weighted, sagittal, gadolinium-enhanced MR image demonstrates a solid (lower arrow) and cystic (upper arrow) component to the tumor. There is enhancement of the tumor and the cyst wall.

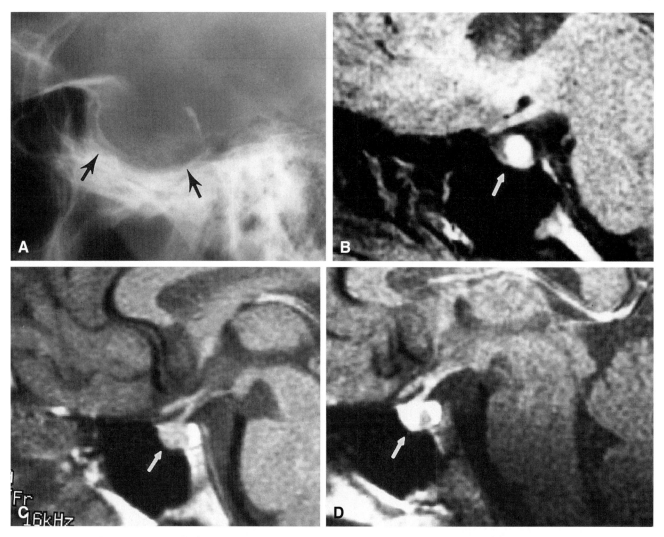

FIGURE 7.127. Pituitary tumors. A. Note the enlarged sella (arrows) resulting from an underlying adenoma. **B.** Note the high signal intensity (arrow) of the pituitary gland in a patient with hemorrhage causing pituitary apoplexy. The underlying lesion was an adenoma. **C. Microadenoma.** Note the relatively normal appearance of the pituitary gland. The anterior lobe (arrow) may be slightly enlarged. **D.** With gadolinium, there is clear-cut enhancement of the anterior lobe (arrow) consistent with an underlying adenoma.

produce bulging of the adjacent calvarium. Otherwise, astrocytomas or gliomas in the supratentorial compartment produce nonspecific findings, except that they often are cystic.

Posterior fossa tumors also are readily identified with both CT and MR. However, the findings often are variable even with the most common posterior fossa tumor, the medulloblastoma. Both gliomas and medulloblastomas may show cystic changes, but gliomas generally show them much more frequently. Ependymomas are intraventricular tumors and tend not to demonstrate cystic change, but they also can be extraventricular (22). Calcifications occur most commonly in slow-growing gliomas, but also can be seen with medulloblastomas and ependymomas. In the end,

therefore, even though one may be able to categorize a good many of these tumors (Fig. 7.129), there is enough overlap that absolute histologic definition on the basis of imaging findings is not possible in all cases.

The benign lipoma of the corpus callosum should be mentioned. This lesion can occur anywhere along the corpus callosum and can be associated with calcification. Occasionally, these lipomas can extend extracranially (23). With lipoma of the corpus callosum an area of fatty radiolucency occasionally can be seen on plain films, but the tumor is more readily demonstrable with CT, ultrasound, or MR. With CT, it is radiolucent, whereas with MRI, it shows high signal intensity on T1-weighted images, and ultrasound demonstrates it to be highly echoic (24, 25) (Fig.

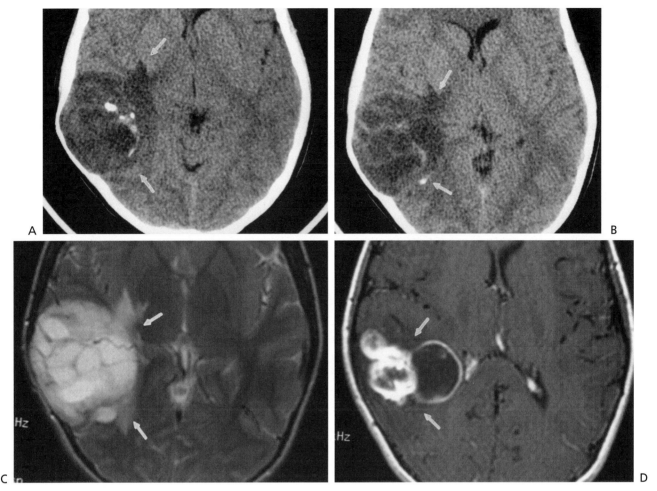

FIGURE 7.128. Supratentorial glioma. A. Low-grade glioma: ganglioglioma. Note the hypodense tumor with calcifications (arrows). It is slow growing and has eroded the calvarium and caused it to bulge. **B.** Another cut demonstrates the multicystic appearance of the tumor (arrows). **C.** T2-weighted MR image demonstrates high signal intensity in the multiple cystic areas in the tumor. **D.** Another T1-weighted image with gadolinium enhancement demonstrates uptake in the nodular tumor (arrows) and enhancement of the wall of one of the cystic components.

7.130). Lipomas of the corpus callosum and pericallosal region also has been documented with frontonasal dysplasia (26).

Meningeal carcinomatosis is not common but does occur (27–29). It has been demonstrated that enhancement of the meninges is best seen on FLAIR (27) or T1 gadolinium-enhanced (28) image sequences. The findings are difficult to differentiate from those of inflammatory meningitis and viral encephalitis (28). Often, they are so diffused that they can be missed (Fig. 7.131).

Spectroscopy in the analysis of brain tumors has recently come on the scene but may be of limited practical value when it comes to differentiating one tumor from another (30). Overall, however, it is CT and especially MRI that are the primary imaging modalities for the investigation of brain tumors. Sonography can be used in the neonate (31).

REFERENCES

1. Ambrosino MM, Hernanz-Schulman M, Genieser NB, et al. Brain tumors in infants less than a year of age. Pediatr Radiol 1988;19:6–8.
2. Buetow PC, Smirniotopoulos JG, Done S. Congenital brain tumors: a review of 45 cases. AJR 1990;155:587–593.
3. Storr U, Rupprecht T, Bornemann A, et al. Congenital intracerebral teratoma: a rare differential diagnosis in newborn hydrocephalus. Pediatr Radiol 1997;27:262–264.
4. Levy ML, Goldfarb A, Hyder DJ. Choroid plexus tumors in children: significance of stromal invasion. Neurosurgery 2001;48: 303–309.
5. Cila A, Ozturk C, Senaati S. Bilateral choroid plexus carcinoma of the lateral ventricles. US, CT and MR findings. Pediatr Radiol 1992;22:136–137.
6. Gubaud L, Rode V, Saint-Pierre G, et al. Giant hypothalamic hamartoma: an unusual neonatal tumor. Pediatr Radiol 1995;25: 17–18.

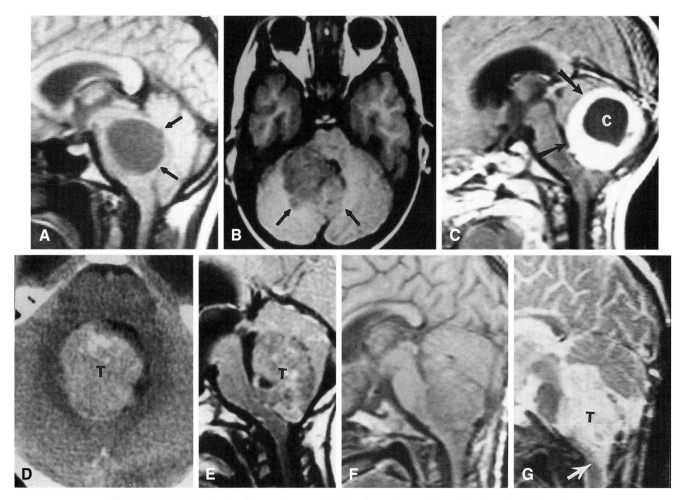

FIGURE 7.129. Posterior fossa tumors. A. Pontine glioma. Note the low-signal-intensity tumor (arrows) in the characteristic location of a pontine glioma. **B. Astrocytoma.** Note the nonspecific features of this lobulated low-signal-intensity astrocytoma (arrows). It is causing some compression of the fourth ventricle, as seen on the T1-weighted image. **C. Cystic astrocytoma.** Gadolinium-enhanced, T1-weighted image demonstrates uptake in a rim of tumor (arrows) surrounding a low-signal cyst (C). **D. Medulloblastoma.** CT study demonstrates the central location of the intraventricular tumor (T) with punctate calcifications. **E.** Same patient demonstrating the tumor (T) on a gadolinium-enhanced image. The tumor shows patchy uptake and is compressing the fourth ventricle anteriorly. **F. Ependymoma.** Note the intraventricular tumor, which appears to be extending into the foramen magnum. **G.** T2-weighted image of the tumor (T) with high signal intensity clearly demonstrates that it has passed through the fourth ventricular foramina and entered the spinal canal (arrow). This is characteristic of ependymomas.

7. Karmazyn B, Michovitz S, Sirota L, et al. Intracranial cavernous hemangioma in a neonate. Pediatr Radiol 2001;31:610–612.

8. Evans A, Ganatra R, Morris SJ. Imaging features of primary malignant rhabdoid tumour of the brain. Pediatr Radiol 2001; 31:631–633.

9. Goldberg RM, Keller IA, Schonfeld SM, et al. Intracranial route of a cervical neuroblastoma through skull base foramina. Pediatr Radiol 1996;26:715–716.

10. Lirng JF, Enterline DS, Tien RD, et al. MRI of papillary meningiomas in children. Pediatr Radiol 1995;25:S9–S13.

11. Starshak RJ. Cystic meningiomas in children: a diagnostic challenge. Pediatr Radiol 1996;26:711–714.

12. Schulman H, Hertzanu Y, Maor E, et al. Primary lymphoma of brain in childhood. Pediatr Radiol 1991;21:434–435.

13. Vazquez E, Lucaya J, Castellote A, et al. Neuroimaging in pediatrics leukemia and lymphoma: differential diagnosis. Radiographics 2002;22:1411–1428.

14. Swischuk LE, Bryan RN. Double midline intracranial atypical teratomas (a recognizable neuroendocrinologic syndrome). AJR 1974;122:517–524.

15. Boyko OB, Curnes JT, Oakes WJ, et al. Hamartomas of the tuber cinereum: CT, MR, and pathologic findings. AJR 1991; 156:1053–1058.

16. Lourie GL, Osborne DR, Kirks DR. Involvement of posterior visual pathways by optic nerve gliomas. Pediatr Radiol 1986;16: 271–274.

17. Pusey E, Kortman KE, Flannigan BD, et al. MR of craniopharyngiomas: tumor delineation and characterization. AJR 1987;149:383–388.

18. Poussaint TY, Barnes PD, Anthony DC, et al. Hemorrhagic

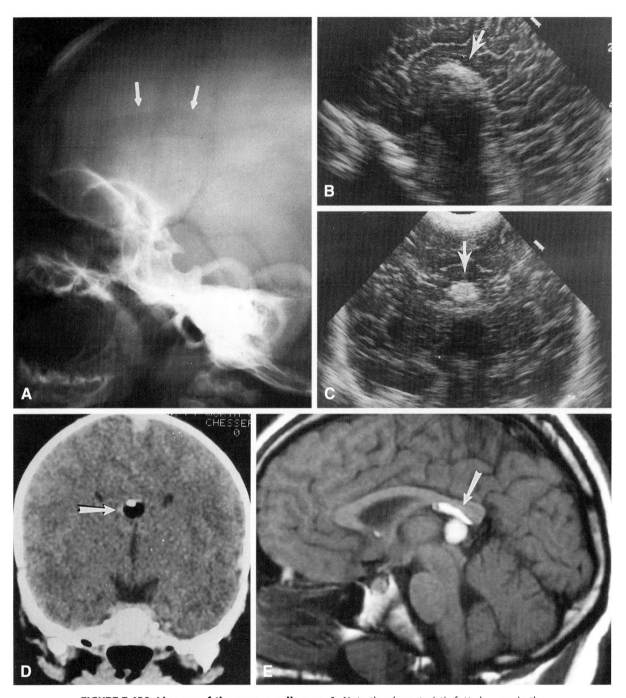

FIGURE 7.130. Lipoma of the corpus callosum. A. Note the characteristic fatty lucency in the anterior portion of the brain (arrows). **B.** Similar findings on ultrasound where the lipoma is very echogenic (arrow). **C.** Frontal view demonstrates the midline position of the lipoma (arrow). **D.** In another patient, a CT scan demonstrates typical lucency of fat in the region of the lipoma (arrow). A punctate calcification is seen in association. **E.** T1-weighted MR image demonstrates a lipoma in the splenium of the corpus callosum (arrow). It has extended into the ambient cistern. (**A** courtesy of R. I. McPherson, M.D.)

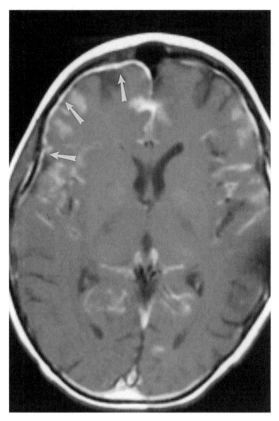

FIGURE 7.131. Meningeal enhancement with metastatic disease. Note the diffuse meningeal enhancement (arrows) in this patient with diffuse carcinomatosis.

MR images of meningitis, viral encephalitis, and leptomeningeal metastasis. AJNR 2002;23:535–542.

30. Norfray JF, Romita T, Byrd SE, et al. Clinical impact of MR spectroscopy when MR imaging is indeterminate for pediatric brain tumors. AJR 1999;173:119–125.
31. Simanovsky N, Taylor GA. Sonography of brain tumors in infants and young children. Pediatr Radiol 2001;31:392–398.

INTRACRANIAL CYSTS

One can encounter a variety of intracranial cysts or cystic structures in infants and children. These include developmental subarachnoid cysts, dermoid cysts, cysts within neoplasms, colloid cysts of the third ventricle, Rathke's pouch cysts, and cysts of the pineal gland. Arachnoid cysts can occur as isolated abnormalities (Fig. 7.132, A and B), both supratentorially and infratentorially, but also can be seen in the Hunter-Hurler syndrome and with agenesis of the corpus callosum in the Dandy-Walker syndrome. Colloid cysts of the third ventricle characteristically are located just anterior to the third ventricle and may produce obstructive hydrocephalus. Because they often have high cholesterol content, they will show increased signal intensity on T1-weighted MR images and decreased signal intensity on T2-weighted images. They can be watched (1) and a case of rupture of a small cyst after trauma has been documented (2).

Rathke's pouch cysts occur just above the sella (Fig. 7.132, C and D) and often are asymptomatic (3). They show enhancement of the wall with gadolinium-enhanced MRI (4) and, when large, can produce symptoms (5). Many have high protein content and therefore show high intensity signal on T1-weighted MR images and low intensity signal on T2-weighted images (6). Some of these cysts also can calcify (7). Overall, these cysts are so benign that, once identified, these patients probably could be followed clinically without further imaging (8). Cysts of the pineal gland usually are innocuous (Fig. 7.132E) but also show enhancement of their rims on MRI with contrast (6). In addition, they have been shown to collapse and disappear on their own (9).

A note regarding porencephalic cysts is in order. These cysts are acquired and the result of destruction of the brain parenchyma from intracranial bleeding, infection, or infarction. They are identified by the fact that they communicate with the ventricular system. The demonstration of any of these intracranial cysts is rather straightforward with all imaging modalities.

REFERENCES

pituitary adenomas of adolescence. AJNR 1996;17:1907–1912.
19. Shah SA, Pereira JK, Becker CJ, et al. Pituitary apoplexy in adolescence: case report. Pediatr Radiol 1995;25:S26–S27.
20. Chang YW, Yoon H-K, Han BK. Suprasellar retinoblastoma in a 5-month-old girl. Pediatr Radiol 2002;32:869–871.
21. Serra A, Strain J, Ruyle S. Case report. Desmoplastic cerebral astrocytoma of infancy: report and review of the imaging characteristics. AJR 1996;166:1459–1461.
22. Fukui MB, Hogg JP, Martinez AJ. Extraaxial ependymoma of the posterior fossa. AJNR 1997;17:1179–1181.
23. Lin K-L, Wang H-S, Lui T-N. Sonographic diagnosis of a corpus callosum lipoma with extracranial extension in an infant. J Ultrasound Med 1995;14:537–541.
24. Auriemma A, Poggiani C, Menghini P, et al. Lipoma of the corpus callosum in a neonate: sonographic evaluation. Pediatr Radiol 1993;23:155–156.
25. Fisher RM, Cremin BJ. Lipoma of the corpus callosum: diagnosis by ultrasound and magnetic resonance. Pediatr Radiol 1988;18:409–410.
26. Alzoum MA, Alorainy IA, Husain MA, et al. Multiple pericallosal lipomas in two siblings with frontonasal dysplasia. AJNR 2002;23:730–731.
27. Tsuchiya K, Katase S, Yoshino A, et al. FLAIR MR imaging for diagnosing intracranial meningeal carcinomatosis. AJR 2001;176:1585–1588.
28. Singh SK, Leeds NE, Ginsberg LE. MR imaging of leptomeningeal metastases: comparison of three sequences. AJNR 2002;23:817–821.
29. Lee JH, Na DG, Choi KH, et al. Subcortical low intensity on

1. Pollock BE, Huston J III. Natural history of asymptomatic colloid cysts of the third ventricle. J Neurosurg 1999;91:364–369.
2. Lipinski CA, Bechtel K, Pollack I. Acute rupture of an arachnoid cyst after a minor head injury. Pediatr Emerg Care 1997;13:27–28.
3. Christophe C, Flameant-Durand J, Hanquinet S, et al. MRI in

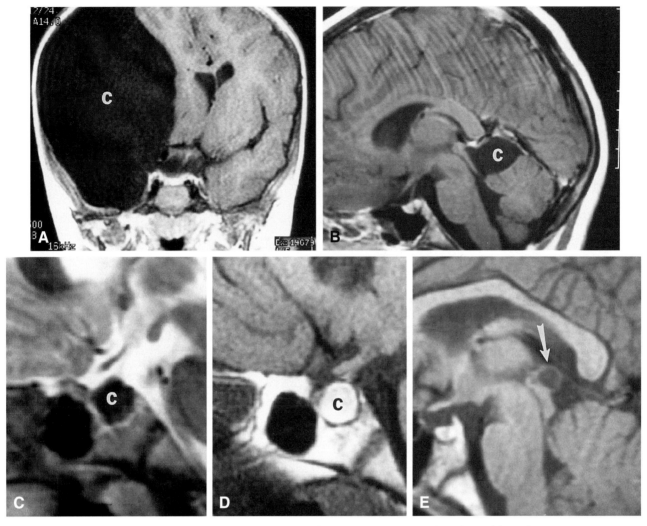

FIGURE 7.132. Intracranial cysts. A. Arachnoid cyst. Large arachnoid cyst (C) producing marked displacement of the brain. **B.** Small arachnoid cyst (C) located in the quadrigeminal plate cistern region. **C. Rathke's pouch cyst.** Note the typical location of the cyst (C). **D.** T2-weighted image demonstrates increased signal intensity in the cyst (C). **E. Pineal cyst.** Note the characteristic location and appearance of a pineal cyst (arrow) on this T1-weighted image.

seven cases of Rathke's cleft cyst in infants and children. Pediatr Radiol 1993;23:79–82.

4. Sumida M, Uozumi T, Mukada K, et al. Rathke cleft cysts: correlation of enhanced MR and surgical findings. AJNR 1994;15: 525–532.

5. Meyer JR, Quint DJ, McKeever PE, et al. Giant Rathke cleft cyst. AJNR 1994;15:533–536.

6. Hayashi Y, Tachibana O, Muramatsu N, et al. Rathke cleft cyst: MR and biomedical analysis of cyst content. J Comp Assist Tomogr 1999'23:34–38.

7. Nakasu Y, Makasu S, Nakajima M, et al. Atypical Rathke's cleft cyst associated with ossification. AJNR 1999;20:1287–1289.

8. Barboriak DP, Lee L, Provenzale JM. Serial MR imaging of pineal cysts: implications for natural history and follow-up. AJR 2001; 176:737–743.

9. Sener RN. The pineal gland: a comparative MR imaging study in children and adults with respect to normal anatomical variations and pineal cysts. Pediatr Radiol 1995;25:245–248.

MISCELLANEOUS ABNORMALITIES OF THE BRAIN

Accessory Ventricles

Accessory ventricles are not true ventricles, but rather potential or actual arachnoid spaces. When encountered, although initially puzzling, they usually are of no particular consequence to the patient. They consist of the cavum septum pellucidum, cavum vergae, cavum interpositum (cisterna interventricularis), and cisterna vena magnae. The cavum septum pellucidum and cavum vergae commonly are seen in premature infants. Occasionally, the septum cavum pellucidum, located in the septum pellucidum between the two lateral ventricles, can become large and cystic, but most often it is small (Fig. 7.133). The cavum

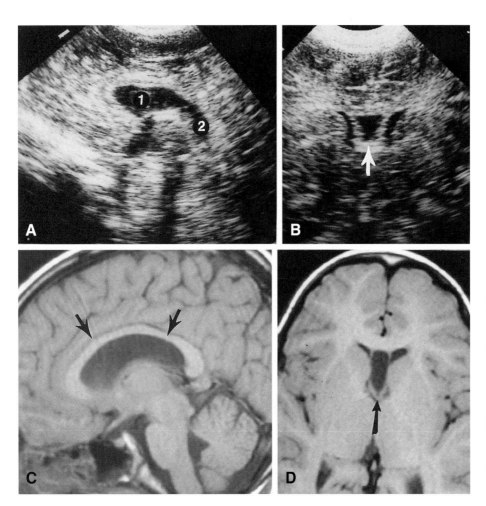

FIGURE 7.133. Accessory ventricles. A. Midsagittal ultrasonogram demonstrates the anterior septum cavum pellucidum (1) and posterior cavum vergae (2). **B.** Coronal image demonstrates the central location of the septum cavum pellucidum (arrow) between the two lateral ventricles. **C.** Sagittal, T1-weighted MR image in another patient demonstrates the low-signal-intensity septum cavum pellucidum located just below the corpus callosum (arrows). **D.** Axial image demonstrates the cavum septum pellucidum (arrow) located between the two lateral ventricles.

vergae lies directly behind the septum cavum pellucidum and above the third ventricle. It usually is seen in conjunction with this latter structure (Fig. 7.133). The septum velum interpositum lies behind the third ventricle; and the cisterna vena magnae, just below the septum velum interpositum. These latter structures were more commonly seen when pneumoencephalography was in vogue.

Absent Septum Pellucidum

Absence of the septum pellucidum, in whole or in part, is not an uncommon anomaly. It is frequently seen with the Arnold-Chiari malformation. It also is a feature of septo-optic dysplasia. In either case, the lateral ventricles assume a heart-shaped configuration, and the septum is absent in whole or in part (Fig. 7.134). In septo-optic dysplasia, smaller than normal optic nerves also are present and can be demonstrated with CT or MRI.

Agenesis of the Corpus Callosum

Agenesis of the corpus callosum can be complete or partial or the corpus callosum simply may be hypoplastic (1, 2).

Although it can be seen as an isolated anomaly, it frequently is associated with other central nervous system congenital abnormalities. It not uncommonly is seen with Dandy-Walker cysts, and even in those patients where no anomalies co-exist, some degree of mental retardation often is present.

The imaging findings are typical and consist of separation of abnormally slanted lateral ventricles by a high-rising third ventricle (Fig. 7.135). The foramina of Monro are somewhat elongated and transversely placed to accommodate the high-rising third ventricle. Overall, the configuration of the third ventricle and slanted lateral ventricles has led to descriptions such as "longhorn" and "happy moose" signs (Fig. 7.135). On lateral view, absence or hypoplasia of the corpus callosum is best identified with ultrasound and MRI. On MRI, the findings are straightforward (Fig. 7.135), while with ultrasound, they consist of absence of the normal echogenic corpus callosum above the third ventricle, elevation of the third ventricle, and a radiating pattern of the pericallosal sulci. Interhemispheric arachnoid cysts can be associated (3), and some can be extremely large (4) (Fig. 7.136).

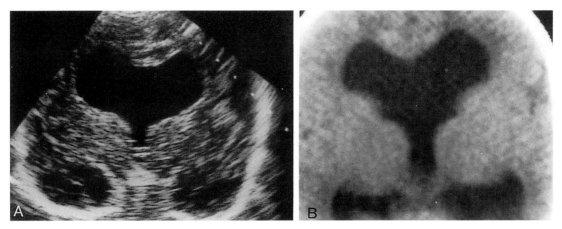

FIGURE 7.134. Absent septum pellucidum. A. Coronal sonogram demonstrates dilated lateral ventricles and absence of the septum cavum pellucidum. The heart-shaped configuration is characteristic. This patient also had hydrocephalus resulting from aqueductal stenosis. **B.** Similar findings on a CT study.

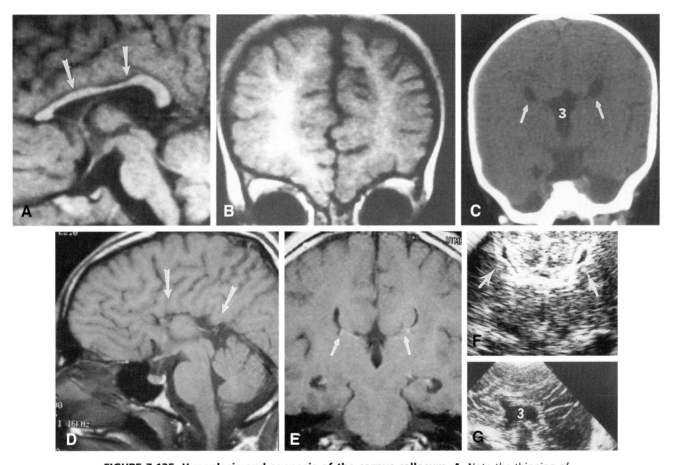

FIGURE 7.135. Hypoplasia and agenesis of the corpus callosum. A. Note the thinning of the corpus callosum (arrows). **B.** Same patient showing associated absence of the falx and interdigitation of the hemispheres. **C.** CT study in another patient demonstrates a high-rising third ventricle (3) and typical horizontal orientation of the lateral ventricles resulting in the "longhorn" sign (arrows). **D.** Midsagittal MR study in another patient demonstrates total absence of the corpus callosum (arrows). Also note how the overlying sulci radiate outward. This is typical of agenesis of the corpus callosum and also is seen with ultrasound. **E.** Coronal view demonstrates the typical "longhorn" sign. **F.** Longhorn sign demonstrated on ultrasound (arrows). **G.** Sagittal ultrasound view demonstrates the high-rising third ventricle (3) and the typical outward radiating pattern of the sulci.

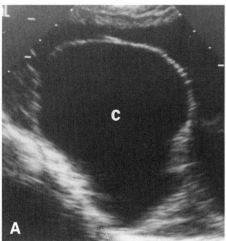 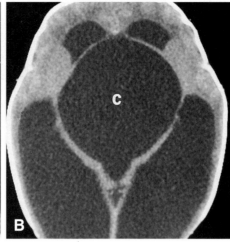

FIGURE 7.136. Interhemispheric cyst with agenesis of the corpus callosum. A. Sagittal sonogram demonstrates the large cyst (C) extending transtentorially into the posterior fossa. **B.** CT study demonstrates large cyst (C) and associated marked hydrocephalus.

REFERENCES

1. Bodensteiner J, Schaefer GB, Breeding L, et al. Hypoplasia of the corpus callosum: a study of 445 consecutive MRI scans. J Child Neurol 1993;9:47–49.
2. Rubinstein D, Youngman V, Hise JH, et al. Partial development of the corpus callosum. AJNR 1994;15:869–875.
3. Swett HA, Nixon GW. Agenesis of the corpus callosum with interhemispheric cyst. Radiology 1975;114:641–645.
4. Mori K. Giant interhemispheric cysts associated with agenesis of the corpus callosum. J Neurosurg 1992;76:224–230.

Anencephaly

Anencephaly is a gross deformity of the brain in which all but a small nubbin of midbrain and/or brainstem is absent. The calvarium is markedly underdeveloped and, except for its basal portions, is virtually absent (Fig. 7.137). Intracranial vessels are also underdeveloped, and considerable variation in the origin of the brachiocephalic vessels can occur.

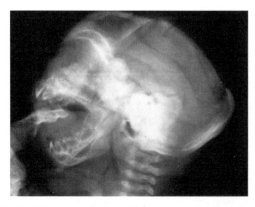

FIGURE 7.137. Anencephaly. Note the extremely small head, which shows development of only the face and base of the skull.

Holoprosencephaly (Arrhinencephaly)

This is a severe deformity of the forebrain (prosencephalon) in which there is failure of development of the interhemispheric fissure associated with abnormal callosal formation. The end result is a single midline ventricle, and the anomaly in its most extreme form is seen in the cyclops abnormality. In milder cases, only some degree of hypotelorism may be noted. Generally, the more severe the abnormality, the less the chance of survival, and infants with cyclops or cebocephalic deformity are either born dead or die shortly thereafter. In the most severe forms there is failure of the forebrain to separate into lobes (alobar holoprosencephaly). Infants with partial or incomplete lobation (semilobar holoprosencephaly) frequently survive, but are usually retarded. Many of these children have associated midline defects such as cleft palate and cleft nose and holoprosencephaly is commonly seen in the trisomy 13–15 syndromes.

Radiographically, in alobar holoprosencephaly the anterior fossa is extremely small (especially from front to back), and the orbital roofs arch higher than normal (Fig. 7.138). On frontal view there is extreme hypotelorism, trigonocephaly, and absence of the nasal bones. Associated intracranial abnormalities consist of absence of the olfactory tracts (arrhinencephaly) and hypoplasia of the internal carotid arteries.

On CT or MR, with holoprosencephaly there is failure of visualization of the falx and a large, fused central single ventricle is seen. The thalami are fused into a solid central mass and only a thin mantle of cerebral tissue remains. The third ventricle is small or absent, but the cerebellum and brainstem, along with the fourth ventricle, are relatively normal. These findings can be demonstrated with any imaging modality (Fig. 7.139). The pancake appearance of the remaining brain tissue in the anterior portion of the calvarium is characteristic (Fig. 7.139). With semilobar holo-

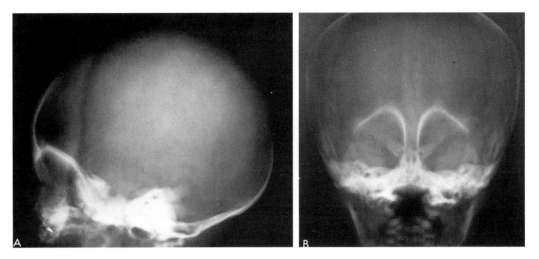

FIGURE 7.138. Arrhinencephaly (alobar holoprosencephaly). A. Lateral view showing extremely shallow anterior fossa. The coronal suture is in a far anterior position. **B.** Frontal view showing extreme hypotelorism commonly seen in these infants.

prosencephaly the single ventricular cavity is not as large, and there is more cerebral tissue remaining. The ventricle dilates more over its posterior aspect. The third ventricle is incorporated into the single ventricle, but the fourth ventricle remains relatively normal (Fig. 7.140). The septum pellucidum is absent in both types of holoprosencephaly.

Iniencephaly

Iniencephaly is a rare abnormality that is usually incompatible with life. There is extensive calvarial deficiency in the region of the occiput, a rather wide cervical spina bifida, and marked backward flexion of the head and cervical spine.

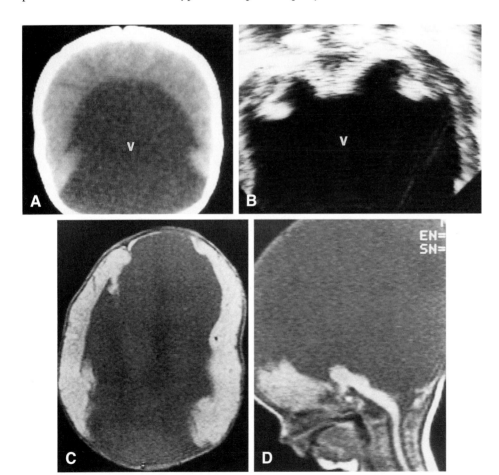

FIGURE 7.139. Alobar holoprosencephaly. A. Note the typical large, single ventricle (V) and characteristic remaining pancake-like cerebral tissue anteriorly. **B.** Ultrasonogram in another patient demonstrates similar findings. Note the large, dilated, single ventricle (V). **C.** Another patient with more pronounced findings of a single ventricle and only a small residual amount of cortex to either side. **D.** Sagittal view of this infant. The T1-weighted image demonstrates the large univentricle and only a small amount of cerebral tissue lying anteriorly. The vermis also is hypoplastic in this patient.

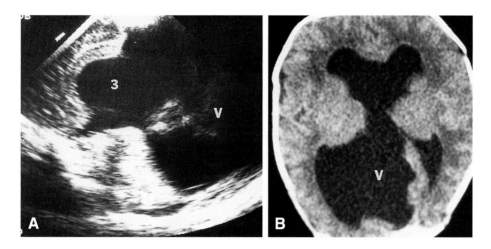

FIGURE 7.140. Semilobar holoprosencephaly. A. Sagittal sonogram demonstrates the large dilated posterior single ventricle (V) and the dilated third ventricle (3). **B.** Axial CT study demonstrates the dilated ventricular system. Note that anteriorly two ventricles are still present but that the septum pellucidum is absent and the third ventricle is dilated. It blends with the large posterior single ventricle (V).

Migrational Disorders

With the advent of MRI, the migrational disorders of the brain have come to be more readily and commonly identified. Normally, there is progressive migration of the neurons from the center of the brain to the outer surface, but in this group of abnormalities there is either total or partial migrational arrest. Total arrest results in lissencephaly or agyria, while other partial arrest abnormalities include pachygyria, polygyria, and micropolygyria. These abnormalities can be focal or diffuse and may be associated with other problems of migration. Deep focal arrest results in heterotopic gray matter nodules, while focal arrests with clefts constitute schizencephaly. When a migrational problem occurs unilaterally and the ipsilateral cerebral hemisphere is enlarged, the condition is known as hemimegalencephaly. With lissencephaly, the brain surface is smooth

with a complete lack of gyri. Only the upper four of the total of six layers of the cortex migrate to the surface, and because the last two do not, there is no induction of gyral formation. The findings are characteristic, consisting of dilated ventricles, often more pronounced posteriorly, a smooth brain surface, poor gray-white matter differentiation, and deficient white matter (1, 2). Calcifications in the septum pellucidum can occur. Examples of lissencephaly are shown in Figure 7.141.

Heterotopic gray matter most commonly occurs in the subependymal region of the lateral ventricles (Fig. 7.142). The nodules can best be demonstrated with CT or MRI (3), where they appear as nodules projecting into dilated ventricles or as masses in the brain substance. They frequently are associated with other brain abnormalities such as agenesis of the corpus callosum and must be differentiated from the subependymal nodules of tuberous sclerosis.

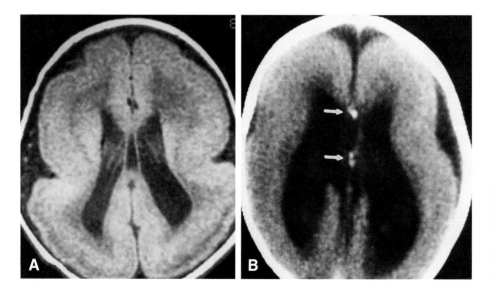

FIGURE 7.141. Lissencephaly. A. Note the smooth appearance of the brain with no gray-white matter organization. The white matter is scant, and the cortex is thick. **B.** Another patient has similar findings in addition to midline calcifications (arrows).

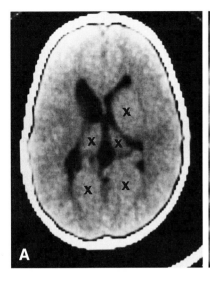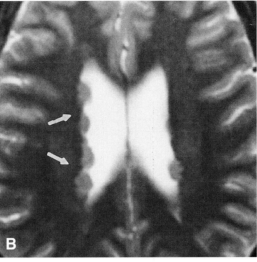

FIGURE 7.142. Heterotopic gray matter. A. Note the heterotopic gray matter nodules (X) of various sizes seen within both lateral ventricles. **B.** T2-weighted MR image of another patient demonstrates a number of nodules lining the subependymal region (arrows). Note that the nodules have the same tissue signal as does normal gray matter.

In terms of their MRI signal, the heterotopic nodules of gray matter behave the same as normal gray matter. They are readily differentiated from tumors, which show increased signal intensity on T2-weighted and FLAIR images. Rarely, heterotopic gray matter can be extracerebral and another form of gray matter heterotopia is referred to as subcortical heterotopia (4) or subcortical dysplasia (5, 6). In this condition a focal, subcortical area of dysplastic brain tissue is present and overall, the findings do not precisely conform to the other forms of migrational abnormality (Fig. 7.143).

Schizencephaly represents a focal abnormality of neuronal migration in which a variably sized cleft is present in

the brain. **Depending on whether the cleft is closed or open, the condition is called "closed or opened lip" schizencephaly**. It is characterized by full-thickness, transcerebral columns of gray matter extending from the subependymal layer of the ventricle to the cortex. Type I schizencephaly is not associated with hydrocephalus and the area of involvement is small. With type II schizencephaly a larger area of involvement is present, and hydrocephalus is associated. The abnormalities can be demonstrated with any imaging modality, but perhaps are best demonstrated with MRI (Fig. 7.144). Schizencephaly also can be seen with septo-optic dysplasia (7).

With pachygyria, there are too few gyri and those remaining are large, flat, and broad (8, 9) (Fig. 7.145A). The problem can be focal or widespread and associated with other neuronal migrational abnormalities. Pachygyria probably is related to lissencephaly and could be considered focal lissencephaly. With polymicrogyria, the normal gyral pattern is replaced by numerous small microgyri and focal abnormality of contour of the cortex.

Hemimegalencephaly is a rare condition (10–12) associated with mental retardation, intractable seizures, and a large hemicranium. The underlying cerebral hemisphere is enlarged with the gray matter distorted so that normal gyri are absent. White matter extends to the cortical surface (Fig. 7.145B). The condition has been treated with embolic hemispherectomy (13).

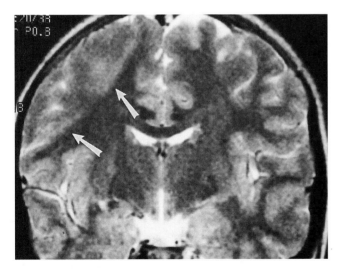

FIGURE 7.143. Subcortical heterotopic gray matter. Note the dysplastic-appearing portion of the frontoparietal area on the right (arrows). Gray-white matter separation is completely distorted, and there is no semblance of normal brain tissue organization.

REFERENCES

1. Barkovich AJ. Subcortical heterotopia: a distant clinicoradiologic entity. AJNR 1996:17:1315–1322.
2. Smith AS, Blaser SI, Ross JS, et al. Magnetic resonance imaging of disturbances in neuronal migration: illustration of an embryologic process. Radiographics 1989;9:509–522.
3. Barkovich AJ, Kjos BO. Gray matter heterotopias: MR charac-

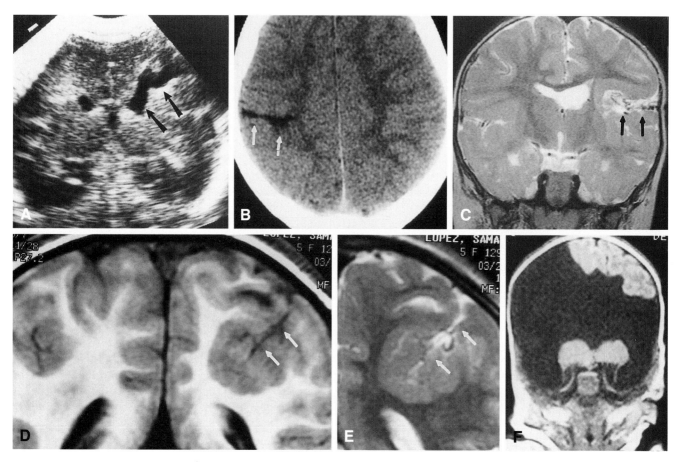

FIGURE 7.144. Schizencephaly. A. Open-lip schizencephaly (arrows) demonstrated with ultrasound. **B.** Similar lesion seen on CT (arrows). **C.** Closed-lip schizencephaly (arrows) on a T2-weighted MR image. **D.** Minimal closed-lip schizencephaly (arrows), T1-weighted image. Note the surrounding gray matter and how deep it extends toward the center of the brain. **E.** T2-weighted image demonstrates the same findings (arrows). **F.** Major open-lip schizencephaly causing a deep cleft in the brain, which communicates with the ventricles.

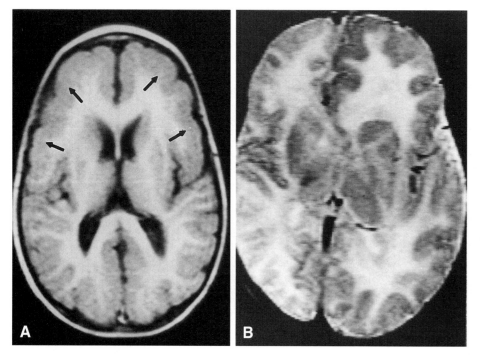

FIGURE 7.145. A. Pachygyria. Note the loss of normal sulci and gyri over the frontal lobes (arrows). The remaining gyri are large and the underlying gray-white matter interdigitation is completely lost. **B. Hemimegalencephaly.** Note the large right hemisphere. Gray-white matter organization is distorted.

TABLE 7.1. CLINICAL SYNDROMES ASSOCIATED WITH VERMIAN HYPOPLASIA

Vermian agenesis
  Consistent component
    Joubert's syndrome
    Walker-Waardenburg syndrome
    Cerebro-oculo-muscular syndrome
  Occasional component
    Meckel-Gruber syndrome
    Coffin-Siris syndrome
    Ellis-van Creveld syndrome
    Fraser cryptophthalmus
Nonmendelian conditions
  Dandy-Walker malformation with facial angioma
  Dominant X-linked Aicardi's syndrome
  Cornelia de Lange syndrome

teristics and correlation with developmental and neurologic manifestations. Radiology 1992;182:493–499.

4. Barkovich AJ. Subcortical heterotopia: a distinct clinicoradiologic entity. AJNR 1996;17:1315–1322.
5. Bronen RA, Vives KP, Kim JH, et al. Focal cortical dysplasia of Taylor, balloon cell subtype: MR differentiation from low-grade tumors. AJNR 1997;18:1141–1151.
6. Yagishita A, Arai N, Maehara T, et al. Focal cortical dysplasia: appearance on MR images. Radiology 1997;203:553–559.
7. Kuban KCK, Teele RL, Wallman J. Septo-optic-dysplasia-schizencephaly. Radiographic and clinical features. Pediatr Radiol 1989;19:145–150.
8. Kao CH, Han NT, Liao SQ, et al. Infantile spasm induced by hemispheric pachygyria ultrasound, MRI and Tc-99m HMPAO SPECT. Pediatr Radiol 1991;21:373–374.
9. Titelbaum DS, Hayward JC, Zimmerman RA. Pachygyric-like changes: topographic appearance at MR imaging and CT and correlation with neurologic status. Radiology 1989;173:663–667.
10. Fariello G, Malena S, Lucigrai G, et al. Hemimegalencephaly: early sonographic pattern. Pediatr Radiol 1993;23:151–152.
11. Lam AH, Villanueva AC, de Silva M. Hemimegalencephaly: cranial sonographic findings. J Ultrasound Med 1992;11:241–244.
12. Wolpert SM, Cohen A, Libenson MH. Hemimegalencephaly: a longitudinal MR study. AJNR 1994;15:1479–1482.
13. Mathis JM, Barr JD, Albright AL, et al. Hemimegalencephaly and intractable epilepsy treated with embolic hemispherectomy. AJNR 1995;16:1076–1079.

Vermian Agenesis

Vermian agenesis is classically associated with the Dandy-Walker syndrome complex of abnormalities, but it also can occur alone. Hypoplasia involves primarily the inferior vermis (1–5), but the midbrain also can be involved. The most common of these conditions, although still rare, are the Joubert's (6), Walker Waardenburg, and cerebro-oculomuscular or oculomotor apraxia syndromes (1, 3, 5). Other conditions in which vermian hypoplasia or agenesis can be encountered are summarized in Table 7.1. In Joubert's syndrome, respiratory compromise and abnormal patterns of breathing are common, and the patients often are retarded. In the Walker-Waardenburg syndrome, cerebellar malformations co-exist as well as do eye abnormalities. Vermian (cerebellar) agenesis also occurs in the syndromes of pontocerebellar hypoplasia (7, 8), carbohydrate-glycoprotein deficiency syndrome (9), and infantile autism (10). The findings of vermian agenesis are best demonstrated with MRI (Fig. 7.146A).

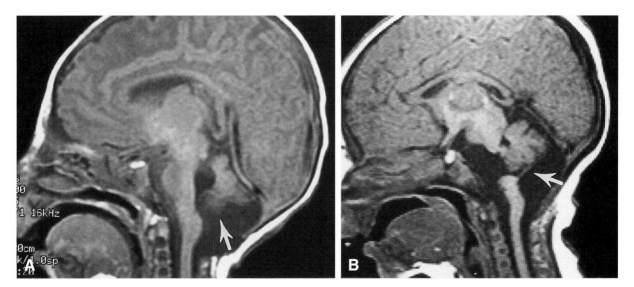

FIGURE 7.146. A. Vermian hypoplasia. Note the hypoplasia of the inferior vermis (arrow). **B. Cerebellar pontine disconnection.** Note the very thin remaining connection (arrow) between the underdeveloped cerebellum and brainstem.

REFERENCES

1. Adamsbaum C, Moreau V, Bulteau C, et al. Vermian agenesis without posterior fossa cyst. Pediatr Radiol 1994;24:543–546.
2. Barzilai M, Ish-Shalom N, Lerner A, et al. Case report. Imaging findings in COACH syndrome. AJR 1998;170:1081–1082.
3. Kollias SS, Ball WS Jr, Prenger EC. Cystic malformations of the posterior fossa: differential diagnosis clarified through embryologic analysis. Radiographics 1993;13:1211–1231.
4. Soto-Ares G, Devisme L, Jorriot S, et al. Neuropathologic and MR imaging correlation in a neonatal case of cerebellar cortical dysplasia. AJNR 2002;23:1101.
5. Whitsel EA, Castillo M, D'Cruz O. Cerebellar vermis and midbrain dysgenesis in oculomotor apraxia: MR findings. AJNR 1995;16:831–834.
6. Sztriha L, Al-Gazali LI, Aithala GR, et al. Joubert's syndrome: new cases and review of clinicopathologic correlation. Pediatr Neurol 1999;20:274–281.
7. Barth PG, Blennow G, Lenard H-G, el al. The syndrome of autosomal recessive pontocerebellar hypoplasia, microcephaly, and extrapyramidal dyskinesia (pontocerebellar hypoplasia type 2): compiled data from 10 pedigrees. Neurol 1995;45:311–317.
8. Uhl M, Pawlik H, Laubenberger J, et al. MR findings in pontocerebellar hypoplasia. Pediatr Radiol 1998;28:547–551.
9. Antoun H, Villeneuve N, Gelot A, Panisset S, et al. Cerebellar atrophy: an important feature of carbohydrate deficient glycoprotein syndrome type 1. Pediatr Radiol 1999;29:194–198.
10. Courchesne E, Townsend J, Saitoh O. The brain in infantile autism: posterior fossa structures are abnormal. Neurology 1995:44:214–223.

Pontomedullary Disconnection

This rare anomaly is believed to result from an intrauterine ischemic insult to the pontomedullary region. Very little tissue remains in the area and the findings, especially as demonstrated with MR, are characteristic (Fig, 7.146B).

REFERENCES

1. Mamourian AC, Miller G. Neonatal pontomedullary disconnection with aplasia or destruction of the lower brain stem: a case of pontoneocerebellar hypoplasia? AJNR 1994;15:1483–1485.

Neurocutaneous Melanosis

In this rare condition (1, 2), melanotic tumors are seen throughout the skin and leptomeninges (3) of the central nervous system. The main feature to be remembered about this condition is that, since melanin is present in these tumors, MRI signals are reversed from ordinary tumors. In other words, these tumors demonstrate increased signal intensity on T1-weighted images and decreased signal intensity on T2-weighted images.

REFERENCES

1. Barkovich AJ, Frieden IJ, Williams ML. MR of neurocutaneous melanosis. AJNR 1994;15:859–867.
2. George JC, Edwards MK, Jakacki RI, et al. Melanotic neuroectodermal tumor of infancy. AJNR 1995;16:1273–1275.
3. Byrd SE, Darling CF, Tomita T, et al. MR imaging of symptomatic neurocutaneous melanosis in children. Pediatr Radiol 1997;27:39–44.

Pituitary Abnormalities

In patients with primary hypopituitarism and idiopathic growth hormone deficiency, it has been demonstrated that a certain combination of findings usually are present. These include smallness of the pituitary gland, absence of the anterior portion, ectopia of the bright posterior portion, and thickening and shortening of the stock of the pituitary (1–5). The findings are illustrated in Figure 6.91 in Chapter 6. In central precocious puberty, the pituitary gland increases both in height and width (7, 8), and frequently a hypothalamic tumor is present. The tumor often is a hamartoma of the tuber cinereum (9). In terms of such tumors, it has been suggested that when one encounters a pituitary gland with absence of the bright signal in its posterior lobe and a thickened stock, one is obligated to search for such a tumor (3).

Traumatic transsection or pathologic infiltration of the pituitary stock can interfere with conduction between the hypothalamus and the gland and result in diabetes insipidus or growth hormone deficiency (10–12). The pituitary gland can hypertrophy and even transform into an adenoma in patients with primary hypothyroidism (13). The same rebound growth phenomenon occurs with ablation of the adrenal glands and is called Nelson syndrome. Tumors of the pituitary gland are less common in children than in adults and include a variety of adenomas, microadenoma, and occasionally a pituitary cyst. These tumors, for the most part, have been discussed earlier.

REFERENCES

1. Abrahamas JJ, Trefelnaer E, Boulware SD. Idiopathic growth hormone deficiency: MR findings in 35 patients. AJNR 1991;12:155.
2. Argyropoulou M, Perignon F, Brauner R, et al. Magnetic resonance imaging in the diagnosis of growth hormone deficiency. J Pediatr 1992;120:886–891.
3. Hamilton J, Blaser S, Daneman D. MR imaging in idiopathic growth hormone deficiency. AJNR 1998;19:1609–1615.
4. Ochi M, Morikawa M, Yoshimoto KE, et al. Growth retardation due to idiopathic growth hormone deficiencies: MR findings in 24 patients. Pediatr Radiol 1992;22:477–480.
5. Ultmann MC, Siegel SF, Hirsch WL, et al. Pituitary stalk and ectopic hyperintense T1-signal on magnetic resonance imaging: implications for anterior pituitary dysfunction. Am J Dis Child 1993;147:647–652.
6. Chen S, Leger J, Garel C, et al. Growth hormone deficiency with ectopic neurohypophysis: anatomical variations and relationship between the visibility of the pituitary stalk asserted by magnetic resonance imaging and anterior pituitary function. J Clin Endocrinol Metab 1999;84:2408–2413.

7. Kao SCS, Cook JS, Hansen JR, et al. MR imaging of the pituitary gland in central precocious puberty. Pediatr Radiol 1992; 22:481–484.
8. Sharafuddin MJA, Luisiri A, Garibaldi LR, et al. MR imaging diagnosis of central precocious puberty: importance of changes of the shape and size of the pituitary gland. AJR 1994;162: 1167–1173.
9. Kornreich L, Horev G, Blaser S, et al. Central precocious puberty: evaluation by neuroimaging. Pediatr Radiol 1995;25: 7–11.
10. Hasegawa T, Hasegawa Y, Yokoyama T, et al. Partial growth hormone deficiency with pituitary stalk transection. Endocrinol Jpn 1991;38:573–575.
11. Tien R, Kucharczyk J, Kucharczyk W. MR imaging of the brain in patients with diabetes insipidus. AJNR 1991; 12:533–542.
12. Yamanaka C, Momoi T, Fujisawa I, et al. Acquired growth hormone deficiency due to pituitary stalk transection after head trauma in childhood. Eur J Pediatr 1993;152:99–101.
13. Kuroiwa T, Okabe Y, Hasuo K, et al. MR imaging of pituitary hypertrophy due to juvenile primary hypothyroidism: a case report. Clin Imaging 1991;15:202–205.

Seizures

Generally, with first onset seizures in infancy, imaging findings are normal (1). This is important to appreciate, because further imaging should be confined to those patients where clinical findings suggest some underlying pathologic focus. This could be a tumor or an area of inflammation or injury. When seizures are confined to the temporal lobe (i.e., temporal lobe seizures), a more definitive imaging protocol should be performed. This requires thin-slice MRI through the hippocampus. The findings are characteristic and consist of hypoplasia of the hippocampus along with increased signal intensity on T2-weighted images (Fig. 7.147), produced by so-called mesial temporal sclerosis (2–8).

REFERENCES

1. Sharma S, Riviello JJ, Harper MB, et al. The role of emergent neuroimaging in children with new onset afebrile seizures. Pediatrics 2003 (in press).
2. Clifford RJ Jr, Krecke KN, Luetner PH, et al. Diagnosis of mesial temporal sclerosis with conventional versus fast spin-echo MR imaging. Radiology 1994;192:123–127.
3. Ende GR, Laxer KD, Knowlton RC, et al. Temporal lobe epilepsy: bilateral hippocampal metabolite changes revealed at proton MR spectroscopic imaging. Radiology 1997;202:809–817.
4. Grattan-Smith JD, Harvey AS, Desmond PM, et al. Hippocampal sclerosis in children with intractable temporal lobe epilepsy: detection with MR imaging. AJR 1993;161:1045–1048.
5. Meiners LC, vanGils A, Jansen GH, et al. Temporal lobe epilepsy: the various MR appearances of histologically proven mesial temporal sclerosis. AJNR 1994;15:1547–1555.
6. Ng TC, Comair YG, Xue M, et al. Temporal lobe epilepsy: presurgical localization with proton chemical shift imaging. Radiology 1994;193:465–472.
7. Oppenheim C, Dormont D, Hasboun D, et al. Bilateral mesial temporal sclerosis: MRI with high-resolution fast spin-echo and fluid-attenuated inversion-recovery sequences. Neuroradiology 1999;41:471–479.
8. Tien RD, Felsberg GJ. The hippocampus in status epilepticus: demonstration of signal intensity and morphologic changes with sequential fast spin-echo MR imaging. Radiology 1995;194: 249–256.

Brain Death

It is important to determine brain death when a decision must be made to discontinue life support. In this regard, this can be accomplished with nuclear scintigraphy, angiography, and Doppler ultrasound (2). Brain death is manifest by absence of flow in the intracranial vessels, no matter which imaging modality is used. However, in this regard, nuclear scintigraphy remains the most direct and expedient imaging modality to secure this information (Fig. 7.148).

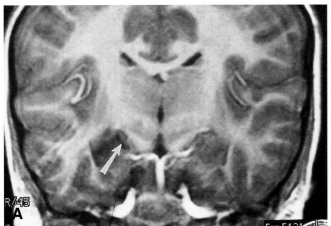
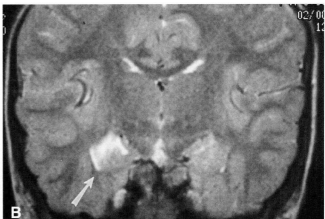

FIGURE 7.147. Mesial temporal sclerosis: temporal lobe seizures. A. Note hypoplasia of the right hippocampus (arrow). **B.** T2-weighted image demonstrates increased signal intensity in the area (arrow).

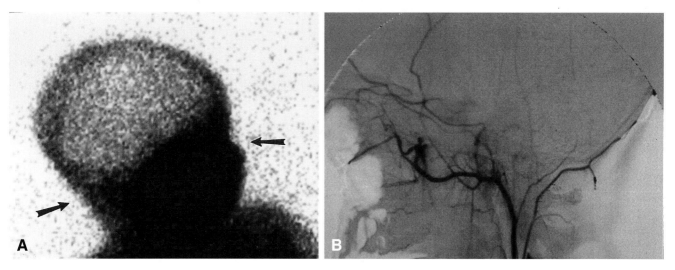

FIGURE 7.148. Brain death. A. Nuclear scintigraphy demonstrates blood flow to the base of the skull and face (arrows), but no flow is seen to the brain. **B.** Angiography demonstrates the same findings.

Neurofibromatosis

The cranial manifestations of neurofibromatosis do not usually become apparent in the neonatal period. In older children one of the bizarre mesenchymal disturbances associated with neurofibromatosis is the presence of a bony defect in the occipital bone along the lambdoid suture (Fig. 7.149). More commonly one sees sphenoid wing dysplasia and enlargement of the orbit (Fig. 7.150). These changes may or may not be associated with plexiform neurofibro-

matosis, a manifestation of the disease where neurofibromatous tissue grows in sheets and creeps relentlessly around and into adjacent structures. As far as sphenoid wing dysplasia is concerned, it usually is associated with enlargement of the orbit, and since the temporal bone is thin or absent, cerebral spinal fluid (CSF) pulsations can be transmitted to the orbit with resulting pulsating exophthalmus.

In addition to the foregoing changes, dysplastic changes in and around the sella can result in a bizarre appearance to this structure (Fig. 7.151A). Macrocrania also occurs and

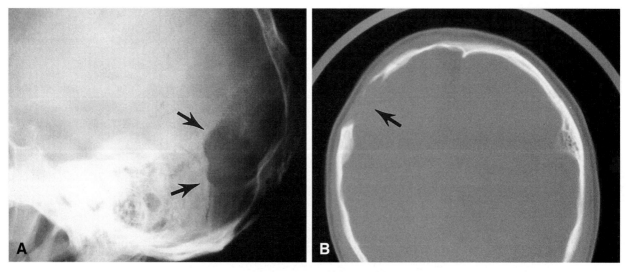

FIGURE 7.149. Neurofibromatosis: calvarial defect. A. Note the typical lucent posterior occipital defect (arrows). **B.** CT study demonstrates the same defect (arrow).

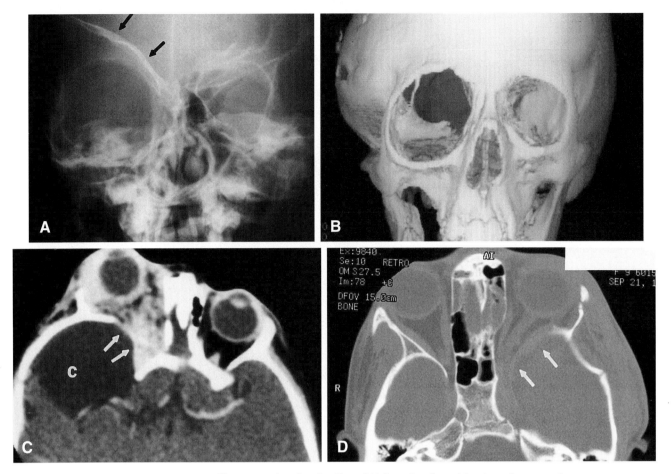

FIGURE 7.150. Neurofibromatosis: dysplastic orbital and sphenoid wing changes. A. Note the characteristically enlarged orbit and elevated sphenoid wing (arrows). **B.** Three-dimensional reconstructed CT in the same patient dramatically demonstrates the enlarged right orbit and absence of the sphenoid wing. **C.** Another patient with sphenoid wing dysplasia (arrows) leading to pulsating exophthalmus. The temporal fossa is enlarged. In this patient, an associated arachnoid cyst (C) is seen. Plexiform neurofibromatosis is present in the retro-orbital region, and there is marked proptosis of the globe. **D.** CT study in another patient demonstrates extensive sphenoid wing dysplasia with virtually no ossification of the bone (arrows). There is bulging into the retro-orbital region. This causes pulsating exophthalmus. The temporal fossa is enlarged.

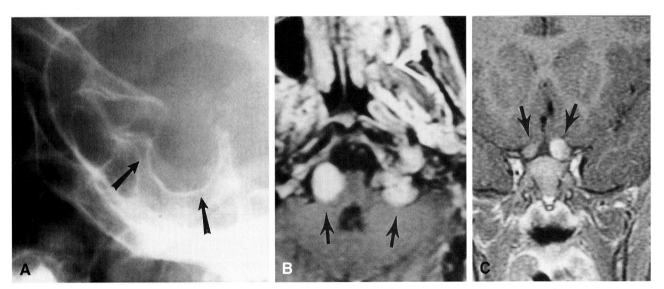

FIGURE 7.151. Neurofibromatosis. A. Sellar dysplasia. Note the enlarged deformed sella and optic chiasm (arrows). **No tumors were present in this area. B. Acoustic neuromas.** Note the bilateral acoustic neuromas (arrows). **C. Bilateral optic gliomas.** Note the round structures (arrows) representing bilateral optic gliomas.

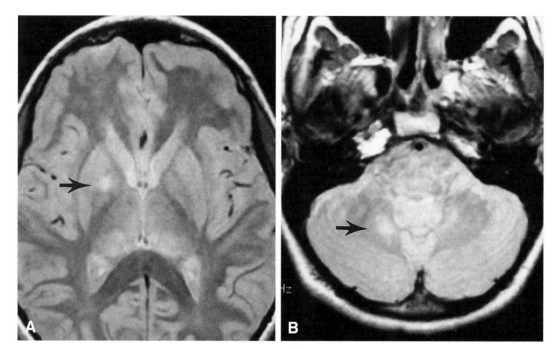

FIGURE 7.152. Neurofibromatosis: white matter lesions. A. Note the high-signal lesion (arrow) in the basal ganglia. **B.** Another high-signal lesion is present in the white matter of the cerebellum (arrow).

dural ectasia without tumor formation can lead to auditory canal expansion (1, 2). The latter phenomenon is similar to that seen in the spinal canal where scalloping of the vertebral bodies occurs but no underlying tumor is present.

Intracranially, arachnoid cysts can develop in the areas of sphenoid wing dysplasia, and stenotic arterial lesions along with small vessel vasculopathy can be encountered (3). Optic gliomas and acoustic neuromas (Fig. 7.151, B and C) also occur, but these tend to be more common in the so-called "type 2" neurofibromatosis. When they occur in type 1 neurofibromatosis, they generally are slow-growing (4). In type 2 neurofibromatosis, the various mesenchymal defects of the calvarium seen with Type I neurofibromatosis, along with dysplastic features such as dysplasia and scoliosis of the spine, dural ectasia, kyphoscoliosis of the tibia and fibula, and extremity gigantism also are not seen.

Another peculiar manifestation of neurofibromatosis type 1 is the presence of cortical and white matter abnormalities resulting in "white spots" on MR studies (5, 6). The etiology of these white spots is not known, but they appear to be innocuous and tend to spontaneously resolve (Fig. 7.152). Some consider them hamartomas.

REFERENCES

1. Egelhoff JC, Ball WS, Towbin RB, et al. Dural ectasia as a cause of widening of the internal auditory canals in neurofibromatosis. Pediatr Radiol 1987;17:7–9.

2. Menor F, Marti-Bonmati L, Mulas F, et al. Imaging considerations of central nervous system manifestations in pediatric patients with neurofibromatosis type 1. Pediatr Radiol 1991;21:389–394.

3. Woody RC, Perrot LJ, Beck SA. Neurofibromatosis cerebral vasculopathy in an infant: clinical, neuroradiographic and neuropathologic studies. Pediatr Pathol 1992;12:613–619.

4. Listrnick R, Charrow J, Greenwald M, et al. Natural history of optic pathway tumors in children with neurofibromatosis type 1: a longitudinal study. J Pediatr 1994;125:63–66.

5. Itoh T, Magnaldi S, White RM, et al. Neurofibromatosis type 1: the evolution of deep gray and white matter in MR abnormalities. AJNR 1994;15:1513–1519.

6. Sevick RJ, Barkovich AJ, Edwards MSB, et al. Evolution of white matter lesions in neurofibromatosis type 1: MR findings. AJR 1992;159:171–175.

Gray Matter, White Matter, and Basal Ganglia Diseases

With the advent of MRI and spectroscopy (1–4), a great deal has been learned regarding diseases affecting the gray matter, white matter, and basal ganglia. This has become a complex and cumbersome subject, which is constantly undergoing change. Many groups of diseases previously of little or no concern for radiologists now have come to haunt us. It would be impossible to discuss all these conditions in detail, and only a summary of their main imaging manifestations is presented. This is further summarized in Table 7.2.

TABLE 7.2. GRAY MATTER/WHITE MATTER AND BASAL GANGLIA DISEASE

Disease	Type	Basal Ganglia	White Matter (Central)	White Matter (Peripheral)	Gray Matter (Cortical)
GM$_1$ gangliosidoses	L				X
Mucolipidoses	L		X	X	X
Mucopolysaccharidoses	L		X	X	
Fucosidosis	L		X	X	
Sialidosis	L		X	X	
Chediak-Higashi disease	L		X	X	
Cockayne's disease	L ?, D	X	X		
MERRF	M				X
Leigh's disease	M	X (P, G, C)	X (Midbrain)		
MELAS	M				X
Methylmalonic acidemia	M	X (G)			
Propionic acidemia	M	X (G)			
Alpers disease	M		X	X	X
Menkes' syndrome (kinky hair)	M		X	X	X
GM$_2$ gangliosidoses	M	X (T)	X	X	
Kearns-Sayre syndrome	M			X	
Glutaric acidurias types I and II	M, Ac	X			
Carbon monoxide poisoning	To	X (P, C, G)			
Kernicterus	To	X			
Wilson's disease	To	X (G)	X	X	
Canavan's disease (large head)	D		X	X	
Alexander's disease (large head)	D			X (Frontal)	
Krabbe's disease	D	X (T, C)	X		
Metachromatic leukodystrophy	D		X		
Pelizaeus-Merzbacher disease	D		X	X	
Adrenoleukodystrophy (X linked)	Pe		X	X (Occipital)	
Zellweger syndrome	Pe		X	X	X
Hyperpipecolic acidemia	Pe		X	X	
Adrenoleukodystrophy (infantile)	Pe		X	X	
Phenylketonuria	Ac		X	X	
Maple syrup urine disease	Ac	X (G)	X (Brainstem)		
Homocystinuria	Ac		X	X	
Multiple sclerosis	Au		X	X	
Lowe's syndrome			X	X	
Acidemias (Table 7.3)			X	X	
Galactosemia				X	
Hallervorden-Spatz syndrome		XX G			
Juvenile Huntington's disease		(P, C)			X

L, lysosomal; M, mitochondrial; D, dysmyelinating disorder; Ac, acidemia; Au, autoimmune; Pe, peroxisomal; To, toxin;
P, putamen; C, caudate nucleus; G, globus palidus; T, thalamus.

Generally, one needs to decide whether primary involvement involves the cortical gray matter, white matter, or the basal ganglia (deep gray matter). Combinations commonly exist, and in terms of white matter involvement, it is important to determine whether the peripheral, subcortical white matter or the deeper white matter (i.e., periventricular and more central white matter) is involved (Fig. 7.153). However, there often is no sharp distinction, and many diseases beginning in the periphery eventually show central involvement.

There are a number of groups of diseases that can be considered: mitochondrial abnormalities (5, 6), lysosomal abnormalities (5), peroxisomal disorders (5), autoimmune diseases, amino and organic acidurias, dysmyelinating leukodystrophies, and toxic destruction of brain tissue. Mitochondrial, lysosomal, and peroxisomal disorders represent inborn, intracellular errors of metabolism. Mitochondrial disorders include the MELAS (mitochondrial encephalomyopathy with lactic acid and stroke) syndrome (7, 8), myoclonic epilepsy with ragged red fibers (MERRF) syndrome, glutaric aciduria, Alpers disease, Menkes' syndrome, and Leigh's disease. These entities involve the gray matter primarily but can involve the white matter (Fig. 7.154).

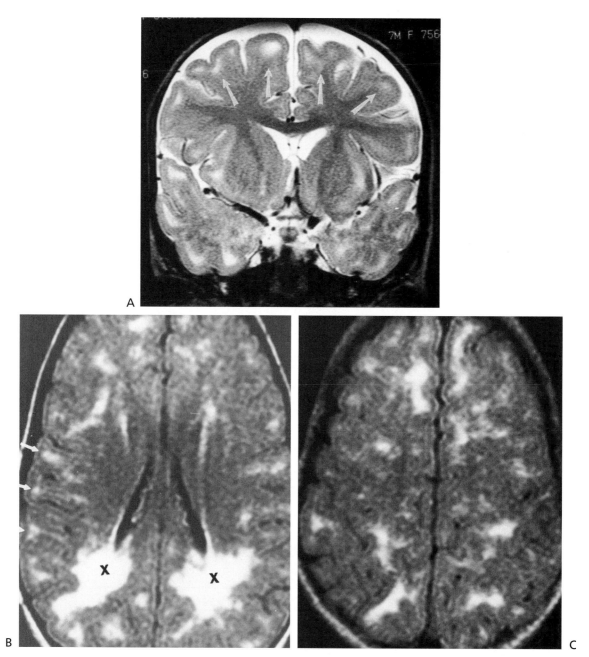

FIGURE 7.153. Deep and superficial white matter disease. A. Typical superficial white matter changes (arrows). **B.** In this patient with an organic acidemia, note the deep periventricular changes (Xs) and superficial subcortical changes (small arrows). These latter changes are seen throughout the brain. **C.** A higher cut demonstrates the subcortical distribution of the white matter changes.

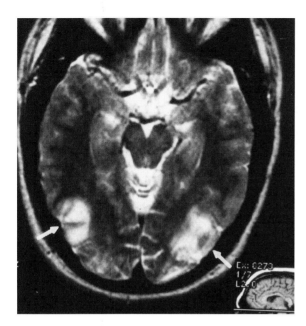

FIGURE 7.154. MELAS syndrome. Note the high-signal-intensity lesions (arrows), primarily in the occipital lobes (arrows). Note that the changes occur both in the white and gray matter, extending to the very edge of the brain surface.

Lysosomal abnormalities generally include the storage diseases (e.g., mucopolysaccharidosis, mucolipidosis) and conditions such as the Chédiak-Higashi syndrome (9, 10), fucosidosis (11), sialidosis, Gaucher's disease, glycogen storage disease, GM₁ gangliosidosis and Salla disease (12). The generalized peroxisomal disorders include Zellweger syndrome, neonatal adrenal leukodystrophy, and hyperpipecolic acidemia (13). The dysmyelinating leukodystrophies include subacute necrotizing encephalomyelopathy or Leigh's disease (14), Alexander's disease (15), sex-linked adrenoleukodystrophy (16–19), Canavan's disease, Krabbe's disease (20), the Pelizaeus-Merzbacher syndrome (21, 22), and metachromatic leukodystrophy. Alexander's disease characteristically produces white matter changes more pronounced in the frontal regions (Fig. 7.155, A and B). Adrenal leukodystrophy first produces changes in the occipital regions (Fig. 7.155C). However, bilateral, frontal involvement (23) as well as unilateral disease (24) can occur. Extension into the pontomedullary cerebrospinal tracts has been noted (25). This form of adrenoleukodystrophy occurs only in males. A further differentiating feature in these conditions is that the head is enlarged in both Canavan's and Alexander's disease. In the Pelizaeus-Merzbacher syndrome both deep and superficial white matter changes are seen, often beginning in the occiput but frequently extending throughout the brain (Fig. 7.156).

With the autoimmune diseases it is multiple sclerosis that is best known (Fig. 7.157). The changes are much the same as those seen in adults, but the spinal cord may be involved a little more often in children (26). The findings consist of patchy white matter changes, primarily peripheral, and similar to those seen with viral encephalitis. The aminoacidurias, including Glutan aciduria type I (27), generally produce nonspecific white matter changes and the most common of these are listed in Table 7.3. In this group, maple syrup urine disease tends to produce more pronounced brainstem changes (28) (Fig. 7.158).

Toxic substances tend to attack the basal ganglia more than the brain parenchyma. Examples of toxic insults to the brain producing such change include carbon monoxide poisoning (29, 30), manganese toxicity with parenteral nutrition (31), methanol intoxication (32), toluene abuse (32), and even though not purely a toxic problem, Wilson's disease (33, 34). In most of these conditions the basal ganglia show increased signal intensity on T2-weighted images. However, with carbon monoxide poisoning, they are basically normal on T2-weighted images but show increased signal intensity on T1-weighted images (Fig. 7.159D). Kernicterus results in the deposition of bilirubin into the basal ganglia (35), and both Huntington's chorea (juvenile form) (Fig. 7.159C) and Sydenham's chorea also involve the basal ganglia (36–39). Basal ganglia changes also can be seen in other myelopathic conditions such as Leigh's disease (Fig. 7.159, A and B). For a more detailed review of the various conditions resulting in basal ganglia changes one is referred to Table 7.2.

Methotrexate (40, 41), Cisplatin (42), and cyclosporin neurotoxicity also produce white matter changes. These are rather generalized and nonspecific (Fig. 7.160). Similarly, hypertensive encephalopathy (43) can produce white matter changes that are nonspecific but often tend to involve the occipital lobes (43) (Fig. 7.161, A and B). Systemic lupus also can involve the white matter, usually in a subcortical distribution (Fig. 7.161C), and widespread deep white matter changes occur with viral encephalitis (Fig. 7.161D).

REFERENCES

1. Barkovich AJ, Good WV, Koch TK, et al. Mitochondrial disorders: analysis of their clinical and imaging characteristics. AJNR 1993;14:1119–1137.
2. Cheon J-E, Kim I-O, Hwang YS. Leukodystrophy in children: a pictorial review of MR imaging features. Radiographics 2002;22:461–476.
3. Hatten HP Jr. Dysmyelinating leukodystrophies: "LACK proper myelin." Pediatr Radiol 1991;21:477–482.
4. Nowell MA, Grossman RI, Hackney DB, et al. MR imaging of white matter disease in children. AJR 1988;151:359–365.
5. Barkovich AJ, Good WV, Koch TK. Mitochondrial disorders:

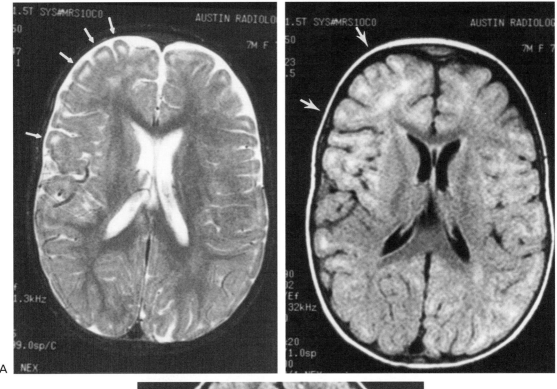

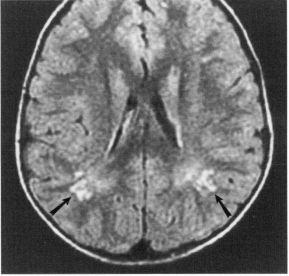

FIGURE 7.155. Alexander's disease. A. Note the superficial white matter changes primarily in the frontal lobes, best seen on the right (arrows). There also is some underlying deeper white matter change. **B.** Similar changes on a FLAIR image (arrows). **C. Adrenal leukodystrophy.** Note the deep white matter changes (arrows) in the occipital lobes.

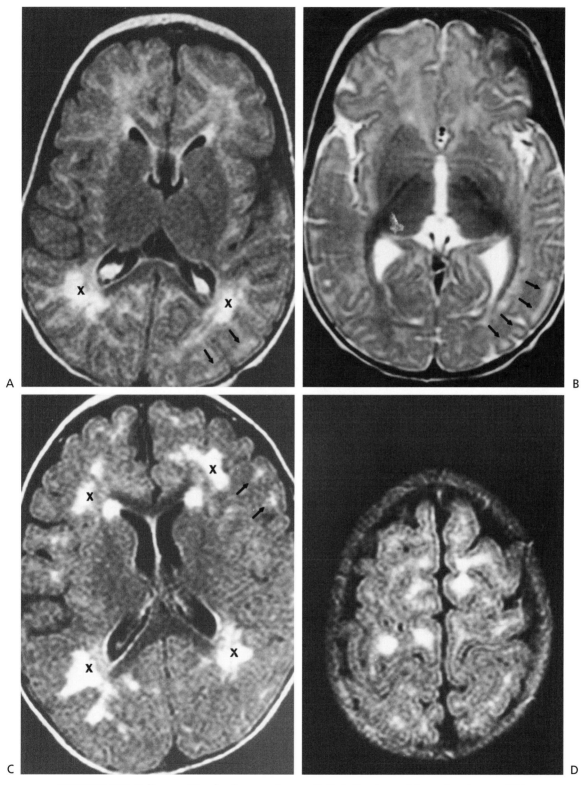

FIGURE 7.156. Pelizaeus-Merzbacher syndrome. A. Note the deep white matter changes (X's) over the occipital regions. Associated superficial white matter changes also are seen (arrows). **B.** Superficial changes more vividly demonstrable (arrows) on a T2-weighted image. **C.** Another patient with more extensive frontal and occipital deep white matter changes (X's). Also note superficial white matter changes (arrows). **D.** Higher cut demonstrates the superficial subcortical white matter changes.

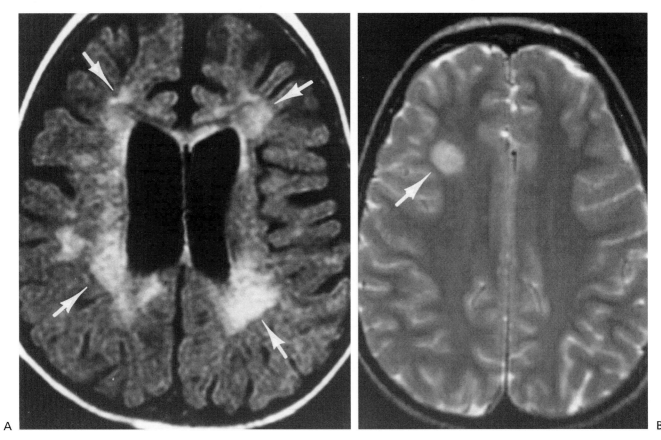

A   B

FIGURE 7.157. Multiple sclerosis. A. Note the diffuse deep white matter change (arrows). **B.** Another patient with a focal deep white matter focus (arrow) of demyelinization.

TABLE 7.3. AMINO AND ORGANIC ACIDOPATHIES

Argininosuccinic aciduria
Citrullinemia
Cystathioninuria
Glutaric acidurias types I and II
Homocystinuria
Hyperargininemia
Hypermethioninemia
Hyperphenylalaninemia
Hyperprolinemia
Maple syrup urine disease
Methylmalonic acidemia
Nonketotic hyperglycinemia
Ornithine transcarbamylase deficiency
Phenylketonuria
Propionic acidemia
Tyrosinemia

From Barkovich AJ. Pediatric neuroimaging, 2nd ed. New York: Raven Press, 1995:101, with permission.

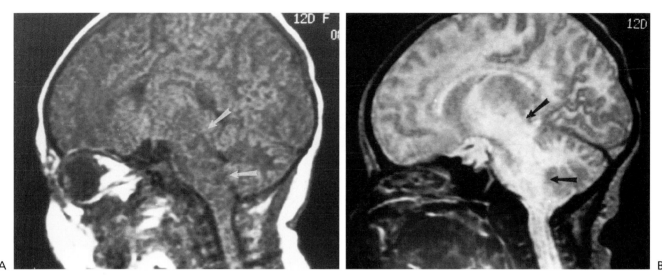

FIGURE 7.158. Maple syrup urine disease. A. T1-weighted, sagittal view demonstrates slight hypodensity through the brainstem (arrows). **B.** T2-weighted image demonstrates markedly increased signal intensity in the brainstem (arrows).

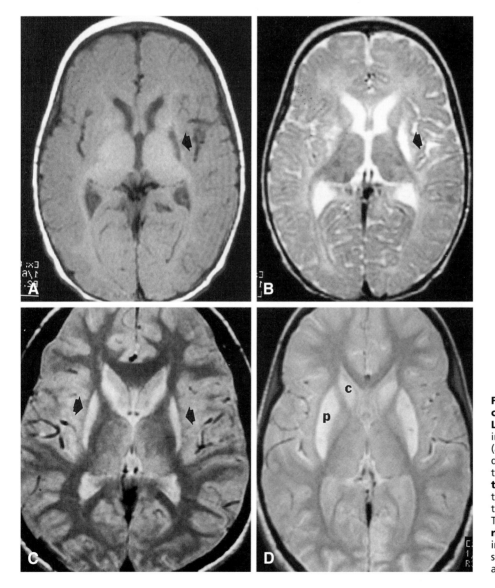

FIGURE 7.159. Diseases producing changes in the basal ganglia. A. Leigh's disease. Note the low signal intensity of the globus pallidus (arrow). **B.** T2-weighted image demonstrates high signal intensity in the same area (arrow). **C. Huntington's chorea, spastic type.** Note the bilateral high signal intensity in the globus pallidus (arrows) on this T2-weighted image. **D. Carbon monoxide poisoning.** Note the increased signal on this protein-density image in the caudate nucleus (c) and putamen (p).

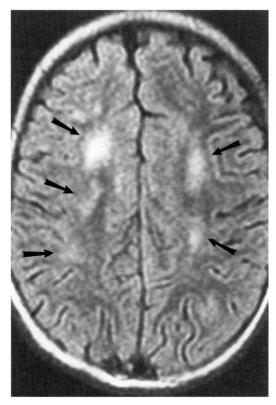

FIGURE 7.160. Cyclosporin myelopathy. Note the deep white matter changes on both sides (arrows).

analysis of their clinical and imaging characteristics. AJNR 1993;14:1119–1137.

6. Valanne L, Ketonen L, Majander A, et al. Neuroradiologic findings in children with mitochondrial disorders. AJR Am J Neuroradiol 1998;19:369–377.

7. Kim I-O, Kim JH, Kim WS, et al. Mitochondrial myopathy-encephalopathy-lactic acidosis and strokelike episodes (MELAS) syndrome: CT and MR findings in seven children. AJR 1996; 166:641–645.

8. Kimura M, Hasegawa Y, Yasuda K, et al. Magnetic resonance imaging with fluid-attenuated inversion recovery pulse sequences in MELAS syndrome. Pediatr Radiol 1997;27:153–154.

9. Ballard R, Tien RD, Nohria V, et al. The Chediak-Higashi syndrome: CT and MR findings. Pediatr Radiol 1994;24:266–267.

10. Herman TE, Lee BP. Accelerated phase of Chediak-Higashi syndrome diffuse white-matter enhancing lesions. Pediatr Radiol 1999;29:527–529.

11. Provenzale JM, Barboriak DP, Sims K. Neuroradiologic findings in fucosidosis, a rare lysosomal storage disease. AJNR 1995;16: 809–813.

12. Sonninen P, Autti T, Varho T, et al. Brain involvement in Salla disease. AJNR 1999;20:433–443.

13. Nelson MD Jr, Wolff JA, Cropss CA, et al. Galactosemia: evaluation with MR imaging. Radiology 1992;184:255–261.

14. Greenberg SB, Faerber EN, Riviello JJ, et al. Subacute necrotizing encephalomyelopathy (Leigh disease): CT and MRI appearances. Pediatr Radiol 1990;21:5–8.

15. Schuster V, Horwitz AE, Kreth HW. Alexander's disease: cranial MRI and ultrasound findings. Pediatr Radiol 1991;21:133–134.

16. Jensen ME, Sawyer RW, Braun IF, et al. MR imaging appearance of childhood adrenoleukodystrophy with auditory, visual, and motor pathway involvement. Radiographics 1990;10:53–66.

17. Melhem ER, Barker PB, Raymond GV, et al. Review. X-linked adrenoleukodystrophy in children: review of genetic, clinical, and MR imaging characteristics. AJR 1999;173:1575–1581.

18. Pasco A, Kalifa G, Sarrazin JL, et al. Contribution of MRI to the diagnosis of cerebral lesions of adrenoleukodystrophy. Pediatr Radiol 1991;21:161–163.

19. Patel PJ, Kolawole TM, Malabarey TM, et al. Adrenoleukodystrophy: CT and MRI findings. Pediatr Radiol 1995;25:256–258.

20. Hittmair K, Wimberger D, Wiesbauer P, et al. Early infantile form of Krabbe disease with optic hypertrophy: serial MR examinations and autopsy correlation. AJNR 1994;15:1454–1458.

21. Spalice A, Popolizio T, Parisi P, et al. Proton MR spectroscopy in connatal Pelizaeus-Merzbacher disease. Pediatr Radiol 2000;30: 171–175.

22. Ziereisen F, Dan B, Christiaens F, et al. Connatal Pelizaeus-Merzbacher disease in two girls. Pediatr Radiol 2000;30: 435–438.

23. Castellote A, Vera J, Vasquez E, et al. MR in adrenoleukodystrophy: atypical presentation as bilateral frontal demyelination. AJNR 1995;16:814–815.

24. Close PJ, Sinnott SJ, Nolan KT. Adrenoleukodystrophy. A case report demonstrating unilateral abnormalities. Pediatr Radiol 1993;23:400–401.

25. Barkovich AJ, Ferriero DM, Bass N, et al. Involvement of the pontomedullary corticospinal tracts: a useful findings in the diagnosis of X-linked adrenoleukodystrophy. AJNR 1997;18: 95–100.

26. Glasier CM, Robbins MB, Davis PC, et al. Clinical, neurodiagnostic and MR findings in children with spinal and brain stem multiple sclerosis. AJNR 1995;16:87–95.

27. Brismar J, Ozand PT. CT and MR of the brain in glutaric acidemia type I: a review of 59 published cases and a report of 5 new patients. AJNR 1995;16:675–683.

28. Fariello G, Dionisi-Vici C, Orazi C, et al. Cranial ultrasonography in maple syrup urine disease. AJNR 1996;17:311–315.

29. Caronia C, Sagy M, Maytal Y, et al. Carbon monoxide poisoning. Arch Pediatr Adolesc Med 1994;148:1307–1308.

30. Rachinger J, Fellner FA, Stieglbauer K, et al. MR changes after acute cyanide intoxication. AJNR 2002;23:1398–1401.

31. Mirowitz SA, Westrich TJ, Hirsch JD. Hyperintense basal ganglia on T1-weighted MR images in patients receiving parenteral nutrition. Radiology 1991;181:117–120.

32. Rubinstein D, Escott E, Kelly JP. Methanol intoxication with putamenal and white matter necrosis: MR and CT findings. AJNR 1995;16:1492–1494.

33. Sener RN. Wilson's disease: MRI demonstration of cavitations in basal ganglia and thalami. Pediatr Radiol 1993;23:157.

34. Sener RN. The claustrum on MRI: normal anatomy and the bright claustrum as a new sign in Wilson's disease. Pediatr Radiol 1993;23:594–596.

35. Martich-Driss V, Kollias SS, Ball WS Jr. MR findings in kernicterus. AJNR 1995;16:819–821.

36. Comunale JP Jr, Heier LA, Chutorian AM. Case report. Juvenile form of Huntington's disease: MR imaging appearance. AJR 1995;165:414–416.

37. Ho VB, Chuang HS, Rovira MJ, et al. Juvenile Huntington disease: CT and MR features. AJNR 1995;16:1405–1412.

38. Kienzle GD, Breger RK, Chun RWM, et al. Sydenham chorea: MR manifestations in two cases. AJNR 1991;12:73–76.

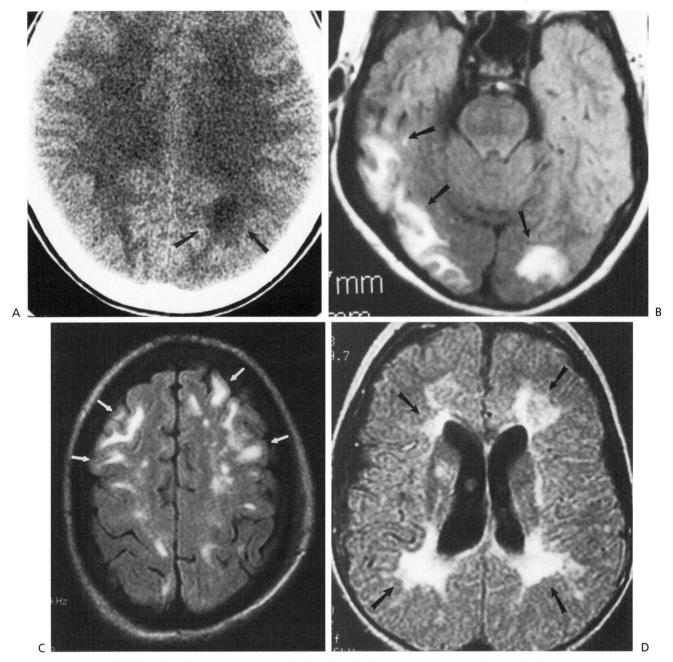

FIGURE 7.161. Hypertensive encephalopathy. A. Note the area of posterior occipital hypodensity (arrows) in a patient with hypertensive encephalopathy. **B.** In another patient, extensive occipital subcortical lesions (arrows) are demonstrated on MRI. **C. Lupus encephalopathy.** Note the widespread deep and superficial white matter change (arrows). **D. Post viral encephalitis.** Note the extensive white matter changes over the frontal and occipital regions (arrows).

39. Savoiardo M, Strada L, Oliva D, et al. Abnormal MRI signal in the rigid form of Huntington's disease. J Neurol Neurosurg Psychiatry 1991;54:888–891.
40. Kim TS, Kim I-O, Kim WS, et al. MR of childhood metachromatic leukodystrophy. AJNR 1997;18:733–738.
41. Lovblad K-O, Kelkar P, Ozdoba C, et al. Pure methotrexate encephalopathy presenting with seizures: CT and MRI features. Pediatr Radiol 1998;28:86–91.
42. Ito Y, Arahata Y, Goto Y, et al. Cisplatin neurotoxicity presenting as reversible posterior leukoencephalopathy syndrome. AJNR 1998;19:415–417.
43. Jones BV, Egelhoff JC, Patterson FJ. Hypertensive encephalopathy in children. AJNR 1997;18:101–106.

SCALP AND MISCELLANEOUS CALVARIAL LESIONS

Infections

Osteomyelitis of the calvarium can result from either calvarial puncture wounds or hematogenous spread of infection from other foci. The roentgenographic findings are not specific and merely consist of irregular foci of destruction of the calvarium. There may or may not be some sclerosis around the margin of the defects, and they are usually easy to differentiate from the round or oval, densely marginated, epidermoid inclusion cyst. Infections that can involve the calvarium include staphylococcal osteomyelitis, congenital lues and, in older infants, tuberculosis.

Tumors and Cysts

Tumors of the calvarium, even such lesions as hemangiomas, lymphangiomas, or benign fibrous tumors, are uncommon in infancy and childhood. One can occasionally encounter an epidermoid inclusion cyst (congenital cholesteatoma) in a young infant's skull, but virtually never in the skull of a newborn. These lesions are characteristic and are usually located in the frontoparietal region. However, they can occur almost anywhere, including the sphenoid wings. They are round or oval and have a discrete, densely sclerotic margin (Fig. 7.162).

Calvarial defects secondary to histiocytosis X are seen in older infants and are well known to all. Multiple destructive foci can also be seen with metastatic neuroblastoma, leukemia, and lymphoma. Hemangiomas and lymphangiomas of the scalp are more common than are their calvarial counterparts and are readily imaged with ultrasound. Lymphangiomas tend to be cystic and avascular, while hemangiomas are solid and have a coarse ultrasonographic texture. Except for capillary hemangiomas, color flow Doppler demonstrates excessive flow within these lesions. Lipomas of the scalp also can occur and ultrasonographically are echogenic with a fine texture pat-

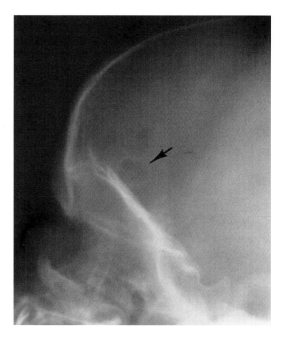

FIGURE 7.162. Epidermoid inclusion cyst (congenital cholesteatoma). Characteristic configuration of cholesteatoma consisting of round or oval radiolucency surrounded by a crisp sclerotic margin (arrow).

tern. All of these features of soft tissue tumors are discussed in Chapter 6.

Primary calvarial hemangiomas characteristically produce an area of bone destruction that at times is somewhat honeycombed. Most often, a vague, peripheral zone of sclerosis is present. Lymphangioma can lead to large areas of bone lysis on Gorham's disease (1). Chordoma of the clivus produces bony destruction and nonspecific calcification and frequently presents as a nasopharyngeal mass with a potential for both extracranial and intracranial extension. This tumor now readily is imaged with CT or MRI (2–4) (Fig. 7.163, A and B). Enchondromas of the base of the skull can be seen with Ollier's disease, but overall this entire problem is uncommon in childhood. Fibrous dysplasia also commonly involves the calvarium. It can produce lytic or sclerotic expansile lesions. Most often, it affects the skull base, and the findings are readily demonstrable with plain films and CT (Fig. 7.163, C and D).

Retinal anlage tumors usually are seen in the first year of life. They are relatively uncommon and most frequently involve the maxilla. Rhabdomyosarcoma of the soft tissues is a common tumor in infancy and childhood. It can arise almost anywhere along the base of the skull, around the orbit, and over the face. Characteristically, a

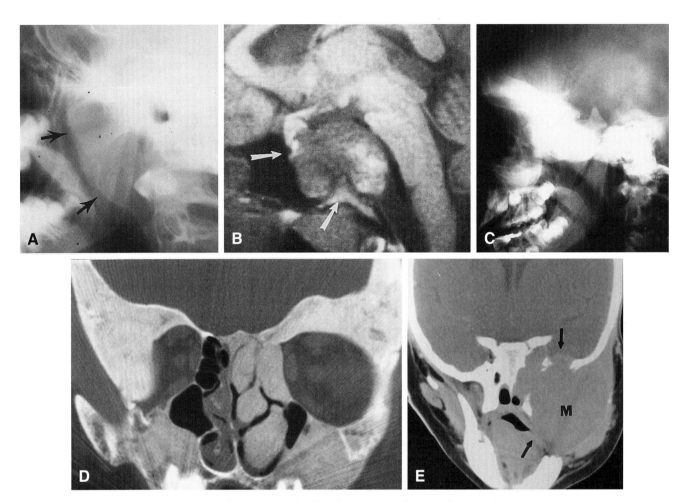

FIGURE 7.163. Calvarial tumors. A. Chordoma. Note the nasopharyngeal soft tissue mass (arrows). **B.** T1-weighted MR image of another patient demonstrates characteristic findings of a chordoma (arrows) of the clivus. **C. Fibrous dysplasia.** Note the characteristic sclerosis and thickening of the base of the skull. **D.** Coronal CT study demonstrates thickening of almost all of the bones, including the sphenoid wings, maxilla, and turbinates. **E. Rhabdomyosarcoma.** Note the extensive soft tissue mass (M) with underlying bony destruction of the face and base of the skull (arrows). Also note that there is a little truncation of the left lateral ventricle and some midline shift to the right. (**B** from Matsumoto J, Towbin RB, Ball WS Jr. Cranial chordomas in infancy and childhood. A report of two cases and review of the literature. Pediatr Radiol 1989:20:28–32, with permission.)

soft tissue mass is seen, and adjacent bony destruction occurs (Fig. 7.163E). The findings are nonspecific, but when one encounters an aggressive soft tissue mass in the areas mentioned, one should think of rhabdomyosarcoma. In addition, rhabdomyosarcoma often arises from the middle ear and causes destruction of the petrous bone.

Dermoid cysts of the scalp also are common in infancy. Generally, they are freely moveable and readily palpable. There really is no need to image such a lesion. However, if needed, ultrasound usually is best and will demonstrate that a cyst is present. If the cysts contain fat, they will be echogenic on ultrasound, radiolucent on CT images, and bright on T1-weighted MR images (Fig. 7.164). If these cysts are not freely mobile, intracranial extension should be considered (5), especially if they are in the midline. Additional imaging in the form of either CT or MRI usually then is employed. Fibrous lesions producing focal lysis of the calvarium also can be encountered (6).

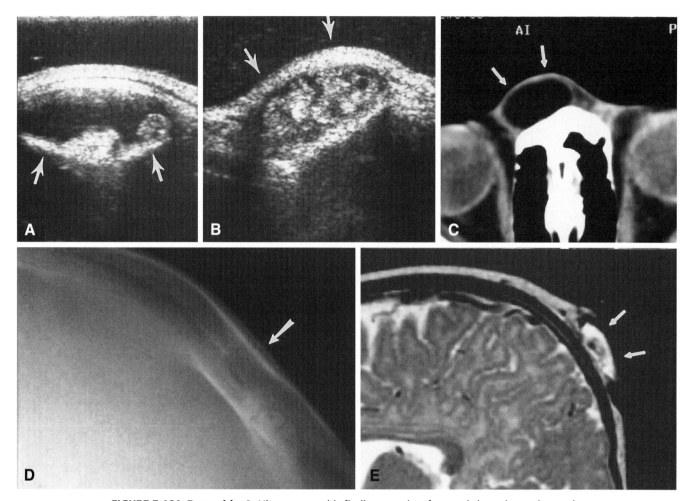

FIGURE 7.164. Dermoids. A. Ultrasonographic findings consist of an oval-shaped mass (arrows) with a hypoechoic center and some nodular debris. **B.** In another patient, mixed echogenicity in a nasal dermoid cyst (arrows) is characteristic of fat. **C.** In the same patient, the CT scan demonstrates typical lucency of fat in the dermoid (arrows). **D.** Another patient with a calvarial defect (arrow) and a clinically present scalp nodule. **E.** T2-weighted MR study demonstrates the nodule to be a dermoid (arrows) located in the scalp but not invading the calvarium. The defect was erosive but not destructive.

REFERENCES

1. Frankel DG, Lewin JS, Cohen B. Massive osteolysis of the skull base. Pediatr Radiol 1997;27:265–267.
2. Matsumoto J, Towbin RB, Ball WS. Cranial chordomas in infancy and childhood. A report of two cases and review of the literature. Pediatr Radiol 1989;20:28–32.
3. Meyers SP, Hirsch WL Jr, Curtin HD, et al. Chordomas of the skull base: MR features. AJNR 1992;13:1627–1636.
4. Sze G, Uichanco LS III, Brant-Zawadzki MN, et al. Chordomas: MR imaging. Radiology 1988;166:187–191.
5. Crawford R. Dermoid cyst of the scalp: intracranial extension. J Pediatr Surg 1990;25:294–295.
6. Queralt JA, Poirier VC. Solitary infantile myofibromatosis of the skull. AJNR 1995;16:476–478.

HEADACHE IN CHILDREN

Most often, headaches in children are the result of migraine or tension. Seldom are they the result of sinusitis. However, imaging of these patients is common and usually is normal. In this regard, predictive factors of significant pathology causing headaches were determined to be sleep related headache and no family history if migraine (1).

REFERENCE

1. Medina LS, Pinter JD, Zurakowski D, et al. Children with headache: clinical predictors of surgical space-occupying lesions and the role of neuroimaging. Radiology 1997;202:819–824.

PARANASAL SINUSES AND MASTOIDS

Paranasal Sinuses

The maxillary sinus cavities usually are roentgenographically visible by 2–3 months of age. They are small and triangular. The ethmoid sinus cavities are much smaller, but usually parallel the maxillary sinuses in development. The sphenoid sinuses usually become aerated and visible at 1–2 years age, but frontal sinus development is delayed into later childhood.

Sinus disease in the neonate is not a real problem, but in older infants sinus infection is coming to be increasingly recognized as a definite clinical problem (1–3). Such ideas as "sinuses are not present in patients under 2 years of age," "sinusitis does not occur in infants under 2 years of age,"

and "the sinuses can be obliterated in association with crying in the infant" are slowly being discarded. It is apparent that maxillary and ethmoid sinus cavities are present in infants (Fig. 7.165), and when they are opacified, they are abnormal (Fig. 7.166). This is not to say that the roentgenogram can define degree or type of abnormality, but only to say that abnormality is present. Furthermore, if one does not see the results of treatment with the sinuses clearing, one will continue to have doubts as to whether sinusitis is a real problem in infants and children (Fig. 7.166). Nonetheless, there is a constant argument based on the premise that maxillary sinus opacification can be seen in asymptomatic children and that opacified maxillary sinuses really do not mean much in the pediatric age group. However, in one series where aspiration of such opacified sinuses

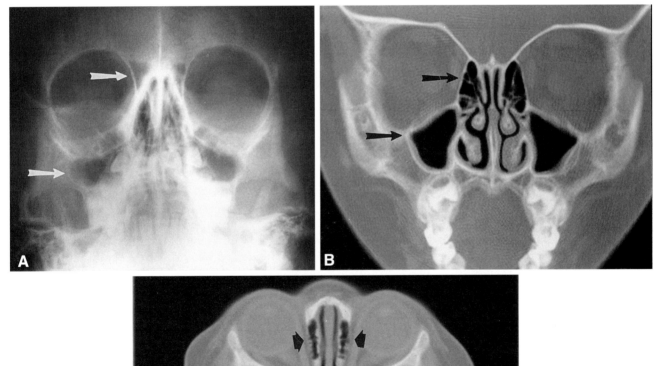

FIGURE 7.165. Normal sinuses. A. Waters' view demonstrates normal maxillary (lower arrow) and ethmoid (upper arrow) sinus cavities. **B.** CT scan demonstrates similar findings (arrows). **C.** Axial view demonstrates aerated ethmoid sinus cavities (arrows) in a 3-month-old infant.

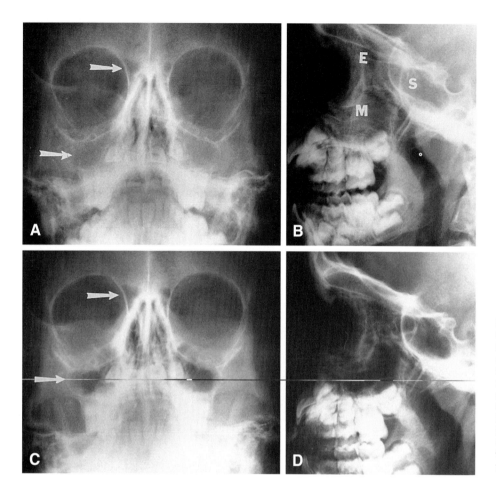

FIGURE 7.166. Sinusitis. A. Note the opacification of the maxillary (lower arrow) and ethmoid (upper arrow) sinus cavities. **B.** Lateral view demonstrates opacification of the maxillary (M), ethmoid (E), and sphenoid (S) sinus cavities. **C.** After appropriate treatment, the maxillary (lower arrow) and ethmoid (upper arrow) sinus cavities are clear. **D.** Lateral view demonstrates that all of these sinus cavities, which were obliterated in **B**, are now clear.

was performed, 70% proved positive for bacterial infection (4), and in another series, nearly 60% proved positive (2).

In terms of understanding sinus disease in children, it must be appreciated that bacterial infection usually is secondary. The most important predisposing factor to sinus infection is poor drainage. This occurs most commonly after viral disease or allergy. In both cases, mucosal edema interferes with drainage through the ostia of the sinus cavities. Thick mucosal secretions as seen in cystic fibrosis also predispose to sinusitis (5). In all these cases as secretions accumulate the sinuses become opacified. Eventually, they can become superinfected with a bacterial infection, but just when this occurs on the basis of the radiographic findings alone is not readily determined. It is only when air-fluid levels are seen that acute bacterial sinusitis can be suggested.

The radiographic findings of inflammatory sinus disease in children include total opacification, mucosal thickening, and air-fluid levels (Fig. 7.167). Total opacification may be the result of fluid accumulation or mucosal thickening, and in terms of mucosal thickening it has been demonstrated in adults that thickening of 3 mm or less is not associated with symptoms (4), but that thickening of 4 mm or greater cor-

relates highly with symptomatic sinusitis. **This has been our experience and we attach little significance to minimal (under 3 mm) mucosal thickening.**

Symptoms of sinusitis in childhood include repeated middle ear infections, a nighttime cough, and chronic nasal discharge. Headaches are not a common feature of sinusitis in children and, when headaches alone are the presenting symptom, or even if they are associated with one other symptom, the yield of positive roentgenograms is less than 5% (3). In terms of the radiograph, it is the Waters' view that is most helpful (6). CT and MRI tend to demonstrate the changes a little more clearly (7), but generally are not needed, especially MRI. CT is helpful in refractory cases and when orbital complications occur. These complications basically take two forms: inflammation without abscess and inflammation with abscess or osteomyelitis (Fig. 7.168, A and B). If the inflammation is confined to the soft tissues over the globe, the term "preseptal cellulitis" is employed (Fig. 7.167C), and if inflammation extends into the orbit (i.e., retro-orbital inflammation), contrast-enhanced CT or MRI can be employed to determine whether an abscess is present. Findings associated with intraorbital inflammation include displacement of the medial rectus muscle and

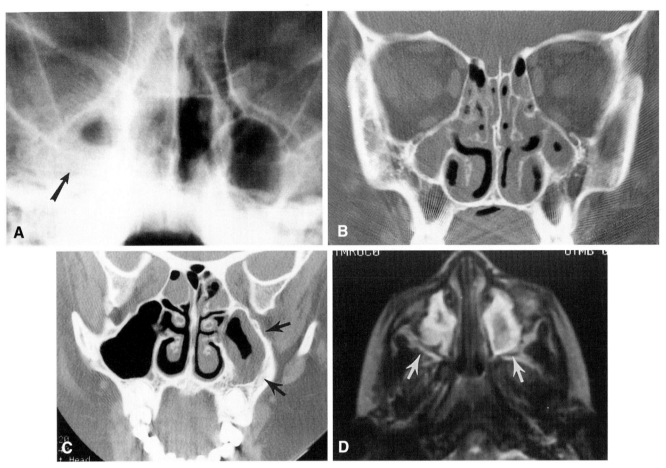

FIGURE 7.167. Sinusitis: various configurations. A. Note the opacified right maxillary sinus (arrow) with an air-fluid level. **B.** Coronal CT in this patient demonstrates almost complete obliteration of the maxillary and ethmoid sinus cavities (i.e., pansinusitis). **C.** Note the mucosal thickening (arrows) in the left maxillary sinus. The ethmoid air cells on both sides also are partially obliterated. **D.** T2-weighted MR study demonstrates high signal intensity in bilateral mucosal thickening (arrows) in the maxillary sinuses.

destruction of the cribriform plate (Fig. 7.168, A and B). The latter is often difficult to determine with certainty, as the cribriform plate is extremely thin and at times irregular, even in normal individuals. Intracranial complications such as meningitis, abscess formation, and epidural or subdural empyemas can occur (8, 9). Orbital pseudotumor mimicking orbital cellulitis is rare (10) as is myositis of the recti muscles leading to rectus muscle palsy (11).

Occasionally, as in adults, rounded filling defects can be encountered in the sinus cavities. The sinus cavities, in these cases, generally are otherwise clear, and the findings represent mucoceles, the aftermath of inflammation causing obstruction of the mucus glands. The findings are characteristic on any imaging modality (Fig. 7.169A). Nasal polyps, allergic or in association with cystic fibrosis can fill and expand the sinuses (Fig. 7.169B). The maxillary and ethmoid sinuses also can be involved with Wegener's granulomatosis in childhood, and the findings are no different from those seen in adults. Similarly, allergic aspergillosis or

other fungal disease can be seen and is associated with polyp formation. The sinuses are totally impacted in these patients and may be expanded. There may be erosion of the skull base (12). The imaging findings on MRI are characteristic in that there is decrease signal on T2-weighted images (Fig. 7.170). We have seen similar changes in chronic *Pseudomonas* infection (Fig. 7.170C).

Tumors of the facial bones and paranasal sinuses are uncommon in infancy, but may include entities such as odontomas, retinal anlage tumors, leukemia, metastatic disease such as neuroblastoma, and histiocytosis X. Rhabdomyosarcoma of the soft tissues also can involve the bones secondarily.

REFERENCES

1. Arruda LK, Mimica IM, Sole D, et al. Abnormal maxillary sinus radiographs in children. Do they represent bacterial infection? Pediatrics 1990;85:553–558.

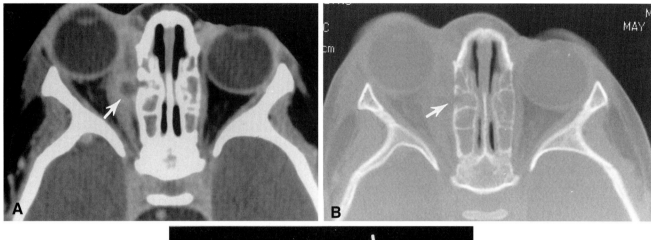

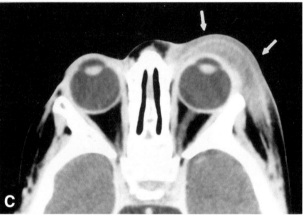

FIGURE 7.168. Sinusitis: orbital complications. A. Orbital abscess. Lucent abscess (arrow) in association with ethmoid sinusitis. The medial rectus muscle is displaced inwardly, and there is considerable soft tissue thickening in the area. Note that there is no soft tissue change anterior to the globe. **B.** Bone window setting demonstrates a defect in the lamina papyracea (arrow) consistent with bony destruction. Note that the ethmoid air cells are totally obliterated on both sides. **C. Preseptal cellulitis.** In this patient, the retro-orbital structures are completely normal but there is extensive swelling of the soft tissues anterior and lateral to the globe (arrows).

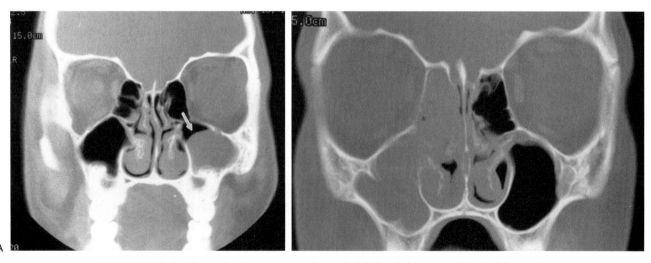

FIGURE 7.169. A. Mucocele. Note the typical rounded filling defect (arrow) in the left maxillary sinus. **B. Nasal polyps.** Note that the right maxillary and ethmoid sinus cavities are completely obliterated (arrows), and there is communication with the nasal passage. The medial bony wall of the maxillary sinus is destroyed.

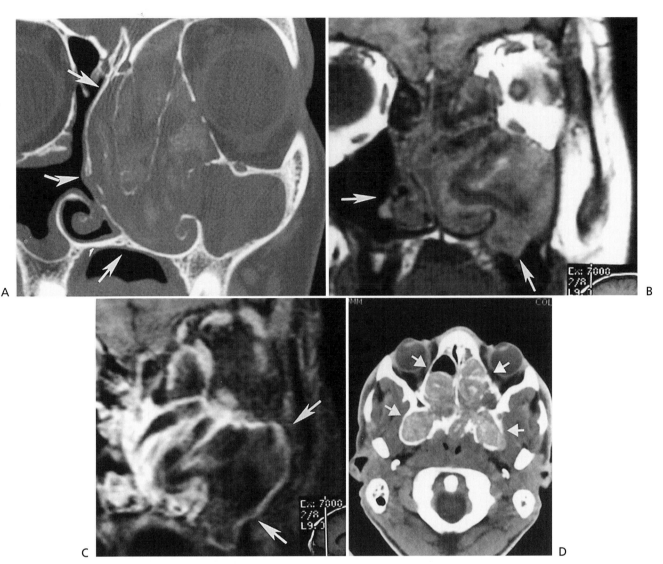

FIGURE 7.170. Chronic sinusitis. A. Fungal sinusitis. CT study demonstrates extensive, expansile opacification of the paranasal sinuses (arrows). **B.** T1-weighted MR image demonstrates the opacified, expanded sinus cavity (arrows). **C.** T2-weighted MR study demonstrates the typical low signal intensity (i.e., black sinus sign) of the involved maxillary sinus (arrows). **D. *Pseudomonas* sinusitis.** The maxillary sinuses are completely obliterated and expanded (arrows) in this patient with underlying cystic fibrosis.

2. Wald ER, Byers C, Guerra N, et al. Subacute sinusitis in children. J Pediatr 1989;115:28–32.

3. McCormick DP, John SD, Swischuk LE, et al. A double-blind placebo-controlled trial of decongestant-antihistamine for the treatment of sinusitis in children. Clin Pediatr 1996;457–460.

4. Rak KM, Newell JD II, Yakes WF, et al. Paranasal sinuses on MR images of the brain: significance of mucosal thickening. AJR 1991;156:381–384.

5. Wiatrak BJ, Myer CM III, Cotton RT. Cystic fibrosis presenting with sinus disease in children. Am J Dis Child 1993;147:258–260.

6. Ros SP, Herman BE, Azar-Kia B. Acute sinusitis in children: is the Waters' view sufficient? Pediatr Radiol 1995;25:306–307.

7. McAlister WH, Lusk R, Muntz HR. Comparison of plain radiographs and coronal CT scans in infants and children with recurrent sinusitis. AJR 1989;153:1259–1264.

8. Gallagher RM, Gross CW, Phillips CD. Suppurative intracranial complications of sinusitis. Laryngoscope 1998;108:1635–1642.

9. Giannoni CM Sewart MG, Alford EL. Intracranial complications of sinusitis. Laryngoscope 1997;107:863–867.

10. Sirbaugh PE. A case of orbital pseudotumor masquerading as orbital cellulitis in a patient with proptosis and fever. Pediatr Emerg Care 1997;13:337–339.

11. Pollard ZF. Acute rectus muscle palsy in children as a result of orbital myositis. J Pediatr 1996;128:230–233.

12. Kinsella JB, Rassekh CH, Bradfield JL, et al. Allergic fungal sinusitis with cranial base erosion. Head Neck 1996;18:211–217.

Mastoids

The antrum of the mastoids is usually visible by 2 or 3 months of age and often even in the neonate. Air cell development proceeds at such a pace that normally air cells become visible by 3–6 months. Mastoid disease, like sinus disease, is not a great problem in neonates, but is very common in infants and children. In mastoid infection (associated with middle ear inflammatory disease), the air cells become hazy (fluid accumulation and mucosal thickening) and the bony walls become indistinct (reactive inflammatory-hyperemic demineralization). The entire process, if unchecked, can progress to coalescent mastoiditis (abscess) and complicating intracranial infection.

With acute mastoiditis, the findings simply consist of increased opacification of the involved mastoid air cells and antral area (Fig. 7.171, A and B). The findings can be seen on plain films, but are more vividly demonstrated with CT or MRI. If infection progresses to a coalescent abscess, bony destruction will be seen and is best assessed with computed tomography (Fig. 7.171C). Because middle ear infections frequently are recurrent, there is concomitant inhibition of mastoid air cell development and aeration. As a result, the number of air cells is diminished. Reactive sclerosis of the petrous bone is seen, and in advanced cases virtually no aeration is present and the petrous bone is very dense. A complication of chronic mastoiditis is the development of an inflammatory cholesteatoma. In the early stages this lesion can be suspected by the presence of tissue in the middle ear involving the space of Prussak, and more specifically, destruction of the scutum (Fig. 7.172A). In more advanced cases extensive destruction of the petrous bone occurs (Fig. 7.172B). Congenital cholesteatomas of the middle ear are rare.

Tumors of the mastoid area and petrous bone are not particularly common in infancy, but it should be remembered that the petrous bone is one of the favorite sites for rhabdomyosarcoma and the problem may masquerade as an infection. Nonspecific bony destruction is seen in this condition, and the findings eventually are best delineated with CT or MRI. Destruction of the petrous bone also occurs with histiocytosis X, lymphoma, and leukemia.

The evaluation of congenital deafness usually is relegated to a study of the internal ear and auditory canal with thin-slice CT. A variety of findings can be encountered, including hypoplasia or atresia of the auditory canal and various malformations, hypoplasia, or entire absence of the auditory ossicles. The entire subject is beyond the scope of this book and only one example is presented in Figure 7.173.

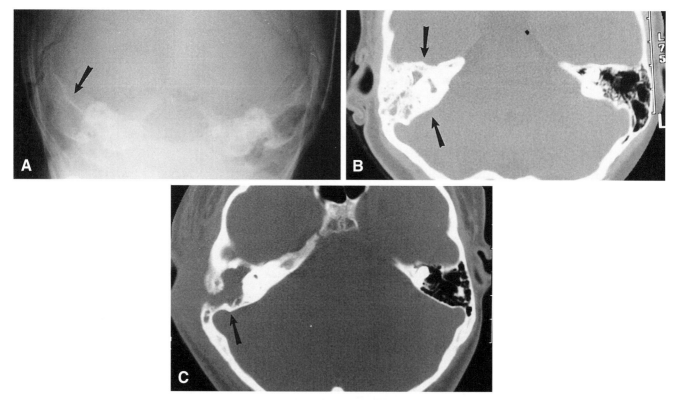

FIGURE 7.171. Mastoid infection. A. Acute mastoiditis. Note that the air cells on the right (arrow) have been totally obliterated as a result of inflammation. **B.** CT study in another patient demonstrates lack of aeration of the right mastoid air cells and increased sclerosis of the petrous bone (arrows). **C. Mastoid abscess** produces destruction of the petrous bone on the right (arrow).

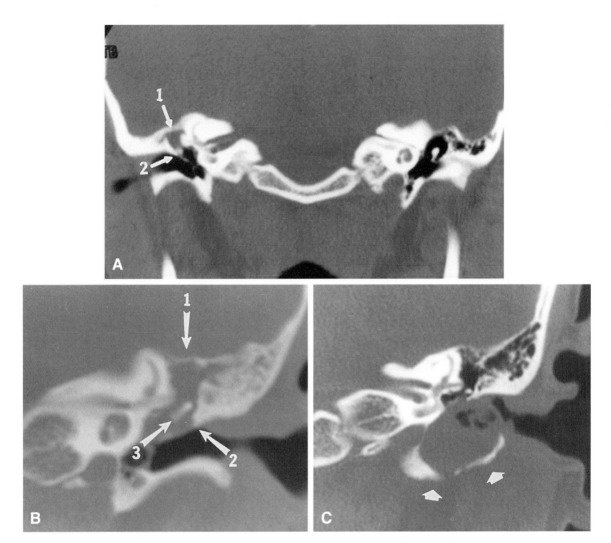

FIGURE 7.172. Cholesteatoma. A. Note the obliteration of Prussak's space (1). The scutum (2), however, still is intact, because it still has a sharp pointed configuration. The auditory ossicles may be displaced. Compare with the normal appearance on the other side. **B.** More advanced changes include obliteration of Prussak's space (1), erosion of the scutum (2), and destruction and dislocation of the auditory ossicles (3). **C.** Advanced case. Note the marked destruction and expansion of the petrous bone by this expanding cholesteatoma (arrows).

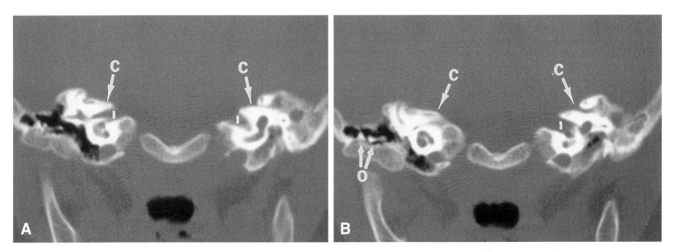

FIGURE 7.173. Congenital deafness. A and B. The internal auditory canals (I) are present, but the external auditory canals are absent. The cochlea (C) on both sides is deformed, but the left is more deformed than the right. On the left, the cochlea lacks all of its normal spirals. On the right, the number of spirals is reduced. No ossicles are present on the left, whereas those on the right (O) are displaced and deformed.

OPHTHALMIC RADIOLOGY

Only a brief summary of ophthalmic imaging is presented here, and for more details one is referred to more comprehensive communications (1–4).

Tumors

The most commonly occurring tumor of the eye is retinoblastoma. Seventy-five percent of these lesions show calcifications, and bilateral tumors can occur. With the latter, a familial incidence has been noted (5), and often, these bilateral tumors are associated with a midline, suprasellar, or pineal tumor (6–8). Radiographically, irregular, granular calcifications can be seen on plain films or CT (Fig. 7.174A), but definitive imaging requires CT or MRI (Fig. 7.174). Behavior of this tumor on MRI is characteristic, because it is one of the few tumors of the body, along with melanoma, that show decreased signal intensity on T2-weighted images (Fig. 7.174F). This is secondary to the hemosiderin present in the pigment. CT is best at demonstrating the calcifications and is especially valuable when the calcifications are small. It also is important, in these tumors, to define whether the optic nerve is involved by tumor spread (Fig. 7.174C). This is important for treatment planning.

Other tumors that can be seen in the orbit include hemangioma, lymphangioma, optic glioma, rhabdomyosarcoma, dermoid, teratoma, and neurofibroma. The latter tumor often is plexiform. All of these lesions are best delineated with CT or MRI (Fig. 7.175), but hemangiomas and lymphangiomas also can be adequately imaged with ultrasound. Optic gliomas commonly occur with neurofibromatosis.

Intraocular Hemorrhage and Orbital Inflammation

Intraocular hemorrhages occur with trauma to the globe and in the more severe cases of head trauma (Fig. 7.176A). Retinal hemorrhages are common in the battered child syndrome, but are not common with ordinary trauma. Orbital abscess, except that which occurs in association with sinusitis, is uncommon. Inflammatory pseudotumors of the retro-orbital region also are uncommon and with MRI can be shown to produce diffuse swelling of the optic nerve muscle and soft tissues in general (Fig. 7.176, B and C).

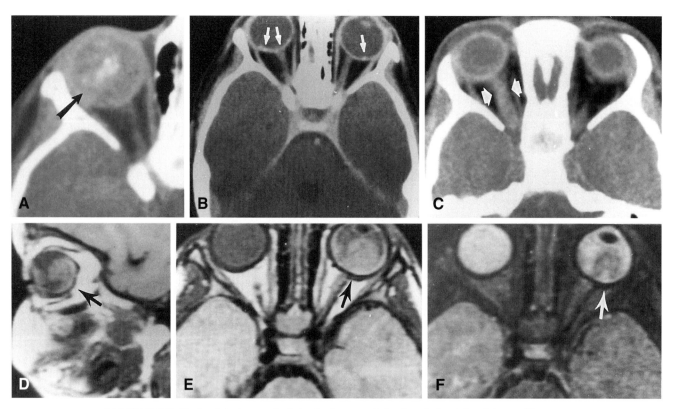

FIGURE 7.174. Retinoblastoma. A. Note the increased density of the right globe and intraocular irregular calcification (arrow). **B.** Small bilateral retinoblastomas (arrows) are present in this patient. **C.** Thickening of the optic nerve (arrows) results from retinoblastoma extending along the optic nerve. **D. MR features of retinoblastoma.** On this T1-weighted image, the retinoblastoma (arrow) produces an area of irregular increase in signal. **E.** Similar findings (arrow) are seen on the axial view. **F.** On the T2-weighted image, the retinoblastoma shows relatively low signal intensity (arrow).

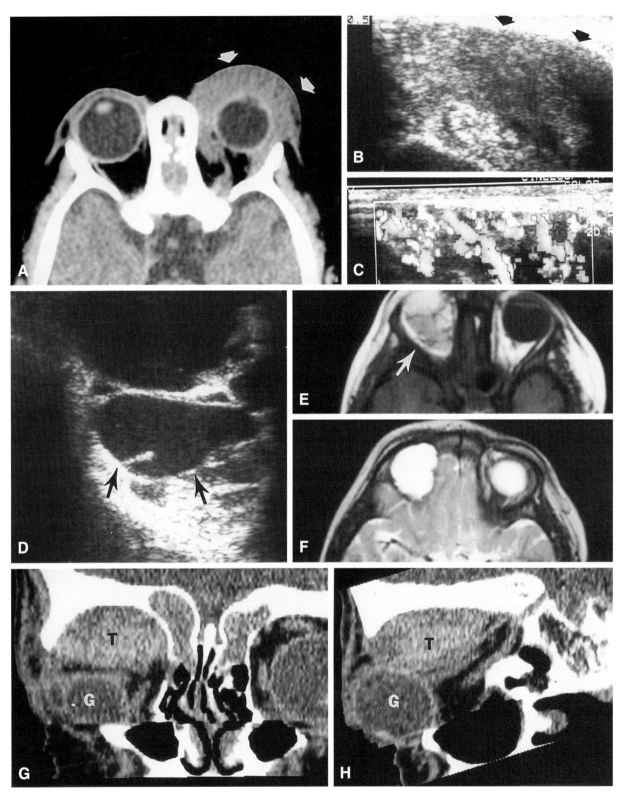

FIGURE 7.175. Orbital tumors. A. Hemangioma. Note the marked thickening of the soft tissues (arrows) over the left globe. There is some retro-orbital extension, and proptosis is present. **B.** Ultrasonogram demonstrates a heterogeneous pattern to the hemangioma (arrows). Punctate densities along the inferior surface probably are areas of calcification. **C.** Color flow Doppler demonstrates markedly increased blood flow to the hemangioma. **D. Lymphangioma.** Ultrasonogram demonstrates characteristic multiloculated cystic appearance (arrows). **E.** T1-weighted MR image demonstrates the relatively low-signal-intensity supraorbital lymphangioma (arrow), surrounded by high-signal-intensity fat. Multiloculation and septa are suggested. **F.** T2-weighted image demonstrates increased signal intensity in the lymphangioma. **G.** Another patient with a lymphangioma whose coronal CT demonstrates the tumor (T) displacing the globe (G) inferiorly. **H.** Similar findings on the lateral view. G, globe; T, tumor.

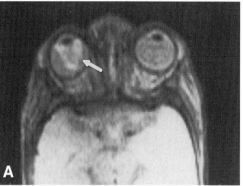

FIGURE 7.176. **A. Intraocular hemorrhage.** Note the area of increased density within the globe (arrow). **B. Pseudotumor.** There is slight proptosis on the right and thickening of the optic nerve and the ocular muscles. **C.** Coronal view demonstrates the enlarged optic nerve and the thickened enlarged muscles. Compare with the normal side.

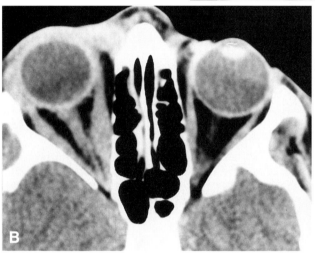
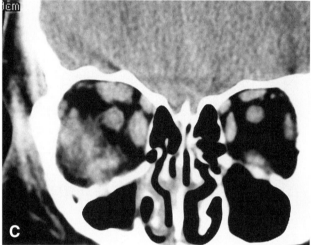

Normal Optic Canal and Optic Nerve

The eye and optic nerve are nearly adult size in the young infant and, as the infant grows older, they undergo proportionately less growth than do other structures. As a consequence, the optic canal is larger than one would expect in the neonate. Normal measurements range from 4 mm in the neonate to 6 mm in the older child. The optic nerves are best visualized with CT or MRI (Fig. 7.177).

Large Optic Canal (Large Optic Nerve)

Enlargement of the optic canal occurs with longstanding intracanalicular expanding tumors such as optic glioma and neurofibroma of the optic nerve. The optic canal also can become ectatic without associated tumor, much the same as the auditory canal does with neurofibromatosis. Enlargement of the optic nerve can occur with inflammation and with inflammatory pseudotumor, but the optic canal does not enlarge.

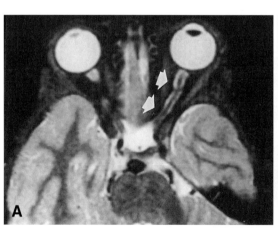
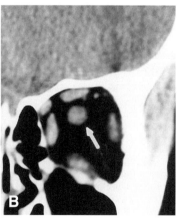

FIGURE 7.177. **Normal optic nerve. A.** T2-weighted MR image demonstrates normal CSF (i.e., high signal intensity) around the optic nerve (arrows) **B.** Coronal CT demonstrates the normal optic nerve (arrow). It is surrounded by the four ocular muscles (i.e., oval densities around the periphery of the orbit).

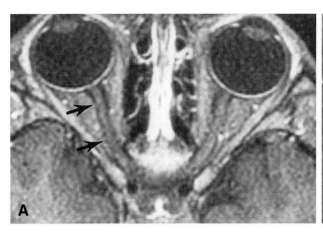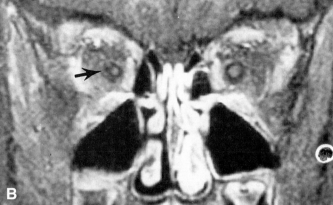

FIGURE 7.178. Small optic nerve: optic nerve atrophy. A. The optic nerve on the right (arrows) is slightly smaller than the left. **B.** Coronal view demonstrates the findings more clearly. The right optic nerve (arrow) now clearly is seen to be smaller than the one on the left. A large optic nerve is illustrated in Figure 7.176.

Small Optic Canal (Small Optic Nerve)

A small optic canal and nerve can be seen with optic nerve atrophy, either as a result of congenital absence of the globe and optic nerve (congenital anophthalmia) or secondary to optic nerve atrophy resulting from early enucleation of an eye (Fig. 7.178). In older children, hyperostosis secondary to certain anemias, hypercalcemia, fibrous dysplasia, and osteopetrosis can lead to encroachment upon the optic canal. Small optic nerves are seen with septo-optic dysplasia.

Large Orbit

Unilateral enlargement of the orbit usually occurs as part of the skeletal dysplasia of neurofibromatosis (Fig. 7.179), but

can also be seen with a rapidly growing orbital tumor in the neonate or young infant. Apart from this, unilateral orbital enlargement is uncommon. With neurofibromatosis, dysplasia of the sphenoid wing also occurs (Fig. 7.150). Orbital enlargement also can be seen with chronic intraorbital, extraocular foreign bodies (9).

Small Orbit

A unilateral small orbit in the newborn or young infant is almost invariably the result of congenital underdevelopment of the globe (congenital anophthalmia). Underdevelopment of the face on the corresponding side is also often present (Fig. 7.180). A small orbit can also be encountered in infants who have had early enucleation of the eye for

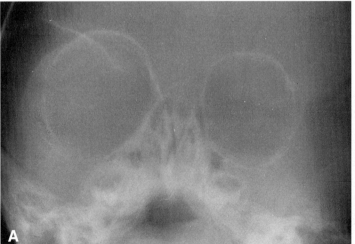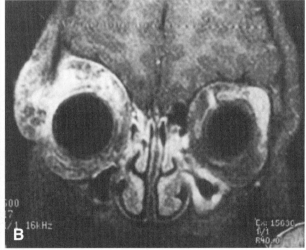

FIGURE 7.179. Large orbit. A. Note the large orbit and elevated sphenoid wing in this patient with neurofibromatosis. **B.** Another patient with an enlarged orbit and elevated sphenoid wing resulting from plexiform neurofibromatosis surrounding the globe. Less pronounced changes are present on the other side.

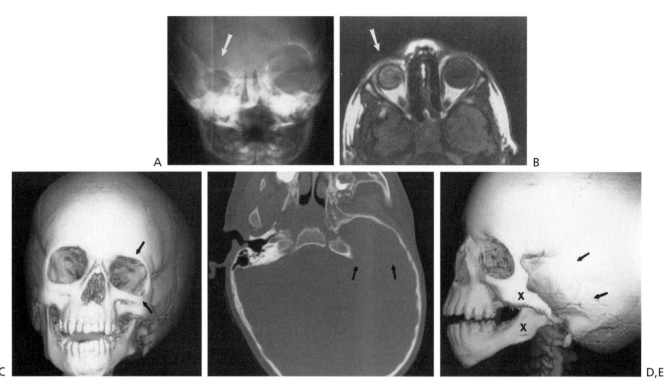

FIGURE 7.180. Small orbit: congenitally hypoplastic. A. Note the congenitally small orbit (arrow). The vertical line is an artifact. **B.** CT study in another patient demonstrates a small orbit and globe (arrow). **C. Hemifacial microsoma.** Note the small orbit on the left (arrows) and generalized smallness of the face. **D.** CT study demonstrates absence of the internal auditory canal and inner ear structures (arrows). **E.** Three-dimensional study demonstrates absence of the auditory canal.

tumor. In older children, the orbit may become small with hyperostosing lesions such as fibrous dysplasia, osteopetrosis, and Cooley's anemia.

Hypotelorism

Hypotelorism of a severe degree is seen with arrhinencephaly. The extremist form is present in the cyclops deformity. Hypotelorism is also seen with simple trigonocephaly secondary to premature closure of the metopic suture. Various degrees of hypotelorism are seen with sagittal craniostenosis and any cause of microcephaly. Normal interorbital distance at birth is approximately 11 mm (6).

Hypertelorism

Hypertelorism occurs as a normal familial variant in some infants. In such cases, it is usually mild. It also occurs sec-

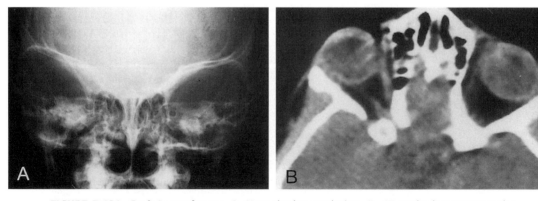

FIGURE 7.181. Greig's syndrome. A. Note the hypertelorism. **B.** CT study demonstrates the same degree of hypertelorism.

ondary to encephalocele of the frontal region, the median cleft face, or Greig's syndrome (Fig. 7.181) and in such bony dysplasias as cleidocranial dysostosis, Crouzon's craniofacial dysotosis, bilateral coronal suture premature synostosis, and in some infants with hypothyroidism. In the median cleft face syndrome, some of these patients demonstrate a peculiar bony spicule in the middle of the frontal portion of the skull. The findings are rather characteristic and are exceptionally well delineated with CT scanning.

Intraorbital Calcifications

Intraorbital calcifications are best assessed with CT. Calcifications are irregular in retinoblastoma, as are they with intraorbital bleeding associated with detached retinas. Calcification of the lens occurs with retrolental fibroplasia, and calcifications are seen throughout the globe. Calcifications in dermoids often are more dense and formed.

Proptosis

Proptosis can occur with intraorbital tumors, orbital infarction in sickle cell disease, intraorbital inflammations secondary to sinusitis, and in some instances with nonspecific inflammation or pseudotumor. In these cases, CT is useful in defining the problem. Pulsating exophthalmus is seen along with proptosis in neurofibromatosis when sphenoid wing dysplasia is present. Proptosis is a common manifestation of hyperthyroidism.

Congenital Nasolacrimal Duct Obstruction

In this condition the lacrimal duct is congenitally stenosed and obstructed (10, 11). Slowly, secretions accumulate and a mucocele develops. These mucoceles can be traced from their origin in the orbit into the nasal cavity. They are best identified with CT (Fig. 7.182) or MRI.

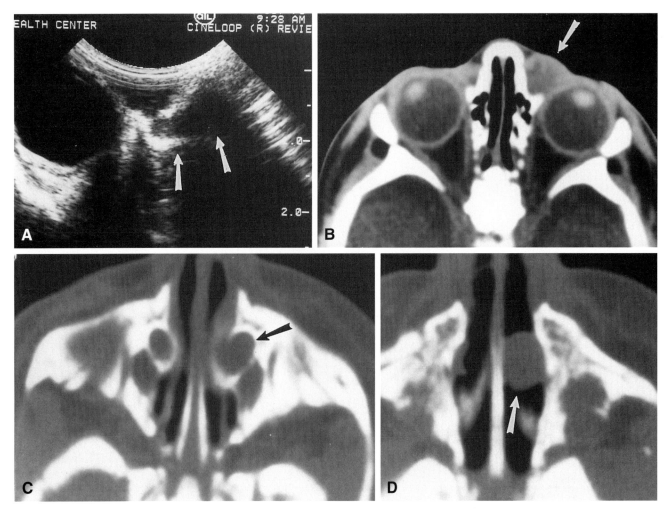

FIGURE 7.182. Nasolacrimal duct obstruction. A. Ultrasound demonstrates the origin of the dilated nasolacrimal duct (arrows). **B.** CT study demonstrates the proximally dilated nasolacrimal duct (arrow) in the same area. **C.** Lower cut demonstrates the dilated canal (arrow). **D.** Still lower, the dilated duct (arrow) is seen in the nasal passage.

REFERENCES

1. Glasier CM, Brodsky MC, Leithiser RE Jr, et al. High resolution ultrasound with Doppler: a diagnostic adjunct in orbital and ocular lesions in children. Pediatr Radiol 1992;22:174–178.
2. Hopper KD, Sherman JL, Boal DKB. Pictorial essay. Abnormalities of the orbit and its contents in children: CT and MR imaging findings. AJR 1991;156:1219–1224.
3. Ramji FG, Slovis TL, Baker JD. Orbital sonography in children. Pediatr Radiol 1996;26:245–258.
4. Wells RG, Sty JR, Gonnering RS. Imaging of the pediatric eye and orbit. Radiographics 1989;9:1023–1044.
5. Judisch G, Patil SR. Concurrent heritable retinoblastoma, pinealoma, and trisomy X. Arch Ophthalmol 1981;99:1767–1769.
6. Finelli DA, Shurin SB, Bardenstein DS. Trilateral retinoblastoma: two variations. AJNR 1995;16:166–170.
7. Provenzale J, Weber A, Klintworth GK, et al. Radiologic-pathologic correlation. Bilateral retinoblastoma with coexistent pineoblastoma (tri-lateral retinoblastoma). AJNR 1995;16:157–165.yy
8. Skulski M. Egelhoff JC, Kollias SS, et al. Trilateral retinoblastoma with suprasellar involvement. Neuroradiology 1997;39:41–43.
9. Swischuk LE. Orbital enlargement secondary to chronic foreign body. Emerg Radiol 2000;7:356–357.
10. John PR, Boldt D. Bilateral congenital lacrimal sac mucoceles with nasal extension. Pediatr Radiol 1990;20:285–286.
11. Ogawa GSH, Gonnering RS. Congenital nasolacrimal duct obstruction. J Pediatr 1991;119:12–17.

SPINE, SPINAL CORD, AND MENINGES

NORMAL SPINE AND VARIATIONS

The normal spine forms around the notochord, and separate vertebrae and intervertebral discs eventually develop. At birth, ossification of the vertebral bodies and neural arches is well underway, and one can readily identify three ossified structures for each vertebra. These include one for the vertebral body and one for each side of the neural arch.

The synchondroses between these ossification centers are usually readily visualized (Fig. 8.1).

Normal curvatures of the spine in the neonate include a **mild** cervical lordosis, dorsolumbar kyphosis, and a lumbosacral lordosis (Fig. 8.1). As the infant grows older, the cervical and lumbosacral lordoses become more pronounced. The individual vertebral bodies are rectangular, especially in the thoracic region. In the lumbar area, normal

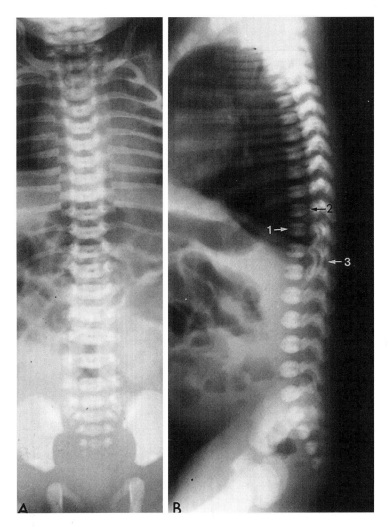

FIGURE 8.1. Normal spine. A. Frontal view. Note the normal diameters of the spinal canal. There is normal widening in the cervical and lumbar regions. The double central vertebral body radiolucencies represent nutrient vessel foramina. The vertebral bodies often appear somewhat bilobed, and the pedicles in the upper lumbar region are flatter and more oval than those in the thoracic area. **B.** Lateral view showing anterior nutrient foramen notches (arrow 1); synchondroses between the vertebral bodies and the well-developed neural arches (arrow 2), and the sometimes puzzling, curvilinear appearance of the normal twelfth ribs (arrow 3). Nutrient vessel notches are also present posteriorly but are less well visualized. Note that the thoracic vertebral bodies are relatively rectangular, while those in the upper lumbar region are more rounded and plump.

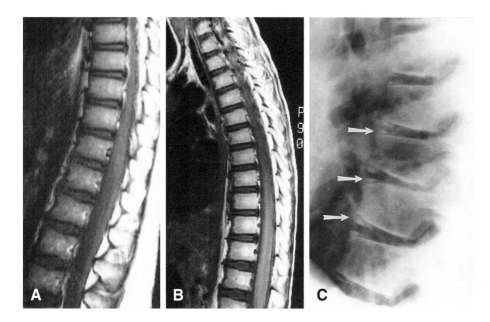

FIGURE 8.2. Normal spine. A. Because the marrow is not fatty in infancy, T1-weighted MR images demonstrate low signal intensity. Note the anterior and posterior notches for the central vein grooves. The posterior ones are more clearly defined. **B.** An older child demonstrates increased signal intensity in the vertebral bodies on this T1-weighted image, indicating fatty replacement of red marrow. Note the configuration of the intervertebral discs. Also note that the central vein grooves are still visible. **C. Ring epiphyses.** Note the normal square appearance of the vertebra and numerous normal ring epiphyses (arrows).

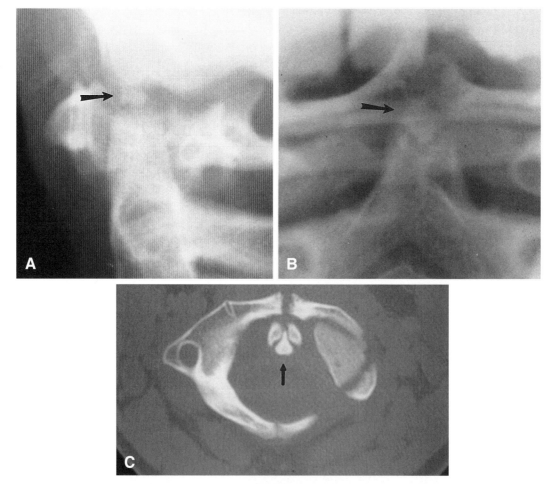

FIGURE 8.3. Os terminale. A. Note the normal os terminale (arrow) on top of a normally developed dens. **B.** Frontal view demonstrates the typical shape of the os terminale (arrow) as it sits in a groove in the dens. **C.** Axial CT study demonstrates the os terminale (arrow) as it sits in the groove of the dens. Note the normal anterior and posterior central defects in the arches of C1.

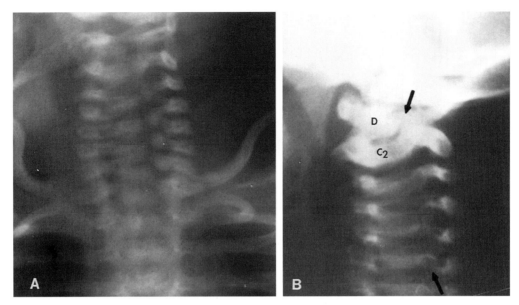

FIGURE 8.4. Normal cervical spine: various normal pitfalls. A. The cervical spinal canal is normally wider than the thoracic spinal canal. With slight degrees of rotation, as in this infant, the canal often appears alarmingly wide. It is normal, however. **B.** Oblique view of the cervical spine demonstrates the synchondrosis between the dens (D) and body of C2. It joins the synchondrosis between the dens and arch of C2 (upper arrow). A synchondrosis in the lower cervical spine is delineated by the lower arrow.

variation includes a slight oval or rounded appearance to the upper lumbar vertebral bodies (Fig. 8.1). Nutrient canals (central vascular grooves) are regularly seen on both frontal and lateral views (Fig. 8.1). Later, these become less prominent, and all the vertebral bodies become more square-cornered. Eventually, the normal ring epiphysis becomes visible (Fig. 8.2C), and then, in adolescence, it fuses with the vertebral body. The vertebra and spinal cord also are readily visualized with magnetic resonance imaging (MRI) (Fig. 8.2 A, and B).

Ossification of the first and second cervical vertebrae is somewhat different from that of the other vertebrae. The first cervical vertebra has no body, but ossification centers for both lateral masses and the posterior aspect of the neural arch are usually present. In approximately 20% of newborn infants, ossification of the anterior arch of the first cervical vertebra is also seen at birth. By 6 months to 1 year of age, all infants show ossification of this latter structure. The body of C2 ossifies in a fashion similar to that of the other vertebral bodies, but the dens arises separately from two ossification centers. At birth, these centers usually have fused into a single structure, but in a few instances, a residual superior cleft may persist. This is often referred to as a bifid odontoid process. Occasionally, an extra, but normal, ossification center is seen just over this midline cleft, the os terminale (Fig. 8.3). **When dens hypoplasia is present, this bone overgrows and becomes the os odontoideum.**

Variation in the diameter of the spinal canal can be problematic because relative proportions usually are different from those in older children and adults. This is especially true of the cervical spine, where the normal interpedicular and sagittal distances can appear alarmingly wide (Fig. 8.4A). A similar problem arises in the lumbar region because the normal canal also widens in this area. Normal interpedicular distances in newborns and young infants are presented in Figure 8.5.

Another normal variation in the lumbar region of older infants and children consists of flattening of the inner aspects of the pedicles and posterior scalloping of the vertebral bodies of the upper lumbar vertebra. These findings are usually more pronounced in older infants and children, and one may falsely suspect an expanding intraspinal lesion in such cases (Fig. 8.6A). One also should be aware of the fact that posterior scalloping is normal in the lumbar vertebra (Fig. 8.6B). It should not be misinterpreted for pathologic scalloping due to an expanding intracanalicular lesion.

In the cervical spine, the various normal synchondroses can pose a problem in differentiation from fracture. Fortunately, fractures of the cervical spine are not particularly common in the neonate and very young infant, but these normal synchondroses should be appreciated (Fig. 8.4B). Most often, one sees these synchondroses on oblique views of the cervical spine, and the synchondroses between the dens and arch of C2 must be distinguished from the hangman's fracture (1).

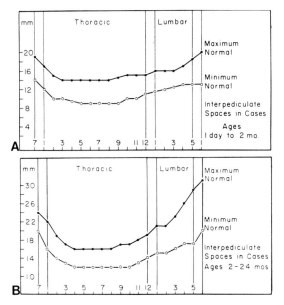

FIGURE 8.5. Normal spinal canal measurements. A. Normal maximum and minimum interpediculate space measurements (in millimeters) in infants 1 day to 2 months of age. **B.** Similar measurements in infants 2 months to 2 years of age. (From Simril WA, Thurston D. Normal interpediculate space in the spines of infants and children. Radiology 1955;64:340–347, with permission.)

Pseudosubluxation of Cervical Spine

With pronounced forward flexion, there is a distinct tendency for the infant's upper cervical spine to appear dislocated or subluxed (2). This is related to generalized laxity of the ligaments in the infant and horizontal positioning of the apophyseal joints. In the older child and adult, the joints become more vertical in position, but in the infant and young child their horizontal attitude predisposes to anterior displacement of the upper vertebral bodies, one on another. Most often, this involves C2 on C3, but pseudo-dislocation of the cervical spine can be seen down to the C4-5 level (Fig. 8.7).

Since the spine must be flexed to produce this pseudoabnormality, the soft tissues anterior to the spine also usually are distorted, and with the airway so buckled, the problem just becomes more confusing. Nonetheless, it is important to appreciate these changes because somewhat similar displacement of C2 on C3 can be produced by a hangman's fracture of C2. Differentiation of the two conditions can be accomplished by use of the posterior cervical line (2). This line, drawn from the cortex of the spinous tip of C1 to the same location on C3, should touch or come within 1–1.5 mm of the anterior cortex of the spinous tip of C2 (Fig. 8.8). It remains normal with pseudosubluxation, but when the hangman's fracture is present the line misses the anterior cortex of C2 by 2 mm or more.

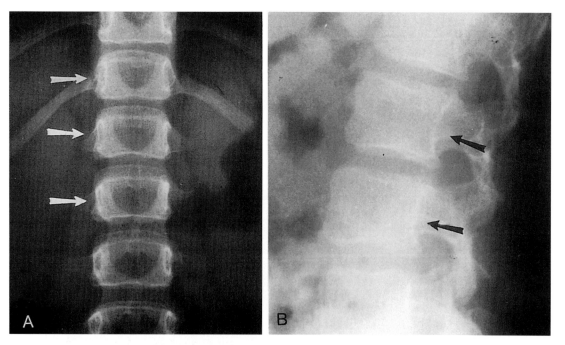

FIGURE 8.6. Normal pedicular flattening. A. Frequently the pedicles are normally flattened in the upper lumbar and lower thoracic regions (arrows). **B. Normal posterior scalloping.** Many children demonstrate scalloping of the posterior vertebral bodies in the lumbar region (arrows), which is completely normal.

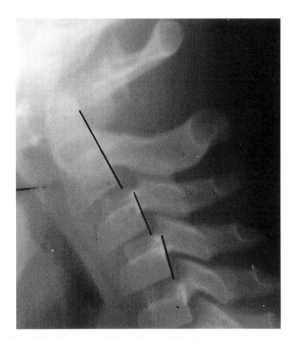

FIGURE 8.7. Pseudosubluxation. With flexion, apparent dislocation of the vertebral bodies in the upper cervical spine is a common normal phenomenon. Lines mark the posterior aspects of the vertebral bodies, and it is easy to see that each is displaced forward on the one underneath it. All of this is normal.

Wedging of C3, and sometimes C4, is another normal variation that commonly is seen in infants and young children (3). It also is associated with normal hypermobility through this area, and it is the chronic, hammering impingement of C2 on C3 that causes C3 to under grow anteriorly. As a consequence, it becomes wedged (Fig. 8.9), and the configuration should not be misinterpreted for a compression fracture (3). Anterior compression fractures of C3 are uncommon in any age group, but if there still is doubt, computed tomography (CT) should be performed because it can clearly establish whether a fracture through the vertebral body exists.

C1-Dens Distance

The distance between the anterior arch of C1 and the odontoid process often appears unduly wide in infants. In adults, maximum normal distance is in the neighborhood of 2 to 2.5 mm, but in young infants, it frequently is 3 mm and can range as high as 4 to 5 mm and still be normal. This latter measurement occurs in less than 5% of cases. Normally, no matter what the original configuration this space, if normal, it does not increase by more than 2 mm during flexion.

Clefts of C1

Since CT was introduced, it has become more and more apparent that normal clefts exist in the anterior and poste-

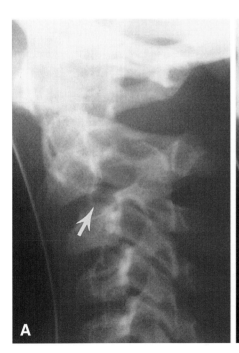

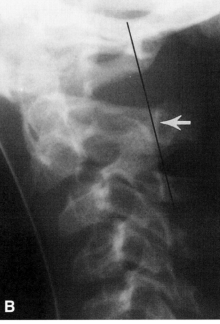

FIGURE 8.8. Pseudosubluxation C2-3: use of posterior cervical line. A. With some forward flexion, this patient demonstrates what appears to be dislocation of C2 on C3 (arrow). A milder degree is suggested at C3-4. **B.** The posterior cervical line drawn from the anterior cortex of C1 to the anterior cortex of C3 passes through the anterior cortex of C2 (arrow). This represents normal alignment of the spinous processes and indicates that dislocation of C2 on C3 is physiologic.

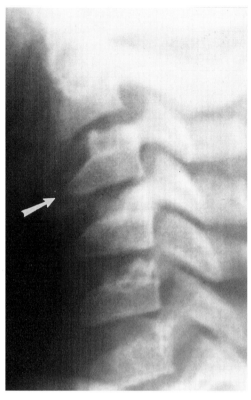

FIGURE 8.9. Normal wedging of C3. Note the marked wedging of C3 (arrow). No fractures were present in this patient.

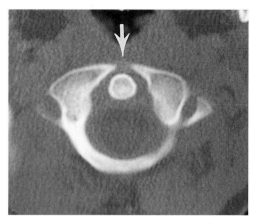

FIGURE 8.10. Anterior defect of C1. Note the anterior defect of C1 (arrow); this is normal. For both anterior and posterior defects, see Figure 8.3C.

rior (4, 5) portions of the ring of C1. These clefts can be identified as being normal and innocuous by their smoothly corticated edges (Figs. 8.3 and 8.10). They must be differentiated from fractures that occur through the ring of C1 in the form of the Jefferson fracture. Fractures generally demonstrate thin radiolucent lines with nonsclerotic bony edges.

Normal Spinal Cord

The normal spinal cord follows the same variations in diameter as does the spinal canal; it is wider in the cervical

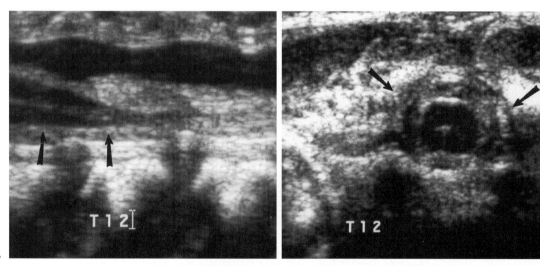

FIGURE 8.11. Normal spinal cord: ultrasound findings. A. Longitudinal view demonstrates the hypoechoic spinal cord and conus (arrows) and the echoic central canal. **B.** Cross section demonstrates the same hypoechoic cord (arrows) with a central echogenic dot (the spinal canal).

region than in the thoracic area. Also recall that the spinal cord ends lower in the newborn infant, but as the infant grows older, the cord migrates towards the head, eventually ending at about L1 (6–8). This level usually is reached in the first few months of life.

The spinal cord is readily evaluated with ultrasound and MRI in infants, and ultrasound is especially useful in the neonate. Normal findings are illustrated in Figure 8.11. On the sagittal view, the normal spinal cord produces three echogenic lines, the outer two of which represent the anterior and posterior aspects of the cord. The cord itself is hypoechoic, and within it lies the third line, the echogenic central canal. The normal conus tapers smoothly and becomes continuous with the filum terminale. Below this level are the fibers of the cauda equina that produce linear echogenicities that blend together and almost totally fill the arachnoid space. Occasionally, one encounters dilation of the distal-most portion of the central canal. The configuration is usually somewhat oval, and the dilated structure is called the "ventriculus terminalis" (9–12). It is a normal finding not to be interpreted for some pathologic problem (Fig. 8.12).

A problem often arises in terms of numbering the vertebral bodies when ultrasound is being used. It has been suggested that the angle that occurs between the lumbar and sacral portions of the spine is consistent and can be used as a marker (13). In other cases, one may match the echogenic vertebra with those seen on plain films and thereby obtain accurate numbering of the vertebral bodies.

Many of the foregoing normal findings can cause problems with diagnosis and differentiation from pathologic conditions. A more comprehensive review (14) of these problems is available.

REFERENCES

1. Swischuk LE, Hayden CK Jr, Sarwar M. The dens-arch synchondrosis versus the hangman's fracture. Pediatr Radiol 1979;8:100–112.
2. Swischuk LE. Anterior displacement of C2 in children: physiologic or pathologic? A helpful differentiating line. Radiology 1977;122:759–763.
3. Swischuk LE, Swischuk PN, John SD. Wedging of C3 in infants and children: usually a normal finding and not a fracture. Radiology 1993;188:523–526.
4. Chambers AA, Gaskill MF. Midline anterior atlas clefts: CT findings J Comput Assist Tomogr 1992;16:868–870.
5. Hosalkar HS, Gerardi JA, Shaw BA. Combined asymptomatic congenital anterior and posterior deficiency of the atlas. Pediatr Radiol 2001;31:810–813.
6. DePietro MA. The conus medullaris: normal US findings throughout childhood. Radiology 1993;188:149–153.
7. Hill CAR, Gibson PJ. Ultrasound determination of the normal location of the conus medullaris in neonates. AJNR 1995;16:469–472.
8. Wolf S, Schneble F, Troger J. The conus medullaris: time of ascendence to normal level. Pediatr Radiol 1992;22:590–592.
9. Coleman LT, Zimmerman RA, Rorke LB. Ventriculitis terminalis of the conus medullaris: MR findings in children. AJNR 1995;16:1421–1426.
10. Kriss VM, Kriss TC, Babcock DS. The ventriculus terminalis of the spinal cord in the neonate: a normal variant on sonography. AJR 1995;165:1491–1493.
11. Kriss VM, Coleman RC. Sonographic appearance of the ventriculus terminalis cyst in the neonatal spinal cord. J Ultrasound Med 2000;19:207–209.
12. Truong BC, Shaw DWW, Winters WD. Dilation of the ventriculus terminalis: sonographic findings. J Ultrasound Med 1998;17:713–715.
13. Beek FJA, van Leeuwen MS, Bax NMA, et al. A method for sonographic counting of the lower vertebral bodies in newborns and infants. AJNR 1994;15:445–449.
14. Swischuk LE. Normal cervical spine variations mimicking injuries in children. Emerg Radiol 1999;6:299–306.

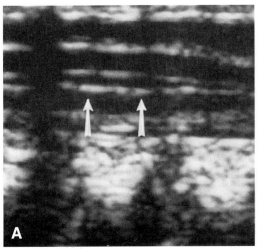
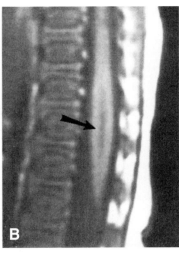

FIGURE 8.12. Ventriculus terminalis. A. Note a slightly dilated distal central canal (arrows). **B.** Similar findings (arrow) on MRI. (From Kriss VM, Kross TC, Babcock DS. Ventriculus terminalis of the spinal cord in the neonate: a normal variant on sonography. AJR 1995;165:1491–1493, with permission.)

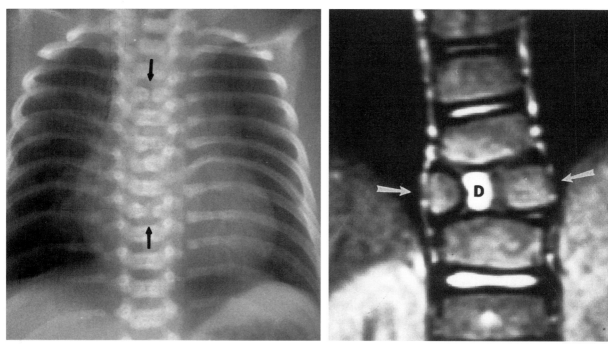

A   B

FIGURE 8.13. Sagittal cleft (butterfly) vertebra. A. Note the sagittal clefts in two thoracic vertebrae (arrows). This probably represents failure of union of the two lateral chondrification centers. Other thoracic vertebrae, in between the two cleft vertebrae, show slight irregularity of shape. **B.** MR study in another patient demonstrates a sagittal cleft vertebra (arrow) with a anomalous central, and displaced intervertebral disc (D).

CONGENITAL ABNORMALITIES OF THE SPINE, SPINAL CORD, AND MENINGES

To completely understand the various congenital anomalies of the spine, one must understand the developmental steps of vertebral body and arch formation. Only a few highlights are considered here, but for more detailed information refer to the classic study of *The Human Spine in Health and Disease* by Schmorl and Junghanns (1).

Early in the development of the vertebral bodies, two lateral chondrification centers are present, one on either side of the notochord. Two ossification centers also eventually appear, one anterior and one posterior. Eventually, the lateral chondrification centers fuse to form a single unit, but if union is incomplete, a sagittal cleft or butterfly vertebra results (Fig. 8.13). If only one of these lateral chondrification centers fails to develop, a hemivertebra results (Fig. 8.14). These hemivertebrae may be single or multiple, and abnormal spinal curvatures often result. There also is an increased incidence of ipsilateral rib anomalies and, in some cases, hypoplasia of the ipsilateral pulmonary artery and lung.

Abnormalities of the dorsal and ventral ossification centers are much less common. However, if one or the other fails to develop, a dorsal (more common) or ventral hemivertebra results (Fig. 8.15A). Underdevelopment of the ventral portion of a vertebral body frequently leads to severe gibbus

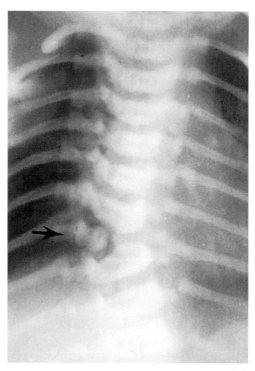

FIGURE 8.14. Sagittal hemivertebra. Note the sagittal thoracic hemivertebra (arrow). There is associated scoliosis, and if the ribs are matched with the adjacent vertebral bodies, it will be noted that one rib is missing on the left.

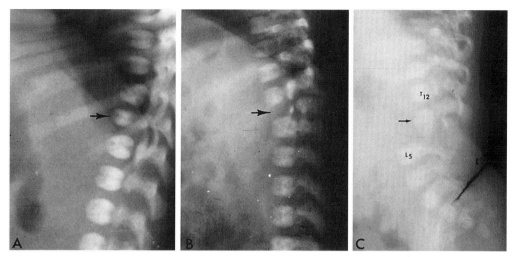

FIGURE 8.15. Hypoplastic and absent vertebra. A. Note hypoplasia of T12 (arrow). The findings also suggest underdevelopment of the dorsal ossification center. **B.** The body of T12 is entirely missing (arrow) in this infant. The ribs and neural arch, however, are present. **C.** Congenital spondylolysis resulting from complex vertebral anomalies. T12 is normal. L1 and L2 are fused to form a single, malformed, blocked vertebra (arrow). The neural arches of these vertebral bodies are visualized as separate structures, but the lower one is deformed. L3 and L4 are completely absent, and L5 is normal.

deformity. Occasionally, an entire vertebral body may fail to develop while the arch develops normally (Fig. 8.15B). In rare instances, both the body and laminal arch are absent (Fig. 8.15C), and in still other instances, only the laminal arches are absent (2). In such cases, instability of the spinal column may be profound, severe curvature abnormalities frequently result, and cord compression can occur (2).

"Blocked" vertebra is the term applied to fusion of one or more adjacent vertebral bodies. The intervening intervertebral discs may be rudimentary or entirely absent. The isolated anomaly usually is of no particular consequence. Blocked vertebrae also are seen as part of the Klippel-Feil abnormality of the cervical spine. In isolated form, they most commonly occur in the cervical spine, and the discs above or below the region of abnormality may be hypertrophied and bulge into the spinal canal. They are, however, innocuous, and the finding is part of the entire anomaly (Fig. 8.16A).

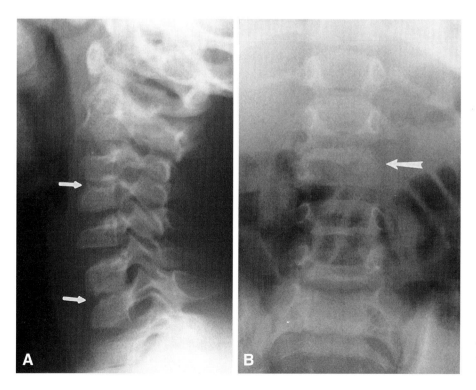

FIGURE 8.16. Other vertebral anomalies: blocked vertebra. A. Note the rudimentary discs at two levels (arrows) and associated fusion or blocking of the vertebral bodies. **B. Absent pedicle**. Note the absence of the left pedicle of L2 (arrow).

Congenital absence of the pedicles (3) also occurs (Fig. 8.16B), especially in the lumbar region (4). They are of no particular consequence, but can be associated with aplastic-hypoplastic anomalies of the spine. They can cause back pain (3), but this is unusual.

REFERENCES

1. Schmorl G, Junghanns H. The human spine in health and disease. Translated from 4th German edition by Wilk SP, Goin LS. New York: Grune & Stratton, 1959:24–59.
2. Hughes LO, McCarthy RE, Glasier CM. Segmental spinal dysgenesis: a report of three cases. J Pediatr Orthop 1998;18:227–232.
3. Wiener MD, Martinez S, Forsberg DA. Congenital absence of a cervical spine pedicle: clinical and radiologic findings. AJR 1990; 155:1037–1041.
4. Polly DW Jr, Mason DE. Congenital absence of a lumbar pedicle presenting as back pain in children. J Pediatr Orthop 1991;11: 214–219.

Spondylolisthesis and Spondylolysis

Spondylolysis and subsequent spondylolisthesis are seldom seen on a congenital basis in infants. If, however, they should occur, severe curvature abnormalities may develop (Fig. 8.15). In older children, the problem is encountered more frequently, and primarily in the lumbar spine. There often is debate as to whether the lesion is congenital or acquired, but most likely it is acquired. However, it also may be, as I have noticed, that the pars interpeduncularis is thinner than usual in these patients. As a result, it would be more susceptible to subclinical or overt trauma. Reactive marrow changes have been demonstrated in the adjacent pedicles with MRI (1), and increased bone activity has been noted with nuclear scintigraphy using SPECT imaging (2, 3). All of this supports a traumatic, rather than a congenital origin. It is a lesion of active children (4), especially those who are athletic, and place excessive strain on the lumbar spine.

The degree of subsequent slippage of the upper vertebral body varies, and while usually the condition is painful (2, 5), it is surprising how often it is discovered as an incidental finding. It is a relatively common cause of low back pain in children, and associated spinal nerve root entrapment has been demonstrated (6). If only a defect exists, the term "spondylolysis" is used, but if there is associated anterior displacement of the upper vertebral body, the condition is called "spondylolisthesis." The defect usually is visible on lateral view but is more exquisitely demonstrated on oblique view (Fig. 8.17). The findings also are vividly demonstrable with CT (Fig. 8.18).

The next most common place for spondylolysis to occur is at the C2 level (7, 8). It is questionable in many cases, however, whether the finding is completely congenital or

actually the result of trauma and representative of a missed hangman's fracture (9). One useful rule in differentiating the two is that, with congenital defects, the margins of the defect are smooth and sclerotic (Fig. 8.19), and the neural arch usually is deformed (10). It is not deformed when the defect is due to a hangman fracture. Congenital defects usually are stable on flexion-extension views, because the defect is replaced by fibrous or cartilaginous tissue. Familial cases have been reported (11).

When a posterior neural arch defect is due to a hangman fracture, the defect is narrow, sharp, and shows no sclerosis of the defect edges. The fracture is unstable and will require surgical intervention. In my experience, hangman fractures of C2 are more common than congenital defects, but they frequently go unnoticed (Fig. 8.20). Because they often are asymptomatic (12), they often are not initially detected, and also for this reason, others (13), as do I, believe that most of these defects are posttraumatic.

REFERENCES

1. Ulmer JL, Elster AD, Mathews VP, et al. Lumbar spondylolysis: reactive marrow changes seen in adjacent pedicles on MR images. AJR 1995;164:429–433.
2. Bellah RD, Summerville DA, Treves ST, et al. Low back pain in adolescent athletes: detection of stress injury to the pars interarticularis with SPECT. Radiology 1991;180:509–512.
3. Anderson K, Sarwark JF, Conway JJ, et al. Quantitative assessment with SPECT imaging at stress injuries of the pars interarticularis and response to bracing. J Pediatr Orthop 2000;20: 28–33.
4. Muschik M, Hahnel H, Robinson PN, et al. Competitive sports and the progression of spondylolisthesis. J Pediatr Orthop 1996; 16:364–369.
5. Lucey SD, Gross R. Painful spondylolisthesis in a two-year-old child. J Pediatr Orthop 1995;15:199–201.
6. Jinkins JR, Matthes JC, Sener RN, et al. Pictorial essay. Spondylolysis, spondylolisthesis, and associated nerve root entrapment in the lumbosacral spine: MNR evaluation. AJR 1992;159:799–803.
7. Fardon DF, Fielding JW. Defects of the pedicle and spondylolisthesis of the second cervical vertebra. J Bone Joint Surg 1981;63: 526–528.
8. Smith JT, Skinner SR, Shonnard NH. Persistent synchondrosis of the second cervical vertebra simulating a hangman's fracture in a child. J Bone Joint Surg Am 1993;75:1228–1230.
9. Konez O, Goyal M, Ciaverella CP. Bilateral absence of para interarticularis of C2: developmental or posttraumatic abnormality. Emerg Radiol 2001;8:48–50.
10. Williams JP III, Baker DH, Miller WA. CT appearance of congenital defect resembling the hangman's fracture. Pediatr Radiol 1999;29:549–550.
11. Nordstrom REA, Lahdenranta TV, Kaitila II, et al. Familial spondylolisthesis of the axis vertebra. J Bone Joint Surg 1986; 68:704–706.
12. Kleinman PK, Shelton YA. Hangman's fracture in an abused infant: imaging features. Pediatr Radiol 1997;27:776–777.
13. Howard AW, Letts RM. Cervical spondylolysis in children: it is posttraumatic? J Pediatr Orthop 2000;20:677–681.

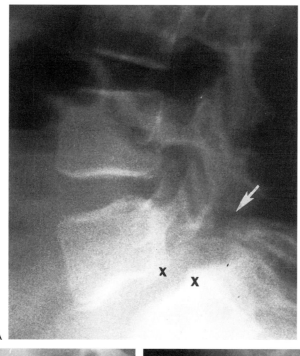

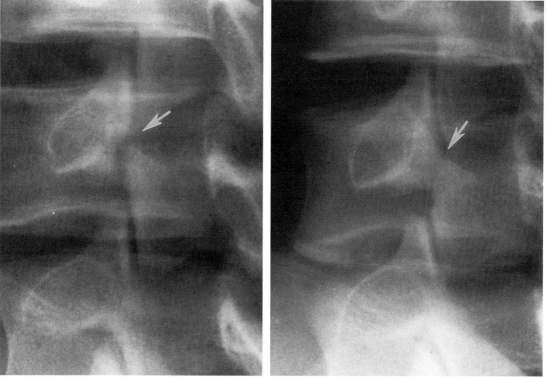

FIGURE 8.17. Lumbar spondylolysis and spondylolisthesis. A. Note the pars defect (arrow). Also note first-degree spondylolisthesis (X's). **B.** Another patient with a frank spondylolysis (arrow) on one side. **C.** On the other side the pedicle is thin and dysplastic (arrow) but spondylolysis has not yet occurred.

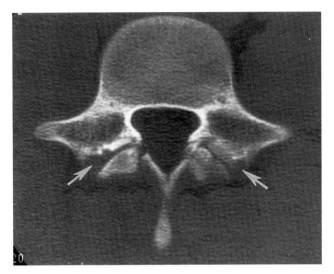

FIGURE 8.18. Lumbar spondylolisthesis: CT findings. Axial view demonstrates bilateral pars defects with sclerotic edges (arrows).

Coronal Cleft Vertebra

Coronal cleft vertebra frequently is found as an incidental finding and usually involves the lumbar vertebrae. Coronal cleft vertebrae can be seen singly or multiply and can occasionally extend into the thoracic region (Fig. 8.21). The defect probably results from tardy union of the anterior and posterior ossification centers.

Coronal cleft vertebrae have been documented with conditions such as imperforate anus, VATER syndrome, spinal meningocele, and chondrodystrophia calcificans, but they are probably just as frequently encountered in the absence of these conditions and in normal infants. Consequently, one must be cautious in assigning any special significance to this anomaly. The clefts usually disappear as the infant grows older, and it is unusual to encounter them after 6 to 12 months of age. Coronal cleft vertebra is more common in males than in females and is common in a number of syndromes (1).

REFERENCE

1. Westvik J, Lachman RS. Coronal and sagittal clefts in skeletal dysplasia. Pediatr Radiol 1998;28:764–770.

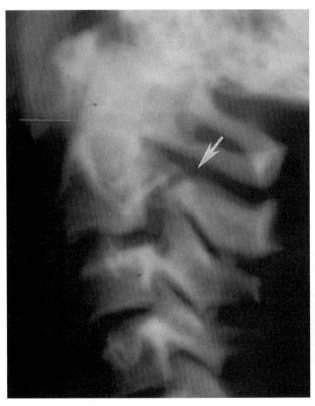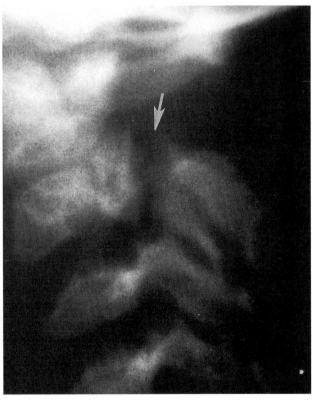

FIGURE 8.19. Congenital defect posterior arch of C2. A. Note the congenital defect (arrow) with sclerotic margins. **B.** Note the defect (arrow) and markedly dysplastic, anomalous posterior arch of C2.

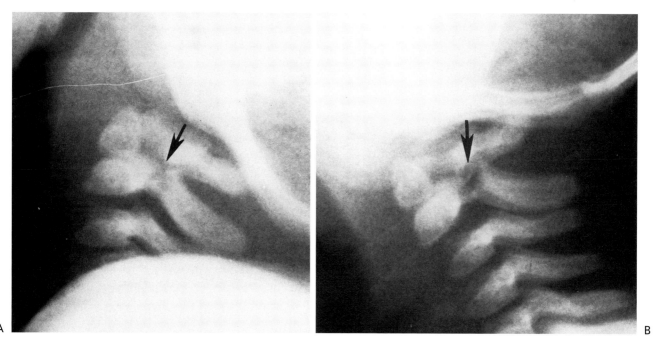

A
B

FIGURE 8.20. Hangman fracture in infant. A. A defect in the posterior arch of C2 (arrow) is barely visible. **B.** With flexion, however, the defect is clearly visible (arrow), constituting a hangman fracture. No anomalous or dysplastic features are pesent. (Courtesy Richard Keller, M.D.)

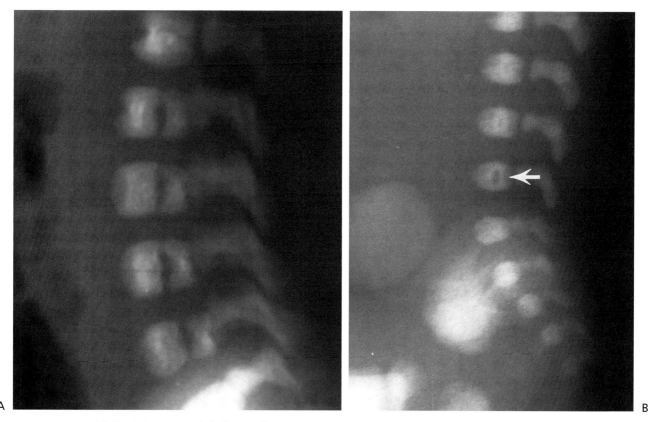

A
B

FIGURE 8.21. Coronal cleft vertebra. A. Note the coronal clefts in the lower lumbar vertebra. **B.** Small radiolucent defect in L5 (arrow), perhaps representing a notochord remnant. A similar but less prominent defect is present in L4.

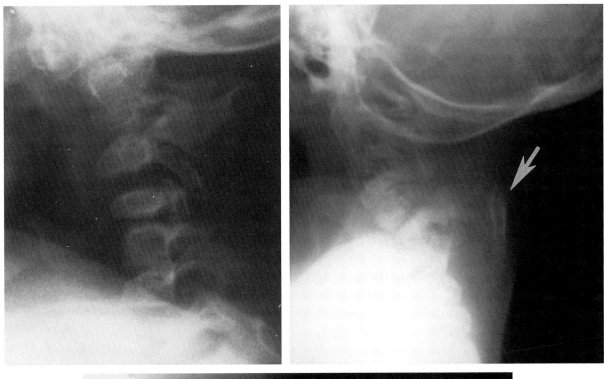

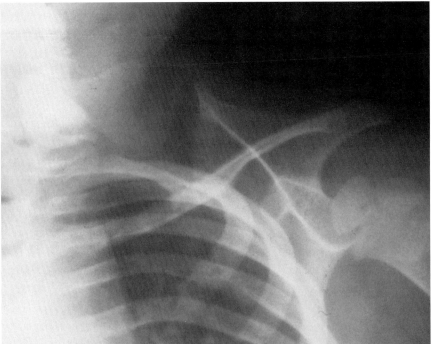

FIGURE 8.22. Klippel-Feil and Sprengel's deformity. A. Note the numerous fusion segmentation anomalies in the cervical spine. Also note that C1 is occipitalized, C2 and 3 are fused posteriorly, C4 is under developed, and C-6 are fused. **B. Patient with Sprengel's deformity.** Lateral view shows multiple fusion-segmentation anomalies of the cervical spine, resulting in marked shortening of the spine. There is also pronounced kyphosis. The arrow points to the omovertebral bone, which is present as part of as associated Sprengel's deformity. **C.** Note that the left shoulder is elevated and that the left scapula is rotated (Sprengel's deformity). The omo vertebral bone (arrows) is not clearly seen. Sprengel's deformity is frequently seen with Klippel-Feil deformity.

Specific Cervical Spine Anomalies

Occipitalization of C1, with or without associated basilar invagination and platybasia, is not usually a problem in the newborn infant. Problems related to these anomalies usually arise later in childhood. Extensive fusion-segmentation anomalies are seen with the **Klippel-Feil syndrome** and are seen in the neonate. This problem is very heterogenous (1), but most infants show marked shortening of the neck, with or without torticollis. Radiographs demonstrate extensive fusion-segmentation and curvature anomalies of the cervical, and at times, the upper thoracic spine (Fig. 8.22A). In some cases, associated upward rotation of the scapula also occurs and results in the so-called Sprengel's deformity (Fig. 8.22B). Rib anomalies also are occasionally encountered, and the Klippel-Feil syndrome can be associated with congenital deafness, renal agenesis, and other anomalies.

Another relatively constant feature of this complex of anomalies is the omovertebral bone. This structure can be seen in the ligament extending from the spine to the abnormally positioned scapula in those patients with associated Sprengel's deformity (Fig. 8.22C). Usually, the cervical spinal cord is normal even though the spinal anomalies may appear alarming. However cord abnormalities can occur (2). In mild cases, only minimal deformity of the cervical vertebral bodies may be seen and no clinical abnormality is detectable. However, neurologic deficits can develop in adulthood (3, 4).

Congenital absence of the odontoid is rare, and absence of the laminal arches and other anomalies were discussed previously. A bifid odontoid is the result of lack of fusion of the two ossification centers of the odontoid (5). **Hypoplasia of the odontoid** is associated with ligament underdevelopment and laxity and formation of the os odontoideum (6). The **os odontoideum** is an overgrown normal os terminale which overgrows when the dens is hypoplastic (6). It also can be acquired after trauma (7, 8). This occurs in infancy but is rare. In infancy in these cases blood supply to the dens is disrupted with severe upper spinal injuries and the dens fails to grow to normal proportions. It then becomes hypoplastic and as such induces the os terminale, on a compensatory basis, to overgrow and form an acquired os odontoideum. In these cases, as apposed to when the os odontoideum is congenital there are no other anomalies of the upper cervical spine. With a congenital os odontoideum, anomalies are numerous and often very bizarre (Fig. 8.23). The os odontoideum can fuse with the anterior arch of C1, and the entire complex of findings is more common in syndromes such as trisomy 21, spondyloepiphyseal dysplasia, and a variety of chondrodystrophies (6). When the posterior arch of C1 is severely hypoplastic or absent, hypermobility is profound (Fig. 8.24). In terms of deficiencies the posterior arch of C1 it should be noted that isolated defects are most common at this level (Fig.

8.25). Furthermore, even though they may appear bizarre and alarming, they are stable unless they are associated with a hypoplastic dens.

REFERENCES

1. Clarke RA, Catalan G, Diwan AD, et al. Heterogeneity in Klippel-Feil syndrome: a new classification. Pediatr Radiol 1998;28: 967–974.
2. Andronikou S, Fieggen AG. Klippel-Feil syndrome with cervical diastematomyelia in an 8-year-old boy. Pediatr Radiol 2001;31: 636.
3. Guiller JT, Miller A, Bowen JR, et al. The natural history of Klippel-Feil syndrome: clinical, roentgenographic, and magnetic resonance imaging findings at adulthood. J Pediatr Orthop 1995;15: 617–626.
4. Ulmer JL, Elster AD, Ginsberg LE, et al. Klippel-Feil syndrome: CT and MR of acquired and congenital abnormalities of cervical spine and cord. J Comput Assist Tomogr 1993;17:215–224.
5. Garant M, Oudjhane K, Sinsky A, et al. Duplication odontoid process: plain radiographic and CT appearance of a rare congenital anomaly of the cervical spine. AJNR 1997;18:1719–1720.
6. Swischuk LE, John SD, Moorthy C. The os terminale os odontoideum complex. Emerg Radiol 1997;4:72–81.
7. Schuler TC, Kurz L, Thompson DE, et al. Natural history of os odontoideum. J Pediatr Orthop 1991;11:222–225.
8. Kuhns LR, Loder RT, Farley FA, et al. Nuchal cord changes in children with os odontoideum: evidence for associated trauma. J Pediatr Orthop 1998;18:815–819.

Sacral Agenesis, Hypoplasia, and Caudal Regression

There is a wide gamut of lower lumbar and sacral spine abnormalities ranging from absence to mild hypoplasia. Hypoplasia may involve the entire sacrum or be more pronounced on one side. In the more severe cases of sacral agenesis, the lower lumbar spine is also usually absent. Absence of the spine above T11 or T12 is usually incompatible with life, and in these more severe cases the lower extremities are often fused in the so-called mermaid deformity. Extensive genitourinary and gastrointestinal anomalies (ectopic anus) are commonly present in such cases. Both of the lower extremities may be absent or underdeveloped, and the entire complex has been referred to as the caudal regression syndrome. These abnormalities are more frequently seen in infants delivered of diabetic mothers.

Generalized sacral hypoplasia, especially if mild, may go unnoticed but in later life may lead to various degrees of bowel, bladder, or motor impairment. In sacral agenesis, on the other hand, neurologic deficit is more profound, and associated clubfoot deformity, wasting of the muscles of the lower extremities, and incontinence of the urinary and anal sphincters are seen. Neurologic deficit in these cases results from underdevelopment of the corresponding nerve roots and distal spinal cord. Innervation usually is intact to the L5-S1 level and, as a result, development of the thigh mus-

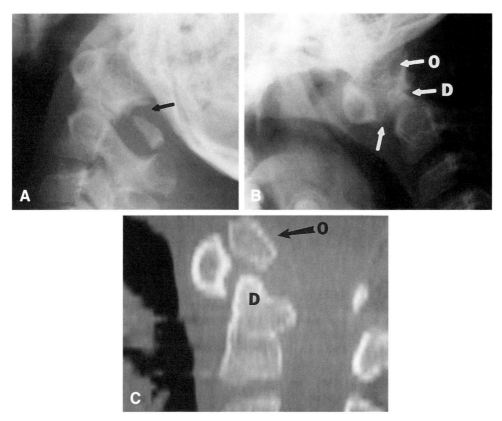

FIGURE 8.23. Os odontoideum. A. On extension, note the defect (arrow) in the underdeveloped posterior arch of C1. The dens is difficult to identify because it is hypoplastic. The anterior arch of C1 is overgrown. **B.** With flexion, the C1-dens distance widens (arrow), and the dens (D) is seen to be hypoplastic. There is vague suggestion of an additional ossicle, the os odontoideum (O), above the hypoplastic dens. **C.** With sagittal, reconstructed CT, the extra ossicle (i.e., os odontoideum) is more clearly visualized (arrow). The dens (D) is deformed and hypoplastic. Note that the anterior arch of C1 is enlarged.

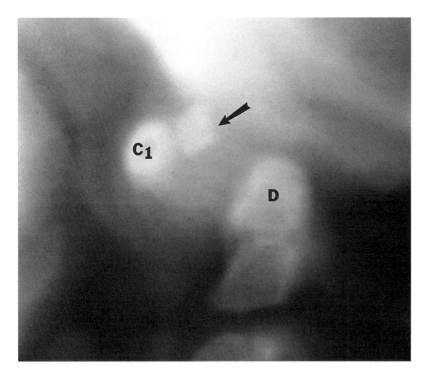

FIGURE 8.24. Os odontoideum with absent posterior arch of C1. In this patient with trisomy 21, there is marked anterior displacement of C1 (C1) from the hypoplastic dens (D). The os odontoideum (arrow) has moved forward with C1.

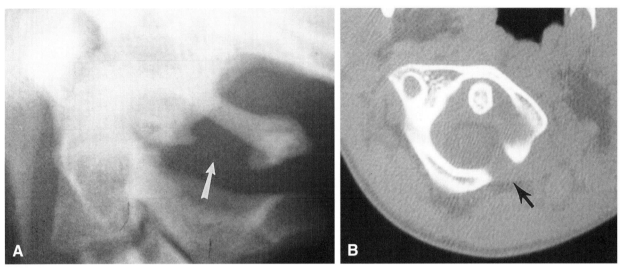

FIGURE 8.25. Congenital defects of C1. A. In this patient, there is unilateral absence of the posterior arch of C1 (arrow). **B.** CT study in another patient demonstrates a partial defect of the posterior arch of C1 (arrow).

cles is relatively normal. This leads to a tapered or cone-shaped appearance of the lower extremities.

Roentgenographically, the sacral anomalies are readily appreciated (Fig. 8.26). The pelvic bones are more closely apposed than normal, and the pelvis often becomes somewhat contracted. Intraspinal lipomas can co-exist, and these infants frequently show cutaneous abnormalities such as tufts of hair, dimples, and subcutaneous lipomas.

Meningocele and Meningomyelocele

Meningocele and meningomyelocele are common abnormalities of the spinal cord and meninges. Meningocele denotes herniation of the meninges only; in meningomyelocele, the sac also contains the spinal cord and nerve roots. Both abnormalities are commonly associated with lacunar skull and the Arnold-Chiari malformation. Most commonly, meningocele and meningomyelocele are encountered in the lumbosacral region, and next most commonly they occur in the lower thoracic spine. Least frequent are cervical defects, and in rare instances, these lesions may be contiguous with a midline posterior occipital encephalocele. Multiple defects also can occur.

There is no difficulty in clinically recognizing this abnormality, because the widened spinal canal and numerous vertebral defects and deformities are readily apparent roentgenographically (Fig. 8.27). In some cases, the neural arches are so defective that only vague vestiges remain. Some of these rudimentary bony structures are so misplaced that one might misinterpret them as representing the bony spicule of diastematomyelia. In other, less common instances there may be a soft tissue bulge only and little in the way of vertebral body or neural arch abnormality. In

more advanced cases, the anterior aspect of the vertebral bodies becomes rounded (Fig. 8.27B). These patients can demonstrate a severe lumbar kyphosis that now is corrected surgically in early infancy (1). This is performed to avoid later severe scoliotic and kyphotic curvature problems.

It is not possible to determine the precise level of communication from plain roentgenograms because it does not necessarily correspond to the area of most severe deformity. The communication may be small but, in any case, if one is interested in obtaining further information regarding these lesions and, more specifically, in outlining the spinal cord and nerve roots, it is best to employ MRI (2–4). This modality most clearly delineates the abnormal underlying anatomy. In the neonate, however, ultrasonography can be useful in delineating the sac of the meningocele, the echogenic neural elements inside, and the presence of associated lesions such as lipomas.

Not uncommonly, the spinal cord in patients with meningomyelocele or meningocele shows widening secondary to hydromelia (3). Lipomas frequently co-exist (1) and on CT studies are of low signal intensity (i.e., radiolucent). On MRI, they produce high T_1 signal intensity, and they are highly echogenic on ultrasonographic studies. Rib anomalies and deformities also commonly co-exist, and with more severe dysraphism, intraabdominal structures such as the aorta and kidneys can be displaced posteriorly and centrally. For this reason, it is often difficult to examine these kidneys with ultrasound. Meningoceles and meningomyeloceles also can be detected in utero with ultrasound.

Although most meningoceles are midline and dorsal in location, one can occasionally encounter a lateral or anterior meningocele. The latter abnormalities most commonly occur in the thoracic or sacral regions. Such meningoceles

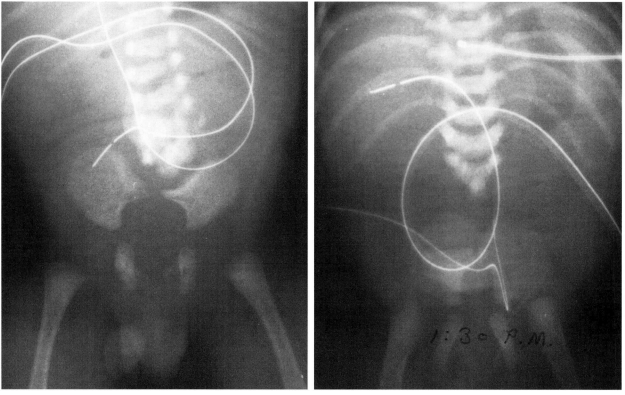

A

B

FIGURE 8.26. Spinal agenesis. A. Agenesis of the sacrum results in a shortened spinal column and pelvic bones that almost meet in the center. **B.** More pronounced spinal agenesis with absence of the vertebral bodies as far up as L3. Note how close together the pelvic bones are positioned. In both infants, umbilical vessel catheters and temperature monitoring devices are present.

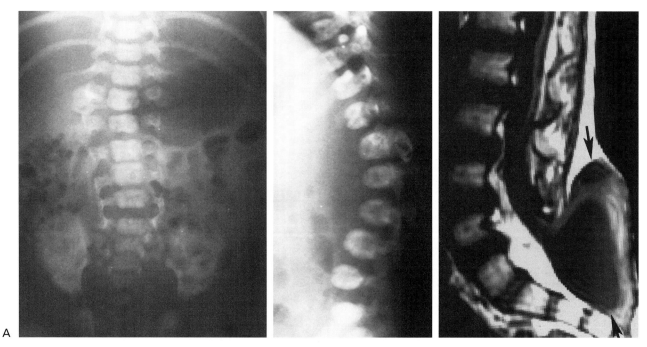

A

B,C

FIGURE 8.27. Meningocele. A. Extensive meningocele producing marked widening of the spinal canal. **B.** Lateral view shows localized kyphosis and deformed, underdeveloped vertebral bodies. **C.** MRI sagittal view in another patient. Note the large sacral meningocele (arrows).

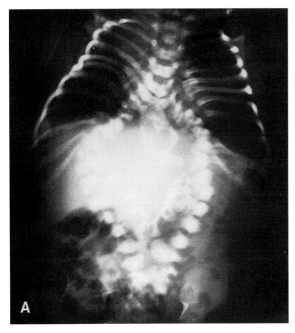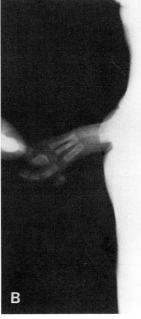

FIGURE 8.28. Total rachischisis or split notochord. A. Note the complete splitting of the spine over the lower thoracic and upper lumbar regions. Formed bony elements are present in the center. This often is also referred to as combined posterior and anterior meningocele and is believed to be one manifestation of the split notochord syndrome. **B.** Lateral view demonstrating a malformed upper extremity (teratoma) extending from the defect. (Courtesy of G. Bess, M.D.)

are frequently associated with neurofibromatosis, and the roentgenographic findings include the presence of a mass (meningocele), a variety of vertebral abnormalities, and in the thorax, thinning of the adjacent ribs.

Anterior sacral meningoceles enter into the differential diagnosis of presacral pelvic masses in newborn and young infants. Primarily, one must differentiate them from presacral teratoma, hydrometrocolpos, ovarian cysts, and pelvic neuroblastoma. Intrasacral or so-called occult sacral meningoceles are not usually detected in the newborn and young infant.

In rare instances, one may come upon a complete midline defect of the spinal column, including the neural arches posteriorly and the vertebral bodies anteriorly (Fig. 8.28). This abnormality has been called "double spine," total rachischisis, split notochord, or combined anterior and posterior meningomyelocele (6, 7). In some instances, dorsal herniation of the gastrointestinal tract through this defect can occur (6). In other instances, associated neurenteric cysts or neurenteric fistulas can be encountered, and yet in other cases the defects may be associated with hamartomas or actual deformed, accessory extremities (8, 9) (Fig. 8.28). Although originally the split notochord syndrome was considered an entity unto itself, more and more it is included in the spectrum of meningocele, diastematomyelia, diplomyelia, and neurenteric cyst (7).

REFERENCES

1. Torode I, Godette G. Surgical correction of congenital kyphosis in myelomeningocele. J Pediatr Orthop 1995;15:202–205.

2. Barnes PD, Lester PD, Yamanashi WS. Magnetic resonance imaging in infants and children with spinal dysraphism. AJNR 1986;7:465–471.

3. Breningstall GN, Marker SM, Tubman DE. Hydrosyringomyelia and diastematomyelia detected by MRI in myelomeningocele. Pediatr Neurol 1992;8:267–271.

4. Szalay EA, Roach JW, Smith H, et al. Magnetic resonance imaging of the spinal cord in spinal dysraphisms. J Pediatr Orthop 1987;7:541–545.

5. Waters KA, Forbes P, Morielli A, et al. Sleep-disordered breathing in children with myelomeningocele. J Pediatr 1998;132:672–681.

6. Fathak VB, Singh S, Wakhlu AK. Double split of notochord with massive prolapse of the gut. J Pediatr Surg 1988;23:1039–1040.

7. Ersahin Y, Mutluer S, Kocaman S. Split spinal cord malformations in children. J Neurosurg 1998;88:57–65.

8. Krishna A, Chandna S, Mishra NK, et al. Accessory limb associated with spina bifida. J Pediatr Surg 1989;24:604–606.

9. Fowler CL. Intraabdominal leg: unique variant of split notochord syndrome. J Pediatr Surg 1998;33:522–524.

Diastematomyelia (Closed Spinal Dysraphism)

Diastematomyelia, or closed spinal dysraphism (1), is a relatively uncommon condition in which there is splitting and transfixing of the spinal cord by an abnormal fibrocartilaginous or bony spicule extending from the dorsal aspect of a vertebral body to the corresponding neural arch. Most frequently the abnormality occurs in the lower thoracic and upper lumbar regions, but it can be seen in other areas. Diastematomyelia at more than one level can occur (2) and, in some cases, the bony spicule can be a massive bar extending over a number of vertebral bodies. **Diastematomyelia is believed to result from faulty notochord development**

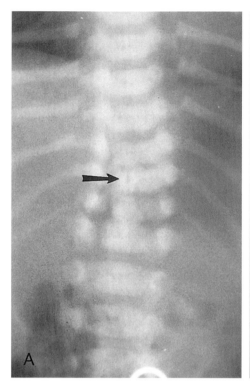
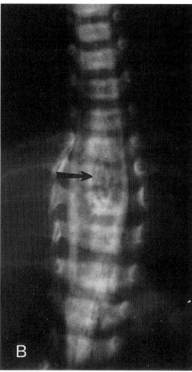

FIGURE 8.29. Diastematomyelia. A. Note the diffuse widening of the spinal canal and a central bony spicule (arrow). **B.** Another patient with a larger bony spicule and marked widening of the spinal canal (arrow). This is a metrizamide myelogram that also demonstrates the widened spinal cord.

and can be considered a form of the split notochord syndrome.

It is important that this condition be recognized early because as the infant grows older, normal ascent of the spinal cord is inhibited by the bony or fibrocartilaginous spicule. As a consequence, there is stretching of the cord (especially during flexion of the spine) and associated downward displacement of the cerebellum and medulla (i.e., Arnold-Chiari malformation). Lower extremity neuro-logic impairment is common and often is the presenting problem. Surgical correction with removal of the bony spicule usually prevents, or at least markedly attenuates, development of neurologic sequelae beyond those present when the condition is diagnosed. The condition should be suspected clinically when lower extremity neurologic deficit, abnormal curvature of the spine, and cutaneous manifestations such as hair tufts, cutaneous dimples, lipomas (3), or even a tail (4) are noted.

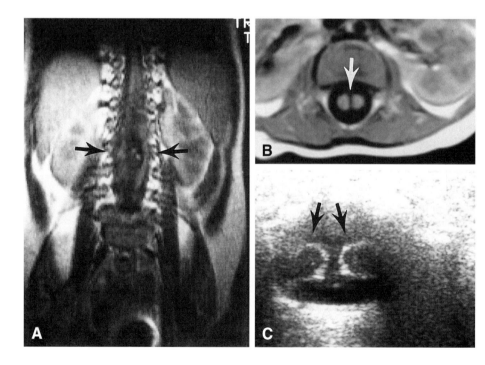

FIGURE 8.30. Diastematomyelia. A. Coronal, T1-weighted MR study demonstrates a central spicule with splitting of the cord (arrows). **B.** Axial MR study of another patient demonstrates a split cord (arrows). **C.** A split cord (arrows) demonstrated on ultrasound.

Roentgenographically, if the spicule is ossified, it is best seen on frontal projection (Fig. 8.29). Associated abnormalities of the vertebral bodies, especially hemivertebra, scoliosis, and widening of the spinal canal, are usually present. Co-existing meningomyeloceles, lipomas, and hydromyelia of the cord can be seen.

Currently, although ultrasound (5) can detect the abnormality in young infants (Fig. 8.30C), the problem is best defined with MRI (6, 7) (Fig. 8.30, A and B). MRI also can define associated problems such as tethering of the cord or the presence of intra-extra spinal lipomas.

REFERENCES

1. Scatliff JH, Kendall BE, Kingsley DPE, et al. Closed spinal dysraphism: analysis of clinical, radiological, and surgical findings in 104 consecutive patients. AJR 1989;152:1049–1057.
2. Herman TE, Siegel MJ. Case report. Cervical and basicranial diastematomyelia. AJR 1990;154:6806–6808.
3. McAtee-Smith J, Herbert AA, Rapini RP, et al. Skin lesions of the spinal axis and spinal dysraphism: fifteen cases and a review of the literature. Arch Pediatr Adolesc Med 1994;148:740–748.
4. Belzberg AJ, Myles ST, Trevenen CL. The human tail and spinal dysraphism. J Pediatr Surg 1991;26:1243–1245.
5. Korsvik HE, Keller MS. Sonography of occult dysraphism in neonates and infants with MR imaging correlation. Radiographics 1992;12:297–306.
6. Han JS, Benson JE, Kaufman B. Demonstration of diastematomyelia and associated abnormalities with MR imaging. AJNR 1985;6:215–220.
7. Roos RAC, Vielvoye GJ, Voormolen JHC, et al. Magnetic resonance imaging in occult spinal dysraphism. Pediatr Radiol 1986; 16:412–416.

Tethered Cord

This condition, which may occur alone or in association with other lower spinal anomalies, consists of failure of the cord to rise to its normal high lumbar position. The cord is tethered at a low lumbar or even sacral level and usually intertwined with lipomatous tissue. The direction of the nerve roots is reversed in that they point obliquely upwardly, and the condition is best demonstrated with MR.

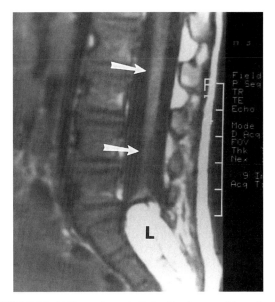

FIGURE 8.31. Tethered cord. Note the low-positioned spinal cord (arrows) attached to an intraspinal lipoma (L). (Courtesy of Dr. James E. Rytting.)

Currently, there is some tendency to include tethered cord under the broad spectrum of the split notochord syndrome, and skin markers such as those seen in other conditions within this syndrome (e.g., hair tufts, lipomas, dimples) commonly are encountered.

Plain films might suggest the abnormality when anomalies of the lower thoracolumbar and sacral spine are visualized. Clinically, many of these patients present with a limp, and after initial plain films the entity can be imaged with any of the available imaging modalities, including ultrasound in infants. Overall, the lesion is best demonstrated with MRI, which exquisitely demonstrates the characteristic low position of the spinal cord and its frequent association with an intraspinal or extraspinal lipoma (Fig. 8.31). Minimal penetration of the tethered cord problem often manifests with simple thickening of the filum terminale (Fig. 8.32). In these cases, the cord is not dramatically displaced.

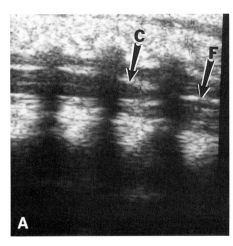
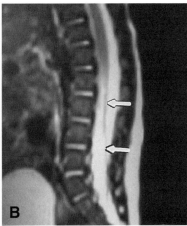

FIGURE 8.32. Thickened filum. A. In this patient, the ultrasonogram demonstrates the conus (C) from which extends a thickened filum (F). **B.** T2-weighted, sagittal MRI demonstrates the thickened filum (arrows).

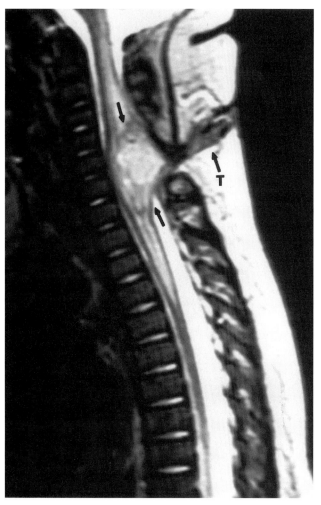

FIGURE 8.33. Congenital dermal sinus. On this T2-weighted image, note the intraspinal, bulbous component of the sinus and the track (T) to the skin.

Congenital Dermal Sinus

Congenital dermal sinus consists of persistence of an epithelium-lined sinus tract extending inward from the skin to the meninges. It most commonly occurs in the lumbosacral region and can be associated with intraspinal or extraspinal lipomas or dermoids. Attention is frequently brought to the lesion by the presence of neurologic deficit, cutaneous dimples, tufts of hair, or an actual sinus tract opening. A variable degree of spina bifida and other vertebral anomalies are also usually present.

As with all spinal anomalies, the findings are best demonstrated with MRI (1) (Fig. 8.33). The sinus tract also can be injected with contrast material, but this generally is discouraged because such an injection can result in a development of meningitis. One of the more important complications of congenital dermal sinus is the development of recurrent attacks of meningitis. Treatment is surgical excision.

REFERENCE

1. Barkovich AJ, Edwards M, Cogen PH. MR evaluation of spinal dermal sinus tracts in children. AJR 1991;156:791–797.

Syringomyelia and Hydromyelia

Syringomyelia occasionally occurs in older children but as an isolated abnormality is uncommon in neonates and young infants. It is, however, seen in this age group in association with anomalies such as the Arnold-Chiari malformation, meningomyelocele, and diastematomyelia. The lesion now is more clearly delineated with MRI (1) (Fig. 8.34), but also is demonstrable with CT.

Recently a hypothesis for the development of syringomyelia in the presence of Arnold-Chiari malformations has been offered (1). In the study just referred to (1), it has been suggested that the piston-like action of the lower tonsils on the cerebrospinal fluid creates pressure waves that propagate fluid caudally within the spinal cord, producing

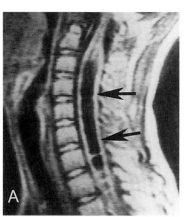
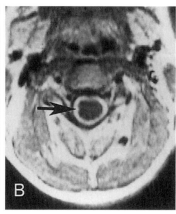

FIGURE 8.34. Syringomyelia. A. In this older patient, the sagittal, T1-weighted MR study demonstrates a large syrinx, producing low signal intensity in the dilated spinal cord (arrows). **B.** Axial view through the same area demonstrates the low-signal-intensity, fluid-filled sac (arrow) of syringomyelia.

dilatation of the central spinal canal and eventually syringomyelia. Syringomyelia is commonly seen with Arnold-Chiari type I and II malformations (Fig. 8.34).

Because the lesion often is longstanding, the spinal canal also is enlarged, and this can be detected on plain films. Often, neurologic findings are confusing in these patients, and it is for this reason that the imaging modalities are so important.

REFERENCE

1. Heiss JD, Patronas N, DeBroom HL. Elucidating the pathophysiology of syringomyelia. J Neurosurg 1999;91;553–562.

Occult Spinal Dysraphism: The Sacral Dimple

Imaging studies often are performed in patients who have simple sacral dimples. Recent studies (1, 2) addressing this problem suggest that simple midline dimples, although most commonly encountered, are associated with a low risk for spinal dysraphism. It was further suggested that only atypical dimples are associated with such abnormality, and these atypical dimples demonstrate the following features: larger than 5 mm in diameter, located high on the back, and may appear in combination with cutaneous lesion such as hemangiomas, masses, tails and hairy patches.

REFERENCES

1. Kriss VM, Desai NS. Occult spinal dysraphism in neonates: assessment of high-risk cutaneous stigmata on sonography. AJR 1998; 171:1687–1692.
2. Sneineh AK, Gabos PG, Keller MS, et al. Ultrasonography of the spine in neonates and young infants with a sacral skin dimple. J Pediatr Orthop 2002;22:761–762.

Hypoplasia and Agenesis of the Spinal Cord

Various degrees of spinal cord underdevelopment occur in association with more severe forms of lumbosacral and lower thoracic vertebral column agenesis. Agenesis of the vertebral column above the level of T11 or T12 is usually incompatible with life; agenesis below this level is associated with various degrees of neurologic deficit.

TRAUMATIC LESIONS OF THE SPINE AND SPINAL CORD

Neonatal Trauma

In the neonate, trauma to the cervical spine or spinal canal is almost always the result of obstetrical trauma. In such cases, the most common predisposing factor is hyperextension of the cervical spine as a result of breech positioning of the fetus (Fig. 8.35). These infants also may show brachial nerve palsies (1) (Fig. 8.36), but most present with generalized floppiness, a bell-shaped chest (as a result of hypotonia), and respiratory distress because of decreased thoracic movement. Generally, bony vertebral abnormalities are lacking but not unheard of (Fig. 8.35D), and it is only with MRI (2, 3) that the extent of the intraspinal injury is delineated. Ultrasonography also can be used (4–7), but overall, MRI is best. Many of these injuries, including transection of the cord, can go undetected for some time after birth because floppiness may be interpreted as resulting from some other problem. Atrophy of the cord and progressive neurologic deficit occur later.

REFERENCES

1. Miller SF, Glasier CM, et al. Brachial plexopathy in infants after traumatic delivery: evaluation with MR imaging. Radiology 1993; 189:481–484.
2. Castillo M, Smith JK. Imaging features of acute head and spine injuries secondary to difficult deliveries. Emerg Radiol 1995;2:7–12.
3. Lanska MJ, Roessmann U, Wiznitzer M. Magnetic resonance imaging in cervical cord birth injury. Pediatrics 1990;85:760–765.
4. Filippigh P, Clapuyt P, Debauche C, et al. Sonographic evaluation of traumatic spinal cord lesions in the newborn infant. Pediatr Radiol 1994;24:245–247.
5. Fotter R, Sorantin EU, Schneider U, et al. Ultrasound diagnosis of birth-related spinal cord trauma: neonatal diagnosis and follow-up and correlation with MRI. Pediatr Radiol 1994;24:241–244.
6. Mills JF, Dargaille PA, Coleman LT, et al. Upper cervical spine cord injury in neonates: the use of magnetic resonance imaging. J Pediatr 2001;138:105–108.
7. Fordham LA, Bell J, Chung CJ, et al. MR imaging of a severe cervical fracture-dislocation after traumatic delivery. Emerg Radiol 1999;6:143–145.

Cervical Spine Trauma in Infants and Older Children

A detailed dissertation of cervical spine and spinal cord injuries will not be presented. Because this topic has been covered elsewhere in considerable detail (1–3) and is available in many other standard textbooks, only a brief account is presented in the following paragraphs.

Injuries to the cervical spine and spinal cord in infants and children generally are the same as those encountered in adults except in infants and young children in whom injuries to the upper cervical spine tend to predominate (1, 3). Otherwise, the same forces are responsible for fractures in older children; flexion, extension, rotation, and axial loading all also are at play in the infant and child.

In the older child, the configuration of fractures is basically no different from that seen in adults (1), but a few differences exist in infants. One of the more common is that fractures through the base of the dens occur through the syn-

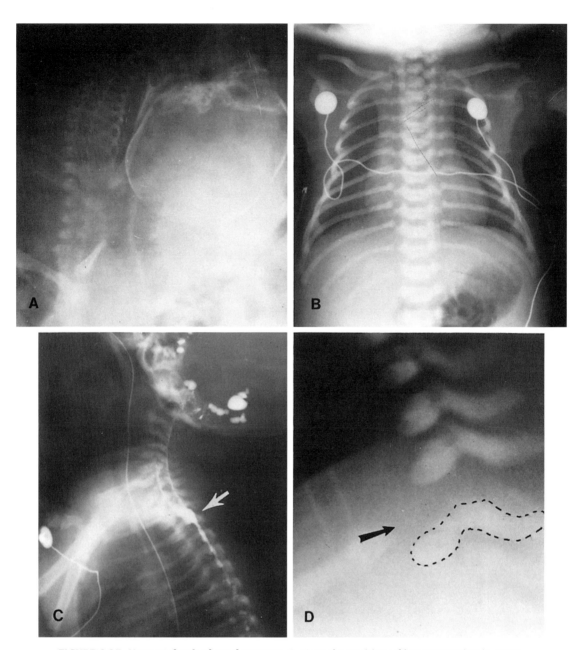

FIGURE 8.35. Neonatal spinal cord trauma. A. Note the position of hyperextension in utero. **B.** Note the slightly bell-shaped configuration of the chest. The lungs are clear. This infant had respiratory distress and was floppy. **C.** Myelogram demonstrates a swollen cord and complete block (arrow) in the lower cervical area. **D.** Another infant, showing complete dislocation of the cervical spine (arrow). (**D** courtesy of Elmer Heimbigner, M.D.)

FIGURE 8.37. Spinal injuries. A. Anterior flexion force. Note anterior displacement of the dens as a result of a fracture through the dens-body synchondrosis (*arrow*). **B. Flexion force injury.** Atlanto-axial dislocation causes widening of the C1-dens distance (*arrow*). **C. Flexion-compression injury of C5** *(arrow)*. Note that the posterior fragment of the vertebral body is displaced into the spinal canal and that the apophyseal joints have become separated. **D. Rotation injury.** In this patient, C5 is displaced forward on C6 (*arrow*). The disc space is narrowed, and the apophyseal joints are open. The spine above this area is rotated. This was the result of a hyperflexion-rotation injury. **E. Compression fracture-dislocation of the lumbar vertebra** *(arrow)*. Note that the posterior aspect of the vertebra has been displaced into the spinal canal. **F.** CT study demonstrates displacement of the fractured vertebral body (*arrows*) into the spinal canal. **G.** Sagittal reconstruction showing same findings (*arrows*). **H. Central cord syndrome (spinal cord injury without bony injury).** This usually results from an extension injury and causes contusion of the lower cervical spinal cord (*arrows*).

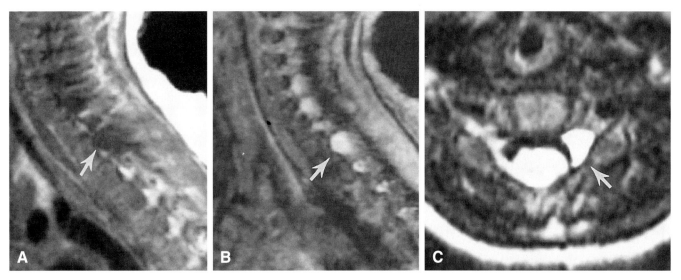

FIGURE 8.36. Brachial plexus injury. A. Obstetric trauma. Sagittal, T1-weighted MR image demonstrates a diverticulum with fluid density (arrow) over one of the lower intervertebral foramina. **B.** T2-weighted study demonstrates high signal intensity in the fluid collection (arrow). **C.** Axial view, T2-weighted, demonstrates the diverticulum along the nerve root (arrow). A smaller one is present on the other side.

chondrosis between the dens and body of C2 (4, 5) (Fig. 8.37A). Most of these injuries result from hyperflexion, rather than hyperextension injuries. Fractures in young infants may remain occult for long periods (6, 7). With flexion injuries, there is compression of the anterior portion of

the vertebral body and distraction of the apophyseal joints and posterior ligaments. With extension injuries, the reverse is true because there is compression of the posterior elements resulting in fractures such as the hangman's fracture of C2 (Fig. 8.20) and the Jefferson fracture of C1. There is disrup-

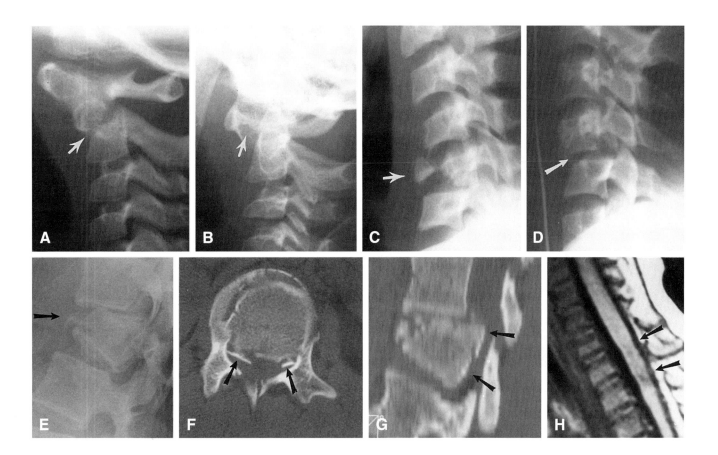

tion of the anterior ligaments, and the involved intervertebral disc space often is wider than normal. With flexion injuries and rotational injuries, disc space narrowing usually is seen.

With rotatory injuries, unilateral dislocation or subluxation of the apophyseal joints occurs, and at the C1-2 level, widening of the C1-dens distance commonly is seen with frank dislocation (8–10). Axial loading (vertical compression) injuries result in bursting of the vertebral bodies, but it should be remembered that, in most cases, more than one injury-causing force is involved. Examples of some of the fractures encountered in the cervical spine are presented in Figure 8.37. An example of atlantooccipital dislocation is presented in Figure 8.38, and rotatory subluxation is demonstrated in Figure 8.39.

Seat belt injuries also occur in children, and pelvic ecchymosis can be a clue to their presence (11). Often, they are missed because only AP views of the abdomen are obtained. This fracture is much more difficult to

detect on this view than on lateral view (Fig. 8.40). In addition to the lumbar seat belt injury, it has become apparent that children, when harnessed in adult seat belts with an oblique band crossing their shoulder, are prone to similar injuries of the cervical spine (12). Odontoid fracture also has been documented as a result of this mechanism (13).

REFERENCES

1. Finch GD, Barnes MJ. Major cervical spine injuries in children and adolescents. J Pediatr Orthop 1998;18:811–814.
2. Roche C, Carty H. Spinal trauma in children. Pediatr Radiol 2001;31:677–700.
3. Swischuk LE. Imaging of the Cervical Spine in Children. New York: Springer-Verlag, 2002.
4. Connolly B, Emery D, Armstrong D. The odontoid synchondrotic slip: an injury unique to young children. Pediatr Radiol 1995;25S:129–133.
5. Odent T, Langlais J, Glorion C, et al. Fractures of the odontoid process: a report of 15 cases in children younger than 6 years. J Pediatr Orthop 1999;19:51–54.
6. Dietrich AM, Ginn-Pease ME, Barkowski HM, et al. Pediatric cervical spine fractures: predominantly subtle presentation. J Pediatr Surg 1991;26:995–1000.
7. Orenstein JB, Klein BL, Ochsenschlager DW. Delayed diagnosis of pediatric cervical spine injury. Pediatrics 1992;89: 1185–1188.
8. Cohen A, Hirsch M, Katz M, et al. Traumatic atlanto-occipital dislocation in children: review and report of five cases. Pediatr Emerg Care 1991;7:24–27.
9. Muniz AE, Belfer RA. Atlantoaxial rotary subluxation in children. Pediatr Emerg Care 1999;15:25–29.
10. Floman Y, Kaplan L, Elidan J, et al. Transverse ligament rupture and atlanto-axial subluxation in children. J Bone Joint Surg Br 1991;73:640–643.
11. Sivit CJ, Taylor GA, Newman KD, et al. Safety-belt injuries in children with lap-belt ecchymosis: CT findings in 61 patients. AJR 1991;157:111–114.
12. Hoy GA, Cole WG. The paediatric cervical seat belt syndrome. Injury 1993;24:297–299.
13. Diekema DS, Allen DB. Odontoid fracture in a child occupying a child restraint seat. Pediatrics 1988;82:117–119.

Flexion-Extension Views and Odontoid Views: Practical Considerations

In terms of the open mouth odontoid view it is questionable and to whether it should be pursued in children 5 years and under (1, 2). If there is any question about the odontoid view one should proceed to CT (3). Because the findings on the open mouth odontoid view often are so difficult to interpret there may be an overuse of CT in these patients, but it is probably warranted in terms of risk and outcome (3). **In the end, however, it will depend on one's experience, one's concern for the patient, and the ever present penumbra of litigation, either warranted or unwarranted.**

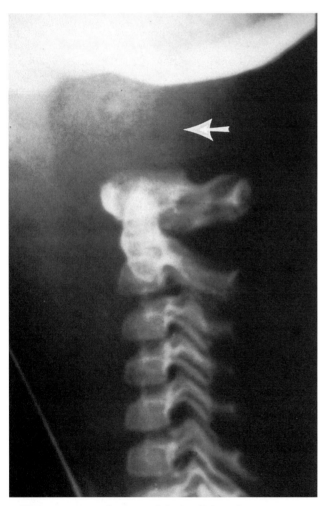

FIGURE 8.38. Atlanto-occipital dislocation. Note the increased distance between the base of the skull and C1 (arrows).

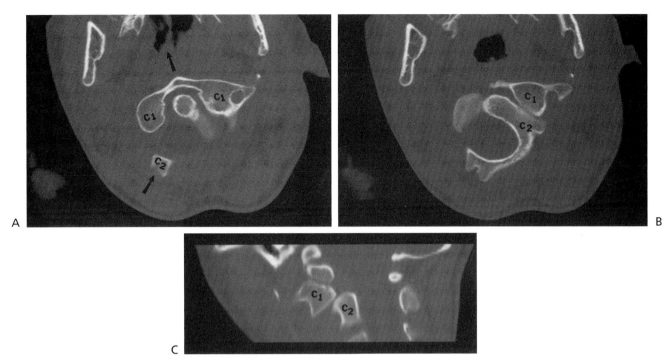

A

B

C

FIGURE 8.39. Rotatory subluxation. A. Note that C1 is pointing (upper arrow) along the sagittal axis of the skull. C2, however is pointing in the opposite direction (lower arrow). **B.** A slightly lower slice demonstrates that the left lateral mass of C1 is anteriorly subluxed on C2. Note the direction in which C2 is pointing. **C.** Sagittal reconstruction demonstrates the anteriorly subluxed lateral mass of C1 on C2.

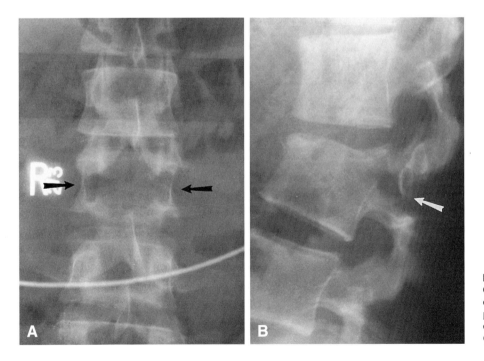

A

B

FIGURE 8.40. Seat belt injury: Chance fracture. A. Frontal view demonstrates fracture through the pedicles (arrows). **B.** Lateral view demonstrates the same fracture (arrow).

Flexion-extension views often are obtained in patients with suspected cervical spine injury. These views are not necessary in every patient and have been determined to be superfluous in children who have normal findings on regular cervical spine radiographs (4). At the same time, this same study (4) indicated that flexion-extension views were valuable when cervical spine radiographs suggested the presented of an abnormality. Flexion-extension views are especially beneficial when there is question about the presence of a hyperflexion cervical spine injury. They are safe (5) as long as the patient is alert and cooperative. In nonalert or even comatose patients, one can still perform these studies if the flexion portion is performed in incriminates. **My approach is to incrementally flex the patient's neck and obtain sequential portable lateral images.** The maneuver is performed by myself to ensure that no cervical cord injury results. This usually takes no more that two or three attempts.

Flexion-extension views are generally used for determining midcervical spine instability and in one study (6) it was determined that flexion-extension studies were requested by consultants rather than by the primary physician (6). This probably is true. Overall, the study is quite useful and rather benign (5), and we frequently use the flexion-extension series in our practice.

REFERENCES

1. Swischuk LE. Pursuing the odontoid fracture in infants. Emerg Radiol 1996;3:54–55.
2. Swischuk LE, John SD, Hendrick EP. Is the open-mouth odontoid view necessary in children under 5 years? Pediatr Radiol 2000; 30:186–189.
3. Buhs C, Cullen M, Klein M, et al. Pediatric trauma C-spine: is the "odontoid" view necessary? J Pediatr Surg 2000;35:994–997.
4. Dwek JR, Chung CB. Radiography of cervical spine injury in children: are flexion-extension radiographs useful for acute trauma? AJR 2000;174:1617–1619.
5. Woods WA, Brady WJ, Pollock G, et al. Flexion-extension cervical spine radiography in pediatric blunt trauma. Emerg Radiol 1998;5:381–384.
6. Brady WJ, Kini N, Duncan C, et al. Flexion-extension cervical spine radiography in blunt trauma: a survey of emergency physicians. Emerg Radiol 1998;5:375–380.

Scheuermann's Disease, Schmorl's Nodes, and Endplate Fractures (Limbus Vertebra)

Scheuermann's disease, Schmorl's nodes, and endplate fractures are probably related, if not the same (1). They most likely result from subclinical trauma, but they also occur with acute trauma (2–4). The end result is that a variety of configurations of disc herniation into the adjacent vertebral

bodies are seen. In terms of degenerative changes in the disc, it has been demonstrated with MRI that these can occur as early as 18 years (5). As a consequence, degenerative disc disease with bulging of the discs into the spinal canal or encroaching on a nerve root can be seen in older children and adolescents (Fig. 8.41F).

Scheuermann's disease usually occurs in the thoracic region at multiple levels and is associated with irregular disc narrowing and kyphosis (Fig. 8.41A). In longstanding cases, anterior vertebral fusion can result. The condition may or may not be painful. **Schmorl's nodes** generally are not painful and tend to occur through the central portions of the vertebral body. Occasionally, however, they are acute and painful (2, 3, 6) and are best demonstrated with plain films and MRI (Fig. 8.41, B and C). The **limbus vertebra** (7, 8) is an anterior herniation of the nucleus through an anterior corner (usually superior) of the vertebra. Occasionally, it can occur posteriorly (8). As with Schmorl's nodes, the condition may or may not be painful and can be detected with plain films and indirectly by nuclear scintigraphy (9). MRI most clearly identifies the abnormality (Fig. 8.41, D and E).

REFERENCES

1. Swischuk LE, John SD, Allbery S. Disk degenerative disease in childhood: Scheuermann's disease, Schmorl's nodes, and the limbus vertebra: MRI findings in 12 patients. Pediatr Radiol 1998; 28:334–338.
2. Hauger O, Cotton A, Chateil J-F, et al. Original report. Giant cystic Schmorl's nodes: imaging findings in six patients. AJR 2001; 176:969–972.
3. Stabler A, Belani M, Weiss M, et al. MR imaging of enhancing intraosseous disk herniation (Schmorl's nodes). AJR 1997;168: 933–938.
4. Wagner AL, Murtagh FR, Arrington JA. Relationship of Schmorl's nodes to vertebral body endplate fractures and acute endplate disk extrusions. AJNR 2000;21:276–281.
5. Erkintalo MO, Salminen JJ, Alanen AM, et al. Development of degenerative changes in the lumbar intervertebral disk: results of a prospective MR imaging study in adolescents with and without low-back pain. Radiology 1995;196:529–533.
6. Walters G, Coumas JM, Akins CM, et al. Magnetic resonance imaging of acute symptomatic Schmorl's node formation. Pediatr Emerg Care 1991;7:294–296.
7. Banerian KG, Wang A-M, Samberg LC, et al. Association of vertebral endplate fracture with pediatric lumbar intervertebral disc herniation: value of CT and MR imaging. Radiology 1990;177: 763–765.
8. Henales V, Hervas JA, Lopez P, et al. Intervertebral disc herniations (limbus vertebrae) in pediatric patients: report of 15 cases. Pediatr Radiol 1993;23:608–610.
9. Mandell GA, Morales RW, Harcke HT, et al. Bone scintigraphy in patients with atypical lumbar Scheuermann's disease. J Pediatr Orthop 1993;13:622–627.

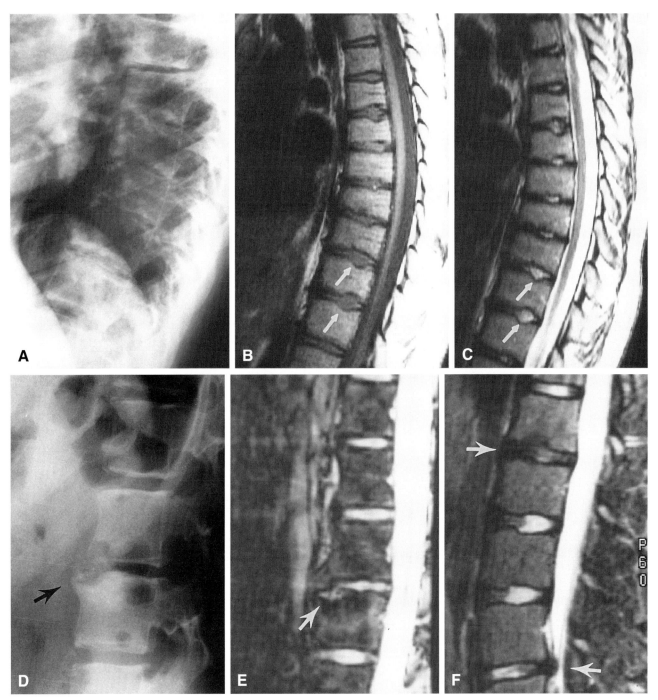

FIGURE 8.41. Disc degeneration. A. Scheuermann's disease. Note the gentle kyphosis and numerous irregular narrowed disc spaces. **B.** Sagittal, T1-weighted MR image demonstrates the ragged intervertebral disc spaces and Schmorl's nodes at least at two levels (arrows). **C.** T2-weighted image demonstrates similar findings and high signal intensity in Schmorl's nodes (arrows) and in the center of the other discs. The remaining portions of the discs show low signal intensity as a result of desiccation. Normal discs show uniform signal from front to back. **D. Limbus vertebra.** Note the characteristic configuration of a limbus vertebra (arrow). There also is reactive sclerosis, some fragmentation, and narrowing of the disc space. **E.** T2-weighted MR image demonstrates extrusion of nuclear material (arrow) into the vertebral body, constituting the so-called limbus vertebra. Note that the involved disc space is narrower and more irregular than normal. The normal discs at the other levels show uniform high signal intensity. **F.** In this patient, advanced disc degeneration with loss of signal has occurred in the disc at the T12-L1 level (upper arrow). There is a small Schmorl's node protruding into T12. The two disc spaces below show loss of signal (i.e., desiccation) and narrowing over their anterior portions. The next disc is narrowed and shows loss of signal as well as posterior bulging (lower arrow).

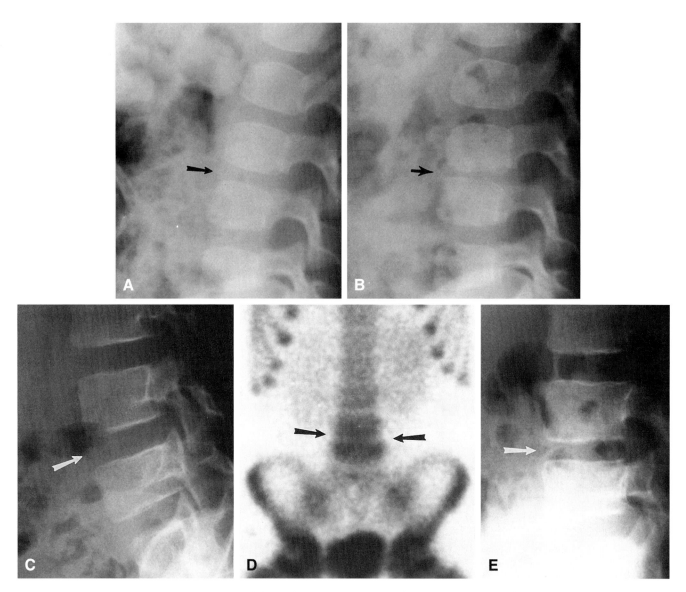

FIGURE 8.42. Discitis. A. Subtle, early change consisting of minimal narrowing of a disc space (arrow). **B.** A few weeks later, clear-cut disc space and vertebral body destruction has occurred (arrow). **C.** Another patient with no abnormalities on plain films. Note specifically that the disc space between L4 and L5 (arrow) is normal. **D.** Nuclear scintigraphy, however, demonstrates clear-cut increased uptake around the disc in L4 and L5 (arrows). **E.** Two weeks later, the disc space between L4 and L5 has become narrowed (arrow).

INFECTIONS OF THE SPINE AND MENINGES

Osteomyelitis and Discitis

Although some consider spinal osteomyelitis and discitis to be separate, there is growing opinion that both basically are the same (1, 2). This has always been my opinion, and it is my belief that so-called discitis, nonspecific discitis, spondylitis, or spondyloarthritis all are the same and are low-grade infections. Most often (1, 2), but not always (3), they are caused by staphylococcal infection. The condition responds well to antibiotic therapy and in the end, it is difficult to argue that it is not caused by infection.

The clinical symptoms in discitis may be subtle and the patient may simply present with a limp. Eventually it may be determined that the problem is in the spine, but if it is not, nuclear scintigraphy is excellent at detecting the problem in its early stages (Fig. 8.42D). Otherwise, plain film findings consist of disc space narrowing with indistinctness of the vertebral endplates on either side of the disc and eventually, destruction of these plates (Fig. 8.42, A and B). With therapy the changes slowly regress, but disc space narrowing and irregularity of the endplates may persist and vertebral fusion can ensue. Discitis also can be a problem in neonates, and overall, it can be fungal or tuberculous (Pott's disease) in origin. The only difference is that tuberculosis tends to involve the thoracic spine, while regular, osteomyelitis and discitis tend to involve the lower thoracic and, even more commonly, the lumbar spine. The cervical spine is not involved by either very often. Because of the chronicity of tuberculosis, it is more apt to show large scalloped areas of vertebral erosion, calcifications, and extradural abscesses (4). In most cases, plain films suffice (Figs. 8.42 and 8.43), but in any case, CT and MRI can be employed for further imaging. In this regard, MRI is probably more rewarding than CT (Fig. 8.44).

REFERENCES

1. Ring D, Johnston CE II, Wenger DR. Pyogenic infectious spondylitis in children: the convergence of discitis and vertebral osteomyelitis. J Pediatr Orthop 1995;15:652–660.
2. Garron E, Viehweger E, Launay F, et al. Nontuberculous spondylodiscitis in children. J Pediatr Orthop 2002;22:321–328.
3. Govender S, Parbhoo AH, Rasool MN, et al. *Salmonella typhi* spondylitis. J Pediatr Orthop 1999;19:710–714.
4. Altieri MF, Watkins T, Hwang G. Pott's disease: an old disease reappears in the pediatric emergency department. Pediatr Emerg Care 1995;11:304–306.
5. Magnus KG, Hoffman EB. Pyogenic spondylitis and early tuberculous spondylitis in children: differential diagnosis with standard radiographs and computed tomography. J Pediatr Orthop 2000; 20:539–543.
6. Song KS, Ogden JA, Ganey T. Contiguous discitis and osteomyelitis in children. J Pediatr Orthop 1997;17:470–477.

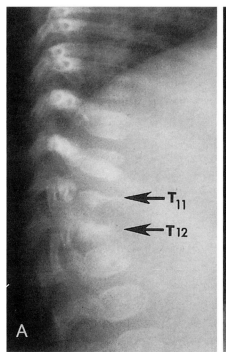
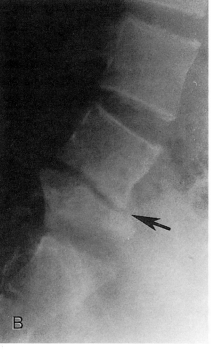

FIGURE 8.43. Osteomyelitis of the spine. A. Note the characteristic destruction of disc space and adjacent vertebral bodies (T11, T12). The disc space below T12 is also slightly narrowed, belying additional involvement at this level. **B.** An older patient with longstanding disc space destruction (arrow) and associated destruction of the underlying vertebral body. This was caused by tuberculosis.

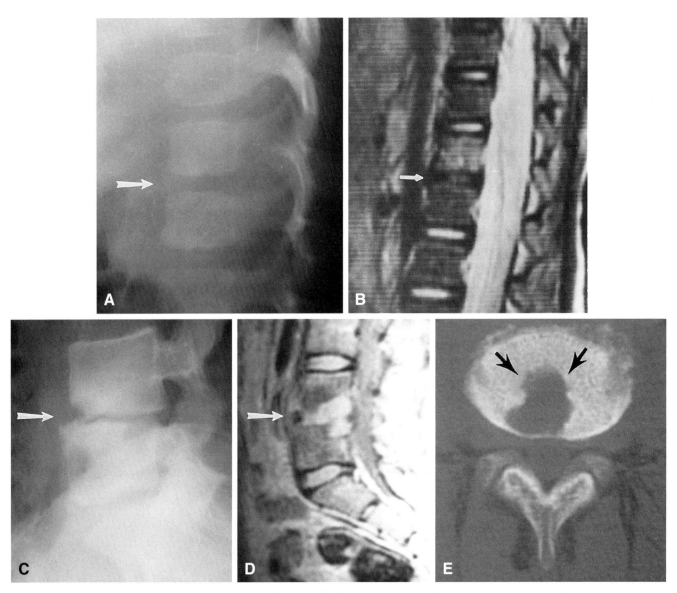

FIGURE 8.44. Discitis-osteomyelitis: MR findings. A. Note the disc space narrowing (arrow). **B.** T2-weighted, sagittal MR image demonstrates loss of signal in the involved disc (arrow) and increased signal intensity in the vertebral body above it. **C.** Chronic infection producing extreme narrowing of the disc space (arrow), some subluxation of the vertebral bodies, vertebral destruction, and a good deal of reactive sclerosis. **D.** Sagittal, T2-weighted MR study demonstrates a completely disrupted disc space (arrow) with herniation of nuclear material posteriorly and into the lower vertebral body. There is extensive loss of signal in both adjacent vertebral bodies. **E.** CT demonstrates bony destruction of the vertebral body (arrows).

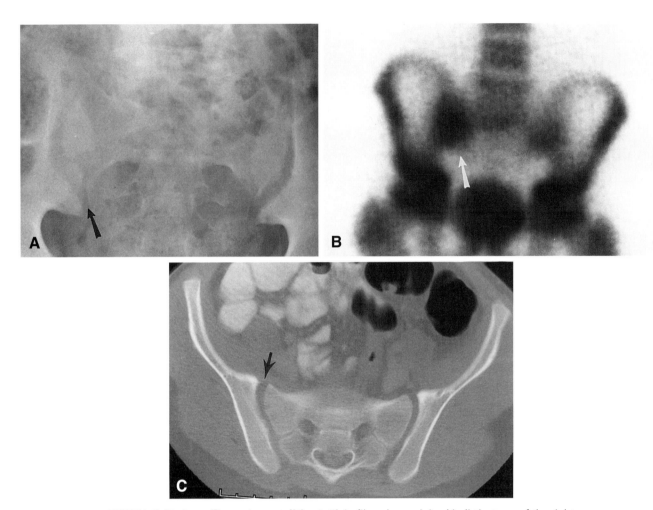

FIGURE 8.45. Sacroiliac osteomyelitis. A. Plain films show minimal indistinctness of the right sacroiliac joint (arrow). **B.** Nuclear scintigraphy clearly demonstrates increased uptake in the area (arrow). **C.** CT demonstrates minimal indistinctness of the bones around the sacroiliac joint (arrow) and some thickening of the soft tissues over the sacroiliac joints.

Osteomyelitis of the Sacroiliac Joints

Osteomyelitis of the sacroiliac joints is not a common problem in infancy but does occur in older children. It may be a cause of limp and onset often is insidious. The problem usually is staphylococcal infection, and bone destruction along the sacroiliac joint often is difficult to detect on plain films (Fig. 8.45A). Nuclear scintigraphy is most rewarding in identifying this condition (Fig. 8.45B), and this is especially important because the findings also are subtle on CT (Fig. 8.45C). MR also is useful, especially with contrast-enhanced imaging (1).

REFERENCE

1. Bollow M, Braun J, Biedermann T. Use of contrast enhanced MR imaging to detect sacroiliitis in children. Skeletal Radiol 1998;27: 606–616.

Infection of the Spinal Cord and Meninges

Spinal epidural abscess is uncommon in infants and children but it is a condition that requires immediate surgical treatment (1–3). The infection arises from hematogenous spread from a distant focus, and unfortunately, plain film roentgenographic findings are normal. There may be some straightening of the spine secondary to muscle spasm, but one must usually resort to CT or MRI to demonstrate the epidural abscess (4). The organism usually is one of the more common pyogenic organisms, but in immunosuppressed patients, aspergillosis or other fungal disease is not uncommon (5).

With MRI, it is possible to image conditions such as transverse myelitis as it occurs with the Guillain-Barré syndrome (6–10). Edema of the cord is best seen on T2-weighted images. Although viral infections are most common, one occasionally encounters bacterial myelitis (11).

REFERENCES

1. Peter JC, Kieck CF, DeVilliers JC. Acute spinal epidural abscess. Pediatr Surg Int 1992;7:284–288.

2. Schweich PJ, Hurt TL. Spinal epidural abscess in children: two illustrative cases. Pediatr Emerg Care 1992;8:84–87.

3. Schneider P, Givens TG. Spinal subdural abscess in a pediatric patient: a case report and review of the literature. Pediatr Emerg Care 1998;14:22–23.

4. Sandhu FS, Dillon WP. Spinal epidural abscess: evaluation with contrast-enhanced MR imaging. AJNR 1991;12:1087–1093.

5. Parker SL, Laszewski MJ, Trigg ME, et al. Spinal cord aspergillosis in immunosuppressed patients. Pediatr Radiol 1990;20:351–352.

6. Baran GA, Sowell MK, Sharp GB, et al. Case report. MR findings in a child with Guillain-Barré syndrome. AJR 1993;161:161–163.

7. Byun WM, Park WK, Park B, et al. Guillain-Barré syndrome: MR imaging findings of the spine in eight patients. Radiology 1998;208:137–141.

8. Delhaas T, Kamphuis DJ, Witkamp TD. Transitory spinal cord swelling in a 6-year-old boy with Guillain-Barré syndrome. Pediatr Radiol 1998;28:544–546.

9. Iwata F, Utsumi Y. MR imaging in Guillain-Barré syndrome. Pediatr Radiol 1997;27:36–38.

10. Tartaglino LM, Croul SE, Flanders AE, et al. Idiopathic acute transverse myelitis: MR imaging findings. Radiology 1996;201:661–669.

11. Friess HM, Wasenko JJ. MR of staphylococcal myelitis of the cervical spinal cord. AJNR 1997;18:455–458.

TUMORS AND CYSTS OF THE SPINE, SPINAL CORD, AND MENINGES

Primary tumors of the spine and spinal cord are extremely uncommon in the newborn and young infant, and not that common in older children. Tumors of the spine include osteoid osteoma or osteoblastoma, chordoma, aneurysmal bone cyst (1), and hemangioma. Chordomas arise from notochordal remnants and most commonly occur around the clivus of the skull or the sacral region of the spine. Characteristically, they produce lytic bone destruction, an associated mass, and in many cases, irregular tumoral calcifications. They may extend into the spinal canal to mimic intraspinal tumors (2).

The cervical spine is a common place for aneurysmal bone cysts to occur. These lesions produce expanding, bub-

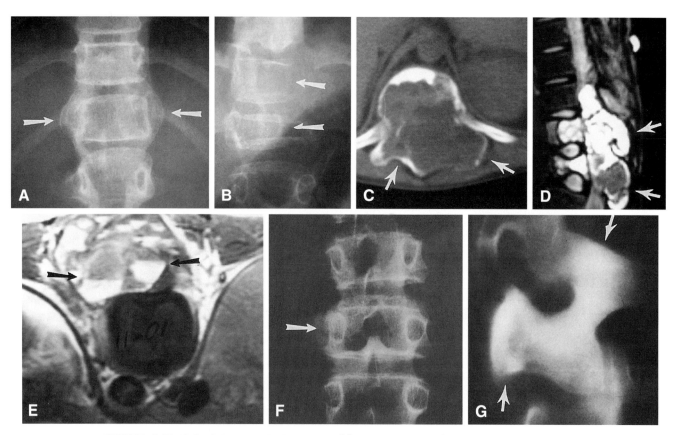

FIGURE 8.46. Spinal tumors. A. Aneurysmal bone cyst. Note the expansile lesion of T12 (arrows). **B.** Another patient with vertebral destruction and collapse of two vertebral bodies (arrows). **C.** Axial CT view through one of the vertebral bodies demonstrates the expansile destructive lesion (arrows). **D.** T2-weighted, sagittal MR image demonstrates the multilobulated, expansile tumor (arrows) invading both vertebral bodies. The lower vertebral body demonstrates collapse. **E.** Axial view demonstrates characteristic blood-fluid levels (arrows). **F. Osteoid osteoma** producing a dense pedicle (arrow). **G.** Lateral view demonstrates the sclerosis (arrows) more clearly. (**E** Courtesy of C. Keith Hayden, Jr., M.D.)

bly configurations of the vertebral bodies, and in some cases, they may extend into the posterior elements (Fig. 8.46, A–E). They may in time be associated with vertebral body fracture-compression and compression of the spinal cord. MRI is excellent for demonstrating aneurysmal bone cysts in which the cystic component and blood-fluid levels are demonstrable (Fig. 8.46E). Hemangiomas also can be encountered (3), and their bubbly appearance may cause confusion with aneurysmal bone cysts (Fig. 8.47, A and B). Osteoid osteomas also can be encountered. This benign lesion usually produces sclerosis of the pedicles and, in some cases, of the vertebral arches (Fig. 8.46, F and G). When they are very large and expanding, they are called "giant osteoblastomas." Bone scintigraphy is helpful in the detec-

tion of osteoid osteoma because the tumor is scintigraphically "hot."

Secondary metastatic tumors of the vertebrae and lymphoma or leukemia (4) vertebral involvement probably are more common than primary tumors, and one of the most common is metastatic neuroblastoma (Fig. 8.47C). Whatever the tumor, however, the vertebral body is destroyed and eventually a pathologic compression fracture is seen. Characteristically, the intervening disc spaces are intact, and this serves to differentiate the findings from those of osteomyelitis. With osteomyelitis, except for fungal infection, the disc spaces are destroyed. Vertebral body destruction with preservation of the disc spaces also occurs in histiocytosis X. In this condition, the destroyed vertebra often

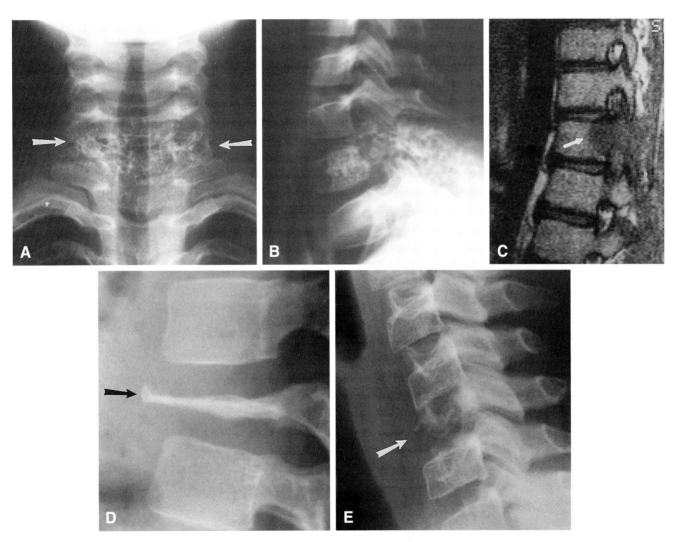

FIGURE 8.47. Spinal tumors. A. Hemangioma. Typical bubbly appearance of a hemangioma (arrows). **B.** Lateral view demonstrates that both the body and neural arch are involved. **C. Metastatic neuroblastoma** (arrow) causing destruction of the vertebral body and associated neural arch. **D.** Typical collapsed vertebra (vertebra plana) in **histiocytosis X** (arrow). **E. Eosinophilic granuloma** in another patient produces complete destruction of the vertebral body of C5 (arrow). There is slight subluxation of the cervical spine.

is compressed and flat and plate-like. It is called "vertebral plana" and is characteristic of histiocytosis X (Fig. 8.47D). In other instances, however, less compression occurs, and pathologic dislocation can co-exist (Fig. 8.47E).

Intraspinal tumors generally produce little change on plain films. If they are longstanding and expanding, they may produce expansile changes on the spinal canal (i.e., flattening of the pedicles, widening of the interpedicular spaces, and posterior scalloping of the vertebral bodies). These tumors, although generally uncommon in children, include gliomas (5, 6), ependymomas, intraspinal neuroblastomas, epidural lymphoma, lipomas of the cauda equina, arteriovenous malformations, and hemangiomas (7). With neuroblastoma (or ganglioneuroma), it also should be appreciated that the problem more often is that of a paravertebral tumor extending into the spinal canal in so-called dumbbell fashion. Teratomas also can present in this manner and occasionally so can lipomas (8) or, retroperitoneal sarcomas, but the neuroblastoma-ganglioneuroma group of lesions is most common. **This "dumbbell" phenomenon in these tumors is important to note because while in adults neurofibroma is the tumor to think of, in children it is neuroblastoma.** A rare problem is that of symptomatic epidural lipomatosis (9).

After plain films, delineation of any intraspinal tumor is best accomplished with MRI, which shows high signal intensity on T1-weighted and low signal intensity on T2-

weighted images with lipomas, and high signal intensity on T2-weighted images with most other tumors (Fig. 8.48). In closing, it might be remembered that intraspinal tumors also can be seen from seeding of intracranial tumors, the most common of which is medulloblastoma, followed by ependymoma.

REFERENCES

1. Caro PA, Mandell GA, Stanton RP. Aneurysmal bone cyst of the spine in children. MRI imaging at 0.5 Tesla. Pediatr Radiol 1991; 21:117–120.
2. Karakida O, Aoki J, Tanikawa H, et al. Epidural dumbbell-shaped chordoma mimicking neurinoma. Pediatr Radiol 1996;26:62–64.
3. Duprez T, Lokietek W, Clapuyt P, et al. Multiple aggressive vertebral hemangiomas in an adolescent: a case report. Pediatr Radiol 1998;28:51–53.
4. Carriere B, Cummins-McManus B. Vertebral fractures as initial signs for acute lymphoblastic leukemia. Pediatr Emerg Care 17: 258–261, 2001.
5. Umemoto M, Azuma E, Ohshima S, et al. Congenital astrocytoma in the cervical spinal cord. Am J Dis Child 1990;144: 744–746.
6. Choi YH, Kim I-O, Cheon J-E, et al. Gangliocytoma of the spinal cord: a case report. Pediatr Radiol 2001;31:377–380.
7. Balaci E, Sumner TE, Auringer ST, et al. Diffuse neonatal hemangiomatosis with extensive involvement of the brain and cervical spinal cord. Pediatr Radiol 1999;29:441–443.
8. Cheng TJ, Wu TT, Hsu JD. A dumbbell spinal lipoma presenting as a neck mass: CT and MR demonstration. Pediatr Radiol 1995; 25:570–571.
9. Munoz A, Barkovich JA, Mareos F, et al. Symptomatic epidural lipomatosis of the spinal cord in a child: MR demonstration of spinal cord injury. Pediatr Radiol 32:865, 2002.

Presacral and Sacrococcygeal Tumors and Masses

Although one can encounter a variety of lesions in the area of the sacrum, in the newborn and young infant, one most commonly is dealing with a teratoma. Other tumors or masses encountered include anterior meningocele, neuroblastoma, and on occasion, chordoma (1), yolk sac carcinoma (2), and ependymoma (3). Although some teratomas are malignant, most are benign and simply cause displacement of the adjacent pelvic structures. Some grow outwardly and present as masses of the perineum, buttocks, or distal sacral region. The tumor can be predominantly intrapelvic, extrapelvic, or both intrapelvic and extrapelvic (Fig. 8.49). Those tumors predominantly extrapelvic seem to be more benign and exhibit a much lesser tendency to metastasize.

Sacrococcygeal teratomas frequently are calcified and in some cases, often the more benign, formed bony or tooth structures are seen. Calcifications probably occur more often in benign lesions, and visualization of these structures clinches the diagnosis (Fig. 8.49). Similarly, if fatty density is seen within the mass, lipomatous tissue is most likely pre-

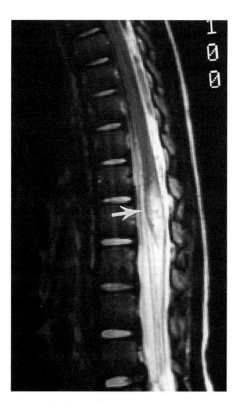

FIGURE 8.48. Spinal cord tumor. Note the increased signal intensity in this oval ependymoma (arrow).

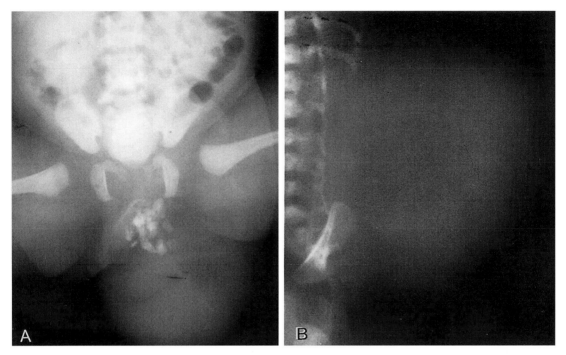

FIGURE 8.49. Presacral teratoma. A. Note the large tumor mass with teeth in it. **B.** Another infant with a large mass showing central lucency caused by fat.

sent, and the diagnosis of teratoma should be confirmed. Although these findings often are visible on plain films, they are more clearly delineated with ultrasound, CT, and MRI (Fig. 8.50). Deformity of the sacral spine can be seen but is less common than with anterior sacral meningocele. High-output cardiac failure as a result of AV shunting in some of these tumors can result (4). A hereditary form of presacral teratoma associated with sacral defects and anorectal stenosis also has been described (5, 6). There seems to be more than a casual relationship between anorectal anomalies, sacral abnormalities, and presacral abnormalities such as tumors, meningoceles, and enteric cysts.

It is not possible to determine whether a teratoma is benign or malignant (although most are benign) on the basis of plain films. Malignancy is more likely to be encountered in predominantly intrapelvic tumors in older infants, and because of this, there is considerable belief that all sacrococcygeal teratomas be considered potentially malignant. Consequently, operative intervention should be employed as soon as possible.

Anterior sacral meningocele is usually associated with some degree of sacral deformity, and anorectal abnormalities such as ectopic anus are not uncommonly associated. Anterior sacral meningocele is also seen with neurofibromatosis. The sacral deformity usually consists of a crescent-shaped sacrum with a large concave defect on the involved side (Fig. 8.51). This has been called the "sickle" sign. It is through this defect that the meningocele arises. No calcifications are present, and the diagnosis should be strongly

suspected when a presacral mass is associated with the typical sacral deformity. MRI readily demonstrates the abnormality.

Neuroblastoma arising anterior to the sacrum is much less common than intraabdominal neuroblastoma. Calcification of a nonspecific, irregular type can point to the proper diagnosis, but confusion with some cases of teratoma can arise. A preoperative diagnosis is not usually made with ease. Spinal column involvement is relatively rare. Neuroblastomas located in this area, much as neuroblastomas located in the chest, appear to carry a better prognosis than do those located in the abdomen.

Neurenteric cysts are occasionally seen in the presacral region. They displace the rectum and, if completely disassociated from the spinal canal, manifest primarily as masses. If they retain a connection with the neural canal, anterior defects in the sacrum may be visualized.

Presacral chordomas are extremely uncommon in infancy, but they can occur, producing destruction and expansion of the sacrum and coccyx. Typically, flocculent cartilaginous calcifications are seen, and the extent of this tumor and all presacral tumors is best demonstrated with CT and MRI.

REFERENCES

1. Cable DG, Moir C. Pediatric sacrococcygeal chordomas: a rare tumor to be differentiated from sacrococcygeal teratoma. J Pediatr Surg 1997;32:759–761.

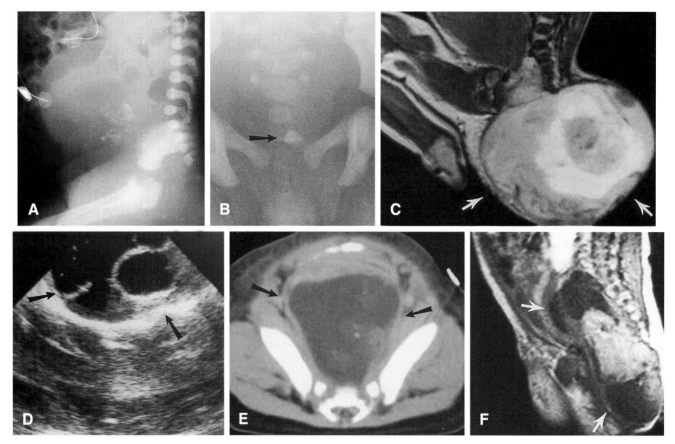

FIGURE 8.50. Presacral teratoma: variable appearances. A. Plain film demonstrates an extensive mass in the presacral region extending into the buttocks and abdomen. Calcifications identify the abnormality, and fatty density is present within the tumor. **B.** Another patient with a small calcific density (arrow). There is little else abnormal to be seen. **C.** T1-weighted MR image in another infant demonstrates a large teratoma extending into the buttocks (arrows). It shows a characteristically heterogeneous signal. **D.** Another patient whose ultrasound demonstrates a multicystic-appearing mass (arrows). **E.** In this patient, a CT study demonstrates a large mass with stippled calcifications and considerable fat (arrows). **F.** T1-weighted, sagittal MR study in the same patient demonstrates the large fluid density mass (arrows) in the center of which is a large echogenic lipomatous mass.

2. Kaste SC, Bridges JO, Marina NM. Sacrococcygeal yolk sac carcinoma: imaging findings during treatment. Pediatr Radiol 1996; 26:212–219.
3. Johnson JM, Jessurun J, Leonard A. Sacrococcygeal ependymoma: case report and review of the literature. J Pediatr Surg 1999; 34:1405–1407.
4. Bond SJ, Harrison MR, Schmidt KG, et al. Death due to high output cardiac failure in fetal sacrococcygeal teratoma. J Pediatr Surg 1990;25:1287–1291.
5. Currarino G, Coln D, Votteler T. Triad of anorectal, sacral, and presacral anomalies. AJR 1981;137:395–398.
6. Sonnino RE, Chou S, Guttman FM. Hereditary sacrococcygeal teratomas. J Pediatr Surg 1989;24:1074–1075.

Neurofibromatosis

Although the bony and other changes in neurofibromatosis occasionally can be encountered in young infants, one is more likely to encounter them in older children and adults. In the spine, these include interpedicular widening, flatten-ing of the pedicles, anterior, lateral, and posterior vertebral scalloping, dysplastic vertebra, dislocations, and scoliosis (1). Scalloping results from an inherent mesenchymal dysplasia of the vertebral bodies and usually is associated with non-tumoral expansion of the spinal subarachnoid space. The vertebrae in neurofibromatosis frequently are dysplastic and scoliosis, angular rather than rotatory can be seen (Fig. 8.52A). In terms of scoliosis, an interesting case of rib displacement causing pressure on the spinal cord in association with severe scoliosis has been documented (2). Neurofibromas and gliomas can be encountered along the spinal nerves, and every so often malignant degeneration can occur (Fig. 8.52, B and C). **Otherwise, most of the bony changes seen in neurofibromatosis are the result of inherent dysplasia rather than the presence of a tumor.**

In patients with neurofibromatosis, high-signal-intensity lesions commonly are seen on FLAIR images of the brain. These have always been a problem, but it seems that they

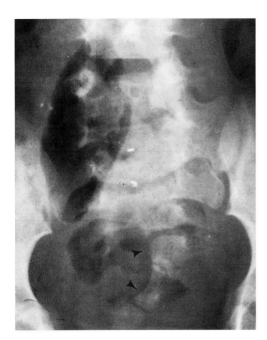

FIGURE 8.51. Anterior sacral meningocele. Note the characteristic scalloped sacrum (arrowheads). This is the most classic type of deformity in anterior sacral meningocele, but in other instances the sacrum may be more disorganized. (Courtesy of D. Harwood-Nash, M.D.)

may represent a hamartomatous abnormality of myeline (3). In addition to this and the preceding considerations of neurofibromatosis, the condition can manifest in sheath-like tumoral growth referred to as "plexiform neurofibromatosis." These lesions can occur almost anywhere in the body (4–6).

REFERENCES

1. Sirois JL III, Drennan JC. Dystrophic spinal deformity in neurofibromatosis. J Pediatr Orthop 1990;10:522–526.
2. Dacher JN, Zakine S, Monroc M, et al. Rib displacement threatening the spinal cord in a scoliotic child with neurofibromatosis. Pediatr Radiol 1995;25:58–59.
3. Eastwood JD, Fiorella DJ, MacFall JF, et al. Increased brain apparent diffusion coefficient in children with neurofibromatosis type 1. Radiology 2001;219:354–358.
4. Fenton LZ, Foreman N, Wyatt-Ashmead J. Diffuse retroperitoneal mesenteric and intrahepatic periportal plexiform neurofibroma in a 5-year-old boy. Pediatr Radiol 2001;31:637–639.
5. Frawley KJ, Cohen R, O'Loughlin EV, et al. Neurofibromatosis of the small intestine mesentery in a child with neurofibromatosis type 1. J Pediatr Surg 1997;32:1783–1785.
6. Nguyen HT, Kogan BA, Hricak H. Plexiform neurofibroma involving the genitourinary tract in children: case reports and review of the literature. Urology 1997;49:257–260.

Intraspinal Cysts

Intraspinal cysts can be extradural or intradural, but both are uncommon in infancy. With extradural cysts, one most

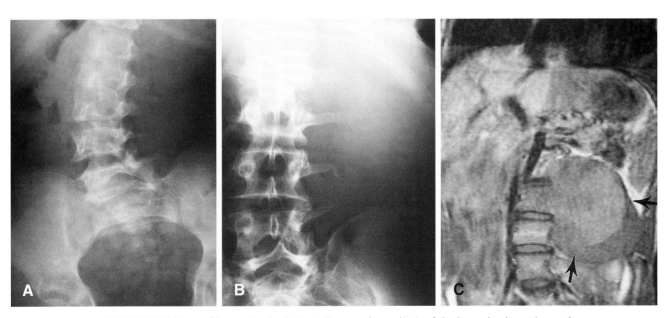

FIGURE 8.52. Neurofibromatosis. A. Note the angular scoliosis of the lower lumbar spine and extensive associated dysplastic changes. **B.** Another patient with dysplastic changes in the lumbar vertebra and transverse processes and a mass in the left abdomen. **C.** T1-weighted, coronal MR image demonstrates the large mass (arrows) invading a vertebral body. This was a large, malignant schwannoma.

commonly sees widening of the interpedicular space, flattening of the pedicles, kyphosis of the spine, and on myelography, evidence of an extradural block. MRI is excellent in defining these lesions, but they also can be demonstrated with CT myelography.

Neurenteric Cyst

This entity has been discussed with mediastinal tumors in Chapter 1 and duplication cysts in Chapter 4. Suffice it to say that the abnormality arises from persistence of the embryonic communication between the gastrointestinal tract and nervous system. Consequently, anterior defects of the vertebral bodies are present, and it is this spinal deformity that is the key to the correct preoperative identification of these cysts. Occasionally, the connecting sinus tract can be seen on plain films (i.e., the canal of Kovalevsky). Neurenteric cysts can also extend into the spinal canal and act as an intraspinal tumor (1). These cysts also can erode so as to create a scalloped lesion of the vertebrae (2). If no connection to the spine exists, the cysts often are called "duplication cysts." Neurenteric cysts are best imaged with MRI. Because they often contain gastric mucosa, nuclear scintigraphy can identify their presence.

REFERENCES

1. Fernandes ET, Custer MD, Burton EM, et al. Neurenteric cyst: surgery and diagnostic imaging. J Pediatr Surg 1991;26:108–110.
2. Ellis AM, Taylor TKF. Intravertebral spinal neuroenteric cysts: a unique radiographic sign—"the hole-in-one vertebra." J Pediatr Orthop 1997;17:766–768.

MISCELLANEOUS ABNORMALITIES OF THE SPINE

Back Pain in Children

Back pain in children usually has a definable cause, but it is becoming apparent that older children and adolescents have presentations and diagnoses similar to those of adults (1). Nuclear scintigraphy is excellent in detecting occult spinal lesions (2), and both nuclear scintigraphy and MR scanning can be used to detect or exclude conditions such as spondylolysis, pathologic fractures, osteomyelitis (discitis), and tumors such as osteoid osteoma. Stress fractures of the sacrum (3) also may be detected.

REFERENCES

1. Combs JA, Caskey PM. Back pain in children and adolescents: a retrospective review of 648 patients. South Med J 1997;90: 89–792.

2. Feldman DS, Hedden DM, Wright JG. The use of bone scan to investigate back pain in children and adolescents. J Pediatr Orthop 2000;20:790–795.
3. Daffner RH, Fedyshin PJ. Insufficiency fractures of the sacrum. Emerg Radiol 2001;8:59–64.

Torticollis

Torticollis can occur on an idiopathic basis in older children and adolescents. The term "wry neck" often is applied to this condition. The problem most likely represents subluxation with pronounced muscle spasm. It is treated symptomatically and usually resolves. Torticollis also can be seen with underlying tumors of the posterior fossa, brainstem, and upper cervical spinal cord and after trauma (i.e., subluxation or dislocation of C1 on C2). In the neonate and young infant, one of the more common causes of torticollis is a fibroma of the sternocleidomastoid muscle, the so-called fibromatosis colli (1). The condition is readily imaged with ultrasound, but the diagnosis usually can be made clinically.

REFERENCES

1. Cheng JCY, Au AWY. Infantile torticollis: a review of 624 cases. J Pediatr Orthop 1994;14:802–808.

Scoliosis and Kyphosis

Scoliosis can result from underlying neuromuscular disease or the presence of vertebral anomalies such as hemivertebra or be idiopathic. Muscle weakness is the cause with neuromuscular disease; with vertebral anomalies, unilateral fusion of vertebral bodies, or the presence of hemivertebrae lead to scoliosis. The precise cause of idiopathic scoliosis is not known but is believed to lie in muscular imbalance (1). The most important point to remember about scoliosis is that, when it is rotatory, it is usually idiopathic (Fig. 8.53A); if it is angular, it usually is the result of some underlying vertebral abnormality or intraspinal problem (Fig. 8.53B). Syringomyelia (2–4) is not uncommonly encountered with angular scoliosis, especially if levoscoliosis is present (Fig. 8.54). Angular scoliosis also occurs with the so-called unilateral bar (Fig. 8.55). This anomaly consists of fusion of the pedicles and transverse processes of the vertebral bodies so that a solid bar exists and impaired growth of the vertebral column occurs. As a result, angular scoliosis is seen (Fig. 8.55). In severe cases and preoperatively, and especially when levoscoliosis is present, it is becoming more and more important to image these patients with MRI (5) because it can disclose underlying spinal cord abnormalities with ease. There are various methods for measuring scoliosis, and two of them are outlined in Figure 8.56.

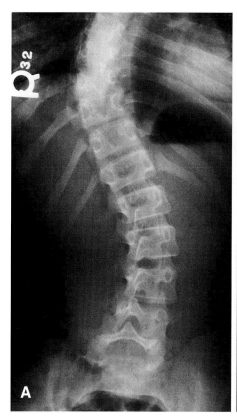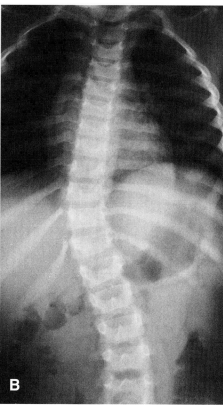

FIGURE 8.53. Scoliosis. A. Rotoscoliosis. Note the double S curve with rotation of the pedicles, especially in the lumbar region. **B. Angular scoliosis.** In this patient, there basically is one curve and there is no rotatory component. Note that the pedicles all are in alignment in this AP view.

Kyphosis is a common feature of Scheuermann's disease (discussed earlier). It also can be seen with meningomyelocele and certain chondrodystrophies, such as achondroplasia. In the latter instances, kyphosis tends to occur in the lower thoracic or lumbar regions. Kyphosis also can result from anterior congenital fusion of the vertebral bodies and after infections such as tuberculous osteomyelitis. The term "gibbus deformity" often is applied to cases of severe angular kyphosis.

Because the radiographic examination of scoliosis entails irradiation to the breasts of adolescent females, it is important to keep the radiation dose as low as possible. Numerous measures are available to accomplish this, including shielding and phosphorplate digital radiography (6–8).

REFERENCES

1. Machida M, Dubousset J, Imamura Y, et al. Pathogenesis of idiopathic scoliosis: SEPS in chicken with experimentally induced scoliosis and in patients with idiopathic scoliosis. J Pediatr Orthop 1994;14:329–335.
2. Charry O, Koop S, Winter R, et al. Syringomyelia and scoliosis: a review of twenty-five pediatric patients. J Pediatr Orthop 1994;14:309–317.
3. Farley FA, Song KM, Birch JG, et al. Syringomyelia and scoliosis in children. J Pediatr Orthop 1995;15:187–192.
4. Tomlinson RJ Jr, Wolfe MW, Nadall JM, et al. Syringomyelia and developmental scoliosis. J Pediatr Orthop 1994;14:580–585.
5. Barnes PD, Brody JD, Jaramillo D, et al. A typical idiopathic scoliosis: MR imaging evaluation. Radiology 1993;186:248–253.
6. Dutkowsky JP, Shearer D, Schepps B, et al. Radiation exposure to patients receiving routine scoliosis radiography measured at depth in an anthropomorphic phantom. J Pediatr Orthop 1990;10:532–534.
7. Kalmar JA, Jones JP, Merritt CRB. Low-dose radiography of scoliosis in children: a comparison of methods. Spine 1994;19:818–823.
8. Stringer DA, Cairns RA, Poskitt KJ, et al. Comparison of stimulable phosphor technology and conventional screen-film technology in pediatric scoliosis. Pediatr Radiol 1994;24:1–5.

Idiopathic Intervertebral Disc Calcifications

Calcification of the intervertebral discs usually is encountered in older children (1–3), where it is idiopathic. There does seem to be some inflammatory etiology involved, however, as these patients present with pain and fever. Treatment is symptomatic, and symptoms usually resolve completely. The calcifications also may disappear with time, and it has been demonstrated that there is little residual change in the vertebral bodies or disc spaces in adulthood.

Herniation of the disc anteriorly or posteriorly also can occur. Most frequently, idiopathic disc space calcification

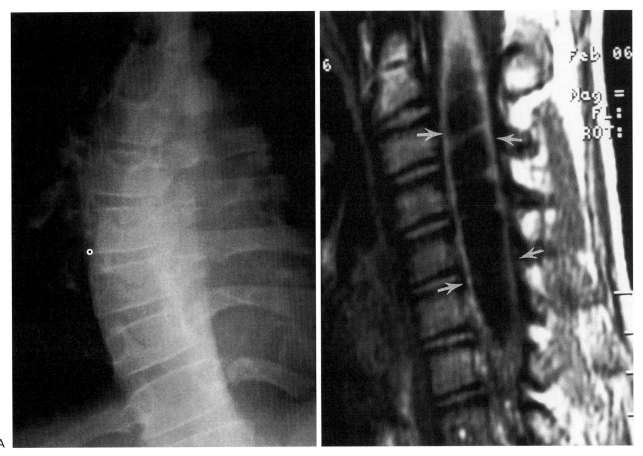

A

B

FIGURE 8.54. Levoscoliosis. A. Patient with levoscoliosis. **B.** MR study demonstrates the presence of a syrinx (arrows).

involves the cervical (Fig. 8.57) and upper thoracic portions of the spine, but disc space calcifications can occur at other levels. In addition to identification on plain films, these calcifications can be demonstrated with CT and MRI (4), and MRI can demonstrate inflammatory changes in the intervertebral discs in the early stages of the condition (4). This can be seen before calcification occurs (Fig. 8.58). In older children, intervertebral disc calcification also can be seen with ochronosis, vitamin D intoxication, idiopathic hypercalcemia, and other causes of hypercalcemia.

REFERENCES

1. Girodias J-B, Azouz EM, Maarton D. Intervertebral disk space calcification. A. report of 51 children with a review of the literature. Pediatr Radiol 1991;21:541–546.
2. Heinrich SD, Zembo MM, King AG, et al. Calcific cervical intervertebral disk herniation in children. Spine 1991;16:228–231.
3. Pattekar MA, Krishnan A, Kazmierczak C. Juvenile intervertebral disk calcification: a cause of painful torticollis. Emerg Radiol 2001;8:338–340.
4. Swischuk LE, Stansberry SD. Calcific diskitis: MRI changes in

disks without visible calcification. Pediatr Radiol 1991;21: 365–366.

Tall Neurogenic Vertebrae

In 1965, Gooding and Neuhauser (1) and then others (2) pointed out that, in the absence of normal vertical stresses, vertebral bodies tend to become taller than normal. This is seen most often in infants with neurologic or neuromuscular deficit (e.g., Down's syndrome, rubella syndrome) because they are unable to maintain the erect posture. Consequently, as time passes, the vertebral bodies assume a tall configuration (Fig. 8.59). However, tall vertebrae also have been seen at birth in flaccid infants (1).

REFERENCES

1. Gooding CA, Neuhauser EBD. Growth and development of the vertebral bodies in the presence and absence of normal stress. AJR 1965;93:388–393.
2. Donaldson JS, Gilsanz V, Gonzalez G, et al. Tall vertebrae at birth:

a radiographic finding in flaccid infants. AJR 1985;145: 1293–1296.

Beaked, Notched, or Hooked Vertebra

The beaked, notched, or hooked vertebra occurs most frequently in the thoracolumbar region involving T11 through L3. I believe it to represent deformity secondary to hyperflexion of the spine, with or without anterior herniation of the nucleus pulposus (1), most times probably without such herniation. Its most frequent occurrence at the thoracolumbar junction is likely related to exaggeration of normal "physiologic" kyphosis commonly seen in this area. It is uncommon to find a hooked vertebra in other than this location. Exaggeration of the curvature can result from acute, overt hyperflexion trauma or subclinical chronic hyperflexion secondary to any cause of generalized muscular hypotonia (1). As a consequence, it is frequently seen in conditions such as mucopolysaccharidosis (1), gangliosidosis (3), mucolipidosis, hypothyroidism, Morquio's disease, and in any hypotonic neuromuscularly handicapped child. In those conditions in which bony dysplasia also is present, it is likely that it further predisposes to anterior notching or compression, but the basic problem is most likely mechanical.

Similar notching can also be seen in infants who are presumably normal (1). In such patients, the notched vertebra is noted as an incidental finding on lateral chest roentgenograms, and in these infants, it is presumed that notching is secondary to subclinical hyperflexion with exaggerated thoracolumbar kyphosis. Such kyphosis is seen in all normal young infants who, because of normal muscular immaturity, are believed unable to remain erect in the sitting position (1).

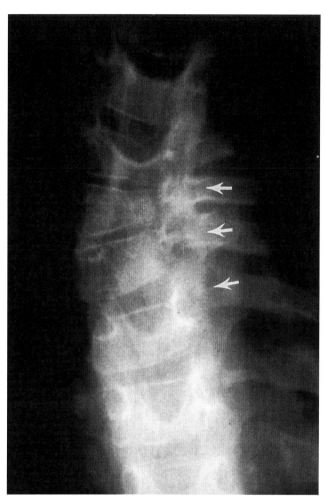

FIGURE 8.55. Scoliosis: unilateral bar. Note the scoliosis with fusion of the bone along the inner aspect (arrows). This constitutes the unilateral bar.

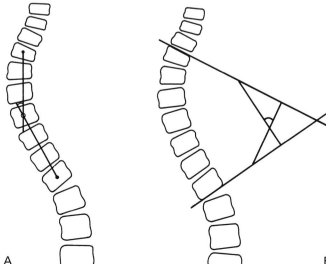

A　　　　　　　　　　　　　　　　　　　B

FIGURE 8.56. Scoliosis: methods of measurement. A. Ferguson method. **B.** Lippman-Cobb method. (Adapted from McAlister WH, Schackleford GD. Measurement of spinal curvatures. Radiol Clin North Am 1975;13:113–121.)

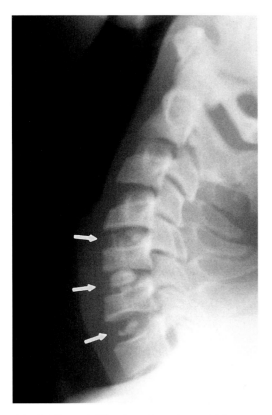

FIGURE 8.57. Disc calcification. Note the variable appearance of disc calcification at three levels (arrows).

Roentgenographically, the findings consist of anterior superior notching or compression of one or more vertebral bodies (Fig. 8.60). Associated intervertebral disc space narrowing may or may not be seen, but there is usually some degree of kyphosis in the region. In some cases, especially those with bony dysplasias, the intervertebral discs are abnormally bulky (e.g., achondroplasia, Hurler's disease), and posterior herniation of the discs can eventually occur. Such herniation is commonly symptomatic in middle-aged achondroplasts.

REFERENCES

1. Swischuk LE. The beaked, notched, or hooked vertebra: its significance in infants and young children. Radiology 1970;95: 661–664.

Platyspondyly

When one or two vertebral bodies are flattened (platyspondyly), one should consider eosinophilia granuloma, histiocytosis X, or metastatic disease. If they are flattened and the intervening disc spaces are destroyed, one should think of infection. Universal platyspondyly or platyspondyly involving more than one vertebra can be seen with conditions in which the bones are softer than normal: osteogenesis imperfecta, rickets, hypophosphatasia, hyperparathyroidism, and Cushing's syndrome. Universal platyspondyly also is a feature of many bone dysplasias, including spondyloepiphyseal dysplasia, Morquio's disease, achondrogenesis, thanatophoric dwarfism, metatropic dwarfism, and Kniest syndrome.

Atlanto-axial and Atlanto-occipital Instability

Atlanto-axial instability can occur after frank trauma to the upper cervical spine but is more commonly seen with hypoplasia of the dens and ligament laxity. This occurs in many chondrodystrophies and storage diseases but it most commonly is seen with trisomy 21 (1–4). In these cases, the problem usually is asymptomatic (Fig. 8.61), but potential injury is always a possibility; therefore, these patients are generally discouraged from participating in active sports. Most often, the entire problem usually is relatively benign, but cerebral and cerebellar infarcts secondary to atlanto-occipital instability has been documented (5). These patients are prone to upper cervical spine anomalies, including hypoplasia of the dens. Hypoplasia of the dens is associated with the formation of the os odontoideum, underdevelopment and laxity of the ligaments, and hypermobility of C1 on C2. The specific anomalous configurations are endless (6), but when the posterior arch of C1 is absent, the problem is compounded (7). In these patients, there is no structural posterior neural arch stability and therefore, severe anterior subluxation of C1 on C2 can occur. Atlanto-axial subluxation also occurs with rheumatoid arthritis and has been documented with systemic lupus erythematosus (8). In these patients, the problem is inflammation-induced ligament laxity.

Cervical-occipital instability or frank dislocation can occur after frank trauma. However, it most commonly occurs with trisomy 21 (4, 9, 10). The degree of instability can be pronounced (Fig. 8.62), but the abnormality usually is detected in asymptomatic individuals. The same precautions applying to patients with atlanto-axial instability applies to these patients.

REFERENCES

1. Committee on Sports Medicine, Fitness. Atlantoaxial instability in Down syndrome. Pediatrics 1995;96:151–154.
2. Tredwell SJ, Newman DE, Lockitch G. Instability of the upper cervical spine in Down syndrome. J Pediatr Orthop 1990;10: 602–606.
3. Uno K, Kataoka O, Shiba R. Occipitoatlantal and occipitoaxial hypermobility in Down syndrome. Spine 1996;21:1430–1434.
4. Stein SM, Kirchner SG, Horev G, et al. Atlanto-occipital subluxation in Down syndrome. Pediatr Radiol 1991;21:121–124.

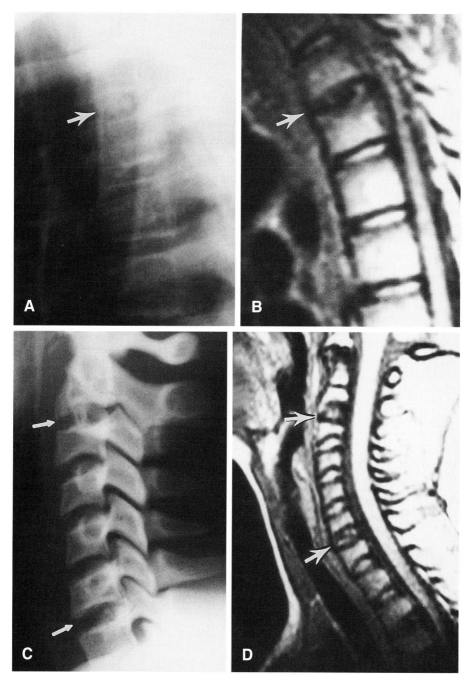

FIGURE 8.58. Disc calcification: MR appearance. A. Note the calcification in the upper thoracic region (arrow). **B.** T1-weighted MR image shows absence of signal in the involved disc space (arrow). **C.** Same patient, who also had neck pain. Note the slight suggestion of calcification at the C6-7 disc level (lower arrow). The disc space between C2 and C3 is bulging (upper arrow), but no calcifications are seen. **D.** MR study demonstrates loss of signal and bulging of the discs at both levels (arrows). (From Swischuk LE, Stansberry SD. Calcific discitis: MRI changes in discs without visible calcification. Pediatr Radiol 1991;21:365–366, with permission.)

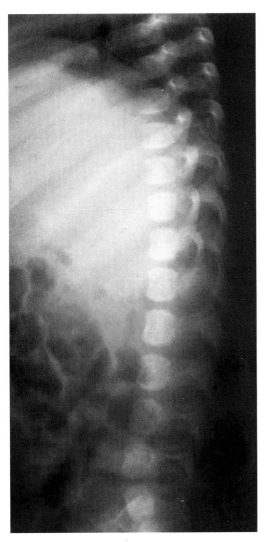

FIGURE 8.59. Tall vertebral bodies. Note how tall the vertebral bodies are, especially those in the lumbar region. These are characteristically seen in hypotonic, neuromuscularly impaired infants who have difficulty maintaining an erect posture.

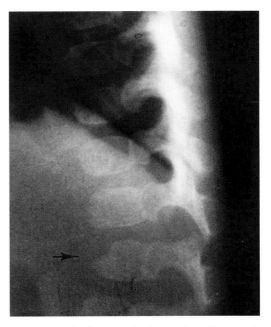

FIGURE 8.60. Hooked or notched vertebra. Note the hooked vertebra (arrow) at the thoracolumbar junction. This was an incidental finding in this infant examined because of an upper respiratory tract infection. Such notching is probably mechanical in origin and secondary to exaggerated local kyphosis and compression. Anterior herniation of the nucleus pulposus may also be present. Such notching can be seen in normal infants and in infants with underlying hypotonia and bone dysplasias.

5. Bhatnagar M, Sponseller PD, Carroll C IV, et al. Pediatric atlantoaxial instability presenting as cerebral and cerebellar infarcts. J Pediatr Orthop 1991;11:103–107.
6. Pueschel SM, Scola FH, Tupper TB, et al. Skeletal anomalies of the upper cervical spine in children with Down syndrome. J Pediatr Orthop 1990;10:607–611.
7. Martich V, Ben-Ami T, Yousefzadeh DK, et al. Hypoplastic posterior arch of C1 in children with Down syndrome: a double jeopardy. Radiology 1992;183:125–128.
8. Babini SM, Maldonado Cocco JA, Babini JC, et al. Atlantoaxial subluxation in systemic lupus erythematosus: further evidence of tendinous alterations. J Rheumatol 1990;17:173–177.
9. Parfenchuck TA, Bertrand SL, Powers MJ, et al. Posterior occipitoatlantal hypermobility in Down syndrome: an analysis of 199 patients. J Pediatr Orthop 1994;14:304–308.
10. Pueschel SM, Scola FH, Pezzullo JC. A longitudinal study of

atlanto-dens relationships in asymptomatic individuals with Down syndrome. Pediatrics 1992;89:1194–1198.

Basilar Impression

Basilar impression most often is associated with congenital occipitalization of C1 onto the base of the skull. In these cases, C1 is underdeveloped and fused with occiput and the dens protrudes into the foramen magnum (Fig. 8.63). These patients may or may not demonstrate brainstem symptoms. Basilar invagination also occurs in patients who have softening of the base of the skull or ligamentous instability in this region. These patients include those with osteogenesis imperfecta, hyperparathyroidism, and rheumatoid arthritis.

Iliac Spur–Sacral Anomaly Syndrome

Iliac spur–sacral anomaly syndrome is characterized by a peculiar iliac bony spur arising from the iliac bone and adjacent to the greater sciatic notch. For this reason, the condition can be associated with sciatic nerve compression; in addition, the sacrum may be malformed, a sacral lipoma may be present, and tethered cord may be seen. The findings on plain films are highly suggestive (Fig. 8.64).

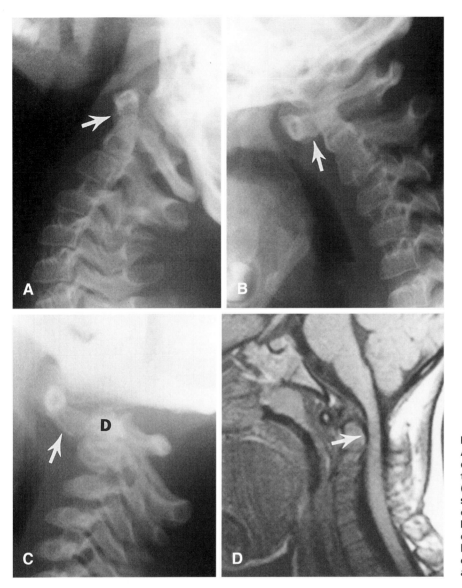

FIGURE 8.61. Atlanto-axial instability. A. Trisomy 21. On extension, note the C1-dens distance (arrow). **B.** With flexion, there is moderate widening of the space (arrow). **C. Spondyloepiphyseal dysplasia.** There is marked anterior displacement of C1 and a wide C1-dens distance (arrow). **D.** MR study demonstrates impingement on the cord by the dens (arrow). Dens hypoplasia also is present. For other cases of atlanto-axial instability, see Figures 8.23 and 8.24.

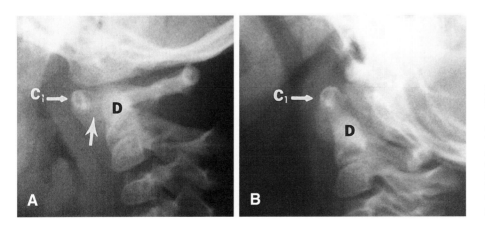

FIGURE 8.62. Atlanto-occipital instability. A. Trisomy 21. With flexion, there is slight widening of the C1-dens distance (arrow). Note the position of the anterior arch of C1 (C1) and the dens (D) and the relationship of both of these structures to the base of the skull. **B.** With extension, there is marked posterior displacement of the skull and C1. Specifically note the new positions of C1 and the dens.

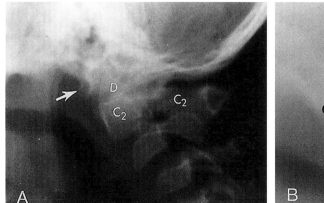
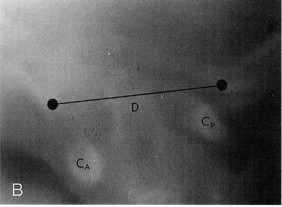

FIGURE 8.63. Basilar invagination and occipitalization. A. In this patient with a short neck, note that the anterior arch of C1 (arrow) is fused with the base of the skull (occipitalization). The posterior arch is underdeveloped and fused to the skull base. The dens (D) is hypoplastic but protrudes slightly into the foramen magnum. Note the body and arch of C2 (C2). **B.** Another patient whose midline tomogram demonstrates that the dens protrudes into the foramen magnum (dots). Also note the anterior arch of C1 (Ca) and the posterior arch of C1 (Cp). The posterior arch is high in position and probably attached to the skull by non–bony union.

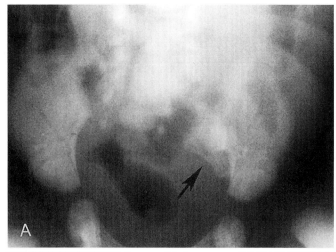

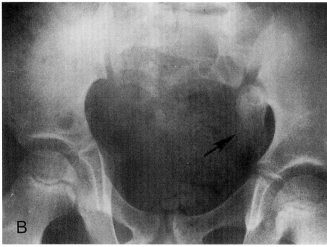

FIGURE 8.64. Iliac spur—sacral anomaly syndrome. A. Infant with bony iliac spur (arrow) and minimally deformed sacrum. **B.** An older child with similar spur (arrow) and more marked deformity of the sacrum.

APPENDIX

These tables are designed to assist one in analyzing certain imaging findings, which require a differential diagnosis that may not be at one's fingertips at any given time. The tables have been designed to reflect possible diagnoses as being most common, moderately common, less common, rare, etc. At times one may have to obtain information from more than one of these tables but it is hoped that these tables will provide an initial starting place for the evaluation of problems which might go beyond the common day-to-day data base that we all have.

CHAPTER 1

TABLE A1.1. LARGE OPAQUE HEMITHORAX

Pus (empyema)	}	Most common
Effusion with lymphoma, neuroblastoma Hemothorax	}	Common
Effusion with tuberculosis Fungal disease Chest tumor Pancreatitis Abdominal tumors and infections Chylothorax	}	Uncommon
Large mass or cyst (fluid filled) Diaphragmatic hernia (airless) Fluid-filled lung (bronchial atresia, congenital lobar enphysema)	}	Rare

TABLE A1.2. SMALL OR NORMAL SIZE OPAQUE HEMITHORAX

Small opaque or hazy hemithorax		
Atelectasis	}	Common
Pulmonary agenesis	}	Rare
Normal size opaque or hazy hemithorax		
Pleural fluid on supine film	}	Common
Developing empyema	}	Moderately common
Total lung consolidation (all lobes on one side)	}	Rare

TABLE A1.3. LARGE HYPERLUCENT (RADIOLUCENT) HEMITHORAX

Obstructive emphysema Compensatory emphysema[a]	}	Common
Pneumothorax	}	Moderately common
Cystic disease of the lung Large pneumatocele Diaphragmatic hernia (stomach)	}	Relatively rare

[a]Changes size on inspiration-expiration.

TABLE A1.4. SMALL HYPERLUCENT HEMITHORAX

Pumonary artery and lung hypoplasia[a] Swyer-James lung[b]	}	Moderately common
Postradiation[b] Pulmonary vein atresia or stenosis[b] Pulmonary embolus[a]	}	Rare

[a]Changes size on inspiration-expiration.
[b]May show scarring or reticulation.

TABLE A1.5. CALCIFICATIONS IN THE CHEST

Flocculent or irregular

Granulomas (nodules) Old inflamed lymph nodes	Common
Old thrombi in IVC or SVC	Moderately common
Necrotic or treated tumor Calcific pericarditis Pleural calcifications Teratoma Old pulmonary hematoma Hamartoma Cardiac valve Myocardial infarction	Rare

Linear and curvilinear

Pleura Pericardium Vascular	Uncommon
Calcification of cyst wall	Rare

Punctate calcifications

Old healed granulomatous disease	Common
Calcification of ligamentum arteriosum Osteogenic sarcoma metastases	Uncommon
Chickenpox pneumonia Pulmonary microlithiasis Hypercalcemia states Sarcoidosis	Rare

IVC, inferior vena cava; SVC, superior vena cava.

TABLE A1.6. PULMONARY CAVITIES

Pneumatocele-inflammatory[a] Pulmonary abscess[a]	Common
Pneumatocele-traumatic[a] Pneumatocele-hydrocarbon pneumonia[b] Echinococcal cyst[c]	Uncommon
Solitary cyst (congenital) Adenomatoid malformation[a] Cavitary tuberculosis Cavitating pneumonia Cavitating hematoma Cavitating infarct Lymphangioma of the lung	Rare

[a]Frequently multiple.
[b]May be multiple.
[c]Common in endemic areas.

TABLE A1.7. LARGE OR PROMINENT HILAR REGIONS

Bilateral
Adenopathy

Viral infection *Mycoplasma pneumoniae* infection	Common
Cystic fibrosis Fungal infection Chronic aspiration Tuberculosis	Moderately common
Sarcoidosis Wegener's granulomatosis Reticuloendothelioses Metastases Leukemia-lymphoma	Rare

Pulmonary artery enlargement

Pulmonary hypertension	Moderately common
Absent pulmonary valve	Rare

Unilateral
Adenopathy

Tuberculosis *Mycoplasma pneumoniae* infection Bacterial pneumonia Superior segment, lower lobe pneumonia artifact	Common
Fungal infections Metastases	Uncommon

Pulmonary artery enlargement

Pulmonary stenosis with left pulmonary artery enlarged	Uncommon
Absent pulmonary valve with unilateral absent pulmonary artery	Rare

TABLE A1.8. PULMONARY NODULES

Solitary Nodule

Granuloma-tuberculosis[a]	}	Common

Granuloma-fungal[a]		
Consolidating pneumonia	}	Moderately common
Metastases[d]		

Small abscess[d]		
Small cyst		
Hamartoma[a]		
Nipple shadow		
Other primary neoplasia		
Sarcoidosis[b,d]		
Pulmonary varix or arteriovenous malformation		
Cutaneous nodules		
Mucous plugs (asthma)	}	Rare
Mucocele (bronchial atresia)		
Healed (posttraumatic) hematoma[b,d]		
Postinfarct		
Collagen vascular disease[d]		
Atypical measles[b]		
Old pneumonia[b]		
Primary tumor		
Multiple nodules		

Multiple Nodules

Granulomas[a] (TB, fungus)	}	Common

Metastases[d]	}	Moderately common

Laryngeal papillomatosis[d]		
Multiple abscesses[c]	}	Uncommon
Multiple emboli[d]		

Wegener's granulomatosis[c]		
Sarcoidosis[b,d]		
Mucous plugs		
Cutaneous lesions (artifact)	}	Rare
Collagen vascular disease[d]		
Lymphoma		
Multiple hamartomas[b]		
Other primary tumors		

[a]Commonly calcify.
[b]May calcify.
[c]Commonly cavitate.
[d]May cavitate.

TABLE A1.9. PULMONARY EDEMA

Cardiac Causes
Left-side cardiac failure

Myocardial disease	}	Common

Valvular disease (obstruction, insufficiency)	}	Uncommon
Vascular obstructive disease (e.g., coarctation)		

Hyperkinetic cardiac failure Left-to-right shunt, admixture lesions	}	Common

Anemia		
Arteriovenous fistula	}	Rare
Thyrotoxicosis		

Noncardiac Causes
Kidney disease

Acute glomerulonephritis	}	Common
Chronic renal failure		

Iatrogenic fluid overload		
Near-drowning	}	Moderately common
Neurogenic (increased intracranial pressure)		

Lung toxicity		
Rheumatic pneumonitis		
Allergic lung		
Toxic inhalants	}	Uncommon
Vasculitis		
Collagen vascular diseases		
Idiopathic hemosiderosis		

Pulmonary vein obstruction (acquired or congenital)	}	Rare
Drug abuse		

TABLE A1.10. PULMONARY INFILTRATE PATTERNS—INFECTIONS

Pattern	Pneumococcus	Staphylococcus	Haemophilus	Streptococcus	Pertussis (Early)	Mycoplasma	Virus	Tuberculosis	Fungus	Pneumocystis carinii
Consolidation	+++	++	+++	+	+/−	+++	−	+	+[a]	+/−
Atelectasis (lobar)	−	−	−	−	+	+++	+++	+++	+	−
Patchy, fluffy										
Bilateral, diffuse	−	+++	+	+	+[b]	+[b]	+[b]	−	+++	++
Lobar	+/−	+++	+	++	−	++	−	−	+	+
Basal, bilateral	−	−	−	−	−	−	+/−[b]	−	−	−
Parahilar-peribronchial	−	−	−	−	+++	+++	+++	−	−	−
Reticulonodular	−	−	−	−	+	+++[c]	+++	+[d]	++	++
Honeycombed	−	−	−	−	−	−	−	−	−	−
Hazy to opaque	−	−	−	−	−	+/−	+	−	−	+++
Hazy (basal)	−	−	−	−	−	+	++	−	−	+
Miliary	−	−	−	−	−	+/−	+	+++	+	−
Diffuse streaks and wedges[b]	−	−	−	−	+	+++	+++	−	−	−

+++, commonly seen in the condition; ++, moderately common in the condition; +, occasionally seen in the condition; +/−, rarely seen in the condition; −, never, or nearly never, seen in the condition.
[a]Especially actinomycosis.
[b]Atelectasis usually.
[c]Often one lobe only.
[d]Usually nodular.

TABLE A1.11. PULMONARY INFILTRATE PATTERNS—NONINFECTIONS

Pattern	Pulmonary Edema	Pulmonary Hemosiderosis	Allergic Lung	Sarcoidosis	Aspiration Pneumonia	Pulmonary Fibrosis	Pulmonary Contusion	Pulmonary Hemorrhage	Reticuloendotheliosis	Leukemia-Lymphoma	Asthma	Cystic Fibrosis	Lymphangiectasia Hemangiomatosis
Consolidate	+	−	−	−	++	−	+++	+	−	−	+[a]	+[a]	−
Atelectasis (lobar)	−	−	−	−	+++	−	−	−	−	−	+++	+++	−
Patchy													
Bilateral	+	+++	+++	+	+++	−	−	+++	+++	−	+/−[b,c]	++	−
Lobar	−	−	+/−	−	+++	−	−	+++	−	−	+++[c]	++[c]	−
Basal	−	−	−	−	+++	−	−	−	−	−	−	−	−
Parahilar-peribronchial	++	−	−	+	+++	−	−	−	+	−	+++	+++	−
Reticulonodular	++	+++	+	++	+	+++	−	−	++	++	+/−[b]	++	+++
Honeycombed	−	+	−	+	−	+++	−	−	+++	−	−	+++[d]	+
Hazy to opaque	+++	++	−	+/−	+	+/−	−	++[e]	−	−	−	−	−
Hazy (basal)	++	+	−	−	−	+++	−	−	−	−	−	−	−
Miliary	−	++	−	−	−	−	−	−	−	+	−	−	−
Diffuse streaks and wedges[c]	−	−	−	−	++	−	−	−	−	−	+++[c]	+++[c]	−

+++, commonly seen in the condition; ++, moderately common in the condition; +, occasionally seen in the condition; +/−, rarely seen in the condition; −, never, or nearly never, seen in the condition.
[a]With superimposed bacterial infection only.
[b]With superimposed virus infection.
[c]Atelectasis usually.
[d]Large honeycomb due to cystic change.
[e]Usually opaque.

TABLE A1.12. SUPERIOR MEDIASTINAL WIDENING

Bilateral and Relatively Symmetric

Normal thymus gland	}	Common
Adenopathy (inflammatory, tumoral) Mediastinal tumor Dilated aorta	}	Moderately common
Persistent LSVC Vein of Galen aneurysm TAPVR-type I ("snowman" or "figure 8") Mediastinitis Thyroiditis Mediastinal hematoma Goiter Mediastinal fat Dilated esophagus	}	Uncommon
Bilateral upper lobe agenesis Aneurysm of great veins	}	Rare

Unilateral

Thymus, normal (R or L)	}	Common
Superior vena cava (R) Dilated ascending aorta (R) Upper lobe atelectasis (R) Adenopathy (R or L) Mediastinal tumor, cyst (R or L) Right-side aorta (R) Dilated esophagus (R or L)	}	Moderately common
Persistent LSVC[a] Mediastinal hematoma (R or L) Goiter (R or L) Mediastinal fat (R or L)	}	Rare

LSVC, left superior vena cava; TAPVR, total anomalous pulmonary venous return.
[a]Usually causes bilateral widening because of normal inferior vena cava on right.

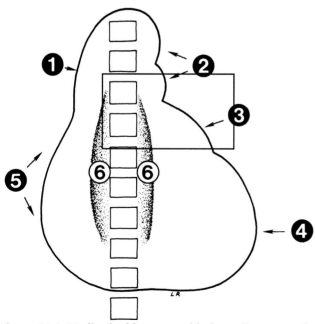

Figure A1.1. Mediastinal bumps and bulges: diagrammatic representation. Lumps, bumps and bulges along the mediastinum can be considered according to location: *location 1*—right paratracheal; *location 2*—left paratracheal; *location 3*—high left upper cardiac border; *location 4*—lower left cardiac border; *location 5*—entire cardiac border; and *location 6*—paraspinal areas.

TABLE A1.13. DISCRETE MEDIASTINAL BUMPS

Location 1

Normal azygous vein Lymph node	}	Common
Right-side aorta Tumor, cyst Compressed thymus with anterior pneumothorax	}	Moderately common
Dilated azygous vein	}	Uncommon

Location 2

Large aorta Ductus bump in neonate	}	Common
Tumor, cyst Compressed thymus with anterior pneumothorax	}	Moderately common
Postcoarctation patch Hemiazygous vein enlarged Aorta, pulmonary artery, ductus aneurysm	}	Rare

Location 3

Thymus Left atrial appendage	}	Common
Congenital corrected transposition Ebstein's anomaly	}	Uncommon
Partial absence of pericardium Single ventricle with transposition Coronary artery aneurysm Juxtaposition of right atrial appendage Postoperative conduits Dilated patch of repaired tetralogy of Fallot	}	Rare

Location 4

Left ventricular hypertrophy Right ventricular hypertrophy	}	Common
Tumor (cardiac, pericardial) Congenital aneurysm of heart	}	Rare

Location 5

Enlarged right atrium Displacement of right atrium by large heart	}	Common
Mesoversion Large thymus	}	Uncommon
Tumor (cardiac or pericardial) Congenital aneurysm of the heart Coronary artery aneurysm (upper border) Pericardial defect (upper border)	}	Rare

Location 6

Long stripes Normal aorta	}	Common
Pleural fluid Dilated aorta	}	Moderately common
Localized bulge Paraspinal abscess Compression fracture with hematoma	}	Common
Spinal or paraspinal tumor Adenopathy; inflammation, tumor	}	Uncommon
Extramedullary hematopoiesis Neuroenteric cyst	}	Rare

TABLE A1.14. MEDIASTINAL MASSES

Anterior

Normal thymus (infants)	}	Common
Lymphoma	}	Relatively
Teratoma		common
Cystic hygroma	}	
Hemangioma		
Germ cell tumor		Uncommon
Enlarged thyroid (goiter, tumor)		
Vascular anomaly, aneurysm		
Morgagni hernia		
Thymoma	}	
Thymic cyst		Rare
Histiocytosis-X		

Middle

Lymphoma, leukemia	}	Common
Lymphadenopathy (inflammatory)		
Lymphadenopathy (metastatic)	}	
Enlarged vessels		Uncommon
Duplication cyst		
Hiatus hernia		
Pericardial cyst or tumor	}	Rare
Cardiac tumor or aneurysm		

Posterior

Neuroblastoma/ganglioneuroma	}	Common
Pulmonary sequestration	}	Moderately
Bochdalek hernia		common
Neurofibroma	}	
Neuroenteric cyst		
Anterior/lateral meningocele		Rare
Teratoma, sarcoma		
Extramedullary hematopoesis		
Spinal tumor, infection, fracture		

CHAPTER 2

TABLE A2.1. CAUSES OF NASOPHARYNGEAL SOFT TISSUES

Increased Thickness

Normal or hypertrophied adenoids	}	Common
Infection		
Nasal polyp	}	
Nasopharyngeal tumors		Uncommon
Nasolacrimal duct mucocele		
Basal encephalocele	}	Rare
Base of skull tumors		

Decreased Thickness

Small, normal (<3 months)	}	Common
Surgical removal	}	Moderately common
Hypo- or agammaglobulinemia	}	Uncommon
Ataxia telangiectasia syndrome		

TABLE A2.2. CAUSES OF RETROPHARYNGEAL SOFT TISSUE THICKENING

Buckling of airway (pseudothickening)	}	
Inflammation (adenopathy)		Common
Retropharyngeal abscess		
Edema with cervical spine injury	}	Moderately
Retropharyngeal tumor		common
Noninflammatory adenopathy	}	
Osteomyelitis of cervical spine		Uncommon
Tumors of cervical spine		
Myxedematous thickening	}	
Edema with obstructed superior vena cava		
Vein of Galen aneurysms		Rare
Enteric cyst		
Goiter		

TABLE A2.3. CAUSES OF EPIGLOTTIC AND ARYEPIGLOTTIC FOLD ENLARGEMENT

Epiglottitis	}	Common
Angioneurotic edema	}	Uncommon
Corrosive burns		
Face and neck edema	}	
Tumor		
Aryepiglottic fold cyst		Rare
Sarcoidosis		
Hemorrhage (hemophilia)		
Radiation		

TABLE A2.4. VOCAL CORD ABNORMALITIES

Indistinct, Fuzzy on Lateral View

Croup	}	Common
Paralysis	}	Moderately common
Trauma	}	
Storage diseases		Rare
Lipoid proteinosis		

Bilateral Cord Thickening and/or Fixation

Croup	}	Common
Trauma (iatrogenic)	}	Moderately
Paralysis		common
Epiglottitis		
Trauma (noniatrogenic)	}	Uncommon
Laryngeal web		
Storage diseases	}	Rare
Lipoid proteinosis		

Unilateral Thickening and/or Fixation

Paralysis	}	Common
Iatrogenic trauma	}	Moderately
Subglottic hemangioma		common
Laryngeal web (unilateral)	}	Rare

Nodules

Papillomatosis	}	Common
Postintubation granuloma	}	Uncommon
Benign and malignant tumors	}	Rare

TABLE A2.5. CAUSES OF SUBGLOTTIC TRACHEAL NARROWING

Circumferential Narrowing		
Croup	}	Common
Subglottic stenosis	}	Moderately
Paradoxic collapse with other glottic obstruction		common
Eccentric Narrowing		
Subglottic hemangioma	}	Moderately
Posttracheostomy fibrosis		common
Intratracheal thyroid	}	
Subglottic mucocele		
Histiocytoma		Rare
Papilloma		
Intratracheal thymus		

CHAPTER 3

TABLE A3.1. BLOCK VERTEBRAE

Congenital—with spinal dysraphism	}	Common
Congenital	}	
Isolated		Moderately
Klippel-Feil syndrome		common
Acquired, after infection		
Acquired—after trauma	}	Relatively
Scheuermann disease		rare

TABLE A3.2. SPINAL CANAL DIAMETER ABNORMALITIES

Enlarged		
Normal, cervical and lumbosacral	}	Common
Meningocele-meningomyelocele		
Diastematomyelia	}	
Intraspinal tumor, cyst		Relatively rare
Syringomyelia, hydromyelia		
Narrowed		
Chondrodystrophies[a]	}	Commonest
Congenital narrowing	}	Rare

[a]For example, achondroplasia.

TABLE A3.3. INTERVERTEBRAL FORAMEN SIZE ABNORMALITIES

Small		
Congenital with other anomalies	}	Common
Posttraumatic	}	Relatively rare
Enlarged		
Congenital with dysraphism anomalies	}	Commonest
Dumbbell tumor	}	Moderately
Neurofibromatosis[b]		common
Intraspinal tumor	}	
Posttraumatic nerve root diverticulum		
Congenital absence or hypoplastic pedicle		
Lateral meningocele		Rare
Interstitial polyneuritis		
Dural ectasia, idiopathic		

[a]Usually neuroblastoma-ganglioneuroma.
[b]Bony dysplasia-dural ectasia.

CHAPTER 4

TABLE A4.1. PRESACRAL MASSES

Sacrococcygeal teratoma	}	Common
Obstructed rectum with fecal material		
Abscess (ruptured appendix, regional enteritis)	}	
Neurogenic tumors		Uncommon
Hematoma with trauma		
Rhabdomyosarcoma	}	
Chordoma of sacrum		Rare
Anterior meningocele		
Duplication cyst		

TABLE A4.2. CYSTIC ABDOMINAL OR PELVIC MASS

Hydronephrosis (severe)	}	
Multicystic dysplastic kidney		Common
Ovarian cyst		
Abscess		
Parasitic cyst	}	
Enteric duplication cyst		
Mesenteric cyst		
Hydrops of gallbladder		
Choledochal cyst		
Urachal cyst		
Pancreatic pseudocyst		
Cerebrospinal fluid pseudocyst		Uncommon
Teratoma or dermoid		
Lymphangioma		
Necrotic tumor		
Adrenal hemorrhage (resolving)		
Biloma		
Renal multilocular cyst		
Mesenchymal hamartoma (liver)	}	
Cystic hepatoblastoma		Rare
Cystadenoma (ovary, biliary)		
Papillary cystic and solid tumor (pancreas)		

TABLE A4.3. LIVER MASSES AND LESIONS

Hemangioma or hemangioendothelioma Hepatoblastoma Infection or abscess Hematoma Metastases	Relatively common
Mesenchymal hamartoma Embryonal sarcoma Hepatocellular carcinoma Lymphoma or leukemia Biliary tract neoplasms	Uncommon
Adenoma Focal nodular hyperplasia Lipoma or angiomyolipoma Peliosis hepatis Rhabdomyosarcoma Mesenchymoma	Rare

TABLE A4.4. INTRAABDOMINAL CALCIFICATIONS AND OPACITIES

Irregular-Flocculent

Tumors (esp. neuroblastoma)[a]	Common
Idiopathic adrenal[b] Foreign material (pica)[a] Meconium peritonitis[a]	Moderately common
Liver, postabscess, after thrombus[b] Papillary necrosis (kidney)[b] Lymph nodes[b] Infarct (spleen, liver, kidney, intestine)	Uncommon
Bladder (schistosomiasis, cytoxan) Oxalosis (kidney) Hamartoma[b] Prostate Necrotic bowel-old[b] Infarcted ovary[b] Infarcted abdominal testes[b] Pancreatitis[a]	Rare

Curvilinear

Cystic tumors Posthemorrhagic outline of adrenal gland	Moderately common
Residual meconium peritonitis from neonate Hydronephrosis Cystic kidney or other cyst Renal cortical necrosis	Relatively rare

Stones or Stone-Like Densities

Fecalith in appendix	Common
Urinary tract stones Gallstones Ingested pebbles Granulomas in spleen, liver	Moderately common
Phleboliths Medullary sponge kidney Ingested mercury, chromium salts	Rare

Formed Calcification

Teratoma, dermoid	Common
Staghorn calculi	Rare
Fetus-in-fetu	Very rare

Miscellaneous—Diffuse of Organ

Milk of calcium gallbladder or hydronephrotic kidney Diffuse kidney (oxalosis, renal tubular acidosis, chronic glomerulonephritis) Wolman disease (adrenal gland) Hemochromatosis (liver)	Rare

[a]Generalized or focal.
[b]Focal.

TABLE A4.5. ASCITES

Hydrops fetalis Liver disease Nephrotic syndrome Portal vein obstruction Hemorrhage	Common
Urinary tract obstruction Neonatal chylous ascites Hypoproteinemia Cardiac disease Peritonitis Ruptured cysts	Uncommon
Intestinal lymphangiectasia Pancreatitis Peritoneal metastasis Vascular emergencies Bile duct perforation Lysomal storage disease	Rare

TABLE A4.6. ABDOMINAL GAS PATTERNS

Distended Stomach

Normal (infants) Hypertrophic pyloric stenosis Pylorospasm	Common
Antropyloric membrane Gastric ulcer disease Gastroenteritis Duodenal obstruction	Uncommon
Antral foveolar hyperplasia (prostaglandin therapy) Duplication cysts (antrum) Ectopic pancreas (antrum) Polyps, tumors (antrum)	Rare

Small Bowel Obstruction (Beyond Neonatal Period)

Perforated appendicitis Intussusception Incarcerated hernia	Common
Postoperative adhesions Regional enteritis Pseudo-obstruction in gastroenteritis	Moderately common
Peritoneal bands Duplication cysts Midgut volvulus Small bowel tumors Chronic pseudo-obstruction syndrome	Rare

Dilated Colon (Beyond Neonatal Period)

Functional (psychogenic) megacolon Hirschsprung's disease	Common
Colonic stenosis Hypothyroidism Chagas' disease Chronic immobilization Medication producing hypotonia Neuronal intestinal dysplasia Plexiform neurofibromatosis of colon Segmental dilation of colon	Rare

TABLE A4.7. ABDOMINAL GAS PATTERNS

Paralytic Ileus

Gastroenteritis	Common
Peritonitis Sepsis Moribund patient	Moderately common
Vascular insult Drug depression Hypokalemia	Rare

Dilated Transverse Colon (Colon Cutoff)

Normal Perforated appendicitis	Common
Pancreatitis	Uncommon
Ischemia, infarct Toxic megacolon	Rare

Sentinal Loop

Appendicitis	Common
Paralytic ileus Pancreatitis	Moderately common
Isolated loop in gastroenteritis Normal, fortuitous Closed-loop obstruction	Uncommon
Intestinal trauma Infarction	Rare

TABLE A4.8. ESOPHAGEAL STENOSIS

Corrosive esophagitis Peptic esophagitis	Common
Posttracheoesophageal fistula repair	Moderately common
Congenital, tracheobronchial remnants Trauma, chronic foreign body Infectious esophagitis Epidermolysis bullosa Barrett esophagus Neoplasm	Rare

TABLE A4.9. GASTRIC MASSES AND THICKENED MUCOSAL FOLDS

Gastritis[a] Polyps[b] Ectopic pancreatic tissue[b] Caustic ingestion[a]	Moderately common
Foreign body, bezoar[b] Gastric duplication[b] Menetrier's disease[a] Crohn's disease[a] Neoplasm[b] Inflammatory pseudotumor[b]	Rare

[a]Gastric masses.
[b]Thickened mucosal folds.

TABLE A4.10 THICKENED SMALL BOWEL MUCOSAL FOLDS

Edema[a]
  Nephrotic syndrome
  Hypoproteinemia
  Portal vein obstruction
  Portal hypertension
Gastroenteritis[a]
Giardiasis[b]
Celiac disease[a]
	Common

Cystic fibrosis[b] Protein losing enteropathy[a] Regional enteritis[a]	Moderately common
Eosinophilic gastroenteritis[a] Intestinal lymphangiectasia[b] Zollinger-Ellison syndrome[a] Cardiac disease[a]	Relatively rare
Behçet syndrome[b]	Very rare

[a]Thick and straight.
[b]Thick and tortuous.

TABLE A4.11. INTESTINAL MASSES AND NODULES

Normal fecal material Lymphoid hyperplasia (colon)	Common
Lymphoid hyperplasia (small bowel) Juvenile polyps: inflammatory, sporadic	Moderately common
Pseudopolyps-ulcerative colitis, regional enteritis Familial polyposis	Uncommon

Other polyposis syndromes
  Peutz-Jeghers syndrome (small bowel)
  Canada-Cronkhite syndrome (colon, stomach)
  Gardner syndrome
Juvenile polyps: inflammatory, familial
Neoplasm
	Rare

CHAPTER 5

TABLE A5.1. RENAL MASSES

Wilms' tumor[a] Mesoblastic nephroma[a]	Common
Lobar neohronia[a] abscess[b]	Moderately common
Simple cyst[b] Multilocular cyst[b] Epithelial nephroblastoma[b] Renal cell carcinoma[a] Lymphoma[a]	Uncommon
Rhabdoid tumor[a] Clear cell sarcoma[a] Angiomyolipoma[a] Juxtaglomerular cell tumor[a] Lymphangioma[b] Teratoma[a]	Rare

[a]Solid or complex.
[b]Cystic.

TABLE A5.2. ADRENAL ENLARGEMENT OR MASS

Adrenal hemorrhage Neuroblastoma or ganglioneuroma	Common
Adrenal cortical hyperplasia	Moderately common
Adrenocortical carcinoma Cortical adenoma Pheochromocytoma Congenital cyst Abscess Wolman disease	Rare

TABLE A5.3. LARGE KIDNEYS

Nephrotic syndrome[a] Acute glomerulonephritis[a] Hydronephrosis Duplication anomaly	Common
Compensatory hypertrophy[b] Fused ectopy[b] Infant of diabetic mother[a] Infantile polycystic kidney[a] Adult polycystic kidney[a] Multicystic dysplastic kidney[b] Leukemia-lymphoma[a] Hemolytic-uremic syndrome[a] Henoch-Schönlein purpura[a] Intrarenal abscess, hematoma[b]	Moderately common
Renal vein thrombosis (acute)[b] Glycogen storage disease[a] Tuberous sclerosis[a] Beckwith-Widermann syndrome[a] Sickle cell disease[a]	Uncommon
Nephroblastomatosis[a] Bile nephrosis[a]	Rare

[a]Usually bilateral.
[b]Usually unilateral.

TABLE A5.4. SMALL KIDNEYS

Chronic pyelonephritis[a] Chronic glomerulonephritis[a] Congenitally hypoplastic[b]	Common
Renal vein thrombosis (chronic with atrophy)[b] Atrophy after obstructive uropathy[a] Reflux nephropathy[a] Renal artery stenosis, occlusion[b]	Moderately common
Postirradiation[b] Papillary necrosis (late)[a] Ask-Upmark kidney[b] Juvenile nephronophthisis (medullary sponge)[a]	Rare

[a]Often or usually bilateral.
[b]Usually unilateral.

TABLE A5.5. ABNORMAL BLADDER SIZE

Small Bladder

Spastic neurogenic Chronic bladder outlet obstruction (hypertrophy)	Common
Severe cystitis (infection, drug-induced) Bladder diversion	Uncommon
Congenital small Surrounding tumor	Rare

Large Bladder

Neurogenic	Common
Prune-belly syndrome Chronic diuretic therapy	Moderately common
Diabetes insipidus Psychogenic water drinking Megacystis-microcolon syndrome Bartter syndrome	Rare

CHAPTER 6

TABLE A6.1. INCREASED BONE DENSITY (GENERALIZED)

Osteopetrosis Chronic renal disease[a]	Common
Idiopathic osteosclerosis of newborn Neonatal intrauterine infections Hypothyroidism Heavy metal intoxication Old periosteal bone deposition	Moderately common
Idiopathic hypercalcemia Storage diseases	Relatively rare
Pyknodysostosis Myelofibrosis Fluorosis Hypervitaminosis D Sclerosteosis and Van Buchem disease Kenny-Caffey syndrome Sarcoidosis Robinow-Silverman-Smith syndrome Pyle's disease	Rare

[a]Treated.

TABLE A6.2. DECREASED BONE DENSITY

Osteoporosis

Disuse[a] Nutritional	Common
Chronic anemia Osteogenesis imperfecta Steroid therapy Collagen vascular diseases Hyperemia with infection, inflammation, arteriovenous fistula[b] Storage diseases	Moderately common
Idiopathic hypocalcemia Cushing's syndrome Idiopathic juvenile osteoporosis Turner's syndrome Hyperthyroidism Sudeck atrophy[b]	Relatively rare
Scurvy Sarcoidosis Progeria Ehlers-Danlos syndrome Homocystinuria Phenylketonuria Fibrogenesis imperfecta	Rare

Osteomalacia

| Rickets[c]
Hyperparathyroidism
Renal osteodystrophy | Commonest |
| Hypophosphatasia, pseudohypophosphatasia
Fibrogenesis imperfecta
Gangliosidosis[d]
Jansen metaphyseal dysostosis[d]
Mucolipidosis II (I-cell disease)[d] | Relatively rare |

[a]Immobilization.
[b]Single bone.
[c]All types.
[d]In infancy, changes resemble hyperparathyroidism.

TABLE A6.3. UNDERTUBULATION: SHORT, SQUAT BONES

Achondroplasia[a] Storage diseases[b,c]	} Common
Metaphyseal dysostosis[a] Pseudoachondroplasia[a] Madelung's deformity[d] Hypochondroplasia[a] Vitamin D-resistant rickets, type B[c] Neonatal dwarfs[a] Chondrodystrophy with immune deficiency[a]	} Moderately common
Rhizomelic punctate epiphyseal dysplasia[a] Diastrophic dwarfism[a,d] Hypophosphatasia[a] Metatropic dwarfism[e] Kniest syndrome[e] Dyggve-Melchior-Clausen[e] Camptomelic dwarfism[b,d] Larsen's syndrome[b,d] Weissenbacher-Zweymuller syndrome[a]	} Rare

[a]Flared metaphyses.
[b]Hypoplastic ends.
[c]No metaphyseal flaring.
[d]Middle segment predominance.
[e]Dumbbell-shaped bones.

TABLE A6.4. OVERTUBULATION: THIN, GRACILE BONES

Neurologic-neuromuscular disease	} Commonest
Osteogenesis imperfecta Arthrogryposis syndromes	} Moderately common
Marfan's syndrome Homocystinuria	} Relatively rare
Cockayne's syndrome Winchester syndrome Progeria Kenny-Caffey[a] Marfan's contractural arachnodactyly Stickler syndrome Hallermann-Streiff syndrome Seckel bird-headed dwarf	} Rare

[a]Medullary stenosis syndrome. Thin bones but thick, sclerotic cortex.

TABLE A6.5. DIFFUSELY BALLOONED BONES (OSTEOECTASIA)

Generalized

Severe anemia	} Common
Familial hypophosphatemia Mastocytosis Craniodiaphyseal dysplasia	} Rare

Asymmetric or localized

Fracture with subperiosteal bleeding[a] Battered child syndrome[a] Hemophilia[a] Neurogenic fracture[a]	} Common
Fibrous dysplasia	} Moderately common
Scurvy[a] Neurofibromatosis[a]	} Rare

[a]Subperiosteal bleed.

TABLE A6.6. BOWED BONES

Generalized bowing

Rickets	} Common
Osteogenesis imperfecta[a] Madelung's deformity[b] Neonatal dwarfs Hyperparathyroidism	} Moderately common
Diastrophic dwarfism[c] Camptomelic dwarfism[c] Larsen's syndrome[c] Neonatal Ellis-van Creveld syndrome[c] Parastremmatic dwarfism Hypophosphatasia Hyperphosphatemia	} Rare

Localized bowing

Plastic bending fracture Normal Bowed legs[d]	} Common
Post trauma or osteomyelitis Neurofibromatosis (tibia, fibula) Fractures in softened bones	} Moderately common
Tibial kyphosis with or without absent fibula	} Relatively rare

[a]Especially congenita form with fracture.
[b]Dyschondrosteosis.
[c]Symmetric middle segment dwarfism predominates.
[d]See Table A6.7.

TABLE A6.7. BOWED LEGS AND KNOCK-KNEES

Bowed legs

Physiologic	
Rickets	
Femoral anteversion	Common
Blount's disease	
Bone dysplasias[a]	
Epiphyseal injuries	
Hypophosphatasia	
Hyperphosphatemia	Relatively rare
Hyperparathyroidism	
Metaphyseal dysostoses	

Knock-knees

Physiologic	Common
Muscular weakness	
Epiphyseal-metaphyseal injuries	Relatively rare
Trevor disease	

[a]See Table A6.6.

TABLE A6.8. COXA VARA AND COXA VALGA

Coxa vara

Idiopathic slipped epiphysis	
Legg-Perthes disease[a]	Common
Rickets	
Fracture or infection of femoral neck	Moderately
Sickle cell disease, steroid therapy (femoral head necrosis)	common
Slipped epiphysis (secondary)[b]	
Radiation therapy[c]	
Gaucher's disease[c]	
Osteogenesis imperfecta[d]	Rare
Metatropic dwarfism	
Storage diseases	
Congenital coxa vara	

Coxa valga

Neurologic disease	Common
Chronic muscle hypotonia	
Turner's syndrome	Moderately
Storage diseases	common
Needles-Melnick syndrome	
Prader-Willi syndrome	
Progeria	Rare
Pyle's metaphyseal dysplasia	
Stickler syndrome	

[a]Healing.
[b]Hyperparathyroidism, hypothyroidism, pseudo- or pseudopseudohypoparathyroidism.
[c]Femoral head necrosis.
[d]Congenita form.

TABLE A6.9. FOCAL BONY HYPOPLASIAS

Radial ray syndrome	
Holt-Oram syndrome	
Poland's syndrome	
Fanconi's anemia	Common
Thrombocytopenia- absent radius syndrome	
VATER syndrome	
Hypoplastic radial head with congenital dislocation	Moderately common
Nonspecific focal hypoplasias[a]	
Proximal focal femoral deficiency	Relatively
Absent fibula	rare
Absent tibia	
Mermaid deformity	Rare
Thalidomide embryonopathy[b]	

[a]Cause unknown.
[b]Currently not seen.

TABLE A6.10. PSEUDOARTHROSES

Postfracture long bones or clavicle	Common
Congenital: clavicle	
Neurofibromatosis: tibia, fibula	Moderately
Post infection, osteomyelitis[a]	common
Osteogenesis imperfecta, fracture[a]	
Congenital: radius, ulna, fibula	
Proximal focal femoral deficiency: upper femur	Rare
Post irradiation[a]	

[a]Pathologic fracture.

TABLE A6.11. SUBPERIOSTEAL BONE RESORPTION

Hyperparathyroidism	Common
Secondary, renal osteodystrophy	
Hyperparathyroidism	Moderately
Secondary, severe rickets	common
Focal, with tendon avulsion	
Hyperparathyroidism	
Primary	
Secondary, in pancreatitis	Relatively rare
Secondary, in neonate	
Focal with subperiosteal hematoma	
Jansen metaphyseal dysostosis[a]	
Generalized gangliosidosis[a]	
Mucolipidoses[a]	Rare
Lipogranulomatosis[a]	
Pseudohypohyperparathyroidism	

[a]Present in infancy.

TABLE A6.12. CORTICAL DEFECTS AND EROSIONS

Benign cortical defect Tendon avulsion injuries	} Commonest

Focal subperiosteal bone resorption[a]
Metaphyseal bone destruction with
   Lymphoma, leukemia
   Metastatic disease
   Infection, infarction, congenital syphilis
Juxtaarticular erosion with
   rheumatoid arthritis
	Moderately
	common

Adjacent soft tissue tumors Humeral notch (Gaucher's disease)	} Relatively rare

[a]See Table A6.11.

TABLE A6.13. FOCAL BONY SCLEROSIS

Stress fracture (healing)	} Common
Healed cortical defect, nonossifying fibroma Fibrous dysplasia Bone infarct Healed histiocytosis X Osteoid osteoma	Moderately common
Idiopathic, bone island Ewing's sarcoma (solitary) Meningioma (skull) Foreign body reaction Osteoma	Relatively rare
Osteogenic sarcoma (multiple) Tuberous sclerosis Healing mastocytosis Osteoblastic metastases	Rare

TABLE A6.14. EXOSTOSES

Osteochondroma Calcaneal spurs: normal neonate Healed avulsion injuries Pronounced medial tibial metaphyseal beaks in conditions with bowed legs	Common
Costoclavicular ligament exostosis, midclavicle Tuberous sclerosis Myositis ossificans progressiva Multiple enchondromatosis[a] Supracondylar spur: humerus Camptomelic dwarfism: calcaneal spur	Relatively rare
Fong's lesion Epiphyseal osteochondroma[b] Hypertrophic degenerative spurs Iliac spur with tethered cord	Rare

[a]Ollier's disease.
[b]Trevor disease.

TABLE A6.15. STIPPLED EPIPHYSES

Punctate epiphyseal dysplasia[a]	} Common
Warfarin embryopathy Fetal alcohol syndrome	Moderately common
Cerebrocostomandibular syndrome Smith-Lemli-Opitz syndrome	Rare

[a]All forms.

TABLE A6.16. IRREGULAR OR FRAGMENTED EPIPHYSES

Normal: distal femur, capitellum Legg-Perthes disease	Common
Aseptic necrosis[a] Rheumatoid arthritis Hemophilic arthritis	Moderately common

Multiple epiphyseal dysplasia
Spondyloepiphyseal dysplasia
Aseptic necrosis
  Collagen vascular disease
  Congenital hip treatment
  Gaucher's disease
  After hip surgery
  After septic hip
  Hip trauma
Hypothyroidism[b]
Frostbite of feet and hands
Osteomyelitis of epiphysis
Pigmented villonodular synovitis
	Relatively
	rare

Morquio's disease
Epiphyseal dysplasia hemimelica:
  Trevor disease
Thiemann disease[c]
Trichorhinophalangeal syndrome:
  femoral head
Dyggve-Melchior-Clausen syndrome
Meyer dysplasia (hips)
Winchester syndrome
Zellweger syndrome
	Rare

[a]Sickle cell disease, steroid therapy.
[b]Epiphyseal dysgenesis.
[c]Hand.

TABLE A6.17. IRREGULAR, FRAGMENTED APOPHYSES

Normal
  Hands, feet
  Distal humerus
  Calcaneus
  Scapula
Osgood-Schlatter disease: tibial tubercle
	Common

Hypothyroidism Trisomy 21: feet	Relatively rare

TABLE A6.18. LARGE, OVERGROWN EPIPHYSES

Rheumatoid arthritis[a,b]	
Hemophilic arthritis[a,b]	
Healed Legg-Perthes disease: coxa plana magna	Common
Chondrodystrophies with short bones and flared metaphyses[c]	
Tuberculous and fungal arthritis[a,b]	Moderately common
Pyogenic arthritis: chronic	
Winchester syndrome[a]	
Epiphyseal dysplasia hemimelica[b]	Rare
Fibrous dysplasia of epiphysis	
Megaepiphyseal dwarfism	

[a]Epiphysis often large and glassy.
[b]Unilateral enlargement usually.
[c]See Table A6.25.

TABLE A6.19. SMALL EPIPHYSES

Generalized

Delayed bone age: any cause	Common
Hypothyroidism	
Dysplasia	Moderately common
Multiple epiphyseal	
Spondyloepiphyseal	
Morquio's disease	Relatively rare

Unilateral

Early Legg-Perthes disease	
Congenital dislocating hip: developmental hip dysplasia	Common
Post infection, injury, etc.	Moderately common
Normal[a]	

[a]Minimal asymmetry, usually hips.

TABLE A6.20. CONE-SHAPED EPIPHYSES

Normal[a]	Common
Trauma	
Infection	Moderately common
Achondroplasia	
Bone infarction	
Sickle cell disease	
Frostbite: hands and feet	
Multiple osteochondromatosis	
Metaphyseal dysostosis-dysplasia	
Metaphyseal and spondyloepiphyseal dysplasia	Relatively rare
Cleidocranial dysostosis	
Acrocephalosyndactyly syndrome	
Asphyxiating thoracic dystrophy	
Osteopetrosis	
Pseudo- or pseudopseudohyperparathyroidism	
Trichorhinophalangeal syndrome	
Vitamin A intoxication: chronic	
Acrodysostosis	
Ellis-van Creveld syndrome	
Nonspecific brachydactyly	
Marchesani syndrome	
Seckel bird-headed dwarf	Rare
Oro-facial-digital syndrome	
Otopalatodigital syndrome	
Ruvalcaba syndrome	
Conorenal syndrome	
Radiation injury	
Hypophosphatasia	

[a]Especially feet.

TABLE A6.21. INDISTINCT AND RINGED EPIPHYSES

Indistinct epiphyseal margins

Rickets	Common
Hyperparathyroidism[a]	
Hypothyroidism	Moderately common
Hyperparathyroidism[b]	
Jansen metaphyseal dysostosis	Relatively rare
Mucolipidosis II	
Gangliosidosis	

Ringed epiphysis

Severe chronic osteoporosis[c]	Common
Healing rickets	Moderately common
Healing hypothyroidism	Relatively rare
Osteogenesis imperfecta	
Scurvy[d]	Rare

[a]Secondary.
[b]Primary.
[c]See Table A6.2 for causes.
[d]Wimberger's ring.

TABLE A6.22. EPIPHYSEAL DEFECTS

Fovea centralis: normal femoral head defect Osteochondritis dissecans: distal femur Avulsion injuries: anterior tibial spine, knee	Common
Normal femoral condyle defects Rheumatoid arthritis Osteochondritis dissecans: other bones Hemophilic arthritis	Moderately common
Tuberculous arthritis Fungal arthritis Other chronic arthritis Osteomyelitis of epiphysis	Relatively rare
Histiocytosis X Synovial tumors Fibrous defects	Rare

TABLE A6.23. TRANSVERSE METAPHYSEAL BANDS

Alternating radiolucent and radioopaque

Severe illness, trauma[a] Battered child syndrome, deprivational dwarf[b]	Common
Healing rickets[a] Healing neonatal infections[a] Chronic diseases[b] Chemotherapy[b]	Moderately common
Osteopetrosis[b] Prenatal stress[a]	Rare

Solitary radiolucent band (no opaque band)

Severe illness, trauma Leukemia, lymphoma[c] Metastatic disease[c] Prematurity[a] Trauma: fracture	Common
Neonatal infections (especially syphilis)[c]	Moderately common
Scurvy[c] Hypermagnesemia	Rare

Solitary radiodense band

Normal, physiologic	Common
Chronic lead intoxication	Moderately common

Other heavy metal or chemical
   intoxication
Radiation injury by bone-seeking isotopes
   Idiopathic hypercalcemia
   Hypervitaminosis D
   Hypothyroidism: treated
   Bisphosphonate therapy
	Relatively
	rare

[a]Single line usually.
[b]Multiple lines.
[c]Fracture (pathologic) may occur.

TABLE A6.24. METAPHYSEAL BEAKING

Normal (knees) in bowed legs
   Other causes of bowed legs[a]
Epiphyseal metaphyseal fractures in normal
   bones and battered child syndrome
Blount's disease
	Common

Epiphyseal metaphyseal fractures in
   Breech delivery
   Rickets
   Hyperparathyroidism
   Neurologic disease
   Leukemia, lymphoma
   Metastatic disease
   Osteomyelitis
   Congenital infections
   Metabolic bone disease (premature)
	Moderately
	common

Menkes' kinky hair syndrome Scurvy (Pelkan spurs) Hypophosphatasia Desbuquois syndrome	Rare

[a]See Table A6.7.

TABLE A6.25. METAPHYSEAL FLARING, WIDENING, AND CUPPING

Metaphyseal flaring and cupping[a]

Rickets	}	Common
Epiphyseal-metaphyseal injury Achondroplasia Metaphyseal dysostosis	}	Moderately common
Hypochondroplasia Pseudoachondroplasia Thanatophoric dwarfism Hypophosphatasia Immunologic diseases Bone infarction	}	Relatively rare
Metatropic dwarfism Kniest syndrome Ellis-van Creveld syndrome Mesomelic dwarfism Short rib-polydactyly syndromes Diastrophic dwarfism Stippled epiphyses congenita Hypophosphatasia Spondylometaphyseal dysplasia Taybi-Lindner syndrome Osteodysplasia: Needles-Melnick Hypervitaminosis A Scurvy Phenylketonuria Weissenbacher-Zweymuller syndrome Achondrogenesis Trichorhinophalangeal syndrome	}	Rare

Metaphyseal widening without cupping[b]

Chronic anemias: sickle cell, Cooley's	}	Common
Pyle's disease Otopalatodigital syndrome Other craniometaphyseal dysostoses Gaucher's disease	}	Relatively rare
Chronic lead intoxication Mastocytosis Weaver syndrome	}	Rare

[a]Also affects anterior rib ends.

TABLE A6.26. METAPHYSEAL DESTRUCTION

Mottled destruction

Leukemia, lymphoma Metastatic disease Osteomyelitis	}	Common
Primary malignant bone tumors	}	Moderately common

Homogeneous destruction: no mottling

Osteomyelitis Congenital syphilis[a]	}	Common
Bone infarction: sickle cell Histiocytosis X Leukemia, lymphoma Metastatic disease	}	Moderately common
Primary malignant bone tumors Scurvy[a] Infantile fibromatosis	}	Relatively rare

Focal cyst-like destruction

Osteomyelitis Histiocytosis X Benign cortical defect: en face	}	Common
Small bone cysts Leukemia[a] Lymphoma Metastatic disease	}	Moderately rare
Primary benign bone tumor	}	Relatively rare

[a]Often through trophic lines.

TABLE A6.27. WIDENED EPIPHYSEAL LINE

Epiphyseal metaphyseal fractures: normal bones	}	Commonest
Epiphyseal metaphyseal fractures: pathologic bones Rickets: any type Hyperparathyroidism: secondary in renal osteodystrophy	}	Moderately common
Hyperparathyroidism: primary Metaphyseal dysostosis	}	Relatively rare
Hypophosphatasia Jansen metaphyseal dysostosis[a] Gangliosidosis[a] Mucolipidosis II[a]	}	Rare

[a]Mimics hyperparathyroidism in infancy.

TABLE A6.28. CLINODACTYLY: FIFTH DIGIT

More Common Conditions	Less Common Conditions
Normal	**Syndromes**
Sporadic	Aarskog syndrome
Syndromes	Bloom's syndrome
Acrocephalosyndactyly	Cerebrohepatorenal syndrome
Camptomelic dwarfism	Cri-du-chat syndrome
Cornelia de Lange syndrome	Hand-foot syndrome
	Nievergelt syndrome
Fanconi's anemia	Oculodentodigital syndrome
Goltz syndrome	Oculodento-osseous dysplasia
Holt-Oram syndrome	Orofaciodigital syndrome I and II
Klinefelter's syndrome	
Laurence-Moon-Biedl-Bardet syndrome	Popliteal pterygium syndrome
	Rieger syndrome
Marfan's syndrome	Senior syndrome
Myositis ossificans progressiva	Seckel bird-headed syndrome
	Thrombocytopenia absent radius syndrome
Noonan's syndrome	
Otopalatodigital syndrome	Trichorhinophalangeal syndrome
Poland's syndrome	
Russell-Silver syndrome	Penta X (XXXXX) syndrome
Trisomy 18	Wolf syndrome: 4p syndrome
Trisomy 21	XXXY syndrome
Trisomy 13	Whistling face syndrome

TABLE A6.29. CAMPTODACTYLY

More Common Conditions	Less Common Conditions
Holt-Oram syndrome	Isolated phalangeal hypoplasia or absence
Arthrogryposis congenita	
Poland's syndrome	Orofaciodigital syndromes I and II
Trisomy 18	Aarskog syndrome
Acquired	Cerebrohepatorenal or Zellweger syndrome
Burns	
Infections	Goltz syndrome
Fractures	Marfan's contractural arachnodactyly
Contractures	Osteo-onychodysplasia
	Popliteal pterygium syndrome
	Trichorhinophalangeal syndrome
	Camptodactyly-ankylosis-pulmonary hypoplasia syndrome

TABLE A6.30. SYNDACTYLY

More Common Conditions	Less Common Conditions
Acrocephalosyndactyly[a]	**Isolated**
Cornelia de Lange syndrome	Sporadic
Fanconi's anemia	**Syndromes**
Holt-Oram syndrome	Aarskog syndrome
Thrombocytopenia absent radius syndrome	Aglossia-adactyly syndrome
Trisomy 13	Bloom's syndrome
Trisomy 18	Carpenter's syndrome
Syndromes with polydactyly[b]	Punctate epiphyseal dysplasia: Conradi's syndrome
	Goltz syndrome
	Laurence-Moon-Biedl syndrome
	Möbius' syndrome
	Nager's syndrome
	Mesomelic dwarfism
	Otopalatodigital syndrome
	Popliteal pterygium syndrome
	Robinow-Silverman syndrome
	Rothmund-Thomson syndrome
	Rubinstein-Taybi syndrome
	Smith-Lemi-Opitz syndrome
	Trichorhinophalangeal syndrome

[a]Including Apert's.
[b]See Table A6.32.

TABLE A6.31. POLYDACTYLY

More Common Conditions	Less Common Conditions
Acrocephalosyndactyly[a]	**Isolated**
Blackfan-Diamond anemia[a]	Sporadic
Dubowitz syndrome[a]	**Syndromes**
Fanconi's anemia[a]	Acropectorovertebral dysplasia[a]
Holt-Oram syndrome[a]	
Rubinstein-Taybi syndrome[b]	Asphyxiating thoracic dystrophy[b]
VATER syndrome[a]	
	Biedmond syndrome[b]
	Bloom's syndrome[a]
	Ellis-van Creveld syndrome[a]
	Goltz syndrome[b]
	Grieg syndrome[b]
	Hereditary hydrometrocolpos:[b] McKusick-Kaufman syndrome
	Kaufman-McKusick syndrome[b]
	Mohr syndrome[a,b]
	Möbius' syndrome
	Myositis ossificans progressiva
	Nager's syndrome[a]
	Orofaciodigital syndrome
	Poland's syndrome[a]
	Short rib-polydactyly syndrome[a,b]
	Smith-Lemli-Opitz syndrome[b]
	Trisomy 13
	Werner mesomelic dysplasia[a]
	Weyer syndrome[b]

[a]Preaxial (radial side).
[b]Postaxial (ulnar side).

TABLE A6.32. DACTYLITIS

Infection: osteomyelitis Infarction: hand-foot syndrome	} Common
Frostbite	} Relatively rare

Radiation injury
Microgeodic syndrome
Tumor mimicking dactylitis
  Ewing's sarcoma
  Hemangioma
  Metastatic neuroblastoma
	Rare

TABLE A6.33. CARPAL-TARSAL COALITION

More Common Conditions	Less Common Conditions
Idiopathic, isolated	Diastrophic dwarfism
Ellis-van Creveld syndrome	Hand-foot-uterus syndrome
Holt-Oram syndrome	Kniest syndrome
Acrocephalosyndactyly	Nievergelt mesomelic
Arthrogryposis congenita	dwarfism
Turner's syndrome	Otopalatodigital syndrome
Dyschondrosteosis:	Frontometaphyseal dysplasia
Madelung's deformity	Stickler syndrome
Acquired	
Trauma	
Inflammation, infection	

TABLE A6.34. SMALL, SQUARED, AND FLARED ILIAC WINGS—DECREASED ACETABULAR ANGLE

Type A
Achondroplasia
Achondrogenesis
Asphyxiating thoracic dystrophy
Ellis-van Creveld syndrome
Short rib-polydactyly syndromes
Metatropic dwarfism
Kniest syndrome
Spondyloepiphyseal dysplasia congenita
Punctate epiphyseal dysplasia: rhizomelic form
Thanatophoric dwarfism
Morquio's disease
Severe metaphyseal dysostoses
Dyggve-Melchior-Clausen syndrome
Immune deficiency syndromes

Type B
Trisomy 21: Down's syndrome
Mucopolysaccaridoses: except Morquio's
Mucolipidoses
Other storage diseases
Cleidocranial dysostosis
Cockayne's syndrome
Acrocephalosyndactyly
Aminopterin-induced syndrome
Arthrogryposis
Cornelia de Lange syndrome
Hypophosphatasia
Popliteal pterygium syndrome
Osteo-onchodysplasia
Prune belly syndrome
Rubinstein-Taybi syndrome
Bladder extrophy
Sacral agenesis
Trisomy 13, 18
Metaphyseal dysostoses: mild cases
Osteogenesis imperfecta
Weissenbacher-Zweymuller syndrome
Larsen's syndrome
Congenital dislocating hip
Needles-Melnick syndrome

TABLE A6.35. RIB ABNORMALITIES

Anterior rib cupping[a]

Anterior rib straightening Hypothyroidism Osteopetrosis Storage diseases	} Common
Rib notching Coarctation of aorta	} Common
Postoperative Blalock-Taussig shunt Normal	} Moderately common
Neurofibromatosis	} Relatively rare
Needles-Melnick osteodysplasia Collaterals with pulmonary valve atresia Superior vena cava obstruction Arteriovenous fistula of chest wall Intercostal nerve tumors Intercostal arteritis Poliomyelitis	Rare

[a]Same as metaphyseal cupping (see Table A6.25).

TABLE A6.36. JOINT SPACE WIDENING AND NARROWING

Joint space widening[a]

Pyogenic arthritis: hip, shoulder Traumatic effusion or hemarthrosis: hip, shoulder Toxic (transient) synovitis: usually hip Developmental hip dysplasia	Common
Rheumatoid arthritis Traumatic dislocation Joint laxity: neurogenic, neuromuscular Tuberculous arthritis Fungal arthritis	Moderately common
Pigmented villinodular synovitis Ligamentum teres rupture: hip Retained cartilage fragment: hip Synovial tumors Winchester syndrome Congenital dislocation—other joints Farber lipogranulomatosis Larsen's syndrome Desbuquois syndrome	Relatively rare

Joint space narrowing

Septic arthritis	Common
Rheumatoid arthritis Hemophilic arthropathy Tuberculous arthritis Fungal arthritis Degenerative arthritis	Moderately common
Slipped capital femoral epiphysis: postoperative Pigmented villinodular synovitis Winchester syndrome Degenerative arthritis: primary Traumatic dislocation Farber lipogranulomatosis	Relatively rare

[a]Also use for joint dislocation.

TABLE A6.37. FRANK JOINT DISLOCATION

Traumatic[a] Developmental hip dysplasia[a] Rheumatoid arthritis[a,b] Neurologic-neuromuscular disease[a,b]	Common
Congenital radial head dislocation[a] Madelung's deformity[a]	Relatively rare
Larsen's syndrome[b] Genu recurvatum[a] Winchester syndrome[a,b] Farber syndrome[b] Werner mesomelic syndrome[b] Stickler syndrome[b]	Rare

[a]Single joint involvement.
[b]Generalized joint involvement.

TABLE A6.38. JOINT CALCIFICATION

Intraarticular

Traumatic avulsion Osteochondritis dissecans	Common
Idiopathic: in infants Synovial chondromatosis Ochronosis Oxalosis Synovial inflammation Synovial tumors	Rare

Periarticular

Collagen diseases: especially dermatomyositis	Common
Trauma Infection Hypervitaminosis D and A Hyperparathyroidism Tumoral calcinosis: large, clumpy	Relatively rare

TABLE A6.39. GAS IN JOINT

Normal vacuum joint	Common
Vacuum joint with hypotonia	Moderately common
Penetrating trauma Infection	Rare

TABLE A6.40. MUSCLE/FAT RATIO ABNORMALITIES

Increased muscle—normal fat
    Muscular dystrophy
    Congenital muscular hypertrophy
    Pyomyositis
    Exercise hypertrophy
Decreased muscle—excess fat
    Neurologic disease: multiple causes
    Arthrogryposis multiplex
    Amyotonia congenita
    Werdnig-Hoffman disease
    Muscular dystrophy
    Prolonged muscle paralysis
Decreased fat—normal muscle
    Malnutrition, cachexia[a]
    Diencephalic syndrome
    Total lipodystrophy
Increased fat—normal muscle
    Exogenous obesity
    Cushing's syndrome
    Laurence-Moon-Biedl syndrome
    Prader-Willi syndrome
    Steroid therapy

[a]In late, severe stages, muscle is also decreased due to protein catabolism.

TABLE A6.41. PERIOSTEAL NEW BONE

Disease	Layered (Single or Multiple)	Solid (Straight, Wavy, Lumpy)	Markedly Elevated (Ballooned)	Spiculated
Infection, inflammation				
Osteomyelitis—neonatal infection (lues, rubella, cytomegalovirus)	++	−	−	−
Bone infarction	++	+	−	−
Cellulitis	++	+	−	−
Caffey's disease	++	++	−	−
Rheumatoid arthritis	+	−	−	−
Fractures, injury				
Fractures (ordinary)	++	++	−	−
Fractures (battered child)	++	++	++	−
Fractures (neurogenic)	++	++	++	−
Fractures (pathologic)	++	+	−	−
Metabolic disease				
Rickets (healing)	++	+	−	−
Scurvy	++	−	+	−
Metabolic bone disease of premature	++	+	−	−
Hypervitaminosis D	++	−	−	−
Hypervitaminosis A	++	−	−	−
Thyroid acropachy	+	++	−	+
Gangliosidosis (infant)	++	−	++	−
Mucolipidosis II (infant)	++	−	++	
Hyperphosphatemia	++	−	++	−
Gaucher's disease	++	+	−	−
Bone tumors and cysts				
Malignant—primary	++	−	−	++
Benign with fracture	++	+	−	−
Bone metastases	++	−	−	+
Leukemia, lymphoma	++	−	−	+
Hemangioma (with or without fracture)	+	+	−	−
Infantile fibromatosis (hamartomas)	++	−	−	−
Miscellaneous				
Osteoarthropathy	++	++	−	−
Pachydermoperiostosis	++	++	−	−
Neurofibromatosis	−	−	+	−
Macrodystrophia lipomatosa	+	+	−	−
Normal infants (prematures)	++	−	−	−
Vascular soft tissue tumors	+	+	−	−
Mastocytosis (early stages)	+	−	+	−
Prostaglandin E treatment	++	−	−	−
Melorheostosis	+−	++	−	−
Venous stasis	+−	+	−	−

(++), quite common; (+), occasional; (−), rare or never.

CHAPTER 7

TABLE A7.1. LARGE AND SMALL HEAD

Large head

Hydrocephalus Subdural hematoma Subdural effusions	Common
Chondrodystrophies Calvarial thickening[a]	Moderately common
Cleidocranial dysplasia Craniometaphyseal dysplasia Pyle's disease Beckwith-Wiedemann syndrome Russell-Silver dwarf Storage diseases Neurofibromatosis	Uncommon
Sotos syndrome Bannayan syndrome Proteus syndrome Robinow syndrome Zellweger syndrome Ruvalcaba-Myhre-Smith syndrome Alexander disease Familial megalencephaly Lipomatosis-hemangiomatosis syndrome Large brain tumor or cyst	Rare

Small head

Brain atrophy Poor brain growth[b]	Common
Universal craniosynostosis	Rare

[a]See Table A7.2.
[b]Multiple causes.

TABLE A7.2. CALVARIAL CONFIGURATIONS IN PRIMARY CRANIOSYNOSTOSIS

Suture	Calvarial Configuration	Descriptive Terms
Sagittal	Long, narrow head	Scaphocephaly or dolichocephaly
Bilateral coronal	Short, wide head, hypertelorism proptosis, small anterior fossa	Brachycephaly or bradycephaly
Metopic	Frontal wedging or keel-shaped head	Trigonocephaly
Bilateral lambdoid	Shallow posterior fossa, prominent bregma	Turricephaly
Unilateral coronal	Unilateral, frontal flattening, uptilting of orbit and tilting of nasal septum	Plagiocephaly
Unilateral lambdoid	Unilateral posterior flattening	Plagiocephaly
All sutures	Small, round head	Microcephaly

TABLE A7.3. GENERALIZED CALVARIAL THICKENING (WITH OR WITHOUT SCLEROSIS)

Homogenous sclerosis

Normal
Decreased intracranial pressure
   Brain atrophy
   Posthydrocephalus shunting
	Common

Dilantin therapy Hypervitaminosis D Hypoparathyroidism Idiopathic hypercalcemia Storage diseases Osteopetrosis Healing rickets[a]	Uncommon
Acrodysostosis Cockayne's syndrome Craniometaphyseal dysplasia[b] Jansen metaphyseal dysostosis Lipodystrophy Osteopathia striata Otopalatodigital syndrome Pyknodysostosis Proteus syndrome Van Buchem osteosclerosis Fluorosis Melorheostosis Kenny-Caffey syndrome[c] Myelosclerosis Myotonic dystrophy	Rare

Nonhomogeneous sclerosis or no sclerosis

Chronic anemia[d] Thalassemia, sickle cell disease, iron deficiency anemia, hereditary spherocytosis	Common
Hyperparathyroidism Active and healing rickets	Moderately common
Dilantin therapy Polycythemia Metastatic disease[e]	Uncommon
Hyperphosphatasia Hypophosphatasia Leukemia, lymphoma[e]	Rare

[a]With bossing.
[b]Pyle disease.
[c]Tubular stenosis of long bones.
[d]Often show vertical striations.
[e]May show vertical striations.

TABLE A7.4. ORBITAL MASSES

Intraocular

Retinoblastoma	}	Moderately common
Medulloepithelioma	}	Rare

Extraocular

Dermoid	}	Moderately common
Hemangioma		
Teratoma	}	Rare
Lymphangioma		
Rhabdomyosarcoma		
Optic glioma		
Neuroblastoma		
Neurofibroma/schwannoma		
Histiocytosis X		
Metastases		
Orbital varix or arteriovenous malformation		
Granulocytic sarcoma		

CHAPTER 8

TABLE A8.1. BONE-IN-BONE AND SANDWICH VERTEBRA

Physiologic in premature infant	}	Common
Healing renal osteodystrophy[a]	}	Moderately common
Osteopetrosis[a]	}	Relatively rare
Chronic lead poisoning[a]		
Hypercalcemia		
Chronic illness, trophic lines[a]		

[a]Usually sandwich vertebra.

TABLE A8.2. FOCAL SCLEROSIS OF VERTEBRA

Osteoid osteoma	}	Common
Sclerosis with apophyseal joint malalignment		
Bone islands	}	Rare
Osteoblastic metastases		
Ewing's sarcoma		
Osteogenic sarcoma		
Lymphoma		
Tuberous sclerosis		
Healed trauma, infection		

TABLE A8.3. ABNORMAL PEDICLE SHAPES

Flattened pedicles

Normal[a]	}	Common
Intraspinal expanding tumor or cyst	}	Relatively rare

Dysplastic pedicle

Part of other spinal anomaly	}	Common
Neurofibromatosis	}	**Moderately common**

[a]Lumbar region.

TABLE A8.4. ABNORMAL PEDICLE SIZE

Enlarged pedicle

Osteoblastoma	}	Relatively rare
Hemangioma		
Lymphangioma		
Other tumor		
Contralateral arch deficiency		

Small pedicle

Congenital with other anomaly	}	Common
Post radiation therapy	}	Moderately common
Congenital absence or hypoplasia	}	Relatively rare

TABLE A8.5. DESTROYED, ABSENT, AND SCLEROTIC PEDICLES

Destroyed or absent pedicles

Metastatic disease	}	Moderately common
Leukemia, lymphoma		
Primary bone tumor	}	Relatively rare
Histiocytosis X		
Congenitally absent pedicle		

Sclerotic pedicle

Osteoid osteoma	}	Common
Stress with abnormal apophyseal joint alignment	}	Moderately common
Ewing's sarcoma	}	Rare
Hodgkin's lymphoma		
Osteogenic sarcoma		

TABLE A8.6. POSTERIOR ARCH DEFECTS OR UNDERDEVELOPMENT

Congenital defects C1	}	Common
Spondylolysis, spondylolisthesis[a]		
Normal synchondroses between body and arches		
Fractures with hyperextension injury[b]	}	Moderately common
Congenital defects with myelomeningocele, etc.		
Neurofibromatosis[c]		
Spondyloepiphyseal dysplasia[c]		
Spondylometaphyseal dysplasia[c]		
Storage diseases[c]		
Congenital defects other than C1	}	Rare
Defects acquired after infection, tumor, etc.		
Chondrodystrophies[c]		

[a]Lower lumbar spine.
[b]Hangman fracture of C2 and other levels.
[c]Underdevelopment.

TABLE A8.7. VERTICAL DEFECTS OF VERTEBRAL BODIES

Pseudodefect, posterior arch synchondrosis Sagittal cleft vertebra	} Common
Compression fractures	} Moderately common
Coronal cleft vertebra	} Relatively rare

TABLE A8.8. PROMINENT CENTRAL VEIN GROOVES

Normal, infants	} Common
Hypothyroidism Osteopetrosis	} Moderately common
Thalassemia major Sickle cell disease Gaucher's disease Leukemia Lymphoma Metastatic neuroblastoma	} Relatively rare

TABLE A8.9. VERTEBRAL SCALLOPING

Posterior

Normal, lumbar	} Common
Intraspinal tumor, cyst Neurofibromatosis[a] Achondroplasia, other chondrodystrophies[b] Storage diseases	} Moderately common
Ehler-Danlos syndrome[a] Marfan's syndrome[a] Hydromyelia, syringomyelia Uncontrolled communicating hydrocephalus	} Rare

Anterior

Normal, lower thoracic and upper lumbar	} Common
Neurofibromatosis[c] Leukemia, lymphoma[d] Metastatic disease[d]	} Moderately common
Adjacent intraabdominal tumors, cysts[e]	} Rare

[a]Dural ectasia.
[b]Small canal.
[c]Dysplastic vertebra.
[d]Destruction.
[e]Erosion.

TABLE A8.10. FLAT VERTEBRAE

Single or multiple but not all vertebral bodies

Fracture Eosinophilic granuloma Histiocytosis X	} Common
Metastatic disease Congenital variation Osteogenesis imperfecta Osteomalacia, osteoporosis Leukemia, lymphoma	} Moderately common

All vertebral bodies

Severe osteoporosis, osteomalacia[a,c] Sickle cell disease[c]	} Common
Severe osteogenesis imperfecta[a,c] Other anemias[a,c] Leukemia, lymphoma[a,c] Spondyloepiphyseal dysplasia[a,b]	} Moderately common
Thanatophoric dwarfism[a] Metatropic dwarfism[a] Morquio's disease[b]	} Relatively rare
Achondrogenesis Kniest syndrome[a] Dyggve-Melchior-Clausen syndrome[b]	} Rare

[a]Uniformly flat.
[b]Pear shaped.
[c]Biconcave.

TABLE A8.11. CUBOID VERTEBRAE

Normal[a] Achondroplasia	} Common
Hypochondroplasia Other chondrodystrophies Storage diseases	} Moderately common
Short rib-polydactyly syndrome	} Rare

[a]Cervical and thoracolumbar spine.

TABLE A8.12. BICONCAVE VERTEBRAE

Sickle cell disease[a] Osteoporosis, osteomalacia	} Common
Osteogenesis imperfecta Renal osteodystrophy Normal Schmorl's nodes	} Moderately common
Thalassemia[b] Gaucher's disease[b] Homocystinuria[b]	} Relatively rare

[a]Often step-like depression.
[b]Occasionally step-like depression.

TABLE A8.13. TALL VERTEBRAE

Trisomy 21 Other causes of hypotonia	} Common

TABLE A8.14. ROUND AND EXPANDED VERTEBRAE

Round vertebrae

Normal neonate[a] Meningocele	} Common
Hypothyroidism	} Moderately common
Short rib-polydactyly syndromes Bone dysplasias[b]	} Rare

Expanded vertebrae

Compression fracture with expansion	} Common
Aneurysmal bone cyst Hemangioma, lymphangioma	} Relatively rare
Osteoblastoma Ewing's sarcoma[c]	} Rare

[a]Especially thoracolumbar junction.
[b]With pear-shaped vertebrae (see Table A8.10).
[c]Sclerotic, treated.

TABLE A8.15. WEDGED VERTEBRAE

Anterior compression fracture Scoliosis[a]	} Common
Kyphosis[b] Scheuermann's disease Normal[c] Hemivertebrae, sagittal[a]	} Moderately common
Hemivertebrae, coronal[d] Gibbus[e]	} Relatively rare

[a]Lateral wedging.
[b]Various causes.
[c]Thoracic spine minimal.
[d]Gibbus.
[e]Other causes.

TABLE A8.16. HOOKED OR BEAKED VERTEBRAE

Normal in infants[a]	} Common
Storage diseases Hypothyroidism Acute and chronic trauma Scheuermann's disease Neurogenic or neuromuscular disease with hypotonia	} Moderately common
Achondroplasia Bone dysplasia in neurofibromatosis	} Relatively rare

[a]Thoracolumbar junction.

TABLE A8.17. BLOCK VERTEBRAE

Congenital, with spinal dysraphism	} Common

Congenital
  Isolated
  Klippel-Feil syndrome
Acquired, after infection
	} Moderately common

Acquired, after trauma Scheuermann's disease	} Relatively rare

TABLE A8.18. INTERVERTEBRAL FORAMEN SIZE ABNORMALITIES

Small

Congenital with other anomalies	} Common
Posttraumatic	} Relatively rare

Enlarged

Congenital with dysraphism anomalies	} Commonest
Dumbbell tumor[a] Neurofibromatosis[b]	} Moderately common
Intraspinal tumor[c] Posttraumatic nerve root diverticulum Congenital absence or hypoplastic pedicle Lateral meningocele Interstitial polyneuritis Dural ectasia, idiopathic	} Rare

[a]Usually neuroblastoma, ganglioneuroma.
[b]Bony dysplasia, dural ectasia.
[c]Other.

TABLE A8.19. DISC ABNORMALITIES

Narrowed discs

Infection[a]	} Common
Scheuermann's disease Congenital narrowing[b] Acute trauma[c]	} Moderately common
Spondyloepiphyseal dysplasia Morquio's disease Cockayne's syndrome	} Relatively rare
Ruvalcaba syndrome Ankylosing spondylitis Kneist syndrome	} Rare

Widened discs

Osteoporosis, osteomalacia Endplate infarction[d]	} Common
Trauma[e]	} Moderately common

Disc calcification

Idiopathic[f]	} Common
Ochronosis Hemochromatosis Hyperparathyroidism Hypervitaminosis D Pseudogout Ankylosing spondylitis	} Rare

[a]Discitis, spondyloarthritis, osteomyelitis.
[b]Blocked vertebra.
[c]Flexion-rotation.
[d]Sickle cell, Gaucher's.
[e]Hyperextension.
[f]Cervical, thoracic.

TABLE A8.20. SCOLIOSIS

Paraspinal muscle spasm Idiopathic rotoscoliosis	Common
Rotoscoliosis with muscle hypotonia Scoliosis with vertebral anomalies Congenital heart disease	Moderately common

Radiation therapy
Scoliosis
    With intraspinal and spinal tumors, cysts
    With neurofibromatosis
    With unilateral bar
	Relatively rare

TABLE A8.21. KYPHOSIS

Normal, thoracolumbar in infants Cervical spine angulation, C2–3, normal	Common
Compression fractures[a] Infection with vertebral destruction Congenital spine anomalies Storage diseases Chondrodystrophies and Scheuermann's disease	Moderately common
Absent vertebral body Spine and spinal cord tumors Radiation therapy Underlying spinal cord disease[b]	Relatively rare

[a]Regular, pathologic.
[b]Other than tumor.

TABLE A8.22. TORTICOLLIS OR WRY NECK

Idiopathic Trauma, spasm	Common
Congenital short muscle Upper cervical or posterior fossa tumor	Moderately common
Sandifer syndrome, gastroesophageal reflux	Rare

TABLE A8.23. HYPOPLASTIC OR ABSENT DENS

Congenital anomaly[a]	Common
Congenital anomaly[b]	Moderately common
Resorption after trauma	Relatively rare

[a]With certain syndromes.
[b]Isolated.

TABLE A8.24. INCREASED C1-DENS DISTANCE

Normal	Common
Congenital hypoplasia of dens and C1[a]	Moderately common

Dislocation of C1–2
    Rotatory
    Anterior
	Relatively rare

Rheumatoid arthritis Morquio's disease Other storage diseases	Rare

[a]Isolated or with syndromes.

SUBJECT INDEX

Page numbers in *italic* denote figures; page numbers followed by "t" denote tables.